Practical Prehospital Care

D1091766

Commissioning Editor: Robert Edwards
Development Editor: Catherine Jackson
Project Manager: Joannah Duncan
Designer: Sarah Russell
Illustration Manager: Merlyn Harvey
Illustrations: Bill Le Fever, David Graham, Chartwell Illustrators, Joanna Cameron

Practical Prehospital Care

The Principles and Practice of Immediate Care

Ian Greaves

OStJ FRCP FCEM FIMC RCS(Ed) DTM&H DMCC DipMedEd RAMC
Defence Consultant Advisor in Emergency Medicine;
Visiting Professor of Emergency Medicine, University of Teesside,
Middlesbrough UK; Consultant in Emergency Medicine, British Army

Keith Porter

MB BS FRCS FRCS(Ed) FIMC RCS(Ed) FSEM FCEM
Consultant Trauma Surgeon, Queen Elizabeth Hospital, Birmingham, UK;
Professor of Clinical Traumatology, University of Birmingham, Birmingham, UK

Jason Smith

MB BS MSc MRCP FCEM DiPIMC RCS(Ed)
Consultant in Emergency Medicine, Royal Navy, Derriford Hospital, Plymouth, UK;
Senior Lecturer in Prehospital and Emergency Medicine, Academic Department of
Military Emergency Medicine, Royal Centre for Defence Medicine, UK

WITHDRAWN

TOURO COLLEGE LIBRARY
Midtown

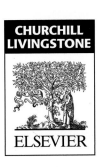

CHURCHILL LIVINGSTONE
ELSEVIER

EDINBURGH LONDON NEW YORK OXFORD PHILADELPHIA ST LOUIS SYDNEY TORONTO 2011

MT

**CHURCHILL
LIVINGSTONE**
ELSEVIER

© 2011 Elsevier Ltd. All rights reserved

No part of this publication may be reproduced or transmitted in any form or by any means, electronic or mechanical, including photocopying, recording, or any information storage and retrieval system, without permission in writing from the publisher. Details on how to seek permission, further information about the Publisher's permissions policies and our arrangements with organizations such as the Copyright Clearance Center and the Copyright Licensing Agency, can be found at our website: www.elsevier.com/permissions.

This book and the individual contributions contained in it are protected under copyright by the Publisher (other than as may be noted herein).

ISBN 978 0 443 10360 5

British Library Cataloguing in Publication Data
A catalogue record for this book is available from the British Library

Library of Congress Cataloging in Publication Data
A catalog record for this book is available from the Library of Congress

Notices
Knowledge and best practice in this field are constantly changing. As new research and experience broaden our understanding, changes in research methods, professional practices, or medical treatment may become necessary.

Practitioners and researchers must always rely on their own experience and knowledge in evaluating and using any information, methods, compounds, or experiments described herein. In using such information or methods they should be mindful of their own safety and the safety of others, including parties for whom they have a professional responsibility.

With respect to any drug or pharmaceutical products identified, readers are advised to check the most current information provided (i) on procedures featured or (ii) by the manufacturer of each product to be administered, to verify the recommended dose or formula, the method and duration of administration, and contraindications. It is the responsibility of practitioners, relying on their own experience and knowledge of their patients, to make diagnoses, to determine dosages and the best treatment for each individual patient, and to take all appropriate safety precautions.

To the fullest extent of the law, neither the Publisher nor the authors, contributors, or editors, assume any liability for any injury and/or damage to persons or property as a matter of products liability, negligence or otherwise, or from any use or operation of any methods, products, instructions, or ideas contained in the material herein.

ELSEVIER your source for books, journals and multimedia in the health sciences
www.elsevierhealth.com

Working together to grow
libraries in developing countries

www.elsevier.com | www.bookaid.org | www.sabre.org

ELSEVIER   BOOK AID International   Sabre Foundation

The Publisher's policy is to use **paper manufactured from sustainable forests**

Printed in China

10/06/11

Dedication

In memory of Peter Baskett
Pioneer, officer, gentleman and friend

Contents

Preface xi

Acknowledgements xiii

Contributors xv

Part 1

1   **Immediate care in the United Kingdom** 3
    R. Fairhurst

2   **Immediate care world-wide** 8
    B. Robertson

Part 2

3   **Basic life support** 17
    A.H. Swain

4   **Airway management and ventilation** 26
    J.M. Elliot

5   **Advanced life support** 48
    C.L. Gwinnutt

6   **Vascular access** 57
    C.L. Gwinnutt and K. J. Souter

7   **Shock** 74
    H.M. Sherriff and D. Walter

Part 3

8   **Understanding the electrocardiogram** 85
    C. Weston

9   **Cardiac emergencies** 104
    C. Weston

10 **Respiratory emergencies** 118
    T. Wardle

Contents

11   The unconscious patient 130
K. Mackway-Jones and S. Maurice

12   Acute abdomen 139
S.W. Metcalf and M. Gavalas

Part 4

13   Therapeutics 151
P.F. Mahoney and P. Haji-Michael

14   Analgesia and pain relief 162
N. Sherwood

15   Substance abuse 173
J. Briscoe and A. Doyle

16   Poisoning 182
P.A. Younge

Part 5

17   Paediatric history and examination 197
T.F. Beattie

18   Paediatric emergencies 209
T.F. Beattie

19   Paediatric life support 220
D.A. Zideman

20   The injured child 230
M. Cooke

Part 6

21   Scene approach, assessment and safety 245
R. Weekes

22   Assessment and management of the trauma patient – the primary and
secondary survey 251
H.M. Sherriff

23   Head and neck injuries 260
D. Gentleman

24   Maxillofacial injuries 272
P.V. Dyer

25   Chest injuries 277
P. Driscoll and J. Nancarrow

26   Spinal injuries 290
A.K. Marsden

27   Abdominal and genitourinary trauma 298
P. Driscoll and J. Nancarrow

28   The prehospital care of bone and joint injuries 305
M.A. Green

29   Prehospital care of soft tissue injuries 315
M.A. Green and K. Allison

30   Gunshot wounds and blast injury 322
J.M. Ryan and L.C. Biant

31   **Thermal injury** 332
       K.C. Judkins

Part 7

32   **The elderly patient** 347
       A. Main

Part 8

33   **Hypothermia** 361
       E.L. Lloyd

34   **Rescue from remote places** 376
       J. Colville Laird

35   **Near drowning** 383
       A.D. Simcock

36   **Heat illness** 389
       P.N. Gillespie

37   **Acute diving emergencies** 398
       P. Grout and G. Laden

38   **Electrocution injury** 405
       J.M. Kendall

39   **Risk of infection in prehospital care** 410
       A.K. Marsden

Part 9

40   **Emergencies in pregnancy** 419
       P.J.P. Holden

41   **Trauma in pregnancy** 433
       V. Argent

42   **Childbirth** 439
       V. Argent

43   **Neonatal resuscitation and transport** 448
       S. Walsh

Part 10

44   **Psychiatric emergencies** 455
       J. Briscoe

45   **Human reactions to trauma: their features and management** 465
       D.A. Alexander and S. Klein

46   **Dealing with the violent or uncooperative patient** 476
       B. Armstrong

Part 11

47   **Major incidents** 483
       T.J. Hodgetts and A. Brett

48   **Triage** 493
       A. Brett and T.J. Hodgetts

Contents

49 Chemical incidents 503
V. Murray and D.J. Baker

50 Radiation incidents 514
C. Kalman

51 Mass gathering medicine 529
J.M. Fisher

52 Medicine at sporting events 534
I.D. McNeil

53 Disaster medicine 540
A.D. Redmond

Part 12

54 Immobilization and extrication 555
J. Scott

55 Transport in prehospital care 568
R. Fairhurst

56 Aeromedical evacuation 572
G. Davies

57 Aviation medicine 581
T.E. Martin

58 Structure and function of the ambulance service 594
C. Carney

59 The fire service: structure and roles 603
S.G. Martin

60 Police force: structure and roles 614
R.F. Evans and R. Michael

61 The role of other agencies at a major incident 625
K.C. Hines

Part 13

62 Legal aspects of immediate care 633
C. Constant

63 Record keeping in prehospital care 653
R. Fairhurst

64 Communications and despatch 656
C. Carney

65 Trauma scoring 661
A. Brett and T.J. Hodgetts

Part 14

66 Training and education 671
J. Scott

67 Immediate care equipment 678
I.D. McNeil

Index 685

Some years ago two of the editors of this book (IG and KP) believed that the time was right for a definitive textbook of prehospital medicine (immediate care). The result was *Prehospital Medicine: the principles and practice of immediate care*, which was published by Arnold in 1999.

Prehospital Medicine (often referred to as 'the big blue book') was very well received but unfortunately its publication in hardback at a high cost put it beyond the pocket of many of those who would perhaps have bought it. When it was subsequently made available at a reduced price the remaining copies sold out very rapidly. Unfortunately the publishers felt that a reprint was not financially viable.

I am delighted that Elsevier have seen the importance of this project and have taken on the preparation and publication of a new edition. *Practical Prehospital Care* is a revised and updated version of *Prehospital Medicine*. The entire text has been reviewed, revised and corrected where necessary. This current book represents, we believe, a modern statement of best practice in prehospital care. We are delighted that such a work will be available in paperback at a price which makes it affordable to the vast majority of those who practice in this area.

The two original editors would like to offer our sincere thanks to Jason Smith, who has joined us for this edition. Without his hard work and attention to detail the production of this volume would not have been possible.

Prehospital care has moved on dramatically since 1999. The Faculty of Prehospital Care is now open to nurses and paramedics, the Diploma in Prehospital Care is universally accepted as the definitive standard for postgraduate training and the first professor of Prehospital Care has been appointed. In addition, the Faculty and BASICS recognize or organize a wide range of courses and support an ongoing active research programme. Before too long, prehospital care will be recognized as a medical sub-specialty throughout Europe and it continues to attract increasing numbers from general practice, emergency medicine, anaesthetics and a range of other specialties. As editors of this book we are convinced that a definitive statement of best practice is as important now as it was when the first edition was published. We hope that this new edition will be an important part of every prehospital care practitioner's bookshelf.

Needless to say we are always delighted to hear from readers with any comments, questions or suggestions and where appropriate we will of course incorporate these in future editions.

I Greaves, 2009

Acknowledgements

We would like to thank all the original contributors to this book, which was first published as *Prehospital Medicine* in 1999, as listed below. Much work has gone into updating the book since, and some of the original contributions have been edited to avoid repetition, particularly due to pressure of space in this paperback edition of the book.

Keith Allison, David A. Alexander, Vincent Argent, Bruce Armstrong, Barry Barrett, Thomas F. Beattie, Leela Biant, A. Brett, James Briscoe, Chris Carney, Christopher R. Constant, Matthew Cooke, Gareth Davies, Anne Doyle, Peter Driscoll, Peter V. Dyer, J. Michael Elliott, R.F. Evans, Richard Fairhurst, Judith M. Fisher, Manolis Gavalos, Douglas Gentleman, Neil Gillespie, Marcus A. Green, Paul Grout, Carl L. Gwinnutt, Philip G. Haji-Michael, Karen J. Heath, Ken Hines, T.J. Hodgetts, Peter J.P. Holden, Keith C. Judkins, Chris Kalman, Jason Kendall, Gerard Laden, J. Colville Laird, Evan L. Lloyd, Kevin Mackway-Jones, Peter F. Mahoney, Alastair Main, Bob Mark, Andrew K. Marsden, Steven Martin, Terry E. Martin, Sue Maurice, Iain D. McNeil, Steven W. Metcalf, Roger Michael, Virginia Murray, Julie Nancarrow, Anthony D. Redmond, Brian Robertson, James M. Ryan, John Scott, Howard M. Sherriff, Nick Sherwood, Anthony D. Simcock, Andrew H. Swain, Mark Tomlins, Darren Walter, Sean Walsh, Simon J. Ward, Terence D. Wardle, Richard Weekes, Clive F.M. Weston, Paul A. Younge, David A. Zideman.

Thanks also to our families for tolerating our absences whilst working on this book.

David A. Alexander MA(Hons) CPsychol PhD FRSM FBPS (Hon)FRCPsych
Professor of Mental Health, Robert Gordon University, Aberdeen Centre for Trauma Research, Faculty of Health and Social Care, Robert Gordon University, Aberdeen, UK

Keith Allison MB ChB MD FRCS FRCS(Plast) FIMC RCS(Ed)
Consultant Plastic Surgeon, South Tees Hospitals NHS Trust, James Cook University Hospital, Middlesbrough, UK; Nuffield Health Tees Hospital, Stockton-on-Tees, UK

Vincent Argent FIMC FRCA FRCOG
Consultant Obstetrician and Gynaecologist, Defence Medical Services, UK

Bruce Armstrong BA(Hons) MSc RGN RMN DipIMC RCS(Ed)
Consultant Nurse, Department of Emergency Medicine, Basingstoke and North Hampshire Hospital, Basingstoke, Hampshire, UK

David J. Baker MPhil DM FRCA FRSM
Consultant Medical Toxicologist, Centre for Radiation, Chemicals and Environmental Hazards (CRCE), Health Protection Agency, London, UK

Thomas F. Beattie MB MSc DCH FRCS(Ed A&E) FCEM FRCPE FFSEM DCH
Honorary Senior Lecturer, University of Edinburgh, Department of Emergency Medicine, Royal Hospital for Sick Children, Edinburgh, UK

L.C. Biant FRCS(Ed Tr&Orth) MS
Consultant Trauma and Orthopaedic Surgeon, Department of Trauma and Orthopaedic Surgery, The Royal Infirmary of Edinburgh, UK; Honorary Senior Lecturer, The University of Edinburgh, Edinburgh, UK

Andrew Brett FRCP FCEM DipIMC
Consultant in Emergency Medicine, Jersey General Hospital, St Helier, Jersey, Channel Islands

James Briscoe MB ChB MRCPsych MMedSci
Consultant Psychiatrist, Midland Psychiatry and Psychology Ltd, Birmingham, UK

Chris Carney MB BS FIMC RCS(Ed)
Former Chief Executive, East Anglian Ambulance Services NHS Trust, Norwich, UK

Christopher Constant MA LLM MCh MB BCh BAO FRCS
Clinical Anatomist, University of Cambridge, Cambridge, UK; Emeritus Consultant Orthopaedic Surgeon and Visiting Specialist in Shoulder and Elbow Surgery, Addenbrooke's Hospital, Cambridge, UK

Matthew Cooke MB ChB PhD FCEM DipIMC
Professor of Emergency Medicine, Warwick Medical School, Coventry, UK

Gareth Davies MB ChB MRCP(UK)
Consultant in Accident and Emergency, Medicine and Pre-Hospital Care, Royal London Hospital, Whitechapel, London, UK

Anne Doyle MB BCh BAO DORCPI MRCPsych PGDip Group Psychotherapy Member IGA
Consultant Psychiatrist, Personality Disorder Service, Birmingham and Solihull Mental Health NHS Trust, Birmingham, UK

Peter Driscoll BSc MD FCEM
Professor, College of Emergency Medicine, Emergency Department, Salford Royal Foundation Trust, Salford, Manchester, UK

Peter V. Dyer MA FFDRCSI FHEA
Maxillofacial Surgeon, University Hospitals of Morecambe Bay NHS Trust, Lancashire, UK

J.Michael Elliot MB BS DipIMC FRCA RCS(Ed)
Consultant in Anaesthesia and Intensive Care, Good Hope Hospital, Sutton Coldfield, West Midlands, UK

R.F. Evans QPM LLB
Former Deputy Chief Constable and Former Chairman of the ACPO Emergency Procedures Sub-Committee, South Wales Police, Mid-Glamorgan, UK

Richard Fairhurst FCEM FIMC RCS(Ed)
Former Medical Director, Lancashire Ambulance Service, Lancashire, UK; Chairman, Training and Standards Board, Faculty of Pre-hospital Care of the Royal College of Surgeons, Edinburgh, UK

Judith M. Fisher MB BS FRCGP FFAEM FIMC RCS(Ed)
Senior Physician, Carnival Cruise Lines, USA

Manolis Gavalas FRCS FFAEM
Senior ED Consultant, Emergency Department, University College London Hospitals, London, UK

Douglas Gentleman BSc MB ChB FRCS(Eng&Glas)
Honorary Consultant Neurosurgeon, Ninewells Hospital, Dundee, UK

P.N. Gillespie OstJ MRCGP FIMC RCS(Ed) DTM&HMSc
Senior Medical Officer, Infantry Training Centre, British Army, Catterick, North Yorkshire, UK

Ian Greaves OStJ FRCP FCEM FIMC RCS(Ed) DTM&H DMCC DipMedEd RAMC
Defence Consultant Advisor in Emergency Medicine; Visiting Professor of Emergency Medicine, University of Teesside, Middlesbrough, UK; Consultant in Emergency Medicine, British Army, Middlesbrough, UK

Marcus A. Green BSC(Hons) MB ChB FRCS FRCS(Tr&Orth) DipIMC
Consultant Orthopaedic Surgeon, Royal Orthopaedic Hospital, Northfield, Birmingham, UK

Paul Grout MBE BM DCH DA FRCS(A&E) FCEM
Head of Medical Training, College of Search and Rescue Medicine; Consultant in Accident and Emergency Medicine, Accident and Emergency Department, Furness General Hospital, Barrow in Furness, Cumbria, UK

Carl L. Gwinnutt MB BS FRCA
Consultant Anaesthetist, Salford Royal Hospital Foundation Trust, Salford, Manchester, UK

Philip Haji-Michael BSc MB BS MRCP(UK) FRCA
Consultant in Critical Care and Anaesthesia, Critical Care Unit, Christie NHS Foundation Trust, Manchester, UK

K.C. Hines MB BS MRCOG MEPS MICPEM FRSH
Former Accredited Immediate Care Practitioner and General Practitioner, London, UK

Timothy J. Hodgetts CBE QHP MMEd MBA CMgr FRCP FRCS(Ed) FCEM FIMC RCS(Ed) FIHM FCMI L/RAMC
Defence Professor of Emergency Medicine, College of Emergency Medicine, Royal Centre for Defence Medicine, Birmingham, UK

Peter J.P. Holden MB ChB FIMC RCS(Ed) MRCGP DRCOG
General Practitioner, Vice Chairman BASICS UK; Immediate Care Physician, East Midlands Ambulance Service NHS Trust; Physician Aircrew, Lincolnshire and Nottinghamshire Air Ambulance; Immediate Care Physician, MAGPAS Emergency Medical Team, UK

Keith C. Judkins MB ChB FRCA
Consultant Anaesthetist, The Burn Centre, Pinderfields Hospital, Wakefield, West Yorkshire, UK

Chris Kalman MSc MB ChB FFOM FRCP(Glas)
Director of Occupational Health and Safety Services, NHS Lothian, Astley Ainslie Hospital, Edinburgh, UK

J.M. Kendall MB ChB MD MRCP DIMC FCEM
Consultant in Emergency Medicine, Frenchay Hospital, Bristol, UK

Susan Klein MA(Hons) Cert(COSCA) PhD
Reader in Trauma Research, Aberdeen Centre for Trauma Research, Faculty of Health and Social Care, Robert Gordon University, Aberdeen, UK

Gerard Laden BSc
Director, Hyperbaric Medical Unit, East Riding Hospital, Hull, UK

J.Colville Laird MB ChB FIMC RCS(Ed)
General Practitioner and Director of Education for BASICS Scotland, UK

Evan L. Lloyd MB ChB FRCPE FRCA FFSEM(I&UK) FISM MFPreHospC DipSportsMed DipIMC
Former Consultant Anaesthetist, Western General Hospital, Edinburgh, UK

Kevin Mackway-Jones MA FRCP FRCS(Ed) FCEM
Professor of Emergency Medicine, Manchester Royal Infirmary, Manchester, UK

Peter F. Mahoney OBE TD FRCA L/RAMC
Defence Professor Anaesthesia and Critical Care, Insititue for Research and Development, Birmingham, UK

Alistair Main MD FRCP
Consultant Geriatrician, Selly Oak Hospital, University Hospitals Birmingham NHS Trust, Birmingham, UK

Andrew K. Marsden MB ChB FRCS(Ed) FFAEM FIMC RCS(Ed)
Medical Director, Scottish Ambulance Service National Headquarters, Edinburgh, UK

Steven G. Martin MSc GIFireE
Former ACO, South Wales Fire and Rescue Service, UK

Terry E. Martin MSc DAvMed FIMC FRCS(Ed) FRCS(Ed) FCARCSI FRCA
Consultant in Anaesthetics and Intensive Care, Medicine, Royal Hampshire County Hospital, Winchester, UK; Associate Professor, Department of Surgery, University School of Medicine, St George's Medical

School of Medicine, Grenada; Senior Medical Advisor (Safety), DERA, Centre for Human Sciences, Farnborough, Hampshire, UK

Ian D. McNeil MB ChB FIMC RCS(Ed) MRCGP AFCEM DRCOG DFFP
Medical Director, Reliance Medical Services; Consultant Medical Adviser, Race Course Association, Bristol, UK

Sue Maurice MB BS FRCS FCEM
Consultant in Emergency Medicine, Emergency Department, University Hospital of South Manchester, Wythenshawe Hospital, Manchester, UK

Steven W. Metcalf BSc(Hons) MB BS MRCP
Consultant in Emergency Medicine, Emergency Department, Queen Elizabeth Hospital, Woolwich, London, UK

Roger Michael
Former Detective Chief Inspector, South Wales Police, UK; former Head of Scientific Support and Head of the Regional Fingerprint Bureau, South Wales Police, Bridgend, Mid Glamorgan, UK

Virginia Murray FFOM FRCP FRCPath FFPH
Consultant Medical Toxicologist, Centre for Radiation, Chemicals and Environmental Hazards (CRCE), Health Protection Agency, London, UK

Julie Nancarrow MB ChB FCEM FRCS(A&E Ed) DA DIMC RCS(Ed) DRCOG
Consultant in Emergency Medicine, Warwick Hospital, Warwick, UK

Keith Porter MB BS FRCS FRCS(Ed) FIMC RCS(Ed) FSEM FCEM
Consultant Trauma Surgeon, Queen Elizabeth Hospital, Birmingham, UK; Professor of Clinical Traumatology, University of Birmingham, Birmingham, UK

A.D. Redmond OBE MB ChB MD FRCP(Glas) FRCS(Ed) FCEM FIMC RCS(Ed)
Professor of International Emergency Medicine, University of Manchester, Salford Royal NHS Foundation, Manchester, UK

B. Robertson OStJ TD MIEM LRCP MRCS
Managing Director, The Event Medicine Company, Aldershot, Hampshire, UK

James M Ryan OStJ MB MCh FRCS HonFCEM DMCC
Emeritus Professor of Conflict Recovery at UCL and University of London, London, UK

John Scott MB ChB FIMC RCS(Ed)
Medical Director, East Anglian Ambulance NHS Trust, UK

Howard M. Sherriff MB ChB FECM FRCS(Ed) FCEM FIMC RSC(Ed) MA
Consultant in Accident and Emergency Medicine, Addenbrooke's Hospital, Cambridge, UK

Nick Sherwood MB ChB FRCA DA(UK)
Consultant, Anaesthesia and Critical Care Medicine, City Hospital, Birmingham, UK

A.D. Simcock MB BS FRCA
Former Honorary Consultant Anaesthetist, Royal Cornwall Hospitals, Cornwall, UK

Jason Smith MB BS MSc MRCP FCEM DipIMC RCS(Ed)
Consultant in Emergency Medicine, Royal Navy, Derriford Hospital, Plymouth, UK; Senior Lecturer in Prehospital and Emergency Medicine, Academic Department of Military Emergency Medicine, Royal Centre for Defence Medicine, UK

Karen J. Souter MB BS FRCA
Associate Professor, Vice Chair for Education and Residency Program Director, Department of Anesthesiology and Pain Medicine, University of Washington Medical Center, Seattle, USA

Andrew H. Swain BSc PhD FRCS FCEM FACEM
Senior Lecturer in Emergency Medicine, Department of Anaesthesia and Surgery, University of Otago, Wellington, New Zealand

Darren Walter MB ChB FRCS(Ed) FIMC FCEM
Consultant in Emergency Medicine, University Hospital of South Manchester, Manchester, UK

Sean Walsh MB DCH MRCPI FCEM
Consultant in Paediatric Emergency Medicine, Our Lady's Children's Hospital, Crumlin, Dublin, Ireland

Terence Wardle BMedSci(Hons) BMBS(Hons) DM FRCP
Professor of Clinical Science, Consultant Physician, Directorate of Medicine, Countess of Chester Foundation Trust, Chester, UK

Richard Weekes MB ChB DFFP DipIMC MRCGP
General Practitioner, Ullapool, UK

Clive Weston MB FRCP
Reader in Clinical Medicine, Swansea University, Swansea, UK

Paul A. Younge BSc BM DA MRCP FCEM
Consultant in Emergency Medicine, Frenchay Hospital, Bristol, UK

David A. Zideman LVO QHP(C) BSc MB BS FRCA FIMC
Consultant Anaesthetist, Imperial College Healthcare NHS Trust, London; Honorary Senior Lecturer, Imperial College, London, UK

Part One

1   Immediate care in the United Kingdom 3
2   Immediate care world-wide 8

Immediate care in the United Kingdom

1

Introduction	3
History	3
The development of BASICS	5
Structure of BASICS	6
National accreditation	6
Immediate care today	6
What for the future?	7
References	7
Further reading	7

Introduction

Immediate care is defined in the Constitution of the British Association for Immediate Care (BASICS) as:

the provision of skilled medical help at the scene of an accident, medical emergency or during transport to hospital.

Although immediate care would appear to fill an obvious need for patients it developed surprisingly late in medical history and indeed is still not part of the statutory response to medical incidents outside hospital in the UK.

History

The first recorded mention of any help for patients outside hospital in the UK was in 1665 when Samuel Pepys described the use of pest coaches. These were used to transport those dying of fever to appropriate institutions. There was no medical provision whatsoever and the vehicles were little better than the charnel wagons available at the time. One has to look to military medicine for further developments, and no significant developments in prehospital care in the UK followed until the early 19th century.

The 19th century saw massive industrialization and a mass movement of the population from the land to cities. This was the time of huge civil engineering projects, and the need for medical help in the large construction projects and the factories became very clear. In 1888 the construction of the Manchester Ship Canal began. This involved linking the Irish Sea at Liverpool with inland Manchester. The project took 5 years and during its construction there were 3000 accidents. Sir Robert Jones was appointed Chief Surgeon and developed an emergency medical system linking the Royal Liverpool Hospital and the Manchester Royal Infirmary by telegraph (Fig. 1.1) (Irving 1989).

A railway was built along the side of the Ship Canal on which the injured could be transported, and two intermediate infirmaries were built and staffed by doctors. It could be said that this was the first development in the world of an integrated emergency medical service bringing together primary care, communication, transport, first-level care and tertiary referral.

The need for first aid in this new environment was self-evident. In 1877 two military medical officers, Surgeon Major Peter Shepherd and Colonel Francis Duncan, began

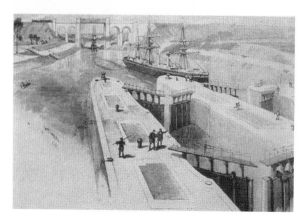

Fig. 1.1 • The Manchester Ship Canal. From Birmingham Accident Hospital Archive. Courtesy of Keith Porter.

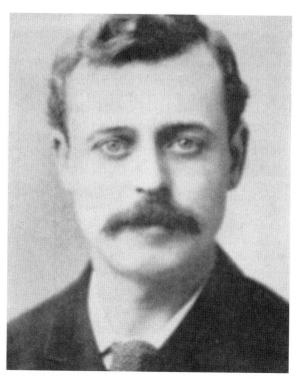

Fig. 1.2 • Sir Robert Jones. From Birmingham Accident Hospital Archive. Courtesy of Keith Porter.

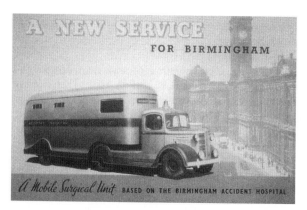

Fig. 1.3 • The Birmingham Accident Hospital mobile surgical vehicle. From Birmingham Accident Hospital Archive. Courtesy of Keith Porter.

to teach first-aid skills to civilians under the auspices of the St John Ambulance Association, which developed from the Order of St John. They drew from their experience in the military and also from the Royal Humane Society, which had been established in 1774 by Drs William Hoars and Thomas Coglan. The Society employed icemen to rescue people from drowning and built more than 250 receiving houses, which were effectively emergency first-aid stations but staffed by doctors.

First aid to the civilian community developed rapidly as a result of the work of the St John Ambulance Association. In industrial areas the Association became very involved in factory health and rescue operations in mines. A further component of the community self-help idea was the development of the panel doctor in coal mining areas. These doctors were actually appointed by the Miners' Association to look after miners and their families, and as a secondary role were expected to be present during colliery accidents. This is well described in A.J. Cronin's novel *The Citadel*, set in the South Wales mining valleys.

The First World War was notable for the introduction in 1915, by Sir Robert Jones (Fig. 1.2), of the Thomas splint (Rang 1966), which reduced the mortality of compound fractures of the femur from approaching 80% to approximately 20% in less than 1 year. Blood transfusion was introduced, and it was observed by Canon et al in 1918 that 'shock hinders bleeding', the first recorded description of hypotensive resuscitation.

In 1937 the General Post Office Telephones introduced the number 999 to be used on automatic dial telephones, which provided a single number access for all the emergency services. By the end of the Second World War this was a national service, not emulated in the USA until the mid-1980s with the 911 number.

In 1941 William Gissane established the concept of the Birmingham Accident Hospital, where there was a trauma team to care for accident victims led by senior clinicians. The Birmingham Accident Hospital, in 1964, was the first in the UK to offer a mobile surgical team delivering prehospital surgical care, mainly to industrial and road traffic accidents (Fig. 1.3). In a ground-breaking paper in 1942, J. Trueta postulated for the first time that immediate medical care made a difference to survivability.

In 1946, in the original National Health Service Act, it was said that the National Health Service would 'provide ambulances wherever necessary' and this was implemented in 1948 by local authorities. In 1974 the 144 local ambulance services were reduced to 64 ambulance services as part of the National Health Service under the Area Health Authorities. Prior to this, in 1966, the so-called Miller Report for the first time introduced a 6-week training period for ambulance employees. In 1969 Baskett introduced Entonox, the first drug to be available to ambulance staff for the control of pain. Finally, in 1976 the Department of Health agreed to recommend the advanced training of ambulance personnel. This had first been described by Haacker in Vietnam in 1966. In 1969 Pantridge & Adgey in Belfast described their mobile intensive care ambulance and Fry et al showed how aggressive resuscitation at the site of a motor vehicle accident could save lives.

Following the Platt Report, the first National Health Service Accident and Emergency (A&E) consultants were introduced in 1970, and after this no major changes were undertaken in the hospital delivery of care until the Royal College of Surgeons' *Report into Trauma* in 1988, which led to the setting up of a pilot trauma centre at Stoke-on-Trent with two comparator sites at Hull and Preston. At the same time a UK trauma registry, the Major Trauma Outcome Study (MTOS), was established at the Academic Department of A&E Medicine at Hope Hospital in Salford. In London, Wilson & Earlam developed the concept of the Helicopter Emergency Medical Service (HEMS) at the Royal London Hospital.

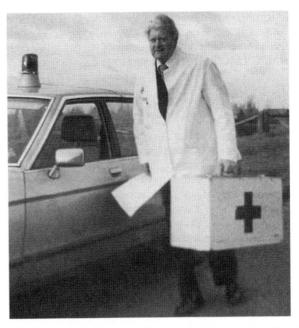

Fig. 1.4 • Ken Easton OBE. From Birmingham Accident Hospital Archive. Courtesy of Keith Porter.

The development of BASICS

Dr Kenneth Easton was an RAF officer in Catterick in the late 1940s who was often asked by the police to attend road accident victims on the A1 road many miles from a hospital. He realized that there was a major therapeutic vacuum between the time of the accident and the time of the first medical treatment in hospital (Fig. 1.4). Easton worked over many years with the then embryonic Royal College of General Practitioners and the Medical Commission for Accident Prevention, headed by Norman Capner, to develop the concept of immediate medical care provided by general practitioners (GPs). He was also at the forefront of pressure for improvement in the hospital accident and emergency services. In 1967 the first immediate care scheme was started at Richmond. In 1971 MAGPAS (Mid-Anglia General Practitioner Accident Service), which was destined to become the biggest immediate care scheme in the country, was established in East Anglia by Derek Cracknall and Neville Silverstone.

BASICS itself was inaugurated on 25 June 1977, operating from an office in the Royal College of General Practitioners. It initially had 1200 doctors and 73 immediate care schemes. At first there were no individual members, the organization being seen as an umbrella for schemes. From its inception it was realized that BASICS doctors needed to be able to share information and a journal was one of the first achievements of the new organization in 1977, acting as a means for the dissemination of information on techniques and equipment. A symposium was also organized in Cardiff to allow members to meet and exchange ideas and to learn of new innovations in the field. By the mid-1980s it was recognized that there was a need for a qualification in immediate medical care and, following discussions with a number of the Royal Colleges, the Royal College of Surgeons of Edinburgh agreed to award the Diploma in Immediate Medical Care, which was first examined in 1990. The Diploma continues to thrive and currently takes place over 2 days with written examinations including short-answer questions, multiple-choice questions, and triage exercises and vivas on trauma, medicine and major incident management.

It rapidly became clear that the Diploma was very much an examination for the competent, experienced immediate care doctor and the need for a basic entry-level exam was soon recognized. Following discussions in 1993 a multidisciplinary Pre-hospital Emergency Care Certificate was introduced. This is a 3–day course with an examination that is uniquely open to doctors, registered nurses and paramedics.

Academic accreditation was gained with the foundation of the Faculty of Pre-hospital Care at the Royal College of Surgeons, Edinburgh in 1995. In 1998 the College Council approved the decision to open the Diploma of Pre-hospital Care to paramedics and nurses, and agreed in principle to establish a College Fellowship in Pre-hospital Care. This will become the academic standard for the specialist in pre-hospital care in the UK. However, examinations are not the whole story. Clearly there needs to be some method of monitoring the activity of individual immediate care doctors. The concept of a log book was discussed by BASICS over many years and the pilot study started in the early 1990s.

In 1997 the *BASICS Journal* was developed into the *Journal of Pre-Hospital Immediate Care* in a cooperative venture between the Faculty of Pre-hospital Care, BASICS and BMJ Publications. This journal has recently joined forces with the *Journal of Accident and Emergency Medicine* to form the *Emergency Medicine Journal* (EMJ), which has a specific section within each issue dedicated to prehospital immediate care.

Structure of BASICS

The BASICS organization consists of a central council, with regional subcommittees. In the case of Scotland, the regional committee has very wide autonomous powers because of the different organization of the health service in that country. The administrative headquarters of BASICS is in Ipswich. There is a series of committees that have progressed much of the work of the organization; these include BASICS Education, which, under the leadership of Dr John Scott, was responsible for a number of innovative educational developments including the 5-day Immediate Care Course at Madingley Hall and the Pre-hospital Emergency Care (PHEC) courses. The equipment committee has not only looked at medical equipment but produced specifications for protective clothing and for the markings for vehicles. Cooperation and team work have always been promoted by BASICS; thus the interservice committee has been a forum for discussion between all the disciplines involved in immediate care and practical evidence of this was seen at major incidents such as the Clapham rail crash. In recent years, the research and development committee has started to work towards establishing an evidence base for immediate care.

National accreditation

For years BASICS sought national recognition for its work and on many occasions was encouraged by politicians, only to see the activities come to nought. This was particularly clear after the Hidden Report into the railway accident at Clapham, despite which no recognition or funding for BASICS was forthcoming. However, with the development of accreditation in the health service, change is beginning. Parliamentary investigations into the health service in Wales and the National Health Service Accreditation Agency have recommended that immediate care doctors and schemes should be accredited. It has now been agreed by the NHS accreditation agency that, in order to work as an agent of the ambulance service, accreditation will be compulsory, the gold standard being the Diploma in Immediate Medical Care and the minimum standard being the Pre-hospital Emergency Care Certificate. From April 1997, a formal accreditation process has been ongoing.

Table 1.1 Historical immediate care milestones

1937	London	GPO	999
1942	Birmingham	W. Gissane	Accident Hospital
1946	UK	Government	Ambulance Service
1949	Catterick	K.C. Easton	Attendance at road traffic accidents
1955	Derby	J. Collins	Hospital Flying Squad
1957	Heidelberg	Gogler	Mobile Operating Theatre
1960	Preston	H.M. Hall	Hospital Flying Squad
1964	Birmingham	Accident Hospital	Mobile Operating Theatre
1967	Bath	R. Snook	Hospital Flying Squad
1967	Catterick	K. Easton	Road Accident Aftercare Scheme
1971	East Anglia	Cracknel and Silverstone	MAGPAS
1972	Bristol	P. Baskett	Mobile Resuscitation Unit
1977			BASICS
1989	UK	JRCALC	Joint Royal Colleges Ambulance Service Liaison Committee
1990	Edinburgh	Royal College of Surgeons	Diploma in Immediate Medical Care
1995	Edinburgh	Royal College of Surgeons	Faculty of Pre-hospital Care
2001	UK		British Paramedic Association
2004	Edinburgh	Royal College of Surgeons	Fellowship in Immediate Medical Care

Immediate care today

Immediate care, having started very much as an initiative from GPs, now encompasses doctors from many other specialities, perhaps especially accident and emergency medicine (Table 1.1). There is a mixture of schemes, from very small GP-based schemes (such as those in the rural areas of Scotland where GPs provide a high standard of immediate care to their own patients) to large schemes such as those in Mid-Anglia, which have a membership that includes hospital accident and emergency staff, a full-time medical director and a training officer (Fig. 1.5).

Throughout the years Hospital Flying Squads have continued to develop. One has seen the development of the

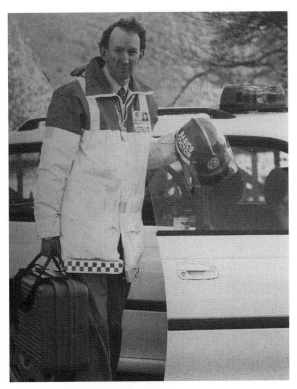

Fig. 1.5 • GP-based immediate care. From Birmingham Accident Hospital Archive. Courtesy of Keith Porter.

PETS system in Preston and the Derby Royal Infirmary Flying Squad. A major development was the introduction of the helicopter with the launch of HEMS at the Royal London Hospital delivering doctor-based medical care to the victims of trauma. An alternative model for the development of immediate care is provided by the CARE (Central Accident Resuscitation Emergency) team in Birmingham. The CARE team, which works alongside the ambulance service and provides medical and nursing pre-hospital skills, has members from both general and hospital practice. All the doctors are required to have passed the Diploma in Immediate Care and a very active training programme is ongoing. Every Friday and Saturday night, training 'slots' are provided for visiting BASICS doctors, which allow supervised hands-on training.

During its short history, BASICS has spawned various special interest groups. The first was the Association of Emergency Medical Technicians, which predated paramedic training. Members of BASICS have campaigned for national paramedic standards and have trained paramedics to this level. The Resuscitation Council has gone from strength to strength and is now accepted as the national body setting standards for resuscitation. Other smaller bodies such as the Association of Rally Doctors and the Medical Equestrian Foundation have done much to improve standards in their areas of interest.

What for the future?

The future shape of emergency services within the health service is far from clear. The bulk of GPs would seem to be withdrawing from emergency care, this work being delegated to cooperatives. This has led to an increasing demand on the ambulance service and an exponential increase in accident and emergency attendances and acute hospital admissions.

An initiative driven by the Faculty of Prehospital Care and involving the Academy of Royal Medicine colleges in 2008 is seeking to create a medical subspecialty of prehospital medicine.

References

Canon WB et al 1918 The preventative treatment of wound shock. Journal of the American Medical Association 70: 618–621

Fry C, Huelke DF, Gikas PW 1969 Resuscitation and survival in motor vehicle accidents. Journal of Trauma 9: 292

Haacker LP 1966 Time and its effects on casualties in World War II and Vietnam. Archives of Surgery 98: 39

Irving M 1989 The evolution of trauma care in the UK. Injury 20: 317–321

Pantridge JF, Adgey AAJ 1969 Prehospital coronary care. American Journal of Cardiology 24: 66

Rang M 1966 In: Anthology of orthopaedics. E. & S. Livingstone, Edinburgh

Trueta J 1942 Treatment of war wounds and fractures. British Medical Journal 1: 616

Further reading

Easton K (ed) 1977 Rescue emergency care. Heinemann Medical, London

Immediate care world-wide

2

Historical background   8

Modern prehospital care   9

Conclusion   13

Further reading   13

Historical background

The first recorded example of prehospital care being practised might be said to be the actions of the good Samaritan on the road to Damascus in New Testament times. The development of prehospital care throughout history has, however, been inextricably linked to warfare. The need to care for and treat the wounded of battle stimulated men such as Baron Dominique-Jean Larrey (1766–1842) (Fig. 2.1) during the Napoleonic Wars. He is credited with the development of the 'flying ambulance' (*ambulance volante*), a lightweight, covered horse-drawn wagon used to collect the wounded from the battlefield and transport them swiftly to the surgeons supporting the armies. He introduced the concept of taking the traditional hospital skills of the period into the field, and he is credited with personally performing 200 amputations in one 24-hour period at the Battle of Borodino. Many lives were undoubtedly saved as a result of his foresight in that campaign and his example has led many to consider him the founder of the modern emergency medical services (EMS) concept.

As the years went by, others took up the cause of the victims of warfare and another milestone was reached after the Battle of Solferino (1859) when Jean Henri Dunant

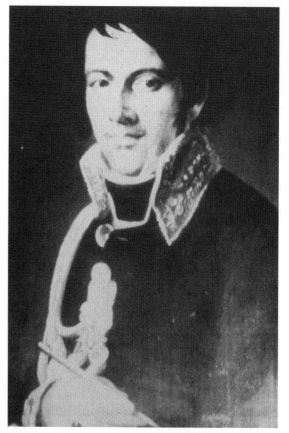

Fig. 2.1 • Baron Larrey. From Birmingham Accident Hospital Archive. Courtesy of Keith Porter.

(Fig. 2.2) called on the international community to recognize and alleviate the suffering of sick and wounded soldiers. His efforts led to the first Geneva Convention of 1864, which gave neutrality to medical personnel on the

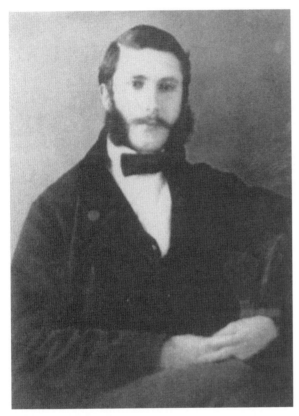

Fig. 2.2 • John Henri Dunant. From Birmingham Accident Hospital Archive. Courtesy of Keith Porter.

battlefield and led to the formation of various national aid societies, and ultimately to the International Red Cross.

The second half of the 19th century saw increasing industrialization, bringing with it increased accident rates and the first ambulance services in the UK were established in 'the potteries' and mining areas under the auspices of the Order of St John. The St John Ambulance Association started training the public in the provision of both aid to the injured and ambulance transport in 1877. The first first-aid manual was published in 1878. The St John Ambulance Brigade was founded in 1887 and London saw its first ambulance service in 1889.

Looking across the Atlantic to the USA, Baron Larrey's example was followed by the surgeons of the American Civil War, but civilian ambulance services were not to appear until the 1890s in Cincinnati and New York.

Many developments in medicine took place during the early part of the 20th century, and the First and Second World Wars continued to provide a stimulus to prehospital care and transportation of the sick and wounded. During the First World War horse-drawn ambulances were being replaced by the internal combustion engine, and by the end of the Second World War the era of aeromedical evacuation had arrived.

The mid-1960s saw a realization of the value of prehospital care in the cardiac sphere, and pioneering work was being done in various centres around the world from Belfast to Seattle.

The Vietnam War became another prehospital care milestone with the development of rapid transportation of the injured from point of wounding to the surgeon by helicopter, with commensurately increased survival rates. The increased levels of prehospital care in Vietnam prompted comments that the soldier wounded by enemy fire had a better chance of survival than the victim of a motor vehicle collision back in the USA.

Modern prehospital care

The provision of prehospital care in the modern world varies from country to country around the world. While many administrations aspire to the very best modern EMS concepts, their financial status does not allow it to be achieved. In some countries topography and demography are the keys, with good quality EMS available in the urban areas and little or no service in the rural districts.

The level of EMS provided in a country will often reflect the general level of secondary hospital care available. There is little point in providing state-of-the-art prehospital expertise if it cannot be followed up and capitalized on following arrival in hospital.

The rest of this chapter will look at prehospital care in contrasting countries from around the world.

PREHOSPITAL CARE IN FRANCE

France, including its overseas territories, is made up of 101 administrative departments. In each department there is an emergency medical assistance service, Service d'Aide Medicale Urgente (SAMU), which is usually attached to a major hospital. A few departments have two SAMUs.

Although not yet universal throughout France, SAMU is generally accessed through a dedicated telephone number 15. The SAMU is a 24-hour control centre that coordinates all medical response (Fig. 2.3). The first SAMU was created in Toulouse in 1967 and the current organization is now based on a legislative decree issued on 16 December 1987 that lays down how SAMUs are to be structured and operated. Each SAMU is under the direction of a 'Chef de Service' who is a doctor of consultant status.

The major functions of the SAMU can be described as:

- the provision of a centralized control room for the receipt of all emergency medical calls
- organization of the appropriate response
- ensuring the rapid arrival of skilled medical assistance
- maintaining radio links with hospitals
- identification of hospital beds for patients

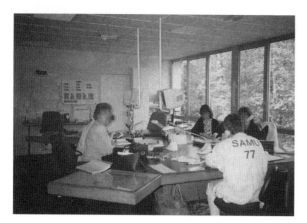

Fig. 2.3 • The SAMU 77 control room.

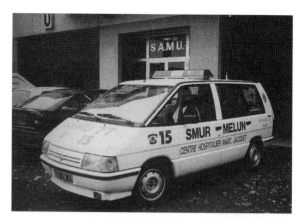

Fig. 2.4 • A typical SAMU rapid response unit.

- organization of interhospital transfers
- promotion of research and teaching of emergency and disaster medicine for medical and nursing personnel.

The SAMU service is physician led and the appropriate response to a request for medical help will be decided by a doctor on duty in the control room. Known as the regulating doctor, he or she will decide whether the response required should be from the general medical services that are equivalent to general or family practitioners. Alternatively, SAMU will despatch a Service Mobile d'Urgence et de Réanimation – Mobile Emergency and Resuscitation Service (SMUR) – team of which there are some 300 allocated to the various SAMUs around France.

The SMUR team consists of a doctor and nurse along with a driver in a fast-response vehicle (Fig. 2.4). Prehospital care is delivered exclusively by doctors and nurses. There are no ambulance paramedics or their equivalent in France. Ambulance services in France are generally seen as private transport agencies with little or no treatment component. Services in Paris and some other areas are provided by the fire brigade. In Marseille, the front-line ambulance service is the Naval Fire Service, as the municipal fire service has historically been provided by the French Navy. This dates from a historical occasion when a major fire in the docks areas was brought under control by French Navy personnel from ships moored in the harbour. As a consequence of this, in SAMU 13 in Marseille a naval doctor is present in addition to the SAMU regulating doctor to undertake the despatch of fire service ambulance resources.

The SAMU will provide and mobilize mobile intensive care ambulances for their SMUR teams to use and also for interhospital transfers.

The doctors working for SAMU have no specialty status so they tend not to stay in the service. Four to five years is the average duration of service before they move on. Throughout France all medical students do a period of secondment with SAMU during their training. The total number of medical students in France is, however, declining so a question mark hangs over the future supply of adequate numbers of SAMU doctors. There is a need to develop the equivalent of the paramedic but so long as there is a doctor-led service there is no establishment desire to change the status quo.

SAMU drivers are trained in basic first aid and have further training to ensure that they can assist the doctors. Legally, however, all interventions must be performed by doctors.

As an example of SAMU activity, SAMU 62 serves the Pas de Calais, a department with a population of 1.5 million people. This SAMU has seven SMUR teams, with the Arras SMUR attending 7000 calls per year. 60% of calls are for assistance with medical rather than trauma cases. In addition to its SMUR teams, this SAMU has two EMS helicopters based in Arras and Lille.

PREHOSPITAL CARE IN THE REST OF EUROPE

The French SAMU model is widely utilized throughout Europe. There are local and regional variations. Belgium has a prehospital care system largely based on the French SAMU concept. Germany also has a physician-led prehospital care service with its high profile network of EMS physician-staffed helicopters.

Portugal is a very good example of the other extreme. It has lagged behind the rest of Europe in its prehospital care provision and at present has a system that is physician-led in the three major cities of Lisbon, Oporto and Coimbra. In these locations there are medical-led 24-hour despatching centres using the single common emergency telephone number 112. These centres are comparatively recent developments based on the SAMU model. The Lisbon service started in 1987 but the Coimbra service only as recently as 1995.

In the more rural areas the ambulance service is less consistent, lacks physician involvement and is usually under

Table 2.1 The 15 components of the role of an EMS system

- Training
- Patient transfer
- Access to care
- Disaster planning
- Public safety agencies
- Communications
- Emergency facilities
- Public information
- Mutual aid
- Consumer participation
- Transportation
- Critical care units
- System evaluation
- Manpower
- Standardized record keeping

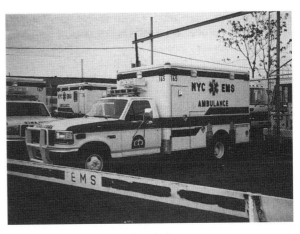

Fig. 2.5 • A New York EMS ambulance.

police despatch. There is no doubt that the concepts established in the three big centres of population will spread once finance and resources are identified and the need fully appreciated.

PREHOSPITAL CARE IN THE USA

The birth of prehospital care in the USA is considered to have occurred in 1965 when there was a realization that motor vehicle accidents were the major cause of death among those under the age of 75 years. The efforts of the next few years were to lay the foundations for the Emergency Medical Services (EMS) as known today throughout the USA.

The Highway Safety Act passed by the United States Congress in 1996 led to the development of a comprehensive Highway Traffic Safety Program, on which individual states were to base their own EMS developments. The federal guidelines defined three objectives for individual states to achieve. These were:

- the provision of a response to road crashes
- the sustaining of life through first aid and emergency care both at the scene and in transit
- provision of the coordination, transportation and communications that will ensure the injured victim reaches definitive medical care in the shortest possible time.

The first state to pass an act providing for paramedics and an emergency medical service was California in 1970. A standardized training curriculum for emergency medical personnel was also developed by the Department of Transportation in 1970. In 1973 the Emergency Medical Services Act specifically focused on EMS developments and redefined the 15 components of an EMS system. These were listed in the 1973 legislation and are given in Table 2.1.

Despite all the detail contained in the 1973 legislation the role of physician involvement in prehospital care in the USA was not defined until a subsequent report in 1981.

It was in the early 1980s that various training programmes were established from which were developed courses that are now well established throughout the

Table 2.2 The 14 components of a modern EMS system

- Medical direction
- Education
- Interfacility transport
- Dispatch
- Disaster planning
- Protocols
- Communication
- Receiving facilities
- Public information
- Mutual aid
- Finance
- Prehospital transport
- Special care units
- Audit

emergency care world. The first such course was the Advanced Cardiac Life Support (ACLS) course from the American Heart Association. This was followed by Basic Trauma Life Support (BTLS) from the American College of Emergency Physicians; Advanced Trauma Life Support (ATLS) from the American College of Surgeons; Prehospital Trauma Life Support (PHTLS) from the National Associations of EMTs and Pediatric Advanced Life Support (PALS) from the American Academy of Pediatrics and the American Heart Association.

A modern EMS system consists of a communication system that initiates a response, vehicles and personnel of appropriate training and qualifications, and an appropriate receiving hospital for the casualty (Fig. 2.5). The size and complexity of an EMS system, with its trauma centres, mobile intensive care units and helicopters, will reflect the geography and demography of the region it serves.

Regardless of their size, all modern EMS systems in the USA are now considered to consist of 14 components. These are listed in Table 2.2.

Medical direction of EMS systems in the USA is one of the major differences between the delivery of prehospital care in the USA and the UK. US law requires all states to have prehospital care under the control and certification of a physician. This physician is usually the medical director of the EMS and is then, in law, ultimately responsible for the care given by the staff employed in his or her EMS.

Medical direction is delivered in two forms, namely off-line medical control and on-line medical direction. Off-line medical control is usually vested in the medical director of the service and consists of the monitoring of all the elements of the EMS system, including protocols, standing orders and continuing educational programmes. Off-line medical control is therefore embodied in several of the 14 components of the modern US EMS system. On-line medical direction is real-time direct doctor/paramedic contact via a radio network usually located in a hospital emergency receiving room (Fig. 2.6). By this means crews in the field can receive physician direction, particularly in relation to drug administration, with the physician at all times retaining medicolegal responsibility. As a consequence of the lack of physicians actually delivering prehospital care in the USA, this means that on-line direction is often being provided by physicians with no prehospital experience. Some EMS organizations train emergency room doctors in the protocols that their personnel will use in the field but this is by no means universal. On-line medical direction is also a feature of several of the 14 components of the modern EMS systems listed in Table 2.2.

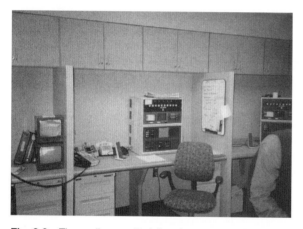

Fig. 2.6 • The on-line medical direction station in the emergency room complex at Parklands Hospital, Dallas, TX, USA.

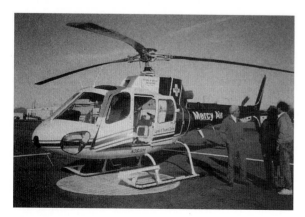

Fig. 2.7 • A typical US EMS helicopter.

The EMS systems in the USA have come a long way comparatively rapidly. One American medical text described the ability of EMS to grow from a gratuitous service provided by funeral directors in most communities to a multibillion dollar industry as quite remarkable. But further change will inevitably occur in the prehospital arena, as it will in the whole of medicine.

The prehospital care world watches the activity in the USA and often follows where the USA leads. Future changes in EMS systems will revolve around research into the clinical effectiveness of prehospital care interventions and the cost-effectiveness of the equipment used to deliver the service. The medical director of an EMS will be pivotal in future changes ensuring that the needs of the patient are paramount.

PREHOSPITAL CARE IN AUSTRALIA

The systems for provision of prehospital care in Australia vary from state to state. All states have a statutory ambulance service, which in some areas has developed from services originally provided by the St John Ambulance Brigade. These services are provided by paramedics. Although doctors are involved in training paramedics, medical directors of services have not yet been appointed. Some ambulance services have paramedics of various levels of training filling the first-responder role, especially in rural environments. Some areas have helicopter emergency medical systems, which are doctor-based. The Royal Flying Doctor Service serves remote areas providing flight nurses and doctors. All states are required to have a statutory voluntary state emergency service manned by civilians trained to ambulance technician status. In addition, there is the Voluntary Rescue Association, providing patient retrieval and care. Both these organizations have medical input to their training but are not staffed or operated by doctors.

PREHOSPITAL CARE IN ISRAEL

Prehospital care arose as a consequence of warfare, and in the modern world conflicts of all types serve to stimulate developments in prehospital care and the organizational aspects of triage, mass casualty handling and evacuation.

Israel is one such country where a number of wars during its comparatively short existence have led to very close integration between military and civilian medical organizations. Israel has both physicians and paramedics in the prehospital arena.

The ambulance service Magen David Adom (MDA) (Red Shield of David) is closely allied with the Israeli Defence Forces. The MDA was originally founded in 1918 by volunteer Jewish women providing care for Jewish fighting units but was disbanded in the 1930s.

Today the MDA has spread throughout the country and has several constituent parts. Its domestic first-aid stations, which provide both first aid and medical services, double as ambulance stations. The vehicle fleet consists of ambulances with paramedic crews and mobile intensive care units that are physician staffed. In addition, MDA runs a blood transfusion service. This national network can rapidly dovetail with the military in the event of conflict or large-scale incidents. For example, there are no military hospitals in Israel and in times of national emergency all hospitals may be put under command of the surgeon-general of the Israeli Defence Forces. Israel is a country that has moulded its prehospital care systems to meet its domestic, political, military and strategic needs.

PREHOSPITAL CARE IN HONG KONG

To complete this brief survey of prehospital care around the world mention should be made of the Far East. Hong Kong has been much in the news with its handback to China in 1997 after more than 150 years of colonial rule. Prehospital care throughout Hong Kong is coordinated by the Ambulance Command of the Fire Services Department. With the exception of the major incident situation there is no routine use of doctors in the prehospital arena in Hong Kong.

Prehospital care in Hong Kong has been influenced by outside countries and it must be wondered whether the return to China will alter or delay the progress being slowly achieved in prehospital care. Emergency Medical Assistant II level training, which includes defibrillation, is being delivered by a joint training programme imported from British Columbia in Canada. In addition, a paramedic level course is being imported from Australia but is in the early stages of implementation.

In addition to search and rescue services, off-shore Hong Kong has two volunteer organizations of particular importance in the field of disaster relief. The Auxiliary Medical Service, consisting of doctors, nurses and other specialists, and the Civil Aid Services both provide volunteers in the event of cyclones, forest fires, refugee influxes and other disasters, both natural and man-made.

Conclusion

There is no one single way of delivering an emergency medical service and it is valuable to study how things are done around the world. While it may be inappropriate to lift an entire service concept from one country to another because of cultural, financial or topographical considerations, they may all contain elements worthy of study that would transfer successfully from one country to another.

Further reading

American College of Emergency Physicians 1993 Medical direction of emergency medical services. ACEP, Irving, TX

Cole-Mackintosh R 1986 A century of service of mankind: the story of the St John Ambulance Brigade. Century Benham, London

Roush WR 1994 Principles of EMS systems. ACEP, Irving, TX

Salluzzo R et al 1997 Emergency department management: principles and applications. Mosby Year Book, St Louis MO

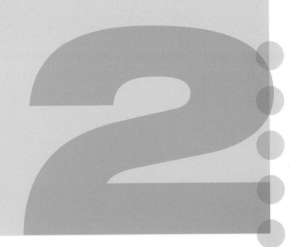

Part Two

3 Basic life support 17

4 Airway management and ventilation 26

5 Advanced life support 48

6 Vascular access 57

7 Shock 74

Basic life support

3

Introduction   17

Indications   17

Limitations   17

Contraindications to BLS   18

BLS – the technique   18

Physiology of BLS   20

Complications   21

The recovery position   21

Choking   22

Summary   23

References   24

Introduction

Basic life support (BLS) can be defined as the establishment of a patent airway, artificial ventilation and circulatory support in a person suffering cardiorespiratory arrest when no resuscitation equipment other than simple airway devices or protective shields is available (European Resuscitation Council 2005). Following a brief clinical assessment of the victim, vital functions are maintained by means of expired air ventilation and chest compressions. When basic airway equipment is employed, the term 'basic life support with airway adjuncts' is often used.

Indications

Once respiratory or cardiac arrest has been established in an unresponsive victim by confirming apnoea and/or the absence of a major pulse, BLS must be started immediately. In monitored arrests in prehospital care, defibrillation (in shockable rhythms) should precede BLS.

Limitations

One of the main factors limiting any improvement in survival following cardiorespiratory arrest is the incidence and variable quality of BLS performed by persons at the scene of collapse. Limiting factors include:

- lack of training amongst rescuers
- failure of untrained laypersons to diagnose cardiorespiratory arrest and to summon help
- failure of trained persons to commit themselves to BLS as a result of perceived inadequacies or unjustified fears of associated risks such as HIV transmission (Brenner et al 1994)
- environmental circumstances which may conspire against effective BLS (e.g. poor access to the patient)
- loss of skills despite the availability of refresher training, as there is no pressure on laypersons or most health workers to keep their skills up-to-date.

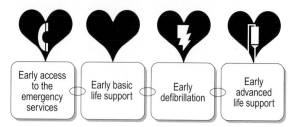

Fig. 3.1 • The chain of survival.

Although thousands of people have taken advantage of community resuscitation initiatives such as Heartstart UK, lack of training remains a problem for laypersons. Unfortunately, it will also continue to be a problem for medical, nursing and paramedical staff unless appropriate training is organized for these groups. BLS certification amongst GPs is usually confined to those who have fulfilled the entrance requirements for the MRCGP examination. Yet patients often collapse in the presence of a GP or close to a health centre (Colquhoun 1988). Good BLS skills are essential for all medical staff, irrespective of their specialty, and this is an obligation that all should accept. Individuals with greater experience of BLS achieve higher cardiac outputs (Fodden et al 1996).

BLS must be started within 3 min of cardiorespiratory arrest to provide a reasonable chance of cerebral recovery, and mortality rises markedly once the delay exceeds 4 min (Eisenberg et al 1979). The failure of bystanders to promptly apply effective BLS before trained staff arrive remains a major barrier to successful resuscitation.

Although BLS plays a vital role in saving life, it must be accepted that even optimal BLS can only restore about *25%* of the normal cardiac output (Del Guercio et al 1963), achieving an average systolic pressure of about 60 mmHg (Von-Planta & Trillo 1994). BLS therefore represents a *holding manoeuvre* designed to perfuse the brain and myocardium with partially oxygenated blood until definitive treatment, usually with a defibrillator, can be instituted. Without definitive treatment, irreversible asystole occurs in the majority of patients after 12 min of BLS (Enns et al 1983). The only aspect of resuscitation that is of greater value than BLS is early defibrillation and this sequence of priorities explains the concept of the chain of survival (Fig. 3.1) (Cummins et al 1991).

Despite these limitations, BLS is the foundation of ALS (advanced life support) and all health professionals need to be well trained in the procedure so that they can:

● institute effective BLS when confronted by an emergency while off duty and without expert assistance or equipment

● assess the competence of bystander BLS at an emergency and assist in improving its performance

● contribute to BLS teaching in the community.

Contraindications to BLS

The first principle of BLS is to protect both the rescuer and the victim from further harm. The absence of a safe environment (e.g. fire, frozen water, poisonous chemicals) is an absolute contraindication to BLS, as is knowledge of any current medical directive that resuscitation is inappropriate because of terminal disease or a similar condition.

Relative contraindications that may influence the application of BLS in the absence of airway adjuncts include contamination of the victim's mouth by poisons such as cyanide, infections such as tuberculosis or meningococcal septicaemia, or bleeding oral wounds in those who are positive for hepatitis B or human immunodeficiency virus (Zideman 1994). These rare circumstances may not be evident to the rescuer so it is always wise to carry an interpositional device such as a purpose-designed membrane (e.g. the Life Key) or a pocket mask with a non-return valve (which is much more bulky). Survival after submersion in water for more than 3 h has not been reported and BLS is normally inappropriate in this situation. Similarly, there is no record of any non-intoxicated normothermic adult surviving an arrest of cardiac origin unless BLS is instituted within 15 min of collapse, but the electrocardiogram should always be checked in such cases (Marsden et al 1995).

Infections, other than those mentioned above, that pose a lesser risk to the rescuer but are said to have been communicated by mouth-to-mouth ventilation include shigella, salmonella and herpes simplex (Zideman 1994).

BLS – the technique

The sequence shown in Table 3.1 is the procedure of BLS as advocated by the Resuscitation Council (UK) and European Resuscitation Council in 2005. It is purposely simplistic to cater for laypersons and the health-care professionals who teach them.

For resuscitation, the priorities are the airway, breathing and circulation – *ABC* (Table 3.2).

First, responsiveness should be assessed by gently shaking the shoulders of the patient and saying 'Are you all right?' If the patient is unresponsive, shout for help and open the airway.

The airway must be opened, either by combining chin lift with head tilt (Fig. 3.2) or applying jaw thrust (Fig. 3.3). Head tilt should always be avoided if trauma to the neck is suspected. For laypersons, it is recommended that these manoeuvres are first performed with the victim in the position found, turning him or her supine in the event of any difficulty.

By placing an ear over the victim's mouth and looking inferiorly along the front of the chest (Fig. 3.4), the presence of *breathing* can be determined in the standard manner

Table 3.1 Assess safety, check responsiveness

- *Ensure safety of the victim and rescuer* – both need to move if in danger
- *Check responsiveness* – stimulate the victim by shaking the shoulders gently and issuing a loud verbal challenge ('Are you all right?' is the standard phrase, even if it is patently inappropriate!)
- *If the victim responds by answering or moving* make a brief assessment and call for assistance if required. Reassess the victim regularly
- *If the victim is unresponsive*, shout or send someone for help.

Table 3.2 Open the airway, check for breathing

- *Open the airway* (see text)
- *Check for breathing* (see text)
- *If breathing is absent or abnormal*, obtain help, then start chest compressions
- *If normal breathing is present*, place the victim in the recovery position (Fig. 3.7) and monitor the breathing and pulse while help is obtained.

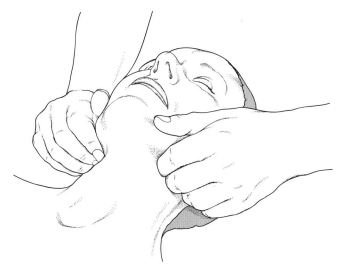

Fig. 3.3 • The jaw thrust manoeuvre.

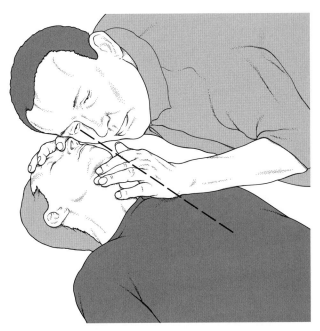

Fig. 3.4 • Checking for breathing.

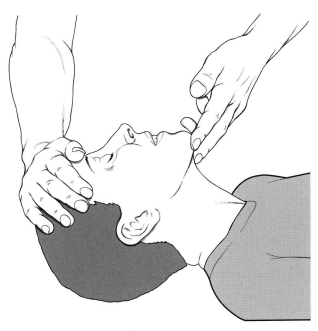

Fig. 3.2 • The chin lift and head tilt manoeuvres.

by *looking* for chest movement whilst *listening* and *feeling* for air on the cheek for up to 10 s. An occasional gasp should be considered no different from apnoea. The new guidelines emphasize that a diagnosis of cardiac arrest should be made if a victim is unresponsive and not breathing normally.

Rescuers are always advised to obtain assistance as soon as possible but the way this is achieved will depend on the situation (Table 3.3).

Once help is on its way, chest compressions should be started. The landmark for hand position has been simplified to the centre of the chest (Fig. 3.5), and 30 compressions should be delivered, depressing the sternum 4–5 cm on each compression, at a rate of about 100 per minute. Compression and release should take equal amounts of time.

After 30 compressions, two *effective expired-air ventilations (rescue breaths)* should be delivered, by opening the

Table 3.3 Obtaining help (call an ambulance)

- *If more than one rescuer is present*, commence resuscitation while the other fetches help
- *If you are alone, after establishing the patient is not breathing normally*, go for help yourself except when the victim:
  - has sustained serious trauma
  - is suffering from near-drowning
  - has suffered from poisoning
  - is a child.
  In these circumstances, there is a better prospect for survival if BLS is maintained for 1 min or so as the heart is usually healthy, cardiac arrest is a secondary event, and BLS alone may revive the victim
- *If none of these situations applies*, it must be assumed that the collapse has resulted from a primary cardiac event, that defibrillation will be the most effective intervention and that the lone rescuer should therefore leave the victim for as short a period as possible to call an ambulance.

Table 3.4 Breathing and circulation (I)

- Commence chest compressions. Place the hands in the centre of the chest. Give 30 chest compressions.
- Open the airway and deliver two rescue breaths.
- *If difficulty is encountered inflating the chest* at the first two attempts, recheck the mouth and remove any airway obstruction (but leave well-fitting dentures in place). Adjust head and jaw positioning but if obstruction persists make five attempts at giving two breaths before assessing the circulation as follows (it may be necessary to perform abdominal thrusts later, see text).
- Continue compressions and ventilations at a ratio of 30:2.

Basic life support is continued until:

- the victim exhibits signs of life, or
- appropriately qualified assistance arrives, or
- the rescuer becomes exhausted.

The use of adjuncts such as pocket masks and oropharyngeal or nasopharyngeal airways is described in the next chapter.

Prolonged BLS is indicated for certain conditions which may cause an otherwise healthy heart to arrest. Full neurological recovery has been reported in adults who received prolonged resuscitation (sometimes over a period of hours) following near drowning (Simcock 1991), hypothermia (Lloyd 1996), poisoning (Henry 1997) or electrical injury (Fontanarosa 1993, Graber et al 1996).

In hypothermia, up to 1 min is allowed to feel a major pulse, which may be very slow and weak. If any pulse is felt, or the cardiac arrest is known or considered to be less than 2 h old, full BLS is indicated (Lloyd 1996). Chest compressions may be less effective because cold tissues are more rigid and the blood is more viscous.

Physiology of BLS

The first attempts at basic life support may have been made in biblical times (Paraskos 1992), and chest compressions were used in the 19th century to try and restore cardiac output. In the early 20th century the only accepted technique for maintaining the circulation in a patient with cardiac arrest was internal cardiac massage through a thoracotomy incision. However, in 1960 Kouwenhoven and colleagues published their seminal paper on external chest compression which forms the basis of current practice (Kouwenhoven et al 1960).

Effective ventilation not only improves oxygen and carbon dioxide levels in the circulation but it also contributes to the forward flow of blood (Thompson & Rockey 1947, Forney & Ornato 1980). High tidal volumes or inflation

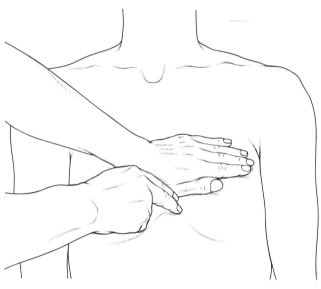

Fig. 3.5 • Correct hand position for cardiopulmonary resuscitation – simplified to the centre of the chest.

airway, pinching the nose and opening the mouth slightly while maintaining chin lift with the other hand. A good seal is made with the lips around the victim's mouth and *two* rescue breaths are given, sufficient to make the chest rise and fall as in normal breathing. Each inflation should be given over 1 s, avoiding high pressure and gastric distension that might result from this (Table 3.4). The chest wall is allowed to fall completely after removing the mouth. Compressions and ventilations should be continued at a ratio of 30:2, as outlined in Table 3.4.

pressures tend to distend the stomach and increase the risk of gastric regurgitation, which would pose a significant threat to the unprotected airway during BLS. It has recently been shown that expansion of the chest can be detected after only 400–600 ml of gas is insufflated (Baskett et al 1996). Carbon dioxide production is significantly reduced during circulatory arrest and further studies may show that a ventilatory volume of 400–600 ml is adequate, produces no additional hypercarbia or acidosis and carries less risk of aspiration.

Some uncertainties persist concerning external chest compression. One cannot tell in an individual case whether the pulses felt during chest compression predominantly represent a shock wave or forward flow, although the latter certainly occurs when effective chest compressions are performed (Del Guercio et al 1963). Forward flow is increased by maintaining pressure on the sternum during compression rather than jabbing at it (Taylor et al 1977) and it is therefore recommended that 50% of each cycle is devoted to compression and 50% to relaxation. Compression rates above $60\,min^{-1}$ fail to increase arterial pressure or end-tidal carbon dioxide levels (Ornato et al 1988), but to allow interruptions for ventilation a compression rate of $100\,min^{-1}$ is recommended.

Two theories have been used to explain the forward flow of blood that occurs during chest compression. It was originally thought that the heart was compressed between the sternum and the thoracic spine, and this 'cardiac pump' theory has been justified by many findings including those obtained by echocardiography (Deshmukh et al 1989, Higano et al 1990). However, as stated above, increases in intrathoracic pressure also generate forward blood flow (Thompson & Rockey 1947, Forney & Ornato 1980) and this has led to development of the thoracic pump theory, that chest compressions produce circulatory flow by generating cyclical increases in intrathoracic pressure. In reality, it is likely that both mechanisms operate (Robertson & Holmberg 1992, Redberg et al 1993, Von-Planta & Trillo, 1994) but whatever the mechanism, the perfusion pressure attained in the coronary arteries is a major determinant of survival (Paradis et al 1991).

The diagnosis of cardiac arrest and the return of spontaneous circulation are not as straightforward as previously believed. The circulatory output may be insufficient to permit the detection of major pulses, but even in healthy and awake patients it has been shown that the carotid pulse is not as easily located as is generally assumed (Mather & O'Kelly 1996, Monsieurs et al 1996).

Various techniques have been used to try and augment the effectiveness of chest compressions, either by using simultaneous compression and ventilation (Chandra et al 1980, Krisher et al 1989), abdominal compression alternating with chest compression (Mateer et al 1985), compression of the chest using a pneumatic vest (Halperin et al 1993) or use of a high compression rate (Maier et al 1984). None of these techniques has improved survival from cardiac arrest, but the latter did increase coronary perfusion pressure and for this reason the recommended rate of chest compressions has been increased to $100\,min^{-1}$.

In 1990, a male patient in the USA was successfully resuscitated with the aid of a sink plunger attached to his chest (Lurie et al 1990). No expired-air ventilations were performed. The device was thought to have worked by actively decompressing as well as compressing the chest and a commercial product (the CardioPump®) was developed based on this principle. The device has now been subjected to several trials but, despite initial optimism, none of these studies has demonstrated improved survival (Steill et al 1996).

There is now evidence that compression-only CPR may be as effective as combined compression–ventilation CPR in the first few minutes of cardiac arrest (Hallstrom et al 2000), and this method is now recommended if the rescuer is unable or unwilling to perform expired air ventilations.

Complications

Many complications have been attributed to external chest compressions. In order of frequency, these include rib fractures, sternal fractures, liver injury, gastric injury, pericardial bleeding and myocardial contusion (Nagal et al 1981). Mediastinal bleeding and emphysema (Powner et al 1984), as well as cardiac lacerations and pulmonary contusions (Beddell & Fulton 1986), have also been described. Emphysema may also extend into the peritoneal cavity (Rainer 1995). There is a strong consensus that the best way to avoid such complications is to perform chest compressions according to the standards taught, focusing on careful hand positioning (as described above).

If vomiting or regurgitation occurs during BLS, the risk of aspiration can be reduced in the absence of trauma by rotating the head fully to one side, allowing fluid material to drain, and residual debris can be cleared from the mouth with fingers, a handkerchief or similar material.

The recovery position

In the unconscious patient, this position is vital for preventing or reducing airway obstruction by the tongue and the aspiration of regurgitated gastric contents. Internationally, a number of slightly different positions have been advocated but the principles are the same and more important than the detail.

The recovery position advocated by the European Resuscitation Council in 1992 has been shown to produce

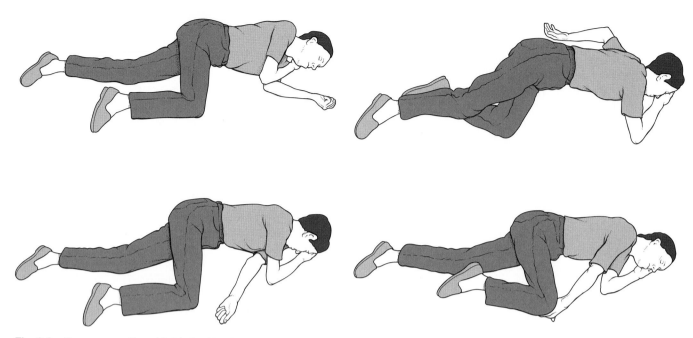

Fig. 3.6 • Recovery positions (a)–(d). Position (a) is that recommended by the European Resuscitation Council. (Redrawn from Rathgeber J, Panzer W, Betthauer M et al 1996 Influence of different types of recovery positions on perfusion indices of the forearm. Resuscitation 32: 13–17, with permission from Elsevier Ireland Ltd.)

arterial compression in the underlying arm (Rathgeber et al 1996). Current recommendations are therefore that:

● the victim should be as close to a true lateral (side) position as possible with the mouth dependent to allow free drainage of fluid from it
● the position should be stable
● it should be possible to turn the victim to or from the supine position whilst maintaining spinal alignment
● the position should permit observation of and access to the airway
● any pressure on the chest which might impair breathing must be avoided.

Four different positions which are said to satisfy these criteria are shown in Figure 3.6 (after Rathgeber et al 1996). The position taught by the European Resuscitation Council is currently used in the UK (Fig. 3.6a).

How to place a patient in the recovery position is illustrated in Figure 3.7 and Table 3.5.

Choking

Many patients will be able to dislodge a foreign body from their airway simply by coughing, and they should initially be encouraged to do so. If the airway obstruction is partial and the patient is still able to breathe, no further action may be necessary other than to arrange hospital transfer.

If the airway obstruction is complete or the patient is becoming exhausted or cyanosed, back blows or chest thrusts can be performed.

BACK BLOWS

Back blows are performed on the conscious patient as follows:

● the rescuer stands behind and slightly to one side of the casualty
● the casualty's chest is supported with one hand and the casualty is leant forward
● five sharp blows are given between the scapulae with the heel of the other hand; all five blows may not be necessary.

ABDOMINAL THRUSTS

If back blows fail, or the patient is unconscious, abdominal thrusts should be carried out.

For the unconscious patient:

● the rescuer kneels astride or to one side of the supine victim
● the rescuer places the heel of one hand over the midline of the upper abdomen (above the navel), with the other hand on top, and thrusts both hands sharply upwards towards the head, five times if necessary.

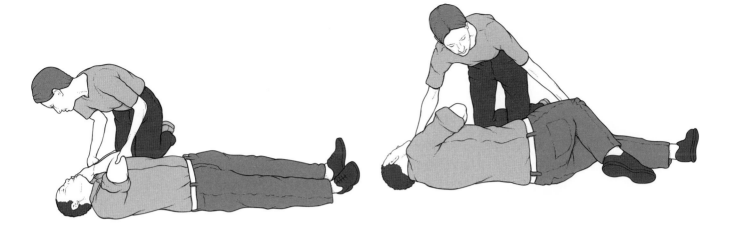

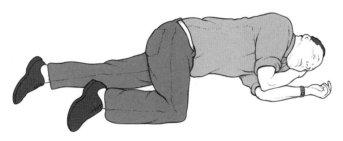

Fig. 3.7 • Putting a patient in the recovery position.

Table 3.5 Putting a patient in the recovery position

- With the casualty flat on their back, place the nearest arm out perpendicular to the body
- Bring the far arm across the chest and hold the back of the hand against the casualty's nearest cheek
- With your other hand grasp the casualty's far thigh just above the knee and raise it, keeping the foot on the ground
- Keeping the casualty's hand against his or her cheek, pull on the leg, rolling the casualty towards you on to his or her near side
- Adjust the upper leg (far leg) so that the hip and knee are bent at right angles
- Tilt the head back to ensure that the airway remains open and adjust the hand under the cheek if necessary.

For the conscious patient:

- in the conscious patient the rescuer stands behind the victim
- the rescuer's arms are put around the casualty
- one fist is clenched against the victim's epigastrium and the fist grasped with the other hand
- pulling sharply upwards and inwards, five abdominal thrusts are given.

Abdominal thrusts are contraindicated in infants because of the risk of visceral damage. In adults abdominal thrusts and back blows may be alternated in sequences of five in an attempt to clear an airway obstructed by a foreign body (Fig. 3.8).

Summary

A universal approach to basic life support in adults and children has now been agreed in accordance with the following sequence:

- check responsiveness
- open airway and check breathing
- start chest compressions
- continue compressions and ventilations at a ratio of 30:2.

To this must be added the prerequisite that safety for the rescuer and the victim are of paramount importance. A number of BLS options that may relieve airway obstruction (e.g. abdominal thrusts and the recovery position) are also important when resuscitation is performed in the absence of specialized equipment or expertise.

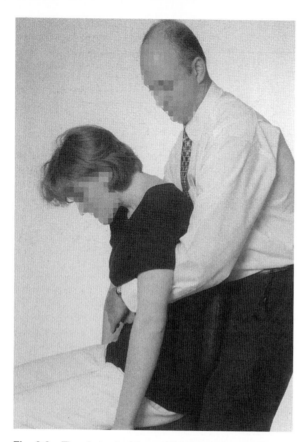

Fig. 3.8 • The abdominal thrust (Heimlich manoeuvre).

All medical and paramedical personnel may be called upon to resuscitate individuals inside and outside their normal clinical environment. Knowledge of the theoretical basis of BLS and competence in its application are essential if our common law obligation to save life is to be met.

References

Baskett P, Nolan J, Parr M 1996 Tidal volumes which are perceived to be adequate for resuscitation. Resuscitation 31: 231–234

Beddell SE, Fulton EJ 1986 Unexpected findings and complications at autopsy after cardiopulmonary resuscitation (CPR). Archives of Internal Medicine 146: 1725–1728

Brenner B, Stark B, Kauffman J 1994 The reluctance of house staff to perform mouth-to-mouth resuscitation in the inpatient setting: what are the considerations? Resuscitation 28: 185–193

Chandra N, Rudikoff M, Weisfeldt ML 1980 Simultaneous chest compression and ventilation at high airway pressure during cardiopulmonary resuscitation. Lancet 1: 175–178

Colquhoun MC 1988 Use of defibrillators by general practitioners. British Medical Journal 297: 336

Cummins RO, Omato JP, Thies WH et al 1991 Improving survival from sudden cardiac arrest: the 'Chain of Survival Concept'. Circulation 83: 1832–1846

Del Guercio L, Coomaraswamy R, State D 1963 Cardiac output and other haemodynamic variables during external cardiac massage in man. New England Journal of Medicine 269: 1398

Deshmukh HG, Weil MH, Gudipati CV et al 1989 Mechanism of blood flow generated by precordial compression during CPR. I. Studies on closed chest precordial compression. Chest 95: 1092–1099

Eisenberg MS, Bergner L, Hallstrom A 1979 Cardiac resuscitation in the community. Journal of the American Medical Association 241: 1905–1907

Enns J, Tweed WA, Donen N 1983 Pre-hospital cardiac rhythm deterioration in a system providing only BLS. Annals of Emergency Medicine 12: 23–26

European Resuscitation Council 2005 Guidelines for Resuscitation. Section 2. Adult Basic Life Support and use of automated AEDs. Resuscitation 67Sl: S7–S23

European Resuscitation Council (Basic Life Support Working Group) 2001 Guidelines 2000 for adult basic life support. Resuscitation 48: 199–205

Fodden DI, Crosby AC, Channer KS 1996 Doppler measurement of cardiac output during cardiopulmonary resuscitation. Journal of Accident and Emergency Medicine 13: 379–382

Fontanarosa PB 1993 Electrical shock and lightning strike. Annals of Emergency Medicine 22: 378–387

Forney J, Ornato JP 1980 Blood flow with ventilation alone in a child with cardiac arrest. Annals of Emergency Medicine 9: 41–43

Graber J, Unmenhofer W, Herion H 1996 Lightning accident with eight victims: case report and brief review of the literature. Journal of Trauma, Injury, Infection, and Critical Care 40: 288–290

Hallstrom A, Cobb L, Johnson E et al 2000 Cardiopulmonary resuscitation by chest compression alone or with mouth to mouth ventilation. N Engl J Med 342: 1546–1553

Halperin HR, Tsitlik J, Gelfand M et al 1993 A preliminary study of cardiopulmonary resuscitation by circumferential compression of the chest with use of a pneumatic vest. New England Journal of Medicine 329: 762–768

Henry J 1997 Poisoning. In: Skinner D, Swain A, Robertson C, Peyton R (eds) Cambridge textbook of accident and emergency medicine. Cambridge University Press, Cambridge, (ch 11)

Higano ST, Ewy GA, Seward JB 1990 The mechanism of blood flow during closed chest cardiac massage in humans: transoesophageal echocardiographic observations. Mayo Clinic Proceedings 65: 1432–1439

Kouwenhoven WB, Jude JR, Knickerbocker GG 1960 Closed chest cardiac massage. Journal of the American Medical Association 173: 1064–1067

Krisher JP, Fine EG, Weisfeldt ML et al 1989 Comparison of pre-hospital conventional and simultaneous compression–ventilation cardiopulmonary resuscitation. Critical Care Medicine 17: 1263–1269

Lloyd EL 1996 Accidental hypothermia. Resuscitation 32: 111–124

Lurie KG, Lindo C, Chin J 1990 CPR: the P stands for plumber's helper. Journal of the American Medical Association 264: 1661

Maier GW, Davis J, Tyson GJ et al 1984 The physiology of external cardiac massage: high-impulse cardiopulmonary resuscitation. Circulation 70: 86–101

Marsden AK, Andre G, Dalziel K, Cobbe S 1995 When is it futile for ambulance personnel to initiate cardiopulmonary resuscitation? British Medical Journal 311: 49–51

Mateer JR, Stueven HA, Thompson BM et al 1985 Pre-hospital IAC-CPR versus standard CPR: paramedic resuscitation of cardiac arrests. American Journal of Emergency Medicine 3: 143–146

Mather C, O'Kelly S 1996 The palpation of pulses. Anaesthesia 51: 189–191

Monsieurs KG, De Cauwer HG, Bossaert LL 1996 Feeling for the carotid pulse: is five seconds enough? Resuscitation 31: 0–8, S3

Nagal EL, Fine EG, Krischer JP, Davis H 1981 Complications of CPR. Critical Care Medicine 9: 424

Ornato JP, Gonzalez ER, Garnett AR et al 1988 Effect of cardiopulmonary resuscitation compression rate on end-tidal carbon dioxide concentration and arterial pressure in man. Critical Care Medicine 16: 241–245

Paradis NA, Martin GB, Rosenberg J 1991 The effect of standard- and high-dose epinephrine on coronary perfusion pressure during prolonged cardiopulmonary resuscitation. Journal of the American Medical Association 265: 1139–1144

Paraskos JA 1992 Biblical accounts of resuscitation. Journal of Medicine and Allied Sciences 47: 310–321

Powner DJ, Holcombe P, Mello L 1984 Cardiopulmonary resuscitation-related injuries. Critical Care Medicine 12: 54

Rainer TH 1995 Pre-hospital cardiopulmonary resuscitation and pneumoperitoneum. Journal of Accident and Emergency Medicine 12: 288–290

Rathgeber J, Panzer W, Betthauer M et al 1996 Influence of different types of recovery positions on perfusion indices of the forearm. Resuscitation 32: 13–17

Redberg RF, Tucker K, Cohen T et al 1993 Physiology of blood flow during cardiopulmonary resuscitation. A transoesophageal echo-cardiographic study. Circulation, 88: 534–542

Resuscitation Council (UK) 2005 Resuscitation guidelines. Resuscitation Council (UK), London

Robertson CE, Holmberg S 1992 Compression techniques and blood flow during cardiopulmonary resuscitation. Resuscitation 24: 123–132

Simcock T 1991 The treatment of immersion victims. Care of the Critically Ill 7: 177–181

Steill IG, Herbert P, Wells G 1996 The Ontario trial of active compres-sion–decompression cardiopulmonary resuscitation for in-hospital and pre-hospital cardiac arrest. Journal of the American Medical Association 275: 1417–1422

Taylor GJ, Tucker WM, Greene HL et al 1977 Importance of prolonged compression during cardiopulmonary resuscitation in man. New England Journal of Medicine 296: 1515–1517

Thompson SA, Rockey EE 1947 The effect of mechanical artificial respiration upon maintenance of the circulation. Surgery, Gynecology and Obstetrics 1984: 1059–1064

Von-Planta M, Trillo G 1994 Closed chest compression: a review of mechanisms and alternatives. Resuscitation 27: 107–115

Zideman DA 1994 Risks to rescuers. In: Handley AJ, Swain AH (eds) Advanced life support manual. Resuscitation Council (UK), London, ch 3

Airway management and ventilation

4

Introduction   26

Assessment   27

Basic airway management   27

Advanced airway management   31

The surgical airway   38

Oxygen therapy   41

Ventilation   43

References   45

Introduction

Patient assessment and resuscitation follow the sequence 'A, B, C' and this is more than just a mnemonic. Airway obstruction is a common and often preventable cause of death in prehospital care (Hussain & Redmond 1994), and can often be relieved by simple measures. The airway is the *first priority*: unless it is cleared, severe hypoxic brain damage can occur within minutes and any further treatment of the patient is futile.

Airway obstruction and poor ventilation lead to hypoxia and hypercarbia. Hypoxia causes ischaemia not only of the brain but also of other organs, particularly the heart and kidneys. Cardiac ischaemia may cause myocardial infarction or arrhythmias (ultimately severe bradycardia leading to asystole); renal ischaemia may contribute to subsequent renal failure. Hypercarbia also causes cardiac arrhythmias, and drowsiness or even unconsciousness. In addition, persisting airway obstruction may result in later pulmonary oedema (Willms & Shure 1988). Both hypoxia and hypercarbia are particularly dangerous in the head-injured patient, in whom they will cause a further rise in intracranial pressure (Ch. 23).

Airway obstruction may be either the cause or the effect of loss of consciousness. Most cases of acute life-threatening airway obstruction occur in the upper airway, i.e. above the thoracic inlet. Common causes are:

- soft tissue obstruction
- foreign bodies or foreign material
- haematoma
- oedema.

Soft tissue obstruction in the pharynx may be due to impaired consciousness and reduced muscle tone. The tongue is often said to fall back and block the pharynx: in fact this is an oversimplification, as the airway may obstruct in any position, including the upright and recovery positions. Nandi et al (1991) showed that the pharynx actually collapses at multiple sites, including the soft palate and epiglottis.

Foreign bodies or foreign material. Children are prone to inhaling peanuts and other food particles, and in adults the 'café coronary' is classically due to an inhaled piece of steak. Teeth or fragments of tissue may be inhaled in victims of facial trauma. The cerebrally obtunded patient may aspirate regurgitated stomach contents, although this usually causes more diffuse lower airway obstruction.

Haematoma, swelling or displacement of tissues may occur as a consequence of facial trauma.

Oedema may occur as a result of burns, anaphylaxis, infection (acute epiglottitis, croup) or trauma. Airway burns in particular can cause very rapid and severe oedema, which may be fatal without early intubation.

The prehospital situation presents its own problems in airway management, for example:

- access to the patient's head may be difficult
- the equipment available may be limited
- environmental difficulties (poor visibility; tracheal and other tubes becoming brittle in the cold; hazards of oxygen in the vicinity of sparks or cutting equipment)
- the cervical spine is at risk in many trauma victims, necessitating in-line immobilization of the head and neck
- aspiration of gastric contents is a risk in patients with a reduced level of consciousness.

This chapter discusses airway management and assisted ventilation by basic and advanced techniques. High-percentage oxygen should be given as soon as possible to patients with major trauma, serious medical conditions or airway compromise, and this is also discussed.

Assessment

After scene safety and evaluation, the airway and breathing are the first priorities for assessment.

INITIAL APPROACH

Clues about possible airway problems may be gained as the incident is approached, for example:

- *Fire*: consider smoke inhalation, carbon monoxide and cyanide toxicity, airway oedema
- *Chemicals*: airway problems from specific agents; for example, organophosphorus pesticides cause respiratory muscle paralysis, bronchoconstriction and pulmonary oedema
- *Trauma*: cervical spine, maxillofacial and chest injuries.

FIFTEEN-SECOND ASSESSMENT

A patient who answers your first questions sensibly must have a clear airway, reasonable breathing and adequate cerebral oxygenation. During this very quick assessment the cervical spine must be controlled and oxygen given if appropriate. Agitation or confusion must be assumed to be due to cerebral hypoxia until proved otherwise.

DETAILED ASSESSMENT

Look at:

- the patient: for cyanosis, respiratory distress or a choking appearance
- the airway: for obvious obstruction, oedema, haematoma, foreign body, trauma or burns
- the neck and chest (fully exposed): for respiratory rate, pattern and depth, use of accessory muscles, tracheal deviation, jugular venous distension, abnormal movement, intercostal or subcostal recession, or visible trauma.

Feel:

- at the mouth: for air movement
- the chest and neck: for tenderness, crepitus, subcutaneous emphysema and wounds.

Listen:

- at the mouth: for stridor (an inspiratory 'crowing' noise signifying upper airway obstruction), hoarseness or laryngospasm
- with a stethoscope: for abnormal or absent breath sounds.

If a problem is found at any stage it must be treated immediately and the patient reassessed until it has been corrected, before moving on to other forms of treatment.

Basic airway management

A summary of basic airway management in the unconscious patient is given in Table 4.1.

RATIONALE FOR BASIC AIRWAY MANAGEMENT

Continual *reassessment* is vital, particularly after every intervention.

In the unconscious patient, check the mouth visually for foreign matter *before* performing head tilt and chin lift. Otherwise, if soft-tissue obstruction is relieved by the latter methods, any foreign matter will be sucked into the trachea if the patient breathes. First-aid manuals often recommend the removal of tight clothing, but it is important not to become too distracted by this: if the patient's clothing did not obstruct his or her breathing before the emergency, it is unlikely to do so afterwards.

Visible foreign material in the airway should be removed. Blind finger sweeps are *not* recommended, as they can impact foreign bodies further down into the larynx and cause trauma and infection (European Resuscitation Council 2001, Kabbani & Goodwin 1995). Back blows or the Heimlich manoeuvre may be used in the conscious choking patient.

Table 4.1 Basic airway management (summary)

Reassess the patient at every stage.

Assess the airway and breathing. If compromised:
- remove obvious external obstruction (for example strangulation; object on chest)
- check the mouth for foreign matter; if present, remove by a finger sweep in adults or suction
- perform head tilt and chin lift, or – if cervical spine injury is suspected – jaw thrust.

If obstruction persists, try:
- increasing head tilt (care in trauma), chin lift or jaw thrust
- an oropharyngeal or nasopharyngeal airway
- if a foreign body is suspected but not visible, abdominal or chest thrusts (see 'Choking' in Chapter 3). Avoid blind finger sweeps.

If facial trauma is present:
- forward traction on a fractured maxilla, mandible or the tongue may relieve obstruction.

If the airway is clear but ventilation inadequate, assist by whatever means is available:
- mouth-to-mouth or mouth-to-nose ventilation
- Laerdal pocket mask
- self-inflating bag/valve/mask device.

Add high-flow oxygen as soon as possible, whether breathing is spontaneous or assisted.

If obstruction is relieved and the patient is breathing but unconscious, turn him/her into the recovery position unless injuries preclude this (Ch. 3).

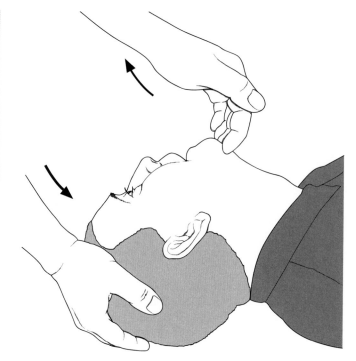

Fig. 4.1 • Head tilt and chin lift.

Head tilt and chin lift are performed by extending the head with one hand on the hairline or occiput and lifting the chin with the fingers of the other hand under the symphysis menti (Fig. 4.1). This pulls the tongue and epiglottis forward, and separates the pharyngeal walls. If cervical spine injury is suspected, a jaw thrust is an alternative method that minimizes cervical spine movement. A jaw thrust may be done in two ways.

- *From above the patient's head or beside his body (e.g. if he or she is trapped sitting in a car):* place your thumb on the patient's zygoma at each side while pushing the angles of the jaw forwards with your fingers
- *From above the patient's head:* open the patient's mouth with both your thumbs anterior to his or her symphysis menti while pushing the angles of the jaw forwards with your fingers (Fig. 4.2).

Another option is the 'trauma chin lift', in which the jaw is lifted between the thumb (inside the patient's mouth) and fingers (under the chin) without moving the head and neck.

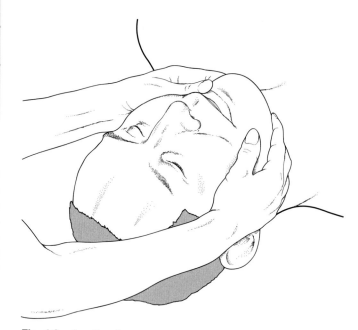

Fig. 4.2 • Jaw thrust.

Although cervical spine movement should be avoided if possible, *the airway always takes priority*, and neck movement must be accepted if the airway cannot be cleared in any other way.

Airway takes priority over cervical spine.

Only a small percentage of unconscious trauma victims will actually have a cervical spine injury and even if one is present neck movement may or may not make it worse. On the other hand, death is certain if the airway remains blocked.

In cases of facial trauma, a fractured maxilla may be displaced backwards and downwards, obstructing the airway by the soft palate contacting the posterior pharyngeal wall. This can be relieved by grasping the maxilla between the thumb (in the arch of the palate) and the fingers (in the alveolar margin) and pulling it forwards (Parkins 1996). A conscious patient can be encouraged to sit with his/her head held forwards, and the lateral or prone position is sometimes recommended (provided spinal immobilization can be maintained). Similarly a bilateral mandibular fracture allows the tongue to ride backwards, as it is effectively attached by the genioglossus muscle to a 'flail segment'. This can be relieved by pulling the segment forwards, or (in the unconscious patient) pulling the tongue forwards by a tongue suture (Ch. 24).

The recovery position (or other lateral position with spinal stabilization) helps to reduce tongue and soft tissue obstruction, as well as allowing vomit, blood and secretions to drain from the mouth. However, *it does not guarantee a clear airway*, and manoeuvres such as chin lift and jaw thrust may still be needed.

BASIC AIRWAY ADJUNCTS

The following devices are used to help clear the airway or to allow ventilation. They are *aids to, and not substitutes for*, the basic positional methods described above. Cervical spine protection must always be remembered.

Oropharyngeal (Guedel) airway

This is a short, curved, hollow tube, flattened in one diameter and with a flange at one end. When inserted into the mouth it is designed to keep the tongue forwards and maintain a clear airway for either spontaneous or assisted ventilation. Various sizes are available:

- neonates/children: sizes 000, 00, 0 or 1
- small adult: size 2
- medium adult: size 3
- large adult: size 4.

Alternatively, the size is chosen that is equal in length to the distance between the corner of the mouth and the angle of the jaw.

Table 4.2 The oropharyngeal airway: indications, contraindications and complications

Indications

- As an aid to airway maintenance in unconscious patients without a gag reflex
- As an adjunct to orotracheal intubation (with a tracheal tube in situ helps to stabilize tube position and stop the patient biting the tube if consciousness returns)

Contraindications

- Presence of a gag reflex

Complications

- Trauma (to teeth, mucosa, etc.)
- Worsening airway obstruction (the tongue may be pushed further backwards, or an oversized airway may lodge in the vallecula)
- Gagging or coughing
- Laryngospasm
- Vomiting

Insertion method

Check correct size, use head tilt if there is no risk of cervical spine injury. Insert the tip of the airway into the mouth, with the airway inverted (convex downwards). Pass the airway backwards into the mouth, rotating through 180° as it goes, until the flange lies anterior to the teeth. It is important to maintain head tilt, chin lift or jaw thrust: an oral airway alone may not be enough to maintain a patent protected airway.

Reassess: if obstruction is worse, remove it. If gagging, coughing, vomiting or laryngospasm occur, remove the airway and consider another method.

Nasopharyngeal airway

These are tubes of approximately 12–17 cm in length, usually made of soft plastic and bevelled at the tip (Fig. 4.3). They have a small flange at the proximal end and usually come packaged with a safety pin for insertion through this end to prevent them being inhaled through the nostril. When inserted through the nose the tip should lie in the hypopharynx, providing a clear passage behind the soft palate and tongue for spontaneous or assisted ventilation. They are better tolerated than oropharyngeal airways in semiconscious patients and are particularly useful when an oropharyngeal airway cannot be inserted because of trismus or facial swelling. Suitable sizes are:

- adult female: 6.0–7.0 mm (internal diameter)
- adult male: 7.0–8.0 mm.

Otherwise choose an external diameter just smaller than the patient's nostril.

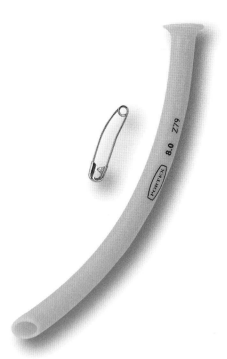

Fig. 4.3 • A nasopharyngeal airway. Reproduced with permission of Smiths Medical International Ltd.

Table 4.3 Nasopharyngeal airway: indications, contraindications and complications

Indications

- As an aid to airway maintenance in unconscious or semi-conscious patients, with or without a gag reflex
- Head-injured patients with clenched teeth

Contraindications

- Suspected base of skull or maxillary fractures are relative contraindications (theoretical danger of the airway penetrating the cribriform plate into the cranial vault)

Complications

- Trauma to turbinates and nasal mucosa
- Bleeding from nasal mucosa (can be severe)
- Coughing, vomiting, laryngospasm and airway obstruction if airway too long: may impact on the epiglottis or lodge in the vallecula (Stoneham 1993)
- Cribriform plate penetration in the presence of basal skull fracture

Cribriform plate penetration is a theoretical possibility, so these should be avoided in patients with severe facial trauma or evidence of basal skull fracture.

Insertion method

Choose the correct size airway, and lubricate it with water-soluble jelly. Insert the airway through a nostril, *directing it*

Table 4.4 Laerdal pocket mask: indications, contraindications and complications

Indications

- Ventilation of an apnoeic casualty, either:
  - as an alternative to mouth-to-mouth ventilation
  - as an alternative to a BVM device, when used by only one rescuer

Contraindications

- Major facial trauma

Complications

- Inadequate ventilation
- Gastric distension
- Hypercarbia, from the rescuer's expired air
- Hypoxia, unless supplemental oxygen is given (expired air contains about 16% oxygen)

posteriorly along the *floor* of the nasopharynx. Rotating the airway from side to side between your thumb and finger may ease its passage. If difficulty is encountered on one side, try the other. It does not matter which side is attempted first.

Continue inserting until the flange lies at the nostril. If coughing, laryngospasm or airway obstruction occur, withdraw by 1–2 cm. Insert the safety pin through the proximal end, close to the nostril.

Reassess airway and breathing.

Laerdal pocket mask

The Laerdal pocket mask is a plastic facemask for ventilation, of similar shape to the anaesthetic type with a flexible cuff to provide a seal around the patient's mouth and nose. It is held in position with both hands by a single rescuer, who gives expired air ventilation through a port at the apex of the mask. It is easier to use than the bag/valve/mask (BVM) device, especially for a single rescuer and for those less experienced in airway management.

With a single rescuer, better tidal volumes are possible than with a BVM device (Lawrence & Sivaneswaran 1985). Oxygen can be added through a nipple on the mask and the transparent plastic allows vomit or blood to be seen through the mask. Mouth-to-mouth contact is eliminated and a one-way valve prevents contamination of the rescuer's mouth by secretions or expired air.

Maximum oxygen concentration is lower than with a BVM device with oxygen reservoir (see below).

Technique

Position yourself behind the patient's head if possible (the mask is not easy to use unless the patient is supine). Use

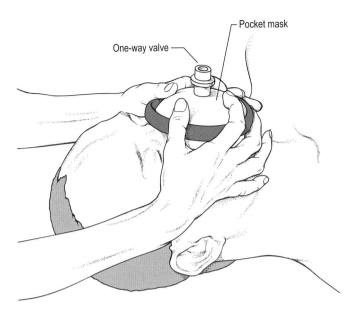

One-way valve — Pocket mask

Fig. 4.4 • Using the Laerdal pocket mask.

head tilt if there is no cervical spine injury. Hold the mask over the mouth and nose, and seal by either:

- holding the mask with both thumbs and index fingers, hooking the other fingers of each hand under the jaw and lifting the jaw into the mask using a 'pincer' movement (Fig. 4.4), or

- holding the mask with the thenar eminences on each side and lifting the jaw as before with the fingers of each hand.

Blow through the one-way valve, and watch for adequate chest movement. High-flow oxygen should always be administered. If ventilation is poor, adjust the mask position for a better seal, or use more head tilt or jaw lift.

Supplemental oxygen
When oxygen is added through the nipple on the mask, the percentage delivered depends on several factors, including the ventilation pattern. It is therefore an over-simplification to quote exact percentages (as some textbooks do), but at flows of around $15\,l\,min^{-1}$ between 35% and 58% oxygen may be delivered (Stahl et al 1992, Thomas et al 1992). If cylinder supplies are limited, lower flows may give lower but still useful concentrations. Flow rates above $15\,l\,min^{-1}$ may further increase the concentration delivered, as well as increasing tidal volumes and diluting carbon dioxide from the rescuer's breath. Therefore, if supplies allow, it seems sensible to use flow rates of at least $10–15\,l\,min^{-1}$, *provided* overinflation and gastric distension are avoided.

Advanced airway management

TRACHEAL INTUBATION

Tracheal intubation is the definitive method of airway control. A cuffed tracheal tube allows:

- a clear passage between the lips and trachea
- ventilation without air leak or stomach distension
- administration of 100% oxygen
- protection of the lungs from aspiration (stomach contents or foreign material)
- bronchial suction
- delivery of drugs during cardiopulmonary resuscitation (CPR).

However, the technique needs training and experience to perform and can have serious complications. It may also be difficult in the prehospital setting, because of poor access and inadequate equipment, and in patients who are not completely unconscious.

Intubation is not difficult to learn but is one of the most potentially dangerous treatments in resuscitation. It should never be undertaken lightly and should never be performed by those who are not properly trained. Patients rarely die from not being intubated but they may die from misplaced attempts.

In the apnoeic patient, unrecognized oesophageal intubation will quickly cause hypoxia and death.

Indications

In general, prehospital intubation may be indicated in:

- unconscious patients who are apnoeic or hypoventilating
- unconscious patients who are unable to maintain or protect their airway and are at risk of aspiration
- actual or potential airway obstruction (e.g. oedema from airway burns)
- significant head injury (Ch. 23).

However, there are few, if any, absolute indications for intubation in prehospital care. Whether or not to intubate depends not only on the patient's condition but also on the environment, the operator's expertise, the transfer time to hospital and the equipment available (particularly alternative airway devices).

Consider a patient with a Glasgow coma score of 8 following an isolated head injury. He is breathing spontaneously and has a gag reflex. In hospital he would be intubated urgently with the aid of anaesthetic drugs but should he be intubated at the scene? In fact, any attempt at intubation (even if nasotracheal) without the aid of such drugs may cause gagging, laryngospasm, hypoxia and raised intracranial pressure, as well as wasting valuable time. Unless anaesthetic drugs and expertise are available it may be best to transport the patient rapidly, maintaining the airway and oxygenation with more basic methods unless further deterioration occurs. Similarly, traumatic intubation attempts in a patient with airway burns may only worsen the oedema, and again rapid transport may be the safest option.

Contraindications

The only absolute contraindication is lack of training in the technique. Otherwise the complications listed below should be considered in the light of the need for airway control.

Complications

- Hypoxia, from prolonged attempts at intubation
- Oesophageal intubation – if unrecognized, leading to anoxia and *death*
- Intubation of a main bronchus, usually the right, if the tube is inserted too far
- Trauma to the teeth, pharynx, larynx or trachea
- Worsening airway obstruction, e.g. in acute epiglottitis, or laryngeal or tracheal trauma
- Exacerbation of cervical spine injury
- Gagging, coughing, laryngospasm, regurgitation or vomiting in the semiconscious patient
- Exacerbation of raised intracranial pressure in patients with head injury
- Cardiac dysrhythmias: tachycardia, bradycardia or extrasystoles. (*Bradycardia* is usually due to *hypoxia*.)

Table 4.5 Equipment for adult endotracheal intubation

- Laryngoscope (e.g. Macintosh, standard and large adult blades) – ideally two
- Cuffed tracheal tubes, sizes:
  - males – internal diameter 8.0–9.0 mm, length 23–24 cm
  - females – internal diameter 7.0–8.0 mm, length 20–22 cm
- Adult-size tubes may be precut but smaller uncut tubes may be needed if the airway is narrowed
- Suction equipment with wide-bore (Yankauer) catheter
- Gum-elastic bougie or intubating stylet
- Water-soluble lubricating jelly
- Magill's forceps (to remove foreign bodies or guide the tube through the cords)
- 10 ml syringe
- Stethoscope
- Adhesive tape or tie
- Ventilating device (self-inflating bag or purpose-designed ventilator) and oxygen
- Catheter mount (not essential)

TECHNIQUE FOR ADULT OROTRACHEAL INTUBATION

The following is a brief description; however, intubation can only be learned by adequate practical training.

1. Position the patient optimally where possible:
   - *No spinal injury*: flex the lower cervical spine and extend the head on the neck ('sniffing the morning air' position)
   - *Possible cervical spine injury*: use manual in-line stabilization (see under 'Difficult intubation').
2. Preoxygenate the patient for at least 30–60 s using high-flow oxygen and a tight-fitting facemask. Ventilate if necessary via a bag–valve–mask device or pocket mask.
3. Check the intubation equipment and suction apparatus.
4. Cricoid pressure (see below) should be applied if possible.
5. Insert the laryngoscope (held in the left hand) into the right-hand corner of the mouth, sliding the blade backwards and downwards towards the midline, so that the tongue is displaced to the left.
6. As the epiglottis comes into view, lift *along the line* of the laryngoscope handle (without levering on the teeth) to show the vocal cords beneath (Fig. 4.5). The tip of the curved blade should be in the vallecula, between the epiglottis and base of the tongue.
7. *If the vocal cords are visible*, insert the tracheal tube via the right-hand side of the mouth, *making sure that you see it pass through the cords*. Otherwise, do not attempt intubation blindly. A stylet or gum-elastic bougie may be used depending on experience.
8. Attach the self-inflating bag to the 15 mm connector on the end of the tracheal tube, either directly or via a catheter mount. Ventilate the lungs with oxygen and inflate the cuff with air until a leak is no longer heard at the mouth.

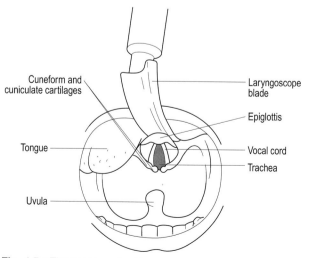

Cuneiform and cuniculate cartilages

Laryngoscope blade

Epiglottis

Tongue

Vocal cord

Trachea

Uvula

Fig. 4.5 • The vocal cords at laryngoscopy.

9. Check the tube position by watching for chest movement, listening with a stethoscope over the axillae and stomach, and other methods if available (see below). Have a high index of suspicion for misplacement. If only one lung inflates, withdraw the tube 1–2 cm and reassess.

If in doubt, take it out.

10. Secure the tube with adhesive tape or a tie. An oropharyngeal airway may also be inserted to prevent biting on the tube if consciousness returns.

11. Continue ventilation, keeping a constant watch to ensure this remains adequate.

Note: intubation should take no longer than 30 s. If unsuccessful within this time, revert to facemask ventilation for another 30–60 s before trying again. *Do not let the patient become hypoxic.*

RECOGNITION OF TUBE PLACEMENT

Clinical

- *See* the tube pass through the cords at intubation
- *Watch* the chest rise and fall with ventilation (both sides equally) and see that the abdomen does not distend
- *Listen* to both lungs (in the axillae, to avoid transmitted large-airway noises) and over the stomach
- *Feel* the self-inflating bag as you ventilate: the lungs often have an 'elastic' feel, whereas the bag usually deflates with a 'squelch' if the tube is oesophageal.

The first of these is the most reliable. However, *watching and listening to the chest are not always reliable*, especially in the obese patient: 'breath sounds' can sometimes be heard when the tube is in the oesophagus (Pollard & Junius 1980). The feel of the bag and the presence of condensation inside the tube can also mislead (Andersen & Hald 1989). By the time the patient becomes cyanosed, it is almost too late. If in doubt, take the tube out and ventilate with oxygen by another method.

Carbon dioxide detectors

Detecting carbon dioxide in expired air is an almost foolproof way of confirming tracheal intubation. A capnograph may be used but these are bulky and expensive (Donnelly et al 1995). Disposable carbon dioxide detectors (Denman et al 1990) are more practical, although the indicator colour change which these rely upon can be contaminated by stomach acid or acidic drugs such as adrenaline (epinephrine). Using either method, low cardiac output states (as in hypovolaemia or during CPR) lead to low carbon dioxide levels in expired air and may make positive confirmation difficult (Macleod et al 1991). Indeed expired carbon dioxide levels may correlate with the effectiveness of CPR (Sanders et al 1989).

Oesophageal detector device

As described by Wee (1988), this is a simple portable device consisting of a 50 ml syringe attached to a catheter mount, which fits over the 15 mm connector on the tracheal tube (Fig. 4.6). Easy aspiration of air from the syringe suggests tracheal placement; failure to aspirate air suggests oesophageal placement, as the walls of the oesophagus collapse around the tube. (It is vital to check the device is airtight before use.) Nunn (1988) described a modification using a self-inflating bulb. The device has been found by paramedics to be accurate and easy to use (Donahue 1994), and is reliable with uncuffed tubes in children above the age of 2 years (Wee & Walker 1991).

CRICOID PRESSURE

Regurgitation of gastric contents in the unconscious or semiconscious patient leads to pulmonary aspiration, with chemical pneumonitis and infection. In patients who may have a full stomach, cricoid pressure is used during intubation (and other forms of airway management) to prevent regurgitation (Sellick 1961). An assistant presses firmly backwards on the cricoid cartilage, usually with thumb and index finger, to occlude the oesophagus against the vertebral column (Fig. 4.7). If active vomiting occurs, the pressure is released to prevent oesophageal rupture (Ralph & Wareham 1991). Although often precluded by lack of available help, cricoid pressure is probably underused in prehospital care. It should be used where possible in any unconscious patient at risk of aspiration, before the airway is secured by intubation. In practice most patients in need of immediate care must be assumed to have a full stomach, unless they are capable of telling you otherwise.

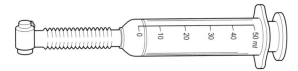

Fig. 4.6 • An oesophageal detector device.

DIFFICULT INTUBATION

Intubation difficulties may be due to:

- poor access to the patient
- persistent muscle tone
- the need for cervical spine stabilization
- the presence of swelling, haematoma or foreign material in the airway
- equipment problems
- anatomical abnormalities.

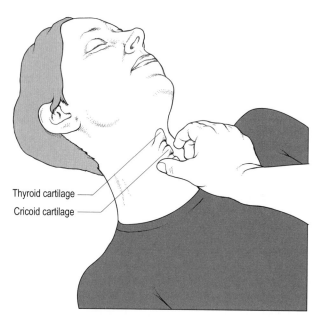

Thyroid cartilage
Cricoid cartilage

Fig. 4.7 • Cricoid pressure.

A patient trapped sitting in a car is a common access problem, in which case a laryngeal mask, Combitube or blind nasotracheal intubation could be life-saving (although every paramedic has his or her story of having intubated through a sunroof). Persistent muscle tone in the patient who is not fully unconscious makes intubation difficult without anaesthetic drugs (see below). Equipment problems may be due simply to lack of equipment or to the environment (for example, tracheal tubes and gum-elastic bougies become much less flexible in the cold).

Anatomical abnormalities are uncommon but Cormack & Lehane (1984) described four grades of laryngoscopic view in normal patients (Fig. 4.8). Grade 1 (full view of the vocal cords) is the most common. In grades 2 and 3 a gum-elastic bougie can be manipulated into the trachea and the tube railroaded over it, or a malleable metal stylet can be inserted into the tube to increase its curvature. In grade 4, intubation is likely to be unsuccessful despite these aids.

If cervical spine injury is suspected, intubation is ideally performed with an assistant maintaining manual in-line stabilization of the head and neck while the anterior portion of any cervical collar is removed (Criswell et al 1994). Semirigid collars make intubation more difficult by limiting mouth opening without giving any better immobilization than the manual method (Majernick et al 1986, Hastings & Marks 1991). If assistance is not available the collar may be left in place and the patient's head stabilized with blocks or the operator's legs. The effect of either method is usually to convert the laryngoscopic view to a higher (more difficult) grade, and a gum-elastic bougie is helpful in this situation (Nolan & Wilson 1993).

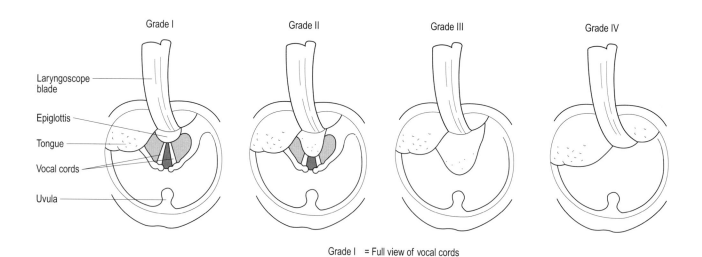

Grade I   Grade II   Grade III   Grade IV

Laryngoscope blade

Epiglottis

Tongue

Vocal cords

Uvula

Grade I = Full view of vocal cords
Grade II = Arytenoid cartilages and very posterior part of cords visible
Grade III = Epiglottis only visible
Grade IV = No laryngeal structures visible

Fig. 4.8 • Grades of laryngoscopic view in normal subjects.

Other aids and intubating techniques are:

- improving the head and neck position, if the patient's condition allows
- using cricoid pressure (see above)
- using a special laryngoscope (e.g. a McCoy laryngoscope) designed to improve the view of the cords
- intubating via a laryngeal mask (see below)
- using a 'light wand' (Vollmer et al 1985)
- tactile digital intubation
- using an alternative technique, e.g. a laryngeal mask, Combitube (see below), *or ventilation with bag, valve and mask device*
- blind nasotracheal intubation (see below).

INTUBATION IN CHILDREN

Despite the anatomical differences in children's airways, paediatric intubation is not usually difficult. However, intubation will not be tolerated and is potentially dangerous unless the child is fully unconscious, and rapid transport is the safest option in most paediatric airway emergencies. Important points are:

1. Pre-oxygenation is essential, as children desaturate very quickly.

2. A standard adult Macintosh blade laryngoscope is adequate for most children over 1–2 years old. Under this age, a straight paediatric blade is preferable (with the tip *posterior* to the epiglottis).

3. *Uncuffed* tracheal tubes are used below the ages of 10–12 years, as the cricoid ring is the narrowest part of the child's airway. A small leak should be present around the tube after intubation (too tight a tube may cause pressure damage, and later subglottic stenosis). (If in doubt, use a tube size similar to that of the child's little finger.) It may be better not to precut paediatric tubes to length, as in some conditions a narrower than usual tube may be needed. Where space to carry equipment is limited, tubes of internal diameter 3.0, 5.0 and 7.0 mm have been recommended as suitable temporarily in most adult and paediatric emergencies (European Resuscitation Council 1996).

As a rough guide to tracheal tube size:

Internal diameter (mm) = 4 + (age/4).

Because of the relatively short trachea, tube displacement and bronchial intubation are likely; therefore tube position and fixation are critical.

ORAL VS BLIND NASOTRACHEAL INTUBATION

In patients with possible cervical spine injuries, nasotracheal intubation (NTI) has been recommended as an alternative to oral intubation as it can be performed without laryngoscopy or neck extension (American College of Surgeons Committee of Trauma 1993). It can also be performed in unconscious or semiconscious patients with a gag reflex. However, *NTI has not been shown to be safer than oral intubation in cervical spine injury* (Wood & Lawler 1992), and it has the following drawbacks:

- the patient must be breathing spontaneously
- gagging, vomiting and laryngospasm may still result if airway reflexes are present
- trauma to and bleeding from the nasal cavity are likely
- a smaller diameter tube is necessary.

Suspected basal skull fracture or middle third facial fractures are relative contraindications, as meningitis is a risk, and intracranial passage of the tube through the cribriform plate has been reported (Horellou et al 1978, Patrick 1987).

Blind NTI is used commonly in the USA and some European countries but has not been popular in the UK. It may have a place in patients trapped in a difficult position (e.g. sitting in a car), when laryngoscopy is not possible. However, many such patients whose condition is serious enough to warrant intubation will have skull or facial fractures such that NTI would theoretically be contraindicated. In situations such as this the benefits of intubation may still outweigh the risks, which some argue have been overstated (Rhee et al 1993). The laryngeal mask airway and Combitube are showing promise in the management of these difficult situations.

Otherwise, it is generally felt that oral intubation is at least as safe as nasal, provided the operator is skilled in the technique, the head is kept in neutral and airway reflexes are absent. Bear in mind that if the patient *is* breathing and *does* have a gag reflex then the need for intubation is not absolute, and attempts may only worsen the situation.

ANAESTHESIA FOR INTUBATION

Oral intubation can only be achieved without anaesthesia in deeply unconscious patients without airway reflexes – in other words, in those who generally have the worst prognosis. Those who would benefit most from intubation are often semiconscious with preserved muscle tone and clenched teeth (e.g. after head injury), which makes any form of airway management difficult. These are the patients who might benefit from anaesthesia and muscle relaxation to allow intubation at the scene.

Indications for prehospital anaesthesia for intubation depend on the operator's expertise and the situation, but might include:

- head injury with reduced level of consciousness
- hypoxia unrelieved by other methods (for example in chest injury)
- actual or potential airway obstruction (but note the danger mentioned below).

The following drugs may be used:

- *Induction agents:*
  - thiopentone, etomidate, propofol, ketamine
- *Muscle relaxants:*
  - short-acting (for intubation): suxamethonium
  - longer-acting (for continued paralysis for ventilation): atracurium, vecuronium, pancuronium
- Maintenance of anaesthesia:
  - benzodiazepines and/or opiates (although these alone may not guarantee unconsciousness), propofol (by infusion).

Anaesthetic drugs should only be given by those who are *properly trained* in their use, and who are *skilled* at intubation. Their greatest danger is that they will easily cause *complete airway obstruction* as well as *apnoea*, turning a manageable situation into a potential disaster. If the operator finds himself or herself unable to intubate or ventilate, then the only option is a hurried surgical airway. Even experienced anaesthetists would think carefully before using such drugs outside hospital.

THE LARYNGEAL MASK AIRWAY

The laryngeal mask airway (LMA) has become widely used in anaesthesia over the last 20 years (Brain 1983). It consists of a wide-bore tube with a large, spoon-shaped inflatable cuff at the distal end (Fig. 4.9). When inserted blindly into the mouth the cuff sits above the laryngeal inlet and seals the pharynx, maintaining a clear airway and allowing spontaneous or controlled ventilation. Different sizes are available, for all ages from neonates to large adults (Table 4.6).

Indications

To provide a clear airway and/or to allow controlled ventilation in patients with decreased levels of consciousness, especially:

- when intubation is impossible because of patient factors (e.g. facial trauma, oedema) or environmental factors (e.g. difficult access to the patient)
- when no-one trained in intubation is present
- as an aid to difficult intubation.

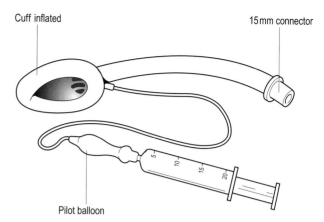

Fig. 4.9 • The laryngeal mask airway.

Table 4.6 Laryngeal mask sizes		
Laryngeal mask size	**Approximate patient weight (kg)**	**Cuff inflation volume (ml)**
1	<5	2–5
1.5	5–10	5–7
2	10–20	7–10
2.5	20–30	12–14
3	30–small adult	15–20
4	Medium adult	25–30
5	Large adult	35–40

Contraindications

- Lack of training in the technique.

Advantages

- Insertion is usually easy.
- It may be tolerated by patients in whom the gag reflex is not completely absent.
- Laryngoscopy is not needed for insertion. Therefore it can be inserted in most positions, e.g. with a patient sitting in a car.
- It may be inserted without neck extension in suspected cervical spine injury.
- It is suitable for all ages.
- It attaches directly to a bag–valve device, with or without a catheter mount.

Disadvantages

- It may stimulate gagging, coughing and vomiting in the semi-conscious patient.

- It does *not* protect against aspiration.

- It does *not* always guarantee a clear airway (it may be misplaced, the tip of the mask may fold or the epiglottis may be folded down inside the opening of the mask).

- It does *not* guarantee adequate ventilation. Ventilation with pressures that are too high may cause gas to escape around the cuff and may lead to gastric distension. Because of this, LMA ventilation must not coincide with chest compression during CPR.

- It can easily be displaced following insertion.

There are now numerous reports of its use in difficult airway problems in anaesthesia and prehospital care (Calder et al 1990, Greene et al 1992, Aye & Milne 1995). During CPR it has been found to be easy to use by nurses and paramedics (Pennant & Walker 1992, Stone et al 1994) and more effective than bag–valve–mask ventilation (Alexander et al 1993, Martin et al 1993). It is now included in the advanced airway management algorithm of the European Resuscitation Council (1996) as an initial alternative to tracheal intubation during CPR.

Intubation using the laryngeal mask

This can be performed in cases of difficult intubation, or where access to the patient is limited. With a size 3 or 4 LMA in situ, a size 6.0 uncut tracheal tube is passed through it into the trachea (Heath & Allagain 1991). Alternatively a gum-elastic bougie is passed through the LMA into the larynx, the LMA is removed and a larger tracheal tube is threaded over the bougie (Chadd et al 1989). An 'intubating laryngeal mask' has recently been developed.

Conclusion

The LMA has a useful place in prehospital care as an alternative to facemask ventilation, or to intubation when this is not possible. It functions as a mask and not a tube, and so does not guarantee ventilation or prevent aspiration.

THE OESOPHAGEAL–TRACHEAL COMBITUBE

The oesophageal–tracheal Combitube is a double-lumen airway, which allows ventilation and protection from pulmonary aspiration (Frass et al 1987). It consists of two parallel lumina, one open at the distal end and the other closed distally but with perforations in its midsection (Fig. 4.10). There is a small distal cuff and a larger proximal (pharyngeal) balloon. As well as sealing the pharynx, the larger balloon helps to keep the device in position. It is designed for use in adults over 1.52 m (5 feet) tall (the smaller Combitube SA can be used in adults between 1.22 and 1.52 m (4 and 5 feet) in height).

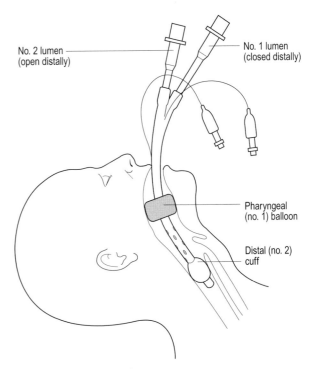

Fig. 4.10 • The Combitube.

Following blind insertion into the pharynx, the proximal balloon is inflated with 100 ml of air, and the distal cuff with 15 ml. In most cases the tube will enter the oesophagus and the lungs can be ventilated via the perforations in the closed lumen. This is confirmed clinically by watching and auscultating the chest and abdomen. (A carbon dioxide detector or self-inflating bulb can also be used to check placement.) If the tube has entered the trachea, ventilation is changed to the open lumen and checked in the same way. In either case the lungs are protected from aspiration.

Indications

To provide a clear airway and allow controlled ventilation in patients with decreased levels of consciousness, especially when:

- intubation is impossible because of patient factors (e.g. facial trauma, oedema) or environmental factors (e.g. difficult access to the patient)
- no-one trained in intubation is present.

In common with the LMA, the Combitube has been used in difficult airway problems (Banyai et al 1993, Staudinger et al 1995), including a patient with neck impalement (Eichinger et al 1992). It is also included in the advanced airway management algorithm of the European Resuscitation Council (1996) as an initial alternative to tracheal intubation, and has been used successfully by paramedics and nurses during CPR (Atherton & Johnson 1993, Staudinger et al 1993).

Ventilation through the Combitube during CPR has been shown to give a slightly higher arterial oxygen partial pressure than with conventional tracheal intubation, of statistical but probably not clinical significance. This was probably due to prolonged expiratory flow through the perforated lumen with the generation of positive end-expiratory pressure (Frass et al 1989).

Contraindications

- Patients with active gag reflexes
- Patients with known oesophageal disease, or who have ingested caustic substances
- Lack of training in the technique.

Advantages

- Insertion is usually easy and laryngoscopy is not needed
- It may be inserted with the neck in neutral alignment
- The inflated pharyngeal balloon helps to anchor the device in position
- It attaches directly to a bag–valve device, with or without a catheter mount
- Intubation is possible past the Combitube by deflating the pharyngeal balloon.

Disadvantages

- The Combitube is bulky
- It is unsuitable for use in children
- It is not tolerated by patients with gag reflexes
- It is inadvisable in cases of foreign body upper airway obstruction (blind insertion may push the object further down)
- Insertion may worsen soft-tissue airway injuries
- Gastric inflation may occur if the tube position is not checked carefully
- The large pharyngeal balloon may be damaged on insertion by sharp teeth
- The Combitube cannot be used for drug delivery during CPR.

Conclusion

The Combitube may prove a useful alternative to intubation when the latter is not possible in prehospital care. Unlike the LMA it may protect against pulmonary aspiration.

The surgical airway

A surgical airway is created by:

- tracheostomy
- cricothyrotomy: either by (a) needle or (b) surgically.

In immediate care a tracheostomy is *inappropriate* as it is technically difficult, time-consuming and has serious complications from injury to adjacent structures (thyroid gland, carotid arteries, jugular veins, pleura and vagus and recurrent laryngeal nerves). However, the cricothyroid membrane is superficial, easily accessible and relatively clear of major vessels and nerves. Therefore, *cricothyrotomy* is the only option in the emergency situation.

Surgical cricothyrotomy involves incising the cricothyroid membrane with a blade and inserting a small tracheostomy or other tube into the trachea. Ventilation can then be controlled or spontaneous, provided that a large enough tube is used. In needle cricothyrotomy the membrane is punctured by a large cannula (12 or 14G), and ventilation must be controlled by the insufflation of oxygen.

'Hybrid techniques' are also possible with devices such as the Nu-Trach or Melker sets, inserted through a cricothyroid puncture but allowing dilation to accommodate a larger tube. However, these methods may be more time-consuming than the standard needle or surgical approaches.

Indications

A surgical airway is indicated when the airway and ventilation cannot be maintained in any other way. This may occur in the presence of:

- severe injury, haematoma or oedema of the face or airway
- foreign body upper airway obstruction
- limited access to the patient's head.

This 'can't intubate can't ventilate' scenario is rare but life-threatening, and demands *immediate treatment* to prevent cerebral anoxia.

Contraindications

As cricothyrotomy is a last resort, there are no absolute contraindications. However, *surgical* cricothyrotomy is not advised in children, as it may cause damage to the cricoid cartilage and upper airway collapse.

COMPLICATIONS

Early

- Hypoxia and hypercarbia (prolonged insertion, failed insertion, misplacement or inadequate ventilation)
- Haemorrhage: external
- Haemorrhage: internal – into the neck tissues, or into the airway (cardiac arrest due to airway obstruction from blood clot has been reported following Mini-Trach insertion (Campbell & O'Leary, 1991)

- Oesophageal perforation
- Surgical emphysema (usually from misplacement of cannula)
- Air trapping due to inadequate exhalation, leading to:
  - pneumothorax, pneumomediastinum
  - surgical emphysema
  - reduced venous return, reduced cardiac output and hypotension.

Late

- Infection
- Subglottic stenosis, especially in children (Burkey et al 1991)
- Voice dysfunction, due to vocal cord or cricothyroid muscle damage.

ANATOMY

The cricothyroid membrane lies between the thyroid and cricoid cartilages on the anterior surface of the larynx (Fig. 4.11). Its upper margin is about 10 mm below the vocal cords. Trapezoid in shape, it measures approximately 30 mm from side to side and 9 mm from top to bottom, with an area of 3 cm^2. The small cricothyroid artery runs transversely across the upper third of the membrane (Burkey et al 1991).

TECHNIQUE

With either technique, *speed is essential*. Irreversible brain damage may occur within a few minutes if the airway is completely obstructed.

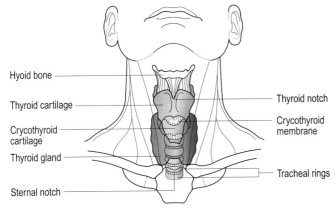

Hyoid bone

Thyroid cartilage

Crycothyroid cartilage

Thyroid gland

Sternal notch

Thyroid notch

Crycothyroid membrane

Tracheal rings

Fig. 4.11 • Anatomy of the cricothyroid membrane.

Needle cricothyrotomy

1. Prepare the equipment: 12 or 14G intravenous cannula, syringe, oxygen source, delivery system and connectors (see below), stethoscope.
2. Position the patient, identify the membrane and stabilize the larynx as described for 'Surgical cricothyrotomy' below.
3. Puncture the skin in the midline over the cricothyroid membrane, using the cannula with syringe attached.
4. Aiming 30–45° caudally, keeping to the midline, advance the cannula towards the lower cricothyroid membrane while aspirating on the syringe.
5. When air is aspirated, advance the cannula over the needle into the trachea.
6. Withdraw the needle and *aspirate again* to confirm tracheal placement.
7. Attach the ventilating system (see below) to the hub of the cannula.
8. Ventilate as appropriate, checking clinically for adequate inflation.
9. Secure the cannula in place: in practice it is easily displaced and the only reliable way is to hold it continually.

Surgical cricothyrotomy

1. Prepare the equipment: scalpel blade, swab, tube (ideally size 6.0 cuffed tracheostomy tube if available, or tracheal tube), self-inflating bag and oxygen source, 10 ml syringe, stethoscope, tape or bandage.
2. Position the patient with his/her head in the midline, and the neck extended if possible.
3. Palpate the cricothyroid membrane between the thyroid and cricoid cartilages.
4. Stabilizing the larynx between thumb and index finger of the non-dominant hand, make a horizontal or vertical midline skin incision over the lower half of the membrane.
5. Incise the membrane horizontally and dilate the opening by inserting the scalpel handle and rotating it through 90° (or using forceps if available).
6. Insert an appropriate tube into the opening.
7. Inflate the cuff and ventilate by attaching a self-inflating bag to the tube connector (directly or via a catheter mount).
8. Check for adequate ventilation.
9. Fix the tube *securely* with tape or a tie, or by holding it.

OXYGEN DELIVERY AND VENTILATION SYSTEMS

Ventilation through a tracheostomy tube can be achieved using a self-inflating bag or a mechanical ventilator. These are not very suitable for needle cricothyrotomy, and a variety of systems have been described for ventilation through a cannula. These systems must be assembled in advance, and include the following:

- A jet injector system using a high-pressure (50–60 psi) oxygen source.
- The following systems connected to a standard oxygen flowmeter, set to 15 l min⁻¹:
  - a length of standard green oxygen tubing. An expansion at the distal end is pushed *firmly* into the barrel of a 2 ml syringe with the plunger removed. A hole is cut across the side of the tubing just before the syringe. The syringe is pushed into the cannula hub and ventilation is achieved by intermittently occluding the hole ('1 s on, 4 s off')
  - an intravenous giving set cut off just below the drip chamber and connected to an oxygen supply. The distal end is attached to a three-way tap, which is attached to the cannula hub. Ventilation is achieved similarly by occluding the open port on the three-way tap.
- A self-inflating bag-valve device attached to:
- a 3 mm endotracheal tube connector, the smaller end of which is pushed into the cannula hub
- a 7 mm endotracheal tube connector, the smaller end of which is pushed into the barrel of a 2 ml syringe, which is attached to the cannula hub
- a suitably sized cuffed tracheal tube. The distal end of the tube is inserted into the barrel of a large syringe and the cuff inflated. The syringe is then attached to the cannula hub.

A high-pressure oxygen source is preferable, and a jet injector system using oxygen at 50 psi has been shown to give good tidal volumes (Benumof & Scheller 1989). However, such systems are not usually available outside hospital. A standard oxygen flowmeter delivers oxygen at lower pressures (even at maximal flow rates), and these pressures may be too low to give adequate tidal volumes through a relatively narrow cannula. Similarly, ventilation with a self-inflating bag may not generate sufficient pressure for adequate tidal volumes. Therefore carbon dioxide will accumulate with the latter two methods, although *oxygenation* may well be adequate. These techniques are therefore thought to give only 20–40 min grace before a better method is established.

Needle cricothyroidotomy provides 20–40 min grace.

Whichever system is used, ventilation will be impaired if exhalation is not adequate. Although *insufflation* is determined by the flow of oxygen under pressure, *exhalation* is driven only by the elastic recoil of the lungs and the upward excursion of the diaphragm. The force generated by these

is unlikely to overcome the high resistance of the relatively narrow cannula, and therefore exhalation is mainly dependent on a patent upper airway. In other words, the upper airway must act as a one-way valve, allowing gas to escape from below although ventilation is impossible from above. If gas cannot escape from below, air trapping and high intrathoracic pressures will occur. As well as compromising ventilation further, this carries the risks of reduced venous return and cardiac output, pneumothorax, pneumomediastinum and surgical emphysema.

Needle or surgical cricothyrotomy?

The relative advantages and disadvantages of these two methods are summarized in Table 4.7.

Ventilation is likely to be better with the surgical technique. The larger tube should allow adequate tidal volumes to be delivered and should also allow complete *exhalation,* preventing the problems of air trapping described above. Spontaneous ventilation may also be possible provided that a short (e.g. tracheostomy) tube of adequate calibre is used. The minimum internal diameter needed for sustained spontaneous breathing is often said to be 6 mm, although smaller tubes may be suitable in the short term (Ooi et al 1993). In addition, tube fixation is easier and ventilation is possible using a standard self-inflating bag, without the special tubing and connectors needed for needle cricothyrotomy.

In favour of needle cricothyrotomy is the fact that it is quicker to perform in a situation where speed is absolutely

Table 4.7 Needle vs surgical cricothyrotomy

Characteristic	Surgical cricothyrotomy	Needle cricothyrotomy
Ease of insertion	Not difficult, but more training needed	Usually easy
Complications	Mainly from trauma at insertion	Mainly from barotrauma or poor ventilation
Ease of ventilation	Easy and effective with standard equipment	Equipment needs special preparation: oxygenation adequate but carbon dioxide removal poor
Duration of effective ventilation	Hours or days	20–40 min only
Spontaneous breathing	Possible	Not possible
Ease of fixation	Easy	Difficult
Use in children	No	Yes

essential. It is also arguably easier to learn, and some UK ambulance services are already using the technique. Needle cricothyrotomy is less traumatic than the surgical approach and in particular minimizes the risk of bleeding (potentially severe) from the cricothyroid artery, which crosses the membrane. In children below the age of 12 years needle cricothyrotomy is the recommended approach.

It must be remembered that needle cricothyrotomy is a *temporary life-saving measure* and must be replaced as soon as possible by intubation or tracheostomy. Any patient after needle cricothyrotomy must undergo *rapid transport to hospital.*

In summary, no comparative trial is available of the success rates and overall complications of the two approaches. Therefore (except in children) no firm recommendations can be made, and each person must decide which method is best in view of his or her own skills, the clinical circumstances and the environment.

Oxygen therapy

Patients with significant trauma or serious medical conditions are at risk of hypoxia for the reasons listed below. Hypoxia means reduced oxygen availability at *tissue* level and is usually due to reduced oxygen content of arterial blood (hypoxaemia). This may be hard to detect clinically: cyanosis occurs only with severe arterial desaturation. Detection is especially difficult in the prehospital setting, where lighting is often poor.

Hypoxia leads to tissue anaerobic metabolism and lactic acidosis, cerebral and cardiac ischaemia, mental confusion and agitation, impaired cardiac contractility, and cardiac arrhythmias (tachycardia, bradycardia, extrasystoles and ultimately cardiac arrest).

Patients with major trauma and serious medical conditions should generally be given high-percentage oxygen as soon as possible, provided it is safe to do so. *Oxygen therapy comes with the 'A' and 'B' of the primary survey.* There are very few medical contraindications to high-percentage oxygen (see below) and if in doubt it is better to give it than to withhold it.

PHYSIOLOGY OF OXYGEN CARRIAGE

Inspired air containing 21% oxygen is normally drawn into the lungs by the process of ventilation (see under 'Ventilation' below). Once in the alveoli, oxygen diffuses across the alveolar–capillary membrane to the blood, while carbon dioxide passes in the reverse direction. In the blood, oxygen is carried almost entirely bound to haemoglobin, although very small amounts are also dissolved in plasma.

From the tissue capillary beds, oxygen diffuses into cells, where it takes part in *aerobic* metabolism. Under conditions of hypoxia, *anaerobic* metabolism occurs: this is less efficient in terms of energy production and also generates lactic acid. The resultant metabolic acidosis is responsible for harmful effects such as impaired cardiac contractility.

The term *oxygen delivery* refers to the quantity of oxygen delivered to the body as a whole per min, and is given by the formula:

Oxygen delivery = Cardiac output × Arterial oxygen content.

Therefore in a patient with both hypoxaemia and reduced cardiac output (as, for example, in cardiogenic shock with pulmonary oedema) these two factors will combine to cause tissue hypoxia and both must be corrected.

Under normal conditions, a small amount of blood (approximately 1–2% of the cardiac output) enters the systemic circulation without having been oxygenated in the lungs. This 'physiological shunt' consists of desaturated blood from the thebesian veins of the heart and the bronchial veins, which drain into the left ventricle and the pulmonary veins respectively. This has the effect of depressing the arterial $P\text{O}_2$ slightly. In conditions such as pulmonary oedema or consolidation, poor oxygenation of blood in the lung capillaries leads to a much greater 'pathological shunt', with potentially serious hypoxia.

CAUSES OF HYPOXIA

Hypoxia may be due to either reduced delivery or increased consumption of oxygen.

Increased consumption will occur in patients who are shivering or restless, or in those who are already pyrexial. *Reduced delivery* may be caused by problems at any stage of oxygen uptake and carriage, as listed in Table 4.8.

Low cardiac output states lead to a reduction in mixed venous oxygen saturation because the body continues to extract the same amount of oxygen from the slower circulation. Therefore the tendency of the normal physiological shunt to lower arterial $P\text{O}_2$ will be increased. Many causes of a low cardiac output (e.g. pulmonary oedema) are also associated with a pathological shunt, and these two problems will combine to give more serious hypoxaemia than either alone would do.

Carbon monoxide has approximately 200 times the affinity of oxygen for haemoglobin and therefore reduces carriage of oxygen to the tissues. Giving high-percentage oxygen will reduce the half-life of carbon monoxide by displacing it from haemoglobin. In anaemia the arterial oxygen *content* will be reduced because of lack of haemoglobin, although the oxygen *saturation* of haemoglobin remains normal.

Table 4.8 Hypoxia due to reduced delivery

- Low partial pressure of inspired oxygen:
  - Smoke inhalation
  - Non-respirable atmosphere
- Airway obstruction
- Hypoventilation or mechanical ventilatory problems – see under 'Ventilation'
- Impaired diffusion across alveolar-capillary membrane:
  - Pulmonary oedema
  - Lung contusion
  - Lung consolidation or collapse
  - Aspiration of fluid, blood or vomit
- Low cardiac output:
  - Hypovolaemia
  - Cardiac failure/cardiogenic shock
  - Cardiac tamponade
  - Tension pneumothorax
- Reduced combination of oxygen with haemoglobin:
  - Carbon monoxide poisoning
  - Anaemia
- Inability of cells to utilize oxygen:
  - Cyanide poisoning
  - Carbon monoxide poisoning

Cyanide and carbon monoxide inhibit the cytochrome system and block cellular metabolism, despite adequate tissue oxygen delivery.

OXYGEN STORAGE

In prehospital care, oxygen is usually carried in cylinders in the form of a compressed gas. Liquid oxygen reservoirs and chemical oxygen generators are also available and offer much greater economy of space for a given volume of oxygen. They are sometimes used for prolonged journeys or special environments, e.g. on aircraft or submarines.

Oxygen cylinders are generally made of molybdenum steel although some (e.g. those supplied with some forms of transport ventilators) are aluminium. In the UK they have the standard colour black with white shoulders but different colours are used in other countries (e.g. blue in Germany, and green in the USA). Different sizes of cylinder are available, and it is important to know the volumes of gas that these contain (Table 4.9). A full D-size cylinder, for example, contains 340 l and at an oxygen flow rate of 15 l min^{-1} will need replacing after only 23 min.

Whatever the size, a full cylinder has a pressure of 137 bar (1987 psi) at 15°C, and this pressure does not vary significantly over normal ambient temperatures in the UK. Because the cylinders contain compressed gas, the pressure decreases in direct proportion to the volume of oxygen used – in other words, a pressure of 68 bar shows that only

Table 4.9 Sizes and capacities of oxygen cylinders

Cylinder size	C	D	E	F	G	J
Height (inches)	14	18	31	34	49	57
Capacity (l)	170	340	680	1360	3400	6800

half the gas remains. These pressures would be dangerously high if transmitted directly to a patient's lungs, so cylinders are fitted with pressure-reducing devices that limit the pressure to about 4 bar. The gas is then supplied to the patient through a flowmeter, which reduces the pressure still further and allows delivery of flow rates typically between 0 and 15 l min^{-1}.

Although oxygen cylinders are very robust they should be handled carefully, as the very high internal pressures could cause cylinders to explode if damaged. Extreme heat (such as in a fire) could cause a dangerous rise in pressure, again with the risk of explosion.

DANGERS OF OXYGEN THERAPY

Scene safety

As well as the above risks, there is also the danger of fire or explosion if oxygen is used close to sparks or a naked flame (cigarettes, fire service cutting equipment), or if oil or grease comes into contact with the cylinder valve or attachments. Burns to a patient have also been reported from ignition of oxygen when a defibrillator was used; therefore the oxygen supply must be kept away from the patient when defibrillating.

Medical

Carbon dioxide retention is a theoretical risk if high-percentage oxygen is given to certain patients with chronic obstructive airways disease (COAD). These are patients who normally retain carbon dioxide and have lost their hypercarbic stimulus to breathing. Their respiratory drive therefore depends solely on hypoxia, and high blood oxygen tensions may lead to hypoventilation and carbon dioxide retention to the point of carbon dioxide narcosis. In a hospital situation these patients would normally be given limited concentrations of oxygen (24% or 28%), via a fixed performance mask (see below) and monitored by blood gas estimation.

In practice, this risk is often overstated. Chronic carbon dioxide retention occurs in only a minority of patients with COAD: it occurs rarely if at all in young people or in pure asthma (unless during a severe attack, when it is a sign of exhaustion). If carbon dioxide retention is seriously thought to be a risk, then low flow rates can be used initially with careful monitoring. But *correction of hypoxia takes priority*: give as much oxygen as is needed to do this, and assist ventilation if necessary.

Cylinder oxygen is a dry gas and has an unpleasant drying effect on the patient's pharynx. Prolonged use of dry oxygen also leads to impaired clearance of sputum and secretions. Ideally, oxygen should be humidified, but this is rarely practicable outside hospital: portable 'bubble humidifiers' are not very effective and need to be kept upright. However, these side-effects are not usually a problem given the short timescales involved in prehospital care.

Oxygen toxicity is a theoretical risk with prolonged administration but can be ignored in immediate care.

OXYGEN DELIVERY SYSTEMS

Devices used for the spontaneously breathing patient are considered here: equipment for ventilation is discussed below.

Oxygen delivery devices are classified into:

- fixed performance (Venturi masks)
- variable performance (Hudson-type mask, nasal cannulae).

The non-rebreather reservoir mask falls between these two categories, and is discussed below.

Variable performance devices deliver an inspired oxygen concentration that varies with the patient's breathing pattern and is hard to predict. Fixed performance devices are designed to deliver a known constant percentage of oxygen whatever the breathing pattern. The difference is rarely important in prehospital care, when the aim is usually to give the highest possible concentration of oxygen. However, in a patient with carbon dioxide retention a fixed performance Venturi mask is preferred, to give a known and limited oxygen concentration. Failing this, a variable performance mask can be used at low flow rates.

The reason for this difference in performance is as follows. Inspired oxygen from a mask will be diluted on inspiration by air entrained around the side of the mask, *unless* the gas flow rate exceeds the patient's inspiratory flow rate. Although a patient's minute volume (see under 'Ventilation') may be only $6–7 \, l \, min^{-1}$, the *peak inspiratory flow rate* (PIFR) may be over $30 \, l \, min^{-1}$. Variable performance devices cannot match these flow rates and so allow dilution of oxygen to an extent dependent on the patient's breathing pattern. The fixed performance Venturi mask is designed so that the oxygen flow entrains large volumes of air *in a known proportion* through a Venturi attachment. Provided the oxygen flow rate is adequate (as written on the mask), the total flow rate is comparable to the PIFR and so gas dilution around the mask is minimized.

Table 4.10 Approximate oxygen concentrations delivered by a Hudson-type mask at different oxygen flow rates

Oxygen flow ($l \, min^{-1}$)	Percentage oxygen
2	24–38
4	35–45
6	51–61
8	57–67

These percentages may be reduced by hyperventilation.

Hudson-type mask

These simple plastic facemasks give variable oxygen concentrations depending on flow rate and breathing pattern (Table 4.10). They can be used if a better device is not available but even high flow rates will give little more than 60–70% oxygen.

Non-rebreather reservoir mask

This consists of a lightweight plastic Hudson-type facemask connected to a plastic reservoir bag via a one-way valve. The reservoir is designed to supply peak inspiratory demands and minimize air entrainment around the mask. Ideally it would function as a fixed performance mask giving 100% oxygen but in practice some entrainment will occur. *This is the preferred device for giving high oxygen concentrations*, and a flow rate of $15 \, l \, min^{-1}$ should give over 85% oxygen.

Venturi mask

These fixed-performance masks are available in 24, 28, 35, 40 and 60% versions. The lower-concentration types may be useful in carbon dioxide retention, but the higher-concentration ones offer no advantage over the Hudson-type mask.

Nasal cannulae

These may be better tolerated by a conscious patient but give relatively low and unpredictable concentrations of oxygen. Their use in immediate care is therefore limited.

Ventilation

'Ventilation' is the process of gas movement in and out of the lungs. It is essential to allow oxygen uptake by and carbon dioxide elimination from the body. Ventilation may be spontaneous, assisted or controlled (i.e. artificial). Next to a clear airway, ventilation is the most important consideration in resuscitation: if it is inadequate, hypoxia and death may ensue.

PHYSIOLOGY

In spontaneous breathing, inspiration occurs when the diaphragm contracts and moves downwards, and the external intercostal muscles swing the ribcage outwards. The resulting expansion of the thoracic cavity causes expansion of the lungs due to the subatmospheric pressure in the closed pleural space, and air is drawn in through the trachea. The diaphragm is the most important muscle, accounting for two thirds of lung expansion, and receives its innervation from cervical segments 3, 4 and 5. The intercostal muscles receive their nerve supply from the corresponding thoracic segments. In respiratory difficulty the accessory muscles (scalene and sternomastoid) help to raise the thoracic cage. By contrast, normal breathing expiration is a passive process caused mainly by the elastic recoil of the lungs.

The volume of gas drawn into the lung with each breath is called the tidal volume and averages 500 ml in the resting adult. The volume of gas exchanged each minute is called the minute volume and at a normal respiration rate of 12 inspirations min^{-1} is about 6 l – in other words:

minute volume = tidal volume × respiration rate.

Causes of inadequate ventilation are listed in Table 4.11.

ASSISTED VENTILATION

When the patient's breathing is inadequate or absent, ventilation must be assisted or fully controlled as appropriate. Devices to achieve this are discussed below. Generally the aim is to provide 'normal' tidal volumes and respiration rates, although hyperventilation may be beneficial in head injury (Ch. 23).

Facemask ventilation is the first-line approach but all types of facemask carry the risks of poor ventilation, gastric inflation and aspiration. Pneumocephalus and meningitis have also been reported after positive pressure applied through a facemask in patients with basal skull fracture (Kitahata & Collins 1970, Klopfenstein et al 1980). Ventilation by any means increases intrathoracic pressure, which reduces venous return and hence cardiac output, and this may be significant in hypovolaemic patients. Positive pressure ventilation may also convert a simple pneumothorax into a tension pneumothorax.

Table 4.11 Causes of inadequate ventilation

- Central hypoventilation:
  - Severe head injury
  - Cerebrovascular accident
  - Drugs (including opiates)
- Airway obstruction:
  - Upper: oedema, haematoma, foreign body, soft-tissue obstruction
  - Lower: diffuse bronchospasm, secretions
- Respiratory muscle weakness/paralysis:
  - Spinal cord injury: affecting thoracic intercostal nerves or diaphragm (C3–5)
  - Diseases of peripheral nerves or muscles
- Chest trauma:
  - Flail chest
  - Pneumothorax (closed, open, tension)
  - Haemothorax
- Pain, from chest injury, abdominal injury or peritonitis, limiting breathing

LAERDAL POCKET MASK

(See under 'Basic airway adjuncts'.) The pocket mask is generally the best device for ventilation of a non-intubated patient by a *single* rescuer, because it gives better tidal volumes under these conditions than a self-inflating bag and mask. However, the oxygen concentration delivered is limited and another method may be substituted if help becomes available.

SELF-INFLATING BAG-VALVE DEVICE

These devices (such as the Ambu bag and Laerdal bag) consist of a self-inflating bag with one-way valves at either end – the patient valve and the gas inlet valve. When the bag is squeezed, gas is delivered through the patient valve while the other valve remains closed. As the bag reflates the expired gas is vented to the atmosphere through the patient valve, while air is drawn in through the inlet valve. Oxygen should be given through the inlet valve if available and a second reservoir bag is attached to this valve to minimize air entrainment and improve the delivered oxygen concentration. Adult and paediatric sizes are available, with some paediatric versions having pressure relief valves set to 40 cmH$_2$O.

These devices can be used for ventilation via a facemask, tracheal tube, laryngeal mask or Combitube. Their main advantages are that oxygen concentrations close to 100% can be given if high-flow oxygen and a reservoir bag attachment are used (Table 4.12), but *ventilation with air is still possible if there is no source of oxygen*. Other advantages are that squeezing the bag gives a 'feel' for the lungs, and carbon dioxide rebreathing is eliminated by the one-way valve.

Table 4.12 Percentage oxygen delivered by a 1600 ml Laerdal resuscitator with a 2600 ml reservoir bag

Oxygen flow (l min^{-1})	Tidal volume (ml) × ventilation rate (min^{-1})					
	Oxygen concentrations (%) using a reservoir (without reservoir in parentheses)					
	500 ml × 12 min^{-1}	500 ml × 24 min^{-1}	750 ml × 12 min^{-1}	750 ml × 24 min^{-1}	1000 ml × 12 min^{-1}	1000 ml × 24 min^{-1}
3	56 (37)	39 (32)	47 (33)	34 (29)	41 (32)	30 (28)
5	81 (52)	52 (38)	62 (41)	42 (33)	52 (39)	38 (31)
10	100 (73)	84 (48)	100 (56)	65 (42)	84 (55)	53 (39)
12	100 (84)	97 (53)	100 (61)	74 (45)	94 (60)	59 (42)
15	100 (89)	100 (59)	100 (69)	86 (48)	100 (69)	66 (44)

Figures are percentages: those in brackets are without the reservoir bag. Reproduced with permission from Davey A, Moyle JTB, Ward CS 1992 Ward's anaesthetic equipment, 3rd edn, WB Saunders, London.

The main disadvantage of these devices is that considerable skill and practice are needed to use them effectively with a facemask. Achieving a good mask seal may be difficult with one hand, and tidal volumes are lower than with a pocket mask when used by one person (Lawrence & Sivaneswaran 1985). Gastric inflation also occurs if ventilation pressures are too high. The European Resuscitation Council (1996) recommends that, if possible, ventilation using the self-inflating bag and facemask is performed by two rescuers (one to hold the mask and the other to squeeze the bag). Another disadvantage is that if used without oxygen in a non-respirable atmosphere, hypoxic gas (and possibly toxic fumes) will be entrained.

OXYGEN-POWERED RESUSCITATORS

These deliver pressurized oxygen via a facemask or tracheal tube, and the supply is activated by pressing a button or lever on the patient attachment. 100% oxygen is delivered and both hands can be used to hold the facemask. However, there is no 'feel' for the patient's lungs, and overinflation and gastric distension may result.

MECHANICAL VENTILATORS

Several compact and robust mechanical ventilators are available for prehospital use. When attached to a tracheal tube, Combitube or LMA, they will deliver a preset tidal volume, rate and oxygen concentration while leaving the operator's hands free for other tasks. Typical settings would be a tidal volume of 10 ml kg^{-1} and a ventilation rate of 10–14 breaths min^{-1}. (If used with an LMA, airway pressures must be kept low to avoid gastric inflation.) Most of these work by a 'pneumatic logic' mechanism (Davey et al 1992),

which does not rely on electrical power but is driven only by cylinder oxygen at a pressure of 4 bar.

Many such ventilators are becoming increasingly sophisticated, giving a wide range of tidal volumes and ventilation rates for adults and children. Many have a 'demand' mode that allows the patient to breathe spontaneously through the ventilator but gives triggered inflations if this becomes inadequate. Some will also give positive end-expiratory pressure (PEEP), which improves oxygenation in conditions such as pulmonary oedema and atelectasis.

When powered by cylinders, it is important to know the oxygen consumption of these ventilators. Most have two concentration settings, typically for 45% or 100% oxygen ('air mix' or 'no air mix'). The 100% setting generally consumes oxygen at a rate slightly above the preset minute volume, e.g. the 'transPAC', 'paraPAC' and 'ventiPAC' ventilators use the set minute volume plus 10 ml cycle^{-1}; the older 'pneuPAC' consumes up to 2 l min^{-1} more than the minute volume (manufacturer's data). The 45% setting uses air entrainment and is much more economical, using only 30% of the set tidal volume plus 10 ml cycle^{-1} with the 'transPAC', 'paraPAC' and 'ventiPAC'. For obvious reasons the 'air mix' setting should not be used in toxic atmospheres.

References

Alexander R, Hodgson P, Lomax D, Bullen C 1993 A comparison of the laryngeal mask airway and Guedel airway, bag and facemask for manual ventilation following formal training. Anaesthesia 48: 231–234

American College of Surgeons Committee on Trauma 1997 Advanced trauma life support student manual, 6th edn. American College of Surgeons, Chicago, IL

Andersen KH, Hald A 1989 Assessing the position of the tracheal tube. The reliability of different methods. Anaesthesia 44: 984–985

Atherton G, Johnson JC 1993 Ability of paramedics to use the Combitube in pre-hospital cardiac arrest. Annals of Emergency Medicine 22: 1263–1268

Aye T, Milne B 1995 Use of the laryngeal mask prior to definitive intubation in a difficult airway: a case report. Journal of Emergency Medicine 13: 711–714

Banyai M, Falger S, Roggla M et al 1993 Emergency intubation with the Combitube in a grossly obese patient with bull neck. Resuscitation 26: 271–276

Benumof JL, Scheller MS 1989 The importance of transtracheal jet ventilation in the management of the difficult airway. Anesthesiology 71: 769–778

Brain AIJ 1983 The laryngeal mask – a new concept in airway management. British Journal of Anaesthesia 55: 801–805

Burkey B, Esclamado R, Morganroth M 1991 The role of crico-thyroidotomy in airway management. Clinics in Chest Medicine 12: 561–571

Calder I, Ordman AJ, Jackowski A, Crockard HA 1990 The Brain laryngeal mask airway. An alternative to emergency tracheal intubation. Anaesthesia 45: 137–139

Campbell AM, O'Leary A 1991 Acute airway obstruction as a result of minitracheotomy. Anaesthesia 46: 854–855

Chadd GD, Ackers JWL, Bailey PM 1989 Difficult intubation aided by the laryngeal mask airway. Anaesthesia 44: 1015

Cormack RS, Lehane J 1984 Difficult tracheal intubation in obstetrics. Anaesthesia 39: 1105–1111

Criswell JC, Parr MJA, Nolan JP 1994 Emergency airway management in patients with cervical spine injuries. Anaesthesia 49: 900–903

Davey A, Moyle JTB, Ward CS 1992 Anaesthetic equipment. WB Saunders, London, ch 12

Denman WT, Hayes M, Higgins D, Wilkinson DJ 1990 The Fenem CO_2 detector device. Anaesthesia 45: 465–467

Donahue PL 1994 The oesophageal detector device. An assessment of accuracy and ease of use by paramedics. Anaesthesia 49: 863–865

Donnelly JA, Smith EA, Hope AT, Alexander RJT 1995 An assessment of portable carbon dioxide monitors during interhospital transfer. Anaesthesia 50: 703–705

Eichinger S, Schreiber W, Heinz T et al 1992 Airway management in a case of neck impalement: use of the oesophageal tracheal Combitube airway. British Journal of Anaesthesia 68: 534–535

European Resuscitation Council 1996 Guidelines for the advanced management of the airway and ventilation during resuscitation. European Resuscitation Council. A statement by the Airway and Ventilation Management of the Working Group of the European Resuscitation Council. Resuscitation 31: 201–230

European Resuscitation Council 2001 Guidelines 2000 for paediatric life support. (Paediatric Life Support Working Group). Resuscitation 48: 223–229

Frass M, Frenzer R, Zdrahal F et al 1987 The esophageal tracheal Combitube: preliminary results with a new airway for CPR. Annals of Emergency Medicine 16: 768–772

Frass M, Rodler S, Frenzer R et al 1989 Esophageal tracheal Combitube, endotracheal airway, and mask: comparison of ventilatory pressure curves. Journal of Trauma 29: 1476–1479

Greene MK, Roden R, Hinchley G 1992 The laryngeal mask airway. Two cases of pre-hospital trauma care. Anaesthesia 47: 688–689

Hastings RH, Marks JD 1991 Airway management for trauma patients with potential cervical spine injuries. Anesthesia and Analgesia 73: 471–482

Heath ML, Allagain J 1991 Intubation through the laryngeal mask. Anaesthesia 46: 545–548

Horellou MF, Mathe D, Feiss P 1978 A hazard of nasotracheal intubation. Anaesthesia 33: 73–74

Hussain LM, Redmond AD 1994 Are pre-hospital deaths from accidental injury preventable? British Medical Journal 308: 1077–1080

Kabbani M, Goodwin SR 1995 Traumatic epiglottitis following blind finger sweep to remove a pharyngeal foreign body. Clinical Paediatrics 34: 495–497

Kitahata LM, Collins WF 1970 Meningitis as a complication of anaesthesia in a patient with a basal skull fracture. Anesthesiology 32: 282–283

Klopfenstein CE, Forster A, Suter PM 1980 Pneumocephalus. A complication of continuous positive airway pressure after trauma. Chest 78: 656–657

Lawrence PJ, Sivaneswaran N 1985 Ventilation during cardiopulmonary resuscitation: which method? Medical Journal of Australia 143: 443–446

Macleod BA, Heller MB, Gerard G et al 1991 Verification of endotracheal tube placement with colorimetric end-tidal CO_2 detection. Annals of Emergency Medicine 20: 267–270

Majernick TG, Bieniek R, Houston JB, Hughes HG 1986 Cervical spine movement during orotracheal intubation. Annals of Emergency Medicine 15: 417–420

Martin PD, Cyna AM, Hunter WAH et al 1993 Training nursing staff in airway management for resuscitation. Anaesthesia 48: 33–37

Nandi PR, Charlesworth CH, Taylor SJ et al 1991 Effect of general anaesthesia on the pharynx. British Journal of Anaesthesia 66: 157–162

Nolan JP, Wilson ME 1993 Orotracheal intubation in patients with potential cervical spine injuries. An indication for the gum elastic bougie. Anaesthesia 48: 630–633

Nunn JF 1988 The oesophageal detector device. Anaesthesia 43: 804

Ooi R, Fawcett WJ, Soni N, Riley B 1993 Extra inspiratory work of breathing imposed by cricothyrotomy devices. British Journal of Anaesthesia 70: 17–21

Parkins DRJ 1996 Maxillofacial injuries in immediate care. Journal of the British Association of Immediate Care 19: 34–36

Patrick MR 1987 Airway manipulations. In: Taylor TH, Major E (eds) Hazards and complications of anaesthesia. Churchill Livingstone, Edinburgh

Pennant JH, Walker MB 1992 Comparison of the endotracheal tube and laryngeal mask in airway management by paramedical personnel. Anesthesia and Analgesia 74: 531–534

Pollard BJ, Junius F 1980 Accidental intubation of the oesophagus. Anaesthesia and Intensive Care 8: 183–186

Ralph SJ, Wareham CA 1991 Rupture of the oesophagus during cricoid pressure. Anaesthesia 46: 40–41

Rhee KJ, Muntz CB, Donald PJ, Yamada JM 1993 Does nasotracheal intubation increase complications in patients with skull base fractures? Annals of Emergency Medicine 22: 1145–1147

Sanders AB, Kern KB, Otto CW et al 1989 End-tidal carbon dioxide monitoring during cardiopulmonary resuscitation. Journal of the American Medical Association 262: 1347–1351

Sellick BA 1961 Cricoid pressure to control regurgitation of stomach contents during induction of anaesthesia. Lancet 2: 404–406

Stahl JM, Cutfield GR, Harrison GA 1992 Alveolar oxygenation and mouth-to-mask ventilation: effects of oxygen insufflation. Anaesthesia and Intensive Care 20: 177–186

Staudinger T, Brugger S, Watschinger B et al 1993 Emergency intubation with the Combitube: comparison with the endotracheal airway. Annals of Emergency Medicine 22: 1573–1575

Staudinger T, Tesinsky P, Klappacher G et al 1995 Emergency intubation with the Combitube in two cases of difficult airway management. European Journal of Anaesthesia 12: 189–193

Stone BJ, Leach AB, Alexander CA et al 1994 The use of the laryngeal mask airway by nurses during cardiopulmonary resuscitation. Results of a multicentre trial. Anaesthesia 49: 3–7

Stoneham MD 1993 The nasopharyngeal airway. Assessment of position by fibreoptic laryngoscopy. Anaesthesia 48: 575–580

Thomas AN, Hyatt J, Chen JL, Barker SJ 1992 The Laerdal pocket mask: effects of increasing supplementary oxygen flow. Anaesthesia 47: 967–971

Vollmer TP, Stewart RD, Paris PM et al 1985 Use of the lighted stylet for guided orotracheal intubation in the pre-hospital setting. Annals of Emergency Medicine 14: 324–328

Wee MYK 1988 The oesophageal detector device. Anaesthesia 43: 27–29

Wee MYK, Walker AKY 1991 The oesophageal detector device. An assessment with uncuffed tubes in children. Anaesthesia 46: 869–871

Willms D, Shure D 1988 Pulmonary oedema due to upper airway obstruction in adults. Chest 94: 1090–1092

Wood PR, Lawler PG 1992 Managing the airway in cervical spine injury. Anaesthesia 47: 792–797

Advanced life support

5

Introduction   48

Advanced airway management and ventilation   52

Defibrillation   52

Conclusion   55

References   55

Introduction

In 1992, the European Resuscitation Council published the first set of internationally accepted Guidelines for Advanced Life Support (Chamberlain et al 1992). These were based on the information available at that time, with acknowledgement that, as further scientific evidence became available, there would be the need for review and updating of the guidelines. In 1997, the International Liaison Committee on Resuscitation (ILCOR) issued a set of Advisory Statements on Advanced life Support (Kloeck et al 1997), which the Resuscitation Council of the United Kingdom decided to adopt and, at the same time, assess on behalf of the European Resuscitation Council (ERC). In Spring 1998, the guidelines were formally approved by the executive committee of the ERC and adopted for use throughout Europe. These have now been revised according to current best evidence, with ILCOR guidelines being issued in 2000, followed by a statement by the ERC in 2001 (European Resuscitation Council 2001) outlining some changes to the way Advanced Life Support is taught throughout Europe. The guidelines were once again updated in 2005 (Resuscitation Council (UK) 2005) and it is upon these guidelines that this chapter is based.

WHAT IS ADVANCED LIFE SUPPORT?

In adults, the majority of cardiac arrests occur outside hospital and the commonest rhythm at the time of arrest is ventricular fibrillation, which may be preceded by a period of pulseless ventricular tachycardia (Sedgewick et al 1994). Patients who arrest in either of these two rhythms have the best chance of surviving if they are defibrillated promptly and effectively with the restoration of a spontaneous circulation (Bossaert & Koster 1992). However, the chances of successful defibrillation diminish rapidly with time (Hargarten et al 1990, Cobbe et al 1991) as myocardial energy reserves are depleted. This process can be slowed, but not halted, by the provision of effective basic life support, BLS (also referred to as cardiopulmonary resuscitation, CPR, see Ch. 3). These are the only two interventions which have been clearly demonstrated to affect outcome after cardiac arrest (Eisenberg et al 1979) (Table 5.1).

If the initial attempts at defibrillation fail or the primary arrest rhythm is other than ventricular fibrillation or pulseless ventricular tachycardia (VF–pulseless VT), then advanced airway and ventilation manoeuvres, accessing the circulation and the administration of drugs (e.g. adrenaline (epinephrine)) may be performed. *Advanced life support* is the term used to encompass the techniques used in resuscitation beyond basic life support and consists of:

- rhythm diagnosis
- defibrillation

Table 5.1 Effect of time to starting cardiopulmonary resuscitation (CPR) and advanced life support (ALS) on survival after cardiac arrest

Time to starting CPR (min)	Time to starting ALS (min)		
	< 8	8–16	> 16
0–4	43%	19%	10%
4–8	26%	19%	5%
8–12	6%	0%	

- advanced airway management and ventilation
- accessing the circulation
- administration of pharmacological agents.

THE RESUSCITATION GUIDELINES 2005

The guidelines are presented as a single algorithm (Fig. 5.1) for the management of VF–pulseless VT and other rhythms. The guidelines cannot and do not attempt to cover all of the eventualities leading to a cardiac arrest. Although the details may need to be modified to maximize the chances of successful resuscitation after cardiac arrest as a result of trauma, drowning, hypothermia, poisoning, pregnancy and anaphylaxis, etc., the principles remain the same. Details of these special circumstances are covered elsewhere.

VF–PULSELESS VT

Emphasis is placed on the early diagnosis and treatment of these two rhythms (Figs 5.2 and 5.3). The most effective treatment of both is the same – defibrillation. Therefore, as soon as the ability to monitor the patient's ECG is available this must take place by attaching a dedicated ECG machine, attaching an automated defibrillator or using the paddles of a defibrillator with an ECG display. Basic life support should be started if there is any delay in obtaining a defibrillator but must not delay defibrillation. If, by chance, the arrest was witnessed or monitored, then this may be preceded by a precordial thump.

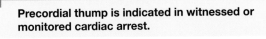

Precordial thump is indicated in witnessed or monitored cardiac arrest.

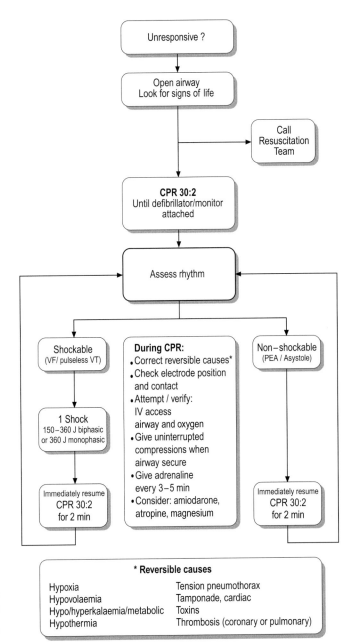

Fig. 5.1 • The ERC universal algorithm for the management of cardiac arrest in adults. (With permission from European Resuscitation Council 2005.)

A sharp blow is delivered to the patient's sternum with a closed fist. This delivers a small amount of mechanical energy to the myocardium and, if soon enough after the onset of VF, may convert the rhythm to one capable of restoring the circulation (Robertson 1992).

In the presence of VF–pulseless VT, a single shock should be delivered, followed by resumption or commencement of basic life support for 2 min at a ratio of 30 compressions to 2 ventilations. The energy level should

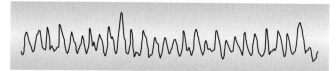

Fig. 5.2 • Ventricular fibrillation.

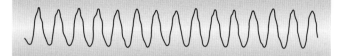

Fig. 5.3 • Ventricular tachycardia.

be 150–200 J if the defibrillator is biphasic or 360 J if monophasic. After 2 min of basic life support, the rhythm should be checked. Palpation of the carotid pulse should only take place if, after the shock, the rhythm changes to one normally capable of supporting the circulation (including ventricular tachycardia). During the period of basic life support the airway is secured and intravenous access obtained.

Tracheal intubation remains the 'gold standard' for securing the airway but requires considerable skill, practice and equipment for success. Acceptable alternatives are insertion of a laryngeal mask airway or a Combitube (Baskett et al 1996). In many situations an airway and bag–valve–mask device will be used, especially in the early stages of resuscitation. Whichever technique is used, the aim should be to deliver the highest possible concentration of oxygen into the patient's lungs, preferably 100%.

Access to the circulation via the central veins is the optimal route during resuscitation after a cardiac arrest, as this allows drugs to be delivered rapidly into the central circulation (Hapnes & Robertson 1992). However, the technique of central venous catheterization has a variety of complications, some of which are potentially life-threatening. Peripheral venous cannulation is quicker, easier to perform and safer, and is the route of choice in prehospital care. Peripheral access via the external jugular vein may be possible and provide access to a large vein near the heart. Drugs administered by any peripheral route must be followed by a flush of normal (0.9%) saline to assist their transfer to the central circulation. Ultimately, the route chosen for access will depend upon the skills and equipment available.

If VF–pulseless VT persists after a second shock, adrenaline (epinephrine) should be administered, at a dose of 1 mg intravenously or 2–3 mg via the tracheal tube. If the latter route is used, the adrenaline should be diluted to at least 10 ml and administration followed by five large tidal volume ventilations to disperse the drug into the peripheral bronchial tree to aid absorption. The role of adrenaline is to improve the efficacy of BLS (Lindner & Koster 1992). Its alpha-adrenergic actions cause arteriolar vasoconstriction, 'diverting' blood away from non-essential organs, i.e. the skin, muscles and viscera, to help maintain myocardial and cerebral perfusion. Although this effect can be demonstrated in vitro there is little good clinical evidence that adrenaline improves survival in humans (Herlitz et al 1995). Furthermore, despite anecdotal reports and animal studies, clinical trials have failed to find evidence to support the use of higher doses of adrenaline and such strategies are detrimental in the postresuscitation phase, increasing the incidence of arrhythmias (Woodhouse et al 1995). Adrenaline should also be used cautiously when the cardiac arrest is associated with solvent abuse or overdose with drugs with sympathomimetic actions, e.g. cocaine.

The loops of the algorithm now continue with each sequence of one shock being followed by CPR for 2 min, during which further attempts can be made to secure the airway or venous access if this has not already been successfully achieved. In addition, 1 mg of adrenaline should be given every 3–5 min during the resuscitation attempt.

When VF is refractory to treatment, and as early as following the third shock, consideration should be given to the use of intravenous amiodarone at a dose of 300 mg. Lidocaine may be used as an alternative if amiodarone is unavailable. The role of alkalinizing agents is not clear. If cardiopulmonary resuscitation is being performed effectively, an acidosis, as determined by analysis or arterial of mixed venous blood samples, does not occur rapidly (Steedman & Robertson 1992). Furthermore, the administration of sodium bicarbonate will result in an increased carbon dioxide load to be excreted via the lungs, requiring an increase in ventilation to prevent accumulation. The current recommendation is therefore to limit the use of bicarbonate in the prehospital environment to those circumstances where the arrest is associated with poisoning due to tricyclic overdose (Nee et al 1994) or possible hyperkalaemia. The position of the paddles can also be changed to anteroposterior and, if easily available, a different defibrillator and paddles can be tried. Finally, it is important to ensure that the potentially reversible causes listed have been eliminated, as any of these can impair the ability to successfully defibrillate VF. It is usually considered worthwhile continuing resuscitation as long as the patient remains in VF or VT.

During the resuscitation of a patient in VF or pulseless VT, if defibrillation results in a change of rhythm that restores the patient's circulation, and the patient then reverts back to VF or pulseless VT, the algorithm should be recommenced from the beginning.

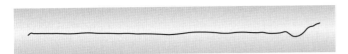

Fig. 5.4 • Asystole.

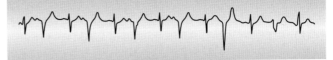

Fig. 5.5 • Electromechanical dissociation.

NON-VF–NON-PULSELESS VT ARREST

Unfortunately, the outcome from these rhythms is relatively poor unless a reversible cause can be found and effectively treated. When secondary to heart disease, survival rates are as low as 5% (Chamberlain et al 1992).

ASYSTOLE (Fig. 5.4)

It is essential that the correct diagnosis is made, the most important problem being misdiagnosis of VF as a result of lead disconnection, incorrect gain setting, movement artefact or equipment failure. If there is any doubt, treatment should be commenced as for VF. The risks of not treating VF, with its greater potential for a successful outcome, are greater than those of unnecessary shocks. Basic life support should now be commenced (or restarted) for 2 min, during which time advanced airway and ventilation techniques are performed, access is gained to the circulation and the first dose of adrenaline (epinephrine) is given. Consideration should also be given to the administration of atropine, 3 mg intravenously or 6 mg via the tracheal tube, to provide complete block of the vagus (Stueven et al 1984).

At the end of this time, the ECG should be carefully checked for the presence of P waves or slow ventricular activity. These may respond to external cardiac pacing, if the equipment is available. Consideration should also be given to percussion 'fist' pacing in those circumstances where the myocardium has not been severely injured (Dowdle 1996). If the rhythm has changed to VF, then the left-hand side of the algorithm is now followed and if the patient remains in asystole, BLS is continued with adrenaline (epinephrine) administered every 3–5 min while resuscitation is considered worthwhile.

ELECTROMECHANICAL DISSOCIATION, EMD (PULSELESS ELECTRICAL ACTIVITY, PEA) (Fig. 5.5)

As the name suggests, this condition comprises the clinical signs of a cardiac arrest but in the presence of an ECG rhythm normally associated with a cardiac output. The patient's best chance of survival in this situation is prompt assessment to identify and treat any underlying cause.

Table 5.2 The four 'H's
● Hypoxia
● Hypovolaemia
● Hyperkalaemia/hypocalcaemia
● Hypothermia

Table 5.3 The four 'T's
● Tension pneumothorax
● Tamponade (cardiac)
● Thromboembolism
● Therapeutic/toxic substances

Treatable causes fall into two main groups, which are listed in Figure 5.1. However, resuscitation must not be withheld while these conditions are sought and the right-hand side of the algorithm is followed. Basic life support is started immediately, advanced airway and ventilation manoeuvres performed as appropriate, and access gained to the circulation. Adrenaline (epinephrine), 1 mg intravenously, is administered every 3 min.

POTENTIALLY REVERSIBLE CAUSES

For ease of memory, these are divided into two groups of four based upon their initial letter – either H or T (Tables 5.2 and 5.3).

The four 'H's

Hypoxia is best eliminated by intubating the patient with a cuffed endotracheal tube and ventilating with 100% oxygen. If this is not possible one of the alternative techniques described in Chapter 4 should be used. *Hypovolaemia* in adults causing EMD is usually secondary to blood loss. Although trauma is an obvious cause, other sources include massive gastrointestinal bleeding or rupture of an aortic aneurysm. The intravascular volume should be restored rapidly with appropriate fluids, coupled with arresting the cause of the haemorrhage. *Hyperkalaemia, hypocalcaemia* and other metabolic disorders may only come to light following biochemical tests. However, some may be suggested by the patient's history, if available, e.g. renal failure (hyperkalaemia, hypocalcaemia), acute pancreatitis (hypocalcaemia), burns or crush injury (hyperkalaemia), or Addison's disease (hyperkalaemia). The ECG may be diagnostic. The use of calcium salts intravenously in EMD is restricted to the treatment of hyperkalaemia and hypocalcaemia. *Hypothermia* should be suspected in any immersion injury and a low-reading thermometer must always be used. It is covered in more detail in Chapter 33.

The four 'T's

A *tension pneumothorax* may be the primary cause of EMD or occur secondary to attempts to insert a catheter into a central vein. The diagnosis is clinical – unilateral absence of breath sounds and hyperresonant percussion note, and tracheal deviation away from the side of the pneumothorax. Rapid decompression should be performed, initially, by needle thoracocentesis followed by insertion of a chest drain (Driscoll et al 1993). Cardiac *tamponade* is a difficult diagnosis as the signs of Beck's triad are obscured by the arrest itself. The history and examination may be helpful if associated with a penetrating wound over the precordium. If suspected, an attempt to relieve the tamponade by needle pericardiocentesis should be made. The commonest cause of *thromboembolic or mechanical obstruction* is pulmonary embolus. The diagnosis is usually suspected from the history. Definitive treatment requires transfer of the patient to a centre with facilities for cardiopulmonary bypass in order to allow operative removal of the clot. The final cause is accidental or deliberate ingestion of *therapeutic* or *toxic substances*. In the absence of a specific history, the cause may only be revealed by laboratory investigations. Where available, the appropriate antidotes should be used but most often treatment is supportive.

Advanced airway management and ventilation

Tracheal intubation remains the standard against which all other techniques must be judged. However, it requires a great deal of skill and practice to remain competent. Other forms of advanced airway management and methods of ventilation are discussed fully in Chapter 4.

Defibrillation

Electrical defibrillation depolarizes a critical mass of the myocardium, allowing the natural pacemaker to take over and restore normal conduction and coordinated contraction. Measurement of the current is difficult but the delivered energy, which is a function of current, can and should

be measured. Factors such as patient size and weight, and thoracic impedance determine current flow through the heart (Sirna et al 1988), the latter being affected by:

- size of the electrodes
- force applied
- use of electrode gel or gel pads
- distance between electrodes
- previously administered shocks
- phase of ventilation.

Adult electrodes are normally 13–14 cm in diameter and should be applied to the chest wall with a force of 12 kg (firm pressure). One paddle should be placed to the right of the sternum, beneath the clavicle, and the other just outside the cardiac apex, the V4–5 position of the ECG (Fig. 5.6). In the female, placement over the breast tissue should be avoided (Pagan-Carlo et al 1996). Although the polarity of the paddles is indicated, each can be placed in either position (Weaver et al 1993); however, the ECG tracing will be inverted if the paddles are used for monitoring. If access to the patient is difficult then they can be placed anteroposterior, the anterior one to the left lower sternal border, the posterior one beneath the left scapula (Kerber et al 1981).

SAFETY

A defibrillator delivers enough current to cause, as well as to treat, VF. It is the responsibility of the operator to ensure that it is used safely, in particular that no one is in contact directly or indirectly (e.g. via spilt electrolyte solution) with the patient as the device is charged or discharged. Before defibrillating a patient, nitrate patches or ointment (Percutol) must be removed, along with any source of high-flow oxygen to prevent any risk of explosion or fire (Stoneham 1996). When placed on the chest the paddles must not be touching or in contact via poorly

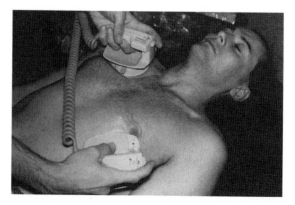

Fig. 5.6 • Paddles correctly placed for defibrillation. (With permission from Gwinnutt CL 1997 Lecture notes on clinical anaesthesia. Blackwell Science, Oxford.)

applied electrode gel as this will cause arcing on discharge and result in insufficient current delivery and burns to the patient. Paddles must not be placed adjacent to a permanent pacemaker, and if gel pads are used they must be replaced every three loops in order to maintain good conductivity. Once a defibrillator is being charged or is fully charged the paddles should either be in their location on the defibrillator or left on the patient's chest. Finally, before each shock is administered a clear, audible, warning must be given and a visual check of the area made.

TECHNIQUE OF DEFIBRILLATION

1. Confirm cardiac arrest. Turn on the defibrillator power switch.
2. Ensure synchronization is set to 'off'.
3. Apply electrode gel or gel pads to the patient's chest wall.
4. Select the appropriate energy level.
5. Place the paddles in the appropriate position on the patient's chest wall with firm pressure.
6. Press the charge button and wait until the defibrillator indicates it is fully charged.
7. Shout 'stand back' and visually check the area to make sure nobody is in contact. Finally check the monitor to make sure the rhythm has not changed.
8. Deliver the shock by pressing the button on each paddle simultaneously.
9. Return the paddles to the defibrillator.

Never hold both paddles in the same hand.

AUTOMATED EXTERNAL DEFIBRILLATORS (AEDS)

Manual defibrillators require the operator to undergo considerable training in both ECG recognition and operation of the defibrillator in order that they are used safely and effectively. This can prevent their use in many areas where these skills are not available. The development of semi-automatic or advisory defibrillators has simplified the process, as these tasks are now performed by the machine. The operator only has to recognize that a cardiac arrest has occurred, attach the semi-automatic defibrillator to the patient and follow the instructions given.

The device is attached to the patient via two large self-adhesive electrodes (placed on the chest in the same area as for standard paddles), which both monitor the ECG and deliver the DC shock. The device is then activated and, following a period during which the patient's ECG is analysed, further instructions are given visually, audibly or both. If a rhythm is recognized for which a shock is indicated, the machine will charge itself to a preprogrammed level and then indicate to the operator when to deliver the shock, having first issued a warning that this is about to happen. Most machines are capable of delivering three shocks in rapid succession, unless a change in rhythm is detected for which a shock would be inappropriate. This is usually indicated by the machine advising either 'check pulse' or 'no shock advised'. It is essential when using one of these devices that there is no rescuer contact with the patient during the initial analysis phase or during the shock sequence (by checking for a pulse). The interference generated on the patient's ECG by contact may prevent analysis and thereby delay the diagnosis and delivery of a shock. There is also a potential risk to the person in contact with the patient were a shock to be delivered (Bossaert & Koster 1992).

All automated defibrillators have a large number of built-in algorithms to allow recognition of the many artefacts that may affect a patient's ECG during resuscitation and ensure that a shock is not administered inappropriately. However, some devices have a manual override facility, which allows the machine to function as a manual defibrillator.

DEVELOPMENTS IN DEFIBRILLATION

In order to try and overcome the problem of variable thoracic impedance, defibrillators are being assessed that can perform automatic measurement of transthoracic impedances. They can automatically adjust the shock energy to minimize the risk of myocardial injury in patients with low impedance and avoid inadequate energy delivery in the presence of high impedance (Kerber et al 1984).

The other major area of interest is the use of defibrillators that deliver the energy using a different waveform. The current generation of defibrillators deliver a high-energy, damped sinusoidal monophasic waveform. To produce this requires an inductor, which is extremely inefficient and increases the capacitor volume and the voltage required. In turn this leads to the need for larger batteries, transformers, insulation and high-voltage mechanical switches. The latest devices deliver the shock energy as a truncated, biphasic waveform (Bardy et al 1995). This waveform is much more efficient at defibrillating the myocardium, allowing lower energies and therefore lower voltages to be used. Practically, this translates as smaller capacitors, batteries and transformers, less insulation and the ability to use solid-state switches. When combined with the fact that the inductor can be removed, the defibrillator can be reduced in both size and weight by more than 50% (Bardy et al 1996). Furthermore, these waveforms, by utilizing lower energies, reduce myocardial injury, particularly when a series of shocks are administered (Reddy et al 1995). Clearly the development of such devices will have a major impact on the availability of defibrillators in the prehospital environment.

ALTERNATIVE TECHNIQUES IN CPR

Open chest or internal cardiac compression

Internal cardiac compression has been well demonstrated experimentally to provide superior cerebral and coronary perfusion than that associated with standard external chest compression techniques. However, there is no good evidence comparing its efficacy with external techniques following cardiac arrest secondary to heart disease. It is likely that the delay in performing a thoracotomy would only exacerbate ischaemic cerebral and myocardial injury, thereby offsetting any potential advantages. The main role at present for this technique is in the management of cardiac arrest following penetrating trauma. It should also be considered in those cases where the conventional technique is ineffective, e.g. following recent sternotomy, in the presence of a fixed rib-cage or gross emphysema, or in patients undergoing thoracic or abdominal surgery (Robertson & Holmberg 1992).

The indications for open cardiac compression in prehospital care are extremely rare. It is not indicated in 'medical' cardiac arrest.

Active compression–decompression CPR

In 1990, a case report appeared describing how a bathroom plunger was used to achieve both compression and active decompression of the chest in a patient who had suffered a cardiac arrest, with successful return of spontaneous circulation (Lurie et al 1990). Subsequent studies using animal and human models of ventricular fibrillation demonstrated improvements in myocardial and cerebral blood flow and perfusion pressures when chest compression was accompanied by active decompression (Cohen et al 1992, Schultz et al 1994). This technique became known as active compression–decompression (or ACD) CPR and led to the development of the Ambu CardioPump™. This consists of a neoprene suction cup, attached to which is a circular handle containing a force gauge. The suction cup is positioned over the patient's midsternum and the handle is gripped with both hands to allow compression and decompression, the force of both being displayed on the gauge to assist the operator (Fig. 5.7). The method by which ACD CPR improves perfusion is not fully understood but it probably augments the return of venous blood into the chest. During standard CPR, venous return is dependent on the natural elasticity of the chest generating a small, transient negative phase on release of compression. ACD CPR increases the magnitude and duration of the negative phase during the active decompression, thereby improving venous return and filling of the ventricles (Lurie et al 1995).

Unfortunately, to date, clinical trials of ACD CPR vs standard CPR have failed to demonstrate any consistent improvement in patient outcome and therefore a change to

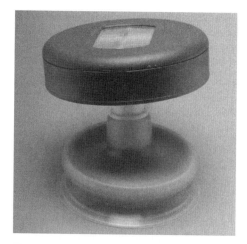

Fig. 5.7 • Active compression–decompression device.

this technique cannot be recommended as yet (Schwab et al 1995, Steill et al 1996).

CARDIAC PACING

A cardiac pacemaker is a device used to deliver an electrical current to the myocardium to initiate depolarization and cardiac contraction. This can be performed by application of the current to the chest wall (external pacing) or directly to the heart (internal pacing). The latter is usually achieved by placing an electrode in the right ventricle via the venous system and often referred to as either transvenous or endocardial pacing. It is not available in the prehospital situation. In advanced life support, the use of pacing is restricted to those patients who:

- are in asystole with P waves
- have a bradycardia with either a risk of asystole or adverse signs and have failed to respond to atropine.

External cardiac pacing

If the patient is conscious, an explanation of events should be given and care must be taken that the patient is electrically isolated, particularly from water. The skin on the chest wall is then cleaned and two large self-adhesive electrodes are applied; the *negative* one to the left anterior chest wall, over the heart (corresponding to V3 of the ECG), and the *positive* one to the left posterior chest wall beneath the scapula (Fig. 5.8). The electrodes are attached to the pacing generator and, if there is no underlying rhythm, the pacing generator is set to 'fixed' mode, 70–90 beats min^{-1} and 2–3 V output or minimum current. The latter is then increased as necessary until ventricular capture occurs, i.e. depolarization of the myocardium, seen on the ECG as a QRS complex. The rate is then

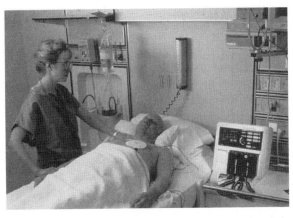

Fig. 5.8 • External cardiac pacing. The negative electrode is visible, the positive electrode is situated posteriorly beneath the scapula. (Reproduced with permission of Medtronic Inc.)

adjusted according to the haemodynamic response. If the patient has some underlying intrinsic rhythm the same preliminary settings are used but the generator should be set to 'demand' mode to avoid the risk of precipitating VF (Millane & Camm 1997). Pacing can therefore be achieved quickly, without the need for X-rays and with few complications. The main problems associated with external pacing are the discomfort and skeletal muscle stimulation experienced by the patient. External pacing should now be considered the technique of choice in the emergency situation until arrangements can be made for the formal insertion of a transvenous system.

Conclusion

As improvement in our knowledge of resuscitation has led to the production of the latest guidelines, the future is likely to see further changes as science and experience dictate the way ahead. It may be that the current guidelines are shorter-lived than their predecessors; however, it is likely that, while the details may change the principles will remain the same. Health-care professionals, whatever their background, who are expected to deal with patients who have suffered a cardiac arrest are encouraged to attend a recognized 'advanced life support' course to stay abreast of the developments and thereby offer their patients the best chance of successful recovery.

References

Bardy GH, Gilner BE, Kudenchuck PJ et al 1995 Truncated biphasic pulses for transthoracic defibrillation. Circulation 91: 1768–1774

Bardy GH, Marchlinski FE, Sharma AD et al 1996 Multicenter comparison of truncated biphasic shocks and standard damped sine wave monophasic shocks for transthoracic ventricular defibrillation. Circulation 94: 2507–2514

Baskett PJF, Bossaert L, Carli P et al 1996 Guidelines for the advanced management of the airway and ventilation during resuscitation. Resuscitation 31: 201–230

Bossaert L, Koster R 1992 Defibrillation: methods and strategies. Resuscitation 24: 211–255

Chamberlain D, Bossaert L, Carli P et al 1992 Guidelines for advanced life support. Resuscitation 24: 111–121

Cobbe SM, Redmond MJ, Watson JM et al 1991 'Heartstart Scotland' – initial experience of a national scheme for out of hospital defibrillation. British Medical Journal 302: 1517–1520

Cohen TJ, Tucker KJ, Lurie KG et al 1992 Active compression–decompression: a new method of cardiopulmonary resuscitation. Journal of the American Medical Association 267: 2916–2923

Dowdle JR 1996 Ventricular standstill and cardiac percussion. Resuscitation 32: 31–32

Driscoll P, Gwinnutt C, Goodall O 1993 Thoracic trauma. In: Driscoll PA, Gwinnutt CL, LeDuc Jimmerson C, Goodall O (eds) Trauma resuscitation: the team approach. Macmillan Press, Basingstoke, pp 67–101

Eisenberg M, Bergner L, Hallstrom A 1979 Cardiac resuscitation in the community. Importance of rapid provision and implications for program planning. Journal of the American Medical Association 241: 1905–1907

European Resuscitation Council 2005 Guidelines for Resuscitation. Section 4. Adult advanced life support. Resuscitation 67Sl: S39–S86

Gwinnutt CL 1996 Alternatives to endotracheal intubation in airway management. Journal of the British Association for Immediate Care 19: 37–41

Hapnes SA, Robertson C 1992 CPR – drug delivery routes and systems. Resuscitation 24: 137–142

Hargarten KM, Steuven HA, Waite EM et al 1990 Prehospital experience with defibrillation of coarse ventricular fibrillation: a ten-year review. Annals of Emergency Medicine 19: 157–162

Herlitz J, Ekstrom L, Wennerblom B et al 1995 Adrenaline in out-of-hospital ventricular fibrillation. Does it make any difference? Resuscitation 29: 195–201

Kerber RE, Grisaille J, Kennedy J et al 1981 Elective cardioversion: influence of paddle electrode location and size on success rates and energy requirements. New England Journal of Medicine 305: 658–662

Kerber RE, Kouba C, Martins J et al 1984 Advance prediction of transthoracic impedance in human defibrillation and cardioversion: importance of impedance in determining the success of low energy shocks. Circulation 70: 303–308

Kloeck W, Cummins R, Chamberlain D et al 1997 The universal ALS algorithm. Resuscitation 34: 109–111

Lindner K, Koster R 1992 Vasopressor drugs during cardiopulmonary resuscitation. Resuscitation 24: 147–153

Lurie KG, Lindo C, Chin J 1990 CPR: the P stands for plumbers helper. Journal of the American Medical Association 264: 1661

Lurie KG, Coffeen P, Schultz J et al 1995 Improving active compression–decompression cardiopulmonary resuscitation with an inspiratory impedance valve. Circulation 91: 1629–1632

Millane TA, Camm AJ 1997 Cardiac arrhythmias. In: Skinner D, Swain A, Peyton R, Robertson C (eds) Cambridge textbook of emergency medicine. Cambridge University Press, Cambridge, pp 897–930

Nee PA, Hodgkinson OW, Gwinnutt CL 1994 Treatment of severe tricyclic antidepressant poisoning alkalinisation. Care of the Critically Ill 10: 125–127

Pagan-Carlo LA, Spencer KT, Robertson CE et al 1996 Transthoracic defibrillation: importance of avoiding electrode placement directly on the female breast. Journal of the American College of Cardiology 27: 449–452

Resuscitation Council (UK) 2005 Resuscitation guidelines. Resuscitation Council (UK), London

Reddy RK, Glevea MJ, Dolack GL et al 1995 Biphasic truncated wave form transthoracic defibrillation results in less post-shock ECG ST segment changes than standard damped sine wave shock. Journal of the American College of Cardiology 405A

Robertson C 1992 The precordial thump and cough techniques in advanced life support. Resuscitation 24: 133–135

Robertson C, Holmberg S 1992 Compression techniques and blood flow during cardiopulmonary resuscitation. Resuscitation 24: 123–132

Schultz JJ, Coffeen P, Sweeney M et al 1994 Evaluation of standard and active compression–decompression CPR in an acute human model of ventricular fibrillation. Circulation 89: 684–693

Schwab TM, Callaham ML, Madsen CD, Utecht TA 1995 A randomised clinical trail of active compression–decompression CPR vs standard CPT in out-of-hospital cardiac arrest in two cities. Journal of the American Medical Association 273: 1261–1268

Sedgewick ML, Dalziel K, Watson J et al 1994 The causative rhythm in out-of-hospital cardiac arrests witnessed by the emergency medical services in the Heartstart Scotland project. Resuscitation 27: 55–59

Sirna SJ, Ferguson DW, Charbonnier F, Kerber RE 1988 Electrical cardioversion in humans: factors affecting transthoracic impedance. American Journal of Cardiology 62: 1048–1052

Steedman DJ, Robertson CE 1992 Acid base changes in arterial and central venous blood during cardiopulmonary resuscitation. Archives of Emergency Medicine 9: 169–176

Steill IG, Herbert PC, Wells GA et al 1996 The Ontario trail of active compression–decompression cardiopulmonary resuscitation for in-hospital and pre-hospital cardiac arrest. Journal of the American Medical Association 275: 1417–1423

Stoneham MD 1996 Anaesthesia for cardioversion. Anaesthesia 51: 565–570

Stueven HA, Tonsfeldt DJ, Thomson BM et al 1984 Atropine in asystole: human studies. Annals of Emergency Medicine 13: 815–817

Weaver WD, Martin JS, Wirkus MJ et al 1993 Influence of external defibrillator electrode polarity on cardiac resuscitation. Pace 16: 285–290

Woodhouse SP, Cox S, Boyd P et al 1995 High dose and standard dose adrenaline do not alter survival compared with placebo, in cardiac arrest. Resuscitation 30: 243–249

Vascular access

6

Intravenous access   57

Access via the peripheral veins   57

Access via the central veins   63

Intraosseous access   66

Fluid flow through cannulas and catheters   67

Crystalloid and colloid fluid therapy   68

Body fluid compartments   68

Fluid therapy   70

The crystalloid colloid controversy   72

References   73

Further reading   73

Intravenous access

INTRODUCTION

The ability to gain intravenous access to the circulation is an essential skill that all those involved in the care of critically ill or injured patients must acquire as it allows a number of important therapeutic options:

- Fluid can be given to restore or maintain a patient's circulation

- Drugs can be given intravenously, the optimum route of administration, eliminating the delay following intramuscular or subcutaneous injection

- Blood can be withdrawn for investigations and cross-matching in advance of the patient arriving at the hospital.

Intravenous access can be achieved in several ways:

- *Percutaneous cannulation of a peripheral vein*. This is the most common and preferred initial technique. If veins are not easily visible or palpable, surgical exposure and cannulation under direct vision can be performed – the venous 'cutdown' technique.

- *Percutaneous cannulation of a central vein*. This route is used when the above methods have failed or are inadequate. It also allows monitoring of the central venous pressure and the infusion of vasoactive drugs, e.g. catecholamines.

- *The intraosseous route*. This requires the insertion of a needle into the marrow cavity of a long bone, a technique gaining popularity for use in children.

Access via the peripheral veins

The veins most commonly used are the superficial peripheral veins in the upper limbs. If these are not accessible, the saphenous vein at the ankle and the superficial external jugular vein in the neck can be used. In most cases, the veins are cannulated percutaneously. In some circumstances, with appropriate experience and training, venous cutdown remains a useful and safe alternative.

ANATOMY OF THE PERIPHERAL VEINS

The veins in the upper limb may appear very variable in their layout, but certain common arrangements are found (Fig. 6.1).

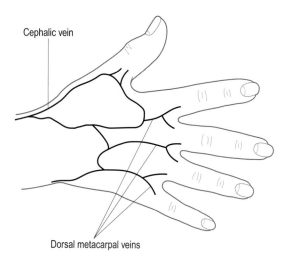

Fig. 6.1 • Typical distribution of veins in the dorsum of the right hand.

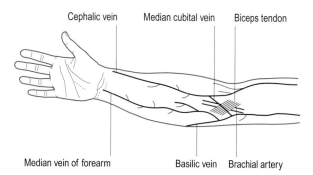

Fig. 6.2 • Major veins, right forearm and antecubital fossa.

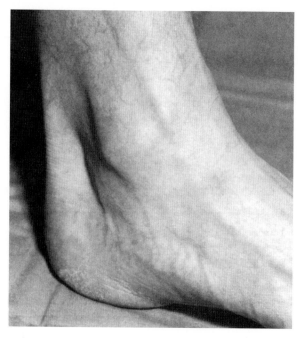

Fig. 6.3 • The long saphenous vein at the ankle, left leg.

- The veins draining the fingers unite to form three *dorsal metacarpal veins*
- Laterally these are joined by veins from the thumb and continue up the radial border of the forearm as the *cephalic vein*
- Medially the metacarpal veins unite with the veins from the little finger and pass up the ulnar border of the forearm as the *basilic vein*
- There is often a large vein in the middle of the ventral (anterior) aspect of the forearm, the *median vein of the forearm*.

In the antecubital fossa (Fig. 6.2):

- The *cephalic vein* passes through the antecubital fossa on the lateral side
- The *basilic vein* enters the antecubital fossa medially, just in front of the medial epicondyle of the elbow
- These two large veins are joined by:
  - the median cubital or antecubital vein
  - the median vein of the forearm.

Although the veins in this area are prominent and easily cannulated, there are many other adjacent vital structures that can be damaged:

- The *brachial artery* which lies beneath the median cubital vein, deep to the biceps tendon. Occasionally the artery is superficial and may be cannulated instead of the vein
- The *median nerve*, medial to the brachial artery
- The *medial cutaneous nerve* of the forearm which is adjacent to the basilic vein
- The *lateral cutaneous nerve* of forearm which is adjacent to the cephalic vein.

At the ankle (Fig. 6.3):

- The most accessible vein is the *long saphenous vein*
- It is very consistent in its location, being found 2 cm in front and 2 cm above the medial malleolus
- It is accompanied very closely by the saphenous nerve.

In the neck (Fig. 6.4):

- The *external jugular vein* is easily identified and accessible
- It runs downwards and forwards from the angle of the mandible and passes behind the middle of the clavicle
- The vein is relatively superficial, covered only by a thin sheet of muscle (platysma), fascia and skin.

EQUIPMENT

A variety of devices of different lengths and diameters are used to secure venous access (Fig. 6.5). The term *cannula*

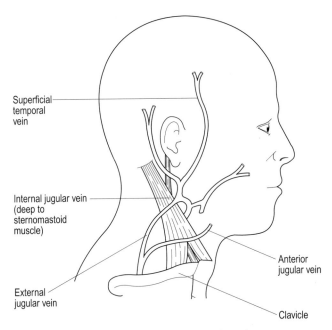

Fig. 6.4 • Anatomy of the right external jugular vein.

Superficial temporal vein

Internal jugular vein (deep to sternomastoid muscle)

External jugular vein

Anterior jugular vein

Clavicle

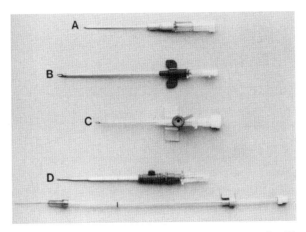

Fig. 6.5 • Intravenous cannulas: (A) cannula over needle; (B) cannula over needle with 'wings'; (C) cannula over needle with injection port; (D) Seldinger type.

is used for those of 7 cm or less in length and *catheter* for those longer than 7 cm. The diameter of the cannula or catheter is often quoted in terms of its *gauge*. The two most common definitions of gauge are:

- Standard wire gauge (SWG) – the number of a particular size of cannula that will fit into a standard orifice. Thus, as the diameter of the cannula increases, the number that fit into the orifice decrease and therefore so does the gauge.
- French gauge (FG) – the circumference in millimetres. Therefore as the diameter increases, so does the gauge.

Increasingly, the external diameter is now quoted in millimetres.

Cannula over needle

This is by far the most popular device for achieving intravenous access and is available in a wide variety of sizes, 12–27 gauge (12–27G). It consists of a plastic (PTFE or similar material) cannula which is mounted on a smaller-diameter metal needle, the bevel of which protrudes from the cannula. The other end of the needle is attached to a transparent 'flashback chamber', which fills with blood indicating that the needle bevel lies within the vein. Some devices have flanges or 'wings' to facilitate attachment to the skin (Figs. 6.5A and B). All cannulas have a standard Luer-lock fitting for attaching a giving set and some have a valved injection port attached through which drugs can be administered (Fig. 6.5C).

Seldinger type

The Seldinger technique (Seldinger 1953) uses a small needle to puncture a vein and introduce a blunt, flexible guide wire. A relatively large cannula is then inserted over the guide wire into the vein. This method allows the insertion of a large-diameter cannula without having to use a large-diameter needle and risk damaging the vein. The devices available consist of a small-diameter needle (a 'search needle') with a flashback chamber at the hub. Mounted on the needle is a larger-diameter vein dilator and on the outside of this the cannula. The final component is the spring-wire guide, which is attached to the needle hub (Fig. 6.5D).

TECHNIQUE

The superficial veins are situated immediately under the skin in the superficial fascia along with a variable amount of subcutaneous fat. The veins are relatively mobile within this layer and are also capable of considerable variation in their diameter. These details are of particular importance when it comes to inserting an intravenous cannula either percutaneously or by a cutdown. The size of cannula used will depend upon its purpose; large diameter ones are required for rapid fluid administration, smaller ones if simply for drug administration.

As with any procedure where there is a risk of contact with body fluids, gloves should be worn by the operator.

Percutaneous cannulation

1. Choose a vein capable of accommodating the size of cannula needed, preferably one that is both visible and

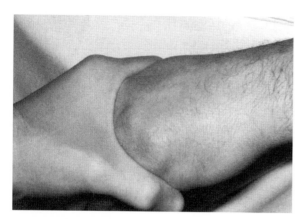

Fig. 6.6 • Vein immobilized prior to cannulation.

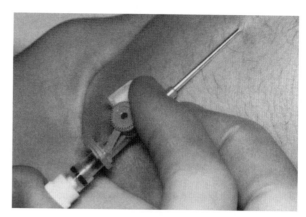

Fig. 6.7 • Vein punctured with flashback of blood.

palpable. The junction of two veins is often a good site as the 'target' is relatively larger. Avoid veins distal to fractures and, if possible, those over joints.

2. Encourage the vein to dilate. In the limb veins this can be achieved by using a tourniquet to stop venous return from the limb. Further dilatation can be encouraged by gently tapping the skin over the vein. In the patient who is cold and vasoconstricted, if time permits, topical application of heat from a towel soaked in warm water can also be useful.

   If cannulating the external jugular vein, and it is safe to do so, the patient can be tipped slightly head-down to encourage the vein to dilate.

3. If time permits, the skin over the vein should be cleaned. Ensure there is no risk of allergy if iodine-based agents are used. If alcohol-based agents are used they must be given time to work (2–3 min). Ensure that the skin is dry before proceeding further.

4. Ideally a small amount of local anaesthetic should be infiltrated into the skin at the point of cannulation, if a > 1.2 mm, 18G cannula is to be used. This reduces the pain of cannulation, making the patient less likely to move, and reduces reluctance to permit further attempts if the first is unsuccessful! However, in the prehospital environment with a desperately injured patient this is rarely if ever possible.

5. If a large cannula is used, insertion through the skin may be facilitated by first making a small incision with either a 19G needle or a scalpel blade. Take care not to puncture the vein.

6. The vein should be immobilized to prevent it being displaced by the advancing cannula. This is achieved by pulling the skin over the vein tight with the operator's spare hand (Fig. 6.6).

7. Hold the cannula firmly, at an angle of 10–15° to the skin and advance it through the skin and then into the vein. Often a slight loss of resistance is felt as the vein is entered. This should be accompanied by the appearance of blood in the flashback chamber of the cannula (Fig. 6.7). However, the appearance of blood only

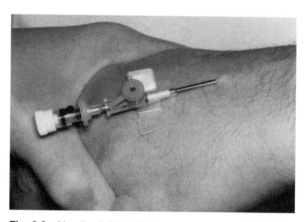

Fig. 6.8 • Needle slightly withdrawn prior to advancing cannula.

indicates that the tip of the needle is within the vein, not necessarily any of the cannula.

8. Keeping the skin taut, reduce the angle of the cannula slightly and advance it a further 2–3 mm into the vein to ensure that the first part of the plastic cannula lies within the vein. Care must be taken at this point not to push the needle out of the back of the vein.

9. Withdraw the needle 5–10 mm into the cannula so that the point no longer protrudes from the end. Often, as this is done, blood will be seen to flow between the needle body and the cannula, confirming that the tip of the cannula is within the vein (Fig. 6.8).

10. The cannula and needle *together* are now advanced along the vein. The needle is retained within the cannula to provide support and prevent kinking at the point of skin puncture (Fig. 6.9).

11. Once the cannula is inserted as far as the hub, the tourniquet should be released and the needle should be completely removed and disposed of safely.

12. Confirmation that the cannula lies within the vein should be made by attaching an intravenous infusion, ensuring that it runs freely, or an injection of saline can be used. The tissues around the site must be observed for any

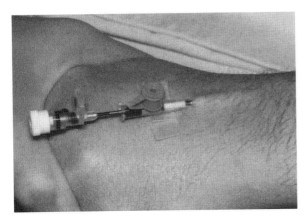

Fig. 6.9 • Cannula fully inserted into vein.

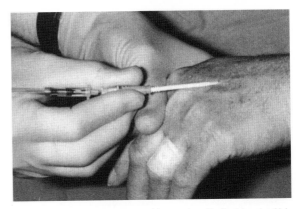

Fig. 6.10 • Needle tip inserted into vein with flashback of blood.

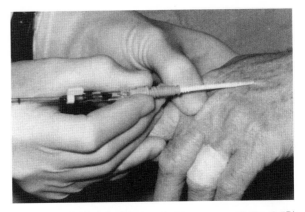

Fig. 6.11 • Guide wire fully inserted (compare with Fig. 6.5D).

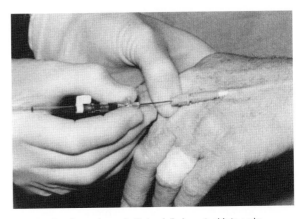

Fig. 6.12 • Cannula and dilator fully inserted into vein.

signs of swelling that might indicate that the cannula is incorrectly positioned. Finally, the cannula should be secured in an appropriate manner.

It is customary in books on the management of trauma to recommend the insertion of 'two large-bore cannulas', 16G or 14G. It must be accepted that this is not always possible and it is often far better to successfully achieve intravenous access with a smaller cannula than to fail repeatedly with a larger one. Once access has been achieved, placement of a proximal tourniquet and infusion into the arm distally will often dilate a vein sufficiently for a large bore cannula to be successfully placed.

Percutaneous cannulation using Seldinger technique

Seldinger-type devices can be used for central and peripheral venous access. The Arrow® device illustrated is useful for gaining access into peripheral veins but the technique requires a greater degree of training and experience than direct percutaneous cannulation. The technique is included as a situation may occasionally arise when such a device is appropriate.

1–7 Identification, preparation and initial puncture of the vein are exactly as described above (Fig. 6.10). Because of the large diameter of the cannula, a nick must be made in the patient's skin to facilitate introduction.

8. Hold the device firmly and advance the spring-wire guide down the centre of the needle into the vein, so that 5–10 cm of wire lies in the vein (Fig. 6.11).

9. Advance the dilator, with the cannula, along the guide wire into the vein using a gentle twisting action (Fig. 6.12).

10. Once advanced as far as the hub, the tourniquet is released and the dilator and guide-wire together are removed, leaving the cannula within the vein.

11. The position of the cannula is checked and it is secured as described above.

A similar technique is used to insert a wire through a small peripheral cannula (21G or larger) already in situ, followed by removal of the cannula and insertion of the dilator and large-bore cannula over the wire.

The venous cutdown technique

The veins most commonly used for this technique are the long saphenous vein at the ankle (Fig. 6.3) and the basilic vein in the antecubital fossa (Fig. 6.2).

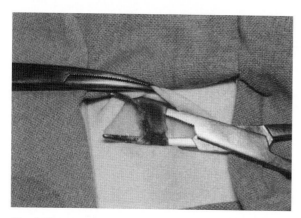

Fig. 6.13 • Vein dissected from surrounding structures.

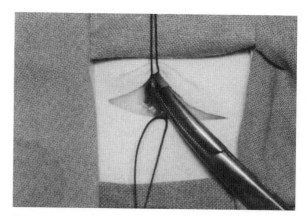

Fig. 6.15 • Venotomy and dilatation.

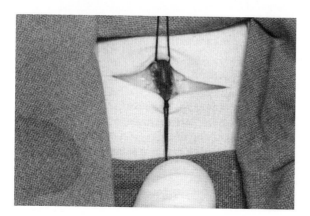

Fig. 6.14 • Ligatures passed under the vein; distal one tied.

1. The skin over the area of the cutdown is sterilized and infiltrated with a small amount of local anaesthetic using a 25G needle, taking care not to puncture the vein.

2. A full-thickness transverse skin incision is made over the vein using a scalpel.

3. The vein is identified and completely freed from the surrounding connective tissue by careful blunt dissection, using a small curved haemostat (Fig. 6.13).

4. Two ligatures are passed underneath the vein.

5. The distal ligature is then firmly tied to prevent back-bleeding from the distal vein (Fig. 6.14)

6. The vein is then gently elevated using both ligatures and a small transverse venotomy is made. This is gently dilated using the haemostat to accept a 14 G cannula (Fig. 6.15).

7. The cannula is advanced into the vein and firmly secured with the proximal ligature (Fig. 6.16). Note, the point of the needle should be withdrawn into the cannula to prevent it cutting and damaging the vein wall as the cannula is advanced.

8. The skin incision is closed and a dressing placed over the site.

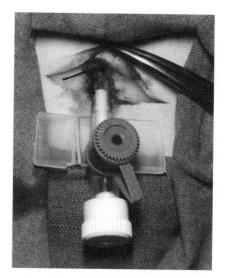

Fig. 6.16 • Cannula in place and secured.

The technical difficulty of performing a venous cutdown, especially in the cold, dark and rain, should not be underestimated. It is not as easy as it would appear to be from practice on training mannequins. In general, any patient in whom a cutdown is contemplated should be transported to hospital urgently so that venous access can be achieved in more conducive surroundings. The only likely exceptions to this are entrapments and very prolonged transfer times.

COMPLICATIONS

There are a large number of complications, both early and late, associated with both percutaneous and cutdown techniques for venous cannulation. Fortunately, most of them are relatively minor. However, this must not be used as an excuse for carelessness and poor technique.

Early complications

- *Failed cannulation.* Usually as a result of pushing the needle completely through the vein. It is experience-related. Wherever possible, it is best to start distally in a limb and work proximally. In this way, if further attempts are required, fluid or drugs will not leak from previous puncture sites.

- *Haematomas.* Secondary to the above, with inadequate pressure applied to prevent blood leaking from the vein. They are made worse by forgetting to remove the tourniquet following percutaneous cannulation!

- *Extravasation of fluid or drugs.* Commonly a result of failing to recognize that the cannula is not within the vein before use. A cannula inserted in the antecubital fossa, or prolonged use to infuse fluids under pressure, predisposes to leakage. Once identified, the cannula must no longer be used. Damage to the overlying tissues will depend primarily upon the nature of the extravasated fluid.

- *Damage to other local structures.* Secondary to poor technique and lack of knowledge of the local anatomy.

- *Air embolus.* Occurs when the pressure in the veins is lower than in the right side of the heart and air is entrained. It is usually prevented from occurring via the peripheral veins as they collapse when empty. However, once a cannula is in place this is prevented. It is most likely to happen in the external jugular vein, particularly if the patient is in a head-up position. If unrecognized it can be fatal.

- *Shearing of the cannula.* This allows fragments to enter the circulation. It is usually a result of trying to reintroduce the needle after it has been withdrawn. The safest action is to withdraw the whole cannula and attempt cannulation at another site.

Late complications

Correct technique at the time of insertion may reduce the incidence of these problems.

- *Inflammation of the vein (thrombophlebitis).* Related to the length of time the vein is in use and irritation caused by the substances flowing through it. High concentrations of drugs, fluids with extremes of pH or high osmolality are the main cause. Once a vein shows signs of thrombophlebitis, tenderness, redness and deteriorating flow, the cannula must be removed to prevent subsequent infection or thrombosis which may spread proximally.

- *Inflammation of the surrounding skin (cellulitis).* Usually secondary to poor aseptic technique initially, prolonged use or leakage from the vein.

Access via the central veins

The central veins are not visible in the same way as the peripheral ones. They are deeper structures and are frequently closely related to major arteries and nerves, which are easily damaged by careless attempts at cannulation.

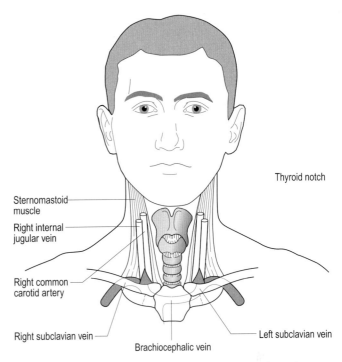

Fig. 6.17 • Anatomy of the internal jugular and subclavian veins.

Consequently, the techniques described below are not recommended as a method of venous access in the prehospital environment except by appropriately trained personnel in circumstances where other methods of vascular access have been unsuccessful. Peripheral cannulation is as effective and associated with fewer complications.

The central veins used most often are:

- the internal jugular vein
- the subclavian vein
- the femoral vein.

ANATOMY OF THE CENTRAL VEINS

The internal jugular vein

The internal jugular vein (Fig. 6.17):

- emerges from the jugular bulb at the base of the skull
- initially lies behind the internal carotid artery
- as it descends in the neck comes to lie lateral to the common carotid artery
- in the lower part of the neck is covered by the sternomastoid muscle
- then passes beneath the triangular interval formed by the sternal and clavicular heads of the sternomastoid muscle
- ends its course by joining with the subclavian vein posterior to the sternoclavicular junction to form the brachiocephalic vein.

The subclavian vein

The subclavian vein (Fig. 6.17):

- commences as the proximal continuation of the axillary vein as it crosses the first rib
- lies posterior to the medial third of the clavicle and anterior to the subclavian artery, from which it is separated by the scalenus anterior muscle
- terminates by joining with the internal jugular vein as described above.

The femoral vein

The femoral vein (Fig. 6.18):

- is the proximal continuation of the popliteal vein, ending at the level of the inguinal ligament

- below the inguinal ligament it occupies the middle compartment of the femoral sheath, medial to the femoral artery
- the femoral nerve lies lateral to the artery, outside the femoral sheath.

EQUIPMENT

Three main types of catheter (i.e. those >7 cm in length) are used to gain access to the central veins. The most basic is a catheter over needle, similar in construction and use to a peripheral intravenous cannula. A syringe is sometimes attached to the hub to allow aspiration of blood to confirm entry into the vein. Alternatively, a large-bore needle can be introduced percutaneously into the vein, through which a catheter is passed and the needle then withdrawn. Increasingly popular is a modification of the Seldinger technique.

- The chosen vein is punctured percutaneously with a metal needle, confirmation given by the ability to freely aspirate blood into an attached syringe.
- The syringe is removed and a flexible metal guide wire is passed down the needle into the vein.
- The needle is withdrawn leaving the wire in situ.
- A dilator is passed over the wire to produce a tract in the skin and subcutaneous tissues, and then removed.
- The catheter is passed over the wire into the vein.
- The wire is removed leaving the catheter in the vein.

At all times care must be taken not to let go of the wire as it may enter the vein completely and cause serious complications.

The needle initially used to puncture the vein is usually 16–18G. The diameter of the catheter inserted will depend on the indication for utilizing the central veins. Single, double or triple lumen catheters, 14–16G, up to 30 cm long, are used to allow monitoring of the central venous pressure and the infusion of drugs. Short 7.5–12G catheters are used when rapid infusion of large volumes of fluid are required.

TECHNIQUE

There are numerous approaches to both the internal jugular and subclavian veins. The following is an outline and not intended as a comprehensive review. The interested reader should consult the references for further details. Whichever vein is chosen:

- an aseptic technique must be used
- the patient is best placed 10–15° head-down to help distend the vein.

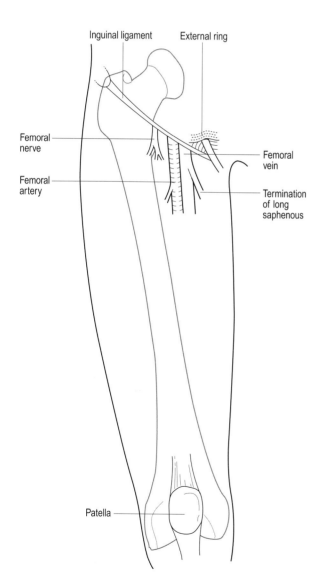

Fig. 6.18 • Anatomy of the right femoral vein.

The internal jugular vein

- The patient's head is turned slightly away from the side to be punctured.
- The apex of the triangle formed by the two heads of the sternomastoid muscle at the level of the cricoid cartilage is identified as the site of insertion of the needle.
- The carotid artery should be lightly palpated medial to the puncture site.
- The vein is fairly superficial (2–3 cm deep) and can be punctured by aiming the needle slightly laterally and caudally (towards the nipple in the male).

Alternatively, the vein may be punctured by the 'low approach'. The advantage of this technique is that it does not rely on identification of the sternomastoid muscle, which may be difficult in obese patients.

- A small sandbag or litre of saline is placed under the patient's shoulders and his/her head is turned away from the side of approach.
- The notch on the superior surface of the medial end of the clavicle is palpated.
- The needle is introduced just above the notch and then raised at an angle of 30–40° to the coronal plane.
- The needle is advanced posteriorly and caudally.
- The vein is usually located at a depth of 1.5–4 cm.

Recently, a technique has been described where the neck remains in the neutral position, and various bony and cartilaginous landmarks are used (Willeford & Reitan 1994). This approach may be advantageous in patients who have potential cervical spine injuries.

The subclavian vein

- The patient's head is turned slightly away.
- The junction of the middle and outer thirds of the clavicle and the suprasternal notch are identified.
- The needle is introduced 1 cm below the junction of the middle and outer thirds of the clavicle, aiming slightly cephalad under the clavicle, towards the suprasternal notch.
- The vein is usually located at a depth of 4–6 cm.

Any technique used for central venous catheterization that involves turning of the patient's head is contraindicated in the presence of a suspected cervical spine injury and/or the presence of a rigid cervical collar. Head-down tilt is contraindicated in patients with head injury.

Do not rotate the neck in suspected spinal injury.

The femoral vein

- The patient is placed in a supine position with the leg on the side chosen slightly externally rotated.
- The femoral artery is palpated just below the inguinal ligament. Remember nerve–artery–vein from lateral to medial.
- The needle is inserted just medially to the artery and advanced cephalad and slightly medially.
- The femoral vein is usually located at a depth of 3–4 cm.

The principal advantages of the femoral approach are the limited possibilities of serious complications and the ability to achieve cannulation using a straightforward cannula and syringe. For these reasons, femoral access must be considered a method of choice if peripheral access cannot be achieved.

COMPLICATIONS OF CENTRAL VENOUS CATHETERIZATION

Early complications

Most are related to damage of associated structures:

- *Arterial puncture.* Not unsurprising, considering the proximity of major arteries to the veins used. Usually seen as pulsatile blood withdrawn into the syringe, the syringe filling unaided or back-flow of the drip even when held well above the patient. The needle should be withdrawn and firm pressure applied over the puncture site for a minimum of 5 min.
- *Haematoma.* This is usually secondary to the above followed by inadequate pressure for insufficient time.

If a haematoma develops in the neck as a consequence of carotid artery puncture, further attempts must not be made on the opposite side as this may lead to tracheal compression and respiratory obstruction.

- *Haemothorax.* May occur secondary to damage to the subclavian artery.
- *Pneumothorax.* Occurs most commonly after using the subclavian approach. In the presence of unilateral chest injury, attempts to insert central venous cannulas, which might result in pneumothorax on the 'good side', are contraindicated.
- *Venous air embolism.* This is often secondary to a poor connection or a three-way tap attached to the catheter being left partly open.
- The thoracic duct can be damaged during approaches to the neck veins on the left side.
- Nerve damage.
- Loss of the guide-wire into the circulation, usually as a result of poor technique.

- *Cardiac arrhythmias*. Due to the guide-line or catheter stimulating the myocardium, having been inserted too far.

Late complications

- These are similar to those following peripheral cannulation with the additional risks of systemic sepsis and the creation of an arteriovenous fistula.

Intraosseous access

The technique is not new and was first described in humans by Josefson in 1934. During the 1940s it was widely used for infusing fluids and drugs, after it was demonstrated that dye solutions infused through the tibial marrow reached the central circulation within 10s, making this route as effective as the intravenous route for rapid drug administration (Tocantins et al 1941). However, with the advent of plastic and polyfluoroethylene venous cannulas the use of the intraosseous route declined, only to be resurrected again in the 1980s as a suitable alternative route for administering drugs to cardiac arrest patients who had no intravenous access. The intraosseous route for fluid and drug administration has recently been reviewed (Sawyer et al 1994) and is increasingly popular in situations where it is difficult to achieve peripheral venous access, especially in paediatric patients.

Intraosseous infusion is used less commonly in adults in whom vascular access by peripheral or central routes is easier to achieve. However, over the last decade it has once again become a standard part of adult as well as paediatric practice, particularly as a rescue procedure in profoundly shocked patients in whom vascular access is not possible. It should be used if peripheral cannulation attempts seem futile, and as the next step after failed peripheral cannulation. There are two basic types of adult intraosseous needles; one type for sternal access and the other for long bone access. Long bone access is straightforward and is not associated with the sometimes serious complications associated with central venous cannulations. Sternal access has been associated with a number of significant complications and is technically more demanding.

ANATOMY

The preferred sites are (Fig. 6.19):

- The *tibia*:
  - proximally, the anteromedial surface 1–2 cm below the tibial tuberosity
  - distally, just proximal to the medial malleolus.
- The *femur*:
  - the anterior surface, in the mid-line 3–4 cm above the femoral condyle.

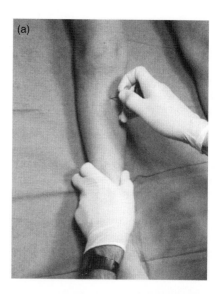

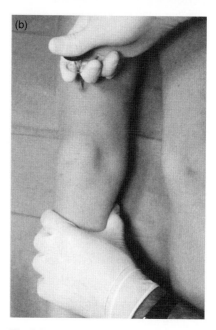

Fig. 6.19 • Sites for intraosseous access, right leg: (a) proximal tibia; (b) distal femur.

These sites are relatively free of other local important structures. The most relevant feature to be borne in mind is the proximity of the epiphyses or growth plates. If damaged, this could interfere with subsequent bone growth and development.

EQUIPMENT

The only needles that should be used for intraosseous access are those specifically designed for the purpose. As a guide, 16–20G needles are used for children less than 18 months old, and 12–16G for children older than 18 months.

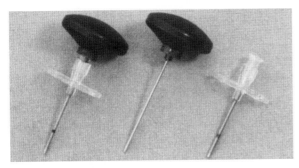

Fig. 6.20 • Paediatric intraosseous needles.

Typically the needle has a short shaft, with a central solid trocar that has a large handle attached. The trocar has to be unscrewed before it can be removed from the needle. Some needles have a screw thread to improve their security within the bone (Fig. 6.20).

TECHNIQUE

- The skin is sterilized when possible.
- A support is placed under the knee to make insertion easier.
- Local anaesthetic may be infiltrated in the skin and deeper tissues including the periosteum at the site of insertion using a fine (23 G) needle.
- The intraosseous needle is inserted perpendicular to the skin until contact with the cortex. It is then angled 10–15° away from the adjacent joint.
- The needle is inserted by firm, twisting motion until the resistance of the bony cortex gives and the needle enters the marrow cavity.
- The central trocar or stylette is withdrawn and aspiration of bloody marrow will confirm the position of the needle in the marrow cavity. Further confirmation is provided by being able to flush 5 ml saline through the needle without resistance or signs of extravasation.
- The needle is then strapped in position and fluids infused using a syringe and three-way tap, as described below.

The sample of bone marrow may be used to cross-match blood and estimate the haemoglobin concentration.

The intraosseous route may be used for up to 24 h for fluid administration; however, it is likely that once initial resuscitation has begun it will then be possible to achieve peripheral or central vascular access. The intraosseous infusion should then be discontinued and the needle removed to reduce the likelihood of complications. If used for the rapid infusion of fluid in a hypovolaemic patient, this is best achieved by attaching a three-way tap to the end of the needle and injecting the fluid as a series of boluses. This also facilitates monitoring of the volume given which is of particular importance in small children. All the common resuscitation drugs can be given by the intraosseous route. An intraosseous needle should not be inserted to a fracture in a long bone. Ideally, no more than one attempt should be made on a single bone in order to avoid the risk of extravasation and consequent compartment syndrome.

COMPLICATIONS

Fortunately, these are relatively rare:

- Failure to enter the bone marrow cavity is the commonest problem. This may occur more often when the distal femur is used due to the difficulty in identifying the correct landmarks. If unrecognized it may lead to extravasation of fluid, and if prolonged could cause a compartment syndrome.
- Infection in the skin, cellulitis or abscess formation. Osteomyelitis is rare (less than 1%) and is associated with long-term use and with administration of hypertonic solutions.
- Damage to the growth plate of the bone used could happen as a result of careless placement and, in very young children, a fracture could occur if excessive force is used.
- Fat and marrow emboli are theoretical problems and have not been reported.

Fluid flow through cannulas and catheters

The flow of fluid through a tube is governed by the Hagen–Poiseuille law:

$$F = \frac{\pi \delta P r^4}{8 \eta l}$$

where F is the flow of the fluid, δP is the pressure difference between the ends of the tubes, r^4 radius of the tube to the power of 4, η is the viscosity of the fluid and l is the length of the tube.

Consequently there are four factors to consider which affect the rate at which fluid will flow through a cannula or catheter:

- The *radius*. This is the most important factor as doubling the diameter increases the flow 16-fold.
- The *length*. Flow is inversely proportional to length, therefore doubling the length will halve the flow.
- The *viscosity*. Flow is inversely proportional to the viscosity, therefore increasing viscosity reduces flow. Colloids and blood are more viscous than crystalloids, especially when cold, and therefore flow more slowly.
- The *pressure applied*. Increasing the pressure will increase the flow of fluid. This may be achieved by elevating the fluid and/or applying pressure bags.

Table 6.1 Rates of water flow through different size cannulas (Venflon®)

Diameter (mm)	Gauge (SWG)	Length (mm)	Flow (ml min^{-1})
1	20	32	54
1.2	18	45	80
1.7	16	45	170
2.0	14	45	270

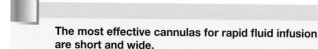

The most effective cannulas for rapid fluid infusion are short and wide.

However, the flow of fluid through veins is not as simple as flow of a fluid through a rigid tube. Veins are living tissues and are neither uniform nor straight; they are also collapsible, and external pressures may result in venous collapse and impede the flow of infused fluids. It has recently been suggested that the use of two smaller intravenous cannulas may be more efficient than a single large one (Elad 1994). An indication of the rate of fluid flow through cannulas of various sizes is shown in Table 6.1.

In the same way that the diameter and length of a cannula or catheter influences the flow of fluid, the diameter and length of the fluid administration tubing (giving set) must also be considered. Standard blood administration sets have an internal diameter of 3.2 mm; however, widebore administration sets are also available ranging from 5.0–6.4 mm (Landlow & Shahnarian 1990). The use of a blood filter will also reduce blood flow.

The flow rates quoted in Table 6.1 are unpressurized and these can be improved by increasing the driving pressure. Various devices are available for pressurizing fluid bags. The simple ones consist of an inflatable bladder within a cloth or plastic bag or rigid box. These need to be operated manually and can be slow to pressurize but are small and light enough to make them useful for out-of-hospital use.

The viscosity of the fluid is inversely proportional to the rate of flow. All fluids will decrease their viscosity when warmed, and warming blood from 4°C to room temperature will more than double its flow through a wide bore infusion set as well as helping to prevent iatrogenic hypothermia.

FLOW THROUGH INTRAOSSEOUS NEEDLES

Using gravity alone, with a 1 m head of pressure, the flow through intraosseous needles in children is similar to that achieved through a cannula of the same diameter. Using a 16G needle, a flow approaching 200 ml min^{-1} is possible in children. With small-diameter needles, fluid (and drugs) can be infused more rapidly by using a syringe and three-way tap.

Crystalloid and colloid fluid therapy

Intravenous fluid resuscitation using salt solutions was first used by O'Shaughnessy in 1831 to resuscitate patients suffering from cholera. However, it was between the major wars in the first half of this century that the use of fluids and blood for the resuscitation of injured, hypovolaemic, patients was developed and refined. Nowadays, a variety of intravenous fluids exist and the controversy over which is the optimal fluid for resuscitation remains unsolved. Interestingly, after 50 years of aggressively resuscitating hypovolaemic trauma patients, it has recently been shown that in penetrating trauma delayed fluid resuscitation may be beneficial (Bickell et al 1994).

In this section the underlying physiological mechanisms governing the distribution of fluid throughout the body will be discussed. The various intravenous fluids that are currently available and some of the newer solutions are described and the main arguments of the crystalloid colloid controversy presented.

Body fluid compartments

In humans, the total body water (TBW) is approximately 60% of the body weight, being slightly greater in infants, and less in females and the obese. The TBW is divided into two main compartments:

- the *intracellular fluid* (ICF), which accounts for *two-thirds* of the TBW
- the *extracellular fluid* (ECF), which accounts for *one-third* of the TBW.

The ECF is further divided into:

- intravascular space comprising one-quarter of the ECF
- the interstitial space comprising three-quarters of the ECF.

To put this into context, in a 70 kg man fluid is distributed as:

- total body water (TBW) = 42.0 l
- intracellular fluid (ICF) = 28.0 l
- extracellular fluid (ECF) = 14.0 l, of which:
  - intravascular fluid (plasma volume) = 3.5 l
  - interstitial fluid (ISF) = 10.5 l.

Total circulating blood volume may be calculated from the plasma volume if the haematocrit (percentage of blood made up of cells) is known:

$$\text{Total blood volume} = \text{plasma volume} \times \left(\frac{100}{100 - \text{haematocrit}} \right).$$

For example, if the haematocrit = 38%:

$$\text{Total blood volume} = 3.5 \times \left(\frac{100}{100 - 38}\right) = 5.6\,l.$$

MOVEMENT OF FLUID BETWEEN COMPARTMENTS

The various compartments are separated from each other by membranes.

- The intracellular fluid is separated from the extracellular fluid by the *cell membrane*.
- The intravascular fluid is separated from the interstitial fluid by the *capillary walls*.

Despite these barriers, there is movement of water and various molecules between the different compartments, the results of which determine the composition of the different body fluids. The main forces producing movement of water and other molecules across these membranes are:

- diffusion
- osmosis
- filtration
- active transport.

Diffusion is the process by which a substance in solution (solute) or a gas expands, due to the movements of the particles (atoms or molecules), to fill all the available volume. By a process of random motion the particles spread from areas of high concentration to areas of lower concentration until their concentration is uniform throughout. Diffusion of solutes occurs both within the various fluid compartments and, provided the membrane is permeable to the particles, across compartments.

Osmosis is the movement of solvent molecules from a region of higher concentration of a solute to a region of lower concentration, across a membrane that is only permeable to the solvent (a semipermeable membrane). This creates a driving force known as the *osmotic pressure* of the solution. The osmotic pressure of a solution depends on the number of particles in solution. The osmotic pressure of plasma is 290 milliosmoles (mosmol) l^{-1}. The term *tonicity* is used to describe the osmotic pressure or *osmolality* of a solution relative to the plasma. Solutions with the same osmolality as plasma are termed *isotonic*, solutions with a greater osmolality *hypertonic* and those with a lower osmolality *hypotonic* solutions.

Plasma proteins and other colloid molecules also generate an osmotic pressure which is much less than that due to the other solutes (for example sodium). This is the *oncotic* or *colloid osmotic pressure* (COP), normally 25 mmHg which is tending to keep water within the intravascular space.

Filtration is the process by which fluid is forced through a membrane by the hydrostatic pressure. The rate of

Table 6.2 Differences in ionic concentrations between intra- and extracellular compartments

Ion	Concentration (mmol l^{-1} water)	
	Intracellular	Extracellular
Na$^+$	15	150
K$^+$	150	5
Cl$^-$	9	125
Ca^{2+} (ionized)	10^{-4}	1.2

movement is proportional to the pressure difference and the surface area of the membrane.

Active transport is the process by which solute particles are moved against the concentration gradient, that is from an area of high to low concentration. The cell membrane that separates the intracellular fluid from the extracellular fluid contains many *active protein channels* that move various ions across the membrane against their concentration gradient, an energy-consuming process. This maintains the differences in ionic composition between the intra- and extracellular fluid compartments. For example, sodium is found in high concentrations in the extracellular fluid while potassium is the major ion in the intracellular fluid (Table 6.2). Failure of tissue oxygenation rapidly causes failure of the active transport of molecules, which then resort to diffusion down their concentration gradients; water and sodium entering the cells resulting in cellular swelling and death.

STARLING'S FORCES

The capillary wall forms the interface between the intravascular and interstitial fluid compartments, between which water and various solutes must move. The majority of solutes (e.g. oxygen, carbon dioxide and glucose) move across the membrane by simple diffusion, but the movement of water is governed by the hydrostatic and osmotic pressure gradient. The latter is generated predominantly by proteins, there being little difference across the capillary wall in ionic concentrations. These are often referred to as Starling's forces.

The hydrostatic pressure at the arteriolar end of the capillary (approximately 35 mmHg) is higher than the colloid osmotic pressure (approximately 25 mmHg); thus there is a tendency for water to move out of the capillary into the interstitium. At the venous end of the capillary, the COP of the plasma exceeds the hydrostatic pressure in the capillary (approximately 10 mmHg) and fluid moves back into the capillary. Any excess fluid accumulating in the interstitium is drained via the lymphatic system back into the blood.

This relationship is summed up in the equation:

$$Q_f = K_f[(P_c - P_i) - O_s(\pi_c - \pi_i)],$$

where Q_f is the net fluid flow across the capillary membrane, K_f is the fluid filtration coefficient, P_c is the capillary hydrostatic pressure, P_i is the interstitial hydrostatic pressure, O_s is a reflection coefficient (a measure of capillary wall permeability to solute), π_c is the capillary colloid osmotic pressure and π_i is the interstitial colloid osmotic pressure.

Consider the situation that occurs in a patient suffering from hypovolaemic shock. The fall in systemic blood pressure will lead to a fall in the hydrostatic pressure in the capillary bed. The COP will be largely unchanged, with the net result being that water is drawn into the intravascular compartment from the interstitial compartment in an attempt to rectify the hypovolaemia. Conversely, if the COP falls (e.g. hypoalbuminaemia) and the hydrostatic pressure is maintained, more water is lost into the interstitial fluid compartment resulting in the formation of oedema.

Fluid therapy

A variety of fluids are available for intravenous administration, however the total volume administered does not necessarily remain within the intravascular compartment. The ultimate distribution will depend on the osmolality of the fluid and the ability of the solutes to pass through the membranes separating the various fluid compartments.

The fluids available are usually divided into three groups:

- crystalloids
- colloids
- blood and blood products.

CRYSTALLOIDS

Crystalloids are solutions of crystalline solids in water. The composition of some of the most commonly used crystalloids is shown in Table 6.3. It is useful to have an understanding of how the various intravenous fluids distribute themselves throughout the body in order to understand their advantages and disadvantages.

Distribution of crystalloids

The capillary membrane is permeable to most electrolytes, therefore fluids that are isotonic to plasma (and therefore interstitial fluid) will distribute themselves throughout the extracellular fluid space. As the plasma volume only represents one-quarter of this volume, only 25% of the volume of an isotonic solution remains intravascular, the rest entering the interstitial space. Consequently, to replace a fluid deficit in the intravascular space with isotonic fluids, between two and four times the volume lost is required to allow for distribution to both parts of the ECF. This process of distribution takes approximately 30 min. For example, after an initial 1 litre bolus of Hartmann's solution, only 250 ml will remain in the intravascular space.

All compartments are freely permeable to water and, if water alone is administered, it will distribute throughout the entire body water. This happens when 5% dextrose is given. Although initially isotonic, the dextrose is rapidly metabolized resulting in a hypotonic solution. The water redistributes throughout the entire body water, and only 85 ml of the 1 litre of the 5% dextrose administered intravenously will remain in the vascular compartment (that is, the same proportion as plasma volume to total body water).

Table 6.3 Commonly used crystalloids

Crystalloid	Na$^+$ (mmol l^{-1})	K$^+$ (mmol l^{-1})	Ca^{2+} (mmol l^{-1})	Cl$^-$ (mmol l^{-1})	HCO$_3^-$ (mmol l^{-1})	Osmolality pH	(mosmol l^{-1})
Hartmann's solution	131	5	4	112	29*	6.5	281
Ringer's lactate	130	4	3	109	28	6.5	273
0.9% sodium chloride ('normal saline')	154	0	0	154	0	5.5	300
4% dextrose and 0.18% sodium chloride ('dextrose saline')	31	0	0	31	0	4.5	284
5% dextrose	0	0	0	0	0	4.1	278

*Present as lactate, which is metabolized to bicarbonate by the liver.

Hypertonic saline

As the name suggests, this fluid has a greater osmolality than plasma. This is achieved by using a much higher concentration of sodium than is normally found in plasma. Sodium is primarily an extracellular ion and the administration of hypertonic saline has a profound osmotic effect, causing a shift of water from the intracellular to the extracellular space. This results in an acute expansion of the plasma volume, which is greater than the volume of saline given. A 7.5% solution of sodium chloride has been shown to be the most effective solution (Traverso et al 1987). Unfortunately, the effects of hypertonic saline in expanding the circulating volume appear too transient to be of clinical value. There is evidence to suggest that the effect might be prolonged by the addition of dextran 6% (hypertonic saline–dextran, HSD) and this area is currently the subject of a great deal of research. Hypokalaemia and metabolic acidosis are significant problems that may occur after the use of hypertonic saline.

COLLOIDS

Colloids are suspensions of molecules of different sizes and are referred to as polydisperse. During resuscitation these substances have been considered to be more efficient than isotonic crystalloids as a higher percentage of the administered fluid volume (approaching 100%) will remain in the intravascular space for longer. In addition, by virtue of their oncotic properties, they also draw water into the intravascular space and therefore act as 'plasma expanders'. The capillary membrane only allows limited passage of colloids; thus the smaller molecules are eliminated rapidly promoting a diuresis and renal perfusion while the larger particles remain within the vascular space for longer periods (hours to days) and maintain plasma volume.

There are a wide variety of colloids available, the most commonly used are derived from *gelatin* (Haemaccel, Gelofusine), *protein* (albumin), *starch* (Hespan, hetastarch) or *polysaccharides* (dextrans). Physical properties of commonly used colloids are shown in Table 6.4. The pharmacokinetic properties of colloids are characterized by their weight-averaged molecular weight, whereas their oncotic pressure is more closely related to their number-averaged molecular weight.

Gelatins

Gelatin is a purified protein derived from bovine collagen. There are two main types:

- *modified fluid gelatin* or succinylated gelatin (Gelofusine)
- *urea-bridged gelatin* or polygelin (Haemaccel).

Gelofusine is available as a 4% solution in 0.9% sodium chloride, and Haemaccel is available as a 3.5% solution in 0.9% saline. Their properties are similar (Table 6.4), although Haemaccel has a higher calcium content and will cause precipitation if mixed in the same giving set as citrated blood. Gelatins may be used in volumes of up to 2500 ml in the treatment of haemorrhage, and act as plasma volume expanders due to their high colloid osmotic pressures. Gelatins have a half-life in the plasma of 2–4 h, with 75% of the infused dose excreted by the kidneys within 24 h. Gelatins do not interfere with blood cross-matching or blood clotting, although they may occasionally affect platelet function.

The main disadvantage of these solutions is the potential for an anaphylactoid reaction. The incidence of severe reactions due to Haemaccel is 0.146% and less with Gelofusine. True anaphylactic reactions may develop secondarily to gelatin–antigelatin antibody reactions in sensitized individuals. Histamine release may occur with rapid infusion of gelatins.

Hydroxyethyl starch (Hetastarch, HES)

This is a synthetic class of molecules similar to glycogen. They consist of a hydroxyethyl-substituted branched chain

Table 6.4 Physical properties of commonly used colloids			
Colloid	**Haemaccel**	**Gelofusine**	**Hetastarch**
Molecular weight (range)	5000–50 000	5000–50 000	10 000–1 000 000
Molecular weight (weight average)	35 000	30 000	450 000
Molecular weight (number average)	24 500	22 600	69 000
Na^+ (mmol l^{-1})	145	154	154
K^+ (mmol l^{-1})	5.1	0.4	0
Ca^{2+} (mmol l^{-1})	6.2	0.4	0
Cl^- (mmol l^{-1})	145	125	154
HCO_3^- (mmol l^{-1})	0	0	0
pH	7.3	7.4	5.5
Osmolality (mosmol l^{-1})	350	465	310

amylopectin and were produced as a result of an effort to find a colloid with minimal side-effects. Solutions contain particles of various molecular weights and degrees of hydroxyethyl substitution, which correlates with its resistance to degradation by serum amylase and therefore the serum half-life.

After intravenous infusion, molecules of less than 50 000 are rapidly excreted unchanged in the urine, with the result that 40% of the administered dose is excreted in this way in 24 h. Larger particles remain in the circulation for longer and are slowly taken up by the reticuloendothelial system, where they remain for long periods but do not appear to have any deleterious effects. Hetastarch exerts a similar colloidal osmotic pressure to human albumin. When given by intravenous infusion, it produces expansion of the plasma volume slightly in excess of the infused volume – the high colloid osmotic pressure of the solution results in water being drawn from the interstitial space into the intravascular space. Its effects last for at least 3 h and up to 24 h. The maximum recommended dose of Hetastarch is 1500 ml or 20 ml kg^{-1} body weight.

Adverse effects of hydroxyethyl starch:

- hypersensitivity
- itching
- coagulopathy and haemorrhage have been reported with Hetastarch in neurosurgical patients (Damon 1987) and in patients who received large volumes for resuscitation (Lockwood et al 1988)
- serum amylase levels may also be elevated after Hetastarch infusion
- Hetastarch is incompatible with a number of injectable antibiotics.

A comprehensive review of Hetastarch may be found in Hulse & Yacobi 1983.

Dextrans

Dextran 70 and Dextran 40 are inert polysaccharides produced by fermentation of sucrose by bacteria *Leuconostoc mesenteroides*. The '70' or '40' denotes the average molecular weight of the molecules. Dextran 40 is presented as a 10% solution in 0.9% sodium chloride or 5% glucose. It produces marked plasma volume expansion when given to patients in hypovolaemic shock. The renal threshold is a molecular weight of 50 000 and consequently Dextran 40 enters the renal tubules and may cause acute tubular necrosis.

Dextran 70 produces a plasma volume expansion effect less than that of Dextran 40. The complication associated with Dextran 70 is in vitro rouleaux formation, which makes blood cross-matching difficult. They may also cause coagulopathy and anaphylactoid reactions, the latter occurring more commonly than with other artificial colloids. Dextrans are no longer used for treatment of hypovolaemia.

The crystalloid colloid controversy

Both crystalloid and colloid solutions are used in the resuscitation of patients suffering from shock, and no particular fluid has been proved to be significantly superior to any of the others. The controversy about which fluid is best continues and is partly fuelled by differences in clinical practice and the availability of products between the USA and the UK. There are several in-depth reviews of the subject (Falk et al 1983, Shires et al 1995). An understanding of the pathophysiology of the causes of the shock and fluid distribution across the body compartments is a useful guide to decide which of the various solutions available is the best for a particular patient.

After haemorrhage there is a shift of fluid from the interstitial fluid compartment into the vascular space. This is due to the alteration in the Starling forces and a decrease in capillary hydrostatic pressure leading to transcapillary influx of interstitial fluid and an increase in the intravascular volume. A reduction in blood viscosity secondary to dilution also occurs. When patients are resuscitated following haemorrhage it is necessary to replace the interstitial water that has been lost, and crystalloid solutions that are distributed to the interstitial compartment are effective for this purpose.

When cardiac parameters and renal function are closely monitored, crystalloid solutions may be used in volumes of between two and four times the amount of blood (or colloid) required to achieve the same improvements in cardiac output and urine output. The majority of patients suffering haemorrhage or other forms of shock may be very adequately resuscitated with crystalloid solutions alone; however patients with major haemorrhage or other severe forms of shock will require very large volumes of crystalloid solutions. In these cases there is concern that the large volumes of crystalloid will distribute throughout the extracellular fluid compartment, ultimately resulting in the formation of tissue and pulmonary oedema.

The formation of pulmonary oedema is a complex process: fluid exchange across the pulmonary capillary membrane depends on the pulmonary interstitial pressure, the intravascular hydrostatic pressure and the plasma oncotic pressure. If the pulmonary capillary membrane is normal, a fall in plasma oncotic pressure resulting from large amounts of crystalloid resuscitation fluid could increase the flux of fluid into the lungs, resulting in pulmonary oedema. Thus, colloid resuscitation is theoretically preferred as it maintains plasma oncotic pressure. This is not the complete picture, however, as the pulmonary capillary membrane may not be normal: it is easily damaged due to trauma or sepsis. If this occurs, fluid translocation across the pulmonary capillary membrane is increased; larger colloid molecules may also cross into the lungs and draw fluid with them, compounding pulmonary oedema. Because of their large molecular size, starches may also reduce fluid translocation through blockage of capillary holes. There is also some evidence to suggest that they reduce the adherence of leukocytes.

The advantages of crystalloid solutions are that they are non-toxic, do not cause allergic or hypersensitivity reactions, have a long shelf-life and are cheap. When compared to colloids for resuscitation they are equally effective for restoring the circulation *provided adequate volumes are used*. The advantages of colloid resuscitation are the maintenance of colloid osmotic pressure and that they may be used in smaller volumes to achieve the same effects on cardiac output and renal function. There are small risks of hypersensitivity reactions to the synthetic colloids and problems with coagulopathy if large volumes are infused. *It must be remembered that neither crystalloid nor colloid solutions have the ability to transport oxygen to the tissues.* For this reason strenuous attempts should be made to commence resuscitation with blood as soon as possible.

In general, the choice of prehospital fluids is likely to remain a matter of personal preference. The key point is that, whatever fluid is chosen, a blood pressure capable of maintaining essential organ perfusion is achieved. The concept of limited resuscitation to achieve a systolic blood pressure of 90–100 mmHg has become widely accepted in prehospital practice.

References

Bickell WH, Wall MJ, Pepe PE et al 1994 Immediate versus delayed resuscitation for hypotensive patients with penetrating torso injuries. New England Journal of Medicine 331: 1105–1109

Damon L 1987 Intracranial bleeding during treatment with hydroxyethyl starch. New England Journal of Medicine 317: 964–965

Elad D 1994 Intravenous infusion: understanding the technical side can improve clinical performance. Journal of Clinical Monitoring 10: 219–221

Falk JL, Rackow EC, Weil MH 1983 Colloid and crystalloid fluid resuscitation. Acute Care 10: 59–94

Hulse JD, Yacobi A 1983 Hetastarch: an overview of the colloid and its metabolism. Drug Intelligence and Clinical Pharmacy 17: 334–341

Josefson A 1934 A new method of treatment: intraossal injection. Acta Medica Scandinavica 81: 550–564

Landlow L, Shahnarian A 1990 Efficacy of large-bore intravenous fluid administration sets designed for rapid volume resuscitation. Critical Care Medicine 18: 540–543

Lockwood DNJ, Bullen C, Machin SJ 1988 A severe coagulopathy following volume replacement with hydroxyethyl starch in a Jehovah's witness. Anaesthesia 43: 391–393

O'Shaughnessy WB 1831 Experiments on the blood in cholera. Lancet 1: 490

Sawyer RW, Bodai BI, Blaisdell FW, McCourt MM 1994 The current state of intraosseous infusion. Journal of the American College of Surgeons 179: 353–358

Seldinger SI 1953 Catheter replacement of the needle in percutaneous angiography: a new technique. Acta Radiology 39: 368–376

Shires GT, Barber AE, Illner HP 1995 Current status of resuscitation: solutions including hypertonic saline. Advances in Surgery 28: 133–169

Tocantins LM, O'Neill JF, Jones HW 1941 Infusions of blood and other fluids via the bone marrow: applications in paediatrics. Journal of the American Medical Association 117: 1229–1234

Traverso IW, Bellamy RF, Hollenbach SJ, Wilcher LD 1987 Hypertonic sodium chloride solutions: effects on haemorrhage in swine. Journal of Trauma 27: 32–39

Willeford KL, Reitan JA 1994 Neutral head position for placement of internal jugular vein catheters. Anaesthesia 49: 202–204

Further reading

American College of Surgeons Committee on Trauma 1997 Advanced trauma life support student manual, 6th edn. American College of Surgeons, Chicago, IL

Atkinson RS, Rushman GB, Alfred Lee J (eds) 1987 Intravascular techniques, infusions and blood transfusions. In: A synopsis of anaesthesia, 10th edn. John Wright, Bristol

Evans RJ, McCabe M, Thomas R 1994 Intraosseous infusion. British Journal of Hospital Medicine 51: 161–164

Resuscitation Council (UK) 2000 Advanced life support course manual, 4th edn (revised). RC(UK), London

Rosen M, Latto IP, Ng WS 1981 Handbook of percutaneous central venous catheterisation. WB Saunders, London

Soni N (ed.) 1989 Intravascular access. In: Practical procedures in anaesthesia and intensive care. Butterworth Heinemann, Oxford

Tonks A 1992 How to put up a drip. Student British Medical Journal 1: 57–59

Warwick R, Williams PL (eds) 1973 Angiology. In: Gray's anatomy, 35th edn. Longman, Edinburgh

Shock

7

Introduction   74

Identification   74

Classification   75

Response to treatment   76

Pathophysiology   76

Management philosophy   77

Intravenous access   78

Fluid administration   78

Hypotensive resuscitation   78

Fluid type   79

Which fluid and how much?   80

Specific management aspects of shock   80

Conclusion   81

References   81

Introduction

The state of shock is the haemodynamic expression of circulatory failure that results in failure of cellular metabolism.

At a clinical level it is defined as inadequate perfusion and oxygenation of the essential organs. Absolute haemodynamic figures for satisfactory tissue perfusion cannot be given as they vary between patients and are affected by the cause of the shock and available organ reserve. Adequacy is best described as the ability to maintain function without long-term organ damage.

This chapter will consider the identification of shock in the prehospital environment, and methods of quantifying and classifying it. It will then consider pathophysiology and the methods of treatment available, and discuss the current controversies regarding the type of treatment and the inherent time delays involved. The appropriateness and types of intervention available for the management of shock in the prehospital environment will be reviewed.

Identification

Current accepted best practice states that the compromised casualty must be assessed and managed properly from the airway and breathing–ventilation perspectives before any assessment of the circulatory state is made. Having adequately managed the A and B of the primary survey, attention turns to the C (circulation).

Often there is an immediate clinical impression of shock based on the patient's appearance, with pallor and cold, clammy skin resulting from peripheral circulatory shutdown. The casualty may be anxious, confused or even agitated.

Peripheral perfusion can be assessed using the capillary refill or blanche test in which a fingernail bed is compressed for 5s and then the time to return of colour is counted. Less than 2s is regarded as normal; longer indicates hypoperfusion. The usefulness of this is compromised by a low ambient temperature, peripheral vasoconstriction occurring in a cold environment and also the adequacy of any lighting.

Normal capillary refill time is less than 2 s.

An assessment of the pulse rate and its volume can also be made. There are many reasons other than shock for a tachycardia in the emergency situation and these should be considered, although in the presence of circulatory compromise its trend in response to treatment is a useful indicator.

A more useful and reproducible indicator is blood pressure. Ideally the non-invasive blood pressure should be measured using a sphygmomanometer (which may be connected to an electronic monitor providing regular readings); however, this is frequently not done because of time pressure or because the environment is too noisy to make an accurate assessment. Under these circumstances an approximation can be made based on the presence or absence of peripheral pulses (assuming the vascular tree is intact) (Table 7.1).

As with the pulse rate, it is the trend over time and in response to treatment, rather than any single reading, that is most useful.

Classification

The shocked state is classifiable both by its degree and by the pathophysiology or mechanism of its origin (Table 7.2). It is also possible to categorize it by the response to treatment.

The most frequently adopted assessment of degree is that taught by the American College of Surgeons' Advanced Trauma Life Support (ATLS) course.

The most important point to note in this system is that the blood pressure does not start to fall until 30% of the circulating volume has been lost.

Blood pressure does not fall until 30% of the circulating volume has been lost.

Pathophysiology allows division into three broad categories:

- hypovolaemic
- vasogenic
- cardiogenic.

HYPOVOLAEMIC SHOCK

In this situation there is an inadequate volume of fluid within the vascular tree. Haemorrhage is the commonest cause in the prehospital environment. In trauma it may result from internal or external haemorrhage, or from fluid shift as a result of injury (e.g. due to burns). Hypovolaemic shock may also occur in acute medical and surgical emergencies such as variceal haemorrhage or rupture of an aortic aneurysm.

If a significant amount of blood is lost then the site should be identifiable clinically. There are five common locations and these should be specifically assessed:

- external or 'on the ground'
- intrathoracic

Table 7.1 Estimating the blood pressure	
Pulse palpable?	**Systolic blood pressure (mmHg)**
Carotid	>60
Femoral	>70
Radial	>80

Table 7.2 A classification of shock (based on a 70 kg male)				
	Class 1	**Class 2**	**Class 3**	**Class 4**
Blood loss (ml)	<750	750–1500	1500–2000	>2000
Blood loss (% blood volume)	<15%	15–30%	30–40%	>40%
Pulse rate (beats min^{-1})	<100	>100	>120	>140
Blood pressure (mmHg)	Normal	Normal	Decreased	Decreased
Pulse pressure (mmHg)	Normal or increased	Decreased	Decreased	Decreased
Respiratory rate (breaths min^{-1})	14–20	20–30	30–40	>35
Mental status	Slightly anxious	Mildly anxious	Anxious and confused	Confused and lethargic

- intra-abdominal and/or retroperitoneal
- pelvis
- long bones (femurs).

'Blood on the floor and four more.'

A less frequently encountered cause of hypovolaemia in British practice is dehydration. This may result from an acute diarrhoeal illness with or without vomiting, from evaporation in heat exhaustion or as a consequence of a metabolic disturbance such as diabetic ketoacidosis.

VASOGENIC SHOCK

As a result of a change in permeability of the vascular tree, or its smooth muscle tone, there is loss of fluid into the interstitial tissues or an increase in the volume of the circulatory space through vasodilatation. Within this category fall anaphylactic and anaphylactoid reactions, septic shock and neurogenic shock.

In anaphylaxis an antigen produces a generalized immune immunoglobulin E (IgE)-mediated release of vasoactive substances from the mast cells. Histamine and kinins cause generalized vasodilatation and an increase in the intravascular space. There is also an increase in capillary permeability with fluid leaking into the extravascular space.

Anaphylactoid reactions present in the same way clinically but the antigen acts directly on the mast cells rather than through an immunoglobulin mediator.

In neurogenic shock there has been an injury to the spinal cord with an interruption to the sympathetic supply. The loss of sympathetic autonomic tone produces an increase in the vascular space. Spinal shock also occurs as a result of local spinal cord injury. It is associated with flaccidity of the limbs and a loss of reflexes, and will resolve over a period of 72–96 h; it is not a vascular condition and the retention of the term causes much unnecessary confusion.

CARDIOGENIC SHOCK

This results from pump failure, and the commonest cause is a consequence of ischaemic heart disease through myocardial infarction, ventricular failure or rhythm disturbance. Cardiomyopathy, myocardial contusion, myocarditis, valvular abnormalities, pericardial tamponade and pulmonary embolism may also cause failure.

As a common pathway, the failure of the circulation from any cause will result in inadequate myocardial oxygenation and the development of cardiac failure as a preterminal event.

Response to treatment

From a prehospital perspective, it is the response to initial treatment, together with consideration of the mechanism of injury, that will have most influence on the management. The ATLS principle advocates the arresting of external haemorrhage and then the replacement of circulating volume by intravenous fluid administration through two large-bore intravenous cannulae. On the basis of response to this dynamic fluid challenge, it is possible to divide patients into the following three groups:

- *Rapid and sustained response* – after a fluid bolus the haemodynamic situation improves and is sustained.
- *Transient response* – while there is an improvement in the clinical condition in response to rapid infusion of fluid, there is a further deterioration after this. This is consistent with ongoing rapid loss such as that found with continued bleeding.
- *Minimal or no response* – there is no significant response to the fluid challenge. This is found in profound hypovolaemia with exsanguinating haemorrhage.

A transient or minimal response will usually be the result of haemorrhage. Other forms of shock will tend to respond to an increase of the circulating volume. The type of response from a patient who is bleeding will be determined by whether the loss is controlled (e.g. a femoral fracture where the leg has been placed in a traction splint) or uncontrolled (e.g. with a splenic tear or unsplinted pelvic fracture).

Pathophysiology

The following discussion of the pathophysiology of shock refers to hypovolaemic shock. As fluid is lost there are a number of cardiac, neuronal and hormonal responses by the body.

CARDIAC

As the fluid loss exceeds 10% of the circulating volume there is a decrease in the venous return to the heart. This is a major contributing factor in the cardiac preload and filling of the ventricles. According to Starling's law of the heart, as the filling decreases there is a negative inotropic effect and the stroke volume, and hence cardiac output, fall (Ganong 1983).

AUTONOMIC

There is a graded increase in activity of the sympathoadrenal axis. The vascular sympathetic tone increases, as does the rate of release of the catecholamines adrenaline (epine-phrine) and noradrenaline (norepinephrine) from the adrenal medullae. This combination of increased sympathetic activity and circulating catecholamines has a positive ino-tropic and chronotropic effect on the heart. It also increases the cardiac afterload by 'tightening' the circulation and increasing the blood pressure (by increasing the systemic vascular resistance), as well as reducing the capacitance of the venous side of the circulation and increasing cardiac return (Cuschieri et al 1988).

HORMONAL

The effects of the catecholamines are augmented by the release of steroids from the adrenal cortex and glucagon from the pancreas. Levels of aldosterone and antidiuretic hormone (ADH) are also raised to promote retention of sodium and water in the kidney.

The fall in renal perfusion stimulates the release of renin from the juxtaglomerular apparatus and the generation of the potent vasoconstrictor angiotensin II.

While these homeostatic mechanisms are quite efficient, they do not restore normality and there is gradual progres-sion to hypoxia. This produces an increase in anaerobic metabolism and the development of a 'sick cell syndrome'. The lactic acidosis alters the vascular reactivity and perme-ability, and fluid shift into the extravascular compartment begins. This is augmented by the release of other local tissue mediators such as histamine and the kinin group (Vary & Littleton-Kearney 1994).

Administration of a high concentration of oxygen and correction of the hypoperfusion should restore the situa-tion to normal, and the severity and duration of the distur-bance ought to influence the morbidity and mortality. The base deficit generated by the lactic acidosis as an indicator of the severity of the oxygen debt has been linked to trans-fusion requirements and outcome (Davis et al 1996).

The physiological consequences of shock have tradition-ally been attributed to cellular ischaemia, however there is also evidence that a sublethal period of hypoxia 'primes' cells and the subsequent reperfusion initiates an inflamma-tory response. The mediators of this are thought to play a part in multiple system organ failure (Waxman 1996).

Management philosophy

In trauma, the loss of circulating volume begins at the point of injury. Even when the prehospital care team rec-ognize that there is a time-critical injury, there is a signifi-cant delay before arrival at a definitive treatment facility (Goodacre et al 1997). As there has to be a loss of 30% of the circulation volume (American College of Surgeons

Committee on Trauma 1997) before there are clear signs of hypovolaemia, it often goes unnoticed in the early stages and the pathological process is well under way before arrival at the point of definitive care.

Should the treatment of the condition begin as soon as possible? This is a subject of ongoing debate, with some parties arguing for a *scoop and run* policy, others for a *stay and play* approach. As with all entrenched views, there is truth in both positions.

The first step in shock management should always be to control any haemorrhage and try to limit the deterioration. If there is obvious bleeding from the skin then the appli-cation of direct pressure should arrest this. In awkward places, such as the scalp, it may be appropriate to consider direct suture of the wound with a heavy thread and a large hand needle or a hair-tie so that pressure at the bleeding skin edges can be generated.

Blood loss from long bone fractures can be limited by improvement in alignment, length and rotation of the frac-tured bone and, in the case of the femur, the application of a traction splint. Management of pelvic haemorrhage might require the use of a sheet, pulled tight to compress the pelvic ring and fastened securely ('sheeting'). The use of a Kendrick (KED) or Russell extrication device (RED) applied around the pelvis is an alternative. Abdominal haemorrhage can only be dealt with effectively in hospital by surgery or angioembolization.

There is little that can be done to arrest significant intrathoracic haemorrhage without thoracotomy, and this is not appropriate in the prehospital situation in a patient with a cardiac output. There is some suggestion that clamping of a chest drain from which the patient continues to bleed catastrophically might provide some degree of tamponade, but this needs to be balanced against the impairment of lung function that might result from a large haemothorax.

In the well-known paper by Bickell et al (1994), for the specific condition of penetrating torso trauma, it was demonstrated that the administration of fluid to a shocked patient before definitive control of the bleeding produced a significant increase in mortality. This paper supports the non-use of fluid resuscitation in the prehospital envi-ronment and augments the recommendation of Gervin & Fischer (1982) of a 'scoop and run' approach. There are a number of caveats with Bickell et al's paper, however, which means that its conclusions cannot be applied to the broad field of prehospital trauma resuscitation (see below).

The accepted and taught standard for trauma resuscita-tion, however, is the American College of Surgeons' ATLS programme, and this requires that the hypotensive and hypovolaemic patient should receive immediate fluid resus-citation to secure adequate perfusion, and so oxygenation of cerebral and myocardial tissue, at the earliest opportunity.

This produces a clinical dilemma within the emer-gency department where there is ready access to definitive operative care. This is complicated further while still some distance from hospital. In Bickell et al's study the interval between injury and surgery was less than 2 h. In the UK, when in the prehospital environment with a hypotensive patient, access to a cardiothoracic surgical facility is unlikely to be achieved, under current levels of service provision, within this 2 h period in the vast majority of cases. In addition, both studies (Gervin & Fischer 1982, Bickell et al 1994) looked at a very specific group of patients with penetrating torso trauma, and in many cases the blood pressure was quite well preserved. This cannot be extrapolated and applied to other forms of trauma such as head injury or blunt trauma, or even to a group of severely hypotensive torso injuries (Bannerjee & Jones 1994).

A compromise philosophy has now arisen, with two stems:

- Intravenous access is obtained while in transit, with no delay on-scene to attend to the circulation beyond assessing it and controlling external haemorrhage.
- Once intravenous access has been obtained, there should be fluid administration aiming for a mildly hypotensive state. The intention is to maintain essential organ perfusion while limiting the increase in bleeding.

Intravenous access

It is generally accepted that securing an airway and optimizing patient ventilation with 100% oxygen offers the best chance of survival, however the benefit of on-scene fluid administration is less than clear (Deakin & Hicks 1994).

The setting up of an intravenous line takes time, varying from 90 s to 12 min (Pons et al 1988). Intuitively, the more critically shocked patient will be the more difficult to cannulate, and the time delay longer. O'Gorman et al (1989) considered these delays in transit and concluded that, in their environment, immediate evacuation produced the best outcome. Obtaining access en route in a moving ambulance has been shown to be a feasible option and does not cause delay (Jacobs et al 1984).

Accepting that access should be obtained in transit, ATLS principles can then be followed, with the use of short, large-bore cannulae to allow for rapid infusion of fluid. The standard approach is two 14 French gauge lines, in separate limbs, avoiding a limb with injury.

Fluid administration

There is a considerable amount of evidence to suggest that the use of prehospital fluid administration does not make a difference. Studies such as those by Champion et al (1981) and Pons et al (1988), where on-scene time was not delayed while access was achieved, showed that fluid infusion did not influence outcome.

A computer model for haemorrhage was presented by Lewis (1985) that predicted an effect from fluid administration only when the rate of infusion was at least equal to the bleeding rate and then the transport time to definitive care longer than 30 min. In the prehospital phase there is a time delay for access to the patient, assessment and intervention (airway and breathing) before the circulation is attended to. If packaging and transport are to be initiated before vascular access is obtained, there will already be significant blood loss.

If hypotension has developed, then, in a 70 kg male, there is a 1500 ml deficit (see Table 7.2) and a large 'catch-up' is going to be required to try to return the haemodynamic state towards normal.

Unfortunately, the beneficial effect of this catch up is difficult to prove in the prehospital phase. Dalton (1995) showed that a mean of 383 ml of fluid was given in a mean of 17 min in 235 consecutive trauma patients. Hypotensive or trapped casualties did not receive more fluid than others and very few in any group received more than 1000 ml. Not surprisingly, no obvious benefit was demonstrated.

The case for normalization of the haemodynamic state remains unproven and benefit has certainly not been clearly shown in the prehospital phase.

Hypotensive resuscitation

The variable case mix in casualties with trauma complicates the analysis of the effect of intravenous fluids. More studies need to be focused, looking at specific patterns of injury (Dick 1997). The assumption is frequently made that different shock states can be treated in the same way.

The group in which fluid resuscitation is going to have the least effect is where there is continued and uncontrolled haemorrhage. If injury type is considered, then benefit from fluid administration may well appear when haemostasis can be achieved (Silbergleit et al 1996). The effect of fluid therapy will be more apparent where the increase in systolic blood pressure permits more efficient essential organ perfusion, such as with maintaining the cerebral perfusion pressure, without greatly increasing the rate of loss from the bleeding sites.

Extrapolating from recent animal work, there has been a move recently towards hypotensive resuscitation. The hypothesis is put forward that standard fluid resuscitation will produce increased bleeding when compared to limited resuscitation or no resuscitation, and that limiting the resuscitation can reduce the blood loss and transfusion requirements (Owens et al 1995, Leppaniemi et al 1996), with less acidaemia and improved survival (Capone et al 1995). There is even evidence to suggest that low-volume fluid resuscitation may produce benefit without a demonstrable increase in blood pressure (Lilly et al 1992).

Intuitively, this is a very acceptable compromise of the two different ends of the spectrum, but the human studies of this have yet to show convincing benefit.

Fluid type

Having decided that intravenous fluids will be given, with due regard to not delaying the transit to hospital and improving the critical organ perfusion without exacerbating the blood loss, the next issue is which fluid.

A great deal of controversy has raged about this for years with the crystalloid–colloid debate. Within the ATLS protocol, an initial fluid bolus of 2000 ml of isotonic crystalloid solution, usually Ringer's lactate or Hartmann's solution, is advised. This equates to $20\,ml\,kg^{-1}$ as a bolus for a child. As already discussed, the patient's response to this is observed to determine the next step.

It is, however, possible to make a rough estimate of the amount that may be required based on the injuries found on examination (Table 7.3).

Large volumes of fluid may be needed. In the prehospital environment there are practical limits to how much can be kept warm, actually given or even carried, and this has led to the consideration of other options.

A multitude of fluids are available, although many are not in general use (Table 7.4). With all colloids there is a small but significant risk of an anaphylactic or anaphylactoid reaction (Table 7.5). This may not be noticed in the critical patient and be interpreted as a further deterioration in the patient's original condition. A discussion of the use of crystalloids and colloids can be found in the previous chapter.

PACKED RED CELLS AND WHOLE BLOOD

Packed red cells are a product supplied by the National Blood Transfusion Service in which a unit of single donor red cells is suspended in approximately 80 ml of a 4:1 mixture of donor plasma and a nutrient–anticoagulant solution. The resultant haematocrit is approximately 70% (Murphy

1992). Each unit of whole blood consists of 450 ml of blood from a single donor, mixed with approximately 60 ml of a nutrient–anticoagulant solution. The haematocrit is approximately 37% (Murphy 1992).

The availability of blood, the ideal replacement solution in massive haemorrhage, in the prehospital environment is extremely limited and requires a great deal of organization to set up a system allowing its availability from a hospital laboratory at short notice. Getting blood to the scene of an incident is really only a practical proposition in long entrapment situations.

With both types of blood there is the need to consider the immunology of transfusion. Is the blood required

Table 7.4 Intravenous fluids currently used in resuscitation

Group	Fluid
Isotonic crystalloids	Ringer's lactate solution Hartmann's solution 0.9% saline
Colloids	Modified gelatin (Haemaccel, Gelofusine) Starch (Hetastarch, Pentastarch) Plasma fraction (4.5% human albumin solution)
Hypertonic solutions	7.5% saline 5% dextrose or 0.9% saline with 10% Dextran 40 5% dextrose or 0.9% saline with 6% Dextran 70
Blood products	Packed red cells Whole blood

Table 7.3 Injury blood loss estimates within the first 4 h (to be doubled if the injury is compound)

Fracture	Estimated blood loss (ml)
Pelvis	2000
Femur	1000
Tibia	650
Rib	150 ml per rib

Table 7.5 Incidence of reactions to colloids. Figures in parentheses indicate the number of severe, life-threatening reactions

Colloid	Number of infusions	Total number of reactions	Incidence (%)
Haemaccel	6151	9 (3)	0.146
Gelofusine	6028	4 (1)	0.066
Hydroxyethyl starch	16405	14 (1)	0.085
Dextran 70	34621	24 (6)	0.069
Albumin	60048	7 (2)	0.011

Reprinted from The Lancet vol 309, Ring J, Messmer K Incidence and severity of anaphylactoid reactions to colloid volume substitutes, pp 466–469, © 1977 with permission from Elsevier.

immediately, in which case the universal donor O negative will be most appropriate (although the transfusion laboratory may supply O positive in a male patient where supplies are short) or can a sample of the casualty's blood be sent from the scene to allow a group-specific typing (taking 10 min) or a full cross-match (taking 45 min)?

As with all the other fluids, blood has its associated problems and there can be immune-mediated reactions to foreign protein, together with disturbance of the coagulation cascade, citrate toxicity and electrolyte disturbances.

Because of the high haematocrit, packed red cells tend to be used for the treatment of the anaemic state rather than resuscitation. With the administration of increasing volumes of the more suitable whole blood, there is development of a dilutional thrombocytopenia and reduced concentration of clotting factors, which are absent from the transfused blood. With large volumes there is the need for the addition of fresh frozen plasma (FFP) and platelets, and this is not practical in the prehospital arena.

Citrate toxicity and an associated hypocalcaemia are a risk – as a result of hypoxia there is impaired metabolism of citrate and lactate, producing an acidosis. There is also a variable potassium load depending on the age of the transfused blood.

FUTURE ADVANCES

Two other means of obtaining efficient resuscitation fluids are in the development stage. Within hospitals it is now standard practice, in some high-blood-loss operations, to use a cell salvage system. While not currently applicable to the out-of-hospital environment, technology may allow this soon.

Another development still in the early stages is the use of haemoglobin solutions and perfluorocarbons. Human trials with polymerized haemoglobin are now being published (Gould et al 1997) and other developments such as liposome-encapsulated haemoglobin are being assessed (Szebeni et al 1997). Animal experiments with an oxygen-carrying perfluorocarbon emulsion in the shock situation have showed promising results (Goodin et al 1994).

Which fluid and how much?

Control of the haemorrhage should be obtained first, if at all possible, on a 'put the plug in the bath before turning on the tap' principle.

There is a general acceptance now that there should not be a delay on-scene for the establishment of vascular access. Access should be obtained while in transit. Once this has been obtained, there needs to be a consideration of the injuries present and an estimate of the amount of blood that has been and may be lost from them.

With this, and an awareness of the late presentation of clear haemodynamic indicators of compromise, fluid losses can be estimated and anticipated. By working in the prehospital environment, it is likely that the carer will be present while the bleeding is ongoing but while the compensatory mechanisms are still effective and the clinical features of shock still subtle.

A decision needs to be made as to whether the problem is one of controlled haemorrhage, in which the ATLS principle of aiming for normal haemodynamic parameters can be applied, or whether there is an uncontrolled situation where the raising of the blood pressure can actually increase the bleeding rate, dilute the clotting factors and exacerbate the situation. Assuming a controlled situation, it is important to get on with administering the fluid without waiting for the clear clinical signs.

According to ATLS principles, the first fluid of choice is isotonic crystalloid, and this should be given rapidly as a dynamic fluid challenge to assess the response. The decisions after this will depend on the practitioner's assessment of the evidence and local policy. A degree of clinical judgement is required (Dick 1997).

The evidence for withholding fluids in penetrating truncal trauma is becoming increasingly accepted when the transit time to definitive care is relatively short. If there is uncontrolled haemorrhage, the current thinking is to aim for essential organ perfusion without reaching normal blood pressure values. The evidence for this is still not categorical (Shoemaker et al 1996).

In the presence of head injury, there is increasing recognition of the need to maintain cerebral perfusion and oxygenation. This may require establishing a blood pressure that is relatively higher than normally recommended in the traumatized and bleeding patient, despite the possibility of exacerbating other bleeding.

Specific management aspects of shock

The general management of the shocked patient requires attention to the airway and breathing–ventilation, with provision of high-concentration oxygen. Having addressed the problems of fluid resuscitation as discussed above, there are a number of specific management aspects for different types of shock that need to be considered.

ANAPHYLAXIS

The UK Resuscitation Council issued guidelines for the emergency treatment of anaphylaxis in 2001 (Project Team of the Resuscitation Council (UK) 2001). If there is significant release of vasoactive substances into the circulation then, in addition to the basic principles, attention should be given to additional forms of therapy (Brown 1998).

Adrenaline (epinephrine)

As there is generalized vasodilatation, it is recommended that a dose of 0.5 ml of 1:1000 adrenaline (epinephrine) should be given intramuscularly. This can be repeated after 5 min if there is no clinical improvement. In a peri-arrest situation, small aliquots of 1:10 000 adrenaline may be given intravenously, depending on the experience of the practitioner.

Chlorpheniramine

10 mg of chlorpheniramine (Piriton) should be given intravenously to counter the effect of histamine (H_1 blockade). Piriton should be given slowly, either diluted or premixed with blood. Rapid administration may result in cardiovascular collapse.

Hydrocortisone

As the substance of the reaction is inflammatory, it is recommended that a dose of steroid is given intravenously (hydrocortisone 100 mg).

Salbutamol

There is frequently a component of bronchospasm, in which case 5 mg of nebulized salbutamol may be given; while the adrenaline (epinephrine) will help, the beta-agonist will also aid the situation.

NEUROGENIC SHOCK

Because of the loss of vascular tone in this type of shock there is warm, pink and dry skin despite the low blood pressure. There may be no sympathetic increase in the heart rate.

While fluid resuscitation may produce a gradual rise in the blood pressure as the increased vascular space is filled, it may take over 3 litres. The ideal treatment is to give a peripheral vasoconstrictor. These agents are not applicable to the prehospital environment. It must be remembered that any patient who is considered at risk of an injury resulting in spinal shock is also likely to have sustained other injuries resulting in significant haemorrhage. In the prehospital environment, unless transfer times are prolonged or the patient is trapped, it is usually safer to assume that the patient has hypovolaemic shock.

CARDIOGENIC SHOCK

If ischaemic heart disease is the cause of the shock, then inotropic support is likely to be required and the use of fluids should be judicious in order to avoid pushing the casualty into cardiac failure. Without accurate and invasive monitoring of the blood pressure and a syringe-driver-controlled rate of infusion, the use of inotropes cannot be supported and they are therefore not indicated in immediate care. Symptomatic treatment and rapid evacuation to a critical care facility is indicated.

If pericardial tamponade is the cause of the failure, then it may be possible to drain the tamponade to good effect, but this should only be done with full cardiac resuscitation equipment to hand and with the facility to continue to drain the sac should the fluid reaccumulate.

Conclusion

After addressing airway and breathing within the primary survey, shock is the third fastest killer of the casualty. While it is thought to be a negative physiological state, there is evidence that it may be protective under some circumstances.

Treatment of shock begins with trying to arrest any further blood loss. Having achieved this, there should be no delay in the transfer of the patient to a place where definitive management can occur. Treatment en route with intravenous fluid may provide significant benefit but requires clinical judgement from the carer, and an awareness that normalization of the parameters may not be the optimum approach.

References

American College of Surgeons Committee on Trauma 1997 Advanced trauma life support student manual, 6th edn. American College of Surgeons, Chicago, IL

Bannerjee A, Jones R 1994 Whither fluid resuscitation. New England Journal of Medicine 344: 1450–1451

Bickell WH, Wall MJ, Pepe PE et al 1994 Immediate versus delayed fluid resuscitation for hypotensive patients with penetrating torso injuries. New England Journal of Medicine 331: 1105–1109

Brown AFT 1998 Therapeutic controversies in the management of acute anaphylaxis. Journal of Accident and Emergency Medicine 15: 89–95

Capone AC, Safar P, Stezoski W et al 1995 Improved outcome with fluid restriction in treatment of uncontrolled haemorrhagic shock. Journal of the American College of Surgeons 180: 49–56

Champion HR, Sacco WJ, Carnazzo AJ et al 1981 Trauma score. Critical Care Medicine 9: 672–676

Cuschieri A, Giles GR, Moosa AR (eds) 1988 Essential surgical practice, 2nd edn. John Wright, Bristol

Dalton AM 1995 Pre-hospital intravenous fluid replacement in trauma: an outmoded concept? Journal of the Royal Society of Medicine 88: 213P–216P

Davis JW, Parks SN, Kaups K et al 1996 Admission base deficit predicts transfusion requirements and risk of complications. Journal of Trauma 41: 769–774

Deakin CD, Hicks IR 1994 AB or ABC: pre-hospital fluid management in major trauma. Journal of Accident and Emergency Medicine 11: 154–157

Dick WJ 1997 Controversies in resuscitation: to infuse or not to infuse (1). Resuscitation 31: 3–6

Ganong WF 1983 The heart as a pump. In: Review of medical physiology. Lange, Los Altos, CA, ch 29

Gervin AS, Fischer RP 1982 The importance of prompt transport in salvage of patients with penetrating heart wounds. Journal of Trauma 22: 443–446

Goodacre SW, Gray A, McGowan A 1997 On-scene times for trauma patients in West Yorkshire. Journal of Accident and Emergency Medicine 14: 283–285

Goodin TH, Grossbard EB, Kaufman RJ et al 1994 A perfluorochemical emulsion for pre-hospital resuscitation of experimental haemorrhagic shock: a prospective, randomised, controlled study. Critical Care Medicine 22: 680–689

Gould SA, Moore EE, Moore FA et al 1997 Clinical utility of human polymerised haemoglobin as a blood substitute after acute trauma and urgent surgery. Journal of Trauma 43: 325–331

Jacobs LM, Sinclair A, Beiser A, D'Agostino RB 1984 Pre-hospital advanced life support: benefits in trauma. Journal of Trauma 26: 779–786

Leppaniemi A, Soltero R, Burris D et al 1996 Fluid resuscitation in a model of controlled haemorrhage: too much too early, or too little too late? Journal of Surgical Research 63: 413–418

Lewis FR 1985 Pre-hospital intravenous fluid therapy: physiologic computer modelling. Journal of Trauma 26: 804–809

Lilly MP, Gala GJ, Carlson DE et al 1992 Saline resuscitation after fixed volume haemorrhage. Role of resuscitation volume and rate of infusion. Annals of Surgery 216: 161–171

Murphy WG 1992 The use of blood and blood products. In: Tinker J, Zapol WM (eds) Care of the critically ill patient. Springer, New York, p 691–703

O'Gorman M, Trabulsy P, Pilcher DB 1989 Zero time pre-hospital IV. Journal of Trauma 29: 84–86

Owens TM, Watson WC, Prough DS et al 1995 Limiting initial resuscitation of uncontrolled haemorrhage reduces internal bleeding and subsequent volume requirements. Journal of Trauma 39: 200–207

Pons PT, Moore EE, Cusick JM et al 1988 Pre-hospital venous access in an urban paramedic system – a prospective on-scene analysis. Journal of Trauma 28: 1460–1463

Project Team of the Resuscitation Council (UK) 2001 Update on the emergency medical treatment of anaphylactic reactions for first medical responders and community nurses. Resuscitation 48: 241–243

Ring J, Messmer K 1977 Incidence and severity of anaphylactoid reactions to colloid volume substitutes. Lancet 309: 466–469

Shoemaker WC, Petitzman AB, Bellamy R et al 1996 Resuscitation from severe haemorrhage. Critical Care Medicine 24(Suppl 2): S12–S23

Silbergleit R, Satz W, McNamara RM et al 1996 Effect of permissive hypotension in continuous uncontrolled intra-abdominal haemorrhage. Academic Emergency Medicine 3: 922–926

Szebeni J, Wassef NM, Hartman KR et al 1997 Complement activation in vitro by the red cell substitute, liposome-encapsulated haemoglobin: mechanism of action and inhibition by soluble complement receptor type 1. Transfusion 37: 150–159

Vary TC, Littleton-Kearney MT 1994 Pathophysiology of traumatic shock and multiple organ system failure. In: Cardona VD, Hurn PD, Mason PJB et al (eds) Trauma nursing from resuscitation through rehabilitation. WB Saunders, Philadelphia, PA

Waxman K 1996 Shock: ischaemia, reperfusion and inflammation. New Horizons 4: 153–160

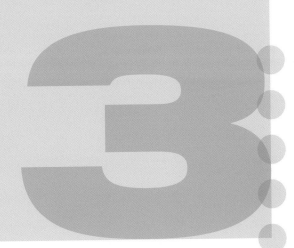

Part Three

8   Understanding the electrocardiogram 85
9   Cardiac emergencies 104
10 Respiratory emergencies 118
11 The unconscious patient 130
12 Acute abdomen 139

Understanding the electrocardiogram

8

Introduction	85
Basic principles	85
Sequence of cardiac activation	86
Electrode placement	87
Abnormalities of rate	88
Tachycardias	88
Bradycardias	93
Atrioventricular block	94
Broad QRS complexes	95
The ECG during chest pain	98
Cardiac pacemakers	102
Further reading	103

Introduction

Monitoring the electrical activity of the heart is an important part of the management of a variety of prehospital emergencies, although it is of most use in cases of cardiac arrest, other cardiac disease, drug intoxication and unconsciousness. This chapter will briefly discuss some basic electrophysiological principles and describe the usual sequence of electrical activation during the cardiac cycle and the corresponding appearance of the normal electrocardiogram (ECG), before presenting examples of some of the more important abnormalities encountered outside hospital. There are no references in this chapter, although a list of sources for further reading is provided at the end.

A number of points should be emphasized to begin with:

- An adequate interpretation requires a technically adequate recording.
- The prehospital environment is not conducive to optimum recording because of movement artefact, skeletal muscle tremor and electrical interference.
- There is no substitute for the recording and interpretation of ECGs from *real* patients; recognition of familiar computer-generated ECG simulations may lead to a false sense of proficiency.
- Although 12-lead ECG machines are increasingly being used outside hospital, most monitoring is performed using systems that use a small number of electrodes attached to the chest, and this may limit the usefulness of such monitoring to anything other than basic interpretation (rate and rhythm).

Esoteric ECG diagnoses have no place in emergency prehospital care. The ECG is only an aid to diagnosis and monitors the response to therapy. It should not deflect the practitioner from the needs of the patient. Patients dying in electromechanical dissociation can have surprisingly normal ECGs!

Basic principles

Resting myocardial cells are polarized (i.e. electrically charged) such that there is a relative negative potential between intracellular and extracellular spaces. This potential is maintained by the cell membrane. Stimulation of the cell leads to abrupt changes in transmembrane permeability for a variety of ions and a rapid, transient reversal of polarity, or depolarization. Depolarization is normally followed by activation of contractile muscle proteins. A more gradual repolarization to the resting potential then occurs. Muscle cells at rest potential can be excited by a neighbouring depolarized cell, allowing a wave of depolarization to spread throughout the myocardium.

This electrical activity (of the myocardium as a whole, rather than of an individual cell) can be recorded on the surface of the body by an exploring electrode. By convention the spread of depolarization towards the electrode results in an upward deflection of the recorder, while spread away leads to a downward deflection. The size of such a deflection depends upon the strength of the source of electrical change (in practice the mass of electrically competent muscle), the angle that exists between the exploring electrode and the direction of the wave of depolarization, and the distance between the source of activity and the electrode. Largest deflections are obtained from electrodes placed close to large masses of myocardium that look along the line of depolarization.

At any moment there may be numerous wavefronts of depolarization travelling in various directions within the heart. The ECG represents the net effect, or sum, of these wavefronts recorded on the skin, using a variety of electrodes. Only 10–15% of the total electrical activity generated by the heart is recorded on the surface ECG.

Sequence of cardiac activation

The shape of the surface ECG is largely determined by the sequence of electrical depolarization and repolarization within the heart (Fig. 8.1).

In health, the origin of cardiac depolarization is a group of cells in the right atrium – the sinoatrial (SA) node – that have an intrinsically unstable resting membrane potential. Activation initiated in the SA node spreads radially throughout the atria at a rate of approximately $1\,\mathrm{m\,s^{-1}}$; cells in the right atrium being depolarized before those in the left. The only electrical connection between the atria and the ventricles is at the atrioventricular (AV) node, which lies in the right atrial free wall above the tricuspid valve and the bundle of His. This bundle of specialized myocardial fibres passes along the posterior interventricular septum before splitting into right and left bundle branches, which in turn give rise to the meshwork of specialized conducting fibres of the Purkinje system.

After a delay at the AV node, depolarization travels rapidly $(4\,\mathrm{m\,s^{-1}})$ through the His–Purkinje system and then spreads from the endocardial to the epicardial ventricular

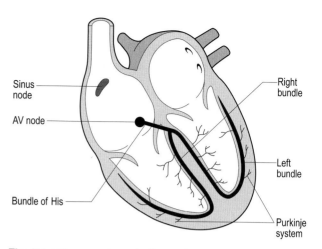

Fig. 8.1 • The normal conducting pathways in the heart.

myocardium (from inside out). Initially activation occurs in the septum, in a rightwards direction, then in the ventricular free wall and finally towards the bases of the ventricles. The surface ECG is influenced more by the left ventricle than the right because of the relatively large muscle mass of the left ventricle. Even though ventricular muscle mass far exceeds that of the atria, the duration of ventricular depolarization is short as long as activation spreads via the specialized conducting fibres. When these fibres are not used, for instance in cases of bundle branch block or a ventricular ectopic focus, ventricular depolarization is prolonged.

Repolarization within the atria probably follows the same path as depolarization, although any deflections due to this are engulfed by the coinciding ventricular activity. In the ventricle, however, repolarization takes place from epicardium to endocardium (from outside in) and such activity is therefore frequently recorded on the surface ECG in the same direction as depolarization.

The shape of the deflections on the ECG is dependent upon the sequence of electrical activation described above. These deflections are arbitrarily labelled P, Q, R, S, T and U (Fig. 8.2).

The P wave, caused by atrial depolarization, is a low-amplitude deflection no longer than 0.1 s in duration. The PR interval represents the time taken for sinus node activity to spread through the atria and reach the ventricular myocardium, normally between 0.12 and 0.2 s. The QRS complex represents ventricular depolarization and may have a number of the following components:

- *R wave*: any positive deflection; any second positive deflection is labelled R′
- *Q wave*: any negative deflection preceding an R wave
- *S wave*: any negative deflection following an R wave.

A negative QRS complex without an R wave is termed a QS wave. In general, large-amplitude deflections (i.e. >0.5 mV) are designated using upper case letters (Q, R, S) while

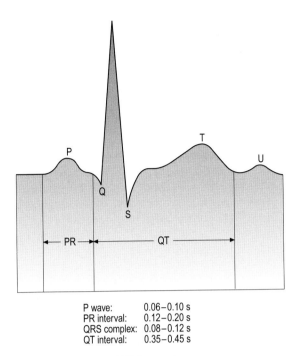

Fig. 8.2 • The normal ECG complex.

P wave:	0.06–0.10 s
PR interval:	0.12–0.20 s
QRS complex:	0.08–0.12 s
QT interval:	0.35–0.45 s

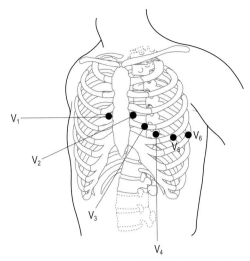

Fig. 8.3 • The positioning of the chest electrodes.

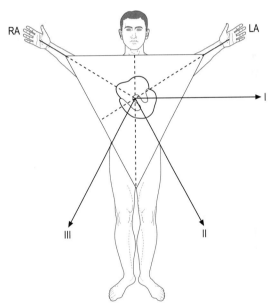

Fig. 8.4 • Bipolar limb leads. Each lead is the sum of the potentials at the positive electrode and at a point 180° opposite the negative electrode. The resulting vector bisects the angle between these two points.

smaller ones are given lower case letters (q, r, s). The QRS complex should not exceed 0.12s in duration. The ST segment represents the period of unchanging potential following ventricular depolarization and is usually on the isoelectric line. The T wave is produced by ventricular repolarization. A further low amplitude deflection, the U wave, occurs in many normal ECGs and is of uncertain cause.

Electrode placement

In the standard 12-lead ECG the heart is viewed in the vertical plane from electrodes attached to the limbs (bipolar and unipolar limb leads) and in the horizontal plane from exploring unipolar electrodes placed in prespecified positions on the chest wall (chest leads) (Fig. 8.3).

Bipolar leads record changes in the potential difference between two electrodes. The bipolar limb leads may be represented as follows:

- *lead I*: potential at the left arm minus that at the right arm
- *lead II*: potential at the left leg minus that at the right arm
- *lead III*: potential at the left leg minus that at the left arm.

The bipolar lead reflects the sum of potentials at the positive electrode and a point 180° opposite the negative electrode, and the viewpoint of the bipolar lead is therefore between these two points (Fig. 8.4).

Unipolar leads record electrical potential at the site of the exploring electrode with respect to the average potential of all three limb electrodes. The three limb electrodes are connected together as a central terminal into the negative pole of the electrocardiograph that is at virtually constant potential throughout the cardiac cycle. Unipolar leads are labelled with the letter V. In the frontal plane the heart is assumed to lie at the centre of an equilateral triangle, with each limb electrode (left arm, right arm and left leg) at an apex. The position of the unipolar limb lead is therefore towards that particular limb. The amplitude of deflection of unipolar limb leads is augmented by 50% by disconnecting the electrode on the limb under study from the central terminal. Augmentation of this type is identified by using the prefix 'a'. Thus, the unipolar limb leads are:

- *aVR*: right arm lead
- *aVL*: left arm lead
- *aVF*: left leg lead.

Chest electrodes are either designated as 'V' leads (American Heart Association) or as 'C' leads (International Electrotechnical Commission). The positions of the chest electrodes are as follows:

- *V1*: fourth intercostal space at right sternal border
- *V2*: fourth intercostal space at left sternal border
- *V3*: mid-way between V2 and V4
- *V4*: fifth intercostal space in left mid-clavicular line
- *V5*: left anterior axillary line, level with V4
- *V6*: left mid-axillary line, level with V4.

In women with pendulous breasts the electrodes should be placed under, rather than on top of, the breast. Other chest electrodes may sometimes be of use, although they have limited potential outside hospital, including:

- *V7*: posterior left axillary line, level with V4
- *V8*: posterior left scapula line, level with V4
- *V9*: left border of spine, level with V4
- *V3R–V9R*: right-sided electrodes in the mirror-image positions to V3–V9.

Significant changes in morphology can occur if electrodes are misplaced. For instance, the positioning of V1 and V2 in the third intercostal space will lead to an rSr pattern (compatible with incomplete right bundle branch block) and inverted P and T waves. Moreover, the practice of placing the limb electrodes on the thorax – commonly seen in prehospital monitoring and exercise electrocardiography – leads to changes in amplitude of deflection. The characteristics of ECG monitors make them less able than a diagnostic electrocardiograph to record detailed waveforms, although more tolerant of electrical interference. These problems are of no importance as long as the prehospital ECG is primarily used to answer the following questions:

- What is the QRS complex rate?
- Are the QRS complexes regular or irregular?
- Are the QRS complexes broad or narrow?
- What is the relationship between the P waves and QRS complexes?

Abnormalities of rate

Modern cardiac monitors automatically display the calculated heart rate on a screen. Misinterpretation of signals can cause spurious results. For instance, a ventricular pacing spike and the following QRS complex may be counted as separate episodes of ventricular activity, leading to a false diagnosis of tachycardia.

A paper record of an ECG signal is made on standard graph paper of feint ('small') 1 mm squares within bolder ('large') 5 mm squares. The vertical axis is a measure of voltage – 10 mm represents 1 mV – and the horizontal axis is a measure of time – 1 mm represents 0.04 s. Thus, one large square is equivalent to 0.2 s and five large squares to 1 s. The approximate heart rate is calculated by dividing the number of large squares between consecutive QRS complexes (or P waves for the atrial rate) into 300.

One large square – rate is 300 min^{-1}
Two large squares – rate is 150 min^{-1}
Three large squares – rate is 100 min^{-1}
Four large squares – rate is 75 min^{-1}
Five large squares – rate is 60 min^{-1}
Six large squares – rate is 50 min^{-1}.

Tachycardias

SINUS TACHYCARDIA

In adults a sinus rate of greater than 100 min^{-1} is regarded as sinus tachycardia, whereas in children this is commonly seen and infants often have rates of around 150 min^{-1}. The commonest symptom is palpitation, which tends to be gradual in onset and to be associated with evidence of an underlying cause such as anxiety, pain, blood loss and hypovolaemia, fever, hyperthyroidism and drug ingestion (e.g. salbutamol for asthma). The ECG shows a rapid (usually <150 min^{-1}) QRS rate, with a P wave preceding each QRS complex (Fig. 8.5). Although the underlying cause may require treatment outside the hospital, it may be harmful to treat sinus tachycardia per se. An exception is in cases of acute myocardial infarction where the appropriate use of intravenous beta-blockers will not only slow the sinus rate but also lead to a reduction in infarct size.

REGULAR, NARROW (QRS)-COMPLEX TACHYCARDIA

The title of this subsection describes what is seen on the ECG and is preferable, in prehospital care, to the broad heading of 'supraventricular tachycardia' (SVT) and to the electrophysiologically precise, and often inaccurate, 'atrial tachycardia'. Patients present with abrupt onset of rapid (140–220 min^{-1}), regular palpitations associated with transient hypotension. Such events tend to recur and the patient may give a history of many episodes of such palpitations,

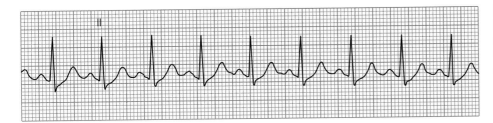

Fig. 8.5 • Sinus tachycardia – in this case due to acute anterior myocardial infarction. Unsurprisingly, there are no diagnostic ST changes in lead II.

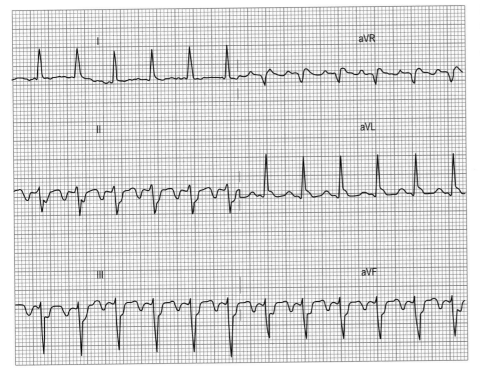

Fig. 8.6 • Atrial flutter with 2:1 conduction. The flutter wave rate is 300 min^{-1} and every other flutter wave is partially obscured by a QRS complex.

some requiring treatment and some stopping spontaneously. Often the patient is otherwise well and tolerates the tachycardia, although in those with significant coronary or valvular disease the tachycardia may lead to angina or haemodynamic collapse. The mechanisms responsible for regular, narrow-complex tachycardia include:

- atrial origin:
  - SA nodal re-entry
  - true atrial tachycardia including atrial automaticity and re-entry
  - atrial flutter with 1:1 or 2:1 conduction
- AV nodal involvement:
  - atrioventricular re-entrant tachycardia (AVRT) including Wolff–Parkinson–White syndrome
  - atrioventricular nodal re-entrant tachycardia (AVNRT).

Atrial flutter, AVRT and AVNRT are relatively common. Atrial flutter with 2:1 conduction is frequently misclassified as sinus tachycardia at a rate of 150 min^{-1} because the atrial flutter rate is around 300 min^{-1} and every second flutter wave is concealed by the QRS complex (Fig. 8.6).

In AVNRT the re-entrant circuit responsible for the arrhythmia lies wholly within the AV node. This causes almost instantaneous depolarization of the atria (retrogradely) and ventricles, and a P wave is difficult to identify because it falls within the QRS complex (Fig. 8.7). In AVRT depolarization passes antegradely from the AV node to the ventricles and thence retrogradely into the atria via an accessory connection.

A P wave following the QRS complex points to the involvement of such an accessory pathway, as does the presence of a short PR interval, slurred delta wave and broad QRS complex in the ECG during normal heart rates; the characteristic findings of the Wolff–Parkinson–White syndrome (Fig. 8.8).

The decision to treat such tachycardias outside hospital depends on a variety of patient and practitioner factors. Because the majority of these arrhythmias involve the AV node, methods that cause varying degrees of AV blockade are likely to be effective. These include the Valsalva manoeuvre, carotid sinus massage and intravenous administration of adenosine (Fig. 8.9). If the AV node is not

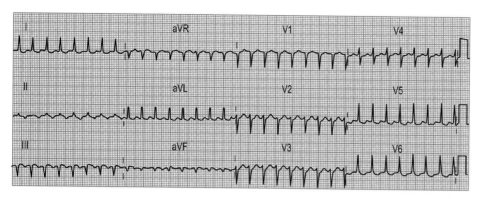

Fig. 8.7 • Regular, narrow-complex tachycardia of 190 beats min^{-1}.

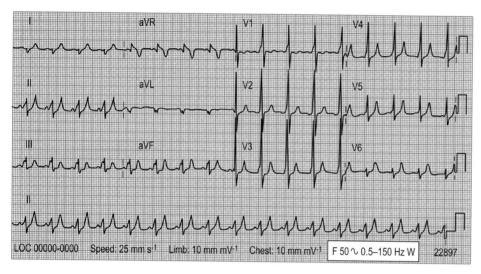

Fig. 8.8 • Wolff–Parkinson–White syndrome. There is pre-excitation shown by a short PR interval (0.08 s) and a delta wave. The delta wave is negative in aVL and results in a Q wave that, taken in isolation, could be mistaken for evidence of myocardial infarction.

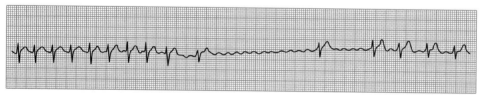

Fig. 8.9 • Intravenous adenosine causes transient slowing of ventricular rate and shows underlying fibrillatory waves. The irregular, narrow-complex tachycardia was therefore atrial fibrillation.

involved in the aetiology of the tachycardia, AV blockade may cause transient slowing of the ventricular rate due to heart block but not restoration of sinus rhythm. Beta-blockers may serve to stabilize atrial activity and a variety of class I and class III agents may also be effective in these cases. Finally, synchronized DC cardioversion can be used outside hospital in life-threatening cases.

RE-ENTRY

Re-entry is thought to be the commonest mechanism involved in the development of tachycardias. A re-entrant circuit consists of two neighbouring, virtually parallel, strips of conducting myocardium, in electrical contact above and below. This anatomical pathway may be small enough to be contained, for example, within the AV node. In order to produce a tachycardia the electrophysiological properties of the two strips of myocardium must differ. One should have a significantly longer *refractory period*, i.e. the interval following depolarization during which another electrical impulse fails to cause another depolarization. The other strip should have a slower conduction velocity. Then, if a premature impulse arrives at the top of the circuit it may fail to excite one of the strips, because it is refractory, yet it may still travel (relatively slowly) down the other strip. By the time the wave of depolarization reaches the bottom of the circuit the neighbouring strip may no longer be refractory and depolarization spreads retrogradely back via this strip to the top of the circuit. A wave of depolarization will therefore circulate around the re-entrant circuit and cause a tachycardia by exciting the surrounding myocardium.

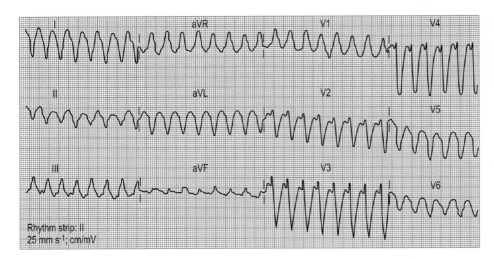

Fig. 8.10 • Ventricular tachycardia. The QRS complexes are extremely broad (almost 0.2 s); there is a right bundle branch block pattern in V1 and a QS wave in V6.

REGULAR, BROAD-COMPLEX TACHYCARDIA

The commonest types of regular, broad (greater than 0.12 s or three small squares)-complex tachycardia are ventricular tachycardia (VT) (Fig. 8.10) and tachycardias of supraventricular origin (SVT) with coexisting or rate-related block of a bundle of His. Much time and effort can be spent trying to distinguish between these two, and various algorithms have been published to aid diagnosis. Occasionally, tachycardias of supraventricular origin may involve antegrade conduction down an accessory AV pathway and retrograde conduction through the AV node. This will also cause regular, broad-complex tachycardia.

In prehospital care the most important factor is to decide whether immediate termination is necessary, for example when the arrhythmia is associated with pulseless cardiac arrest or significant hypotension. In these cases synchronized DC cardioversion is the therapy of choice. When less urgent treatment is required outside hospital, intravenous adenosine has been advocated because of its short duration of action and efficacy in terminating arrhythmias that are dependent upon the AV node for their propagation. While it is unlikely to be effective in the treatment of VT, it is also very unlikely to cause significant deterioration when so given. Intravenous verapamil, on the other hand, should not be given to patients with broad-complex tachycardia unless the diagnosis is certain and VT has been excluded. Intravenous lidocaine is still recommended for the treatment of VT outside hospital.

Verapamil is contraindicated in VT.

If it is deemed necessary outside hospital to differentiate between VT and SVT with bundle branch block, the following points may be useful. First, the clinical state of the patient is of no value: patients with VT may look surprisingly well.

Table 8.1 ECG features suggestive of ventricular tachycardia (VT) (12-lead trace)

- Capture beats
- Fusion beats
- QRS width >0.14 s
- Right bundle branch block pattern in V1 and R taller than R′
- QRS complexes in chest leads predominantly all upwards or downwards

Second, children and young adults are more likely to have SVT than VT. Third, SVT is often found in the presence of an otherwise normal heart, while VT more frequently occurs where there is underlying ventricular disease (e.g. previous or acute myocardial infarction, dilated or hypertrophic cardiomyopathy). Fourth, a 12-lead ECG should be recorded if at all possible. VT is the most likely diagnosis if: there is dissociation of P waves and QRS complexes; there are occasional 'capture' or 'fusion' beats – narrow or intermediate QRS complexes caused by dissociated atrial activity conducting down the normal ventricular-conducting pathways; the QRS width is greater than 0.14 s; there is a right bundle branch block pattern in V1 and R is taller than R′; or the QRS complexes in the chest leads are predominantly all upwards or all downwards (Table 8.1). Fifth, if in doubt treat as VT.

VT that lasts for over 30 s is defined as 'sustained'. If there is no variation in the morphology of the QRS complexes, other than occasional fusion or capture beats, the VT is said to be 'monomorphic'. A rare form of VT is ventricular flutter (Fig. 8.11). Here the QRS complexes blend into the T waves leading to large-amplitude, sine-like wave forms that usually degenerate into ventricular fibrillation (VF).

IRREGULAR, NARROW-COMPLEX TACHYCARDIA

This is most often due to atrial fibrillation (AF) with a rapid ventricular response rate. Atrial activity is chaotic,

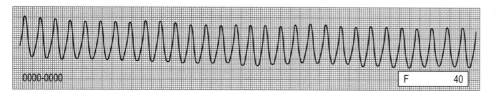

Fig. 8.11 • Ventricular flutter.

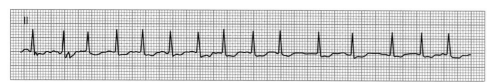

Fig. 8.12 • Rapid atrial fibrillation.

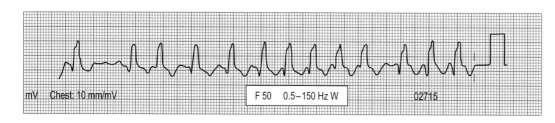

Fig. 8.13 • Irregular, narrow-complex tachycardia due to atrial flutter with variable block.

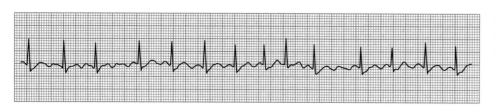

Fig. 8.14 • Atrial fibrillation with coexisting bundle branch block.

with multiple, small re-entrant circuits producing wavelets of activity that are independent of each other. This fragmented activity may be seen in some leads as small irregular 'f' waves at rates of up to 600 min^{-1}, appearing almost like electrical interference. Many or most of these wavelets fail to reach or to excite the AV node because of conduction block and refractoriness. The findings then are of totally irregular, narrow QRS complexes, usually at rates of 100–160 min^{-1} (Fig. 8.12). At faster ventricular rates the 'f' waves may not be apparent and even the QRS irregularity becomes difficult to identify. Carotid sinus massage may cause a slight slowing of the ventricular rate and intravenous adenosine will cause transient AV block, which, while not terminating the arrhythmia, may allow more certain diagnosis.

Conversion of the heart to sinus rhythm (with synchronized DC shock) is usually unnecessary in prehospital care and should not be attempted unless there is a clear understanding of the cause of AF, its duration and its contribution to the present illness/emergency. Slowing of the ventricular rate may be achieved using intravenous verapamil, diltiazem or esmolol. Intravenous digoxin takes effect too slowly.

Whereas atrial flutter may present as regular tachycardia when there is a fixed relationship between the atrial rate and the ventricular response (e.g. 1:1, 2:1, 3:1), atrial flutter with varying AV block is a cause of irregular, narrow-complex tachycardia (Fig. 8.13). The diagnosis is more obvious than in cases of fixed 2:1 block because the classic 'sawtooth' pattern of atrial flutter waves is seen during intermittent slowing of the ventricular response or following carotid sinus massage. Drugs that slow AV nodal conduction will reduce the ventricular response rate. Once again, it is unusual to need to attempt electrical cardioversion outside hospital, even though atrial flutter is less resistant to such treatment than AF.

IRREGULAR, BROAD-COMPLEX TACHYCARDIA

Atrial fibrillation with a rapid ventricular response and coexisting bundle branch block will present as an irregular, broad-complex tachycardia (Fig. 8.14). Again, at fast rates the irregular nature of the QRS complexes may not be obvious, leading to a misclassification as VT. In practice

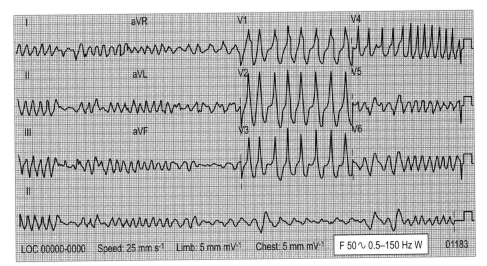

Fig. 8.15 • Atrial fibrillation in Wolff–Parkinson–White syndrome showing irregular, broad-complex tachycardia. In this case the delta wave is apparent in V1–V3 while in the remaining leads electrical activity resembles ventricular fibrillation. This patient remained conscious, although hypotensive.

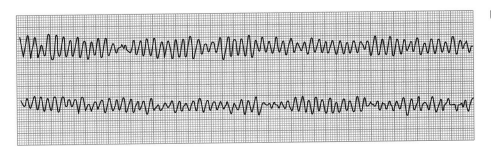

Fig. 8.16 • Torsade de pointes.

this is rarely a problem but can be overcome by scrutiny of a paper printout of the ECG and by noting the effects of either carotid sinus massage or intravenous adenosine.

If atrial fibrillation develops in a patient who has one or more accessory pathways that are capable of conduction antegradely (from atria to ventricles), a rapid, irregular and bizarre ECG appearance results. The QRS complexes have varying morphologies and the tracing may resemble VF (Fig. 8.15). This is a life-threatening situation and is a cause of sudden death in patients with Wolff–Parkinson–White syndrome. If the patient is unconscious the prehospital treatment should be DC shock (as per the VF protocol). If the patient is conscious, although compromised, it is probably best to transport him or her rapidly to hospital while monitoring the ECG.

In polymorphic ventricular tachycardia the shape of the broad QRS complexes varies and there appears to be slight irregularity. This arrhythmia is known as *torsade de pointes* (twisting of the points) (Fig. 8.16) and may present as short-lasting, self-terminating episodes or may progress to VF. It may complicate periods of bradycardia and is associated with electrolyte disturbances and the use of a variety of drugs, including many antiarrhythmic agents. As such, it may be prudent not to treat short-lasting episodes of polymorphic VT outside hospital, reserving DC shock for episodes

that are sufficiently prolonged to cause loss of consciousness. If prehospital prophylaxis *is* thought necessary, intravenous magnesium has been useful. Paradoxically, increasing the resting ventricular rate, by pacing or with isoprenaline, may also help. A marker for patients at risk of torsade de pointes is QT interval prolongation.

Ventricular fibrillation is seen as totally chaotic, rapid, irregular, electrical activity. It is a cause of sudden death and requires emergency defibrillation.

Bradycardias

These are due to either a reduction in the rate of SA nodal discharge or a failure of conduction of SA nodal impulses into the ventricles, or both.

SINUS BRADYCARDIA

This is a sinus rhythm at a rate of less than $60\,\text{min}^{-1}$. It may be physiological, for instance in athletic individuals, or occur as a result of increased vagal tone, hypothermia, hypothyroidism, raised intracranial pressure and some drugs, especially beta-blockers.

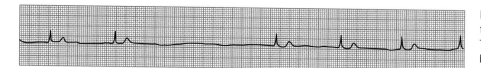

Fig. 8.17 • Sinus arrest leading to a pause of a little over 3 s. The background rhythm is sinus bradycardia.

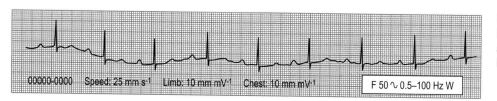

Fig. 8.18 • First-degree heart block with a PR interval of approximately 0.34 s. The QT interval is 0.44 s.

SINUS ARREST AND SA NODAL BLOCK

In cases of sinus arrest there is failure of SA nodal depolarization resulting in a pause of variable duration, which may or may not cause symptoms, during which time there are no P waves visible on the ECG (Fig. 8.17). If SA nodal block occurs, the SA nodal cells depolarize but this fails to excite adjacent atrial myocardial cells. Consequently there is a pause without P waves, the duration of which (between consecutive P waves) is a multiple of the P wave cycle length during sinus rhythm. Both these abnormalities are commonly due to degenerative disease and rarely need specific treatment in the absence of symptoms. However, they may be associated with dizziness, blackout – the *Adams–Stokes attack* – or near-blackout, in which case the prehospital treatment includes cardiac monitoring, administration of atropine or (if life-threatening) isoprenaline, external cardiac pacing and rapid transport to hospital.

Patients manifesting some or all of the above features of sinoatrial disease, with no obvious reversible cause, are said to have the *sick sinus syndrome*. These individuals are usually elderly and are candidates for permanent pacing. Long-term monitoring often reveals intermittent bradycardias and tachycardias (commonly atrial fibrillation or atrial tachycardia). The termination of the tachycardia is frequently followed by a significant period of sinus arrest.

Atrioventricular block

This term is used to denote any delay in conduction of atrial impulses into the ventricles. There are a wide variety of causes, symptoms, electrophysiological sites and prognoses of such blocks. Although AV block often presents with bradycardia, this is not invariable and the hallmark on the ECG is an abnormal relationship between the P waves and the QRS complexes.

FIRST-DEGREE AV BLOCK

This is an asymptomatic ECG finding of prolongation (greater than 0.2 s) of the PR interval. Each atrial depolarization is conducted to the ventricles and no treatment is required outside hospital. Progression to more serious types of heart block is rare (Fig. 8.18).

SECOND-DEGREE AV BLOCK

This occurs when there is intermittent failure of atrial impulses to reach the ventricles. The ECG shows that some P waves are not followed by QRS complexes. There are two types. In both cases, symptoms depend partly upon the ventricular rate and partly upon the underlying cause. *Mobitz type 1* or *Wenckebach* block is characterized by progressive prolongation of the PR interval prior to the failure of conduction and the absence of a QRS complex (Fig. 8.19). The following PR interval returns to normal. The pulse feels irregular and the QRS complexes appear to be grouped on either side of short pauses. The usual site for the block is within the AV node itself, and this has a benign prognosis.

In *Mobitz type 2* block there are episodes of abrupt failure of conduction between atrial and ventricles without the preceding PR interval prolongation. The site of the block is lower in the conduction system, within the His–Purkinje fibres, and there is a greater likelihood that symptomatic complete heart block may develop. The ECG shows either a fixed or varying ratio of P waves to QRS complexes. When there is 2:1 conduction it is impossible to determine whether the block is Mobitz type 1 or type 2 because there is no opportunity to see progressive PR prolongation. Type 2 block often fails to respond to atropine, which may even worsen the conduction ratio. Emergency prehospital treatment may include adrenergic agents and external cardiac pacing (Fig. 8.20).

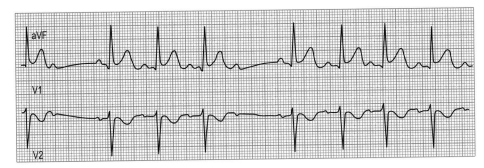

Fig. 8.19 • Mobitz type 1 second-degree block (Wenckebach block). The third, fourth and fifth PR interval are, respectively, 0.18, 0.21 and 0.24 s before a failure of AV nodal conduction.

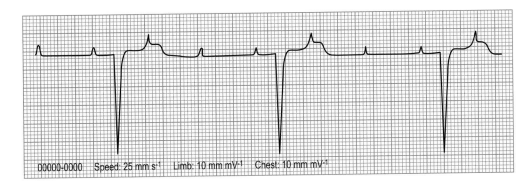

Fig. 8.20 • Mobitz type 2 second-degree block. The ratio of P waves to QRS complexes is 3:1.

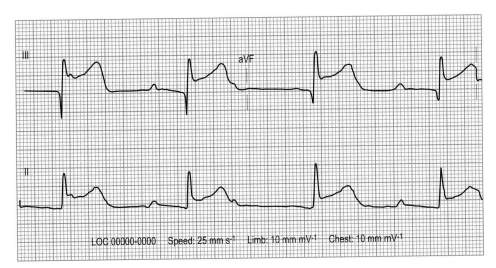

Fig. 8.21 • Third-degree AV block complicating acute, inferior myocardial infarction. The QRS complexes are narrow, at a rate of 42 min^{-1}.

THIRD-DEGREE AV BLOCK

In this case there is a complete interruption in conduction of impulses from atria to ventricles (complete heart block) and ventricular activity is dependent upon an 'escape' rhythm. This is an example of AV dissociation (other examples include cases of ventricular tachycardia and rapid junctional rhythms). The hallmark on the ECG is a regular QRS complex rate that is independent of the P wave rate. If the site of the block is in the AV node, the focus of the escape rhythm is often within the bundle of His, leading (in the absence of a bundle branch block) to a narrow QRS complex that tends to be reasonably fast (e.g. 40–50 min^{-1})

and reliable (Fig. 8.21). If the site of the block is just below the AV node the escape rhythm is slower (e.g. 30 min^{-1}) and less reliable; the QRS complexes are broad. This may lead to ventricular standstill (Fig. 8.22).

Broad QRS complexes

When the QRS complexes are broad the cause usually lies within the ventricles. The prolongation of ventricular depolarization (greater than 0.12 s) may result from:

● an ectopic focus within the ventricles, e.g. ventricular ectopics, idioventricular rhythm, VT

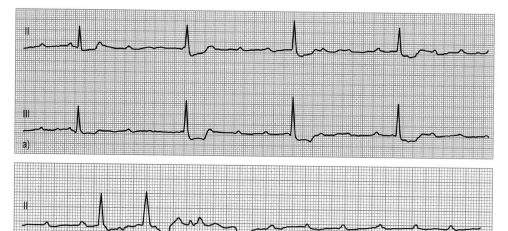

Fig. 8.22 • Third-degree AV block (a) with a regular, slow QRS complex escape rhythm and (b) leading to ventricular standstill.

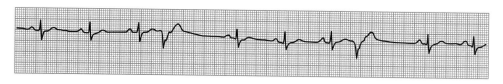

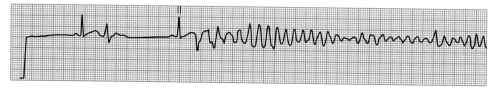

Fig. 8.23 • Ventricular premature complexes followed by a compensatory pause.

Fig. 8.24 • An R-on-T ventricular ectopic (after the second sinus beat) leads to the initiation of ventricular fibrillation. The preceding rhythm was sinus bradycardia.

- a failure of conduction within a branch of the bundle of His, e.g. left or right bundle branch block (LBBB or RBBB)
- pre-excitation of part of the ventricle in Wolff–Parkinson–White syndrome
- drug or metabolic effects, e.g. hyperkalaemia
- ventricular pacing.

VENTRICULAR ECTOPICS

These are broad, bizarre QRS complexes followed by a T wave that is in the opposite direction to the main component of the QRS complex. They are of varying degrees of prematurity, although rarely preceded by a P wave, and may be followed by a pause before the next sinus beat (Fig. 8.23). When the ectopic occurs very early after a sinus beat the QRS complex appears to fall during the preceding T wave. This is termed an *R-on-T ectopic* and as such may be associated with the initiation of VT or VF (Fig. 8.24). If all the ectopics have the same shape they are assumed to originate from a single focus and are *unifocal*; if there is more than one shape they are described as *multifocal*. An alternating rhythm of a sinus beat followed by an ectopic beat is called *bigeminy, coupling* or a *bigeminal rhythm*. Two consecutive ventricular ectopics are a *couplet* and more than two consecutive ectopic beats are called a *salvo* or *non-sustained VT*.

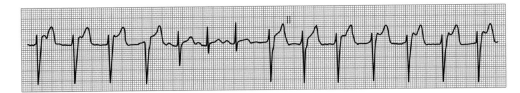

Fig. 8.25 • Idioventricular rhythm developing after a short sinus pause.

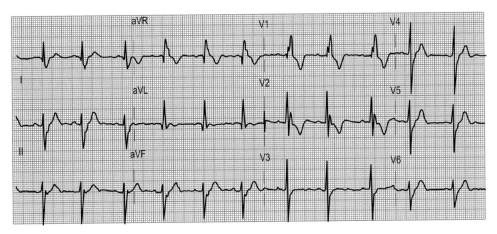

Fig. 8.26 • Right bundle branch block with an RSr' pattern in lead V2, and an RS wave in leads V6 and I. There is also left-axis deviation (not discussed in the text).

Ventricular ectopics may be felt at the wrist as an irregular pulse, or even as a bradycardia if frequently occurring ectopics fail to generate sufficient pulse pressure. The patient is frequently unaware. In normal individuals the presence of ventricular ectopics is almost always of no consequence. However, when occurring in patients with heart disease they are associated with a poorer prognosis, especially if they are frequent, multifocal or occur in salvos. Whilst the prehospital use of intravenous lidocaine has been advocated to suppress such patterns of ventricular ectopics, there is no convincing evidence that this suppression is of long-term benefit.

IDIOVENTRICULAR RHYTHM

The inherent rate of depolarization of ventricular myocardial cells may, under certain circumstances, become enhanced until the rate is faster than the sinus node depolarization rate. At this point there appears a regular, broad-complex rhythm that is slightly faster than the preceding sinus rhythm rate (although no more than $120 \, \text{min}^{-1}$) (Fig. 8.25). No specific treatment is required. Such a rhythm is frequently seen during the early stages of acute myocardial infarction, where it may be a marker of reperfusion of infarcting myocardium, and after defibrillation from VF.

BUNDLE BRANCH BLOCK

If either branch of the bundle of His fails to conduct, ventricular depolarization is prolonged in the appropriate ventricle, and the QRS complex is consequently broad. Bundle branch block may be permanent, intermittent or rate-related, complete (QRS greater than 0.12s) or incomplete.

In right-bundle branch block there is an RSR' pattern in the chest leads facing the right ventricle (V1 and V2) and an S wave in those leads facing the left ventricle (V5, V6, I and aVL) (Fig. 8.26).

In left-bundle branch block there is a deep QS wave in V1, an rS wave in V2 and an RsR', plateau-shaped or 'M'-shaped complex in V5, V6, I and aVL (Fig. 8.27).

The bundle branch blocks do not require specific treatment but are of importance in prehospital care for the following reasons. First, by definition they indicate the presence of conduction abnormality, particularly when associated with AV delay (so-called *bifascicular block*), and identify patients who may be at high risk of syncope due to Adams–Stokes attacks. Second, left bundle branch block is often caused by significant cardiac disease. Third, they may be confused with ventricular rhythms. Fourth, left-bundle branch block in particular interferes with the ECG diagnosis of acute myocardial infarction.

PRE-EXCITATION (Figs 8.8 and 8.15)

As discussed above, patients with the Wolff–Parkinson–White syndrome have one or more accessory pathways that bypass the AV node and allow the premature depolarization of a segment of the ventricular myocardium. The accessory pathway does not necessarily conduct every atrial depolarization and hence the ECG may be entirely normal. When pre-excitation occurs there is a short PR interval

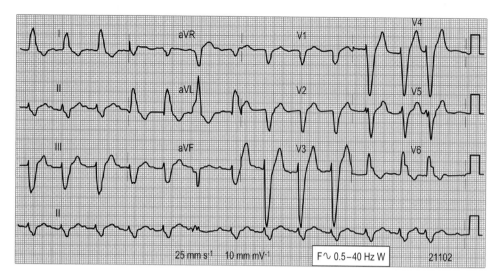

Fig. 8.27 • Left bundle branch block with a wide QS wave in V1 and RSr pattern in V6. There is also first-degree heart block (prolonged PR interval) and occasional premature ventricular and atrial ectopics.

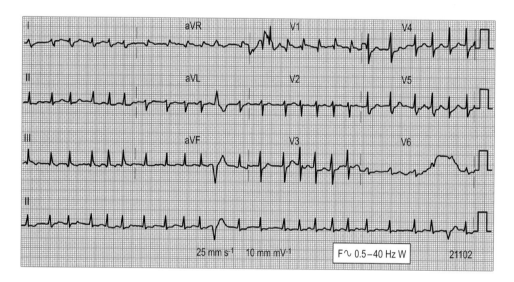

Fig. 8.28 • Acute pulmonary embolus. There is atrial fibrillation with a rapid ventricular rate, a right-bundle branch block pattern and the 'S1, Q1, T3' appearance.

(<0.12 s), and a slurred beginning of the broad QRS complex, the delta wave. Wolff–Parkinson–White syndrome is of importance in prehospital care because it is a cause of narrow-complex, regular tachycardias or, during atrial fibrillation, may present with life-threatening, irregular, broad-complex tachycardia. Moreover, the delta wave may change the shape of the QRS complexes, leading to a false diagnosis of acute myocardial infarction.

The ECG during chest pain

The 12-lead ECG is useful in the diagnosis and management of a variety of causes of chest pain. These include acute pulmonary embolism, pericarditis, aortic stenosis and the manifestations of coronary artery disease: angina and acute myocardial infarction. Again, it must be stressed

that cardiac monitors are of less value than the standard 12-lead ECG and that a normal ECG appearance does not rule out significant pathology. Prehospital care is about the management of patients and is aided, not superseded, by ECG recordings.

ACUTE PULMONARY EMBOLISM (Fig. 8.28)

In mild cases of pulmonary embolism the only ECG change may be a sinus tachycardia, which may merely be a manifestation of the pain. In more severe cases changes occur that reflect dilatation of the right heart chamber, namely the 'S1, Q3, T3' pattern (an S wave in lead I, and both a Q wave and inverted T wave in lead III), right bundle branch block, a peaked P wave or atrial fibrillation, and T wave inversion in leads V1–V3. These changes are often transient. The combination of such T wave inversion in

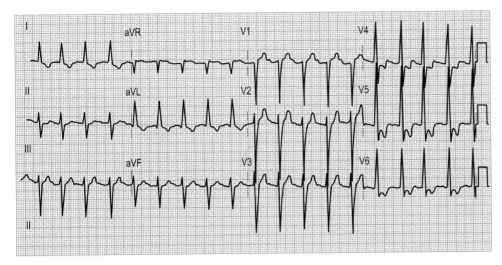

Fig. 8.29 • Left ventricular hypertrophy with strain – with tall R waves in left ventricular leads (V5, V6, I and aVL), and deep S waves in V1 and V2. There is also a widening of the QRS complexes, depressed ST segments and inverted T waves in the lateral leads, left-axis deviation and prolongation of the PR interval.

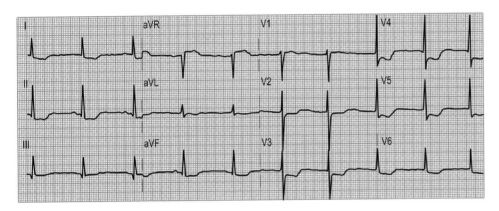

Fig. 8.30 • Acute myocardial ischaemia associated with sinus bradycardia. This patient had stenosis of the left main coronary artery, causing widespread ischaemia.

V1–V3 and in lead III may suggest a combination of both anteroseptal and inferior myocardial infarction.

PERICARDITIS

The pericardium is not thought to be electrically active and so ECG changes seen during acute pericarditis are likely to result from associated injury to the epicardial surface of the heart. The importance of this condition outside hospital is that it may be misdiagnosed as acute myocardial infarction, especially as its hallmark is ST segment elevation above the isoelectric line. In pericarditis the ST elevation tends to be widespread, appearing in most of the leads, except aVR and lead III, and has a concave (upwards) rather than convex shape.

AORTIC STENOSIS (Fig. 8.29)

Patients with aortic stenosis may develop anginal chest pain in the absence of coronary artery disease. The ECG findings are those of *left ventricular hypertrophy*, namely an accentuation of those parts of the QRS complex associated with left ventricular depolarization. Those leads facing the left ventricle (leads I, aVL, V5 and V6) will have tall R waves, and those facing the right ventricle (leads V1 and V2) will have deep S waves. The 'strain' pattern – T wave inversion in the left ventricular leads – may also occur, as may left bundle branch block.

ANGINA (Fig. 8.30)

The ECG may be entirely normal during an episode of angina, although there may be ST segment or T wave abnormalities of varying duration. The ST segment overlying the ischaemic part of the myocardium develops a horizontal or down-sloping depression below the isoelectric line. The junction between the ST segment and the T wave becomes more clearly defined. Occasionally the T waves become flattened or deeply inverted.

TOURO COLLEGE LIBRARY

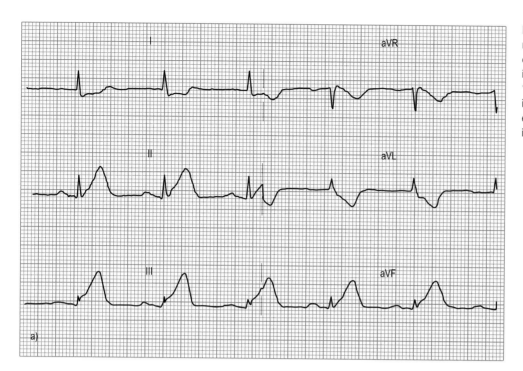

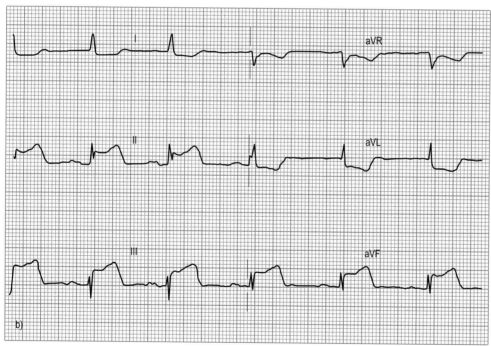

Fig. 8.31 • Acute, inferior, myocardial infarction. (a) The earliest changes include peaked T waves in II, III and aVF, while there are 'reciprocal' ST and T wave changes in I and aVL. (b) Later ST segment elevation becomes prominent in the inferior leads.

ACUTE MYOCARDIAL INFARCTION
(Figs 8.31–8.33)

The ECG may be abnormal to a variable degree, although a prehospital ECG recorded soon after the onset of symptoms may fail to show diagnostic changes. The classic changes evolve over a matter of hours and include:

● an early transient 'hyperacute' phase of widening and peaking of T waves

● ST segment elevation that is initially concave and blending into the peaked T wave before becoming convex

● T wave inversion, which may become deep

● Q wave development.

Q waves are, of course, seen in some leads of the normal ECG. In order to be defined as pathological they should be at least 2 mm deep and longer than 0.04 s in duration. Furthermore, myocardial infarction may be categorized as

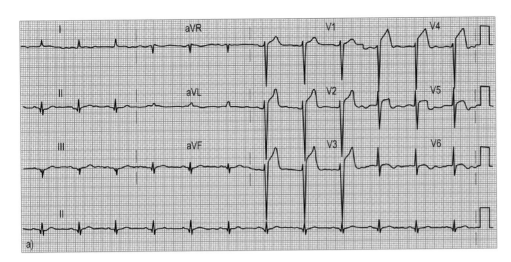

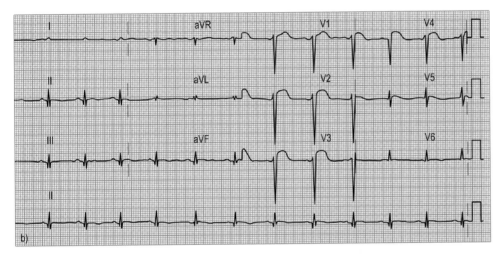

Fig. 8.32 • Acute, anterior, myocardial infarction. (a) Within 1 h of onset of symptoms there are tall T waves in V2–V4, ST segment elevation in V1–V6, and T wave inversion in V5 and V6. There are no pathological Q waves, although there is loss of R wave height in V2–V4. (b) After a further 30 min the ST segment elevation appears more obviously convex upwards and the T wave height has reduced.

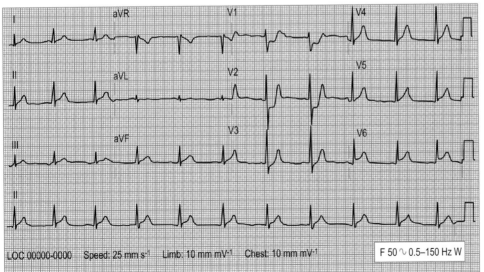

Fig. 8.33 • Acute, posterior myocardial infarction demonstrating the 'mirror-image' changes of infarction in leads V1 and V2, namely the development of tall R waves, ST segment depression and upright T waves. There is also some ST segment elevation on the inferolateral leads.

'Q wave' or 'non-Q wave'. Simplistically, the Q wave is said to indicate myocardial necrosis, ST segment elevation indicates myocardial injury and T wave inversion represents ischaemia. In prehospital care it is the presence of ST segment elevation that is of most importance with respect to decisions regarding the administration of thrombolytic drugs.

The presence of bundle branch block, particularly left-bundle branch block, interferes with the ECG diagnosis of

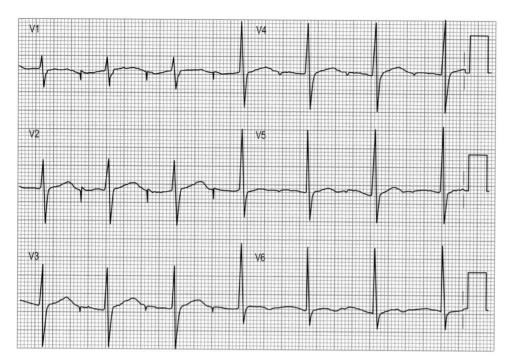

Fig. 8.34 • Atrial pacing. A small pacing spike is followed immediately by atrial depolarization. There is also prolongation of the PR interval.

myocardial infarction, and a high index of suspicion should be exercised when dealing with such patients presenting with cardiac-like chest pain. A variety of arrhythmias are also seen in the early stages of myocardial infarction and have been described above.

The classic infarct pattern gives information as to the location of the myocardial infarction, as follows:

- anteroseptal: V1–V4
- anterolateral: V4–V6, leads I and aVL
- extensive anterior: V1–V6, leads I (II) and aVL
- inferior: leads II, III and aVF
- inferolateral: leads II, III, aVF, V5 and V6 (I and aVL)
- right ventricular: V3R and V4R
- posterior: V8 and V9 with 'mirror image change' in V1–V3.

In posterior infarctions the anteroseptal leads show the development of ST segment depression with tall T waves and a tall R wave. This results in an appearance that is the mirror image of the classic infarct pattern.

Cardiac pacemakers

Because increasing numbers of patients are fitted with permanent artificial cardiac pacemakers, a short introduction to the ECG appearances encountered while managing such patients is useful. The indications for pacing are extensive. In the UK few pacemakers are inserted for (overdrive) tachycardia control and most are of use in the management of symptomatic bradycardia, such as sick sinus syndrome or AV block.

The pacemaker generator box is implanted subcutaneously, usually over the pectoral muscle, although occasionally in the abdominal wall, and connected to the heart by pacing leads that are inserted inside one or both of the right-heart chambers via the venous system. The leads have a dual role: to sense cardiac electrical activity and to stimulate ('pace') the myocardium. Depending upon the placement of the leads and the properties of the generator, a variety of pacing functions are possible.

For example, if a single lead is inserted into the right atrium, the generator can sense atrial activity and, when appropriate, pace the atria. This may be of benefit in cases of sinus node disease (in the presence of normal AV nodal function). The paced atrial beat will appear as an abnormal P wave immediately after a small pacing spike, and the resulting QRS complex will be the same as during sinus rhythm (Fig. 8.34). A single lead in the right ventricle may sense or stimulate ventricular activity. The paced QRS complex will follow a pacing spike and be broad (Fig. 8.35). Some ventricular leads also have sensors along their length that allow for atrial sensing (without atrial pacing), leading to the advantage of ventricular pacing that tracks atrial activity. In a patient with a third-degree AV block, not only is AV synchrony re-established but increases in sinus rate during exercise lead to increases in paced ventricular rate. If both an atrial and a ventricular lead are used the above advantage is achieved, as well as the potential to pace the atria in cases of combined SA and AV nodal disease.

Modern pacemakers are programmed to pace as required and are capable of switching from one mode of pacing to another and of increasing the pacing rate (rate responsiveness)

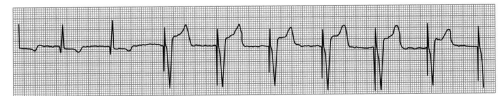

Fig. 8.35 • Ventricular pacing. The atrial rhythm is atrial fibrillation. After two beats conducted via the bundles of His there is a pause that is sensed by the pacemaker and pacing ensues. Each pacing spike is followed by a broad QRS complex.

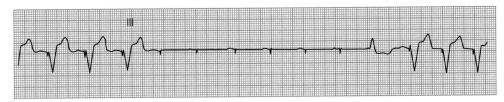

Fig. 8.36 • Failure to capture. Six pacing spikes fail to cause ventricular activation and only atrial activity is apparent. A ventricular escape beat occurs prior to satisfactory capture.

as the patient begins to exercise. This may lead to confusion in the unwary, who may expect to see pacing activity on the ECG at all times and who may interpret the normal variation between sinus rhythm, atrial pacing and ventricular pacing as a type of pacemaker malfunction.

In general, the important pacemaker malfunctions to be aware of in prehospital care are:

- *Failure to sense*: pacing spikes appear too soon after a normal depolarization
- *Failure of capture*: pacing spikes are seen but fail to cause myocardial depolarization (Fig. 8.36)
- *Pacemaker-mediated tachycardia*: the paced ventricular activity is transmitted retrogradely through the AV node, where it is sensed by the atrial wire, leading to further ventricular pacing at increasing rates.

Failure to sense may lead to dangerous 'R-on-T' ectopics and the initiation of VT or VF. Failure of capture, which is usually intermittent, allows the underlying cardiac rhythm, or lack of it, to be manifest.

Further reading

Bennett DH 2002 Cardiac arrhythmias: practical notes on interpretation and treatment, 6th edn. Arnold, London

Fogoros RN 1991 Electrophysiologic diagnosis. Blackwell Scientific, Boston, MA

Hampton JR 2003 The ECG made easy, 6th edn. Churchill Livingstone, Edinburgh

Levy S 1994 Differentiating SVT from VT – a personal viewpoint. European Heart Journal 15(Suppl A): 31–38

Rowlands DJ 1993 Electrocardiography handbook. Kluwer, Dordrecht

Schamroth L, Schamroth C 1990 An introduction to electrocardiography, 7th edn. Blackwell Scientific, Oxford

Wellens HJJ 1996 The value of the ECG in the diagnosis of supraventricular tachycardias. European Heart Journal 17(Suppl C): 10–20

Cardiac emergencies

Introduction   104

Acute myocardial infarction and unstable angina
pectoris   105

The electrocardiogram (ECG)   106

Treatment   107

Anti-arrhythmics   108

Bradycardia and heart block   108

Prehospital thrombolysis   109

Percutaneous coronary intervention   109

Acute pulmonary oedema   110

Arrhythmias   111

Supraventricular tachycardia   112

Atrial fibrillation and atrial flutter   113

Ventricular tachycardia   114

References   114

Introduction

Cardiac diseases commonly present with chest pain, syncope, breathlessness or palpitations, although these symptoms are not specific and the differential diagnosis is extensive. The differential diagnosis of chest pain is given in Table 9.1. Ambulance paramedics are more likely to be called upon to provide advanced skills for patients with such symptoms than for any other group (Weston & McCabe 1992). In a series of almost 7000 people attended to by a Canadian paramedic ambulance service, only 851 required 'special procedures' but 74.1% of these had suspected cardiac disease (Vertesi 1978).

Like many other areas of emergency care, the greatest potential benefit occurs soon after the onset of symptoms. Effective prehospital management offers opportunities for more significant reductions in the burden of cardiac disease than, for example, alterations in the type, or delivery method, of thrombolytic agent to relatively low-risk patients within hospital (GUSTO Investigators 1993).

Unfortunately the beneficial impact of prehospital care upon cardiac mortality and morbidity is diluted by the problems of uncertain diagnosis and lack of, or delayed access to, adequate emergency care. For example, most cardiac fatalities occur outside hospital, the call for emergency aid is usually made after the fatal collapse, and when it is made before the collapse it is most frequently the GP rather than a paramedic ambulance crew who is called (Leslie et al 1996). Compared with ambulance paramedics, GPs should have a wider knowledge base, access to a greater variety of drugs and important insight into the past medical history of the patient. However, while they can provide effective resuscitation when properly equipped (Colquhoun & Julian 1992), it is still unusual for GPs to take a defibrillator with them when attending patients with chest pain. Conversely, while the ambulance service provides a more consistent advanced life support capability and rapid transport to hospital, ambulances only attend about half of all coronary heart disease deaths in the community

Table 9.1 Common causes of chest pain

Cardiac

- Angina pectoris:
  - Coronary atheroma
  - Aortic stenosis/regurgitation
  - Hypertrophic cardiomyopathy
- Myocardial infarction
- Pericarditis

Dissection of the aorta

Pulmonary

- Pneumothorax
- Pneumonia
- Pleurisy
- Pulmonary embolism
- Pulmonary malignancy

Alimentary

- Oesophageal
  - Reflux oesophagitis
  - Oesophageal spasm
- 'Referred' pain cholecystitis
  - Peptic ulcer disease
  - Pancreatitis

Musculoskeletal

- Arthritis with muscle spasm
- Thoracic intravertebral disc disease
- Costochondritis
- Rib fracture

Neurological

- Herpes zoster

(Rowley et al 1990). The potential of prehospital care of patients with heart disease will not be realized until there is better patient education and closer collaboration between GPs, ambulance services and admitting hospitals.

Acute myocardial infarction and unstable angina pectoris

Unstable angina is a syndrome of chest pain due to myocardial ischaemia occurring in a crescendo pattern, at rest or on minimal exertion. Myocardial infarction is heart muscle cell death due to prolonged and complete ischaemia. The two conditions are discussed together because usually they share the same pathophysiology, the same symptoms and, to a large degree, the same early management. Furthermore, the hallmark of acute myocardial infarction – death of heart muscle – has been shown, by sensitive muscle enzyme estimations, to occur to a lesser amount in some cases of unstable angina (Conti 1996). In the very early stages of these two acute coronary events it is often impossible to determine which is occurring and many patients pass through a phase of unstable angina prior to infarction (Falk 1985).

PATHOPHYSIOLOGY

Most cases are accompanied by disruption of the coronary artery endothelium, with resultant thrombosis at the site of pre-existing atheroma (Davies & Thomas 1985). This fissuring of an atheromatous plaque is related to the nature of the plaque constituents and possibly other factors such as endothelial function, vasomotor tone, changes in coronary blood pressure, blood flow dynamics and macrophage activity (Fuster et al 1992).

The thrombus may be restricted to the intima, where it may lead to an abrupt change in plaque configuration and the local release of vasoconstricting factors from aggregating platelets (reversible coronary artery spasm is seen in some patients undergoing coronary angiography at the time of acute myocardial infarction (Oliva & Breckinridge 1977)) or it may protrude into the lumen of the artery, restricting or totally obstructing blood flow distally and allowing platelet aggregates to embolize downstream. The progression from ischaemia to myocardial cell death is dependent upon the abruptness, completeness and duration of coronary occlusion, the presence of any collateral circulation (Habib et al 1991), the protective effect of ischaemic preconditioning (Murry et al 1986) and the oxygen demands of the heart during the acute event. The management of both unstable angina and myocardial infarction is, to a large degree, based upon an understanding of these processes.

Because of the complex interaction between all these factors, there is a large variation in the speed of progression of myocardial infarction and the natural history of coronary thrombosis in humans does not always follow that predicted from animal models of coronary occlusion (Tiefenbrunn & Sobel 1992).

Evidence of an imbalance of the autonomic nervous system is very common in patients who are seen within 30 min of the onset of myocardial infarction. Almost half manifest transient excessive parasympathetic activity – bradycardia, atrioventricular block or hypotension (Webb et al 1972). Sympathetic nervous activity can reduce the threshold for malignant ventricular arrhythmias, such as ventricular fibrillation, whereas parasympathetic activity appears to exert a protective effect (Schwartz et al 1992). In general, these neurally-mediated complications of acute myocardial infarction are seen early in the course of the condition (Table 9.2) and are thus more likely to be witnessed and managed in the prehospital phase than on the cardiac care unit.

Table 9.2 Frequency of arrhythmias within 4 h of myocardial infarction (all figures are percentages)

Arrhythmia	% within		
	0–1 h	1–2 h	2–4 h
Ventricular ectopics	58	27	8
Ventricular fibrillation	9.5	4.5	1.5
Ventricular tachycardia	2	1.5	0.5
Supraventricular tachycardia	1.5	2.5	2
Bradycardia	28	3.5	2.5
Heart block	6	0	0.5

After Pantridge et al 1974

AIMS OF MANAGEMENT

The aims of prehospital management are to rapidly provide resuscitation skills and equipment, adequate analgesia, accurate diagnosis, recognition and treatment of complications and rapid transfer to hospital. Where appropriate, management may include the administration of thrombolytic agents before or during transfer (Weston et al 1994). There is no one prehospital system that is best suited for delivering such care.

DIAGNOSIS

A definite diagnosis of acute myocardial infarction is often delayed, even in hospital (Lee et al 1987) and is based upon a typical history, appropriate abnormalities or serial changes on electrocardiography, and evidence of myocardial damage from measurements of cardiac enzymes. Health-care professionals involved with the prehospital management of patients with suspected myocardial infarction or unstable angina do not have the opportunity to record more than one 12-lead electrocardiogram (ECG), nor are they assisted by knowledge of cardiac enzyme levels (which may be normal in the early phase of infarction in any case). Moreover, diagnostic algorithms derived from quite simple models based upon clinical and electrocardiographic variables that accurately predict the diagnosis of myocardial infarction within hospital (Tierney et al 1985, Kennedy et al 1996) are unsuitable in the prehospital setting (Grijseels et al 1995). Thus, a working diagnosis of myocardial infarction is realistically often the best that can be achieved.

While recognizing the great variation in the presentation of myocardial infarction, this working diagnosis is usually based upon a history of severe retrosternal chest pain, poorly responsive to nitroglycerine, lasting for at least 30 min or until analgesia is provided, often described as 'heaviness' or 'tightness', frequently with radiation to the neck, jaw or arms. In some patients there is also a history of hours or days of unstable or rapidly worsening stable angina. In those with a prior diagnosis of angina, the discomfort of a myocardial infarction is often significantly worse than their usual symptoms.

There is no pathognomonic physical sign and in the prehospital setting the physical examination should take second place to attaching a cardiac monitor/defibrillator. Examination should be aimed at rapidly assessing the need for resuscitation, observing associated sweating (diaphoresis) and vomiting and obtaining measurements of blood pressure, pulse rate and rhythm and evidence of left-ventricular failure (see below). Auscultation of the heart may occasionally be useful. While the detection of a fourth heart sound may rightly be viewed as too esoteric by providers of prehospital care, the presence of a pericardial rub or an aortic diastolic murmur may point towards a diagnosis of pericarditis or aortic root dissection respectively. If prehospital thrombolytic treatment is being considered such an examination is mandatory.

The electrocardiogram (ECG)

A series of ECGs recorded following admission to the cardiac care unit is of great value in identifying patients with myocardial infarction. In one study, 83% of all patients with definite infarction were identified after serial tracings were recorded, whereas only 49% of initial tracings had been considered diagnostic (McGuinness et al 1976). More importantly, the likelihood that a patient admitted to a cardiac care unit will have confirmation of myocardial infarction is virtually 100% if there is significant ST segment elevation on the first tracing, compared with 68.5% if there is another abnormality such as T wave inversion, ST depression or bundle branch block, and 39.7% if the initial ECG is normal (Yusuf et al 1984). Given that patients with myocardial infarction are concentrated within cardiac care units, the prevalence of myocardial infarction among patients with chest pain in emergency departments or in the community will, by comparison, be far lower. The predictive accuracy of any test is determined not just by its sensitivity and specificity but also by the pretest probability (prevalence) of the condition being sought. Not surprisingly, therefore, the interpretation of an ECG recorded in the prehospital phase is less clear-cut, particularly as patients generally will be at an earlier stage in the acute coronary event when the patterns of changes are less well defined.

A definite diagnosis of acute myocardial infarction is difficult to make in the prehospital phase. A strong clinical suspicion, based upon a history and physical examination alone, may be accurate in under half of cases attended (Herlitz et al 1995), the availability of an ECG improves this accuracy to between 60 and 80% (GREAT Group 1992, Hannaford et al 1995) and the use of strict ECG criteria and a screening checklist allows an accuracy of up to 98% (Weaver et al 1990, 1993). A normal ECG makes the final diagnosis of myocardial infarction very unlikely. The recording of an abnormal ECG outside hospital has been shown to accelerate subsequent in-hospital management (Weaver et al 1993).

Treatment

Ideally, those attending cardiovascular emergencies should be equipped with a cardiac monitor, a defibrillator, an oxygen delivery system and facilities for gaining venous access, administering drugs and performing advanced life support (including airway management) as described in Chapter 5. If the patient is conscious the first priority is to provide reassurance and encourage rest, while giving oxygen, obtaining a brief history, attaching monitoring devices and cannulating a large peripheral vein in readiness for any intervention.

MONITORING

Cardiovascular monitoring outside hospital is nearly always non-invasive. It should, however, when combined with simple observation and physical examination, be perfectly adequate to achieve the aims of management, although it may be suboptimal in a moving vehicle or aircraft en route to hospital (Hunt et al 1994). Continuous single-lead ECG monitoring via self-adhesive chest electrodes will allow detection of arrhythmias, conduction abnormalities and ST segment changes (albeit to a limited degree). Automated blood pressure monitors via programmed inflation of a sphygmomanometric cuff are also useful, freeing the attending physician or paramedic to perform other tasks. In the absence of profound hypotension, pulse oximetry provides an assessment of arterial blood oxygen saturation (Yelderman & New 1983).

OXYGEN

Even patients with uncomplicated infarction have been reported to show mismatching of pulmonary ventilation and perfusion (Fillmore et al 1970). More severe ischaemic left ventricular dysfunction may lead to signs and symptoms of heart failure, in which case oxygen therapy becomes mandatory. However, there is experimental evidence that oxygen supplementation reduces ischaemia (Madias & Hood 1976) and infarct size (Maroko et al 1975), and so all patients should be offered oxygen therapy.

NITRATES

Glyceryl trinitrate should be given by sublingual spray (e.g. 400 µg) or tablet (e.g. 300 µg by sublingual tablet, 3 mg by buccal tablet) to patients experiencing cardiac pain, unless the patient has already taken large doses or if there is hypotension (e.g. systolic blood pressure of less than 90 mmHg). In some patients with unstable angina the administration of nitrates may give temporary relief of symptoms. The mechanism of action is to reduce ischaemia by dilatation of veins, arterioles and coronary arteries and collaterals, and there is even evidence that nitrates interfere with platelet aggregation (Loscalzo 1992), and so may be useful in acute infarction. However, high doses, particularly in combination with other potentially hypotensive agents, may cause hypotension leading to reduced coronary perfusion and a reflex tachycardia (Jugdutt 1983). However, such unwanted effects are rare and nitroglycerine is one of the most commonly administered drugs in emergency prehospital care (Abarbanell 1994).

ANALGESIA AND ANTI-EMETICS

The rapid relief of cardiac pain is a humane objective and may also lead to a reduction of sympathetic nervous overactivity, which should reduce cardiac workload during the acute event and the likelihood of ventricular arrhythmias. Parenterally administered drugs should be given intravenously rather than intramuscularly in order to achieve more predictable blood levels and more rapid effect. The drugs of choice for analgesia in suspected acute myocardial infarction remain the opiates diamorphine (usually up to 5 mg) and morphine sulphate (usually up to 10 mg), which should be titrated against the degree of residual pain by using small repeated doses of $1–2\,mg\,min^{-1}$. These opiates also have potentially beneficial haemodynamic effects (Zelis et al 1974, Lee et al 1976), which may be particularly useful in those patients with pulmonary oedema. However, in patients with decreased blood volume due to vomiting or profuse sweating, the combination of morphine and other vasodilators such as nitrates may lead to severe postural hypotension. Opiates are also likely to aggravate vomiting and may depress the ventilatory response to hypoxia and hypercapnia. This latter problem is unusual and may be reversed by the intravenous administration of naloxone (0.8–2.0 mg at intervals of 3 min). A suitable anti-emetic is metoclopramide (10–20 mg).

While ambulance paramedics have been shown to administer morphine safely with little risk of respiratory depression (Bruns et al 1992), ambulance services in the UK have historically been prevented from giving opiates. Alternative therapies include nitrous oxide with oxygen via a facemask (Baskett & Withnell 1970, Thompson & Lown 1976), which has been shown to reduce myocardial oxygen demand

(Wynne et al 1980), or the opioid nalbuphine (10–20 mg intravenously at a rate of about 4 mg min^{-1}) (Troughton & Adgey 1989, Chambers & Guly 1994). Occasionally, especially in patients with hypertension and tachycardia, intravenous beta-blockers such as atenolol (Ramsdale et al 1982), propranolol (Gold et al 1976) and metoprolol (Herlitz et al 1984) have been shown to reduce ischaemic chest pain. Their use is not common practice because of concerns about effects on heart rate and atrioventricular (AV) conduction, yet there is good evidence that intravenous beta-blockade reduces infarct size and mortality if given soon after the onset of symptoms (MIAMI Trial Research Group 1985, ISIS-1 Collaborative Group 1986). Certainly the use of such drugs should not be restricted to hospitals.

ASPIRIN

The precise mechanism by which aspirin exerts its beneficial effects upon mortality after acute myocardial infarction (ISIS-2 Collaborative Group 1988) is unknown; it does not appear to be via improved early coronary patency and is more likely to result from reduced reocclusion and recurrent ischaemia (Roux et al 1992, Norris et al 1993). Even though it is commonly given outside hospital there does not appear to be an important time relationship between aspirin administration and benefit, and limited studies of early aspirin treatment by ambulance paramedics show no significant improvement over delayed in-hospital treatment (Greenbaum et al 1995). Nonetheless, there is evidence of a synergistic effect between aspirin and streptokinase when both drugs are given early (Babinski & Naylor 1991) and it is reasonable for all patients with suspected myocardial infarction to be given 150–300 mg of aspirin during transfer to hospital, unless there is a history of allergy to salicylates. This dose can be chewed in order to increase the rate of absorption and may be delayed in those patients who are vomiting.

Anti-arrhythmics

Arrhythmias classically related to acute myocardial infarction include ventricular ectopics, ventricular tachycardia and fibrillation, atrial fibrillation and idioventricular rhythms following myocardial reperfusion. In 294 patients seen within the first 4 h of myocardial infarction, 46 (15.5%) had ventricular fibrillation; 28 of these within the first hour (Pantridge et al 1974). The treatment of ventricular fibrillation is outlined in Chapter 5 and the management of ventricular tachycardia is described later in this chapter. The frequency of these arrhythmias may be reduced by administration of beta-blockers (ISIS-1 Collaborative Group 1986). Ventricular ectopics and so-called warning arrhythmias,

such as R-on-T ectopics, are common (Campbell et al 1981) but they are not sufficiently powerful predictors of lethal arrhythmias to warrant specific treatment.

Ventricular ectopics (including R-on-T ectopics) do not require specific treatment.

The management of atrial fibrillation during the prehospital phase of acute myocardial infarction is complicated. In those who tolerate the arrhythmia well it is often self-terminating and of little haemodynamic significance, and therefore does not require treatment, while in those who are unwell, atrial fibrillation may be a marker of decompensated heart failure and will be unlikely to convert to sinus rhythm until the heart failure is treated.

Bradycardia and heart block

Julian et al (1964) reported first-, second- and third-degree AV block in 13%, 10% and 8% respectively of patients in the early phase of acute myocardial infarction. In another study, sinus bradycardia occurred in 82 (34%) and second-degree or complete heart block in 16 (6.5%) of 240 patients within 4 h of infarction; most commonly seen with infero-posterior territory infarction (Pantridge et al 1974). This may be of greater importance in the prehospital phase than within hospital, as these slow rates may allow the breakthrough of ventricular ectopics and the development of ventricular fibrillation. Furthermore, when associated with hypotension there may be a significant reduction in coronary perfusion with worsening ischaemia. Bradycardia may be caused by parasympathetic overactivity, ischaemia or infarction of conducting tissues and treatment with opiates and, paradoxically, nitrates.

The need to treat bradycardia is related to the degree of hypotension and the clinical status of the patient. If already administered, sublingual or buccal nitrate tablets should be removed. Lidocaine should *not* be given for ventricular arrhythmias that appear to complicate bradycardia. Intravenous atropine (0.5 mg repeated every few minutes to a dose of 3.0 mg) may reverse both bradycardia and hypotension, although it has been reported to cause ventricular fibrillation in such patients (Massumi et al 1972). Cardiac pacing is the definitive treatment. Transvenous pacing is not an option in the prehospital environment but external transthoracic pacing may be used if the equipment is available. If this is not available an adrenaline (epinephrine) infusion in the range of 2–10 µg min^{-1} may be used and titrated to response as a temporizing measure (European Resuscitation Council 2001).

Finally, patients experiencing heart block in hospital are more likely to exhibit persistent coronary artery occlusion soon after thrombolytic therapy (Berger et al 1992), and thrombolytic treatment strategies resulting in more rapid reperfusion are associated with a lesser frequency of second- and third-degree block (GUSTO Investigators 1993). Early (prehospital) thrombolytic treatment could theoretically reduce the incidence of bradycardia due to heart block and should not be avoided because of the presence of this abnormality.

Prehospital thrombolysis

The benefit of thrombolytic treatment diminishes as a function of the time that has elapsed after the onset of symptoms. The Fibrinolytic Therapy Trialists' Group (1994) described a linear relationship between lives saved and delay to treatment; 35 lives per 1000 when treated within 1 h compared with 16 per 1000 if treatment was received 7–12 h after onset, a loss of benefit of 1.6 lives per 1000 patients treated for each hour's delay. By including smaller trials in an analysis, others have argued against such a linear relationship, describing even greater benefits following very early treatment (Boersma et al 1996).

Prehospital thrombolysis saves lives, but may not have as good an outcome as primary PCI.

A Task Force on the Management of Acute Myocardial Infarction of the European Society of Cardiology (1996) and the British Heart Foundation Working Group (Weston et al 1994) sanctioned the use of thrombolytic agents outside hospital, while the American College of Emergency Physicians (1994) discouraged their use and consider such treatment as investigational. All bodies recognize the importance of early administration of thrombolytic therapy. Studies of prehospital thrombolysis have clearly demonstrated its feasibility and the time savings inherent in this approach (Weston & Fox 1991, Vincent 1994). However, the difference of opinion is related to concerns regarding the accuracy of diagnosis and specificity of ECG changes outside hospital (as described above), together with the safety of use of these agents by practitioners who may not regularly attend suitable patients. Doctors onboard MCCUs (European Myocardial Infarction Project Group 1993), ambulance paramedics (Weaver et al 1993) and general practitioners (GREAT Group 1992) have all been subjected to randomized controlled trials. An overview of these trials suggests that prehospital thrombolytic treatment does more good than harm, although ventricular fibrillation occurs more commonly soon after thrombolytic treatment is given; regardless of where it is given (European

Table 9.3 Dosages of commonly prescribed thrombolytic agents

Agent	Dose	Heparin
Streptokinase*	1.5 million units in 100 ml 5% dextrose or 0.9% saline over 30–60 min	None required
Anistreplase*	30 units by bolus injection over 3–5 min	
Alteplase (t-PA)	15 mg intravenous bolus then 0.75 mg kg^{-1} over 30 min then 0.5 mg kg^{-1} over 60 min (not exceeding 100 mg total)	Intravenous infusion for 48 h
Urokinase	2 million units by intravenous bolus or 1.5 million units as bolus and 1.5 million units over 1 h	Intravenous infusion for 48 h

*Streptokinase and anistreplase are likely to prove ineffective if either agent has been administered more than 5 days previously

Myocardial Infarction Project Group 1993). The beneficial effects appear to be long-lasting (Rawles 1994b). Diagnosis has been augmented by the use of on-board computers capable of ECG interpretation (Bouten et al 1992), by cellular telephonic relay of 12-lead ECGs to a base hospital and by specific educational initiatives (Rawles 1994a).

GPs, in particular, appear uninterested in providing thrombolytic treatment outside hospital (Round & Marshall 1994), although this may be because they are discouraged from doing so by hospital colleagues (Rawles 1994a). If they, or others, are to deliver this therapy (for dosages see Table 9.3), they should have the ability to record and interpret a 12-lead ECG, provide rapid defibrillation, be aware of the indications and contraindications of the agent they choose to use (Table 9.4) and demonstrate that prehospital therapy in their area leads to significant time savings when compared to in-hospital treatment.

Percutaneous coronary intervention

Percutaneous coronary intervention (PCI) has replaced thrombolysis as the gold standard by which to revascularize affected vessels in STEMI. Over and above the goal of salvaging viable myocardium, its main benefit over thrombolysis is stroke prevention. The main question to be considered in the prehospital context is whether the patient is to be transported to a hospital offering such services. If they are, proceeding directly to PCI will avoid the significant stroke risk seen in thrombolysis.

Table 9.4 Use of thrombolytic agents in acute myocardial infarction

- Indications
  - Typical chest pain and associated symptoms for a duration of up to 12 h
  - ST segment elevation >1 mm in two contiguous ECG leads
  - Left bundle branch block
- Absolute contraindications
  - Active bleeding
  - Gastrointestinal bleeding within the last month
  - Major trauma, surgery, head injury within the last 3 weeks
  - Suspected dissecting aortic aneurysm
  - Previous stroke known to be haemorrhagic
- Relative contraindications
  - Transient ischaemic attack or stroke within the last 6 months
  - Warfarin therapy
  - Pregnancy
  - Traumatic resuscitation
  - Hypertension with systolic blood pressure >180 mmHg
  - Recent laser retinal treatment

Source: adapted from Antman 1994 and Task Force on the Management of Acute Myocardial Infarction of the European Society of Cardiology 1996

Acute pulmonary oedema

Pulmonary oedema is a widespread exudation or transudation of fluid into the alveolar walls and spaces from the pulmonary capillaries, due to an imbalance between hydrostatic and osmotic pressures across, or damage to, the capillary membrane. While in this chapter only cardiac causes will be discussed, it should be remembered that pulmonary oedema may be observed in a wide variety of conditions, including fluid overload following blood transfusion, inhalation of toxic agents, acute mountain sickness and adult respiratory distress syndrome.

PATHOPHYSIOLOGY

The normal left-atrial pressure is between 5 and 10 mmHg. As the pulmonary veins and capillaries are in continuity with the left atrium, any increase in left-atrial pressure is associated with a similar rise in pulmonary capillary hydrostatic pressure. At pressures of 25–30 mmHg or greater, the plasma oncotic pressure is overcome and oedema may develop. The likelihood that this will occur is related to the efficiency of pulmonary lymphatic drainage and also to the rate of rise of left atrial pressure. If this pressure rises quickly, for instance in cases of acute myocardial infarction or rupture of a mitral valve chorda, life-threatening pulmonary oedema is seen rapidly. Conversely, if the rate of rise is slow, as in long-standing mitral stenosis, structural changes take place in the alveolar wall that have the effect of protecting from oedema while

leading to fibrosis and reduced lung compliance. Thus, there is no simple relationship between the absolute level of left-atrial pressure and the presence of interstitial or alveolar oedema (nor for that matter the presence of breathlessness on exertion – Lipkin et al 1986).

While cardiac arrhythmias and conduction defects may occasionally be the primary cause of acute heart failure presenting with pulmonary oedema, the commonest precipitating event is a relatively abrupt reduction in left ventricular stroke volume secondary to myocardial disease, rather than pericardial or valvular disease. Apart from the increased left atrial pressure described above, neuroendocrine activation leads to greater sympathetic nervous activity and activation of the renin–angiotensin system. The net result is venous and arterial vasoconstriction with redistribution of blood to the thorax and brain, increased left-ventricular filling pressure and systemic vascular resistance, and salt and water retention (Braunwald 1981).

DIAGNOSIS

Even in hospital practice the diagnosis of acute pulmonary oedema can be difficult because many of the symptoms and signs are also seen in patients with other acute and chronic respiratory diseases, particularly those with an acute exacerbation of chronic obstructive airways disease. Moreover, there is wide interobserver variation in eliciting some of the physical signs (Ishmail et al 1987, Spiteri et al 1988).

Classically, the patient with acute pulmonary oedema is found sitting upright, appears anxious and sweating and is cold to touch (because of cutaneous vasoconstriction) with rapid respiratory rate and pulse rate. The jugular venous pressure is usually elevated but this is extremely difficult to visualize in the distressed patient because the accessory muscles of respiration are prominent and obscure the jugular pulsations. Likewise, important cardiac auscultatory signs such as a third heart sound or a systolic murmur, neither of which are pathognomonic of heart failure (Folland et al 1992), may be totally inaudible in the presence of noisy respiration. Auscultation of the lungs reveals wheezes and fine crackles (crepitations) from both lung bases upwards. In severe cases the patient may expectorate pink frothy sputum and this may be a prelude to respiratory arrest (Jones et al 1995).

The patient with acute severe LVF is usually cold, clammy and sweaty.

An ECG may be useful in demonstrating arrhythmias, conduction abnormalities or evidence of acute or chronic left ventricular damage.

There is evidence from observational studies that the accurate diagnosis of acute pulmonary oedema is important. Those patients who were correctly identified and treated outside hospital by paramedics received medication earlier and had a lower mortality rate than those who were transported to hospital without prehospital treatment. This was most obvious in the subgroup with the most severe presentation. However, treatment after a misdiagnosis (in cases of asthma, chronic airways disease, pneumonia or bronchitis) was associated with increased mortality (Wuerz & Meador 1992). Ten of 84 patients treated with morphine by paramedics for either ischaemic chest pain or pulmonary oedema were felt to have an alternative diagnosis by admitting doctors and one of these had significant respiratory depression and hypotension (Bruns et al 1992). Drug treatments aimed at reducing left ventricular filling pressure and afterload may have profoundly deleterious effects in patients who require high filling pressures (e.g. in pulmonary embolus or right ventricular infarction) or who have obstructing valve lesions.

TREATMENT

The patient requires rapid assessment, reassurance and treatment, and swift transfer to hospital. Cardiac monitoring should be instituted as soon as possible and any significant arrhythmias treated accordingly (see below). Because many of the drugs used to treat ventricular tachycardia are negatively inotropic, great caution should be exercised if the decision is made to treat such an arrhythmia associated with pulmonary oedema outside hospital. Oxygen saturation may be monitored by oximetry. Venous cannulation should be performed prior to transfer.

The recommended treatment of acute pulmonary oedema includes oxygen, a loop diuretic, a nitrate vasodilator and an opiate. Unless there is a history of chronic airways disease, high concentrations of oxygen should be administered. However, a facemask is often poorly tolerated. Diamorphine (up to 5 mg) or morphine (up to 10 mg) with an anti-emetic (not cyclizine – Tan et al 1988) reduces subjective breathlessness and has potentially advantageous haemodynamic effects (Zelis et al 1974). If the diagnosis is correct, respiratory depression is seldom a problem, although doses may need to be reduced in elderly patients (Chambers & Baggoley 1992).

Northridge (1996) has argued persuasively that the treatment of choice is a nitrate vasodilator rather than furosemide, particularly in cases occurring soon after acute myocardial infarction when the acute heart failure is less likely to be associated with fluid retention. This is because nitrates have more predictable haemodynamic effects, have additional anti-ischaemic effects and are available in a variety of easily administered preparations. At lower doses they cause venodilatation, reducing preload and myocardial oxygen demand, and at higher doses they cause coronary and peripheral arterial vasodilatation reducing afterload. Patients with the most severe degrees of left-ventricular dysfunction derive most benefit from these changes (Flaherty 1992). High doses may result in systemic hypotension and reflex tachycardia, and idiosyncratic bradycardic–hypotensive episodes have been reported following nitrate use outside hospital (Wuerz et al 1994). Conversely, the beneficial effects of furosemide (or bumetanide) are less clearly understood. There appear to be venodilator effects but whether these are independent of (Dickshit et al 1973) or dependent upon (Kiely et al 1973) the diuretic effects is uncertain. In a randomized comparison of intravenous furosemide (1 mg kg^{-1}) with an infusion of isosorbide dinitrate in patients with heart failure after myocardial infarction, left ventricular preload fell by 17%, afterload increased by 7% and cardiac output fell by 12% following furosemide; the corresponding figures for nitrate therapy were 30% reduction for preload and 13% reduction in afterload, without change in cardiac output (Nelson et al 1983).

Therefore, in patients with sudden onset of pulmonary oedema, without a preceding history of congestive heart failure and without evidence of peripheral oedema, nitrates should be given. There are advantages in administering sublingual glyceryl trinitrate tablets (300 µg) or buccal tablets (2–5 mg) because they have a rapid onset of action and their effects disappear quickly if the tablets have to be removed because of unwanted effects. Hypotension (e.g. systolic pressure less than 90 mmHg) precludes the use of nitrates. In patients who are known to have chronic heart failure an episode of acute pulmonary oedema is very likely to be related to worsening fluid retention and these patients should also receive intravenous furosemide (40 mg).

Within hospital the aggressive treatment for patients with combined acute pulmonary oedema and hypotension includes invasive monitoring, intravenous infusions of inotropic agents, mechanical circulatory support and urgent revascularization or corrective surgery. However, this is outside the scope of emergency prehospital care.

Arrhythmias

A description of the various electrocardiographic features of both bradycardias and tachycardias are to be found in the previous chapter. Moreover, the management of bradycardias is described in the section dealing with acute myocardial infarction (above). This section will therefore describe the management of tachycardias (greater than 100 beats min^{-1}) in adult patients presenting outside hospital.

While the ECG is essential for correct diagnosis and treatment, it should be emphasized that the cornerstone of management includes a rapid assessment of the patient that includes a measurement of the vital signs (pulse, blood pressure, respiratory rate), as well as a search for possible (cardiac and non-cardiac) causes of the tachycardia. Venous access should be obtained and cardiac monitoring quickly instituted. Unless there is a life-threatening need for immediate treatment, a (paper) record of the ECG should be obtained and kept for future reference. Most importantly, an *ability* to treat is not synonymous with a *need* to treat. Many arrhythmias, particularly narrow complex tachycardias, are well tolerated and may not require emergency treatment outside hospital. Moreover, the arrhythmia may itself be a manifestation of another underlying problem (e.g. sinus tachycardia may be a sign of haemorrhage, atrial fibrillation may complicate pulmonary embolism). The necessity to treat depends mainly on the haemodynamic status of the patient during the arrhythmia.

The need to treat arrhythmias depends mainly on the haemodynamic status of the patient.

PATHOPHYSIOLOGY

The precise electrical mechanisms responsible for arrhythmogenesis are incompletely described. They include disorders of impulse formation, such as an increased or abnormal cellular automaticity and abnormal pacemaker activity triggered by after-depolarizations, and disorders of impulse propagation such as re-entry and reflection (Naccarelli et al 1995). These electrophysiological changes can occur for a variety of reasons, including abnormal autonomic nervous activity, ischaemia, hypoxia, electrolyte imbalance, drug treatment and myocardial scarring. Thus, tachycardias may occur in spite of a structurally normal heart and in the absence of acute ischaemia, even in patients with coronary heart disease or previous myocardial infarction (Meissner et al 1991, Weston 1993).

ANTIARRHYTHMIC DRUGS

Antiarrhythmic drugs should only be administered in an environment that allows cardiac monitoring, a recording of the resultant rhythm and resuscitation. This latter point is most important because existing arrhythmias may occasionally be exacerbated and new arrhythmias unearthed by the proarrhythmic effects of these drugs.

Such compounds were originally classified according to their effects upon the cardiac action potential by Vaughan Williams (1984) (Table 9.5). All class I drugs block sodium channels and slow the maximum rate of depolarization (with variable effects on action potential duration), the class II drugs block adrenergic receptors, class III drugs prolong the action potential without altering the rate of

Table 9.5 The Vaughan Williams classification of anti-arrhythmic drugs

Class I: IA:	Membrane-stabilizing drugs (sodium channel blocking) Prolongs repolarization (quinidine) Procainamide Disopyramide
IB:	Shortens repolarization (lignocaine) Mexiletine
IC:	Unchanged repolarization (flecainide) Propafenone
Class II:	Anti-sympathetic beta-blockade
Class III:	Prolongation of action potential duration (i.e. prolongs repolarization) Amiodarone Sotalol Bretylium
Class IV:	Calcium channel blockers Verapamil Diltiazem

depolarization and class IV drugs inhibit the inflow of calcium into cells. Certain antiarrhythmic agents (e.g. digoxin, adenosine) do not fit into this classification.

A more user-friendly classification distinguishes antiarrhythmic agents by their site of action (Aronson 1985). An extensive classification – the Sicilian Gambit – has been introduced by a Task Force of the Working Group on Arrhythmias of the European Cardiac Society (1991), based upon the effects of each drug on ion channels, membrane receptors and pumps. While this is a more logical approach, it has not yet achieved wide use outside specialist centres. Those involved in prehospital care of cardiac emergencies would be well advised to avoid complex classifications and concentrate on becoming proficient in the use of a small number of drugs aimed at managing specific tachycardias.

Supraventricular tachycardia

As discussed in Chapter 8, such tachycardias have a variety of causes, although the majority involve the AV node either in a micro re-entrant circuit (AV nodal re-entrant tachycardia) or a macro re-entrant circuit (Wolff–Parkinson–White syndrome). The arrhythmia, unless a compensatory sinus tachycardia, is abrupt in onset with a rate of between 140 and 220 beats min^{-1}. In patients with coexisting coronary heart disease it may lead to angina and hypotension that is reversed by conversion to sinus rhythm (McCabe et al 1992). It is usually very well tolerated but has been identified as a trigger for ventricular fibrillation (Hayes et al 1989).

Once monitoring is established, intravenous access secured and oxygen given if required, vagal manoeuvres, such as the Valsalva manoeuvre or carotid sinus massage, may be attempted (Mehta 1988), although with caution, especially in the elderly (Bastuli & Orlowski 1985). The pharmacological therapy of choice is adenosine (6 then 12 mg followed by another 12 mg dose at 2-min intervals) by rapid intravenous injection. This naturally occurring purine nucleoside has a rapid onset of action, few side-effects, a good safety profile, even when given in the presence of ventricular arrhythmias, and is very effective in terminating paroxysmal supraventricular tachycardia (Garratt et al 1992). In prehospital use by paramedics its efficacy ranged from 68% (Lozano et al 1995) to 90% (Furlong et al 1995) and it was as effective as verapamil (Madsen et al 1995). Short-lasting side-effects such as flushing, wheezing and chest pain are common, and adenosine administration has rarely been associated with the development of atrial fibrillation (Cowell et al 1994), polymorphic ventricular tachycardia and ventricular fibrillation (Ben-Sorek & Wiesel 1993). Adenosine is relatively contraindicated in asthmatic patients and in those taking dipyridamole, which enhances its effects in blocking AV nodal activity and significantly prolongs its action; theophylline antagonizes its effects.

Patients in whom adenosine proves ineffective should be reassessed both in terms of the need for prehospital treatment and in terms of the original diagnosis. The calcium antagonist verapamil (5–10 mg IV) may be useful (Shaw 1986). However, its effects are longer-lasting, they tend to cause hypotension (often reversed by intravenous calcium chloride, e.g. 0.5–1.0 g) and they may interact with beta-blockers. Verapamil is particularly hazardous if given to patients with ventricular tachycardia (Rankin et al 1987). The short-acting beta-blocker esmolol (e.g. 40 mg over 1 min) is also effective in the management of narrow-complex tachycardia, although like other beta-blockers it is negatively inotropic, causes dose-dependent hypotension and should not be given to asthmatic patients (Anderson et al 1986, Turlapaty et al 1987). Another useful alternative is to start amiodarone, 300 mg given over an hour (European Resuscitation Council 2001).

Intravenous magnesium infusions are also sometimes of benefit and are very safe but are not a practical proposition outside hospital. Finally, if drug treatment fails or in cases of haemodynamic instability or critical ischaemia, synchronized DC cardioversion, preceded if time allows by sedation with a benzodiazepine, is required, using increasing energies from 100 J, 200 J then 360 J as required.

Atrial fibrillation and atrial flutter

Re-entry is the likely mechanism for these atrial arrhythmias, with a single organized circuit maintaining flutter and multiple circuits being responsible for fibrillation. The ventricular activity in flutter is frequently regular at a set fraction of the atrial rate (i.e. atrial flutter with 2:1 conduction has a

Table 9.6 Common causes of atrial fibrillation

- Coronary heart disease
- Hypertension
- Acute and chronic alcohol ingestion
- Thyrotoxicosis
- Rheumatic heart disease
- Sick sinus syndrome
- Dilated cardiomyopathy
- Hypertrophic cardiomyopathy
- Acute pulmonary embolism

ventricular rate of approximately 150 beats min^{-1}) while in atrial fibrillation such activity is grossly irregular. When the ventricular rate is particularly rapid it may be difficult to establish the precise rhythm. Under these circumstances carotid sinus massage or intravenous adenosine may briefly interrupt AV nodal conduction, allowing the underlying atrial rhythm to be identified (Gausche et al 1994). Atrial flutter is usually a complication of underlying heart disease. Common causes of atrial fibrillation are listed in Table 9.6.

Consider atrial flutter if the ventricular rate is 150.

Patients with these arrhythmias may be asymptomatic or may have palpitations, shortness of breath, dizziness or chest pain. There may be evidence of the heart disease that underlies the arrhythmia, exacerbated by the speed of the ventricular response and the loss of the atrial component of ventricular filling. This may lead to the sudden development of left ventricular failure and pulmonary oedema.

The prehospital management is predominantly aimed at controlling the rapid ventricular rate and only rarely at converting the rhythm. Digoxin, often the first-line therapy within hospitals, acts too slowly to be of use outside hospital in the acutely compromised patient. In the prehospital setting, patients should be assessed according to their heart rate and the presence of additional signs and symptoms, and placed into either high-, intermediate- or low-risk groups (European Resuscitation Council 2001). If the patient has ongoing chest pain, or critical perfusion with a heart rate above 150 beats min^{-1}, immediate DC cardioversion should be attempted, following intravenous heparinization and appropriate sedation. If none of these high-risk features is present, the safest thing to do is facilitate rapid transfer to definitive medical care, where further assessment can be made. Drug treatments for atrial fibrillation are split into those that control rate (e.g. digoxin, beta-blockers) and those that attempt to chemically cardiovert into sinus rhythm (e.g. amiodarone, flecainide).

Ventricular tachycardia

The mechanisms responsible for this tachycardia include re-entry and enhanced automaticity. Whereas the trigger for the tachycardia involves ischaemia, autonomic nervous activity or electrolyte imbalance, there is usually a fixed 'arrhythmic substrate', for instance a previous myocardial infarction. However, it may occur in individuals with otherwise normal hearts, when it appears to be a benign condition (Gill & Camm 1994). The ECG characteristics of ventricular tachycardia, namely broad-complex tachycardia, monomorphic or polymorphic, sustained or non-sustained, have been described in Chapter 8. The patient may present with palpitations, dizziness, breathlessness or chest pain. Pulseless ventricular tachycardia should be treated as ventricular fibrillation (Ch. 5). The severity of symptoms is a poor guide in differentiating between supraventricular and ventricular tachycardias, although profound collapse is unusual in association with supraventricular tachycardia (Kapoor et al 1983) and a history of prior myocardial disease favours a ventricular focus.

Non-sustained polymorphic ventricular tachycardia is commonly seen during acute myocardial infarction (Campbell et al 1981) and only warrants treatment if there is haemodynamic compromise. Sustained (>30s) monomorphic forms may be seen in up to 5% of survivors of myocardial infarction and predict a poor prognosis (Swerdlow et al 1983); this is the commonest type of ventricular tachycardia requiring treatment outside hospital (Brady et al 1995) and is of significance because it may degenerate into ventricular fibrillation (Leclercq et al 1988).

Where possible, a 12-lead ECG recording should be made before any treatment. Caldwell et al (1985) have advocated that patients be asked to cough forcibly, and if this fails a precordial thump may be delivered. These manoeuvres were responsible for terminating 17 of 68 episodes of sustained ventricular tachycardia.

In cases of haemodynamic compromise, synchronised DC cardioversion at 100J, 200J then 360J should be attempted following appropriate sedation. If there is no haemodynamic compromise, pharmacological cardioversion may be attempted using either intravenous amiodarone 150mg over 10minutes or lignocaine (e.g. 50mg over 2min, repeated every 5min up to a total dose of 200mg, with or without an infusion at a rate of $1-4\,mg\,min^{-1}$). Rapid transfer to hospital should be undertaken.

References

Abarbanell NR 1994 Pre-hospital pharmacotherapeutic interventions: recommendations for medication administration by EMT-A and EMT-I personnel. American Journal of Emergency Medicine 12: 625–630

American College of Emergency Physicians 1994 Pre-hospital use of thrombolytic agents. Annals of Emergency Medicine 23: 1146

Anderson S, Blanski L, Byrd RC et al 1986 Comparison of the efficacy and safety of esmolol, a short-acting beta blocker with placebo in the treatment of supraventricular arrhythmias. American Heart Journal 111: 42–48

Antman EM 1994 General hospital management. In: Julian. DG, Braunwald E (eds) Management of acute myocardial infarction. WB Saunders, London, p 29–70

Aronson JK 1985 Cardiac arrhythmias: theory and practice. British Medical Journal 290: 487–488

Babinski A, Naylor CD 1991 Aspirin and fibrinolysis in acute myocardial infarction: meta-analytic evidence of synergy. Journal of Clinical Epidemiology 44: 1085–1096

Baskett PJF, Withnell A 1970 The use of Entonox in the ambulance service. British Medical Journal 2: 41–42

Bastuli JA, Orlowski JP 1985 Stroke as a complication of carotid sinus massage. Critical Care Medicine 13: 869

Ben-Sorek ES, Wiesel J 1993 Ventricular fibrillation following adenosine administration. A case report. Archives of Internal Medicine 153: 2701–2702

Berger PB, Ruocco NA, Ryan TJ et al 1992 Incidence and prognostic implications of heart block complicating inferior myocardial infarction treated with thrombolytic therapy: results from TIMI II. Journal of the American College of Cardiology 20: 533–540

Boersma E, Maas ACP, Simoons ML 1996 Early thrombolytic treatment in acute myocardial infarction: reappraisal of the Golden Hour. Lancet 348: 771–775

Bouten MJM, Simoons ML, Hartman JAM et al 1992 Pre-hospital thrombolysis with alteplase (rt-PA) in acute myocardial infarction. European Heart Journal 13: 925–931

Brady W, Meldon S, DeBehnke D 1995 Comparison of pre-hospital monomorphic and polymorphic ventricular tachycardia: prevalence, response to therapy, and outcome. Annals of Emergency Medicine 25: 64–70

Braunwald E 1981 Heart failure: pathophysiology and treatment. American Heart Journal 102: 486–490

Bruns BM, Dieckmann R, Shagoury C et al 1992 Safety of pre-hospital therapy with morphine sulfate. American Journal of Emergency Medicine 10: 53–57

Caldwell G, Millar G, Quinn E et al 1985 Simple mechanical methods for cardioversion: defence of the precordial thump and cough version. British Medical Journal 291: 627–630

Campbell RWF, Murray A, Julian DG 1981 Ventricular arrhythmias in first 12 hours of acute myocardial infarction. Natural history study. British Heart Journal 46: 351–357

Chambers JA, Baggoley CJ 1992 Pulmonary oedema: pre-hospital treatment. Caution with morphine dosage. Medical Journal of Australia, 157: 326–328

Chambers JA, Guly HR 1994 Pre-hospital intravenous nalbuphine administered by paramedics. Resuscitation 27: 153–158

Colquhoun MC, Julian DG 1992 Treatable arrhythmias in cardiac arrests seen outside hospital. Lancet 339: 1167

Conti CR 1996 Unstable angina: can early decisions about diagnosis and therapy be made using troponin T values? Clinical Cardiology 19: 445–446

Cowell RPW, Paul VE, Ilsley CDJ 1994 Haemodynamic deterioration after treatment with adenosine. British Heart Journal 71: 569–571

Davies MJ, Thomas AC 1985 Plaque fissuring – the cause of acute myocardial infarction, sudden ischaemic death, and crescendo angina. British Heart Journal 53: 363–373

Dickshit K, Vyden JK, Forrester JS et al 1973 Renal and extrarenal haemodynamic effects of furosemide in congestive heart failure after acute myocardial infarction. New England Journal of Medicine 288: 1087–1090

European Myocardial Infarction Project Group 1993 Pre-hospital thrombolytic therapy in patients with suspected acute myocardial infarction. New England Journal of Medicine 329: 383–389

European Resuscitation Council 2001 Guidelines 2000 for adult advanced life support. Resuscitation 48: 211–221

Falk E 1985 Unstable angina with fatal outcome: dynamic coronary thrombosis leading to infarction and/or sudden death. Circulation 71: 699–708

Fibrinolytic Therapy Trialists' Group 1994 Indications for fibrinolytic therapy in suspected acute myocardial infarction: collaborative overview of early mortality and major morbidity results from all randomised trials of more than 1000 patients. Lancet 343: 311–312

Fillmore SJ, Shapiro M, Killip T 1970 Arterial oxygen tension in acute myocardial infarction: serial analysis of clinical state and blood-gas change. American Heart Journal 79: 620–629

Flaherty JT 1992 Role of nitrates in acute myocardial infarction. American Journal of Cardiology 73: 73B–81B

Folland ED, Kriegel BJ, Henderson WG et al 1992 Implications of third heart sounds in patients with valvular heart disease. New England Journal of Medicine 327: 458–462

Furlong R, Gerhardt RT, Farber P et al 1995 Intravenous adenosine as first-line pre-hospital management of narrow-complex tachycardias by EMS personnel without direct physician control. American Journal of Emergency Medicine 13: 383–388

Fuster V, Badimon L, Badimon JJ, Chesebro JH 1992 The pathogenesis of coronary artery disease and acute coronary syndromes. New England Journal of Medicine 326: 242–250

Garratt CJ, Malcolm AD, Camm AJ 1992 Adenosine and cardiac arrhythmias. British Medical Journal 305: 3–4

Gausche M, Persse DE, Sugarman T et al 1994 Adenosine for the pre-hospital treatment of paroxysmal supraventricular tachycardia. Annals of Emergency Medicine 24: 183–189

Gill JS, Camm AJ 1994 Is there a benign form of ventricular tachycardia? In: Jackson G (ed) Difficult concepts in cardiology. Martin Dunitz, London, pp 139–155

Gold HK, Leinbach RC, Maroko PR 1976 Propanolol-induced reduction of signs of ischemic injury during acute myocardial infarction. American Journal of Cardiology 38: 689–695

GREAT Group 1992 Feasibility, safety, and efficacy of domiciliary thrombolysis by general practitioners: Grampian region early anistreplase trial. British Medical Journal 305: 548–553

Greenbaum RA, Sherringham P, Flaherty M, Chan KL 1995 Pre-hospital administration of aspirin to patients with suspected acute myocardial infarction does not improve outcome. British Heart Journal 73: 80

Grijseels EWM, Deckers JW, Hoes AW et al 1995 Pre-hospital triage of patients with suspected myocardial infarction. Evaluation of previously developed algorithms and new proposals. European Heart Journal 16: 325–332

GUSTO Investigators 1993 An international randomized trial comparing four thrombolytic strategies for acute myocardial infarction. New England Journal of Medicine 329: 673–682

Habib GB, Heibig J, Forman SA et al 1991 Influence of coronary collateral vessels on myocardial infarction size in humans. Circulation 83: 739–746

Hannaford P, Vincent R, Ferry S et al 1995 Assessment of the practicality and safety of thrombolysis with anistreplase given by general practitioners. British Journal of General Practice 45: 175–179

Hayes LJ, Lerman BB, DiMarco JP 1989 Non-ventricular arrhythmias as precursors of ventricular fibrillation in patients with out-of-hospital cardiac arrest. American Heart Journal 118: 53–57

Herlitz J, Hjalmarson A, Holmberg S et al 1984 Effect of metoprolol on chest pain in acute myocardial infarction. British Heart Journal 51: 438–444

Herlitz J, Karlson BW, Karlsson T et al 1995 Diagnostic accuracy of physicians for identifying patients with acute myocardial infarction without an electrocardiogram. Experiences from the TEAHAT Study. Cardiology, 86: 25–27

Hunt RC, Carroll RG, Whitley TW et al 1994 Adverse effect of helicopter flight on the ability to palpate carotid pulses. Annals of Emergency Medicine 24: 190–193

Ishmail AA, Wing S, Ferguson J et al 1987 Interobserver agreement by auscultation in the presence of a third heart sound in patients with congestive heart failure. Chest 91: 870–873

ISIS-1 Collaborative Group 1986 Randomised trial of intravenous atenolol among 16,027 cases of suspected acute myocardial infarction. Lancet 2: 57–66

ISIS-2 Collaborative Group 1988 Randomised trial of intravenous streptokinase, oral aspirin, both or neither among 17,187 cases of suspected acute myocardial infarction: ISIS-2. Lancet 2: 349–360

Jones SD, Donnelly PD, Bewley J, Weston CFM 1995 Respiratory arrest outside hospital. Resuscitation 29: 107–111

Jugdutt BI 1983 Myocardial salvage by intravenous nitroglycerin in conscious dogs. Loss of beneficial effect with marked nitroglycerin-induced hypotension. Circulation, 68: 673–684

Julian DG, Valentine PA, Miller GG 1964 Disturbances of rate, rhythm and conduction in acute myocardial infarction. American Journal of Medicine 37: 915–927

Kapoor WN, Karpf M, Weisand S et al 1983 A prospective evaluation and follow up of patients with syncope. New England Journal of Medicine 309: 197–204

Kennedy RL, Burton AM, Fraser HS et al 1996 Early diagnosis of acute myocardial infarction using clinical and electrocardiographic data at presentation: derivation and evaluation of logistic regression models. European Heart Journal 17: 1181–1191

Kiely J, Kelly DT, Taylor DR, Pitt B 1973 The role of furosemide in the treatment of left ventricular dysfunction associated with acute myocardial infarction. Circulation 48: 581–587

Leclercq JF, Maisonblanche P, Cauchemez B, Coumel P 1988 Respective role of sympathetic tone and of cardiac pauses in the genesis of 62 cases of ventricular fibrillation recorded during Holter monitoring. European Heart Journal 9: 1276–1283

Lee G, DeMaria A, Amsterdam E et al 1976 Comparative effects of morphine, meperidine, and pentazocine on cardiocirculatory dynamics in patients with acute myocardial infarction. American Journal of Medicine 60: 949–955

Lee TH, Rouan GW, Weisberg MC et al, the Chest Pain Study Group 1987 Sensitivity of routine clinical criteria for diagnosing myocardial infarction within 24 hours of hospitalization. Annals of Internal Medicine 106: 181–186

Leslie WS, Fitzpatrick B, Morrison CE et al 1996 Out-of-hospital cardiac arrest due to coronary heart disease: a comparison of survival before and after the introduction of defibrillators in ambulances. Heart 75: 195–199

Lipkin DP, Canepa-Anson R, Stephens MR, Poole-Wilson PA 1986 Factors determining symptoms in heart failure: comparison of fast and slow exercise tests. British Heart Journal 55: 439–445

Loscalzo J 1992 Antiplatelet and antithrombotic effects of organic nitrates. American Journal of Cardiology 70: 18B–22B

Lozano M, McIntosh BA, Giordano LM 1995 Effect of adenosine on the management of supraventricular tachycardia by urban paramedics. Annals of Emergency Medicine 26: 691–696

McCabe JL, Adhar GC, Mengazzi JJ, Paris PM 1992 Intravenous adenosine in the pre-hospital treatment of supraventricular tachycardia. Annals of Emergency Medicine 21: 358–361

McGuinness JB, Begg TB, Semple T 1976 First electrocardiogram in recent myocardial infarction. British Medical Journal 2: 449–451

Madias JE, Hood WB 1976 Reduction of precordial ST segment elevation in patients with anterior myocardial infarction by oxygen breathing. Circulation 53(Suppl 1): 198–200

Madsen CD, Pointer JE, Lynch TG 1995 A comparison of adenosine and verapamil for the treatment of supraventricular tachycardia in the pre-hospital setting. Annals of Emergency Medicine 25: 649–655

Maroko P, Radvany P, Braunwald E, Hale S 1975 Reduction in infarct size by oxygen inhalation following acute coronary occlusion. Circulation 52: 360

Massumi RA, Mason DT, Amsterdam EA et al 1972 Ventricular fibrillation and tachycardia after intravenous atropine for treatment of bradycardias. New England Journal of Medicine 287: 336–338

Mehta D 1988 Relative efficacy of various physical manoeuvres in the termination of junctional tachycardia. Lancet 1: 1181–1185

Meissner MD, Akhtar M, Lehmann MH 1991 Nonischemic sudden tachyarrhythmic death in atherosclerotic heart disease. Circulation 84: 905–912

MIAMI Trial Research Group 1985 Enzymatic estimation of infarct size. American Journal of Cardiology 56: 27G–29G

Murry CE, Jennings RB, Reimer KA 1986 Pre-conditioning with ischaemia: a delay of lethal cell injury in ischaemic myocardium. Circulation 74: 1124–1136

Naccarelli GV, Willerson JT, Blomqvist CG 1995 Recognition and physiologic treatment of cardiac arrhythmias and conduction disturbances. In: Willerson JT, Cohn JN (eds) Cardiovascular medicine. Churchill Livingstone, New York, pp 1282–1295

Nelson GIC, Silke B, Ahuja RC, Hussain M 1983 Haemodynamic advantages of isosorbide dinitrate over frusemide in acute heart failure following myocardial infarction. Lancet 1: 730–732

Norris RM, White HD, Cross DB et al 1993 Aspirin does not improve early arterial patency after streptokinase treatment for acute myocardial infarction. British Heart Journal 69: 492–495

Northridge D 1996 Frusemide or nitrates for acute heart failure. Lancet 347: 667–668

Oliva PB, Breckinridge JC 1977 Arteriographic evidence of coronary arterial spasm in acute myocardial infarction. Circulation 56: 366–374

Pantridge JF, Webb SW, Adgey AAJ, Geddes JS 1974 The first hour after the onset of acute myocardial infarction. In: Yu PN, Goodwin JF (eds) Progress in cardiology. Lea & Febiger, Philadelphia, PA, pp 173–187

Ramsdale DR, Faragher EB, Bennett DH et al 1982 Ischaemic pain relief in patients with acute myocardial infarction by intravenous atenolol. American Heart Journal 103: 459–467

Rankin AC, Rae AP, Cobbe SM 1987 Misuse of intravenous verapamil in patients with ventricular tachycardia. Lancet 2: 472–474

Rawles J 1994a Attitudes of general practitioners to prehospital thrombolysis. British Medical Journal 309: 379–382

Rawles J, (for the GREAT Group) 1994b Halving of mortality at one year by domiciliary thrombolysis in the Grampian Region Early Anistreplase Trial (GREAT). Journal of the American College of Cardiology 23: 1–5

Round A, Marshall AJ 1994 Survey of general practitioners' pre-hospital management of suspected acute myocardial infarction. British Medical Journal 309: 375–376

Roux S, Christeller S, Ludin E 1992 Effects of aspirin on coronary reocclusion and recurrent ischaemia after thrombolysis: a meta-analysis. Journal of the American College of Cardiology 19: 671–677

Rowley JM, Garner C, Hampton JR 1990 The limited potential of special ambulance services in the management of cardiac arrest. British Heart Journal 64: 309–312

Schwartz PJ, La Rovere MT, Venoli E 1992 Autonomic nervous system and sudden cardiac death. Circulation 85(Suppl I): I-77–I-91

Shaw LC 1986 Pre-hospital use of intravenous verapamil. American Journal of Emergency Medicine 5: 207–210

Spiteri MA, Cook DG, Clarke SW 1988 Reliability of eliciting physical signs in examination of the chest. Lancet 1: 873–875

Swerdlow CD, Winkle RA, Mason JW 1983 Determinants of survival in patients with ventricular tachyarrhythmias. New England Journal of Medicine 308: 1436–1442

Tan LB, Bryant S, Murray RG 1988 Detrimental haemodynamic effects of cyclizine in heart failure. Lancet 1: 560–561

Task Force of the Working Group on Arrhythmias of the European Cardiac Society 1991 The Sicilian Gambit. A new approach to the classification of antiarrhythmic drugs based on their actions on arrhythmogenic mechanisms. Circulation 84: 1831–1851

Task Force on the Management of Acute Myocardial Infarction of the European Society of Cardiology 1996 Acute myocardial infarction: pre-hospital and in-hospital management. European Heart Journal 17: 43–63

Thompson P, Lown B 1976 Nitrous oxide as an analgesic in acute myocardial infarction. Journal of the American Medical Association 235: 924–927

Tiefenbrunn AJ, Sobel BE 1992 Timing of coronary recanalization: paradigms, paradoxes, and pertinence. Circulation 85: 2311–2315

Tierney WM, Roth BJ, Psaty B et al 1985 Predictors of myocardial infarction in emergency room patients. Critical Care Medicine 13: 526–531

Troughton TG, Adgey AAJ 1989 High dose nalbuphine in acute myocardial infarction. International Journal of Cardiology 23: 53–57

Turlapaty P, Laddu A, Murthy S et al 1987 Esmolol: a titratable short acting intravenous beta-blocker for acute critical care settings. American Heart Journal 114: 866–885

Vaughan Williams EM 1984 A classification of antiarrhythmic actions reassessed after a decade of new drugs. Journal of Clinical Pharmacology 24: 129–147

Vertesi L 1978 The paramedic ambulance: a Canadian experience. Canadian Medical Association Journal 119: 25–29

Vincent R 1994 Pre-hospital management. In: Julian DG, Braunwald E (eds) Management of acute myocardial infarction. WB Saunders, London, pp 3–28

Weaver WD, Eisenberg MS, Martin JS et al 1990 Myocardial triage and intervention project – phase I: patient characteristics and feasibility of pre-hospital initiation of thrombolytic therapy. Journal of the American College of Cardiology 15: 925–930

Weaver WD, Cerqueira M, Hallstrom AP et al 1993 Pre-hospital initiated vs. hospital initiated thrombolytic therapy. The Myocardial Infarction and Triage Intervention Trial. Journal of the American Medical Association 270: 1211–1216

Webb SW, Adgey AAJ, Pantridge JF 1972 Autonomic disturbance at onset of myocardial infarction. British Medical Journal 3: 89–92

Weston CFM 1993 The pathophysiology of sudden death in atherosclerotic heart disease. Resuscitation 26: 111–123

Weston CFM, Fox KAA 1991 Pre-hospital thrombolysis: current status and future prospects. Journal of the Royal College of Physicians of London 25: 312–320

Weston CFM, McCabe MJ 1992 Audit of an emergency ambulance service: impact of a paramedic system. Journal of the Royal College of Physicians of London 26: 86–89

Weston CFM, Penny WJ, Julian DG, on behalf of the British Heart Foundation Working Group 1994 Guidelines for the early management of patients with myocardial infarction. British Medical Journal 308: 767–771

Wuerz RC, Meador SA 1992 Effects of pre-hospital medications on mortality and length of stay in congestive heart failure. Annals of Emergency Medicine 21: 669–674

Wuerz R, Swope G, Meador S et al 1994 Safety of pre-hospital nitroglycerin. Annals of Emergency Medicine 23: 31–36

Wynne J, Mann T, Alpert J et al 1980 Hemodynamic effects of nitrous oxide administered during cardiac catheterization. Journal of the American Medical Association 243: 1440–1443

Yelderman M, New W 1983 Evaluation of pulse oxymetry. Anesthesiology 59: 349–352

Yusuf S, Pearson M, Sterry H et al 1984 The entry ECG in the early diagnosis and prognostic stratification of patients with suspected acute myocardial infarction. European Heart Journal 5: 690–696

Zelis R, Mansour EJ, Capone RJ, Mason DT 1974 The cardiovascular effects of morphine: the peripheral capacitance and resistance vessels in human subjects. Journal of Clinical Investigation 54: 1247–1258

Respiratory emergencies

10

Introduction 118

Primary assessment 118

Secondary assessment 120

Re-assessment 121

Documentation 122

Transportation 122

Summary 122

Specific conditions 122

Pulse oximetry 127

Summary 129

References 129

Further reading 129

Introduction

Respiratory emergencies are common. They may arise in patients with previously healthy or diseased lungs, or as a consequence of extrapulmonary pathology. Relevant triggers include infection, exposure to noxious compounds or following trauma. Management of a patient with a respiratory emergency necessitates rapid assessment and may require immediate medical intervention.

The aim of the primary assessment is to identify and treat any immediately life-threatening conditions. This needs to be repeated frequently so that appropriate resuscitative measures can be commenced and their effect monitored.

Primary assessment

In the severely ill patient a rapid examination of vital functions is required and, where appropriate, resuscitation must be instigated before a more detailed secondary assessment can be performed. During the primary assessment life-threatening conditions are treated as soon as they are identified (Table 10.1).

The key components of the primary assessment are:

A Airway
B Breathing
C Circulation
D Disability
E Exposure.

Although each of these components will be considered in the context of acute respiratory emergencies the main focus will be B.

A – AIRWAY

The objective is to provide and maintain a clear and secure airway.

Table 10.1 Immediately life-threatening respiratory emergencies (excluding trauma)

- Airway compromise
- Pulmonary embolus
- Pulmonary oedema – acute
- Asthma – acute severe
- Respiratory failure – acute ± chronic
- Tension pneumothorax

Assessment

The patency of the airway must be assessed. An appropriate response to the simple question 'Are you OK?' indicates that the airway is patent, breathing is occurring and there is adequate cerebral perfusion. In addition, if the patient can speak more than 10 words a significant respiratory problem is unlikely. There is no reason for complacency, however, as an acute airway problem may develop. Thus, the initial airway assessment will also provide baseline information for future comparison.

Resuscitation

If no answer is forthcoming then appropriate manoeuvres to ensure airway patency must be instigated. If available in the prehospital setting, supplemental oxygen should be administered.

Never assume that noisy, difficult breathing is due to 'asthma'. Always exclude stridor, which is a loud, high-pitched whoop due to restricted airflow, reflecting incomplete or impending upper airway obstruction. Stridor is loudest on inspiration as the negative airway pressure causes collapse of the extrathoracic airway. In addition, patients with either severe airway obstruction or bronchospasm can develop paradoxical respiration (where the chest wall moves out on expiration – the opposite of normal).

B – BREATHING

A patent airway does not necessarily ensure adequate ventilation. The latter requires an intact respiratory centre and adequate pulmonary function augmented by the coordinated movement of the diaphragm and chest wall.

Assessment

This should include *inspection* for the presence of cyanosis, respiratory rate and respiratory effort, including accessory muscle use and intercostal recession. *Palpation* of the trachea will detect any tug or deviation. Remember, however, that tracheal deviation does not always indicate mediastinal

shift away from the lesion as seen in a tension pneumothorax. It can also be pulled to the affected side, as exemplified by loss of lung volume with fibrosis. The anterior chest wall should be *percussed* in the upper, middle and lower zones, comparing the difference in percussion note between the left and right hemithoraces. If possible, this procedure must be repeated on the posterior chest wall and also in the axillae to detect areas of hyperresonance, dullness or stony dullness. *Auscultation* over the three zones and the axillae will establish whether breath sounds are either absent, present or masked by added sounds such as wheezes. It is important to remember that a silent chest is not a good prognostic sign as it reflects insufficient air movement to generate a wheeze.

It is important to examine for a pattern of physical signs. Tachypnoea does not always imply a B problem, as exemplified by patients who are bleeding. Acute asthma should not be diagnosed simply on the basis of wheeze. There are many causes of bronchospasm or wheeze (e.g. acute severe left ventricular failure (LVF)) and other clues must be sought to establish the underlying diagnosis.

Tachypnoea may be a sign of shock.

Resuscitation

Once definitive control of the airway has been achieved, supplemental oxygen, if available, should be given to all patients who have respiratory difficulty. Under ideal circumstances, if the patient is not intubated, oxygen should be delivered using a non-rebreathing mask and reservoir to ensure an inspired oxygen concentration of at least 85%. Even patients who have respiratory failure (e.g. due to chronic bronchitis or emphysema) should receive high-flow oxygen; this can subsequently be reduced according to its clinical effect and arterial blood gas results. It is important to remember that hypoxia kills.

If a tension pneumothorax is suspected, it requires urgent decompression with a needle thoracentesis. This is then followed by intravenous access and chest drain insertion.

Life-threatening bronchospasm should initially be treated with nebulized beta-2-agonists. Further clues as to the underlying cause may be gained from examination of the circulation.

C – CIRCULATION

Assessment

Rapid assessment of the patient's haemodynamic status is mandatory. A central pulse, ideally the carotid, should be assessed for rate, rhythm and character. A tachycardia will usually accompany any respiratory emergency. The blood pressure should be taken and peripheral perfusion should be assessed. It is important to remember that hypovolaemia can impair consciousness through reduced cerebral perfusion.

Resuscitation

Ideally, all acutely ill patients should be transferred immediately to the nearest hospital. If this is not possible then intravenous access should be secured and fluid resuscitation should be commenced as necessary.

D – DISABILITY

Assessment

Rapid evaluation of the nervous system is performed towards the end of the primary assessment. This comprises pupillary size and reaction to light, along with assessment of conscious level using the AVPU system.

Resuscitation

Confusion, coma and fits are associated with hypoxia. In most instances, provided that A, B and C are managed correctly, D should not require active intervention.

MONITORING

The effectiveness of resuscitation is measured by an improvement in the patient's clinical status. It is therefore important that this is assessed frequently and the results recorded. The following should be considered as a minimum level of monitoring:

- respiratory effort (by the number of words of a standard sentence)
- respiratory rate
- pulse rate
- conscious level.

If possible, the following should also be monitored:

- oxygen saturation
- blood pressure, ideally monitored automatically
- continuous electrocardiogram (ECG) monitoring.

The most important assessment is the reassessment.

Table 10.2 Potentially life-threatening causes of breathlessness

- Asthma – severe
- Chronic airflow limitation (COPD) exacerbation
- Embolism (pulmonary)
- Drug use – amphetamines, Ecstasy, salicylate overdose
- Oedema (pulmonary)
- Pneumonia
- Effusion (pleural)
- Simple pneumothorax
- Metabolic acidosis – diabetic ketoacidosis
- Pontine haemorrhage

This type of monitoring must continue until more sophisticated equipment is available. If any deterioration is noted the primary assessment must be repeated.

Secondary assessment

The object of the *secondary assessment* is to identify and treat potentially life-threatening conditions.

This occurs only after vital functions have been stabilized and any immediately life-threatening conditions have been treated. Usually, most medical patients will not require any immediate resuscitative measures. Thus, one can take a comprehensive medical history and perform a relevant clinical examination to identify potentially life-threatening conditions (Table 10.2) and then instigate appropriate treatment.

HISTORY

A medical diagnosis or differential diagnosis depends on a good history. Occasionally, for a variety of reasons, the patient is unable to provide this. Therefore information should be sought from relatives, medical notes, general practitioner, friends, or even the police and ambulance service. A well-'PHRASED' history is mandatory and serves as a useful mnemonic to remember the key features (Table 10.3).

EXAMINATION

Overview

This is the overall appearance of the patient from the proverbial 'end of the bed', looking for cyanosis, signs of respiratory distress and abnormal movements, as well as noting

Table 10.3 Key features in the medical history

- P = Problem
- H = History of presenting problem
- R = Relevant medical history
- A = Allergies
- S = Systems review
- E = Essential family and social history
- D = Drugs

Table 10.4 Relevant pulse abnormalities

Pulse	Significance
Tachycardia	Any respiratory compromise
Paradoxical	Severe bronchospasm Cardiac tamponade
Bounding	Carbon dioxide retention Septicaemia

Table 10.5 Relevant jugular venous pulse (JVP) abnormalities

Height	Pulsatile	Effect of inspiration	Significance
Raised	Yes	Falls	Bronchospasm
	Yes	No change	Severe bronchospasm
	Yes	No change	Pulmonary embolus
	Yes	No change	Tension pneumothorax
	Yes	Increases	Cardiac tamponade
	No	No change	Mediastinal obstruction
Low	Yes	Falls	Hypovolaemia*

*This refers to both actual and relative hypovolaemia

Table 10.6 Causes of tachypnoea

- Hypoxia
- Hypovolaemia
- Pneumonia
- Pulmonary emboli
- Bronchospasm (irrespective of cause)
- Brainstem pathology
- Metabolic acidosis (irrespective of cause)
- Medicines/drugs

the patient's response to questions, which may give clues as to underlying pathology.

Hands

The hands should be inspected for stigmata of carbon dioxide retention (flapping tremor, venous dilatation, warm, sweating). The radial pulse can then be palpated for rate, rhythm and character (Table 10.4).

Face/neck

The face should be examined for cyanosis, plethora and venous engorgement. The height, wave form and characteristics of the internal jugular venous pulse (JVP) must be assessed (a detailed list of potential findings is given in Table 10.5). Remember that on inspiration the JVP should fall. Both internal carotid arteries should be palpated in turn to compare and determine the pulse character. The trachea is palpated to assess deviation, tug and the distance between the sternal notch and the inferior border of the thyroid cartilage. This space should admit three fingers but it is markedly reduced when the chest is hyperexpanded in chronic airflow limitation. Lymphadenopathy should be noted.

Chest

Inspection of the chest must determine the respiratory rate and effort, along with intercostal recession and the presence of surgical scars. The causes of tachypnoea are shown in Table 10.6. The precordium should be palpated to determine the site and character of the apex beat, as well as the presence of a left or right ventricular heaves. The precordium should also be palpated for the presence of thrills. The anterior and posterior chest walls should be percussed bilaterally in the upper, middle and lower zones, comparing a percussion note from the left and right hemithoraces. Auscultation of these areas should determine the type and quality of breath sounds, as well as any added sounds. The first and second heart sounds and any added sounds or murmurs should be noted.

The remainder of the secondary assessment is considered elsewhere.

Re-assessment

The patient should be monitored to assess the effect of treatment as well as any deterioration in their condition. If this occurs then reassessment is mandatory, recommencing the primary assessment.

Documentation

It is mandatory to record the findings of the primary and secondary assessment. All notes should have a clearly recorded date and time and a legible signature or name. They should also contain a management plan, details of any treatment instituted and the patient's response. This will not only provide an aide-mémoire but will also enable the patient's condition to be monitored. In addition, it will provide hospital colleagues with an accurate account of prehospital care.

Transportation

Immediate transfer to hospital is often required. This will depend upon the number and location of the patients, as well as the type and severity of their conditions. Triage will facilitate catagorization according to transfer needs: thus, some patients may have to be managed in the prehospital environment, in adverse conditions, for prolonged periods. In the presence of *unilateral* pulmonary pathology, and provided that there are no contraindications, ensure that the patient is placed in the lateral position, where the 'good lung is kept down', during transportation (Macnaughton 1994, Donnelly et al 1995). This manoeuvre will provide optimum ventilation and perfusion. The majority of patients, however, will be most comfortable sitting up.

Summary

Any patient with a respiratory emergency must be evaluated quickly and accurately. The clinician must develop a structured method for assessment and treatment. In most acutely ill medical patients the primary assessment is rapid and resuscitation is rarely required. Diagnosis is frequently based on a well-'PHRASED' medical history obtained from the patient. If this is not possible, further information must be sought from medical records, relatives, general practitioners or the emergency services (Table 10.7).

Specific conditions

ASTHMA

Asthma is a common condition that affects approximately 5% of the population. It can occur for the first time at any age and there is an inherited component. Although there are many potential triggers, asthma is characterized by wheezing and dyspnoea due to widespread narrowing of the peripheral airways. This is frequently associated with an increase in sputum volume and viscosity. Occasionally

Table 10.7 Summary of assessment and treatment

Assessment and treatment are divided into four key phases:

Primary assessment
- Identify and treat immediately life-threatening problems including
  - Clearing the airway
  - Oxygenation and ventilation
- Monitoring
  - Respiratory effort, rate, pulse and blood pressure

Secondary assessment
- General overview
- Hands and radial pulse
- Facial appearance
- Neck – jugular venous pulse, carotid pulse, trachea
- Chest – precordium and both lungs

Documentation

Transportation

a nocturnal cough will be more prominent than wheezing and patients may describe tightness in the chest or a sensation of choking. Furthermore, exposure to irritants such as cold air, cigarette smoke and paint fumes may induce an acute attack. This does not indicate an allergic response but demonstrates that the airways are hyperreactive and produce an exaggerated response to non-specific irritants.

Pathophysiology

Asthma is a chronic inflammatory condition of the airways.

Although acute attacks of asthma may be precipitated by immunoglobulin E (IgE)-mediated mast-cell degranulation, the airways of known asthmatics are chronically narrowed by mucus secretion, oedema and smooth-muscle contraction, as well as collagen deposition under the basement membrane. This results in increased airflow resistance. As resistance is inversely proportional to the fourth power of the radius (Poiseuille's law), a small decrease in airway diameter will have a marked effect on airway resistance and therefore reduce airflow. Changes in airway diameter are usually due to bronchial muscle contraction but in the asthmatic this is exacerbated by mucosal oedema, increased mucus production and epithelial cell damage, which reduces elastic recoil of the neighbouring airways, further exacerbating the narrowing.

This disturbed and decreased airflow is manifest clinically as audible wheeze and reduced peak expiratory flow rate (PEFR). Because of increased airway resistance the work of breathing is increased and the patient feels breathless.

In an acute asthmatic attack some of the airways become blocked by mucus plugs resulting in hypoxia due to ventilation–perfusion ($\dot{V}/\dot{Q}$) mismatch. As a consequence, the work of breathing is increased even further by hyperventilation in an attempt to reverse the hypoxaemia. Failure to sustain this increased respiratory effort, usually in a severe exacerbation, will be manifest by a silent chest, hypoxaemia and a rising carbon dioxide partial pressure ($P_a\text{co}_2$). Unfortunately, deaths from acute asthma still occur and, although they are preventable, any delay in treatment can be fatal.

Life-threatening asthma

Assessment

Life-threatening asthma is characterized by cyanosis, exhaustion, minimal respiratory effort, silent chest, bradycardia or tachycardia (greater than 130 beats min^{-1}). It is important to remember that a silent chest is not a good prognostic sign as it reflects insufficient air being moved in and out of the airways to generate a wheeze. This is manifested by a peak expiratory flow rate that is less than 33% of either the predicted or the patient's best.

Immediate treatment

This comprises high-flow oxygen and nebulized beta-2-agonist (salbutamol 5 mg) combined with an anticholinergic (ipratropium bromide 0.5 mg) driven by high-flow oxygen. In addition, oral or intravenous steroids (prednisolone 40 mg PO or 100 mg of hydrocortisone IV) should be considered.

If the patient is not settling, intravenous administration of magnesium (1.2–2 g infusion over 20 min) and either salbutamol (200 μg over 10 min) or aminophylline (250 mg over 30 min) may be necessary (British Thoracic Society 2003). Ideally, the patient should have continuous ECG monitoring while these drugs are administered. Furthermore, the dose of aminophylline may have to be amended if the patient is already taking oral theophyllines. These precautions are not always possible in the prehospital arena. Thus, the doctor will have to decide whether the patient's clinical condition merits the use of such drugs in the context of their side-effects.

It is important to remember that an asthmatic can develop a pneumothorax, which can further embarrass the respiratory system. Thus, regular reassessment is required. Furthermore, intravenous fluids should be administered as most patients have coexisting dehydration. Correction of dehydration also helps to render the sputum less tenacious. Hypokalaemia can be a consequence of either asthma or beta-2-agonist therapy. Careful monitoring and appropriate replacement therapy may be required in hospital.

If the patient becomes exhausted or has clinical features of carbon dioxide retention or inadequate oxygenation, then intubation and ventilation will be required. This must only be attempted if appropriate training has been received.

Table 10.8 Causes of acute respiratory failure

- Cardiac – dysrhythmia, failure, arrest
- Pulmonary – asthma, pulmonary embolism
- Neurological – status epilepticus, loss of consciousness
- Neuromuscular – myasthenia gravis
- Trauma – head, neck and chest

Acute severe asthma

Assessment

The patient will usually be unable to complete sentences; tachypnoea (in excess of 25 breaths min^{-1}) and tachycardia (pulse of 110 beats min^{-1} or more) are invariably present (British Thoracic Society 2003).

Immediate treatment

This includes high-flow oxygen, nebulized salbutamol and either oral prednisolone or intravenous hydrocortisone. If the patient does not improve within 10–15 min, nebulized ipratropium bromide and intravenous bronchodilators should be administered, as described above. Patients who respond well to nebulized therapy and who have not previously had steroids can be subsequently started on a reducing course of prednisolone.

Moderate asthma

Assessment

The patient is not distressed or cyanosed and can speak in complete sentences. The respiration rate is less than 25 breaths min^{-1} and the pulse is less than 100 beats min^{-1} In addition, the peak flow is usually greater than 50% of either the predicted or the patient's best (British Thoracic Society 2003).

Immediate treatment

Most of these patients will respond to nebulized beta-2-agonists augmented, on occasion, by oral steroids. If the patient fails to respond, however, treatment should be instituted as described in the subsection on 'Acute severe asthma'.

RESPIRATORY FAILURE

Acute respiratory failure

This is not an uncommon encounter in prehospital care. The management, irrespective of the cause (Table 10.8), is to clear and secure the airway followed by ventilation with high inspired oxygen concentrations, as described earlier.

Chronic respiratory failure

Most patients present with an acute exacerbation of their chronic pulmonary disease. The underlying causes are listed in Table 10.9.

Chronic bronchitis and emphysema (chronic obstructive pulmonary disease, COPD), pulmonary fibrosis and pulmonary vascular disease are frequently encountered medical emergencies. All three can cause hypoxic (type 1) respiratory failure, while COPD is the commonest cause of hypercapnic (type 2) respiratory failure.

PATHOPHYSIOLOGY

Chronic obstructive pulmonary disease

This is a collective term referring to patients who have chronic bronchitis and/or emphysema, most of whom will have a mixture of both conditions. Chronic bronchitis is a common disorder manifested by chronic inflammation both in the bronchi and bronchioles. The major stimulus to this chronic inflammation is cigarette smoking, although inhalation of other gases may cause a similar problem. These noxious compounds stimulate increased mucus production and airway narrowing secondary to mucous gland hypertrophy, mucosal oedema, bronchoconstriction and subepithelial airway fibrosis. Furthermore, the chronic chemical irritant increases the volume of mucus produced and also impairs the ciliary escalator, preventing clearance. As a result of this, coughing is a major symptom.

In contrast, emphysema affects alveolar walls and is attributed to enzyme degradation of both collagen and elastin. This, in turn, destroys the alveolar walls and as a consequence the alveolar spaces coalesce. This disease is also attributed primarily to cigarette smoking. While the changes induced are patchy throughout the lung, they mainly affect the apex. This is attributed to greater mechanical stress due to the weight of the remaining lung tissue. In comparison,

however, alpha-1-antitrypsin deficiency (a rare condition) causes similar changes in the dependent areas. This is likely to reflect higher blood flow and unchecked enzyme degradation because of the lack of the protective antiprotease compound alpha-1-antitrypsin.

In chronic bronchitis the inflammatory changes affecting the large airways have minimal effect but those affecting the smaller airways produce a fixed obstruction affecting both inspiration and expiration. These patients often hypoventilate, predisposing to an elevated $P_a\text{CO}_2$. In addition, chronic hypoxia will lead to increased erythropoietin production by the kidneys, culminating in secondary polycythemia. The combination of pulmonary vasoconstriction and increased blood viscosity adversely influences right heart function. It is not surprising, therefore, that pulmonary hypertension and right heart failure are common sequelae.

In emphysema the enlarged parenchymal air spaces cause two major structural problems. The first is loss of elastic recoil and hence increased compliance. The second is destruction of the framework that attaches the alveoli to the airway. Normally this framework exerts traction to maintain a patent airway. Therefore its destruction increases the susceptibility to airway collapse and hence a reduction in airflow.

Pulmonary fibrosis

Diseases associated with diffuse pulmonary fibrosis are shown in Table 10.10. (C-CODES is a useful mnemonic.)

Interstitial fibrosis is the final stage of a large number of inflammatory processes that relentlessly progress to chronic, extensive deposition of collagen in the alveolar walls. The consequences are very similar, irrespective of the aetiology.

Collagen deposition within the alveolar walls causes thickening, rigidity and microvascular destruction. The increased distance between the alveolar epithelium and the capillary endothelium impairs oxygen diffusion, producing hypoxia. This is exacerbated by marked parenchymal distortion. Furthermore, the elastic recoil of the lung is increased, lung compliance is reduced and the work of breathing is increased. The result of these changes is a restrictive ventilatory defect.

Table 10.9 Causes of chronic respiratory failure

- Parenchymal disease
  - Chronic bronchitis
  - Emphysema
  - Bronchiectasis
  - Pulmonary fibrosis
  - Pulmonary vascular disease
- Obstructive sleep apnoea
- Neuromuscular disorders
  - Motor neurone disease
  - Cervical cord lesion
- Thoracic wall problems
  - Kyphoscoliosis
  - Extreme obesity

Table 10.10 Diseases associated with diffuse pulmonary fibrosis

- Cryptogenic fibrosing alveolitis
- Connective tissue diseases
  - Rheumatoid disease
  - Systemic sclerosis
  - Systemic lupus erythematosus
- Occupation, e.g. asbestosis/pneumoconiosis
- Drug, e.g. busulfan, bleomycin, paraquat
- Extrinsic allergic alveolitis (usually upper lobe and late in the disease)
- Sarcoid

The combination of alveolar wall thickening and microvascular destruction also increases pulmonary vascular resistance. This will be exacerbated by hypoxia, which induces pulmonary vasoconstriction. Consequently pulmonary hypertension will develop, eventually leading to right heart failure. The fibrotic process therefore influences both ventilation and perfusion.

Hypoxia is often severe and present at rest, while the $P_a\text{co}_2$ is generally normal or low. The latter is attributed to hyperventilation. In view of the pathophysiology of diffuse interstitial fibrosis, the diffusing capacity for carbon dioxide is reduced. This is attributed not only to the increased thickness of the interface between alveolar gas and intracapillary red cells but also to the reduced volume of both capillary load and capillary wall surface area.

Bronchiectasis

This is a condition characterized by chronic dilatation of some of the bronchi. The bronchial wall is irreversibly damaged as a consequence of early inflammation or infection of either the bronchus or adjacent lung parenchyma. The normal transport of mucus is impaired and chronic local suppuration ensues.

A variety of conditions are associated with bronchiectasis; they are shown in Table 10.11.

The pathophysiology of bronchiectasis is poorly understood. Despite the wide variety of conditions associated with bronchiectasis, there are certain common features.

First, a severe infection causes extensive tissue damage mediated by persistent inflammation. The repair processes, however, are inadequate with, for example, immunoglobulin deficiency or lack of major inhibitors of proteolytic enzymes (i.e. alpha-1-antitrypsin deficiency). If the inflammation is left unchecked, extensive tissue destruction occurs and inadequate repair results in scarring and tissue distortion. As focal areas of the lungs framework are destroyed the associated bronchoalveolar units become dilated.

Management of chronic respiratory failure

Immediate management

In all these patients it is important to:

- treat the hypoxia
- identify and treat the reason for the acute exacerbation
- assess the severity of the respiratory failure
- monitor the response to treatment.

Hypoxia kills; therefore, patients should receive high-flow oxygen, especially when the underlying cause of their breathlessness is unknown. If ventilatory capacity is sufficient and carbon dioxide sensitivity is maintained (type 1 respiratory failure) oxygen can be given at high concentration. In contrast, patients with severe COPD usually have poor ventilatory capacity and a blunted response to carbon dioxide (type 2 respiratory failure). As a consequence, oxygen therapy may reduce the hypoxic stimulus to ventilation and exacerbate both hypoventilation and carbon dioxide retention. Therefore, oxygen therapy should be given to ensure a saturation of 90–92% and adjusted later in hospital according to arterial blood gas results. If life-threatening hypoxia persists, on arrival in hospital the patient may require either a ventilatory stimulant or ventilation.

Hypoxia kills.

The reason for clinical deterioration is usually bronchospasm resulting in increased resistance of the remaining airways, which will adversely influence ventilation. Nebulized beta-2-agonists will reduce this burden, as will therapy with steroids (to reduce the luminal inflammatory response) and antibiotics (to target infected luminal secretions). Aminophylline is often beneficial in patients who have an acute exacerbation of COPD. Not only does it produce bronchodilatation and inotropic stimulation but it also improves renal perfusion and cardiac output. This is of particular benefit in patients who have coexistent ventricular failure.

In chronic respiratory compromise, especially COPD, the ventilatory load is high but the capacity is impaired. As a consequence, the central nervous system drive to respiration

Table 10.11 Conditions associated with bronchiectasis
Infection
● Measles–pneumonia
● Whooping cough
● Tuberculosis
Immune-related
● Immunoglobulin deficiency
● Complement deficiency
Inhalation
● Gastric aspiration
● Ammonia inhalation
● Foreign body inhalation
Others
● Immotile cilia
● Kartagener's syndrome
● Alpha-1-antitrypsin deficiency

is increased. If the patient does not respond appropriately to treatment, reassessment is required to identify possible causes; these are listed in Table 10.12 (a succubus was a demon in female form).

PNEUMOTHORAX

A pneumothorax results from air entering the potential space between the visceral and parietal pleura. In medical cases this may arise spontaneously from the rupture of a bulla or cyst on the lung surface, allowing alveolar air to enter the pleural space. The integrity of the pleural space can also be disrupted either by a penetrating chest wall

wound allowing atmospheric air entry or via damage to the visceral pleura (as a result of penetrating or blunt injury) allowing alveolar gas to enter the pleural space. Underlying lung disease is an important predisposing factor in the development of spontaneous pneumothoraces.

Pathophysiology

The outward recoil of the chest and inward elastic recoil of the lung result in a negative pressure in the potential space between the visceral and parietal pleura. This pressure becomes more negative during inspiration. Furthermore, because of the elastic recoil of the lung, pleural pressure is always less than alveolar pressure. Following a breach of the visceral pleura, air preferentially moves from the alveolus into the pleural space until these pressures equilibrate and as a result the lung collapses, resulting in a simple pneumothorax. If, however, the breach in the pleura acts as a one-way valve, air will preferentially enter the pleural space during inspiration. Thus, the intrapleural pressure rises above atmospheric pressure. The resulting hypoxia acts as a respiratory stimulus, causing deeper inspiratory effort, which in turn further increases the intrapleural pressure. The result is a tension pneumothorax (Fig. 10.1). Hypoxia is exacerbated by kinking of the great vessels due to mediastinal

Table 10.12 Causes of treatment failure
● Sputum retention
● Untreated bacterial infection
● Coexistent pneumothorax
● Coexistent pulmonary oedema
● Underlying dysrhythmia
● Bronchodilator therapy inadequate
● Unnecessary sedation
● Spurious diagnosis

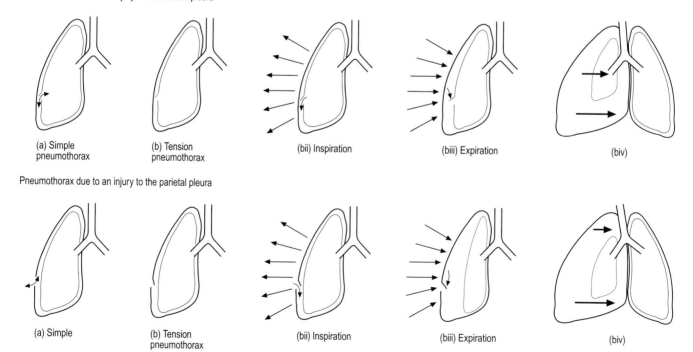

Pneumothorax due to an injury to the visceral pleura

(a) Simple pneumothorax   (b) Tension pneumothorax   (bii) Inspiration   (biii) Expiration   (biv)

Pneumothorax due to an injury to the parietal pleura

(a) Simple   (b) Tension pneumothorax   (bii) Inspiration   (biii) Expiration   (biv)

Fig. 10.1 • The development of a tension pneumothorax.

shift, interference with venous return and compression of the opposite lung. Electromechanical dissociation (pulseless electrical activity) ensues if untreated. Tension pneumothorax is a clinical diagnosis that warrants urgent decompression by needle thoracocentesis.

- Primary pneumothorax is relatively uncommon, affecting about nine people in 100 000, with a male to female ratio of approximately 4:1. It occurs in previously normal lungs. About 20% of patients will have a recurrence of pneumothoraces not only on the ipsilateral but also on the contralateral side.
- Secondary pneumothorax is characterized by pre-existing lung disease (Table 10.13).

A pneumothorax may complicate an acute exacerbation of asthma because of increased intra-alveolar pressures due to air trapping. Malignant disease causing either bronchial obstruction or infiltration of the pleura or subpleural tissues can also predispose to pneumothorax.

Intermittent positive pressure ventilation and attempted subclavian or internal jugular access are also associated with the development of pneumothoraces.

Assessment

Simple pneumothorax

Symptoms and signs may be absent but commonly the patient will present with breathlessness and pleuritic chest pain localized to the affected side. Breathlessness may be related to pain, size of pneumothorax or pre-existing lung disease.

Clinical signs are difficult to detect when the pneumothorax is small or when there is coexistent emphysema. Often there is reduced chest expansion on the affected side (usually due to pain). The percussion note may be resonant – hyperresonance is very difficult to detect even when in comparison with the non-affected side. The most consistent sign is a reduction in breath sounds over the pneumothorax.

Table 10.13 Pre-existing lung conditions associated with pneumothoraces

- Infections
  - Staphylococcal pneumonia
  - Empyema
  - Tuberculosis
- Chronic bronchitis
- Emphysema
- Cystic fibrosis
- Acute exacerbation of asthma
- Neoplasia

Tension pneumothorax

This is manifested as acute respiratory distress. Initially there may be absence of movement on the affected side, increased respiratory effort and rate, hyperresonant percussion note and absent breath sounds. Tracheal deviation, jugular venous distension and cyanosis are late, often preterminal, manifestations.

Management

Simple pneumothorax

It is unlikely that this diagnosis will be made in the prehospital environment unless the patient presents with pleuritic pain. Frequently, the patient is asymptomatic as there is only partial lung collapse. Spontaneous resolution will occur at a rate of approximately 1.25% of the volume of the hemithorax per day. Occasionally, pain relief is required in the form of non-steroidal anti-inflammatory analgesics.

Aspiration of air from a pneumothorax should only be attempted when the patient is in hospital.

In general, formal tube thoracostomy is not performed in the prehospital environment except in cases of prolonged transfer where access to the chest may be difficult or impossible. Conventional helicopter transfer does not mandate the insertion of a chest drain.

Tension pneumothorax

This necessitates immediate needle thoracocentesis to relieve the tension. This should be followed by formal chest drain insertion, after ensuring intravenous access.

Pulse oximetry

PRINCIPLES

In blood, haemoglobin exists in two forms:

- *oxygenated* (HbO_2) with loosely bound oxygen molecules
- *reduced* (Hb) with no bound oxygen molecules.

Thus, arterial oxygen saturation is defined as the ratio of oxygenated haemoglobin (HbO_2) to the total haemoglobin (HbO_2 + Hb + others, e.g. carboxy-, met- and sulphhaemoglobin). As carboxyhaemoglobin, along with other pigments, cannot be measured by the standard pulse oximeter, the internationally recognized denotation for arterial saturation is S_pO_2.

Oximetry is based on the following facts:

- Light 'energy' is attenuated by all tissues.
- Arterial blood flow is pulsatile, unlike other fluids and tissues.
- Oxygenated haemoglobin (HbO_2) and reduced haemoglobin (Hb) absorb different wavelengths of light.

HOW THE PULSE OXIMETER WORKS

The pulse oximeter comprises a peripheral probe connected to a microprocessor unit. It provides a digital display of oxygen saturation ($S_pO_2\%$), pulse rate (beats min^{-1}) and the pulse waveform. The peripheral probe is usually placed on a digit or occasionally the ear lobe or nose. It consists of two light-emitting diodes (LEDs) producing red (660 nm) and infrared (940 nm) light, and a 'photodetector' that produces an electric current proportional to the light intensity. These two beams of light pass through the tissues and are received by a detector. Oxygenated haemoglobin (HbO_2) and reduced haemoglobin (Hb) exhibit different absorption characteristics to red and infrared light. The remaining contribution of other absorbers (e.g. carboxy-, met- and sulph-haemoglobin) is therefore eliminated. The LEDs are switched on and off (approximately 600 times per second) in rapid sequence so that the detector receives an estimate of transmitted red, infrared and ambient light. This transmission is influenced by arterial pulsation but not by tissues or by blood in other vessels.

Therefore, comparing light absorbance at one point of the pulse wave with another ensures that the difference between the values reflects arterial blood saturation alone. This information is converted by the microprocessor to provide mean saturation values and the pulse rate is calculated from the number of LED cycles between successive pulse signals.

Pulse oximeters provide a non-invasive method of monitoring a patient's cardiorespiratory status. They measure:

- the oxygen saturation of haemoglobin in arterial blood; this is a reflection of the average amount of oxygen bound to each haemoglobin molecule
- the pulse rate in beats min^{-1}.

Unfortunately, there are many misconceptions concerning pulse oximeters. They *do not* measure any of the following:

- oxygen content of the blood
- partial pressure of oxygen in arterial blood (P_aO_2)
- amount of oxygen dissolved in the blood
- respiratory rate
- blood pressure
- cardiac output.

OXYGEN SATURATION, CYANOSIS AND THE OXYHAEMOGLOBIN DISSOCIATION CURVE

The oxygen saturation of arterial blood is the average percentage saturation of the population of haemoglobin molecules in a blood sample. It is important to remember

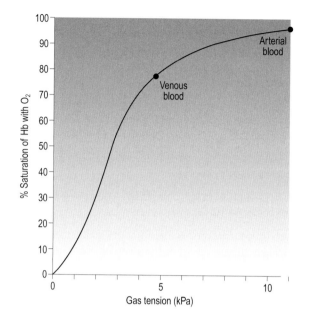

Fig. 10.2 ● The haemoglobin dissociation curve.

that one molecule of haemoglobin can carry a maximum of four molecules of oxygen, when it is referred to as *fully saturated*.

Pulse oximetry is a reliable method of detecting hypoxia. Unfortunately, clinical indicators of hypoxia are less than ideal. Cyanosis, traditionally defined as more than 5 g per 100 ml of reduced haemoglobin in capillary blood, depends on arterial oxygenation, haemoglobin content and skin perfusion. In contrast to peripheral cyanosis, central cyanosis of the mucous membranes does not reflect poor perfusion. With a normal haemoglobin concentration, central cyanosis can occur with an oxyhaemoglobin saturation of less than 85%. Furthermore, examination of the haemoglobin dissociation curve (Fig. 10.2) shows that below 90% oxyhaemoglobin saturation decreases rapidly as oxygen tension declines. Thus, oxygen saturation should be maintained in excess of 92%.

PRACTICAL APPLICATIONS OF PULSE OXIMETRY

The practical applications of pulse oximetry are shown in Table 10.14.

LIMITATIONS OF PULSE OXIMETRY

Although the pulse oximeter has revolutionized clinical practice, there are certain conditions that limit its use. An appropriate probe position can be difficult to find in critically

Table 10.14 Practical applications of pulse oximetry

- Transport of critically ill patients
- Monitoring high-dependency patients
- Limb viability assessment
- Reducing blood gas analysis
- Limiting oxygen toxicity in premature infants

Table 10.15 Practical tips for pulse oximetry

- Always ensure that the batteries are fully charged
- Prevent accidental damage by packing or positioning securely
- Only use the autocalibration
- Select an appropriate probe site that is clean and warm
- Ensure that the probe is secure
- Allow time for the pulse oximeter to detect the pulse and calculate the saturation
- Ensure a wave form is displayed; without this any reading is meaningless
- Wild fluctuations in either pulse rate or saturation should always be interpreted with caution
- Always treat the patient and not the pulse oximeter values
- Ensure that the oximeter probe and sphygmomanometer cuff are not placed on the same limb

ill patients who have poor tissue perfusion. Cardiac dysrhythmias interfere with the pulsatile signal of the oximeter, as can shivering, motion effect (tremor or pulsatile wave forms and saturation values when there is no pulse, i.e. during cardiopulmonary resuscitation) and profound venous pulsation (right-sided heart lesions, e.g. tricuspid regurgitation, may impart venous pulsation and this is recorded by the oximeter). Probe function can also be influenced by bright overhead lighting, dyes, pigments and nail varnish (metallic types only). Furthermore, it is important to realize that the pulse oximeter does not measure carboxy-, met- and sulph-haemoglobin. The pulse oximeter may therefore give reassuringly high values for oxygen saturation in the presence of a high and rising $P_a\text{co}_2$. Remember that the $S_p\text{O}_2$ may be 100% following extensive carbon monoxide poisoning. In contrast, oxygen saturation values of less than 70% are inaccurate.

Table 10.16 Summary

- Respiratory emergencies are common
- Always ensure your safety as well as that of the patient(s)
- A primary assessment is the minimum required in the prehospital environment
- Most respiratory emergencies can be initially managed with ease in the prehospital environment
- Hypoxia is common
- All patients will need supplemental oxygen to maintain a saturation of 92%
- Clear and concise documentation is mandatory

Pulse oximetry gives no measure of $P_a\text{co}_2$.

MISCONCEPTIONS RELATING TO PULSE OXIMETRY

There are many misconceptions regarding pulse oximetry. This technique will not determine the adequacy of ventilation. Furthermore, age, sex, anaemia and skin pigmentation have little or no affect on oximetry function. The standard pulse oximeter does not measure carboxyhaemoglobin.

Practical tips for pulse oximetry in a prehospital environment are given in Table 10.15.

Summary

A summary of the prehospital management of respiratory emergencies is given in Table 10.16.

References

British Thoracic Society 2003 British guideline on the management of asthma. Thorax 58(Suppl 1): 1–83

Donnelly JA, Smith EA, Tullet WM 1995 Inter-hospital transfer of a ventilated patient. British Journal of Intensive Care June: 200–201

Macnaughton PD 1994 Posture and lung function in health and disease. British Journal of Intensive Care December: 133–137

Further reading

Brewis RAL 1991 Lecture notes on respiratory disease. Blackwell Scientific, Oxford

Oh TE 2003 Intensive care manual, 5th edn. Butterworths, London

West JB 1991 Pulmonary physiology. Williams & Wilkins, Baltimore, MD

The unconscious patient

11

Introduction   130

Primary assessment   130

Diagnostic clues from the primary assessment   132

Secondary assessment   133

Specific syndromes   135

Summary   138

Reference   138

Further reading   138

Introduction

An unconscious patient is at some considerable risk. The risk arises both from the consequences of the unconscious state and from the underlying cause of the unconsciousness. In the prehospital environment the primary aim of a rescuer must be to protect the patient from immediately life-threatening consequences of unconsciousness and then to establish whether there are any underlying treatable causes. Appropriate emergency treatment for such causes should be given before further assessment is carried out.

The management of the unconscious patient in the prehospital environment therefore follows the standard approach: a primary assessment is carried out and any threat to the airway, breathing or circulation is managed in the resuscitation phase. Once this is over a secondary assessment may be undertaken and underlying causes amenable to emergency treatment are sought and treated. Following this the patient is moved safely to an environment where more detailed assessment can be carried out and definitive care provided.

Primary assessment

Unconscious patients may be in a variety of dangerous situations and it is always important to ensure that the rescuer is not in danger. Having minimized the dangers to the rescuer and the patient, a patient assessment should be undertaken.

RESPONSIVENESS

First of all, attempts should be made to rouse the patient. This is traditionally done by gently shaking or otherwise stimulating the patient and asking 'Are you all right?'. In patients who have suffered trauma, care should be taken not to disturb the neck during such manoeuvres. Patients who fail to respond to this question are either deaf or suffering from some decrease in the level of their consciousness. It is likely that deaf patients will respond to the shaking even if they do not respond to the shouting.

AIRWAY AND BREATHING

In patients in whom there is no response, the next move is to open the airway. This can be achieved either by head tilt and chin lift in patients in whom there is no danger of cervical spine trauma, or by jaw thrust in others. Any obvious foreign material in the mouth should be removed.

Once the airway is opened then the rescuer can assess for the presence of breathing using the familiar look, listen, feel technique. No more than 10 s should be spent on this assessment and if breathing is either inadequate or absent then respiratory support (including high flow supplemental oxygen) should be given.

CIRCULATION

Following the assessment and resuscitation of breathing, circulation should be assessed. The first part of this assessment involves the palpation of a central pulse. In adults the carotid pulse is preferred, while in small children the brachial pulse may be felt. If a pulse is present then the adequacy of the circulation should be determined by assessing pulse rate, volume and capillary refill time.

Intravenous access should be obtained as soon as possible in all unconscious patients. Once this has been obtained a small amount of blood should be drawn and an urgent glucose estimation should be done. Hypoglycaemia is a treatable cause of unconsciousness and it should be specifically sought and urgently treated during the primary assessment and resuscitation phase.

SIMPLE NEUROLOGICAL ASSESSMENT

Assuming that problems with airway, breathing and circulation have been detected and resuscitation has been commenced where appropriate, then a simple assessment of neurological status should be undertaken. This consists of placing the patient on a simple conscious level scale (Table 11.1) and undertaking an assessment of pupil size, equality and reactiveness.

The AVPU scale is used as a simple alternative to the Glasgow coma scale (GCS) (see below). Both hospital and prehospital carers have difficulty in remembering the full GCS without an aide-mémoire. Furthermore, in the prehospital environment during the early stages of assessment, carrying out an assessment of the GCS can be very time-consuming and is difficult to do accurately. It is more suited to the secondary assessment, when more time is available.

Pupils are assessed for equality (by opening both eyes at once and seeing whether the pupil sizes are the same), reactiveness (by shining a light at them from the side to see whether constriction occurs in both the pupil in which the light is shone and the opposite pupil) and size. The latter can be described either descriptively (pinpoint, dilated) or more accurately in terms of millimetres.

This simple neurological examination in the primary assessment is effective enough to allow changes in conscious level to be detected and to allow some specific diagnoses to be made.

HISTORY

While the primary assessment is being carried out, a simple history can be taken either from relatives or from witnesses. Specific points to be sought in the history include the presence or absence of a traumatic cause, known predisposing conditions such as diabetes, epilepsy or drug abuse, and any available descriptions of the event that led to unconsciousness. The primary assessment and resuscitation of the unconscious patient is summarized in Table 11.2.

Table 11.1 A simple conscious level scale

- **A**lert
- Responds to **V**oice
- Responds to **P**ain
- **U**nresponsive

Table 11.2 Summary of primary assessment and resuscitation of an unconscious patient

- Approach with care
  - If danger is present, identify dangers
    - If possible to minimize dangers, do so
    - If not possible to minimize dangers, then move patient from danger
  - If no danger is present then assess responsiveness
- Assess responsiveness by shaking and shouting
  - If patient responds then act appropriately
  - If no patient response then proceed to open airway
- Open airway
  - If no chance of trauma, use head tilt and chin lift
  - If trauma possible ensure cervical stabilization then use jaw thrust
  - Use airway adjuncts as necessary
  - Once airway opened proceed to assess breathing
- Assess breathing by looking and feeling, listening
  - If no breathing provide respiratory support
  - If breathing adequate proceed to assess circulation
- Assess circulation
  - If no circulation or if circulation inadequate give circulatory support
  - Establish intravenous access
  - Take blood for venous glucose estimation
    - If hypoglycaemic give 50 ml 50% dextrose
    - If normoglycaemic then proceed to simple neurological assessment
- Assess neurology simply
  - Assess conscious level AVPU
  - Assess pupils for size equality and reactivity
- Proceed to secondary assessment
- If any deterioration then return to primary survey

Diagnostic clues from the primary assessment

The cause of unconsciousness may have become apparent from the history given by relatives or witnesses. On other occasions investigations such as the glucose stick test carried out during the assessment will reveal the underlying cause. Often, the underlying cause will not be found and the rescuer will have to look out for clues that will become apparent during the examination of airway, breathing, circulation and neurological status undertaken as part of the primary assessment. These are considered below.

AIRWAY

Airway obstruction or compromise may be either a primary or secondary event when associated with unconsciousness. Complete airway obstruction as a primary event will eventually lead to unconsciousness and then death. If examination reveals a foreign body obstructing the airway then this may itself be the cause of unconsciousness.

BREATHING

There are a number of causes of changes in breathing pattern that may be associated with unconsciousness. A decreased rate of breathing (bradypnoea), in this context, is, usually caused by poisoning (deliberate or accidental, the commonest group of drugs implicated being the opiates) or by head injury.

Tachypnoea (rapid breathing) may be caused by metabolic acidosis. Again, poisoning can be an underlying cause (salicylates and ethylene glycol being common poisons causing acidosis). Metabolic causes such as diabetic ketoacidosis will also produce tachypnoea and this may have particular forms such as the deep, sighing Kussmaul respiration. A further cause of tachypnoea is hypovolaemia, which can be due to trauma, medical conditions (e.g. diarrhoea) and surgical conditions (e.g. ruptured aortic aneurysm).

Changes in the patterns of breathing may also be seen. Cerebrovascular accident (stroke) can result in both Cheyne–Stokes breathing (a pattern of breathing characterized by alternating periods of bradypnoea and tachypnoea) or by irregular breathing interspersed by short periods of apnoea.

Patients will be apnoeic during the tonic phase of a grand mal convulsion and also following cardiorespiratory arrest.

CIRCULATION

There are few specific circulatory signs in the unconscious patient. Tachycardia may indicate hypovolaemia or other causes of shock, or may be a specific effect of ingested or injected drugs such as tricyclics and sympathomimetics. Similarly, bradycardia may reflect an underlying cardiac complaint or may be associated with drugs such as beta-blockers. Bradycardia in association with raised blood pressure is associated with coning (Cushing's response).

Hypertension and hypotension are too non-specific to be of use in this regard.

The diagnostic clues available from examination of the airway, breathing and circulation are summarized in Table 11.3.

SIMPLE NEUROLOGICAL EXAMINATION

As discussed above, the simple neurological assessment consists of AVPU scaling and pupillary examination. Conscious level gives no clues about cause but pupillary findings can be of great value. The pupils are examined for equality, reactivity and size.

Unequal pupils associated with signs of head trauma are suggestive of intracranial haematoma causing tentorial herniation and third nerve palsy. Bilateral dilated pupils are often found in cases of tricyclic overdose but are also present in severe hypothermia. Bilateral pinpoint pupils are suggestive of opiate overdose. Pupillary changes are summarized in Table 11.4.

Table 11.3 Summary of diagnostic clues from the primary assessment

Airway	Breathing	Circulation
Foreign body	Obstructed	Apnoea
Poisoning		
Opiate	Bradypnoea	Hypotension
Ethylene glycol	Tachypnoea	
Beta-blockers		Bradycardia
Tricyclics		Hypotension
Sympathomimetics		Tachycardia
Gamma-hydroxybutyrate	Bradypnoea	Tachycardia
Salicylates	Tachypnoea	
Cerebrovascular accident	Cheyne–Stokes Irregular	
Rising intracranial pressure		Bradycardia Hypertension
Diabetic ketoacidosis	Kussmaul	Tachycardia Hypotension
Hypovolaemia	Tachypnoea	Tachycardia Hypotension

Table 11.4 Summary of pupillary signs in unconsciousness

	Equal	Unequal
Large		
Reactive	Tricyclics Sympathomimetics Hypothermia	Holmes–Adie
Unreactive		Tentorial herniation Mydriatics Local injury
Small		
Reactive	Opiates	Argyll Robertson
Unreactive	Pontine haemorrhage	Miotics Horner's syndrome

Table 11.5 The Glasgow coma scale (GCS)

Eye opening	Spontaneous	4
	To voice	3
	To pain	2
	None	1
Verbal response	Orientated	5
	Confused	4
	Inappropriate words	3
	Incomprehensible sounds	2
	None	1
Motor response	Obeys commands	6
	Purposeful movements	5
	Withdrawal	4
	Flexion	3
	Extension	2
	None	1

EXTERNAL APPEARANCE

By the end of the primary assessment the patient should be appropriately exposed and certain other diagnostic clues may become apparent at this stage. Needle marks overlying veins in any part of the body are suggestive of intravenous drug abuse. Dependent blisters in a patient who is deeply unconscious are strongly suggestive of a barbiturate overdose. Signs of urinary incontinence during removal of lower garments may indicate that the patient has had a grand mal convulsion.

The hypothermic patient may have either a primary or secondary cause of the hypothermia. Hypothermia itself may cause unconsciousness if profound. Certain overdoses and recreational drugs are associated with disordered thermoregulation. Chlorpromazine and MDMA (Ecstasy) can both cause either hypo- or hyperthermia.

Secondary assessment

Once the primary assessment and resuscitation phases have been completed and life-threatening causes of unconsciousness have been identified and treated where possible, the patient may be reassessed in a structured way if circumstances allow. This secondary assessment includes a medical history, a clinical examination and investigations as indicated. It is not designed to provide a definitive diagnosis and treatment plan but rather to identify which emergency treatments might further benefit the patient.

The need for early transfer to a facility able to provide definitive care should be considered at the end of the primary assessment. If transfer is indicated then this must not be delayed by attempts at fuller examination. In such cases transfer should be started and a limited secondary assessment carried out en route.

HISTORY

It is often the history that gives the most important clues to the underlying pathology. This history may be obtained from friends and relatives, bystanders and other witnesses. The patient may carry clues on their person if they have an underlying condition such as epilepsy or diabetes. This may either be a regular prescription card or even a MedicAlert bracelet. The history can often be taken at the same time as the examination is being carried out.

ESTABLISHING CONSCIOUS LEVEL

The Glasgow coma scale was first introduced in 1974. Since that time its use has spread worldwide and it has become an established method of describing conscious level. The scale runs from 3 to 15 and is made up of independent ratings for eye opening, best verbal response and best motor response. The patient's best score is recorded. The GCS is shown in Table 11.5.

Accuracy of scaling is important if the scale is to be of benefit, and users must be properly trained if this is to be achieved. Inexperienced users frequently have trouble deciding where the patient's response falls on the scale, and often use inappropriate painful stimuli during scaling. The scale is described in detail below.

Painful stimuli

Both the method of application and the nature of the painful stimulus are important if coma scaling is to be accurate. This point was emphasized in the initial description of the coma scale and remains as true today. The significance of the response to pain is difficult to interpret unless a standard painful stimulus is applied and maintained until a maximum response is obtained.

Two standard modes of stimuli are used, the first is an upper limb stimulus applied to the fingernail beds. A pencil is used to apply pressure. This stimulus should not be applied to the toes because the spinal reflex may cause flexion even in cases of brain death. The second is a stimulus applied to the face in the supraorbital region. This supraorbital ridge pressure is applied firmly and can be used to assess localization of pain. Supraorbital ridge pressure should not be used to test for eye opening as reflex grimacing may occur. Painful stimuli should only be applied if the patient does not respond to voice. It is often necessary to apply both central and peripheral stimuli to determine the response.

In the presence of a spinal injury, the painful stimulus must be applied above the neck (pressure on supraorbital ridge)

Eye opening

There are four levels of eye opening in the scale. Spontaneous eye opening indicates that the brain-stem arousal mechanisms are working. It does not imply awareness. Eye opening in response to speech is present if the eyes are opened as the result of any verbal stimulus. It is not necessary for the patient to obey a direct command to open their eyes for this level to have been reached. Eye opening in response to pain is tested using finger bed pressure. If both verbal and painful stimuli fail to cause eye opening then no eye opening response is present.

Verbal response

The best verbal response to a number of stimuli is scored independently of the other two responses. Oriented patients know who they are, where they are in time and space, and what has happened to them. It may be possible to hold a conversation with a confused patient but his/her replies will indicate a degree of disorientation and confusion. Inappropriate speech is often exclamatory and random – words are recognizable but they are not in context. A patient using incomprehensible sound may moan and groan but no words are recognizable. Patients who do not vocalize despite the use of both verbal and painful stimuli are said to show no verbal response.

Motor response

A patient who obeys commands will move (e.g. lift a limb) when told to do so. If no movement is elicited by command then a painful stimulus is applied. As mentioned above, the nature of the applied painful stimulus is extremely important

in eliciting motor responses. Patients who can localize pain will make an effort to remove the painful stimulus (e.g. by moving their arm during cannula insertion). If fingernail bed pressure elicits a response then a central (supraorbital) stimulus should be applied to test for localization. In cases of withdrawal there is no localization of a subsequently applied central stimulus – this response is occasionally termed 'normal flexion'. If there is no response to nail bed pressure, application of a supraorbital stimulus will assist in determining the absence of a cervical cord injury.

When the upper limb assumes the decorticate posture (adduction of the shoulder and flexion of the elbow) in response to a painful stimuli then a flexion response is said to be present. This response is sometimes termed 'abnormal flexion'. If, on the other hand, the upper limbs assume a decerebrate posture (adduction and internal rotation of the shoulder and extension of the elbow) then an extension response is said to be present. If despite verbal and painful stimuli no movement is elicited then no motor response has occurred.

OTHER NEUROLOGICAL ASSESSMENT

The Glasgow coma scale is a useful way of communicating a patient's neurological state. Taken together with a neurological examination looking for lateralizing signs, it can be extremely useful in determining the underlying cause of unconsciousness. While a full neurological examination may be possible and necessary in the hospital environment it is rarely possible to achieve this during prehospital care. Despite this, patients who are unconscious should be examined for any evidence of lateralizing signs. These may consist of inequality of the pupils, or obvious flaccidity or spasticity down one side or in a single limb. Furthermore, it may become obvious that patients are in the tonic or clonic phase of a grand mal convulsion or that they are suffering from focal epilepsy following a more generalized convulsion.

RESPIRATORY ASSESSMENT

Unconscious patients may have underlying respiratory problems and a brief respiratory examination should be undertaken as part of the secondary assessment. Specifically, the position of the trachea should be assessed and both lung fields should be auscultated. Any asymmetry in breath sounds or additional sounds such as crackles or wheezing should be noted.

Wheezing may indicate asthma or pulmonary oedema, and unconsciousness in this state would be a preterminal sign. The patient who is cold, clammy and sweaty is more likely to be suffering from left ventricular failure than asthma. Breathing should be supported if possible but increased airway pressure may make this technically difficult – these patients should be moved very rapidly to an advanced facility.

Patients with severe anaphylaxis may also be wheezing, as well as unconscious, secondary to their collapsed circulation. Emergency treatment with adrenaline (epinephrine) is appropriate, followed by rapid transport.

CARDIOVASCULAR ASSESSMENT

Cardiovascular secondary assessment consists of establishing the pulse rate and volume, the blood pressure and auscultating the heart. Patients may be unconscious secondary to hypovolaemia or other causes of shock, and circulatory support may be necessary. Intravenous access will have been established, signs of shock noted and intravenous infusion started in the primary assessment/resuscitation phase. Similarly, life-threatening dysrhythmias should have been discovered and treated at that time.

During secondary assessment stage hypotension or hypertension may be noted together with other cardiac signs. The presence of any of these should indicate the need for urgent transfer to hospital.

Specific syndromes

TRAUMA

Injury may lead to unconsciousness either as a direct result of trauma to the head or following airway, breathing and circulatory compromise. Head injury will usually be diagnosed following an appropriate history together with signs of external head trauma. A head injury that is serious enough to cause persisting unconsciousness is associated with primary brain injury, which may be focal or diffuse. Focal injury may consist of lacerations to the brain substance and haematomas within the brain. These may be complicated by bleeding outside the brain, which can be external to the dura (extradural), between the dural layers (subdural) or in the subarachnoid space. Both extradural and subdural bleeds can increase the intracranial pressure and cause brain compression. As the intracranial pressure rises, the cerebral perfusion pressure will fall and secondary injury to the brain will occur. This injury will be exacerbated by hypoxia and hypovolaemia.

The main aim of care following head injury is to prevent secondary injury and to deliver the patient to a facility able to deal with primary injury as soon as possible. Prevention of secondary injury involves maintenance of airway, breathing and circulation (including delivery of the highest possible fractional inspired concentration of oxygen and ensuring that the minute volume is maintained). The latter is important if partial pressure of carbon dioxide in the arterial blood is to be kept at low normal values, as this in itself helps to reduce intracranial pressure.

There is an association between head injury and cervical spine injury. Unconscious patients who have sustained a traumatic head injury must have full spinal control maintained at all times.

Patients who are unconscious as a result of either breathing or circulatory compromise are in a preterminal state. Standard trauma protocols should ensure that problems with airway, breathing and circulation are diagnosed and that management is commenced during the primary assessment and resuscitation phase. In such cases the unconsciousness is a marker of the general physiological derangement rather than a specific condition in its own right.

CEREBROVASCULAR EVENT (STROKE)

The commonest cerebrovascular event resulting in unconsciousness is stroke due to thrombosis or haemorrhage. Patients may suffer a sudden complete loss of consciousness with or without fitting, or may suffer progressive neurological signs or symptoms prior to the onset of unconsciousness.

Once the patient is unconscious the diagnosis of a cerebrovascular cause can be a difficult. The approach in the prehospital environment is to maintain the airway, breathing and circulation until such time as a formal diagnosis can be made. Secondary assessment may reveal loss of tone in the limbs on one side and this may give some clue to the diagnosis.

The advent of thrombolysis for non-haemorrhagic stroke and the evidence that this might be beneficial in terms of outcome has meant that patients suffering cerebrovascular accidents should have high priority for delivery to definitive care. In the USA there is a move to develop the concept of 'brain attack', similar to that of heart attack, so that the public realize the importance of getting patients with stroke to hospital as soon as possible.

Patients with spontaneous non-traumatic subarachnoid haemorrhage have most commonly suffered the rupture of a cerebral aneurysm. A small number (around 15%) will have sustained the rupture of an arteriovenous malformation while in a further 15% the cause will be idiopathic. Rarely these patients may have suffered complications of vasculitis, neoplasm, bleeding disorders, infection or spinal vascular malformation. Patients with a markedly reduced conscious level (GCS <12) have a worse prognosis than those who have mild alterations in conscious level with symptoms.

The diagnosis of subarachnoid haemorrhage in an unconscious patient can be extremely difficult. If the patient has had a prodromal bleed or if the sudden onset of headache and neck pain preceded the onset of coma then this diagnosis may be suggested. Sudden onset of headache during sexual intercourse, followed by loss of consciousness, is commonly due to subarachnoid haemorrhage. There is no specific emergency treatment but maintenance of airway, breathing and circulation are paramount if the best possible outcome is to be obtained. Patients should be moved to a centre capable of definitive investigations and care.

EPILEPSY

Patients suffering from epilepsy may be unconscious both during and after a fit. Most epileptic fits are short lived. They involve an initial tonic phase with general stiffening of the muscles followed by a clonic stage characterized by rhythmic jerking of the limbs and body. Following a fit (particularly a prolonged one) there may be a period of postictal unconsciousness of varying length.

Short-lived fits (those lasting less than 5 min) require no treatment as they are usually self-limiting. Fits that are prolonged (status epilepticus) should be treated with specific anti-epileptic medication as uninterrupted fits may be fatal – either due to complications of the convulsion (airway obstruction, aspiration of vomit, respiratory insufficiency) or secondary to the underlying disease process. It should be remembered that overmedication can also kill, and the minimum amount of medication necessary to control the fit should be given. The drug of choice for status epilepticus is lorazepam (Cock & Shapira 2002) or, if this is unavailable, diazepam may be given in a titrated dose until control is achieved. Diazepam can be administered rectally (Stesolid) if intravenous access is unavailable, in the dose of $0.4 \, \text{mg} \, \text{kg}^{-1}$.

Achieving control of difficult epileptic seizures is not a priority in the prehospital environment. Basic treatment as outlined above should be given and patients who continue to fit should be moved urgently to a facility that can provide definitive care.

POISONING

Poisoning is a common cause of unconsciousness in the UK. It may be accidental or deliberate and may involve prescribed medication, recreational drugs or other chemicals.

As with other causes of unconsciousness, the primary task of the prehospital provider is to ensure that airway, breathing and circulation are maintained while the patient is moved to a facility able to provide appropriate care.

Opiates

Opiate overdoses commonly occur in drug addicts and less commonly in terminally ill patients who have decided to end their own lives. A specific antagonist, naloxone, is available, and its administration intramuscularly or intravenously can rapidly reverse the effects of opiates.

Naloxone has a shorter half-life than most opiates and a considerably shorter half-life than methadone. While administration of intravenous naloxone will produce an almost instantaneous effect on conscious level, it has to be remembered that this effect is short-lived and that the underlying effects of the background opiate may return, resulting in a relapse of coma at a later time. Most authorities recommend the concurrent administration of an intramuscular dose of naloxone at the time that the intravenous dose is given.

Many patients will become severely agitated when the effects of opiate are rapidly reversed with the use of naloxone. Some may become violent and aggressive. Addicts will frequently seek to discharge themselves from the care of their rescuers as soon as possible because naloxone produces a rapid-onset withdrawal reaction. It may be argued that non-iatrogenic opiate overdose should not be pharmacologically treated in the prehospital environment but that patients with this condition should be moved to a facility where adequate monitoring is available after drug administration. This is particularly the case in overdoses of longer-acting opiates such as methadone. If such a policy is adopted then prehospital care consists of maintenance of the airway and breathing with supplemental oxygen and ventilation while the patient is moved to an appropriate facility.

Benzodiazepines

Benzodiazepines taken in overdose (often in association with alcohol) produce reduction in conscious level and may reduce airway protective reflexes. A specific antidote (flumazenil) is available but the most appropriate treatment prehospital, if any is required, is maintenance of the airway and support of respiration if this is compromised. Patients who are unconscious but breathing normally should simply be transported to hospital under close observation.

Administration of flumazenil in a mixed overdose may cause fitting. This is particularly the case when benzodiazepines have been combined with tricyclic antidepressants (where the former are 'treating' the epileptogenic effect of the latter). Prehospital care in these cases consists of maintenance of the airway, breathing and circulation during transfer to an appropriate facility.

Tricyclic antidepressants

Tricyclic antidepressants are commonly taken in overdose and may be fatal. Patients suffer cardiovascular and neurological symptoms and may become unconscious secondary to cardiac dysrhythmias or to fits. Unconsciousness may, however, be the result of the other components of a mixed overdose.

There is no specific treatment for tricyclic antidepressant overdose in the prehospital environment, and patients should have their airway, breathing and circulation maintained while they are transported to hospital for definitive care. Underlying causes of unconsciousness, such as fitting, should be treated en route if possible. If cardiac arrest occurs then normal advanced life support protocols should be followed and, in addition, sodium bicarbonate (repeated doses of 50 ml of an 8.4% solution) should be given early to achieve alkalinization.

Alcohol

Patients who are unconscious because of ingestion of alcohol require no specific treatment. They are, however, as prone to airway compromise as any other unconscious patient and should be cared for appropriately. Airway and breathing should be maintained and patients should be kept in the recovery position until such time as they are delivered to an appropriate facility for their care. Hypoglycaemia should be specifically sought in all cases of unconsciousness thought to be due to alcohol.

DIABETIC EMERGENCIES

Patients with diabetes suffer a number of complications that can render them unconscious. Diabetic patients may become hypoglycaemic as a result of their insulin therapy or may be hyperglycaemic if their diabetes is not properly controlled.

Patients who are hypoglycaemic initially have altered level of consciousness and finally become unconscious. This condition is often characterized by pallor and sweating but can be notoriously difficult to diagnose. As patients are often described as having slurred speech and staggering prior to becoming unconscious a misplaced diagnosis of alcohol poisoning can be made. Marked aggression may occur in the patient developing hypoglycaemia. Any patient who is unconscious should have their blood sugar checked by glucose stick test to ensure they are not hypoglycaemic. Patients who are hypoglycaemic should be given 50 ml of 50% dextrose intravenously or 1 mg of glucagon intramuscularly. Children should be given $0.5\,g\,kg^{-1}$ $(5\,ml\,kg^{-1})$ of 10% dextrose intravenously. Hypostop (glucose for buccal absorption) can be used as an alternative treatment in this situation.

A patient who has become unconscious as a result of poor diabetic control may be in either ketoacidotic or hyperosmolar coma. In both cases there is likely to be a history of a prodromal illness, often involving vomiting and malaise, whereas hypoglycaemia is much more rapid in onset.

These patients should be moved, with due regard to airway, breathing and circulation, to a facility appropriate for their care. Intravenous access may be obtained en route and an infusion of physiological (0.9%) saline commenced.

CARDIAC CAUSES

A patient who has neither a cardiac output nor spontaneous respiration has suffered a cardiorespiratory arrest and advanced life support protocols should be used. Patients who have poor cardiac output secondary to poor cardiac function or cardiac dysrhythmia may require specific treatment to restore their circulation. Tachyarrhythmias, both narrow-complex and broad-complex, can be associated with poor cardiac output and thus with unconsciousness. These patients should be cardioverted. If a patient has a GCS of less than 8 then additional sedation is not necessary prior to cardioversion.

HYPOTHERMIA

Patients who have been exposed to the elements for a period of time may become hypothermic and will eventually become unconscious. The sudden onset of unconsciousness in a hypothermic patient should suggest that an additional event such as the onset of a dysrhythmia has occurred. Gradual onset of unconsciousness is part of the natural progression of hypothermia and the normal treatment regimen for this condition should be followed (Ch. 33).

Hypothermia may be associated with drug overdose or with other underlying diseases such as hypothyroidism. In the elderly, a simple fall coupled with immobility can result in significant hypothermia. As with all other causes of unconsciousness, the primary responsibility of the prehospital provider is to maintain airway, breathing and circulation while seeking any other conditions that are amenable to immediate treatment.

PSYCHIATRIC

There is a small incidence of psychiatric pseudocoma presenting either as pseudocoma itself or as pseudofit. This can be particularly difficult to diagnose even in the hospital environment and prehospital providers should not attempt to make a definitive diagnosis of a psychiatric cause of coma but should rather perform a primary assessment and maintain the airway, breathing and circulation while transporting the patient to hospital.

Even patients who have a history of pseudocoma or pseudofit may occasionally have a real cause for unconsciousness, such as drug overdose, and the definitive diagnosis of pseudocoma or pseudofit is therefore one of exclusion and cannot be made in the prehospital environment.

Summary

The unconscious patient is at risk of complications in both the prehospital and hospital environments.

Application of simple principles of primary assessment and resuscitation will not only ensure that these patients do not suffer complications but will also ensure that they arrive at an appropriate facility in the best possible condition.

While there are large numbers of conditions that can underlie unconsciousness, their diagnosis can be time-consuming and may involve a considerable number of more advanced investigations. Prehospital providers should seek and treat the immediately treatable causes only. Under no circumstances should the prehospital practitioner delay the transfer of a patient with unexplained unconsciousness to definitive care while a search is made for conditions that are untreatable in the prehospital environment.

Reference

Cock HR, Schapira AH 2002 A comparison of lorazepam and diazepam as initial therapy in convulsive status epilepticus. Quarterly Journal of Medicine 95: 225–231

Further reading

Chem TH, Hu SC, Lee CH et al 1994 The role of flumazenil in the management of patients with acute alterations of mental status in the emergency department. Human and Experimental Toxicology 13: 45–50

Jennett B 1992 Coma. Medicine International 99: 4120–4123

Moulton C, Pennycook AG 1994 Relationship between Glasgow coma score and cough reflex. Lancet 344: 195

Nielson E 1996 Drugs in blood samples from unconscious drug addicts after the intake of overdose. International Journal of Legal Medicine 108: 248–251

Weinbrown A, Rudick V, Vorkine P et al 1996 Use of flumazenil in the treatment of drug overdose: a double-blind and open clinical study in 110 patients. Critical Care Medicine 24: 199–206

Acute abdomen

12

Introduction	139
History	140
Physical examination	142
Common causes of an acute abdomen	143
Reaching a diagnosis	146
Management	147
References	148
Further reading	148

Introduction

The term *acute abdomen* refers to any abdominal condition that is of recent onset, is potentially fatal and may need surgery to preserve life. Although this would appear to be an easy diagnosis to make, in practice it can be one of the most challenging clinical decisions to decide whether abdominal findings constitute serious pathology. This is in part because of the way the abdomen responds to noxious stimuli and also because associated symptoms are often features of non-serious illnesses.

Whereas the shocked patient with a pulsatile mass in the abdomen presents an obvious diagnosis of ruptured abdominal aortic aneurysm, devastating intra-abdominal events such as mesenteric infarction may present with few symptoms and signs, resulting in a delayed or missed diagnosis.

Unrelated conditions may give rise to a similar presentation and the true diagnosis and severity of the condition may only become apparent over time. In addition, the same disease can present in multiple ways. The difficulty in reaching a working diagnosis is further complicated by the fact that abdominal examination is much less precise than examination of other organ systems. Even with the benefit of diagnostic facilities within hospital, the diagnosis can be difficult and patients are often admitted for observation without a definitive diagnosis having been made. The difficulties in reaching a diagnosis in abdominal cases have long been recognized and attempts have been made to aid diagnosis using computers and clinical policies (American College of Emergency Physicians 1994).

Against this background, the main objective of the prehospital physician is to identify the acute abdomen from the mass of patients presenting with abdominal complaints that are non-serious. Besides prompt recognition, immediate care requires resuscitation, stabilization where possible, and transfer to the appropriate facility.

Despite the difficulties alluded to in both the recognition and diagnosis of the acute abdomen, most cases can be diagnosed from the history alone. In prehospital care the history assumes an even greater importance as it may be inappropriate, impracticable or impossible to carry out a complete assessment in the field. Therefore, prehospital involvement should be brief and should concentrate on obtaining a concise history followed by a brief but thorough examination.

The complete list of possible causes of abdominal pain, which is the predominant symptom of most cases of acute abdomen, is extensive and is beyond the scope of this chapter. In one study 41.3% of patients seen in the Emergency Department with the chief complaint of abdominal pain were discharged with the diagnosis of 'abdominal pain of unknown aetiology' (Brewer et al 1976). Rather than attempt to obtain a definitive diagnosis, the prehospital physician must make the diagnosis of acute abdomen, which by itself defines the patient as having a potentially life-threatening acute illness.

Common diseases are common and, although the diagnosis of an acute abdomen is often fraught with difficulty, a difficult case is far more likely to be due to a common disease presenting atypically than to a rare disease presenting typically. Abdominal pain is far more likely to have an underlying serious cause in the elderly, and it is vital that one always approaches the older patient considering possible leaking abdominal aortic aneurysm or mesenteric infarction as the cause of that patient's abdominal pain. With this in mind, when dealing with the elderly patient one should always have a higher index of suspicion for serious illness and a lower threshold for referral to hospital.

As well as the elderly, special groups of patients mandate special attention, such as the immunocompromised (either due to drugs, such as corticosteroids, or acquired immune deficiency syndrome, AIDS), as serious and often unusual abdominal conditions may have subtle presentations. Chronic alcohol misuse may be the aetiological basis for an acute abdomen and patients may present atypically.

There are no golden rules in the diagnosis of acute abdomen and no single sign must be regarded as pathognomonic of a particular diagnosis. A holistic approach is advised and one must exercise judgement, which may only develop through experience. When considering abdominal trauma the approach is different and this area is discussed in a separate chapter. In all cases of acute abdomen a history of trauma must always be specifically asked for.

History

The history should concentrate on pain, its location, nature, mode of onset and duration, and relieving or aggravating factors. Other salient features include vomiting, diarrhoea or constipation, and whether fresh or altered blood has been passed from either end.

Features of abdominal pain:

- Location
- Nature
- Mode of onset
- Duration
- Precipitating and relieving factors
- Aggravating factors.

PAIN

Abdominal pain is the predominant feature in most cases of acute abdomen, representing between 5 and 10% of patients attending accident and emergency departments; of these up to 40% have an underlying surgical cause. However, pain is also the major feature of most minor abdominal illnesses. Fortunately, good clues to the underlying diagnosis can be gleaned by taking a good pain history.

Pain is a subjective experience and the severity of pain expressed by the patient is often a poor guide to the severity of the underlying pathology. Cultural, ethnic and individual factors greatly modify the degree of pain felt. Often the most severely ill are the quietest. The very young are even less able to communicate pain.

Different organs give rise to pain in different areas of the abdomen. For example, pain in the epigastrium suggests a gastric cause, while pain in the right upper quadrant indicates gallbladder or liver pathology. Although each area tends to exhibit pain arising from particular organs, different organs may cause pain in the same location. Pancreatitis can give rise to pain in the epigastrium and/or in either upper quadrant. Because there is considerable overlap between differing organs, and since pain may be referred to or from distant areas, undue diagnostic emphasis should not be placed on the location of the pain alone. In addition, the same structure may give rise to pain in other areas in different patients; extra-abdominal pathology such as myocardial infarction may give rise to such severe abdominal pain as to mimic an acute abdomen. However, the location of the pain does help to *suggest* the involved structure.

Abdominal pain is traditionally divided into two types, visceral or parietal. Visceral pain arises from nociceptors found in structures enveloped by visceral peritoneum; these pain nociceptors are activated in response to distension, ischaemia or inflammation. Impulses are transmitted via small C afferents carried in autonomic nerve trunks that reach the spinal cord through several midline nerve trunks, with different viscera sharing the same spinal segments. Typical visceral pain is dull, aching or cramping, and poorly localized, although it is generally felt in the midline. It is also often variable in intensity. There may be accompanying autonomic phenomena such as pallor, sweating, nausea, vomiting and changes in pulse rate. Ischaemia can cause very intense visceral pain. The degree of pain is often disproportionately greater than the degree of tenderness elicited by the examiner.

Parietal peritoneum is innervated by both C fibres and somatic A fibres that travel to specific cord segments between levels T6 and L1. Parietal nociceptors also innervate the abdominal wall and the diaphragm. Parietal pain is usually felt in response to parietal peritoneal irritation by pus, urine, blood or bile. In contrast to visceral pain, parietal pain is sharper and is usually well localized, overlying the source of the irritation. Tenderness on palpation is usually prominent and approximately indicates the organ involved. Spinal reflexes give rise to secondary signs such as guarding.

Parietal pain may be the only type of pain perceived or it may follow visceral pain as in classic appendicitis, where dull, periumbilical visceral pain migrates to the right iliac fossa, changing in quality to sharp, parietal pain.

Pain may be felt distant from the source of the noxious stimulus, giving rise to referred pain. In this situation pain is perceived in dermatomes of the same segment as that of the involved organ, with pain felt distantly from the site of stimulation. For example, diaphragmatic pain from splenic injury may be felt over the left shoulder because of sensory afferents following the phrenic nerve (C3, C4, C5) causing pain to be felt in the sensory dermatome, C3. Extra-abdominal illness such as myocardial infarction or lower lobe pneumonia may give rise to abdominal pain that may be mistaken for an acute abdomen.

TIME OF ONSET

Abdominal pain that is of sudden onset suggests a serious cause such as viscus perforation, torsion or vascular accident. However, such clinical scenarios may present far less dramatically in the elderly and the young. Pain that wakes a patient from sleep should always be regarded as significant, and pain that persists continuously for more than 6 h often has a surgical cause. A less dramatic onset of pain that tends to increase in severity is a feature of conditions such as acute cholecystitis and bowel obstruction. Changes in the perceived nature and distribution of pain may aid diagnosis, as in acute appendicitis, where early paraumbilical visceral pain may develop into parietal pain in the right iliac fossa. Pain that was initially intermittent and subsequently becomes continuous should alert one to the possibility of ischaemia and may represent an ominous development. Pain that is slow in onset but gradually increases suggests an inflammatory cause such as pancreatitis or acute cholecystitis.

TYPE OF PAIN

True colicky pain is spasmodic in nature and is truly intermittent, with pain-free intervals. It is characteristic of an obstructed viscus such as in ureteric colic and small bowel obstruction. Although simple gastroenteritis may give rise to colicky pain, other features of the history and examination will usually allow differentiation. Contrary to popular belief, biliary colic is not colicky pain but is continuous with superimposed spasmodic exacerbations. Continuous pain suggests peritonitis, ischaemia or strangulation. Tearing pain is classically described in dissecting aortic aneurysm.

VOMITING

Vomiting is a common feature of a multitude of illnesses affecting different organ systems and is a non-specific feature of abdominal disease. However, the history will usually identify whether the vomiting has an abdominal cause. Vomiting is often preceded by pain and is usually the result of stimulation of visceral afferents. Vomiting is a major symptom of upper gastrointestinal pathology and is particularly notable in acute pancreatitis. Although often incorrectly used to describe copious vomiting, true projectile vomiting results in vomitus being expelled some distance and is characteristic of pyloric stenosis. Bilious vomiting is seen in proximal small bowel obstruction, whereas distal small bowel obstruction or large bowel obstruction may give rise to faeculant vomiting. Significant amounts of blood in vomitus mandates the speedy transfer of a patient to hospital.

Haematemesis may be the sole feature of a ruptured aortic aneurysm in the elderly, following the formation of an aortoenteric fistula. It may be modest initially, lulling one into making an erroneous diagnosis.

DIARRHOEA

Diarrhoea is not a major feature of most cases of acute abdomen. However, the presence of bloody diarrhoea, although often of infective origin, should alert one to the possibility of colitis, which may be ischaemic rather than due to inflammatory bowel disease.

CONSTIPATION

Prehospital medical personnel should be wary of accepting constipation as the cause of abdominal pain, especially in the elderly. Constipation should always be a diagnosis of exclusion. Absolute constipation to both faeces and flatus is diagnostic of bowel obstruction. Although patients may have a long history of constipation, serious disease may supervene and faecal impaction may ultimately cause perforation. Each patient and every presentation must always be assessed in an objective manner. In the absence of a previous history of constipation one should err on the side of caution and transfer the patient to hospital for further assessment. Patients with continuing pain who are not admitted should be reviewed.

OTHER FEATURES

Haematuria suggests disease of the genitourinary tract. However, haematuria may be a manifestation of disease of other systems. In the absence of gross haematuria, urine should be dipsticked for blood. A pregnancy test is mandatory in any woman presenting with an acute abdomen despite any assurances from the patient that pregnancy is an impossibility. Modern pregnancy tests are simple to use, rapid and extremely accurate.

Anorexia is a common feature of so many illnesses as to be unhelpful. However, in the child with suspected appendicitis, lack of anorexia virtually excludes the diagnosis.

The past medical history must be sought, and no history is ever complete without a drug history, including alcohol intake. If possible, medication should be collected and taken to the emergency department.

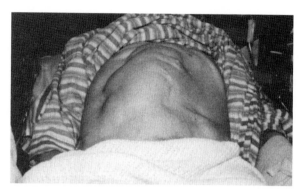

Fig. 12.1 • Visibly distended loops of bowel in acute intestinal obstruction.

Physical examination

Examination always begins with the general observation of the patient in order to establish whether the patient looks ill. Initial assessment must follow first principles, with attention to the airway, breathing and circulation. The pulse, blood pressure and respiratory rate must be recorded and rechecked periodically. The patient must be fully exposed, remembering that the surface markings of the abdominal cavity extend from the fourth to fifth intercostal space to the anus.

Although the patient with generalized peritonitis often lies motionless and quiet, while the patient with ureteric colic writhes and screams, pain is a such a subjective experience that one should not gauge the severity of the underlying diagnosis from the degree of expressed patient discomfort. Patients with peritonitis occasionally gain some relief by flexing their legs, whereas patients with pancreatitis often lie in the fetal position, thus relaxing the psoas muscles.

Signs of hypovolaemic shock with hypotension, tachycardia and tachypnoea suggest intraperitoneal haemorrhage. In an elderly male this should suggest ruptured aortic aneurysm, and in every female of childbearing age the diagnosis is ruptured ectopic pregnancy until proven otherwise. Ribcage excursions are often reduced because of chest wall splinting when peritonitis is present.

Fever is usually present in peritonitis but not invariably so. Rigors are suggestive of Gram-negative septicaemia. This is most commonly seen in acute pyelonephritis, which may present as an acute abdomen. Rigors may also be a feature of advanced peritonitis or ascending cholangitis.

Jaundice is usually obvious but assessment of anaemia is notoriously difficult. Cyanosis may be present, especially if the patient has severe pancreatitis. Signs of chronic liver disease may suggest alcohol abuse and direct one to a

particular diagnostic possibility such as perforation or pancreatitis. Patients occasionally categorically deny alcohol abuse but this possibility should always be considered.

The abdomen should be inspected carefully. Its shape may yield clues. The abdomen has been said to develop a scaphoid contracted shape following perforation of a peptic ulcer. A visible distended bowel obviously suggests bowel obstruction (Fig. 12.1) and visible peristaltic waves may be seen. The measurement of abdominal girth should be avoided as it is useless in the acute setting.

The presence of previous surgical scars may suggest adhesions as a cause for obstruction, and a previous appendicectomy scar allows one to narrow the differential diagnosis, particularly in young females. Evidence of retroperitoneal bleeding such as Cullen's sign and Grey Turner's sign may be apparent and indicate ruptured abdominal aortic aneurysm or pancreatitis.

The male genitalia must always be examined. Testicular torsion may cause high abdominal pain that may be periodic or disappear altogether. Abdominal examination may be otherwise normal and the diagnosis may be missed, with catastrophic results.

AUSCULTATION

In the acute setting, auscultation yields little additional information and undue emphasis is often placed on it. However, certain auscultatory findings may be indicative of certain pathologies. For example, a silent bowel is indicative of peritonitis or late bowel obstruction, and tinkly bowel sounds suggests small bowel obstruction. On the other hand, non-surgical causes producing high-pitched, hyperperistaltic sounds are a finding in gastroenteritis and inflammatory bowel disease. In traumatic abdominal injury, bowel sounds may be present for a time, even in the presence of severe intra-abdominal bleeding. The best information that one should hope to obtain is whether bowel sounds are present or not, and one should listen for at least 90 s before deciding that they are absent.

PALPATION

Palpation should be gentle. It is often necessary to draw up the patient's knees to reduce voluntary guarding. Additional relaxation may be obtained by encouraging the patient to speak while the examination is being performed.

The abdomen is examined systematically, assessing the degree of tenderness and its specific location. Localized tenderness is usually a feature of acute appendicitis, acute cholecystitis, acute diverticulitis and acute salpingitis. Pelvic inflammatory disease does not usually cause unilateral pain, as the disease process is diffuse. Guarding is an important distinguishing sign and is usually absent in conditions that may mimic acute abdomen, such as gastroenteritis.

Visceral peritoneal irritation such as bowel obstruction or mesenteric infarction may give only vague tenderness and is often unaccompanied by guarding. Consequently, the absence of guarding does not exclude life-threatening abdominal conditions. A classic sign of peritonitis is rebound tenderness, although undue emphasis should not be placed on its absence. It may be difficult to elicit in the patient with guarding, either voluntary or involuntary, and it is also very painful and unpleasant for the patient. In general, the same information can be obtained by more gentle means. Gentle percussion of the abdomen that elicits pain suggests peritonitis and is more sensitive in detecting it. In addition, hyperresonance may be elicited in cases of obstruction, and the bladder may be outlined in urinary retention. Although shifting dullness is a sign of intraperitoneal fluid, it may be difficult to elicit, particularly in the elderly.

An old-fashioned technique is to gently shake the patient's bed. If the patient finds this painful, it is highly indicative of peritonitis. A more acceptable approach is to ask the patient to cough; if this causes abdominal pain it is almost diagnostic of peritonitis.

Once seen, the board-like abdomen of generalized peritonitis is never forgotten; however, less severe or more localized peritonitis may be much more difficult to establish. One should always elicit physical signs using the minimum of stimulation. This is more gentle to the patient and positive findings are more meaningful.

The hernial orifices must be specifically examined: strangulated femoral hernia in females may be quite difficult to detect. Although an abdominal examination is never complete without a rectal examination, this is often impracticable or inappropriate in the prehospital setting.

The presence of any masses should be noted. An expansile abdominal mass indicates an abdominal aortic aneurysm and palpation should not be deep or unnecessarily repeated, for obvious reasons.

Murphy's sign is positive when inspiration is stopped by the tender and inflamed gallbladder contacting the palpating hand, and is highly suggestive of acute cholecystitis.

Psoas abscess, although rare, may give rise to pain when the hip is passively flexed or extended. Bowel trapped in the obturator canal may elicit pain on internal and external hip rotation.

Common causes of an acute abdomen

ABDOMINAL AORTIC ANEURYSM

Abdominal aortic aneurysm is one of the most deadly emergencies. It is usually heralded by acute abdominal and/or back pain. 90% of patients with ruptured abdominal aortic aneurysm die before reaching hospital (D'Angelo et al 1993). Of those that reach hospital, mortality approaches 50–75% in the shocked patient and 20% if the patient is not shocked (Aburahma et al 1991). The incidence of ruptured abdominal aortic aneurysm has increased, as has its mortality, despite increased awareness and improved diagnostic modalities. Around 80% of patients with ruptured abdominal aortic aneurysm have never been previously diagnosed as having an abdominal aortic aneurysm. The diagnostic triad of back/abdominal pain, hypotension and a pulsatile mass is diagnostic, but is only present in up to 42% of patients (Banerjee 1993). In a recent series, only 36% of patients developed a systolic pressure of less than 100 mmHg and tachycardia on arrival at the emergency department (Zimmer 1988). The symptoms and signs of an expanding or ruptured abdominal aortic aneurysm may be subtle and most patients have no prior knowledge of their aneurysm. Less common presentations include haematemesis (5%) secondary to aortoenteric fistula and neurological symptoms such as cord ischaemia below T10–T12 due to interruption of flow in the artery of Adamkeiwicz. Up to one-third of cases are misdiagnosed, most commonly as renal colic, acute diverticulitis and gastrointestinal haemorrhage (Marston 1992). Urological symptoms occur in up to 10% of patients because of retroperitoneal compression of sympathetic ureteric pain fibres, and haematuria may manifest as a result of ureteric irritation or renal parenchymal damage.

Ruptured abdominal aortic aneurysm should always be considered as a cause for syncope in the elderly. Between 75% and 90% of abdominal aortic aneurysms rupture into the left retroperitoneal space, which tamponades and may allow containment of bleeding, with potential for survival. It may also give normal vital signs. Rupture directly into the peritoneal cavity usually causes rapid death.

Prehospital fluid replacement for shocked patients must not be too vigorous as this may be detrimental. The presence of a radial pulse should be maintained. The most important step is to convey the patient to an emergency department without delay. The receiving hospital should be alerted as soon as possible so that the surgical team is ready and operating theatres are prepared. In shocked patients diagnostic tests are unnecessary and immediate operation offers the only prospect of salvage. Even if the diagnosis of ruptured abdominal aortic aneurysm is incorrect, around 75% of these patients still have serious intra-abdominal pathology requiring laparotomy (Valentine et al 1993).

ACUTE APPENDICITIS

The classic presentation is of dull periumbilical pain that migrates to the right iliac fossa, becoming sharp in nature. There is accompanying anorexia, nausea and vomiting. Local peritonitis overlying the inflamed appendix gives rise to guarding and rebound tenderness in the right iliac fossa.

McBurney's point is 4–5 cm (1.5–2 inches) above the anterior superior iliac spine on a straight line to the umbilicus, and is the surface landmark that traditionally defines the appendix. However, up to 41% of appendices are mobile and 70% lie inferior to this point. Therefore, the diagnosis must not be based purely on the location of the pain at an exact site in the right iliac fossa.

Abdominal pain occurs in almost 100% of patients, is epigastric in onset in 74%, migrating to the right iliac fossa in 50%. Anorexia is present in 92% and is accompanied by nausea and vomiting in 78% and 54% respectively (Jotte 1996).

In acute appendicitis 19% of all cases perforate with an associated increased morbidity and mortality (Addis et al 1990). Perforation leads to generalized peritonitis or to localized abscess formation. The mortality from ruptured appendix is 1.66%, seven times the mortality for those undergoing appendicectomy for acute appendicitis, and therefore the clinician must aim to diagnose acute appendicitis before perforation occurs (Velanovich et al 1992). The mortality of perforated appendix is 23 times higher in the patient over 60 years of age. Appendicitis is more difficult to diagnose in women, and there is a 35% false-negative appendicectomy rate in young women. Pregnancy increases the perforation rate to 43% (Tamir 1990) but the mortality remains low at 0.7%. However, fetal mortality approaches 8.5%.

Overall diagnostic accuracy averages approximately 85%. The most reliable sign is right iliac fossa tenderness, which is present in nearly all patients. Guarding is seen in around one-third. Rovsing's sign, which is right iliac fossa pain caused by palpation in the left iliac fossa, is seen in 25% of patients and further supports the diagnosis. Special care must be taken with children, gravid females and the elderly, as the diagnosis may be missed and the morbidity and mortality are so much higher. Only 20% of patients over 60 years of age with appendicitis present with the classic symptoms and signs. Perforation may be difficult to distinguish from uncomplicated appendicitis, although more generalized peritonitis is clearly indicative of the former.

GALLBLADDER DISEASE

Gallstones are quite prevalent, occurring in 25% of women and 15% of men. Most are asymptomatic. The commonest complication is biliary colic, which is usually benign and self-resolving. However, life-threatening complications can occur and a high level of suspicion must be maintained. Biliary colic presents with continuous pain in the mid-epigastrium or right upper quadrant. The pain may radiate to the back and scapula. Pain that persists for more than 4 h should suggest that acute cholecystitis or acute pancreatitis may be present. With biliary colic there is often a minor degree of nausea and vomiting, and physical findings are usually sparse. There may be tenderness in the left upper quadrant but Murphy's sign is negative. Acute cholecystitis usually presents with much sharper and more localized pain, which may radiate to the epigastrium or scapula. Nausea and vomiting are usually more pronounced and the patient generally looks unwell. There is usually a low-grade fever. Local peritonism is evident and Murphy's sign is usually positive.

Gallbladder perforation is usually seen in the elderly, infirm or diabetic. The signs are usually more florid and more generalized depending on whether the leakage is contained locally. Jaundice, fever, rigors and right upper quadrant pain are features of ascending cholangitis; the patients usually appear septic but the presentation may be more subtle. Overall mortality for this condition approaches 40%.

Special attention must be paid to patients with AIDS, as acute cholecystitis may be secondary to cytomegalovirus and *Cryptosporidium* infection. This acute acalculous cholecystitis has a mortality approaching 67%.

ACUTE PANCREATITIS

Acute pancreatitis may be a life-threatening condition characterized by haemorrhagic necrosis of the pancreas with severe multiorgan dysfunction and death in up to 10% of cases.

Abdominal pain is the most characteristic feature. The pain is typically severe, although it may be poorly localized in the epigastrium and left upper quadrant. The pain often radiates to the back, and is often aggravated by lying down with the patient gaining partial relief by sitting forward. These patients often look quite unwell. Vomiting is often a prominent feature and may be copious. The abdominal findings are often not striking, but signs of peritonism such as guarding and rebound tenderness may be seen. Tenderness is usually diffuse and may be surprisingly mild. Patients may be shocked and the presentation may suggest intraperitoneal haemorrhage. These severe cases involving haemorrhagic necrosis of the pancreas may give rise to retroperitoneal haemorrhage seen as bruising in the flanks (Grey Turner's sign) or around the umbilicus (Cullen's sign). It should be noted that these signs may also be seen in ruptured aortic aneurysm, and their presence always signifies severe disease.

MESENTERIC INFARCTION

Despite an increased awareness of this condition and its poor outcome, the mortality still exceeds 50%, primarily due to delayed diagnosis. Ischaemia is followed by fluid losses and ultimately gangrene. There are no reliable diagnostic criteria for the condition, and florid signs indicating a major intra-abdominal catastrophe often supervene when the patient is unsalvageable. The condition is seen primarily in the elderly and patients usually have a long history of cardiac disease, most often left-ventricular failure or atrial fibrillation. Pain is almost always present but is of the visceral type and variable in nature. Although often variable in onset, sudden abdominal pain should alert the clinician to the possibility of this diagnosis. Patients often look very sick and up to 40% are obviously volume-depleted (Andersson et al 1984). Abdominal examination is almost never normal but often yields few signs and appears at odds with the pain expressed by the patient. Nausea and vomiting feature in 50–75% of cases and in 25% macroscopic blood is present in the stool or vomitus. Approximately 10% of patients present shocked in extremis, with near uniform mortality.

PEPTIC ULCER DISEASE

Peptic ulcer disease is very common, affecting up to 3% of the population (Kurata & Haile 1984). Although mortality rates have fallen overall over the past few decades, they remain very high for the elderly, being 50–100 times greater at the age of 75 years than at 35 years (Walt et al 1986). It should be remembered that up to one-third of patients with perforated peptic ulcer give no previous history of ulcer disease. Although the pain of peptic ulcer and gastritis is often severe, perforation is suggested by the sudden onset of severe upper abdominal pain associated with signs of peritonitis. For previously symptomatic patients with ulcer pain, a significant change in the pain pattern should suggest that perforation may have occurred. Minor perforations or posterior perforation may result in more gradual symptoms and a slower development of signs. Posterior perforation may also be suggested by severe pain radiating to the back. Although patients with peptic ulcer disease may express very severe abdominal pain, signs of peritonitis such as involuntary guarding and rebound are absent. Shock obviously suggests perforation, and the peritonitis evoked usually forces patients to lie still.

RENAL CALCULUS DISEASE

Renal colic occurs when a calculus obstructs the renal pelvis and upper ureter. The pain is visceral and is felt in the loin and flank, often radiating around into the groin. As the stone migrates down the ureter the pain tends to radiate to the genitalia. The pain of ureteric colic is often agonizing and patients may scream and writhe around. This is in contrast to most cases of peritonitis, when patients tend to lie motionless. Gross haematuria is often absent, but blood is almost invariably present on dipstick testing. Patients often sweat profusely and have nausea and vomiting. The loin is usually tender and signs of peritonism such as guarding may be present, especially if there is superadded infection of the kidney.

It may be impossible to examine the patient without first administering analgesia; diclofenac is highly effective and should be given before opiates. Nitrous oxide is useful and often allows adequate analgesia until the diclofenac takes effect. Although not a life-threatening condition, the patient should be urgently investigated, as obstruction of a single kidney is potentially catastrophic and should be excluded without delay. Moreover, abdominal aortic aneurysm can masquerade as renal colic in older patients and thus aneurysm needs to be excluded in any male over the age of 40 years.

ECTOPIC PREGNANCY

This remains one of the leading causes of maternal death in the UK. In the USA the frequency of ectopic pregnancy has increased fivefold since 1970. Haemorrhagic shock is the cause of death in the majority of cases, and misdiagnosis contributes to 50% of the fatalities (Dorfman et al 1984). The classic presentation of ectopic pregnancy is amenorrhoea, vaginal bleeding and abdominal pain. However, this triad is only seen in 15% of patients, and only 14% of patients with this triad actually have ectopic pregnancy. However, abdominal pain is almost universal and occurs without bleeding in up to one-third of patients. Up to one-third of patients give a normal menstrual history. The pain is hugely variable, both in terms of onset, character and location.

The diagnosis must be excluded in any woman of childbearing age who presents with abdominal pain. The absence of shock is, unfortunately, often interpreted as a signal that investigation can proceed in a leisurely manner. This complacency can be catastrophic, as deterioration may be sudden and absolute, leading to rapid death despite vigorous circulatory support. As a rule, a positive pregnancy test and abdominal pain must be regarded as an ectopic pregnancy until the gestation sac can be shown to be intrauterine.

OTHER GYNAECOLOGICAL CAUSES

Sudden abdominal pain is also a feature of ovarian cyst disease. Pain may be due to rupture, distension or torsion. This diagnosis can only be *suspected* in the prehospital setting. Local peritonitis may be evident at an early stage. Ovarian torsion usually presents dramatically with sudden and extreme pain. The pain may radiate to the back or even the thigh. There is often associated nausea and vomiting. The appearance may resemble renal colic or acute appendicitis. Severe pelvic inflammatory disease can present with severe pain, although the onset is usually more gradual. It should be remembered that tubo-ovarian abscess can occur in pelvic inflammatory disease and may rupture, so even patients with a long history of pelvic inflammatory disease should be carefully examined.

BOWEL OBSTRUCTION

Most cases of small bowel obstruction are secondary to adhesions from previous surgical operations, and the presence of surgical scars on the abdominal wall is highly significant. Other causes include intussusception (which may be seen in the older patient), malignancy, diverticulitis and hernias. Overall mortality is up to 10%.

Although simple obstruction may follow a relatively slow course, leading to gradual fluid losses and volume depletion, strangulation leads to bowel ischaemia and necrosis. Therefore, the diagnosis of bowel obstruction warrants immediate transfer to hospital in anticipation of life-threatening complications. Abdominal pain is usually the predominant feature of bowel obstruction. It is visceral in nature and is often severe, although usually bearable. It is usually accompanied by nausea and vomiting, especially if the small bowel obstruction is proximal, in which case it is usually an early feature. Faeculant vomiting is unusual and is suggestive of distal small bowel obstruction. Moreover, vomiting may be completely absent in distal small bowel and large bowel obstruction.

Constipation is variable and the inability to pass flatus is more significant, although this may be a late finding. Some degree of abdominal distension is usually present, although this may be surprisingly difficult to detect in the obese and elderly. Auscultation adds little additional information, is time-consuming and should be avoided. High-pitched tinkling bowel sounds support the diagnosis of obstruction, but the absence of bowel sounds is more ominous, suggesting bowel strangulation. Palpation is usually tender and the hernial orifices must be examined carefully.

DIVERTICULAR DISEASE

Most patients with colonic diverticulosis remain asymptomatic but the older a patient becomes the more likely are complications. The main complications are acute diverticulitis and rectal bleeding.

Diverticulosis per se may present as dull, crampy pain in the left iliac fossa. The patients look systemically well and relief may be obtained by bowel opening. Acute diverticulitis may present with gradual onset of pain or even abrupt pain in the left lower quadrant with signs of local peritonism. Nausea and vomiting are often present, and patients usually look quite unwell, with signs of infection such as fever and tachycardia. Rectal bleeding, which may be massive, can occur without associated pain. A mass suggests diverticular abscess or perforation that has been contained locally. Patients with diverticulitis often give a history of previous attacks. As these patients are elderly, signs of perforation may be subtle, especially if the patient is taking corticosteroids for another medical condition. All patients with suspected diverticulitis should be taken to hospital for formal investigation and management.

MEDICAL CAUSES OF SEVERE ABDOMINAL PAIN

Myocardial infarction and pneumonia can both give rise to severe abdominal pain, but signs of peritonitis are absent. However, because catastrophic intra-abdominal events such as mesenteric infarction can present with few signs, the true diagnosis may be impossible to establish out of hospital. Therefore, patients should be transported with continuous cardiac monitoring. Diabetic ketoacidosis can present as very severe abdominal pain, and it is always worth measuring the patient's blood sugar while in transit. When the degree of pain is disproportionately greater than the physical findings, one should consider a medical cause.

Reaching a diagnosis

Medical teaching instructs one to reach a diagnosis as a consequence of sequential analysis of information obtained in a logical vertically ordered path. However, in real practice, diagnosis is reached by horizontal cluster analysis, whereby all available information is simultaneously processed. This results in pattern spotting, where certain features of the clinical presentation and findings indicate a likely diagnosis. This allows one to reach rapid working conclusions about the likely diagnosis without ploughing through long lists of differential diagnoses.

First, immediately consider the age of the patient when formulating the likely diagnosis. As can be seen in Table 12.1, age stratifies probable diagnosis in a most helpful manner. For example, for a child under 2 years old approximately 95% of cases of abdominal pain fall into three groups: non-specific, appendicitis and intussusception. In

Table 12.1 Underlying diagnosis with acute abdominal pain

Children aged under 2 years	Adolescents	Adults aged under 50 years	Adults aged over 50 years
Non-specific (61%)	Acute appendicitis	Non-specific (39%)	Cholecystitis (21%)
Acute appendicitis (32%)	Ectopic pregnancy	Appendicitis (32%)	Non-specific (15.7%)
Intussusception (1.3%)		Cholecystitis (6.3%)	Appendicitis (15.2%)
Others:		Bowel obstruction (2.5%)	Bowel obstruction (12.5%)
Non-accidental		Pancreatitis (1.6%)	Pancreatitis (7.3%)
Toxins (5.5%)		Diverticular disease (<0.1%)	Diverticular disease
Primary enterocolitis		Hernia (<0.1%)	Malignancy (4.1%)
		Cancer (<0.1%)	Hernia (3.1%)
		Vascular (<0.1%)	Vascular (2.3%)

Table 12.2 Features and suggested diagnosis

Finding	Consider
Severe abdominal pain radiating to back	Active labour Aortic aneurysm Acute cholecystitis Acute pancreatitis Peptic ulcer disease
Flank pain radiating to groin	Aortic aneurysm Testicular torsion Pyelonephritis Renal/ureteric colic
Pain out of proportion to physical examination	Aortic aneurysm Mesenteric infarction Renal colic Porphyria
Collapse or signs of shock	Aortic aneurysm Ectopic pregnancy Gastrointestinal bleed Myocardial infarction
Distension	Bowel obstruction Ascites Mass Pregnancy
Abdominal bruising	Trauma Aortic aneurysm Acute pancreatitis Coagulopathy
Haematemesis or melaena	Aortic aneurysm (aorto-enteric fistula) Ulcer Diverticular disease Angiodysplasia Malignancy Varices
Constipation	Bowel ischaemia Bowel obstruction Diverticular disease Volvulus

the adolescent, for the diagnosis one must always approach the patient thinking 'Does this patient have appendicitis?'.

The older a patient is, the higher is the probability that abdominal pain, and therefore the acute abdomen, has a vascular origin. However, illness does not always respect age and unusual diagnoses should be considered in difficult cases. For example, torsion does occur in the elderly.

At the extremes of age the history may not be forthcoming and one must be more objective. Moreover, age significantly modifies the response to illness, and the young and the elderly may not respond in the classic manner.

Second, certain features of the case should trigger certain considerations. These are detailed in Table 12.2. It should be noted that this concise list covers all the abdominal illnesses that are immediately life-threatening.

Management

The most important management decision for the prehospital physician is to determine the presence or absence of an acute abdomen and to arrange transfer to hospital where appropriate.

Resuscitation follows first principles and begins with the airway. All patients should receive maximal supplemental oxygen. The respiratory system and circulation should then be assessed and any identified problem should be dealt with. Vital signs, including respiratory rate, must be recorded repeatedly. A large-bore cannula should be inserted into the antecubital fossa. Prehospital care must address volume replacement, as early death from acute abdomen usually results from fluid loss. Although controversy rages around which type of fluid to give, in practice it is unimportant as long as volume expansion occurs. Vigorous fluid administration should be avoided if ruptured abdominal aortic aneurysm is suspected. Attempts to restore a normal circulation may lead to a loss of the retroperitoneal tamponade, leading to further bleeding, worsening shock and death. Normovolaemia should only be obtained in the operating theatre once haemostasis is obtained. As long as the patient is conscious and has adequate peripheral circulation, this is sufficient volume resuscitation (Ernst 1993). There must be continuous electrocardiographic monitoring with non-invasive blood pressure measurement and continuous pulse oximetry.

Pain relief must be addressed. It is wrong to withhold analgesia from patients with severe pain. Giving analgesia does not mask the signs of an acute abdomen; on the contrary, diagnosis may be facilitated (Attard et al 1992). Opiates are the preferred analgesics for severe pain, except for renal colic, where diclofenac is the first choice. Morphine or diamorphine should be used in preference to pethidine. Pethidine confers no clinical benefit whatsoever over morphine with regard to often quoted effects on sphincter contractility. The preferred route for analgesia is intravenous, and opiates should be titrated to the patient's needs. Intramuscular injections are painful, and drugs have a delayed onset of action and unpredictable effect. The elderly are much more susceptible to respiratory depression and smaller aliquots should be given. An anti-emetic should also be given.

Pregnant patients in the third trimester should be transported in the left decubitus position where possible, as should unconscious patients or patients who are vomiting. Airway control is essential.

If the diagnosis of ruptured abdominal aortic aneurysm is suspected, the receiving hospital must be informed so that appropriate preparations can be made for immediate surgery.

References

Aburahma AH, Woodruff BA, Stuart SPL et al 1991 Early diagnosis and survival of ruptured abdominal aortic aneurysm. American Journal of Emergency Medicine 9: 118–121

Addis DG, Shaffer N, Fowler S, Tauxe RV 1990 The epidemiology of appendicitis and appendectomy in the United States. American Journal of Epidemiology 132: 910

American College of Emergency Physicians 1994 Clinical policy for the initial approach to patients presenting with a chief complaint of non-traumatic acute abdominal pain. Annals of Emergency Medicine 23: 906–919

Andersson R, Parsson H, Isaksson B, Nagren L 1984 Acute intestinal ischaemia. Acta Chirurgica Scandinavica 150: 217

Attard AR, Corlett MJ, Kidner NJ et al 1992 Safety of early pain relief for acute abdominal pain. British Medical Journal 305: 554–556

Banerjee A 1993 Atypical manifestations of ruptured abdominal aortic aneurysms. Postgraduate Medical Journal 69: 6–11

Brewer RJ, Golden GT, Hitch D et al 1976 Abdominal pain: an analysis of 1,000 consecutive cases in a university hospital emergency room. American Journal of Surgery 131: 219–223

D'Angelo F, Vaghi M, Martassi R et al 1993 Changing trends in the outcome of urgent aneurysm surgery. A retrospective study on 170 patients treated in the years 1966–1990. Journal of Cardiovascular Surgery 34: 237–239

Dorfman SF, Grimes DA, Cates W et al 1984 Ectopic pregnancy mortality, United States 1979 to 1980: clinical aspects. Obstetrics and Gynecology 64: 386

Ernst CB 1993 Abdominal aortic aneurysm. New England Journal of Medicine 328: 1167–1172

Jotte R 1996 Acute appendicitis. In: Harwood-Nuss AL (ed) The clinical practice of emergency medicine, 2nd edn. Lippincott-Raven, Philadelphia, PA, p 155–159

Kurata JH, Haile BM 1984 Epidemiology of peptic ulcer disease. Clinical Gastroenterology 89: 289

Marston WA, Ahlquist R, Johnson G Jr, Meyer AA 1992 Misdiagnosis of ruptured abdominal aortic aneurysms. Journal of Vascular Surgery 16: 17–22

Tamir HL, Bongard FS, Klein SR 1990 Acute appendicitis in the pregnant patient. American Journal of Surgery 160: 571

Valentine RJ, Barth MJ, Myers SI, Clagett GP 1993 Nonvascular emergencies presenting as ruptured abdominal aortic aneurysms. Surgery 113: 286–289

Velanovich V, Satava R 1992 Balancing the normal appendectomy rate with the perforated appendicitis rate: implications for quality assurance. American Surgeon 58: 264

Walt RP, Katschinski B, Logan R et al 1986 Rising frequency of peptic ulcer perforation in elderly people in the United Kingdom. Lancet 1: 489

Zimmer T 1988 Absence of back pain and tachycardia in the emergency presentation of abdominal aortic aneurysm. American Journal of Emergency Medicine 6: 316–321

Further reading

Carson SA, Buster JE 1993 Ectopic pregnancy. New England Journal of Medicine 329: 1174

Scheeres DE, DeKryger LL, Dean RE 1987 Surgical treatment of peptic ulcer disease before and after introduction of H_2-blockers. Annals of Surgery 53: 392

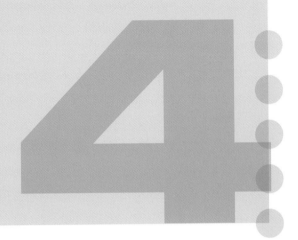

Part Four

13 Therapeutics 151
14 Analgesia and pain relief 162
15 Substance abuse 173
16 Poisoning 182

Therapeutics

13

Introduction	151
Why use drugs in prehospital care?	151
When to use drugs	151
Drug descriptions	156
Summary	160
References	160

Introduction

The 1995 *Oxford English Reference Dictionary* defines 'therapeutics' as 'the branch of medicine concerned with the treatment of disease and the action of remedial agents'.

This chapter presents an overview of the action of drugs and outlines factors relevant to immediate care that influence their selection, dosage and route of delivery.

Why use drugs in prehospital care?

The aims of prehospital care are to save life, preserve function and relieve suffering.

Drugs allow us to achieve these aims in a number of ways, for example:

- *saving life*: by treating hypoxia with oxygen, by beginning antibiotic treatment in bacterial meningitis
- *preserving function*: initiating thrombolysis in myocardial infarction
- *relieving suffering*: by using systemic analgesics, local anaesthesia or general anaesthesia.

Drugs may also be used to allow therapeutic intervention. An example is using intravenous anaesthetic agents and muscle relaxants to allow endotracheal intubation, which in turn allows airway control and oxygen administration.

When to use drugs

All prehospital interventions need to be seen as a balance between providing necessary care at the incident scene and not delaying the patient's onward movement to definitive care (Johnson & Guly 1995). Timely on-scene care may, however, allow the patient to avoid going to hospital altogether.

The choice of drug, the dose and the route of administration depend on a number of factors. These include:

- the suitability of the drug for field use
- the experience and training of the practitioner in using a particular drug
- the clinical condition of the patient, including any pre-existing illnesses and allergies
- the speed of onset required for the drug's action
- the legal classification of a drug and the entitlement of a particular practitioner to use it.

These are considered in turn below.

THE SUITABILITY OF A DRUG FOR FIELD USE

The potential characteristics of an ideal analgesic for use in the field are listed in Table 13.1.

THE EXPERIENCE AND TRAINING OF A PRACTITIONER IN USING A PARTICULAR DRUG

The prehospital environment is not the place to begin using an unfamiliar drug. Training should take place in a more controlled environment (such as the emergency department, intensive care unit or operating theatre) by a practitioner skilled in that drug's use. The individual learning about the drug needs to understand how drug dosage and administration have to be altered depending on the patient's condition.

THE CLINICAL CONDITION OF THE PATIENT, INCLUDING PRE-EXISTING ILLNESSES AND ALLERGIES

Where possible patients should be questioned about pre-existing medical conditions, allergies and drug sensitivities prior to their being given a drug. Even if the patient is unconscious, friends and relatives at the incident scene may know about any medical problems. It is important to check for MedicAlert® bracelets or medallions and medicines carried by the patient. In the absence of any information and if drugs have to be given (e.g. providing rescue anaesthesia in the trapped, unconscious patient) drugs least likely to cause allergic reaction should be selected.

Two situations need special consideration: the shocked patient and the pregnant patient.

The shocked patient

In haemorrhagic shock a number of compensatory responses occur. These include progressive vasoconstriction of skin, muscle and some internal organs to preserve blood flow to the brain, heart and kidneys (American College of Surgeons Committee on Trauma 1997). In some internal injuries, tension in the abdominal muscles ('abdominal splinting') adds to this compensation. The use of drugs such as anaesthetic agents, muscle relaxants and analgesics has the potential to interfere with these compensations and to cause a fall in blood pressure.

This *does not* mean that analgesia and anaesthesia should be withheld. It does mean that analgesics should be given in small intravenous doses titrated to clinical effect while the patient's overall state is monitored and changes managed appropriately. Smaller doses of intravenous anaesthetic drugs will be needed to produce anaesthesia than in an uninjured patient.

This serves to emphasize the need for training in using drugs safely and appropriately prior to deploying into the prehospital environment.

The pregnant patient

The pregnant patient needs special consideration for two reasons:

- Pregnancy involves a number of physiological changes. These include changes in liver metabolism, in renal blood flow and in the concentration of serum proteins relevant to drug binding, as well as an increase in total body water. These lead to a change in the way the body handles certain drugs, and dose adjustments may be required (Rubin 1995, Consumers Association 1996).
- Drugs can have harmful effects on the fetus at any time during pregnancy (British National Formulary 2004).

Medicines taken at or around conception or during pregnancy can harm the fetus (Consumers Association 1996). The effects can vary with the stage of pregnancy:

- During the first trimester drugs can cause congenital malformations (British National Formulary 2004). The type of malformation will depend on which organs are most susceptible at the time of exposure (Consumers Association 1996).
- During the second and third trimesters drugs may affect the growth and development of the fetus or have toxic effects on fetal tissues (British National Formulary 2004).
- Drugs given around the end of pregnancy or in labour may affect the labour or have effects on the baby after delivery (British National Formulary 2004).

Therefore, the benefits of using a particular drug must be greater than the potential risks posed to the mother and fetus.

Table 13.1 The ideal prehospital analgesic

- Powerful action
- Rapid onset and speedy recovery
- Non-depressant on the cardiovascular and respiratory system
- Free from unwanted side effects such as nausea and vomiting
- Portable
- Non-addictive
- Available for safe and easy use by both physicians and non-physicians
- Presented in a form ready to use (rather than having to be mixed on site)
- Presented in robust, non-shattering containers
- Where appropriate, easy to reverse using an antagonist

Reprinted with permission from Baskett PJF 1992 Emergency medicine's involvement in disaster medicine. Baillière's Clinical Anaesthesiology 6(1): 193–207

The *British National Formulary* (2004) recommends that drugs that have been extensively used in pregnancy and appear to be safe should be prescribed in preference to new or untried drugs, and the smallest effective dose should be used. Appendix 4 of the *British National Formulary* provides a table of drugs to be avoided or used with caution in pregnancy and indicates the trimester of risk.

Manufacturers' data sheets provide information about known or likely effects of their drugs, and further information can be obtained from local and national drug information services.

THE SPEED OF ONSET REQUIRED FOR THE DRUG ACTION

The speed of onset will depend on the route of administration of the drug, the preparation of the drug used and the site of action of the drug.

Routes of administration

Routes of drug administration are shown in Table 13.2 and are discussed below.

Intravenous administration
A drug given directly into a vein will be carried within the blood around the body and distributed to different organs and tissues. A proportion will arrive at the target organ or tissue. To cause an effect the drug may need to be actively or passively transported from the blood into the relevant structure. Intravenous administration requires the person giving the drug to be able to locate and cannulate a vein.

Intramuscular administration
A drug given by an injection into muscle (intramuscularly) or under the skin (subcutaneously) relies on the drug being removed from this area by the local blood supply and then distributed by the circulation. This can be a slow process, as the drug needs to get from the tissue into the blood. The local blood supply may be reduced if that area is cold or if the patient is shocked. Resuscitation and rewarming of

the patient with improved perfusion to the area where the drug has been given may result in the drug rapidly entering the circulation, with the risk of overdose. However, intramuscular administration of morphine (into the forearm) was used at the Moorgate underground train disaster, where access to some casualties was too poor to allow intravenous administration (Finch & Nancekievill 1975). In general, however, intramuscular administration has several limitations in prehospital care and therefore intravenous administration is preferable.

Local infiltration
Local infiltration of a drug is a means of delivering the drug to a specific area (e.g. a local anaesthetic into skin to block nerves). Some local anaesthetic preparations (currently EMLA® and Ametop®) can be used as topical ointments to cause anaesthesia over a limited area of skin.

Subcutaneous administration
The drug is absorbed via the subcutaneous tissues. The same problems occur as identified for *intramuscular administration* above.

Transdermal administration
Transdermal delivery is used for drugs such as glyceryl trinitrate, and some analgesic and hormone preparations. The drug is absorbed via the skin into the circulation.

Intraosseous administration
Drugs and fluid given by the intraosseous route into active marrow are carried from the medullary sinusoids to a central venous canal and then into the venous system via the nutrient veins, and can enter the circulation almost as quickly as an intravenous injection (Cooke 1993).

Inhalational administration
A drug given by inhalation may be used to produce a local effect within the lungs (as with an inhaled bronchodilator) or may use the large surface area provided by the alveoli in order to gain access to the circulation. This large surface area usually allows rapid absorption and rapid onset of action. Inhalational general anaesthetics are given this way.

Rectal and sublingual administration
Use of the rectal and sublingual routes tends to avoid the 'first pass effect' (discussed below).

Oral administration
A drug taken by mouth needs to be absorbed via the gastrointestinal tract and then carried by the blood to the site of action. This requires the drug to be dissolved (usually in the stomach) and then absorbed either in the stomach or elsewhere in the intestine. Reduced gastric emptying or reduced gut blood supply can decrease the rate and

Table 13.2 Routes of drug administration	
Injection	**Other**
Intravenous	Intraosseous
Intramuscular	Transdermal
Infiltration	Inhalational
Subcutaneous	Sublingual
Epidural and subarachnoid	Oral Rectal

amount of drug absorption. A proportion of drug will be metabolized in the gut wall. The blood from the intestine drains via the portal system to the liver where further drug metabolism takes place. The gut wall and liver metabolism is known as the *first-pass* effect.

Epidural and subarachnoid drug administration

Epidural and subarachnoid drug administration involves introducing drugs into the epidural or subarachnoid spaces via a needle or catheter system to allow rapid access to the central nervous system (CNS). The intention is usually to block pain signals being transmitted in the spinal cord. Although these methods have been used under field conditions for analgesia (Bull et al 1983, Jowitt & Knight, 1983) this is not common in current UK prehospital care.

Drug action

Drugs are given to cause an effect in an organ or tissue. Consider a drug being carried by the circulation around the body: some drugs tend to become concentrated in a particular tissue or organ, others reach tissues with a large blood supply first but are subsequently moved on to tissues with a lower blood supply (redistribution). A proportion of the drug originally given reaches the organ or tissue of interest (the 'target'). The drug then has to move from the blood into the target organ or tissue. The amount available to do this will depend on whether the drug was being carried bound to a protein or another carrier within the blood or whether it was free. Generally, it is the free portion that is available to move into the target organ or tissue. As the amount of free drug decreases in the blood, 'bound' drug can dissociate from the carrier.

The study of drug absorption, distribution, metabolism and excretion is known as *pharmacokinetics* and can be thought of as 'what the body does to a drug'. A number of mathematical models have been developed to explain these processes. *Pharmacodynamics* (what the drug does to the body) is the study of the pharmacological effects of the drug (Nimmo 1990).

Pharmacokinetics: what the body does to the drug.

A drug works by interacting with 'biological targets' that are chemical components of the body (Foster 1996). Such components include cell membranes, enzyme systems, receptors and transport carriers. The effects of a drug on the body are known as pharmacodynamic effects.

Pharmacodynamics: what the drug does to the body.

In addition to the desired effect, drugs can have unwanted actions, or side effects, such as the nausea associated with opiate analgesia. Side effects are one of the factors to be considered in drug selection. Another problem is producing an exaggerated response to a drug. For example, most intravenous general anaesthetic agents cause a fall in blood pressure. If they are given to a patient suffering from shock they may produce a large fall in blood pressure.

Drugs are described as being *contraindicated* in certain circumstances. Contraindications are divided into absolute and relative. An *absolute* contraindication means the drug should never be given in these circumstances, such as when a person has had a severe allergic reaction to the drug in the past. A *relative* contraindication indicates that significant harm may come to the patient from using the drug but certain circumstances may justify this risk.

Termination of a drug's action can be due to redistribution of the drug to other areas of the body or by drug breakdown (metabolism) in the liver and other organs. The breakdown products of drugs may themselves have pharmacological effects. The breakdown products (and some unchanged drug) are eventually eliminated from the body in urine, bile and, to a lesser extent, saliva and breast milk. The majority of the dose of an inhalational anaesthetic agent is exhaled.

Agonists, partial agonists and antagonists

These concepts are useful when considering using agents such as naloxone or flumazenil to reverse the effects of, respectively, opioids and benzodiazepines.

Consider a drug interacting with a receptor:

- An *agonist* interacts with the receptor to cause an active response within the cell, e.g. morphine causing respiratory depression at the μ-opioid receptor.

- An *antagonist* interacts with the receptor but does not cause an active response. It stops the agonist gaining access to the receptor and thus prevents the effect of the agonist, e.g. naloxone reversing the respiratory depressant effects of morphine.

- A *partial agonist* can be thought of as a drug with properties in between these. When given on its own the drug causes an active response but not as great as the full agonist. If given with the full agonist it competes with it for receptors, thus reducing (antagonizing) the effect of the full agonist; e.g. buprenorphine is a partial agonist at μ-opioid receptors.

The situation in practice can be much more complicated. Drugs having agonist properties at one type of receptor may be antagonist at another. Drugs acting as an antagonist may not last as long as the drug they are trying to antagonize. For example, naloxone does not last as long as many of the opioids, so repeat doses may be required.

Drug dosage

Recommended drug dosages are given on manufacturers' data sheets and in the *British National Formulary*. Dosage may have to be altered depending on the patient's general state of health (particularly cardiac, respiratory, renal and liver diseases) and the presence of injuries.

Drug doses are expressed in a number of different ways including dose per kilogram body weight or dose according to age.

In paediatric practice calculating the correct dose for a patient can be greatly assisted by using the Oakley chart (Oakley 1988, Oakley et al 1993) or the Broselow tape (Luten et al 1992).

THE LEGAL CLASSIFICATION OF A DRUG AND THE ENTITLEMENT OF A PARTICULAR PRACTITIONER TO USE IT

The following section gives a brief outline of the law relating to drugs in the UK. It is strongly recommended that practitioners consult local pharmacists and steering committees if advice is needed regarding the storage, security and appropriate use of drugs. This is also important if the practitioner is using a drug for a purpose outside that drug's product licence (Consumers Association 1992). Use of some drugs outside hospital is a use outside the product licence.

The Medicines Act 1968 and its secondary legislation provides a regulatory scheme of licences, registrations and exemptions that control all aspects of the production and distribution of all medicinal products (Association of Anaesthetists of Great Britain and Ireland 1995).

The Medicines Act 1968 classifies drugs as:

- general sales list (GSL) medicines, suitable for unsupervised sale in shops or supermarkets
- pharmacy-only (P) medicines, which can only be sold or supplied in a pharmacy under the direct supervision of a pharmacist
- prescription-only medicines (POM), which can only be sold or supplied in accordance with a prescription of a registered practitioner (Foster 1996).

The Misuse of Drugs Act 1971 provides the basis of control for certain drugs. Drugs are placed into Class A, B or C based on the harmfulness attributable to a drug when it is misused (British National Formulary 2004). The penalties for unlawful possession of the more harmful drugs are more severe than for those considered less harmful (Cahal 1974a).

The Misuse of Drugs Regulations 1985 define the classes of person authorized to supply and possess controlled drugs while acting in their professional capacities. Conditions are laid down under which these activities may be carried out (British National Formulary 2004).

Drugs are divided into five schedules (Association of Anaesthetists of Great Britain and Ireland 1995, British National Formulary 2004):

- Schedule 1 contains drugs with no recognized medicinal use, including cannabis, hallucinogens, raw opium and coca leaf. These are the most tightly controlled.
- Schedule 2 covers pharmaceutical opioids, amphetamines and cocaine. These are subject to the full controlled drug regulations relating to prescriptions, safe custody and the need to keep registers.
- Schedule 3 contains barbiturates and some slimming preparations.
- Schedule 4 contains benzodiazepines.
- Schedule 5 includes products containing low concentrations of drugs that would be in Schedule 2 if in a stronger preparation.

The Safe Custody Regulations 1973 define the type of cabinet or safe that should be used to store controlled drugs securely. These regulations refer to Schedule 2 and 3 drugs (but many Schedule 3 drugs are exempted) (Association of Anaesthetists of Great Britain and Ireland, 1995, British National Formulary 2004). Effectively this means that specified controlled drugs need to be kept in a locked receptacle which can only be opened by somebody authorized to do so.

Cahal (1974b) felt that, based on previous legal judgements, a locked car did not count as a locked receptacle for the purposes of these regulations.

Paramedic practice

The Joint Royal Colleges and Ambulance Liaison Committee (JRCALC), the Professional Advisory Group to the Scottish Ambulance Service and the Northern Ireland Ambulance Advisory Panel have agreed a list of medicines appropriate for use by extended trained ambulance personnel (Welsh Affairs Committee 1996).

Local paramedic steering committees can decide which of the listed drugs will be used by paramedics operating in their area. They can also recommend for local use drugs that do not appear on the list but that can be administered under the direction of a doctor (in accordance with the Medicines Act 1968) as set out in locally agreed protocols.

In December 1992, a Prescription-only Medicine Amendment Order was passed to allow National Health Service Training Directive (NHSTD) paramedics to administer, on their own initiative, certain POMs parenterally for emergency treatment of the sick and injured. This was in addition to the ability to administer parenteral POMs on a doctor's instructions (Welsh Affairs Committee 1996).

The Home Office has authorized a 'group authority' under the Misuse of Drugs Regulations 1985 for NHS paramedics serving or employed at an approved ambulance station within the NHS to administer diazepam (a controlled drug) in immediate care (Welsh Affairs Committee 1996).

Drug packs in use

Realistically, there is a limit to what can be carried for a given situation and choices need to be made. This will be influenced by the tasks required of the individual or team, their training and the drugs they are legally entitled to use. A family doctor carrying drugs to treat a range of illnesses has a different requirement from a team responding primarily to trauma. In addition, content may be influenced by the conditions in which the drug pack or bag is going to be stored. Even storage in a bag in a car in the UK can expose drugs to temperatures outside that needed for optimum storage (Rudland & Jacobs 1994).

A number of authors have described drug and equipment packs suitable for prehospital and field use. This has included drugs for a mobile anaesthetic service (Roux et al 1992), for GPs (Consumers Association 1989, 1995) and for displaced populations (Hogerzeil & Pinel 1991).

The drug pack from the London Helicopter Emergency Medical Service (HEMS) is given as an example in Table 13.3. The Helicopter Emergency Medical Service has been operating from the rooftop helipad at the Royal London Hospital since August 1990. The present medical crew consists of a doctor (either a post-fellowship anaesthetist, surgeon, physician or emergency medicine specialist) and a paramedic. This combination allows use of a much broader group of drugs than would be the case for a paramedic crew alone. The quantities described are for the drug pack carried in the HEMS rucksack and, like all equipment carried on a helicopter, are a compromise between what is desired and what is essential given weight and space limitations. After a call-out the drug packs are replenished. Other medical equipment carried on the aircraft included intravenous fluids, portable monitors and a defibrillator. The pack described below allows the team to perform resuscitation, provide analgesia, give a general anaesthetic and comply with other locally agreed protocols. The contents of the pack are changed, however, as these guidelines and protocols are revised.

Drug descriptions

The following descriptions of drugs are intended to give a basic outline of drug action and use in prehospital care. In-hospital uses are mentioned for some drugs but this is not intended to be comprehensive, rather to put the drug into context.

Table 13.3 The HEMS London drugs pack (2007)

i. Resuscitation drugs
- Adrenaline (epinephrine): six 10 ml of 1:10 000 dilution (1 mg in 10 ml)
- Atropine sulphate: three 10 ml of 100 µg ml^{-1} (1 mg in 10 ml)
- Lidocaine: one 100 mg vial
- Amiodarone: one 300 mg vial
- Furosemide: 80 mg (one 8 ml of 10 mg ml^{-1})
- Glucose: one 50 ml of 50% (500 mg ml^{-1})
- Sodium bicarbonate. one 50 ml of 8.4%
- (Above as IMS Min-I-Jet®)
- Hydrocortisone: two 100 mg ampoules

ii. Anaesthetic drugs
- Propofol: three 20 ml ampoules (10 mg ml^{-1})
- Midazolam: four 5 ml ampoules (2 mg ml^{-1})
- Ketamine: two 1 g vials
- Etomidate: 10 ml ampoule (2 mg ml^{-1}). One carried in the drug pack, one carried drawn up and labelled in the fluid pack*
- Suxamethonium chloride: 2 ml ampoules (50 mg ml^{-1}). Three carried in the drug pack plus one carried drawn up and labelled in the fluid pack*
- Pancuronium: 2 ml ampoules (2 mg ml^{-1}). Three carried plus one carried drawn up and labelled in the fluid pack*

iii. Analgesic
- Morphine: five 1 ml ampoules (10 mg ml^{-1})

iv. Antiemetic
- Cyclizine: two 50 mg ampoules

v. Antagonist
- Naloxone: two 1 ml ampoules (400 µg ml^{-1})

vi. Other
- Diazemuls: two 10 mg ampoules
- Saline 0.9%: five 10 ml ampoules

*Drugs carried 'drawn up' are prepared in a labelled and capped syringe at the beginning of a shift and, if unused, disposed of at the end of the shift

---

RESUSCITATION DRUGS

Adrenaline (epinephrine)

Adrenaline (epinephrine) is a naturally occurring catecholamine. It works directly on alpha- and beta-adrenoreceptors. It is used to enhance the effectiveness of basic life support in the cardiac arrest treatment algorithms for asystole, electromechanical dissociation and ventricular fibrillation by its action on peripheral alpha-receptors, causing vasoconstriction, raising pressure in the aorta and increasing coronary perfusion (Colquhoun 1995).

In paediatric cardiac arrest, doses are based on body weight (Advanced Life Support Group 2001) and are considered in Chapters 18 and 19.

Adrenaline is also the mainstay of treatment for anaphylaxis. Anaphylaxis is a medical emergency and occurs when substances (such as histamine) are released as part of a hypersensitivity reaction (Consumers Association 1994). Clinical features include urticaria, oedema and itching (which may occur early and warn the patient that an attack is starting), flushing, dyspnoea (due to swelling of the upper airway, tongue and larynx and bronchospasm), hypotension (often a later sign, and due to vasodilation and plasma loss from increased capillary permeability) and tachycardia.

The alpha-agonist actions of adrenaline reverse the peripheral vasodilation, reducing oedema and urticaria. The beta-agonist actions dilate the airways, increase the force of contraction of the heart and suppress the release of further inflammatory substances (Consumers Association 1994).

Atropine

Atropine acts as a competitive antagonist of acetylcholine at muscarinic receptors. The effects caused include tachycardia, dry mouth and reduced sweating. Atropine is first-line treatment for organophosphorus and nerve agent poisoning (Marrs et al 1996).

Furosemide

Furosemide is a rapidly acting diuretic used in prehospital care to treat left ventricular failure, pulmonary oedema and fluid overload. In addition to the diuretic action, it reduces left ventricular filling pressure by a dilator action on veins (Foster 1996). When given intravenously diuresis occurs within a few minutes and lasts around 2 h (Sasada & Smith 1990). It is also used in the treatment of high blood pressure. Side effects include hypokalaemia.

Dextrose 50%

Intravenous 50% dextrose is used in the emergency treatment of adult hypoglycaemia.

Children are treated with 10% glucose at a dose of $5\,ml\,kg^{-1}$ (Advanced Life Support Group 2001). Concentrations of glucose higher than 10% may cause hyperglycaemia in children.

Sodium bicarbonate 8.4%

Intravenous sodium bicarbonate is an alkalinizing agent and is used in the treatment of tricyclic antidepressant overdose (Resuscitation Council (UK) 2000), the emergency management of hyperkalaemia and to treat severe metabolic acidosis (pH < 7.1). It dissociates to produce bicarbonate ions, the predominant extracellular buffer system (Sasada & Smith 1990). In the UK it is no longer used early

in the management of cardiac arrest unless hyperkalaemia or acidosis were known to be present at the time of arrest (Colquhoun 1995), but should be considered after three loops of the ventricular fibrillation protocol. It may also be useful in some instances of electromechanical dissociation. The management of severe acidosis needs to be guided by arterial and central venous blood gas analysis in hospital.

The mainstay of acidosis management is, however, the correction of hypoxia, ventilation abnormalities and fluid balance. Sodium bicarbonate is physically incompatible with calcium salts (causing precipitation) and may cause inactivation of coadministered adrenaline (epinephrine), isoprenaline and suxamethonium.

Hydrocortisone

Hydrocortisone is a glucocorticosteroid used in the treatment of anaphylaxis and allergy, and as replacement therapy in adrenocortical deficiency. Its main action is anti-inflammatory. Hydrocortisone acts via intracellular receptors and influences the rate of protein production, carbohydrate metabolism, vascular permeability and inflammatory cell recruitment (Sasada & Smith 1990). Its onset of action is delayed by several hours (British National Formulary 2004) so, in the management of acute emergencies, it should be given to prevent later deterioration while immediate management is carried out using oxygen, adrenaline (epinephrine), antihistamines and other therapy as indicated.

DRUGS USED FOR GENERAL ANAESTHESIA

The *Oxford English Reference Dictionary* (1995 edition) defines anaesthesia as 'the absence of sensation, especially artificially induced insensitivity to pain'.

General anaesthesia can be thought of as having three main components: producing a state of altered consciousness (being 'put to sleep'), muscle relaxation and pain control. This can be achieved by many different methods including administering drugs by the intravenous, intramuscular and inhalational routes.

The drugs described are divided into anaesthetic agents, muscle relaxants and analgesics. The purist may argue that these are simplistic divisions, as there is overlap between some of the drugs' properties but this is a useful basis on which to consider their use in prehospital care.

We emphasize that these drugs must only be used by practitioners with the appropriate anaesthetic training.

INTRAVENOUS INDUCTION AGENTS

Propofol

Propofol is used for the intravenous induction of anaesthesia, for maintenance of general anaesthesia and for sedation in intensive care. It provides rapid induction of anaesthesia with rapid recovery. In common with other intravenous anaesthetic agents, it can cause apnoea and should only be used by trained individuals able to provide the appropriate airway and ventilatory support. In fit patients it causes a decrease in blood pressure mainly due to vasodilation but also associated with bradycardia. These effects mean it is likely to cause profound hypotension in patients who are hypovolaemic. Its use in prehospital care has been described (Heath et al 1994) to provide anaesthesia and attenuate the hypertensive response to intubation in head-injured patients. Following primary survey and fluid resuscitation the authors used small incremental doses of propofol until the patients were unconscious, gave suxamethonium and performed intubation. The authors found that, in their hands, propofol given in doses of $1.18\,\text{mg}\,\text{kg}^{-1}$ (for isolated head-injured patients) and $1.25\,\text{mg}\,\text{kg}^{-1}$ (for multiply injured patients) did not cause clinically important hypotension. These doses are below the range recommended for anaesthetizing fit patients (2–$2.5\,\text{mg}\,\text{kg}^{-1}$). They stressed that propofol should only be used by doctors with suitable anaesthetic and prehospital experience.

Etomidate

Etomidate is a relatively cardiostable intravenous induction agent. This means that it is likely to cause less hypotension than propofol or thiopentone if used to anaesthetize shocked patients. It can also cause apnoea. In some patients it is associated with involuntary muscle movements. An unwanted effect of etomidate is suppression of adrenocortical function (production of cortisol and aldosterone). It is no longer used for sedation, as etomidate infusions were associated with increased mortality.

Its use in combination with fentanyl for anaesthesia of the head-injured patient during extrication has been described (Ummenhofer et al 1995). The standard induction dose for etomidate by slow intravenous injection is $0.3\,\text{mg}\,\text{kg}^{-1}$ but this is reduced in high-risk patients.

Ketamine

Ketamine is used both as an anaesthetic and an analgesic. In prehospital care it is used intravenously and intramuscularly, and in war has been given intrathecally (Bion 1984). It has a number of properties that make it of value in prehospital care. A comparison of midazolam and ketamine for in-hospital sedation found better airway maintenance with ketamine (Drummond 1996). Ketamine causes sympathetic stimulation (resulting in increased heart rate and blood pressure) and when compared with other anaesthetic agents usually causes less hypotension on induction of anaesthesia, although it can cause a fall in blood in shocked patients (Hirota & Lambert 1996). Disadvantages include nausea,

vomiting, increased salivation and hallucinations (Sasada & Smith 1990). There has also been concern about the non-medical use of ketamine as a 'street drug' (Jansen 1993). In-hospital practice premedication with antisialogues (to dry secretions) has been recommended prior to using ketamine, and benzodiazepines have been used to decrease the incidence of unpleasant dreams. Neither are likely to be practical in the acute prehospital care situation, particularly as using a benzodiazepine may increase the incidence of airway compromise. Ketamine anaesthesia has been described for entrapments (Ummenhofer et al 1995). Ketamine is contraindicated in patients with hypertension (British National Formulary 2004). It has also been avoided in head-injured patients because of concern that it might further increase intracranial pressure, although some authorities use ketamine in haemodynamically compromised patients with or without a head injury (Kerz & Dick 1995).

The doses for anaesthesia are intravenous 1–$3\,\text{mg}\,\text{kg}^{-1}$ (slow injection over $60\,\text{s}$) and intramuscular 6.5–$13\,\text{mg}\,\text{kg}^{-1}$ (British National Formulary 2004). Doses for analgesia are 0.25–$0.5\,\text{mg}\,\text{kg}^{-1}$ intravenously or 0.5–$1\,\text{mg}\,\text{kg}^{-1}$ intramuscularly (Kerz & Dick 1995).

In the prehospital environment we have used smaller doses ($10\,\text{mg}$ intravenous boluses) titrated to effect in adult patients to allow short procedures (such as straightening a limb).

Midazolam

Midazolam is a water-soluble benzodiazepine used for sedation, anxiolysis and premedication. It can be given intramuscularly or intravenously. As with other benzodiazepines it can cause apnoea.

Fentanyl

Fentanyl is a synthetic opioid analgesic. In hospital practice it is used during general anaesthesia (both as an analgesic and to obtund the cardiovascular response to laryngoscopy and intubation), and both intrathecally and epidurally for intra- and postoperative analgesia. It is also available as a sustained-release transdermal patch for treatment of chronic, intractable cancer pain.

Intravenous fentanyl is relatively cardiovascularly stable, although it can cause bradycardia. It is a powerful respiratory depressant and can cause apnoea. Its use as both an analgesic agent and as part of an anaesthetic technique in prehospital care have been described (Ummenhofer et al 1995).

MUSCLE RELAXANTS

Muscle relaxants can be divided into two groups; depolarizing and non-depolarizing.

Suxamethonium

Suxamethonium is a depolarizing muscle relaxant that, when given intravenously, produces rapid relaxation (onset within 30 s). It is used to facilitate endotracheal intubation. The depolarizing agents such as suxamethonium chemically resemble acetylcholine and interact with the cholinergic receptor. The receptor is stimulated (hence the muscle fasciculations seen) and the block lasts 3–5 min. Side effects include an increase in serum potassium (this is exaggerated in casualties with burns or denervation injuries and can cause cardiac arrest) and bradycardia. In hospital practice the drug used is a solution of suxamethonium chloride, which needs to be stored at 4°C. For field and remote locations suxamethonium bromide (which comes as a powder that stores well) may be more appropriate (King 1986, Dobson 1988, Fenton 1993).

Pancuronium

Pancuronium is a non-depolarizing muscle relaxant. It works by competing with acetylcholine at the post-synaptic membrane of the neuromuscular junction. Onset is slower than suxamethonium (90–150 s to provide intubating conditions). It causes an increase in heart rate, blood pressure and cardiac output. A single dose lasts around 45–60 min.

Note: muscle relaxants are not anaesthetic agents. They do not put the patient to sleep. In UK practice muscle relaxants are usually given with anaesthetic, sedative and/or analgesic drugs as part of an anaesthetic induction sequence.

ANALGESICS

Morphine

Morphine is an opioid analgesic agent. Under the Misuse of Drug Regulations 1985 it is classified as a Schedule 2 drug. It is used in prehospital care for both analgesia and in the treatment of left-ventricular failure. It can be administered by oral, intramuscular and intravenous routes. Intravenous titration to obtain the required effect is the optimum route in prehospital care. Intramuscular administration will have a longer time onset and, if the drug is given into poorly perfused muscle, may have little obvious effect. There is the potential risk of 'overdose' when blood supply is improved to a muscle containing a depot of drug. Intramuscular administration may be the only option, however, in certain field situations (Jowitt & Knight 1983) and if there is poor access to a patient (Finch & Nancekievill 1975).

Morphine acts via a number of opioid receptors. There are several subclasses of opioid receptor. Analgesia is mediated by the μ-receptor. Interaction with the receptor causes changes in cell function, which in turn influence processing and transmission of the pain signal.

Unwanted effects of morphine include respiratory depression, nausea and vomiting. Practitioners giving morphine and related drugs must have the ability to control the patient's airway and ventilation. Respiratory depression can be treated using naloxone, a specific antagonist, but this may also antagonize the analgesia. Treatment and prevention of nausea and vomiting includes giving antiemetics either with, before or after the morphine.

Morphine can legally be given by non-medical members of mountain rescue teams, and by paramedics in some ambulance services within the UK.

ANTIEMETICS

Prochlorperazine

Prochlorperazine is a phenothiazine drug. It works by blocking central dopamine receptors at the chemoreceptor trigger zone. Side effects include extrapyramidal reactions (a movement disorder), which are more common in children and elderly patients. It also has blocking actions at adrenergic, cholinergic and histaminergic receptors. It can be given by mouth, by suppository and by deep intramuscular injection in adults, but only by the oral route in children.

ANTAGONISTS

Naloxone

Naloxone is an antagonist at the μ-opioid receptor and is used to reverse opioid-induced respiratory depression and sedation. It is also used to treat opioid overdose. It should be given intravenously in small incremental doses, the aim being to reverse the respiratory depression without reversing analgesia.

The duration of action of the opioid drug causing the problem may be longer than that of naloxone. The casualty will need appropriate monitoring and further doses of naloxone may be needed. Intramuscular naloxone should be given to patients who are unlikely to comply with repeated intravenous doses.

The adult dosage for treating overdose is intravenous 0.8–2 mg repeated at intervals of 2–3 min to a maximum of 10 mg.

The adult dosage to reverse opioid-induced respiratory depression is intravenous injection of 100–200 μg then further doses of 100 μg (if response is inadequate) at 2 min intervals. Further doses can be given by intramuscular injection after 1–2 h if required (British National Formulary 2004).

OTHER DRUGS

Methylprednisolone

Methylprednisolone is a corticosteroid used to suppress inflammatory and allergic disorders, and in the treatment of cerebral oedema (British National Formulary 2004).

High doses given in the first 8 h after spinal cord injury may improve neurological recovery, although this is still a matter of considerable debate. The drug and dosage should be agreed with the local spinal injury centre (Swain et al 1996).

The majority of spinal cord injuries attended by HEMS are incomplete (Wilmink et al 1996). Methylprednisolone is given by intravenous infusion during patient transport after immobilization and extrication. Rapid intravenous injections of large doses of methylprednisolone has been associated with cardiovascular collapse (British National Formulary 2004).

Mannitol

Mannitol is an alcohol, and is available as an intravenous solution of 10% or 20% mannitol in water. Its action is as an osmotic diuretic. It is given as an intravenous infusion.

Mannitol is used to reduce intracranial pressure. This occurs by withdrawing brain extracellular water across the blood–brain barrier into plasma. It should be seen as a means of 'buying time' for the head-injured patient prior to definitive management (Bullock & Teasdale 1996) and, ideally, protocols for use should be agreed with receiving neurosurgical units.

Summary

This chapter has given an outline of drug action and some of the factors that influence drug selection and use in pre-hospital care. The decision to give any drug to a patient must be taken in the context of the overall care plan for that individual.

ACKNOWLEDGEMENT

The authors thank Mr A. W. Wilson for original permission to describe the contents of the 1995 HEMS drug pack and Dr S. Bland for providing an update.

References

Advanced Life Support Group 2001 Advanced paediatric life support: the practical approach, 3rd edn. BMJ Publishing, London

American College of Surgeons Committee on Trauma 1997 Advanced trauma life support student manual, 6th edn. American College of Surgeons, Chicago, IL

Association of Anaesthetists of Great Britain and Ireland 1995 Controlled drugs. Association of Anaesthetists, London

Baskett PJF 1992 Emergency medicine's involvement in disaster medicine. Baillière's Clinical Anaesthesiology 6: 193–207

Bion JF 1984 Intrathecal ketamine for war surgery. A preliminary study under field conditions. Anaesthesia 39: 1023–1028

British National Formulary 2004 London: British Medical Association and the Royal Pharmaceutical Society of Great Britain (This is revised twice yearly and the most recent edition should be consulted)

Bull PT, Merril SB, Moody RA et al 1983 Anaesthesia during the Falklands campaign: the experience of the Royal Navy. Anaesthesia 38: 770–775

Bullock R, Teasdale G 1996 Head injuries. In: Skinner D, Driscoll P, Earlam R (eds) ABC of major trauma, 2nd edn. BMJ Publishing, London, p 28–35

Cahal DA 1974a Misuse of Drugs Act 1971. British Medical Journal 1: 70–72

Cahal DA 1974b Misuse of Drugs Regulations 1973. British Medical Journal 1: 73–75

Colquhoun MC 1995 Drugs and their delivery. In: Colquohoun MC, Handley AJ, Evans TR (eds) ABC of resuscitation, 3rd edn. BMJ Publishing, London, p 74–76

Consumers Association 1989 Drugs for the doctor's bag. Drug and Therapeutics Bulletin 27: 17–19

Consumers Association 1992 Prescribing unlicensed drugs or using drugs for unlicensed indications. Drug and Therapeutics Bulletin 30: 97–99

Consumers Association 1994 Adrenaline for anaphylaxis. Drug and Therapeutics Bulletin 32: 19–21

Consumers Association 1995 Drugs for the doctor's bag. Drug and Therapeutics Bulletin 33: 3–5

Consumers Association 1996 Preconception, pregnancy and prescribing. Drug and Therapeutics Bulletin 34: 25–27

Cooke MW 1993 Intraosseous vascular access in pre-hospital care. Journal of the British Association for Immediate Care 16: 5–7

Dobson MB 1988 Anaesthesia at the district general hospital. World Health Organization, Geneva

Drummond GB 1996 Comparison of sedation with midazolam and ketamine: effects on airway muscle activity. British Journal of Anaesthesia 76: 663–667

Fenton PM 1993 Africa anaesthesia: a training and practice manual for anaesthetists in developing countries. Montford Press, Malawi

Finch P, Nancekievill DG 1975 The role of hospital medical teams at a major accident. Anaesthesia 30: 666–676

Foster RW (ed) 1996 Basic pharmacology, 4th edn. Butterworth Heinemann, Oxford

Heath KJ, Samra GS, Davies GE et al 1994 Blood pressure changes in head injury patients during pre-hospital anaesthesia with propofol. Injury 25(Suppl 2): S-B7–S-B8

Hirota K, Lambert DG 1996 Ketamine: its mechanism(s) of action and unusual clinical uses. British Journal of Anaesthesia 77: 441–444

Hogerzeil HV, Pinel J 1991 The new emergency health kit. Tropical Doctor 21(Suppl): 47–50

Jansen KLR 1993 Non-medical uses of ketamine. British Medical Journal 306: 601–602

Johnson GS, Guly HR 1995 The effect of pre-hospital administration of intravenous nalbuphine on on-scene times. Journal of Accident and Emergency Medicine 12: 20–22

Jowitt MD, Knight RJ 1983 Anaesthesia during the Falklands campaign: the land battles. Anaesthesia 38: 776–783

Kerz T, Dick WF 1995 Analgesia and sedatives in emergencies. In: Goris RJA, Trentz O (eds) The integrated approach to trauma care. Update in intensive care and emergency medicine, vol 22. Springer, Berlin, p 62–77

King M (ed) 1986 Primary anaesthesia. Oxford University Press, Oxford

Luten RC, Wears RL, Broselow J et al 1992 Length-based endotracheal tube and emergency equipment in paediatrics. Annals of Emergency Medicine 21: 900–904

Marrs TC, Maynard RL, Sidell FR 1996 Chemical warfare agents: toxicology and treatment. John Wiley, Chichester

Nimmo WS 1990 Principles of general pharmacology and pharmacokinetics. In: Aitkenhead AR, Smith G (eds) Textbook of anaesthesia, 2nd edn. Churchill Livingstone, Edinburgh

Oakley PA 1988 Inaccuracy and delay in decision making in paediatric resuscitation, and a proposed reference chart to reduce error. British Medical Journal 297: 817–819

Oakley PA, Phillips B, Molyneux E, Mackway-Jones K 1993 Updated standard reference chart. British Medical Journal 306: 1613

Resuscitation Council (UK) 2000 Advanced life support course manual, 4th edn (revised). Resuscitation Council (UK), London

Roux A, van Heerden P, Alper J, Boffard R 1992 The Johannesburg Hospital mobile anaesthesia service. Injury 23: 251–255

Rubin PC (ed) 1995 Prescribing in pregnancy, 2nd edn. BMJ Publishing, London

Rudland SV, Jacobs AG 1994 Visiting bags: a labile thermal environment. British Medical Journal 308: 954–956

Sasada MP, Smith SP 1990 Drugs in anaesthesia and intensive care. Castle House Publications, Tunbridge Wells

Swain A, Dove J, Baker H 1996 Spine and spinal cord injury. In: Skinner D, Driscoll P, Earlam R (eds) ABC of major trauma, 2nd edn. BMJ Publishing, London, p 41–48

Ummenhofer W, Pargger H, Boenicke U, Scheidegger D 1995 Extrication and immobilisation of the severe trauma victim: how is it done? In: Goris RJA, Trentz O (eds) The integrated approach to trauma care. Update in intensive care and emergency medicine, vol 22. Springer, Berlin, p 25–39

Welsh Affairs Committee 1996 Third report. The training of ambulance paramedics. HMSO, London, p 21–22

Wilmink ABM, Samra GS, Watson LM, Wilson AW 1996 Vehicle entrapment rescue and pre-hospital trauma care. Injury 27: 21–25

Analgesia and pain relief

14

Introduction   162

Neural transmission and modulation   162

Analgesia in practice   163

Prehospital practicalities   163

Pharmacology of analgesics   163

Opioids   163

Antipyretic and anti-inflammatory drugs   167

Nitrous oxide in oxygen (Entonox)   169

Ketamine   169

Local anaesthesia   170

References   172

Introduction

Pain management is a common problem frequently faced by the prehospital physician. Pain itself is a complex, multivariable phenomenon and the same stimulus will produce markedly different results not only between different individuals but also in the same individual in different circumstances. Management of this variability is compounded by the ever-increasing variety of analgesics and techniques, with most of which an individual practitioner will have limited experience.

Despite these problems, extrication following vehicle accidents, reduction of fractures and dislocations may all require potent analgesics. Analgesia may also be required for medical emergencies such as ischaemic chest pain (Wyllie & Dunn 1994) and sickle-cell crisis. The prehospital doctor must be able to provide appropriate analgesia for all these situations.

Historically, analgesia has been withheld in many of these situations for fear of masking subclinical signs of occult injury, depression of respiration and protective airway reflexes. Recent studies have shown that patients arriving in emergency departments often have poor prehospital pain control (Chambers & Guly 1993). The adaptation of didactic trauma systems and in-hospital imaging mean that analgesia can now be given more freely than previously, and the improved training of prehospital doctors has led to greater confidence in airway management.

Provision of analgesia should therefore be the norm rather than the exception, but careful patient assessment, selection of the most appropriate analgesic and close monitoring for clinical and adverse affects are mandatory. It should always be borne in mind that, although there are many good humanitarian and physiological reasons for relieving pain, more morbidity and indeed mortality has probably occurred through imprudent use of analgesics than from pain per se. The prehospital physician must always be aware of the adage 'first do no harm'.

Neural transmission and modulation

A painful stimulus activates peripheral nociceptors, specific pain receptors composed of myelinated and unmyelinated nerve fibres. The sensory impulse is transmitted centrally by myelinated Aδ-fibres (conduction velocity 10–20 m s^{-1}) carrying sensations of sharp localized pain, or slow unmyelinated C fibres (conduction velocity 1 m s^{-1}) carrying slow-onset, burning, diffuse pain. These afferent fibres synapse in the dorsal horn of the spinal cord projecting both centrally and to local motor and sympathetic fibres, producing such phenomena as reflex muscle spasm and vasoconstriction.

The synapse in the dorsal horn can be influenced by other afferent nerves. Large diameter Aβ-fibres transmitting sensations of touch, pressure and vibration can interfere with nociceptive transmission – this is the underlying principle of 'gate control'. Similar controls operate centrally to influence pain perception, explaining situations when significant injuries are ignored by the individual.

Analgesia in practice

Pain is a complex interaction of environmental stimulus, nociceptive stimulation, feedback regulation and emotional overlay producing the final sensation. There are obviously a number of points at which analgesic interventions are possible:

- *Environment*: securing the scene to prevent further injury and removing the noxious stimulus
- *Physical*: reduce fractured limbs and dislocated joints, and cover burns with sterile dressings
- *Psychological*: reduce anxiety by giving clear explanations of any problems and how they will be overcome. Fear and ignorance greatly amplify perceived pain
- *Systemic analgesics*: analgesics that are inhaled or given parenterally
- *Regional analgesia*: plexus, field or individual nerve blocks.

Prehospital practicalities

The prehospital physician must be familiar with a wide range of drugs to deal with a variety of medical problems. A small pharmacology text (such as the *British National Formulary*) is a useful addition to the myriad of equipment carried by many physicians. Drugs must be kept in a protective bag, clearly labelled with the owner's contact details in case of loss or theft. As most drugs are still presented in glass ampoules, internal padding and numerous small pockets or elastic straps are useful to limit breakages. Drugs should be organized using a system familiar to the user – alphabetical or drug groups (i.e. analgesics, sedatives, anaesthetics, etc.) are good examples. Members of large teams may find it helpful to standardize both the contents and layout of their drug bags. Certain drugs may be subject to statutory regulations regarding supply, storage and administration (i.e. many of the potent opioids in the UK). The individual must be aware of local regulations and adhere to them, particularly those regarding secure storage, to prevent potentially lethal drugs finding their way on to the open market. Some physicians now avoid 'controlled' drugs altogether and rely on non-controlled opioids for intermediate pain and non-opioids (e.g. ketamine) for many cases of severe pain. Potent opioids have the potential to induce respiratory depression and, occasionally, cardiac decompensation. Users must be competent in advanced airway management in a wide variety of situations and be able to recognize and have the equipment to deal with any potential side effects induced by the agents detailed in this chapter.

Pharmacology of analgesics

An analgesic is a drug that relieves pain non-specifically without depressing conscious level or having a direct physiological action. The definition thus excludes anaesthetic agents (apart from those having genuine analgesic activity at subhypnotic concentrations) and drugs such as glyceryl trinitrate, which relieve ischaemic chest pain by venodilation.

Analgesics can be classified by type:

- opioids, which predominantly act centrally on defined opiate receptors
- anti-inflammatory drugs, which interfere with prostaglandin production and have a predominantly peripheral action
- antipyretics, which lack the anti-inflammatory action of the above group but produce analgesia and lower temperature
- anaesthetic gases, such as nitrous oxide
- anaesthetic vapours, such as ether
- anaesthetic agents, such as ketamine.

Opioids

An *opioid* is a naturally occurring or synthetic compound that will bind to and stimulate an opiate receptor. An *opiate* is a drug structurally related to the opium alkaloids. The term *narcotic* is largely redundant, referring only to the sedative properties of this group of compounds. To confuse the picture further, new drugs such as tramadol have been introduced that structurally resemble opioids but rely on non-opioid-mediated mechanisms for some of their action.

The existence of specific opiate receptors has been postulated for many years but it is only in comparatively recent times that the current classification has been used (μ, κ and δ receptors). Agonists are drugs that bind to and stimulate an opioid receptor – this response increases with the dose of drug administered. In the case of the μ-receptor, stimulation produces an increase in intracellular calcium which, in turn, increases potassium conductance and hyperpolarizes the excitable neuronal tissue, leading to decreased transmission of nociceptive impulses.

Although many drugs may bind to a single receptor group they often produce different levels of response – this phenomenon is known as efficacy. For example, morphine is more efficacious than codeine and will produce greater analgesia. Partial agonists bind to and stimulate opioid receptors but are limited by a ceiling of action. For example, increasing the dose of nalbuphine beyond 30 mg produces no increase in analgesia, or respiratory depression. Antagonists bind to opioid receptors and produce no clinical effect – for example, naloxone binds to μ-receptors and reverses the respiratory depression (and analgesia) produced by μ-agonists such as morphine.

Some drugs, such as nalbuphine, act as agonists at one receptor group (in this case κ-receptors, producing analgesia) and antagonists at other groups (μ-receptor). This has advantages and disadvantages. The disadvantage is that pain that is not controlled by nalbuphine will be difficult to treat with morphine, as the former will antagonize the action of the latter. However, the converse is that respiratory depression produced by excessive doses of morphine can be reversed by nalbuphine (μ-antagonist) while preserving analgesia (κ-agonist).

PHYSICAL PROPERTIES

For an opioid to act on a receptor it must first leave the blood and diffuse through tissue membranes. The ability of any drug to diffuse through membranes is a function of:

- *lipid solubility*: increasing lipid solubility increases diffusive capacity. Opioids with high lipid solubility, such as fentanyl, will have rapid onset due to tissue penetration and a short duration of action due to redistribution throughout body fat stores. Repeated doses or infusions may lead to a longer duration of action due to cumulation of drug in the fat stores and saturation of the elimination capacity of the liver
- *molecular size*: smaller molecules have increased diffusive capacity. Low-molecular-weight opioids, such as alfentanil, have a rapid onset.

ADMINISTRATION

Some of the very lipid-soluble opiates (such as fentanyl and diamorphine) may be given via the intranasal route. This often results in rapid systemic levels and may be preferable to intramuscular administration when intravenous access has not been established.

Intravenous opiates are the analgesic of choice for severe pain in prehospital care.

The gold standard in opiate administration is the intravenous route. Systemic levels are rapidly established allowing frequent, small aliquots of diluted opiate to be given until the desired level of analgesia has been reached. The dose of opiate required to reach an identical level of analgesia may vary by a factor of 10 between individuals. Fractionating the dose takes such variability into account, and minimizes the incidence and severity of side-effects. In an ideal world analgesia is best maintained by a controlled, or patient-controlled, infusion, as this produces the best analgesia with least side-effects. However, infusions are rarely used in the prehospital environment, except by ambulance- and helicopter-based medical teams who do not have the same constraints on space and power supply that face many prehospital physicians. Analgesia is therefore usually maintained by further small intravenous boluses of opiate.

The dose of opiate required to reach an identical level of analgesia may vary by a factor of 10 between individuals.

SIDE-EFFECTS

Opioids that rely on μ-receptor activation for their action show similar side-effect profiles at equianalgesic doses. Tramadol, nalbuphine and pentazocine use different receptor subgroups (see Table 14.1) and therefore have slightly different profiles. The incidence of adverse effects is greatly increased in the hypovolaemic patient – particular care should be taken in this situation.

Respiratory

The principal adverse effect of most opioids is respiratory depression, with a decreased central ventilatory response to hypercapnia and hypoxia. This often leads to hypercapnia, which may lead to adverse effects on intracranial pressure in head-injured patients. Respiratory depression may be life-threatening. Depression of the cough reflex is common (particularly with morphine) and some opiates cause the release of significant amounts of histamine, leading to bronchospasm. Chest wall rigidity may result if high doses of opioids (particularly alfentanil and fentanyl) are given.

Cardiovascular

Most opiates have a minimal effect on the cardiovascular system. Pain produces sympathetic activation leading to vasoconstriction and an increase in afterload and myocardial work. Effective analgesia may thus improve cardiovascular function. Large doses of opioids may lead to bradycardia and hypotension due to vasodilation. Histamine release (particularly with morphine) may result in hypotension.

Central nervous system

Potent opioids often produce sedation, euphoria and anxiolysis. Miosis occurs as a result of stimulation of the Edinger–Westphal nucleus. Long-term use may lead to tolerance, dependence and withdrawal symptoms. Short-term use does not produce these phenomena.

Gastrointestinal

Opioids decrease gastric motility and increase common bile duct pressure. Nausea and vomiting are common adverse effects due to stimulation of the chemoreceptor trigger zone. Constipation may occur with long-term use.

Urogenital system

Ureteric spasm occurs after many opioids. Although uterine contractions are not affected, opioids readily cross the placenta and may cause respiratory depression in the neonate.

CONTRAINDICATIONS

Opioids should be avoided in the following situations:

- pre-existing respiratory depression with a respiratory rate of less than 10 breaths min^{-1}. However, carefully titrated administration of opioids may improve respiratory function following rib fractures or in patients with chronic pulmonary disease complicated by pain following trauma
- raised intracranial pressure in unventilated patients. Opioids may reduce intracranial pressure in head-injured patients, providing end-tidal carbon dioxide levels are controlled (usually by positive pressure ventilation)
- status asthmaticus in unventilated patients
- where expertise and equipment for treatment of overdose (airway and ventilatory management and naloxone) is not available
- opioids should be used with extreme caution in cases of hypovolaemia, central nervous system depression, pulmonary, cardiovascular, renal and hepatic disease.

INDIVIDUAL OPIOIDS

There are many areas of similarity between the potent opiates. Unless otherwise stated, all agents suffer from the above side-effects. The individual subsections will illustrate the areas of contrast. All doses should be given slowly and the clinical response should be monitored.

Morphine

Morphine is the standard opioid against which all others are compared (Bruns et al 1992). Drowsiness is common, and histamine release may be a problem in large doses and in atopic individuals. The usual intravenous dose is 0.1–0.2 mg kg^{-1} given in a number of small aliquots. Onset is within 15–20 min and duration of action is 2–4 h. The relatively slow onset, even after intravenous administration, may lead to difficulties in establishing adequate analgesia rapidly without overdose. Morphine is metabolized to morphine-6-glucuronide, an active metabolite, which may accumulate in the presence of renal failure.

Diamorphine

Diamorphine (heroin) is a semisynthetic morphine derivative. It is much more lipid-soluble than morphine and therefore has a more rapid onset (10–20 min) but shorter duration of action (1–2 h). The usual intravenous dose is 0.1 mg kg^{-1}. It may produce less nausea and vomiting than morphine.

Pethidine

Pethidine is a synthetic opioid with a chemical structure similar to atropine. The usual intravenous dose is 1 mg kg^{-1}, onset is within 10 min and duration of action of 1–2 h. It has a similar side-effect profile to morphine at equianalgesic doses but may produce greater hypotension due to alpha-blockade, tachycardia and more euphoria. Histamine release is less than with morphine and it reduces uterine tone. It is contraindicated in patients receiving monoamine oxidase inhibitors. It is not recommended for prehospital use.

Fentanyl

Fentanyl is a potent synthetic opioid commonly used by anaesthetists. It is rapidly gaining popularity in accident and emergency medicine. It is extremely lipid-soluble with an onset of only 2–5 min and duration of 30–60 min. The short onset time facilitates rapid analgesia with the minimum of adverse effects; however, frequent supplemental doses are required and may lead to accumulation and prolongation of action. The usual intravenous dose is 1 μg kg^{-1}. The same dose is used if the drug is given via the nasal route. Higher doses (10–50 μg kg^{-1}) may be used to obtund the stress response to intubation in critically ill patients. The duration of action may be 4–6 h after this higher dose. Histamine release is extremely uncommon, and there are less marked effects on intracranial pressure than with other opioids. Fentanyl often produces a brady-cardia of vagal origin but blood pressure and cardiac output are maintained.

Alfentanil

Alfentanil is another synthetic opioid used mainly by anaes-thetists. Its onset is even more rapid (90 s) than fentanyl and its duration of action only 5–10 min. These character-istics make alfentanil the ideal drug for use where there is a requirement for intense analgesia of short duration (i.e. during endotracheal intubation). The intravenous dose is 10 μg kg^{-1}. Other effects are similar to fentanyl except that it has a smaller protective effect on intracranial pressure.

Remifentanil

Remifentanil is a new ultra-short-acting synthetic opi-oid in anaesthetic usage. Its onset is within 60 s. The half-life of remifentanil is so short that the drug must be given by intravenous infusion – no residual opioid activity is present within 5 min of discontinuation, even after high doses are used. It is particularly suited to obtunding pressor responses to intubation and surgery. The usual dose is 1 μg kg^{-1} as a bolus, followed by an infusion of 0.5–1.0 μg kg^{-1} min^{-1}. Respiratory depression is common, as is muscular rigidity. Despite its unique pharmacology, the necessity for administration by infusion will limit its use. It is also expensive.

Nalbuphine

Nalbuphine is a synthetic partial κ-agonist and μ-antagonist (Eggers & Power 1995). It is currently in use with a number of UK ambulance services (Chambers & Guly 1994, Johnson & Guly 1995). The onset time is 2–3 min and dura-tion of action is 3–4 h. The intravenous dose for an adult is 10–20 mg. Nalbuphine is as potent as morphine (30 mg nalbuphine is equivalent to 10 mg morphine). Nalbuphine demonstrates a ceiling level of analgesia and increasing the dose above 30 mg produces no further analgesia. However, the ceiling also applies to respiratory depression (Hannhart et al 1992, Vickers et al 1992). Sedation, nausea and vomit-ing are all less frequent than with morphine. It is extremely cardiovascularly stable and is licensed for use in ischaemic chest pain. However, psychomimetic effects may occasion-ally complicate its use. Owing to its μ-receptor antagonism, nalbuphine may complicate the subsequent administra-tion of morphine and other μ-agonists. It has a low risk for inducing dependency and at present is not a controlled drug in the UK.

Pentazocine

Pentazocine is a synthetic partial κ-agonist with weak μ-antagonist activity (Bion 1984). Onset times and dura-tion of action are similar to nalbuphine. The intravenous dose is 0.5–1.0 mg kg^{-1}. It is subject to ceiling analgesia and respiratory depression at doses in excess of 60–90 mg. Although there is a low incidence of euphoria, there is a relatively high incidence of dysphoria, which limits its use.

Meptazinol

Meptazinol is a synthetic opioid related structurally to pethi-dine. The intravenous dose is 1.0–1.5 mg kg^{-1}, the onset time is less than 10 min and the duration of action 2–4 h. It produces less respiratory depression than pethidine.

Buprenorphine

Buprenorphine is a semisynthetic partial μ-agonist and parv-tial κ-antagonist. It has a high μ-receptor affinity producing prolonged receptor binding and duration of action (6–8 h). The drug can be given intravenously (dose 0.3–0.6 mg) or sublingually (dose 0.2–0.4 mg). Onset is within 15 min. It exhibits ceiling analgesia and respiratory depression; however, if respiratory depression does occur it may be difficult to treat because of buprenorphine's high recep-tor affinity. Naloxone may be ineffective but doxapram, a direct respiratory stimulant, may be of use. As with most strong opioids, there is a high incidence of nausea and vomiting if used in ambulant patients and it is not recom-mended for prehospital use.

Codeine

Codeine is a naturally occurring alkaloid. It is only suita-ble for mild to moderate pain because of its low potency. Codeine does not have a licence for intravenous use. The usual intramuscular dose is 30–60 mg. Onset is within 20–30 min and duration of action 3–4 h. Historically, it has been the preferred analgesic for head-injured patients because of its minimal effects on conscious level and pupil reflexes; however, this is simply a reflection of its low potency.

Tramadol

Tramadol lies outside the traditional classification of opi-oid analgesics (Raffa 1996). It is a non-selective μ-, κ- and δ-receptor agonist but has maximal affinity for the μ-receptor (Dayer et al 1994). It also relies on non-opioid mechanisms, such as inhibition of neuronal reuptake of noradrenaline (norepinephrine) and enhancement of 5-hydroxytryptamine (serotonin) release, for a significant portion of its action. The intravenous dose is an initial bolus of 100 mg followed by supplemental doses of 50 mg at 20 min intervals up to a maximum of 250 mg. Subsequent doses should be 50–100 mg every 4–6 h up to a maximum of 600 mg d^{-1}. Tramadol has the least respiratory depressant effect of any opioid, and it also has minimal effects on the cardiovascular system – hypertension is an occasional finding. Studies have shown that it is less suitable for use as part of a balanced anaesthetic technique due to an increased incidence of awareness. The incidence of nausea is also relatively high. Tramadol is best avoided in prehospital practice because of its high incidence of side effects and highly variable efficacy.

TREATMENT OF OPIOID OVERDOSE

Opioid toxicity is either absolute, where an excess of drug has been administered to a fit patient, or relative, where a 'normal' dose has been given to a hypovolaemic or physiologically compromised patient, producing excessive plasma levels. The symptoms are identical in both cases: sedation, respiratory depression and miosis. Left untreated, respiratory and cardiac arrest may occur.

Opioid toxicity should be treated by standard resuscitative measures, including securing the airway, supplying supplemental oxygen and supporting respiration, and with naloxone, the competitive μ-receptor antagonist. Given intravenously the dose is 5–6 μg kg^{-1} – twice this amount may be needed for neonates. Naloxone has a rapid onset of 2–3 min but has a duration of action of only 20 min. This is likely to be far shorter than the duration of action of the depressant opioid. Frequent monitoring is mandatory and supplemental doses of naloxone, or a naloxone infusion, may be required.

Reversal of respiratory depression is usually accompanied by reversal of analgesia. Nalbuphine may reverse moderate levels of respiratory depression while maintaining analgesia. Otherwise a non-opioid, such as ketamine, or a partial opioid, such as tramadol, may be used. The sudden reversal of opioid analgesia in opioid-dependent patients may produce arrhythmias, hypertension, convulsions and even cardiac arrest.

ANTIEMETICS

Nausea and vomiting frequently accompany opioid administration. A past history of postoperative vomiting and motion sickness increases the likelihood of opioid-induced nausea. Nausea is upsetting for the patient but vomiting may jeopardize airway integrity, particularly where lack of access or injury limits placing the patient in the recovery

position. Emesis is produced by a number of mechanisms including:

- action on the chemoreceptor trigger zone located in the floor of the fourth ventricle
- direct action on the vomiting centre in the medulla oblongata
- by vestibular stimulation.

There are many groups of drugs that have an antiemetic action. Those most suitable for prehospital use are reviewed below. Metoclopramide is ineffective in opioid-induced emesis and should not be used for this purpose.

Prochlorperazine

This is a phenothiazine derivative. It is relatively effective in opioid-induced emesis. The intramuscular dose is 12.5 mg for an adult and duration of action is 8 h. It cannot be given intravenously as alpha-blockade may induce severe hypotension. It occasionally produces electrocardiogram (ECG) changes and mild respiratory depression. Extrapyramidal reactions are not uncommon.

Cyclizine

Cyclizine is an antihistamine and is relatively effective in opioid-induced emesis. It may be given intravenously; the adult dose is 50 mg and duration of action is 8 h. The drug has mild anticholinergic properties and tachycardia may be a problem. Mild sedation is also common.

Ondansetron

Ondansetron is a 5-hydroxytryptamine (5-HT$_3$) antagonist. This group of drugs is the most effective in alleviating opioid-induced emesis. They were originally developed for use in nausea associated with chemotherapy. The adult intravenous dose is 4 mg, duration of action is 6–8 h. Bradycardia, hypotension and hypersensitivity reactions may be seen occasionally. Ondansetron does not produce extrapyramidal effects. All 5-HT$_3$ antagonists are considerably more expensive than the other groups of antiemetics.

Antipyretic and anti-inflammatory drugs

Paracetamol and non-steroidal anti-inflammatory drugs (NSAIDs) are useful in treating mild to moderate pain. However, their use in prehospital medicine is limited by route of administration, potency and adverse effects.

PARACETAMOL

Paracetamol (acetaminophen) is a central inhibitor of cyclooxygenase, the enzyme responsible for the production of prostaglandins and prostacyclins. Although prostaglandins have no direct nociceptive action, they sensitize peripheral nerve endings to the effects of other nociceptive mediators released during the inflammatory process such as bradykinin and histamine.

The maximum analgesic effect of paracetamol appears to be greater than any of the non-opioid analgesics. It is a potent antipyretic but does not have any anti-inflammatory properties. The adult dose is 0.5–1.0 g up to four times daily. There is no parenteral preparation but it may be given rectally.

It is metabolized by conjugation with glucuronic and sulphuric acids. This pathway is easily saturated and doses in excess of 10 g may be fatal, leading to hepatorenal failure.

NSAIDs

Unlike paracetamol, NSAIDs have peripheral cyclooxygenase inhibitory activity. They also have other effects, such as free radical scavenging and membrane stabilizing activity, which contribute to their mechanism of action. In adequate doses (which may be higher than those usually needed for analgesia) they are anti-inflammatory, and will reduce swelling and joint tenderness. There are many subgroups of NSAIDs and patients may respond to some better than others. However, many NSAIDs do not have a parenteral formulation and the frequency and severity of adverse effects, and in some cases the slow duration of onset, limits their use in prehospital medicine.

Salicylates

Aspirin is the standard NSAID against which others are compared. The adult dose is 300–900 mg up to four times daily. A minimum of $3.6\,g\,d^{-1}$ is needed for anti-inflammatory activity. A parenteral preparation is not available but there are dispersible tablets that can be chewed and retained in the mouth. The antiplatelet action is beneficial in coronary artery occlusion. Side-effects are common (see below) and frequently limit dose and duration of treatment. Aspirin is associated with Reye's syndrome and is contraindicated in children under 12 years of age.

Phenyl acetic acids

Diclofenac is the most commonly prescribed drug in this group. It is available in a parenteral preparation but must be given by deep intramuscular injection, which is frequently painful and may be accompanied by sterile abscess formation. The adult dose is 75 mg and duration of action

12 h. It may be given by intravenous infusion but only after buffering with sodium bicarbonate. It is used for moderate postoperative pain and renal colic.

Propionic acids

Propionic acids include ibuprofen, naproxen and ketoprofen. The latter is available in an intramuscular parenteral form – the dose is 50–100 mg every 4 h (maximum 200 mg in 1 d) – but the incidence of side-effects is greater than ibuprofen.

Pyrazoles

Ketorolac is a parenteral pyrazole. It can be safely given by slow intravenous injection. The adult dose is 10 mg initially, then 10–30 mg every 4 h up to a maximum of 90 mg in 1 d (60 mg in the elderly and those weighing less than 50 kg). Analgesia may be delayed for up to 30 min after injection.

Oxicams

Piroxicam is available in a deep intramuscular parenteral formulation or as a dispersible tablet designed to dissolve in the mouth. It has a long duration of action and the dose is 20 mg once daily.

ADVERSE EFFECTS OF NSAIDs

Side-effects are variable in frequency and severity between both individuals and drugs. At equianalgesic doses side-effects are similar, but not identical. Short courses of NSAIDs are accompanied by less adverse effects than when used chronically but they should still be used with care in the prehospital environment because of adverse effects.

- *Renal function*: reversible acute renal failure may be precipitated by NSAIDs, particularly when given to individuals with pre-existing renal dysfunction, or in cases of suboptimal renal perfusion (i.e. hypovolaemia).
- *Asthma*: approximately 10% of asthmatics experience bronchospasm after the administration of NSAIDs.
- *Gastrointestinal*: discomfort is common and life-threatening gastrointestinal bleeding may occur in cases of pre-existing peptic or duodenal ulcer disease.
- *Bleeding*: the antiplatelet effect may adversely affect coagulation.
- *Hypersensitivity*: uncommon but life threatening.
- *Fluid retention*: may exacerbate poor ventricular function.
- *Elderly*: all of the above effects are more common in the elderly.

In view of this NSAIDs should be used with extreme caution in the prehospital environment, particularly in the elderly or hypovolaemic patient. Ibuprofen is the NSAID with the most favourable side-effect profile.

Nitrous oxide in oxygen (Entonox)

PHYSICAL PROPERTIES

Nitrous oxide is a colourless, sweet smelling, non-irritant gas that is heavier than air. It is neither flammable nor explosive but will support combustion of other agents at temperatures above 450°C as the gas decomposes into oxygen and nitrogen. It gives a rapid clinical effect. It is not metabolized in the body and is eliminated unchanged via the lungs. It is 15 times more soluble than nitrogen in plasma and will thus rapidly diffuse into any air-filled body cavity (i.e. middle ear, gut, pneumothorax, cranial cavity, air emboli) with a corresponding increase in cavity volume or pressure.

ENTONOX

Entonox is a commercially available 50:50 mixture of nitrous oxide in oxygen. It is supplied as a gas in French blue cylinders with a white shoulder. At room temperature the oxygen and nitrous oxide remain as a homogenous mixture but if the cylinder temperature drops below −7°C some of the gas will separate, producing initial high concentrations of oxygen followed by high concentrations of nitrous oxide later. This low temperature is often achieved in the boot of many vehicles parked out in the open in the British winter. Cylinders can be rewarmed by storage at room temperature for 2 h, or by immersion in water at 50°C for 10 min. The gas is usually self-administered via a patient-demand valve. It is important that patients are correctly instructed on how to breath the gas – slow, large-volume breaths are more effective than rapid, shallow ones. The onset time in correct use is within 60 s, although maximum analgesia takes 3–4 min. The offset after discontinuation is similarly rapid. In long-term use (>12 h) there is a risk of bone marrow depression. It is a relatively potent analgesic (Johnson & Atherton 1994) and is approximately equivalent to 10 mg morphine. It may be used for application of splints, reduction of fractures and dislocations (although muscle spasm may necessitate the use of other agents), extrication from vehicles and as a supplement to other forms of analgesia. It is usually cardiovascularly stable and does not cause respiratory depression; however, prolonged use may cause sedation and confusion.

COMPLICATIONS OF ENTONOX USE

As it displaces nitrogen in any air-filled cavity there is an increase in cavity volume. If the volume of the cavity is fixed or reaches a maximum limit there will be an increase in cavity pressure. Entonox is contraindicated in decompression sickness and should be avoided in cases of suspected bowel obstruction and it is contraindicated in chest injuries, but could theoretically be used after formal tube drainage of pneumothoraces.

Ketamine

Ketamine (2-O-chlorophenyl-2-methylaminocyclohexanone hydrochloride) is a white, water-soluble, crystalline substance and is a parenteral general anaesthetic. It is supplied as a solution containing 10, 50 or 100 mg ml^{-1}, the latter two containing benzethonium chloride as a preservative.

It is an anaesthetic agent, derived from phencyclidine ('angel dust') and was first used in 1965. It has a unique mode of action producing dissociative anaesthesia – the sleep produced is different from other anaesthetic agents and patients frequently keep their eyes open, move and may vocalize. It is a profound, effective analgesic in sub-anaesthetic concentrations.

PHYSIOLOGICAL EFFECTS

Ketamine has a sympathomimetic effect producing tachycardia and hypertension without rhythm disturbance, which may be beneficial in the shocked patient. However, in isolated heart preparations it is a direct myocardial depressant and should be avoided in patients with high spinal cord injuries (above T2). It is a mild respiratory stimulant with relative preservation of protective airway reflexes and bronchodilation. Cerebral blood flow and intracranial pressure are both increased. Although nausea and vomiting are uncommon, salivation is increased and may lead to airway compromise.

ADVERSE EFFECTS

The hypertension and tachycardia produced by ketamine make it unsuitable for use in patients with uncontrolled hypertension (including pre-eclampsia) and ischaemic heart disease. The changes in intracranial blood flow preclude its use in head-injured patients at risk from increases in intracranial pressure. As mentioned above, salivation may be problematic – an antisialagogue such as atropine or glycopyrrolate may be of use.

There is a significant incidence of emergence delirium – vivid, unpleasant dreams and hallucinations – which may persist for several weeks even after a single dose. The reported incidence is lowest in children and the elderly. They can be reduced by leaving the patient to recover in a quiet, dark environment (not often practical in the prehospital setting) or by using small amounts of diazepam or midazolam at the end of the procedure.

The incidence of all the above side-effects is less when the drug is used in the reduced quantities required for analgesia.

KETAMINE AS AN ANALGESIC

The intravenous dose required for analgesia is $0.25-0.5\,mg\,kg^{-1}$ (compared to the anaesthetic dose, which is $1.0-2.0\,mg\,kg^{-1}$), and has an onset time of 2 min and a duration of action of 10–20 min. It also has analgesic activity if given intramuscularly ($1-4\,mg\,kg^{-1}$), orally ($5-10\,mg\,kg^{-1}$) or intranasally ($6-8\,mg\,kg^{-1}$). As with other agents, the intravenous dose should be fractionated. Sedation is common, but respiration is not depressed.

Ketamine for analgesia $0.25-0.5\,mg\,kg^{-1}$.

Ketamine has been used for analgesia during vehicle extrication (Cottingham & Thomson 1994), reduction of fractures and dislocations (although increased muscle tone may require the co-administration of a benzodiazepine), polytrauma (Beliakov et al 1993), transportation (Notcutt 1994), acute war injuries (Bion 1984) and minor surgical cases. Despite its origins as an anaesthetic agent, it has been used successfully by non-anaesthetists on many occasions and is rapidly gaining favour as a prehospital analgesic for severe pain.

Ketamine for anaesthesia $1.0-2.0\,mg\,kg^{-1}$.

Local anaesthesia

Local anaesthesia has much to commend it (Desai et al 1990). It can produce excellent-quality analgesia without sedation, nausea or depression of respiration. However, in inexperienced hands it can be lethal. As with many other aspects of prehospital medicine there is a very fine line between benefit and risk. What is perfectly safe and feasible in hospital may not be so outside of it.

PHARMACOLOGY

Local anaesthetic drugs reversibly interrupt axonal conduction by blocking sodium channels. They are divided into two groups by the type of linkage between the aromatic ring and amino element: esters, e.g. cocaine, procaine and amethocaine; and amides, e.g. lidocaine, bupivacaine, prilocaine and ropivacaine (Table 14.1). Amides are far less likely to trigger hypersensitivity reactions.

There is a wide variation in the clinical effects of each agent related to their unique physiochemical properties. Potency is directly proportional to lipid solubility, speed of onset is inversely related to degree of ionization, and duration of action increases with increased protein binding and intrinsic vasoconstriction. Most local anaesthetics (with the exception of cocaine and ropivacaine) are intrinsic vasodilators and have a shorter duration of action unless exogenous vasoconstrictors (i.e. adrenaline (epinephrine), octapressin, etc.) are added. Adrenaline concentrations of greater than 1:200 000 should be avoided, and no more than 500 μg of adrenaline-containing solution should be injected (50 ml of a 1:200 000 solution). Vasoconstrictors should be avoided near any end artery (digits, penis, nose and ear) to avoid potential ischaemia. Methylhydroxybenzoate is often added as a preservative in multidose vials of local anaesthetic. It may produce hypersensitivity reactions.

METABOLISM

Ester local anaesthetics are rapidly metabolized by the liver and plasma cholinesterase. Amides are broken down by hepatic microsomes and are potentially more toxic as these pathways are subject to saturation. Prilocaine is metabolized in the liver, kidney and lungs to toluidines, which oxidize haemoglobin to methaemoglobin. Large doses ($>6\,mg\,kg^{-1}$) may produce methaemoglobinaemia.

CLINICAL CONSIDERATIONS

Local anaesthetics will work on all nerves. However, the type of nerve and its location will determine the speed of onset and duration of action irrespective of the individual agent used.

- Unmyelinated fibres are blocked before myelinated fibres. Sympathetic block occurs before sensory block which precedes motor block.
- Peripheries of nerves are blocked before the inner core (which carries the fibres supplying the more distal parts of a limb). Blockade of large, myelinated nerve trunks may take 45–60 min; blockade of isolated, small, distal peripheral nerves may take 5 min.
- Central blockade affects a wider anatomical area than peripheral blockade.
- Vascular areas (such as the intercostal space) will absorb large quantities of local anaesthetic with correspondingly high plasma concentrations and short duration of action. Systemic absorption from subcutaneous injection is minimal and duration of action is prolonged.

Table 14.1 Characteristics of amide local anaesthetics

Amide	Onset – peripheral (min)	Onset – plexus (min)	Duration	Relative toxicity	Dose – plain (mg kg^{-1})	Dose with adrenaline (epinephrine) (mg kg^{-1})
Lidocaine	5	20	Medium	Medium	3	7
Prilocaine	5	20	Medium	Low	5	8
Bupivacaine	20	45	Long	High	2	2
Ropivacaine	10	30	Long	Medium	3	Not applicable

COMPLICATIONS OF LOCAL ANAESTHESIA

Toxicity

Local anaesthetic toxicity is either relative, where a 'normal' dose of anaesthetic has been injected either intravascularly or into a highly vascular space with rapid systemic absorption, or absolute, where a miscalculation results in the injection of an inappropriately large dose of anaesthetic. Toxicity can be avoided by scrupulous attention to detail, particularly aspiration before injection, and careful dosage calculations.

> **Toxicity can be avoided by scrupulous attention to detail, particularly aspiration before injection, and careful dosage calculations.**

The main toxic effects are on the central nervous system, followed by the cardiovascular system. They may occur within 2 min of intravascular injection but absolute overdose may take up to 30 min to manifest itself.

The progressive signs and symptoms are as follows:

- perioral numbness with a metallic taste
- light-headedness, tinnitus and visual disturbances
- slurring of speech
- hypertension and tachycardia
- muscular twitching and convulsions
- coma and apnoea
- hypotension and bradycardia
- ventricular arrhythmias
- cardiac arrest.

Treatment is prioritized on the standard advanced life support (ALS) resuscitation protocol of airway, breathing and circulation. Hypoxia and acidosis from inadequate basic and advanced life support potentiate toxicity.

- Stop injecting the local anaesthetic.
- Assess and treat airway obstruction.
- Assess ventilation and support if needed, give supplemental oxygen.
- Gain intravenous access.
- Attach monitoring and record baseline observations.
- Convulsions – treat with diazepam 0.1 mg kg^{-1}.
- Hypotension – elevate patient's legs, give intravenous fluid boluses as needed.
- Arrhythmias – treat only if life threatening as many are self-limiting. Cardiac pacing may be required for heart block.

Hypersensitivity reactions

Fortunately, severe anaphylactoid and anaphylactic reactions are uncommon. They are more common with ester-based local anaesthetics, but these are used infrequently. It is important to exclude toxicity and simple fainting before instituting treatment, which is based on standard therapy for hypersensitivity reactions.

Nerve damage

Nerves are delicate structures and may not recover from direct trauma. Sharp needles intended for intravenous, intramuscular and subcutaneous injection are not suitable for neural blockade. Nerve penetration is a real possibility and nerve transection with permanent disability is not uncommon. Short, bevelled, atraumatic needles specifically designed for nerve blockade should be used if possible. Conscious patients will complain bitterly if a nerve is penetrated – blocks should be avoided on unconscious patients.

Failed nerve block

Blocks fail for many reasons, including incorrect injection site, injection of an inadequate dose or volume of local anaesthetic and failing to allow adequate time for the onset of the block.

Patchy analgesia may be supplemented by more peripheral blocks, or the use of Entonox or opioids. Patients should not be left in pain.

PREHOSPITAL CONSIDERATIONS

Local analgesia can provide excellent analgesia without respiratory depression and cardiovascular instability. However, any block will complicate the future assessment of peripheral neurological function. This should be done before the block is instituted and recorded in the prehospital record. It should also be noted that evolving problems in an anaesthetized limb, such as pressure sores and compartment syndromes, will be masked. Frequent examination of any limb at risk is required, and abnormal pressure and position avoided.

LOCAL ANAESTHETIC AGENTS

Esters have limited use as surface anaesthetic agents (i.e. respiratory tract and cornea) but are limited by the higher incidence of hypersensitivity reactions. Amide local anaesthetics are widely used but have different characteristics – agent selection will vary depending on the patient, required speed of onset and duration, site of injection, and dose and volume of anaesthetic needed (Table 14.1).

Lidocaine

Lidocaine is the 'standard' amide anaesthetic. It is extremely versatile and can be given for all axial, plexus and nerve blocks, and subcutaneous infiltration. It is rapidly acting and lasts for 60–90 min. Speed of onset and duration of action may be increased by the addition of adrenaline.

The safe dose of lidocaine for an average adult is 20 ml of 1% (10 ml of 2%, etc.).

Prilocaine

Prilocaine is similar to lidocaine but has a better safety profile. In doses above 600 mg it can produce methaemoglobinaemia. This can be treated with $2 \, mg \, kg^{-1}$ of methylene blue. Again, it can be used for all common blocks and intravenous regional anaesthesia.

Bupivacaine

Bupivacaine is a long-acting agent – plexus blocks may last for up to 24 h. It is approximately 20 times as toxic and tends to produce greater motor block than lidocaine. These features make it less suitable for prehospital use.

References

Beliakov VA, Sinistyn LN, Maksimor GA et al 1993 Analgesia and anesthesia in the pre-hospital stage of mechanical trauma. Anesteziologiia i Reanmatologiia 5: 24–32

Bion JF 1984 Infusion analgesia for acute war injuries. Anaesthesia 39: 560–564

Bruns BM, Dieckman R, Shagoury C et al 1992 Safety of pre-hospital therapy with morphine sulphate. American Journal of Emergency Medicine 10: 53–57

Chambers JA, Guly HR 1993 The need for better pre-hospital analgesia. Archives of Emergency Medicine 10: 187–192

Chambers JA, Guly HR 1994 Pre-hospital intravenous nalbuphine administration by paramedics. Resuscitation 27: 153–158

Cottingham R, Thomson K 1994 Use of ketamine in prolonged entrapment. Journal of Accident and Emergency Medicine 11: 189–191

Dayer P, Collart L, Desmeules J 1994 The pharmacology of tramadol. Drugs 47(Suppl 1): 3–7

Desai SM, Bernhard WN, McAlary B 1990 Regional anesthesia: management considerations in the trauma patient. Critical Care Clinics 6: 85–101

Eggers KA, Power I 1995 Tramadol. British Journal of Anaesthesia 74: 247–279

Hannhart B, Bailanger G, Audubert G, Laxenaive MC 1992 Nalbuphine analgesia preserves ventilation after thoracotomy despite a reduction in respiratory drive. Respiration 59: 159–163

Johnson JC, Atherton GL 1994 Effectiveness of nitrous oxide in a rural EMS system. Journal of Emergency Medicine 9: 45–53

Johnson GS, Guly HR 1995 The effect of pre-hospital administration of nalbuphine on on-scene times. Journal of Accident and Emergency Medicine 12: 20–22

Notcutt WG 1994 Transporting patients with overwhelming pain. Anaesthesia 49: 145–147

Raffa RB 1996 A novel approach to the pharmacology of analgesics. American Journal of Medicine 101: 40S–46S

Vickers MD, O'Flaherty D, Szekely SM et al 1992 Tramadol: pain relief by an opioid without respiratory depression. Anaesthesia 47: 291–296

Wyllie HR, Dunn FG 1994 Pre-hospital opiate and aspirin administration in patients with suspected myocardial infarction. British Medical Journal 308: 760–761

Substance abuse

15

Introduction 173

Terminology associated with substance misuse 173

Alcohol and alcohol dependence 174

Management of non-alcohol substance misusers 177

Commonly misused substances 177

References 181

Introduction

Problems related to use of alcohol, drugs and solvents are increasing in the UK. This reflects both an increase in incidence and greater awareness of such behaviour by medical, paramedical and lay people. Among teenagers the rising incidence of substance misuse is particularly worrying.

Drug dependence is a socio-psycho-biological syndrome, the key feature being the priority given to drug-seeking behaviour over other behaviours. Drug or alcohol use does not always lead to dependence, and a problem substance taker is someone who experiences social, physical or legal sequelae related to intoxication with, excessive consumption of or dependence on drugs, alcohol or other substances.

Terminology associated with substance misuse

SUBSTANCE MISUSE

Substance misuse covers a spectrum ranging from adverse effects of intoxication through to hazardous use, abuse and dependence. Diagnostic criteria have been drawn up for these different classifications. Substance misuse can be defined as substance use where there is a risk or presence of harmful consequences.

ABUSE AND HARMFUL USE

These terms describe individuals who are manifesting problems related to substance use but who do not meet the criteria for a diagnosis of substance dependence and have never done so in the past. These patients have a better prognosis than those with alcohol dependence, respond better to brief interventions and may be more suited to approaches centring on controlling substance use than abstinence. Examples are a daily drinker in a stable social situation, not dependent on alcohol, who develops liver disease, or an intermittent cocaine user arrested after a car accident while under the influence.

HAZARDOUS USE

This is defined by the World Health Organization (1992) and some national diagnosis systems as a repetitive pattern of use that confers a risk of harmful physical and psychological consequences. It includes binge use, when the individual is intoxicated and has a reduced capacity for self-care, and use in unsafe settings, e.g. before or while driving a motor vehicle, operating machinery or in situations where it would be physically dangerous.

ACUTE INTOXICATION

This is a reversible syndrome that is caused by the recent use of a psychoactive substance. The symptoms and signs are directly related to the physiological effects of the substance on the central nervous system (CNS). It causes impairment in cognition, behaviour, coordination, ability to self-care and, if severe, impairment of vital centres. There is complete recovery except when a specific complication of intoxication (e.g. hypoxic brain damage or aspiration pneumonia) has arisen. The severity of intoxication is related to the dose taken but clinical features are influenced by the presence of organic disorders. The features of intoxication do not always reflect the primary actions of the substance.

WITHDRAWAL

A withdrawal state reflects the absence of a psychoactive substance in a neuroadapted individual. The syndrome results in symptoms and signs that are the opposite of those that occur in intoxication. Withdrawal states last from several hours to several days depending on the biological duration of action of the substance and the severity of the underlying dependence.

WITHDRAWAL STATES AND REBOUND PHENOMENA

It is important to distinguish between a withdrawal state and the rebound phenomenon, which can occur in any individual. A rebound state in the form of a hangover may occur after heavy alcohol consumption. A withdrawal state is diagnosed only if there is a sufficient clustering of symptoms that are of sufficient severity and duration. Usually, the symptoms should last at least 24h or be aborted by further substance use. A withdrawal syndrome can be induced as a conditioned response in the absence of recent substance use. This can occur when, for example, a person returns to an environment that was previously associated with drug use (Grant et al 1990).

DEPENDENCE

Dependence is determined by factors such as amount and frequency of drug use, development of tolerance and withdrawal, inability to abstain and degree of physical, social and personal damage. Physical dependence is caused by alterations in brain function that lead to the experiences of withdrawal. Psychological dependence describes repeated drug seeking and taking in the absence of withdrawal.

Alcohol and alcohol dependence

PREVALENCE OF PROBLEM DRINKING

1.5 million people in Britain are drinking at levels that are definitely harmful (50 units a week or more for men, 36 units a week or more for women), while 7 million people are drinking more than is regarded as sensible. 25% of males are said to be problem drinkers at some point in their lives and approximately 25% of general medical admissions have alcohol-related problems. The male:female ratio is 4:1 but the female rate is increasing.

EFFECTS OF ALCOHOL INGESTION AND ACTIONS OF ALCOHOL

The most important actions of alcohol are on the CNS, in which it causes depression. Low doses cause disinhibition, resulting in hyperactivity and lack of judgement. Alcohol induces peripheral vasodilatation by depressing the vasomotor centre and acts as a diuretic. In moderate concentration it increases secretion of gastric acid. Alcohol initially increases blood glucose, leading to increased glucose metabolism, and inhibits gluconeogenesis. Lactic acidosis occurs with even a moderate dose and this is associated with reduced elimination of uric acid, leading to hyperuricaemia, which may precipitate gout.

SHORT-TERM CONSEQUENCES OF ALCOHOL INTAKE

Acute intoxication

Acute intoxication may lead to physical injury from trauma or head injury. It is important always to look for evidence of injury or illness in an intoxicated patient before putting their clinical state down to alcohol intoxication. Intoxication may cause hypoglycaemia or metabolic acidosis. Severe intoxication with alcohol can cause death often from vomiting leading to asphyxiation, but also directly related to alcohol poisoning.

LONG-TERM PHYSICAL CONSEQUENCES OF ALCOHOL DEPENDENCE

- Gastrointestinal tract:
  - Oesophagitis and gastritis causing vomiting and retching

- Mallory–Weiss tear in lower oesophagus causing haematemesis
- Portal hypertension causing oesophageal varices and possible massive haematemesis
- Peptic ulceration
- Acute and chronic pancreatitis (acute has a mortality of 10–40%)
- Carcinoma of the upper gastrointestinal tract
- Liver damage:
  - Alcoholic hepatitis
  - Fatty liver
  - Cirrhosis
  - Liver failure and hepatic encephalopathy
- Cardiovascular:
  - Cardiac arrhythmias
  - Cardiomyopathy
  - Coronary artery disease, hypertension, cerebrovascular accident
- Metabolic:
  - Hypoglycaemia
  - Ketoacidosis
- Haematological:
  - Anaemia
  - Thrombocytopenia
- Nervous system:
  - Diffuse brain damage from cortical shrinkage and ventricular dilatation
  - Alcoholic dementia
  - Wernicke–Korsakoff syndrome – caused by deficiency of thiamine (vitamin B_1). In acute Wernicke's encephalopathy, symptoms include alteration in level of consciousness, nystagmus, external ophthalmoplegia, ataxia and peripheral neuropathy. A glucose load can precipitate Wernicke's encephalopathy in a malnourished thiamine-deficient patient
  - Epilepsy from withdrawal fits.

PSYCHOLOGICAL PROBLEMS OF ALCOHOL DEPENDENCE

Alcoholic hallucinosis

Hallucinations of voices in the third person, usually derogatory, occur in clear consciousness either when alcohol levels are increasing or decreasing. There is no disorientation.

Affective symptoms

Changes in mood occur in 90% of problem drinkers. Other common symptoms associated with problem drinking include sleep disturbance, change in appetite with weight loss, poor concentration, irritability and anxiety. Taken together with the emotional lability, an initial impression of clinical depression may be formed. However, unless alcohol misuse is secondary to depression and the individual is not dependent on alcohol, antidepressant treatment is not indicated until steps have been taken to treat the alcohol dependence.

Suicide

There is a 10–15% risk of successful suicide in alcohol-dependent people and consideration must be given to whether there is an underlying depressive illness. Admission to a psychiatric hospital for assessment may be appropriate and, if there is good evidence of a depressive or other mental illness coexisting with alcohol dependence, the Mental Health Act 1983 can be used for compulsory admission.

Pathological jealousy

Pathological jealousy (also known as morbid jealousy or Othello syndrome) manifests as a morbid, delusional belief that a partner is being unfaithful. It is twice as common in men and is associated with alcohol dependence. The partner and/or the purported lover may be at risk of serious violence.

SOCIAL PROBLEMS OF ALCOHOL DEPENDENCE

Although the association of drinking with traffic accidents and violence is well known, it is only in the last decade that these topics have been systematically researched. Estimates of the proportion of deaths that occur in people who have been drinking range from 35–63% for falls to 21–47% for drownings and 12–61% for burns, with lower figures for non-fatal accidents (Hingson & Howland 1993). There is a strong association between violent crime and alcohol intoxication. In an examination of more than 9000 crimes reported in 11 countries, nearly two-thirds of violent offenders were drinking at the time of the crime and nearly half of the victims were intoxicated when they were victimized. Drinking to excess takes its toll on relationships, employment and financial state.

PREHOSPITAL MANAGEMENT OF ALCOHOL-RELATED DISORDERS

Assessment

Given that a quarter of general medical admissions have alcohol-related problems, all patients presenting to GPs and

Box 15.1

CAGE questionnaire

Alcohol dependence is likely if the patient gives two or more positive answers:

1. **Have you ever felt you should Cut down on your drinking?**
2. **Have people ever Annoyed you by criticizing your drinking?**
3. **Have you ever felt bad or Guilty about your drinking?**
4. **Have you ever had a drink first thing in the morning to steady your nerves or get rid of a hangover (Eye-opener)?**

emergency departments should be screened for a history of alcohol use and excessive use. Pointers in the history include absenteeism, unstable work, domestic violence, alcohol problems in the family, repeated accidents, and evasiveness when questioned about alcohol use. Symptoms of withdrawal should be sought. Examination may reveal tremor, bruising, rib fractures or signs of liver disease such as spider naevi and liver palms. Depressed mood may be secondary to alcohol misuse and alcohol use should be routinely assessed after any attempted suicide. Enquiry should be made as to the quantity, type and pattern of drinking in the previous week. A simple screening interview such as the CAGE questionnaire (Mayfield et al 1974) should be administered. Laboratory tests such as raised mean corpuscular volume (MCV), raised gamma-glutamyl transferase (γ-GT) taken together with two or more positive answers on the CAGE interview should detect about three-quarters of individuals with an alcohol problem.

Specific medical presentations that particularly affect those dependent on alcohol and that may aggravate or develop during a withdrawal syndrome include hypoglycaemia, dehydration, renal impairment, upper gastrointestinal bleeding, hepatic encephalopathy, rib fractures, subdural haematoma, pneumonia, arrhythmias, alcoholic cardiomyopathy, subacute pontine myelinosis and Zieve's syndrome. The CAGE questionnaire is set out in Box 15.1.

EMERGENCIES RELATED TO ALCOHOL DEPENDENCE

Acute alcohol withdrawal

Alcohol withdrawal occurs in someone dependent on alcohol. The risk of withdrawal does not depend on intake. It may begin within 6h of cessation or reduction of alcohol and peaks by 48h, subsiding over the next 7 days. Early symptoms include anorexia, nausea, vomiting, tremors, anxiety, insomnia, excessive sweating and tachycardia.

Alcohol withdrawal may be associated with hallucinations in clear consciousness and grand mal epileptic seizures 10–60h after drinking. After 72h some patients may go on to develop delirium tremens.

Delirium tremens

Delirium tremens (DTs) occurs on days 3–5 following cessation or significant reduction of drinking in an alcohol-dependent person. It is characterized by confusion, agitation, disorientation, delusions, hallucinations and vivid imagery (often of insects, but not pink elephants), together with intense tremulousness. There is often a marked lability of emotions and autonomic dysfunction. There is no craving for alcohol. Admission must be to a medical ward for rehydration, sedation and nutrition. In 50% of cases DTs are precipitated by an intercurrent infection. Other precipitants include hypoglycaemia, hypokalaemia (with respiratory alkalosis) and hypocalcaemia. Mortality is up to 10%.

Management

Unplanned alcohol withdrawal in someone with a history of withdrawal complications, and certainly delirium tremens, should be managed in a hospital setting. Clearly, if there is a high risk of withdrawal seizures, or incipient or actual delirium tremens, the setting should be a general medical ward. If withdrawals are mild with no history of complications, detoxification can be managed either at home (with appropriate community support) or in a psychiatric inpatient setting, but the likelihood is that if a person is dependent on alcohol and withdrawal is unplanned and unforeseen, he is unlikely to be able to resist the cravings and compulsion to drink and may discharge themselves from hospital. Sufferers of delirium tremens do not have cravings. Alcohol or drug addiction is not a mental disorder as recognized by the Mental Health Act 1983 and individuals with changes in behaviour related to alcohol or drug misuse cannot be admitted compulsorily to hospital under its provisions.

Immediate management of all heavy drinkers should include vitamins B and C daily for a few days. If there is a history of withdrawal seizures carbamazepine 200mg twice daily should be prescribed. For alcohol withdrawal seizures or status epilepticus intravenous benzodiazepines will be required.

If disorientation has developed or is incipient, admission to hospital will be necessary. In these cases other diagnoses such as subdural haematoma, pneumonia and meningitis should be considered. For severe agitation haloperidol or droperidol 10mg intramuscularly may be needed, but a benzodiazepine should also be given for its anticonvulsant effect.

Management of non-alcohol substance misusers

EPIDEMIOLOGY

Unlike the stereotypical image of a drug addict as a dishevelled, unwashed, young man with rather staring eyes and an aggressive manner, people who misuse drugs or other substances come from all walks of life and there is no particular personality profile, ethnic group, class or profession that determines who are characteristic substance misusers.

PREVALENCE

Obtaining statistics

Because drug abuse is illegal it is not easy to determine the numbers of those who misuse substances. The Home Office Addicts Index is the main source of data for the UK but it only includes those who have attended doctors and who have been diagnosed as dependent on controlled drugs. The doctor notifies the Home Office of the addict's name, sex, mode of drug use and type of drug prescribed. Only certain drugs such as heroin, cocaine and certain opiates are notifiable. It is estimated that only about 20% of opiate and cocaine users are notified to the Home Office.

The Misuse of Drugs Act 1971 is detailed in Box 15.2.

Prevalence

Official figures of substance misusers relate to those seeking treatment or those notified to the Home Office and do not reflect the extent of use. A 1995 survey of 15- and 16-year old-pupils in the UK showed that 42.3% had at some time used illicit drugs, mainly cannabis. Glues and solvents had been used by 20.4%, and Ecstasy (3,4-methylenedioxymethamfetamine – MDMA) by 7.3% of girls and 9.2% of boys. Few reported having used drugs such as cocaine and heroin. For all types of drug experimentation there seemed to have been a large rise since 1989.

ASSESSMENT

Unusual behaviour of any sort could be due to substance misuse, and it is important to note that substance misusers may often use more than one substance at a time, causing a mixture of symptoms and signs. Whenever assessing anyone whose behaviour is suggestive of substance misuse, check their arms and legs for evidence of injection sites. Misusers of volatile solvents often smell of glue or aerosol and may have a rash around their mouth and nose where there has been contact with an inhalation bag.

There are few specific antidotes for most substances of abuse, and the basic ABC approach is essential. Specific details of treatment required within the hospital environment have been excluded unless they can be started during prehospital treatment.

When confronted with a person whom you suspect of abusing drugs it is useful to assess the extent of the problem. Enquiry should be made regarding the length of the history of drug abuse, the types and quantities of drugs used and the route of administration. It is important to note any history of intravenous drug use and whether shared needles were used. Information should be sought regarding any psychological or physical problems linked to drug abuse. Intravenous drug users should be asked about previous testing for hepatitis B, hepatitis C and HIV. Current daily supply in terms of amount used and whether prescribed or bought on the street should be noted. Commonly, more than one drug is used at the same time.

Physical examination should check for needle marks, usually on the arms or antecubital fossa but also in the groin area, the femoral vein, or on the legs or ankles. Tender or swollen lymph nodes may be found in the axilla or groin. The examination should also include a check for the presence of any drug-specific effects or drug withdrawal effects.

Commonly misused substances

Cannabis (marijuana)

Street names: dope, grass, joint, joy sticks, Mary Jane, pot, reefers.

Cannabis is the most commonly used illicit drug in the world with about 200–300 million people using it regularly. It is a derivative of the plant *Cannabis sativa*. The preparations in common use are marijuana, hashish and the Indian forms (ganja and bhang). The resin, which contains the tetrahydrocannabinoids (THCs), is the most pharmacologically active part of the plant. Cannabis is most often smoked but can be taken orally and is of relatively low toxicity (unless ingested by children, when coma may ensue). The symptoms of toxicity include excitement, euphoria, drowsiness, panic attacks, toxic psychosis and rarely coma and dilated pupils.

Tetrahydrocannabinol is absorbed into body stores. In humans, chronic use causes accumulation and effects persist for several weeks after stopping the drug. Cannabis has three times the tar content of ordinary cigarettes and is potentially carcinogenic. Because the inhaled smoke is retained longer than smoke from a normal cigarette, the blood carbon monoxide level is, on average, five times the level found from smoking ordinary cigarettes. Use may lead to a persistent tachycardia, which is dose related and

Box 15.2

The Misuse of Drugs Act 1971

Section 1 provides for the establishment of an Advisory Council on the Misuse of Drugs whose purpose is to advise ministers on a range of issues relating to drugs.

Section 2 deals with the classification of controlled drugs according to their perceived harmfulness to society and to the individual. There are three classes: Class A (the most harmful), which includes natural and most synthetic opiates, cocaine, LSD, injectable amfetamine and cannabinol; Class B, which includes oral amfetamine, phenmetrazine, cannabis resin, codeine, dihydrocodeine and certain barbiturates; and Class C which contains methaqualone and certain amfetamine-like drugs.

Section 10 confers powers on the Home Secretary to make various regulations for preventing the misuse of controlled drugs.

Possession, supply and production

A doctor must not administer or supply heroin, cocaine or dipipanone to anyone whom he or she believes or has reasonable grounds to suspect is dependent on any notifiable drug unless he or she has a special licence to do so granted by the Home Office.

Heroin, cocaine and dipipanone may be administered or supplied if they have been authorized by another appropriately licensed doctor.

A doctor may prescribe heroin, cocaine or dipipanone to someone who is dependent on a notifiable drug if the treatment is for organic disease or injury.

Prescriptions

All prescriptions for controlled drugs: must be written in ink, entirely in the doctor's own handwriting, dated and signed. The form of the preparation (e.g. tablets, linctus or capsules), the dose and the strength of the preparation must be specified; the total quantity or the total dosage units must be written in words and figures.

Registers

Doctors are obliged to keep registers recording all transactions relating to Schedule 2 drugs.

Destruction

GPs are not allowed to destroy any controlled drugs except in the presence of one of the following authorized people:

- any police officer
- a Home Office Drugs Branch inspector
- a Pharmaceutical Society inspector
- a Regional Pharmaceutical Officer
- a Regional Medical Officer.

Notification

A doctor has to notify the Chief Medical Officer at the Home Office within 7 days if he or she believes or suspects that the person he or she is attending is dependent on one of the following drugs:

- Cocaine
- Dextromoramide (Palfium)
- Diamorphine (Heroin)
- Dipipanone (Diconal)
- Hydrocodone
- Hydromorphone
- Levorphanol
- Methadone (Physeptone)
- Morphine
- Oxycodone
- Pethidine
- Phanaxocin
- Piritramide.

The address for notifications is: The Chief Medical Officer, Drugs Branch, Home Office, Queen Anne's Gate, London SW1 9AT.

The details supplied should be the name, address, date of birth, sex and NHS number. Having notified the patient to the Home Office does not imply that prescribing is appropriate.

The Addicts Index is strictly confidential and no other agency, such as the police, has access to it.

---

can be blocked by propranolol. Bronchial irritation and dilatation follow acute inhalation. The dilatation of superficial blood vessels leads to red eyes.

Psychological effects of cannabis

Psychological effects include depersonalization and derealization, short-lived psychotic episodes in clear consciousness after acute cannabis intoxication and severe panic. It is now accepted that cannabis use may precipitate relapse of an existing functional psychosis but it is worth noting that the drug may be a symptom rather than a cause of the illness, as patients in the early stages of psychotic relapse may try to treat themselves with illegal drugs.

Management

In the prehospital setting there are no specific treatments required apart from supportive measures. Psychotic symptoms should be treated with antipsychotic medication (e.g. chlorpromazine 50 mg or haloperidol 5 mg twice daily) and the patient should be followed up as appropriate.

STIMULANTS

Stimulants such as amphetamines and cocaine arouse and activate the user in much the same way as natural adrenaline (epinephrine). Breathing and heart rate speed up, the pupils widen and appetite lessens. The user feels more energetic, confident and cheerful. Because of these effects there is risk of psychological dependence.

Cocaine

Street names: blow, coke, crack, dust, freebase, ice, koks.

Cocaine use is still increasing in the UK. Cocaine is an alkaloid found in the leaves of the coca bush, grown in South America. It is usually snorted into the nose through a straw or rolled paper. It may also be injected either alone or with heroin. Crack is cocaine that has been chemically altered into a smokeable crystalline form. These crystals may be placed in a small pipe and heated from below by a match. A cracking sound is produced as the substance vaporizes, which is the origin of its name. Crack differs from cocaine in that the initial rush from crack is much more pleasurable and intense, and its effects are of very rapid onset and a shorter duration (no longer than 15 min). Owing to the powerful emotional effects of crack, there is a high risk of dependence.

Acute administration typically causes an increase in heart rate and blood pressure, sometimes accompanied by pupillary dilatation, perspiration or chills, nausea or vomiting, and chest pain. Cardiac arrhythmias, seizures, dyskinesias and dystonias can occur. Sudden death, probably due to arrhythmias or respiratory arrest, has been observed in otherwise healthy people, as have non-fatal myocardial infarctions and cerebrovascular accidents. An unusual but serious medical complication is pneumothorax resulting from performing Valsalva-like manoeuvres in order to better absorb cocaine that has been inhaled. Cocaine use is associated with irregularities in placental blood flow, abruptio placentae, and premature labour and delivery. These problems can result in very low birthweight infants.

Psychological effects include elation, excitement, restlessness and reduced hunger. The heavy user may experience weight loss with nutritional deficiencies. Snorting may lead to ulceration or perforation of the nasal septum.

High or toxic doses may lead to anxiety or panic, or florid psychosis with paranoid experiences, the experience of imaginary bugs under the skin with itching, severe scratching and self-mutilation. When the high wears off, a crash follows, symptoms of which include irritability that may lead to aggression and depression that may be so severe as to induce a suicidal crisis.

The management consists of general supportive measures and treatment of symptoms, e.g. benzodiazepines if convulsing or very agitated. There is no specific treatment. Psychiatric assessment may be required.

Crack cocaine

Crack cocaine (street name 'crack') is a processed crystalline form of the drug, which is usually smoked through a pipe and inhaled. The name crack originates from the sound made by the heating crystals as they are smoked. It delivers high concentrations of cocaine to the lungs giving a feeling of intense euphoria. Other common effects are hyperactivity, restlessness, hyperthermia, tachycardia and increased blood pressure. Side-effects include cardiovascular (dysrhythmias, acute myocardial ischaemia), neurological (headache, seizures, stoke) and gastrointestinal (nausea and abdominal pain).

Treatment is supportive, and similar to treatment of other forms of cocaine abuse. Intravenous benzodiazepines may be of benefit in overdose or in the presence of myocardial ischaemia.

Amphetamine

Street names: speed, sulphate, uppers, whizz.

Amphetamine (α-methylphenethylamine, phenylpropan-2-amine) was first synthesized in 1887 by Edeleano. Modern amphetamine sulphate may only be 20–30% pure and costs around £10–15 per gram. A heavy user may use several grams a day. Dexamphetamine (Dexedrine – 'dexies') and amphetamine-like drugs, such as methylphenidate (Ritalin) and diethylpropion (Tenuate), are also taken.

Acute effects include euphoria, anxiety, increased energy, reduced need for sleep, oversensitiveness, risky behaviour, miosis and tachycardia. Amphetamine psychosis mimics acute symptoms of schizophrenia and manifests with paranoid delusions, auditory, visual and tactile hallucinations, and increased arousal and irritability. Consciousness is unimpaired.

Toxicity produces a life-threatening state of overactivity of the sympathetic nervous system. Symptoms include high blood pressure, seizures, increase in body temperature, muscle rigidity and profound sweating. Some cases progress to the point of severe muscle damage with subsequent acute renal failure or disseminated intravascular coagulation. Between 15% and 20% of the toxic overdoses of amphetamine have been attributed to cerebrovascular accidents.

Withdrawal effects include dysphoria, fatigue, lassitude and depression.

Opiates

Commonly abused opiates include opium (big 'O', brown stuff, China white, dust), heroin (brown sugar, horse shit, rock, smack), and methadone (doll, dollies, Dolophine).

Opiate overdose is an acute life-threatening event. Overdosage or ingestion of opiates is characterized by altered level of consciousness, respiratory depression and pinpoint pupils. Fits occur less commonly. Other signs include euphoric or stuporose mental state, convulsions, hypotension and hypothermia (Table 15.1). In general, addicts can tolerate higher doses than non-addicts before manifesting the effects of toxicity, but it is important to be aware of addicts who have had a period of abstinence (e.g. in prison) and whose tolerance is therefore markedly reduced.

Table 15.1 Opiate overdose

- Severity:
  - Related to dose, interaction with other drugs (e.g. alcohol, benzodiazepines), time since consumption, patient's general condition
- Signs:
  - Decreased respiration
  - Blue lips
  - Pale or blue skin
  - Pinpoint pupils (unless there is brain damage in which case pupils are dilated)
  - Pulmonary oedema
  - Shock
- Management:
  - Intravenous naloxone 0.4–1.2 mg repeated in 3–10 min up to a dose of 10 mg
  - Suspect additional drug or alternative cause if no response
  - Monitor for 24–72 h post-recovery

The initial management of an opiate overdose or respiratory depression due to opiate ingestion is maintenance of the airway and oxygenation followed by the rapid administration of naloxone. Indeed, naloxone should be administered on the least suspicion of opiate ingestion. The adult dose is 0.4–1.2 mg repeated at intervals of several minutes up to a dose of 10 mg. Failure to respond to a total dose of 10 mg indicates that the respiratory depression and altered conscious level is due either to another drug or alternatively to coadministration of another CNS-depressant drug. It is important to remember that naloxone has a short half-life and that recurrence of respiratory depression or altered conscious level may occur. In such cases further doses are required. The dose of naloxone for children is $0.01\,mg\,kg^{-1}$ repeated as necessary. The patient should be monitored for at least 24 h for heroin and 72 h for methadone. Additional intramuscular naloxone should be considered in patients who are unlikely to be prepared to allow ongoing observation in case of loss of effectiveness of intravenous doses.

HALLUCINOGENS

Lysergic acid diethylamide (LSD)

Street names: acid, blotter acid, paper acid, purple haze, white lightning.

LSD is a synthetic psychedelic drug of low toxicity. Symptoms include confusion, agitation, hallucinations, dilated pupils, piloerection, coma and respiratory arrest. LSD does not cause physical dependence. No fatalities can be directly attributable to LSD but haemorrhage (thought to be due to the action on platelet serotonin function) has been described. Supportive measures only are required.

Psilocybin (magic mushrooms)

Street name: shrooms.

Ingestion of magic mushrooms is a seasonal problem, usually well known in particular localities where the mushrooms can be picked. Cases may occur in small epidemics. The fatal dose is unknown.

Euphoria, anxiety, depression, illusions and psychosis are all common manifestations. Hyperthermia, tachycardia, tremors and dilated pupils are characteristic. There is no specific treatment in the prehospital setting but efforts should be made to calm the victim and give reassurance that the effects are self-limiting. Panic attacks can be treated with diazepam 20 mg by mouth.

Phencyclidine

Street names: angel dust (or dust), busy bee, embalming fluid, PCP, superweed.

Phencyclidine is a psychedelic drug, fatal dose unknown. Symptoms include anxiety and psychosis, ataxia, paraesthesia, catatonic movements, fits, coma, hypotension, respiratory impairment, Cheyne–Stokes breathing and respiratory arrest. Treatment is supportive.

Amyl nitrate

Street names: poor man's cocaine, poppers, snappers, sweat.

Amyl nitrate is toxic by ingestion and inhalation. Its principal mode of toxicity is by the formation of methaemoglobin. The fatal dose is unknown but even small amounts can cause symptoms. Symptoms occur within a few seconds of inhalation but may be delayed with ingestion.

Headache, nausea and vomiting occur, along with sweating and flushing. Tightness of the chest is common, as is confusion and occasionally fits. Cyanosis due to methaemoglobinaemia may occur. There is no specific treatment in the prehospital setting apart from maintenance of the airway and administration of oxygen to treat cyanosis.

Ecstasy (MDMA)

Street names: Dennis the Menace, 'E', white dove.

A semi-synthetic amphetamine (3,4-methylenedioxymethamfetamine), Ecstasy has become notorious in recent years as the cause of deaths that have occurred in otherwise healthy teenagers. Two causes of death are commonly recognized: early deaths are due to arrhythmias and late deaths are due to an effect on muscles associated with a fatal rise in body temperature (a similar condition, neuroleptic malignant syndrome, occurs rarely as a side-effect of antipsychotic drugs). Deaths can occur after exposure to doses previously tolerated and are thought to be due to an idiosyncratic reaction. Symptoms range from mild to life-threatening and include muscle spasms, dilated pupils, anxiety, tachycardia, increased temperature, abdominal pain, hypotension, fits, coma and stroke. The fatal dose is unknown but is close to the 'therapeutic' dose. There are no specific treatments other than supportive measures in the prehospital setting.

Ephedrine

Street names: uppers, ups.

Ephedrine is a sympathomimetic drug with a fatal dose of 200 mg in children and over 2 g in adults. It causes restlessness, tachycardia, dilated pupils, arrhythmias and hallucinations. Apart from treating fits with diazepam, there is no specific prehospital treatment required and supportive measures should be instituted.

Caffeine

Street names: uppers, ups.

Similar in side-effects to ephedrine; the fatal dose is 10 g. Treatment is as for ephedrine.

SEDATIVES

Barbiturates

Street names: barbs, bennies, black beauties, bluebirds, downers, sodies.

Symptoms include ataxia, dysarthria, decreased conscious level, coma, respiratory depression, hypothermia and hypotension. There are no specific treatments apart from general supportive measures. Withdrawal seizures may occur and should be controlled with diazepam.

VOLATILE SOLVENTS

Volatile solvents may be sniffed directly from the container but higher concentrations may be achieved by holding a rag soaked in the substance to the face or by inhaling from a plastic bag containing the substance. Vehicles for such solvents include cleaning fluids, adhesives, typewriter correction fluid, lighter fluids and glues.

Blood levels of most inhalants peak within minutes and are soon sequestered in adipose tissue, so blood assay may not be a reliable indication of brain concentrations.

Inhalant intoxication resembles alcohol intoxication with initial disinhibition and behavioural stimulation followed by depression at higher doses. The user may demonstrate muscular uncoordination and present to medical attention after sustaining trauma from motor vehicle accidents, falls or burns.

Headaches, diplopia, tinnitus, palpitations, abdominal pain, and nausea and vomiting may be reported. On examination the odour of paint or solvents may be apparent on the user's clothes or breath. A characteristic papular rash around the nose and mouth may be observed. Mydriasis, nystagmus and slurred speech may be evident.

Emergency complications include 'sudden sniffing death' (Bass 1970). This is believed to result from cardiac arrhythmia and may occur several hours after sniffing. 20% of such deaths occur in first-time users. 20% of deaths are estimated to be due to aspiration of vomit or anoxia when the bag is placed over the head to enhance inhalation, and respiratory depression may result directly from the CNS-depressant qualities of the substance used.

Glue

Toluene is the commonest solvent used in glues available over the counter. Effects include excitement, chest tightness, fits, coma, arrhythmias and death. Supportive measures should be instituted, with particular emphasis on oxygenation to reduce the likelihood of arrhythmias.

BUTANE

Butane is a colourless, odourless gas commonly used as the propellant in ozone-friendly sprays but available in cigarette lighters; it is generally inhaled from a bag. Symptoms include respiratory depression, coma, hypotension and arrhythmias. Treatment is supportive only.

BUTYL NITRATE

Street names: liquid incense, locker popper, locker room, room deodorizer, rush.

Butyl nitrate is an industrial solvent also used as a room deodorizer. It is fatal when ingested in even small quantities; the fatal dose is unknown. Symptoms include flushing, tachycardia, hypotension, confusion, shortness of breath and cyanosis (from the formation of methaemoglobin), coma and fits. Treatment is supportive.

References

Bass M 1970 Sudden sniffing death. Journal of the American Medical Association 212: 2075–2077

Grant KA, Hoffman PL, Tabakoff B 1990 Neurobiological and behavioural approaches to tolerance and dependence. In: Edwards G, Lader M (eds) The nature of drug dependence. Oxford University Press, Oxford, pp 135–165

Hingson R, Howland J 1993 Alcohol and non-traffic intended injuries. Addiction 88: 877–883

Mayfield D, McLeod G, Hall P 1974 The CAGE questionnaire: validation of a new alcoholism screening instrument. American Journal of Psychiatry 131: 1121–1123

World Health Organization 1992 The ICD-10 classification of mental and behavioural disorders: clinical descriptions and diagnostic guidelines. Geneva, WHO

Poisoning

16

Introduction   182

Epidemiology   182

When to suspect poisoning   183

Toxic syndromes ('toxidromes')   183

Management priorities   183

Decontamination   185

Use of antidotes   186

Specific poisons   186

Poisonous plants and fungi   190

Bites and stings   193

Poisons information services   194

References   194

Introduction

Self-administered drug poisoning accounts for 10% of acute medical admissions to hospital in the UK. These and many other toxic exposures are first attended by prehospital doctors and emergency service personnel.

The majority of patients require no prehospital interventions. Basic and advanced life support with rapid transport to the emergency department are the mainstay of management in cases where treatment is required. The emphasis of this chapter is therefore on the general approach to the poisoned patient. The more common poisons and those important in the prehospital environment are described in more detail.

Epidemiology

Data from the UK on poison centre enquiries, hospital admissions and mortality from specific poisons is not published in a comprehensive form. One can, however, piece together information from regional studies.

Most poisonings occur in the home. The majority are accidental ingestions in children. Ferguson (1992) found that, of 6562 hospital admissions in children, 56.4% were due to ingestion of medicines and 43.6% to ingestion of other substances. Of the ingestions of non-medicinal substances, most were plant material and 22% were corrosive acids and alkalis. Analgesics accounted for 28% of the admissions.

Adults are more likely to deliberately ingest poisons and account for the majority of hospital admissions. It is estimated that adult overdoses account for 100 000 hospital referrals per annum in England and Wales. Attempted suicide rates in Oxford between 1976 and 1990 were highest in 20–34-year-old men followed by 15–19-year-old women (Hawton & Fagg 1992). There was an alarming rise in the use of paracetamol, which accounted for 42% of parasuicides by 1990 (Box 16.1). Other studies have shown that this corresponds to a reduction in the use of benzodiazepines.

Carbon monoxide is probably the most common cause of suicide in males and is increasingly used in adolescent suicide (McClure 1994). Other serious causes of mortality include

Box 16.1

Poisoning epidemiology

- Most poisonings occur in the home
- Most accidental poisonings occur in children
- Adult poisonings more commonly occur in women, are intentional and require hospital admission
- Paracetamol is the most common medicinal overdose
- Successful suicide is much more common in men, carbon monoxide poisoning probably being the most common method

Box 16.2

Suspect poisoning in patients with:

- altered levels of consciousness
- arrhythmia, especially if young
- multiple trauma
- bizarre clinical presentations

Box 16.3

In patients presumed poisoned exclude:

- prehospital
  - hypoxia
  - hypotension
  - hypoglycaemia
  - hypothermia
  - head trauma
  - stroke
  - postictal state
  - Infection
  - electrolyte disturbance
  - subarachnoid haemorrhage

analgesics, antidepressants, cardiovascular drugs, stimulants, sedative antipsychotics, alcohols, chemicals, insecticides, cleaning products and hydrocarbons, in that order. The antidepressants responsible for most fatalities in the UK are amitriptyline and dothiepin (Henry & Antao 1992).

When to suspect poisoning

It is essential never to presume that poisoning is just poisoning or that patients with other presumed diagnoses, such as head injury, are not poisoned. It is helpful to keep an open mind and make sure other differential diagnoses such as hypoxia are excluded. The best way to do this is to follow a system of management priorities that will identify and treat most of these. The most common presentations of poisoning that may be misdiagnosed or coexistent with other conditions are outlined in Boxes 16.2 and 16.3.

Toxic syndromes ('toxidromes')

Poisoning may present with any of a confusing multitude of symptoms and signs. However, there are some common patterns that may be discerned and that may suggest possible toxins and appropriate management. These are listed in Table 16.1.

Management priorities

Many poisonings can cause any combination of respiratory depression, circulatory collapse, fitting or metabolic disturbance. The most important first step, therefore, is to assess and resuscitate the patient using the ABCDE system. Many situations may not be what they seem at first, so a useful maxim is 'treat the patient not the drug'.

The most important initial consideration is safety. If poisoning has occurred through toxic inhalational or skin contact then appropriate protective clothing should be worn by all emergency personnel and the patient must be moved away from further contamination. Contaminated clothing can be removed during the initial resuscitation. Appropriate protocols should be followed, usually under the guidance of the fire service.

Assessment and appropriate care of the airway and ventilation will treat and exclude hypoxia. All patients should receive high-flow oxygen via a reservoir mask. Despite seemingly marked reduction in conscious levels and resultant airway obstruction, oral airways are often poorly tolerated. In this situation a nasopharyngeal airway may be useful. If there is any possibility of trauma, full cervical spine protection must be applied.

Circulatory assessment, vascular access and appropriate support will aid adequate oxygen delivery. Provided there are no signs of heart failure or arrhythmia, judicious use of colloid or crystalloid can be used to treat hypotension. Fluid administration is also important in patients who have been immobile for long periods and thus are at risk of developing rhabdomyolysis. Monitoring, including pulse oximetry, electrocardiogram (ECG) and blood pressure, should be attached whenever possible.

When gaining circulatory access it is helpful to think that after ABC comes 'Don't Ever Forget Glucose'. It is safer to make someone hyperglycaemic than to miss hypoglycaemia. 'D' also stands for disability. A rapid neurological assessment, including a search for lateralizing signs, is useful as a baseline

Table 16.1 Toxic syndromes (toxidromes)

Syndrome	Causes	Symptoms and signs	
Narcotic	Heroin Morphine Methadone Codeine	Reduced level of consciousness Pinpoint pupils Respiratory depression Hypotension Response to naloxone	
Anticholinergic	Atropine Cyclopentolate Tropicamide Tricyclics Phenothiazines *Atropa belladonna*	*Central*: lethargy, confusion, ataxia, hallucinations, seizures, cardiac and respiratory failure	*Peripheral*: dry skin and mouth, blurred vision, dilated pupils, urinary retention, tachycardia, abdominal distension, flushing
Cholinergic	Organophosphates Acetylcholine	*Muscarinic*: sweating, excessive salivation, pupil constriction, blurred vision, wheezing, vomiting, diarrhoea, tachycardia, hypotension or hypertension	*Nicotinic*: striated muscle cramps, weakness, fasciculations and paralysis, respiratory failure *Central*: ataxia, seizures, coma
Sympathomimetic	Aminophylline Amphetamine Caffeine Cocaine Phencyclidine	Excitation Seizures Hypertension Tachycardia	
Extrapyramidal	Phenothiazines Butyrophenones Metoclopramide	*Parkinsonian features*: dysphonia, dysphagia, oculogyric crises, rigidity, tremor, torticollis, opisthotonos, trismus	
Haemoglobinopathies	Carbon monoxide	Headache Nausea, vomiting Dizziness Seizures, coma	
Withdrawal	Alcohol Benzodiazepines Barbiturates Cocaine Opiates	Diarrhoea, mydriasis, piloerection, hypertension, tachycardia, insomnia, restlessness, hallucinations	

and will help to determine the need for airway protection, as well as identifying seizures and suggesting the possibility of head injury and stroke. If an appropriate history and pupillary signs are present naloxone should be given.

A patient with a Glasgow coma scale (GCS) of 8 is at risk of airway compromise. Owing to the fluctuating conscious level of many poisoned patients this decision is difficult. If anaesthetic agents are required for a rapid sequence induction in this situation, a poisoning may be complicated. This should only be used as a last resort. Unless cervical spine trauma is suspected, patients should be transported in the left lateral decubitus position head down to prevent aspiration. There is evidence that transport in this position delays transit from stomach to small bowel, thus decreasing absorption of ingested poisons.

Fitting can cause hypoxia, metabolic upset and difficulty in management of resuscitation. For prolonged or recurrent seizures, most authors recommend first-line treatment with diazepam or lorazepam. This will terminate seizures in at least 80% of patients. Benzodiazepines may cause and

Box 16.4

Management priorities

- Remove yourself and the patient from danger
- Airway and oxygen
- Breathing
- Circulatory access and support
- Identify and treat hypoglycaemia
- Measure GCS and assess pupils
- If in doubt give naloxone
- If GCS ≤8 consider intubation
- Treat prolonged or recurrent fitting
- Ask: What? How much? When? What else?
- Consider head trauma and carbon monoxide
- Consider decontamination
- Contact Poisons Centre
- Liaise with Emergency Department

Box 16.5

Prehospital decontamination

- Remove patient from contaminated area
- Remove contaminated clothing
- Gastric lavage is contraindicated
- Consider ipecacuanha within 30 min of ingestion in children
- Consider activated charcoal within 30 min of ingestion
- Administration of activated charcoal or ipecac should not delay transfer to hospital
- Decontamination is contraindicated if the airway is at risk
- For caustic ingestions give milk

exacerbate cardiorespiratory collapse in any patient; it is therefore important to be ready to resuscitate.

During resuscitation it cannot be over emphasized that a good history is essential. The main questions about the ingestion are:

- what?
- how much?
- when?
- what else?

It is also worth asking why the poison was ingested, as any evidence of suicidal intent affects later management. How long the patient has been lying immobile should be estimated so that they can be screened for rhabdomyolysis. If there is no clear history of an ingestion the most important things to suspect are hypoglycaemia, carbon monoxide poisoning and head trauma.

The next steps in prehospital management are to consider gut decontamination and contacting the nearest poisons centre for advice. Unless a situation arises in which the transfer of a patient to hospital is likely to be delayed or very prolonged, appropriate consideration of both these aspects can usually wait until arrival in hospital. A list of management priorities is given in Box 16.4.

Decontamination

Decontamination refers to poison removal. Where necessary, the patient should first be removed from a contaminated area, resuscitated and affected clothing removed. If appropriate, methods of gut decontamination, such as using activated charcoal, should be undertaken (Box 16.5). This section discusses the prehospital limitations of these methods (Henry &

Hoffman 1998). Dilution is mentioned with reference to caustic ingestions. If protocols for prehospital decontamination are developed they should be coordinated with the local emergency department and poisons information service.

GASTRIC LAVAGE

In the emergency department setting there has been a move away from performing gastric lavage. Perrone et al (1994) reviewed the evidence for gastric lavage and concluded that it was only indicated in the very early stages following a life-threatening ingestion and that endotracheal intubation was sometimes necessary to accomplish this safely in patients at risk of airway compromise. A joint statement by the American Academy of Clinical Toxicology and the European Association of Poison Control Centres and Clinical Toxicologists (1997) states that 'Gastric lavage should not be employed routinely in the management of poisoned patients'. This follows data from a randomized controlled prospective study of 1000 overdose patients in Australia showing no benefit from gastric lavage with activated charcoal versus activated charcoal alone (Pond et al 1995). Therefore gastric lavage is not indicated in the prehospital environment.

EMESIS

Reviews of studies (Jawary et al 1992) consistently show that, in the emergency department setting, use of syrup of ipecac to induce vomiting only reduces absorption by about 30% if given within 1 h of ingestion and may interfere with the efficacy of activated charcoal or other orally administered antidotes. It is not indicated in the routine treatment of poisoning. Emesis is contraindicated with caustic and hydrocarbon ingestions, and in patients with an existing or potential reduced level of consciousness.

ACTIVATED CHARCOAL

Activated charcoal is widely accepted as the agent of choice for gastrointestinal decontamination in most acute poisonings; this view follows work suggesting that it is superior to other methods alone. Tenenbein et al (1987) studied ampicillin absorption following administration of activated charcoal, ipecac or gastric lavage within 30 min in adult volunteers and found that activated charcoal had the greatest effect in reducing drug absorption. Other volunteer studies have suggested benefit up to 1 h (Burton 1984). In addition to direct drug binding, it is thought to generate a gut plasma concentration gradient that enables continued resorption from the circulation. Its efficacy is both time- and drug-dependent. It is not recommended for heavy metals, including iron, lithium and cyanide, strong acids or bases, alcohols and hydrocarbons. The earlier it is given the more effective activated charcoal is likely to be, thus there may be a case for prehospital administration in certain circumstances. The recommended dose is 50 g for the average adult. Drugs particularly well absorbed by activated charcoal include digoxin, aspirin, tricyclic antidepressants, carbamazepine, theophyllines, barbiturates and quinine. The only contraindication to its use is in patients with an existing or potential reduced level of consciousness. Aspiration pneumonitis following its use has been reported (Harsch 1986).

If activated charcoal is to be used in the prehospital situation, a protocol should be agreed with the local emergency department, and its use must not cause delay in transport to hospital.

CAUSTIC INGESTIONS

Chemicals that cause direct injury to tissues include strong acids and alkalis. Some toilet cleaners contain sulphuric acid and bleaches may contain sodium hypochlorite, a strong alkali. Paint removers and drain cleaners contain particularly strong alkalis such as sodium or potassium hydroxide. Cleaning substances account for over 10% of all poison exposures and are even more common in young children. Rarely, such patients will have a compromised airway but for most the mainstay of initial treatment is dilution. 'Neutralizing substances' are not recommended because if a weak acid buffer, such as vinegar, is added heat will be generated, causing more damage. Milk is the diluent of choice, 250 ml for a child and 500 ml for an adult. If this is not available, water will help.

Giving activated charcoal is ineffective and complicates later management, which may include endoscopy.

Use of antidotes

Antidotes are chemical or physiological agents that reverse or prevent the toxic effects of specific poisons. Activated

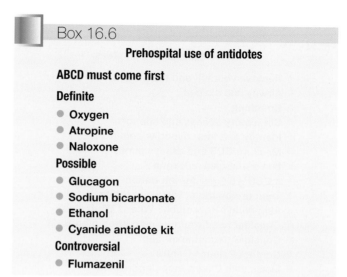

Box 16.6

Prehospital use of antidotes

ABCD must come first

Definite
- Oxygen
- Atropine
- Naloxone

Possible
- Glucagon
- Sodium bicarbonate
- Ethanol
- Cyanide antidote kit

Controversial
- Flumazenil

charcoal may be considered to be an antidote but the term is usually used to refer to specific treatments for specific classes of drug or toxin. They are available for only a limited number of poisons, and in most cases decontamination and supportive care are the mainstay of treatment. Thus, attention to basic resuscitation is far more important in the prehospital phase.

The American Association of Poison Control Centres (AAPCC) recommends a list of stock antidotes. Most of these are items rarely used even in emergency departments and are listed in Table 16.2 along with their uses and doses for completeness only. Naloxone and atropine are carried by most prehospital personnel but there are others that warrant consideration. These are highlighted in Table 16.2. Their use is discussed below in the 'Specific poisons' section.

Specific poisons

Included below are some of the most common poisonings and others amenable to antidote and other treatment in the prehospital phase. Most are highlighted in Table 16.2. It is worth remembering that about 10% of adult drug overdoses are mixed and simultaneous consumption of alcohol is common.

PARACETAMOL

Paracetamol is the most commonly reported overdose. It has no immediate effects that require resuscitation. If symptoms other than nausea and vomiting are present, suspect the ingestion of other drugs. As little as 10 g of paracetamol can be fatal.

There is a risk of hepatotoxicity if more than $100 \, \text{mg kg}^{-1}$ is ingested. In these cases it seems reasonable to consider giving activated charcoal to patients up to 4 h from ingestion.

Table 16.2 Emergency antidotes (shaded poisons are discussed in the text)

Poison	Antidote	Initial adult dose
Adder bite	Zagreb antivenom	see 'Bites and stings' section
Atropine	Physostigmine	0.5–2 mg intravenously
Benzodiazepines	Flumazenil	0.2 mg intravenously
Beta-blockers	Glucagon	3 mg intravenously
Carbon monoxide	Oxygen	100%
Cyanide	Amyl nitrate Sodium nitrate Sodium thiosulphate	Commercially available kit (Eli Lilly)
Digoxin	Digoxin specific Fab	Based on total body load; contact poisons centre
Iron	Desferrioxamine	$15\,mg\,kg^{-1}\,h^{-1}$ intravenously
Lead, cadmium, copper, zinc	Calcium disodium edetate	One 250 ml ampoule ($250\,mg\,ml^{-1}$) over 1 h
Mercury, arsenic, gold	Dimercaprol (BAL)	$5\,mg\,kg^{-1}$ intramuscularly
Methyl alcohol, ethylene glycol	Ethanol	$1\,ml\,kg^{-1}$ of 100% ethanol in glucose solution
Metoclopramide	Procyclidine	5–10 mg intravenously for dystonia
Nitrites	Methylene blue	$0.2\,ml\,kg^{-1}$ 1% solution intravenously
Opiates	Naloxone	0.4–0.8 mg intravenously
Organophosphates	Atropine	2–5 mg intravenously
Paracetamol	N-acetylcysteine (NAC)	$140\,mg\,kg^{-1}$ intravenously or orally
Paraquat	Fuller's earth	200 ml of 30% suspension
Tricyclic antidepressants	Sodium bicarbonate	50 ml of 8.4% solution

In-hospital antidote treatment uses N-acetylcysteine, which is thought to act by replenishing glutathione stores depleted by the overdose. These bind and inactivate the toxic metabolite formed by the P_{450} cytochrome system. It is equally effective by oral or intravenous routes and more effective if given within the first 8 h, although the oral preparation is not currently available in the UK. Indications for urgent treatment with N-acetylcysteine before plasma levels are available include patients in whom more than $140\,mg\,kg^{-1}$ has been ingested or who are more than 8 h post-ingestion. There is a lower threshold for treatment in patients taking cytochrome-P_{450}-inducing drugs such as antihistamines, barbiturates, carbamazepine, phenytoin, rifampicin and griseofulvin, or in patients with a high alcohol consumption. Other in-hospital indications rely on plasma levels taken at or beyond 4 h post-ingestion and the use of the paracetamol treatment graph. In the prehospital environment, use of the oral antidote methionine (2.5 g every 4 h up to a total of 10 g) should be considered if circumstances render a patient geographically remote from

in-hospital treatment. In such circumstances, an appropriate protocol should be developed in conjunction with the local hospital services. There is no evidence that methionine is effective if more than 10 h has passed since the overdose.

SALICYLATES

Although now less common, aspirin overdose remains a significant problem. Historical data suggest that salicylates were responsible for 6% of fatal poison exposures in the USA in 1995. Ingestions of under $150\,mg\,kg^{-1}$ can cause vomiting and gastric irritation. Above this level tinnitus, sweating and tachypnoea can occur. Moderate plasma levels stimulate the respiratory centre, leading to a respiratory alkalosis. At higher levels aspirin's effect of uncoupling oxidative phosphorylation and stimulating lipolysis then leads to a metabolic acidosis. In severe cases a pyrexial, profusely sweating, tachycardic patient who is prone to convulsions and respiratory arrest is seen. They may be hyper- or hypoglycaemic, and later cerebral and pulmonary oedema may supervene.

Immediate care involves treatment of any life-threatening respiratory depression. All those with a reduced level of consciousness or seizures should be presumed to be hypoglycaemic and treated accordingly. Those who are symptomatic are usually dehydrated and will benefit from intravenous fluids to help renal excretion. Aspirin is well absorbed by activated charcoal. All patients should be assessed in the emergency department. A suggested flow-chart for the management of salicylate poisoning can be found in a paper by Dargan et al (2002).

OPIATES

Overdose with opiates often causes coma and respiratory depression. Both readily respond to the pure opiate antagonist naloxone, which can be given subcutaneously, intramuscularly, via an endotracheal tube, or intravenously. The preferred route is intravenously at a dose of 0.4–0.8 mg in adults or 0.01 mg kg^{-1} in children. Often higher doses are needed and up to 20 mg can be given safely. It is important to remember that opiate action is likely to significantly outlast the 1 h half-life of naloxone. Repeat doses (or an infusion in hospital) are often necessary. It is virtually without adverse effects, although administration can occasionally precipitate acute withdrawal symptoms in opiate addicts. Naloxone should be carried by all prehospital practitioners and must be available if opiates are carried.

ORGANOPHOSPHATES

Toxins with anticholinesterase action include the many and varied organophosphate pesticides. Similar effects can also be produced by the rarely ingested topical eye preparations such as acetylcholine and pilocarpine. In severe cases organophosphate exposure results in the easily recognizable 'cholinergic syndrome' (see Table 16.1). First-line therapy is resuscitation and decontamination. It is important to remember that organophosphates are well absorbed dermally and are therefore a risk to medical attendants; all contaminated clothing should therefore be removed.

Atropine administration blocks the effects of excess acetylcholine at muscarinic receptors, and thus helps the respiratory distress caused by copious oropharyngeal secretions and bronchospasm. It can reverse life-threatening bradycardia as well as the less serious cholinergic effects. In conscious patients with mild to moderate poisoning 1–2 mg of atropine given slowly intravenously every 15–30 min is an appropriate dose, with further 5 mg aliquots being required in severe poisoning. Enough atropine has been given when there is drying of excessive secretions. Reversal of the nicotinic and central effects such as muscle paralysis and coma

is achieved with pralidoxime, which is more appropriately given in the emergency department.

BETA-BLOCKERS

Although relatively rare, severe beta-blocker overdose can cause life-threatening bradycardia, heart block and cardiac failure. In addition to its use in reversing hypoglycaemia, glucagon is considered by many to be the drug of choice for the management of these patients. It stimulates the production of adenosine monophosphate (AMP), which beta-blockers reduce and which in turn enhances myocardial contractility, heart rate and atrioventricular conduction. It is anecdotally considered more efficacious than atropine or other inotropes such as dobutamine. Bolus doses of 3–10 mg intravenously have been successful. This is a larger dose than the 0.5–2 mg often carried for treatment of insulin-induced hypoglycaemia. If the diagnosis is certain, and a patient is exhibiting hypotension or heart failure, glucagon should be considered if atropine fails.

ANTIDEPRESSANTS

Antidepressants were the second most likely fatal toxic exposure in the AAPCC data. About 30% of all such overdoses were fatal. Although the newer selective serotonin uptake inhibitors such as fluoxetine (Prozac) are often taken in overdose, they have a high toxic to therapeutic ratio and rarely result in more than nausea, tremor, tachycardia and drowsiness. Reported deaths are thought to be due to simultaneous ingestion of other drugs. The tricyclic antidepressants (TCAs) are far more dangerous.

Perhaps the only definite acute indication for sodium bicarbonate, now that its general use in cardiac arrest is no longer recommended, is in the treatment of the complications of tricyclic antidepressant overdose. This subject has been well reviewed by Pimentel & Trommer (1994). More deaths have resulted from amitriptyline overdose than any other antidepressant and many fatalities occur before reaching hospital. It causes a combination of central nervous system, anticholinergic and direct cardiotoxic effects. Depressed conscious level and convulsions are common, and therefore airway protection is often needed.

Most deaths are due to cardiac toxicity and there is much evidence that sodium bicarbonate reverses the cardiotoxic effects of TCA overdose. Clear indications for its use include marked acidosis, refractory hypotension, prolonged cardiac conduction, ventricular dysrhythmias and cardiac arrest. All but the first of these should be recognizable in the prehospital phase. Following correction of hypoxia, intermittent doses of 1 mEq kg^{-1} (1 ml of 8.4% solution kg^{-1}) are recommended to keep the QRS duration less than 0.16 s. Hyperventilation also helps induce systemic alkalinization. Second-line therapy for ventricular dysrhythmias is lidocaine. The early use of sodium bicarbonate in those with life-threatening cardiac compromise should be considered. The treatment of fits is with diazepam.

ALCOHOLS

Ethanol is the most frequently used and abused drug in the world with significant acute and chronic results. The general effects of acute intoxication are known only too well by all evolved in the emergency services. However, it is easy to assume that a drunk is just drunk. They may be poisoned with something else, head injured or hypoglycaemic as a result of inhibition of glyconeogenesis by ethanol. High plasma levels can cause loss of protective reflexes, airway obstruction and respiratory depression. Following resuscitation the blood glucose level must be checked and restored. There is a risk of permanent cerebral damage following Wernicke's encephalopathy caused by thiamine deficiency in alcoholics, which is precipitated by binges. Thiamine (50 mg intravenously) should be given in hospital to all patients exhibiting any of the typical triad of nystagmus, ataxia and confusion. Some authors advocate its administration to all obtunded patients. Other more dangerous alcohols may mimic ethanol.

When ingested accidentally or deliberately, ethylene glycol, contained in antifreeze and cooling systems, results in toxicity due to the formation via alcohol dehydrogenase of two metabolites, formaldehyde and formic acid. A potentially lethal dose is as little as 2 ml kg^{-1}. It is highly water-soluble and is rapidly absorbed from the stomach. Within 1–12 h patients appear drunk but without the odour of ethanol on their breath, which may give a clinical clue to this poisoning. Hallucinations, seizures and coma can also occur in this phase. Between 12 and 24 h following ingestion congestive cardiac and circulatory failure can occur, with renal failure following at 24–72 h.

Methyl alcohol, also contained in antifreeze, is used as an industrial solvent and is present in many paint removers. Its mode of toxicity is the same as that for ethylene glycol. Clinically this ingestion can be distinguished from ethanol or ethylene glycol by the distinctive odour and the presence of visual disturbances. These take the form of blurred vision, photophobia or blindness, and are present in approximately 50% of patients.

Because of rapid absorption and high toxicity, both these agents need urgent treatment.

With a good history and either of the above clinical states one should not wait for a biochemical diagnosis. Alcohol dehydrogenase has a much higher affinity for ethanol than either of these agents and prompt oral or intravenous administration of ethanol slows the production of toxic metabolites and reduces toxicity. Most fully conscious patients will accept the oral dose suggested in Table 16.2. If this is not available, whisky or similar is an effective substitute. This treatment is normally only given in hospital.

BENZODIAZEPINES

Serious complications from benzodiazepine overdose are rare but the newer short-acting derivatives such as temazepam have been reported to cause cardiorespiratory depression in addition to the more common depression of conscious level and slurred speech. All effects can be augmented by the concomitant ingestion of alcohol which is so often found.

Flumazenil is a unique selective antagonist to the central effects of benzodiazepines. It is not licensed for use following overdose. Its current main use is in reversal of benzodiazepines administered to facilitate emergency procedures. At a dose of 0.2 mg min^{-1} intravenously up to 3 mg, its duration of action is variable and shorter than that of most benzodiazepines. It has been reported to cause seizures in those also ingesting tricyclic antidepressants and in patients already dependent on benzodiazepines (Spivey 1992). In selected difficult cases its use may obviate the need for airway maintenance and ventilation, and may be of diagnostic value. Its use for these purposes is controversial and thus at present its prehospital use cannot be endorsed.

CARBON MONOXIDE

Carbon monoxide (CO) poisoning is among the leading causes of toxin-related death in the Western world. It accounts for about 1800 deaths in the UK annually, with only about 400 occurring in hospital as most are successful suicides. The byproduct of incomplete combustion of organic fuels, it is colourless, odourless, non-irritant and tasteless. This, combined with its vague presentation, means that carbon monoxide leaking from a faulty home heating system is often not detected until it is too late. It is also produced in significant quantities by internal combustion engines, as well as by controlled and uncontrolled household and industrial fires.

With a high affinity for haemoglobin, carbon monoxide displaces oxygen to form carboxyhaemoglobin (COHb) as well as shifting the oxygen–haemoglobin curve to the left, rendering the victim hypoxic. It also has direct toxic effects on the myocardium and cellular respiration, with an even higher affinity for cytochromic P$_{450}$.

The multisystem effects of carbon monoxide mean that clinical presentations are many and varied. Symptoms usually start with headache, drowsiness, weakness and nausea, and progress to confusion, seizures, coma, respiratory

---

Box 16.7

Effects of carbon monoxide poisoning

- Headache
- Seizures
- Drowsiness
- Coma
- Weakness
- Respiratory failure
- Nausea
- Confusion
- Death

---

failure and death. Carbon monoxide poisoning has been misdiagnosed as influenza, gastroenteritis and psychiatric disorder. Among other presentations are visual disturbance and cardiac ischaemia, producing angina and infarction in patients with no pre-existing heart disease. The classic 'cherry red' skin appearance is very rare and cyanosis can occur if respiratory failure supervenes.

Treatment initially involves removal of the victim from the source and attention to airway (A), breathing (B) and circulation (C). The half-life of carboxyhaemoglobin with the patient breathing air is 4–5 h. Breathing 100% oxygen reduces this to 50–80 min. As near 100% oxygen as possible should therefore be administered immediately, followed by rapid transport to the emergency department where the decision to refer for hyperbaric oxygen therapy can be made.

Remove the patient from the CO source and give high-flow oxygen.

Note the length of exposure and activity level during exposure, as these factors are taken into account when considering hyperbaric therapy. It is essential to have a high index of suspicion for carbon monoxide poisoning.

CYANIDE

Cyanide is ubiquitous, it is a precursor and by-product in the manufacture of plastics, solvents and pesticides, and is also contained in plants (see the following section). The most common mode of exposure is during the combustion of nitrogen-containing polymers such as wool, silk or vinyl, but ingestion and cutaneous exposure also occur. Along with carbon monoxide it has been implicated in fire-related deaths.

By inhibiting cytochrome oxidase, which is involved in oxidative phosphorylation, cyanide poisoning can cause a predominantly anaerobic metabolic state despite the presence of oxygen. This results in metabolic acidosis and

a clinical state mimicking hypoxia but without cyanosis. Initially patients present with headache, breathlessness and anxiety, which often resolve on withdrawal from exposure. In more severe cases this may be followed by a reduction in conscious level, seizures and coma. There is often the classic smell of bitter almonds on the patient's breath.

Patients with inhalational exposure usually only require removal from the source, high-flow oxygen and close monitoring. Where there is a clear history of cyanide ingestion and a comatose bradycardic patient, antidotal therapy is indicated. Nitrites, through the formation of methaemoglobin, prevent cyanide binding to cytochrome oxidase. Inhalation of amyl nitrite by the patient is therefore used in the early treatment of cyanide poisoning and it should be available in all areas where cyanide exposure is considered to be a risk. Out of hospital this is only advised in severe cases of clear poisoning. If combined with carbon monoxide poisoning, formation of methaemoglobin could exacerbate hypoxia; thus resuscitation must always take priority. Immediate transfer to hospital is essential.

PARAQUAT

Paraquat is a herbicide found in a number of branded weedkillers. Accidental paraquat poisoning is now rare in the UK and its use in deliberate self-harm has reduced. Fatal systemic poisoning can occur following percutaneous absorption, but this is rare. Most poisonings are due to ingestion. Serious poisoning has not been recorded as a result of inhalation of sprayed solutions that include paraquat. Lethal poisoning can occur with ingestion of as little as 1.5 g of paraquat (one sachet of Weedol). There are many symptoms, depending on the type and quantity of the exposure. These range from sore throat and epistaxis (inhalation) through skin and corneal ulceration (from splashes) to fulminating multisystem failure.

Treatment of paraquat poisoning concentrates on administration of an absorbent in order to reduce the amount of paraquat absorbed. In hospital, fuller's earth, bentonite or activated charcoal can be used. For this reason, the correct prehospital management of these patients is immediate evacuation to hospital. If evacuation to hospital is likely to be delayed, the case should be discussed with the local poisons unit. Antiemetics and analgesia (for mouth and laryngeal burns) are appropriate and intravenous fluids should be given, although none of these measures should be allowed to delay transfer to hospital.

Poisonous plants and fungi

Despite the existence of over 100 known poisonous plants and fungi in the UK, serious toxicity is very rare among humans with only two deaths being recorded in a 15-year period. However, 10% of calls to poison centres concern plant ingestions. Toxins range from the irritant formic acid in nettles to atropine in deadly nightshade berries. The definition of a poisonous plant or non-poisonous plant is difficult as they may vary seasonally, by variety, by plant part and in their effects on different individuals. It is also important to remember that plants are often coated with pesticides. In addition to the two most important groups of plant toxins, the alkaloids and the glycosides, there are viscotoxins, resins, phototoxins and fungal hallucinogens. These cause symptom complexes similar to some of those described in Table 16.1. These categories, their general effects and causative plants and fungi are listed in Table 16.3. Many plants not listed cause gastrointestinal upset when ingested.

GENERAL PRINCIPLES OF MANAGEMENT

As with any poisoning, attention should first be paid to administering oxygen, airway care and ventilatory support if needed, with intravenous access in severe poisonings (see 'Management priorities' section). Cautious fluid replacement can be commenced in those dehydrated from diarrhoea and vomiting, and the blood glucose should always be checked. Cardiac monitoring will be needed if there is a possibility of glycoside ingestion or muscarinic effects. Seizures may be expected with some mushroom ingestions.

Gut decontamination follows the same principles as for most ingestions. Plant alkaloids are particularly well absorbed by activated charcoal, although this should be administered in hospital wherever possible. Induced eme-

Table 16.3 Overview of poisonous plants and fungi detailing toxin types and main clinical features

Toxin	Plant or fungal species	Comments
Plants		
Nicotinic alkaloids		
Nicotine, coniine, cytosine, lupinine	Hemlock Laburnum Broom-seeds Lupins	Moderate toxicity. Low dose causes muscarinic type effects. Higher doses cause nicotinic effects (see Table 16.1)
Antimuscarinic alkaloids		
Atropine, hyoscine, hyoscyamine	Deadly nightshade Jimson weed	Moderate toxicity. Antimuscarinic syndrome (see Table 16.1)
Gastric irritants		
Glycoalkaloids, coumarin glycosides, oxalates, viscotoxins	Yew Potatoes – green/sprouted Monkshood Horse chestnut Spurge laurel berries Araceae Mistletoe berries	Gastrointestinal upset with all. Also burning of the lips, oral swelling. Muscarinic effects occur with higher doses
Cardiac glycosides		
Digitalis	Foxglove leaves/flowers Lily of the valley leaves/flowers Oleander	Moderate toxicity. Gastrointestinal symptoms, visual disturbance, cardiac arrhythmias, confusion
Cyanogenic glycosides		
Amygdalin	Elderberry Cotoneaster – unripe berries Apricot, peach, plum and cherry kernels	Toxicity rare. Gastrointestinal symptoms common. For severe poisoning see cyanide in the 'Specific poisons' section

(Continued)

Table 16.3 (*Continued*)

Toxin	Plant or fungal species	Comments
Plants		
Central nervous system resins		
Cicutoxin, oenanthotoxin	Cowbane Hemlock Water dropwort	Highly toxic. Gastrointestinal symptoms followed by hypersalivation and central nervous system effects: trismus, opisthotonus and convulsions
Oxalates	Primula Narcissi	Can cause acute blistering dermatitis
Phototoxic chemicals		
Furanocoumarins	Giant hogweed Parsnips	Sensitize skin to ultraviolet light, causing sunburn
Fungi		
Muscarine	*Inocybe* *Clitocybe*	Within 30 min. Muscarinic effects (see Table 16.1)
5-hydroxytryptamine (serotonin)	*Psilocybe* (magic mushrooms) derivatives (psilocin) *Panaeolus*	Within 2 h. Hallucinations, mydriasis, tachycardia, flushing
Ibotenic acid	*Amanita muscari*	Within 2 h. Pantherine syndrome: euphoria, ataxia, coma, hallucinations, convulsions
Muscimol Monomethylhydrazine	*Amanita pantherina* *Gyromitra esculenta*	6–8 h. Gastrointestinal symptoms, haemolysis, hepatorenal failure
Amatoxins	*Amanita phalloides*	At 12 h gastrointestinal upset. At 24–48 h hepatorenal failure
Coprine	*Coprinus atramentarius*	Disulfiram reaction with alcohol
Cyclopeptides	*Cortarius speciosissimus*	Gastrointestinal upset, thirst, polyuria, myalgia, rarely renal failure

Many other plants may cause mild gastrointestinal upset when ingested

sis is contraindicated if there is any suspicion that hemlock is involved, as it may cause seizures. Owing to the complex effects of alkaloids causing rapidly changing clinical pictures, antidotes can be counterproductive and are not generally recommended, although the rare life-threatening bradycardias and muscarinic syndrome should be treated with atropine.

Any questions pertaining to the poisonous potential of plants and fungi can be obtained from the nearest poison information centre but they may not be able to identify the plant over the telephone. It is very useful to keep a pictorial guide close at hand for such occasions (Cooper & Johnson 1988, Bresinski & Besl 1990). With this in mind it is important to obtain a sample of the offending plant in a paper bag and take it to the emergency department.

Frozen vomit samples have been used to identify fungi. Computer programs are now available in some emergency departments for the identification of plants and fungi using a Windows-based system. These programs require a sample of the plant ingested.

Fungi rarely account for poisonings and most serious problems occur with one species, *Amanita phalloides*. A very useful guide is that if the onset of symptoms is delayed for more than 5 h following ingestion then serious toxins are a possibility. Poisonous fungi with their time interval to symptoms are detailed in Table 16.3.

Space does not permit an extensive review of this subject and the reader is referred to more comprehensive texts (Cooper & Johnson 1984, Ramrakha & Moore 2004, Greaves & Porter 2006).

Bites and stings

Mortality from bites and stings is relatively rare with about five deaths per annum in the UK. These are mostly due to anaphylaxis from insect bites. There is, however, significant morbidity associated with bites and stings from domestic animals, insects, marine animals, and rarely indigenous and imported snakes. The background and immediate management of these is discussed below. For a more detailed account Warrell (1996) is recommended.

DOMESTICATED ANIMALS

An estimated 200 000 patients attend hospital in England and Wales per annum with dog bites. Most wounds themselves are not serious but left untreated about 15% will develop *Pasteurella multocida* infection. These and any other bites from cats, rodents, farm animals and humans should be referred to the emergency department or general practice treatment room for thorough wound toilet and antibiotics. Tetanus status must also be checked.

SNAKE BITES

World-wide, snake bite is a significant problem, with some of the worst affected areas in the tropics, such as Burma, experiencing 2000 deaths per annum as a result. 14 deaths have been recorded in the UK since 1876 due to Britain's only poisonous snake, *Vipera berus*, the European adder. 50% of snake bites do not result in envenomation. Occasionally, bites are reported from non-indigenous snakes. About 100 people suffer snake bite per year in the UK.

Snakes can be divided into three main groups: the Elapidae include cobras, mambas and coral snakes and secrete venom containing a paralysing neurotoxin; the Hydrophiidae or sea snakes envenomate a myotoxin causing myoglobinuria and renal failure; the Viperidae include the true vipers such as the European adder, pit vipers and rattlesnakes.

In contrast to the first two groups and in addition to coagulopathy and hypovolaemic shock, envenomation by the Viperidae can cause a marked local reaction resulting in necrosis. If adder envenomation has occurred, two adjacent puncture wounds are present with immediate pain and rapid swelling. Regional lymphadenopathy is followed by the development of progressive limb oedema over the next 48 h. Systemic complications can occur in the absence of a local reaction.

On-scene treatment of any snake bite includes full evaluation and resuscitation of life-threatening problems.

In all cases a check at the nearest emergency department is required. The bite should be left and covered with a dry dressing. Incision and suction of the wound should not be attempted as absorption of the poison may be promoted. The limb should be immobilized and kept dependent. A firm, continuous pressure bandage, not obstructing arterial supply, should be applied, starting proximally and covering the whole limb. This should be left in place until a full evaluation and blood profiles have been completed. A window may be cut to expose the bite site. Tourniquets occluding arterial supply have resulted in unnecessary limb loss and should not be used. Dead snakes should be taken to the emergency department for identification, bearing in mind that reflexes resulting in bites can still be present. All snake bites should be observed in hospital where, if necessary, antivenom can be given. The emergency department should be warned that adder bite is probable so that antivenom delivery can be arranged.

MARINE ANIMALS

British beaches, especially in the south-west, are inhabited by the lesser weaver fish, which possess venomous spines in their dorsal fins. The toxins, including serotonin, cause intense local pain and oedema, usually in the feet of bathers. Rarely, local necrosis occurs and even more rarely systemic symptoms develop. As the toxins are heat-labile, immersion of the affected part in just bearable hot water can relieve symptoms. Locals in Cornwall advise running up and down on hot sand.

Most jellyfish in British waters do not sting but a few, such as the bright yellow lion's mane jellyfish and blue sea nettle, do. These usually only result in transient local reaction but anaphylaxis has been reported.

The Portuguese man-of-war is very occasionally seen. From its blue, central, gas-filled body trail tentacles of up to 30 m in length. Thousands of nematocysts situated on the outer tentacle surfaces are triggered by any contact, releasing many vasoactive chemicals and proteases. Contact leaves intensely painful purple tentacle prints, which can blister and exhibit petechial haemorrhages. Local necrosis and delayed systemic reactions including anaphylaxis can occur. Wounds should be rinsed gently with sea water and remaining tentacles very carefully removed with gloved hands. Too much disturbance causes remaining nematocysts to fire. Application of vinegar and hot sea water can help inactivate the toxin. Emergency department review is appropriate.

INSECTS

The honey bee and wasp both envenomate via stings located at the posterior end of their abdomens. The toxins include

Table 16.4 National poisons information services

United Kingdom	
National Poisons Information Service (NPIS)	0844 892 0111
Eire	
National Poisons Information Centre (NPIC) Dublin	00 353 1 809 2566

histamine and serotonin, and cause intense pain and variable local inflammation. Bees leave a sting in place, which should be removed. Occasionally a local reaction from a sting on the pharynx can cause airway obstruction but the more frequent serious complication is anaphylaxis, which can occur in the 0.5% of the population hypersensitive to these stings. Risk factors for allergy include regular use of non-steroidal anti-inflammatory medication, age over 25 years and atherosclerosis. Anyone exhibiting signs of generalized pruritus, erythema or urticaria, wheeze or hypotension should be strongly suspected of developing anaphylaxis.

Poisons information services

National poisons information services provide a 24 h service and are able to provide advice on all types of poisoning and ingestion. Telephone numbers and locations are given in Table 16.4.

References

American Academy of Clinical Toxicology/European Association of Poison Centres and Clinical Toxicologists 1997 Position statement: gastric lavage. Clinical Toxicology 35: 711–719

Bresinski A, Besl H 1990 A colour atlas of poisonous fungi. Wolfe Publishing London

Burton BT 1984 Comparison of activated charcoal and gastric lavage in poisoned patients. Journal of Emergency Medicine 1: 411

Cooper MR, Johnson AW 1984 Poisonous plants in Britain and their effects in animals and man. HMSO, London

Cooper MR, Johnson AW 1988 Poisonous plants in Britain, a pictorial guide. HMSO, London

Dargan PI, Wallace CI, Jones AL 2002 An evidence based flowchart to guide the management of acute salicylate (aspirin) overdose. Emergency Medicine Journal 19: 206–209

Greaves I, Porter KP 2006 Oxford handbook of prehospital care. Oxford University Press, Oxford

Ferguson JA, Sellar C, Goldacre MJ 1992 Some epidemiological observations on medicinal and non-medicinal poisoning in pre-school children. Journal of Epidemiology and Community Health 46: 207–210

Harsch H 1986 Aspiration of activated charcoal. New England Journal of Medicine 314: 318

Hawton K, Fagg J 1992 Trends in self-poisoning and self-injury in Oxford, 1976–90. British Medical Journal 304: 1409–1411

Henry JA, Antao CA 1992 Suicide and fatal antidepressant poisoning. European Journal of Medicine 1: 343–348

Henry JA, Hoffman JR 1998 Continuing controversy on gut decontamination. Lancet 352: 420–421

Jawary D, Cameron PA, Dziukas L 1992 Drug overdose – reducing the load. Medical Journal of Australia 156: 343–346

McClure GM 1994 Suicide in children and adolescents in England and Wales 1960–1990. British Journal of Psychology 165: 510–514

Perrone J, Hoffman RS, Goldfrank LR 1994 Special considerations in gastrointestinal decontamination. Emergency Medicine Clinics of North America 12: 285–299

Pimentel L, Trommer L 1994 Cyclic antidepressant overdoses: a review. Emergency Medicine Clinics of North America 12: 533–547

Pond SM, Lewis-Driver DJ, Williams GM 1995 Gastric emptying in acute overdose: a prospective randomized controlled trial. Medical Journal of Australia 163: 345–349

Ramrakhra P, Moore K 2004 Oxford handbook of acute medicine, 2nd edn. Oxford University Press, Oxford

Spivey WH 1992 Flumazenil and seizures: analysis of 43 cases. Clinical Therapy 14: 292

Tenenbein M, Cohen S, Sitar DS 1987 Efficacy of ipecac-induced emesis, orogastric lavage and activated charcoal for acute drug overdose. Annals of Emergency Medicine 16: 838–841

Warrell DA 1996 Injuries, envenoming, poisoning and allergic reactions caused by animals. In: Weatherall DJ, Ledingham JGG, Warrell DA (eds) Oxford textbook of medicine, 3rd edn. Oxford University Press, Oxford

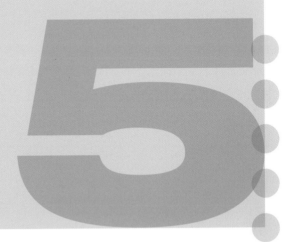

Part Five

17 Paediatric history and examination 197
18 Paediatric emergencies 209
19 Paediatric life support 220
20 The injured child 230

Paediatric history and examination

17

Introduction   197

The normal child   197

Neurological and emotional development   200

History in the critically ill child   200

Symptoms of respiratory disease in childhood   202

Symptoms associated with circulatory problems   203

Examination of the critically ill child   204

Further assessment and management   206

Assessment of the unwell child   207

Non-accidental injury   207

References   208

Further reading   208

Introduction

In the Western world critical illness is rare in children compared with the adult population. In poor and developing countries, by contrast (and in earlier generations in the West), childhood mortality is exceptionally high. Improved sanitation, vaccination and advances in the treatment of infectious illness have all led to an improvement in paediatric mortality and morbidity. Outside the neonatal period accidents and infection account for the vast majority of critical illness encountered in the paediatric population (Table 17.1). A smaller number of children have significant illness arising from underlying congenital abnormalities or problems developing around the perinatal period. For the rest, the problems will arise de novo.

The normal child

From the moment they are born, children develop and progress. They develop physically, physiologically and emotionally, and each of these has to be taken into consideration when assessing the well-being of any child.

It is traditional to refer to children in the first weeks of life as neonates, to those under 1 year old as infants and those over 1 year of age as children. Further divisions can be made (Table 17.2).

Children who have reached the early stages of puberty are usually referred to as adolescents. These definitions will be adhered to for the subsequent portions of this chapter. Problems in the neonatal period will be covered elsewhere (Ch. 43). The rest of this chapter will refer to infants and children up to adolescence.

That children start small and get bigger is a fact. However, this difference has a significant impact on the management of critical illness in childhood. The first difference between infants and children is the relative proportions of the different parts of the body. In early life the head can account for one-quarter of the total length of the body and much of the total surface area. This large head has many implications for management of paediatric injury and illness. First of all, children will fall head first because

Table 17.1 Causes of death by age in declining order of frequency (Scottish national figures for 2004)

<1 year	1–4 years	5–9 years	10–14 years
Perinatal conditions	Malignant neoplasms	Accidents	Malignant neoplasms
Congenital abnormalities	Congenital abnormalities	Malignant neoplasms	Accidents
Nervous system	Infectious diseases	Nervous system	Congenital abnormalities
Malignant neoplasms	Endocrine, nutritional, metabolic and blood diseases	Digestive diseases	Nervous system
Other causes		Infectious diseases	Endocrine, nutritional, metabolic and blood diseases
	Nervous system	Other causes	
	Other causes		Other causes

Source: General Register Office for Scotland Childhood Death Statistics 2004

Table 17.2 Classification of children by age

Neonate	0–6 weeks
Infant	6 weeks–1 year
Toddler	1–3 years
Pre-school	3–5 years
School age	5–12 years
Adolescent	12–16 years

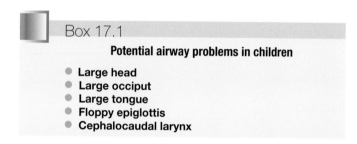

Box 17.1

Potential airway problems in children

- **Large head**
- **Large occiput**
- **Large tongue**
- **Floppy epiglottis**
- **Cephalocaudal larynx**

remove foreign bodies should not include abdominal thrusts, e.g. the Heimlich manoeuvre or paediatric equivalent, as organ damage will occur.

The Heimlich manoeuvre is contraindicated in infants and small children.

of the higher centre of gravity, making head injuries a frequent occurrence in childhood. Second, within the head region the relatively large occiput adds further problems, particularly with regard to airway care. The large occiput tends to force the neck into flexion when the child is supine. Thus, some degree of movement is necessary to extend the neck to ensure that airway opening manoeuvres are adequate. This can be facilitated by placing a small pad underneath the child's shoulders.

With regard to the paediatric airway, infants and young children have a large tongue, a 'floppy' epiglottis and a cephalocaudal larynx. These are all sufficiently different from the adult to make intubation a special skill in the infant population. Practitioners unfamiliar with this anatomy but who may be regular practitioners of airway care in the adult population may find themselves in difficulties if these differences are not appreciated (Box 17.1).

Heart position is different in infants and children to adults (Philips & Zideman 1986). The high heart in the infant means that cardiac compressions are applied at the midpoint of the sternum just below the internipple line. In the older child, the hand position is lower, to reflect the change with age. One, can often palpate the liver below the ribcage in infants. This liver edge disappears as the child gets older. The position of the liver and spleen in infancy makes them vulnerable to blunt trauma to the abdomen, especially from non-accidental injury. Manoeuvres to

SURFACE AREA

Surface area in children is important. Infants have relatively large total body surface areas compared to older children and adults. As described above, a large proportion of this is taken up by the head and neck region. Similarly, the trunk and the limbs have different proportions in childhood than in adulthood and these change with age. This is important when thinking about heat loss. Heat is lost from a larger area and therefore children will cool down very rapidly. This is particularly so in neonates and infants who can get very cold very quickly. If they need resuscitation great care must be taken to ensure their warmth, particularly if they are being resuscitated having been exposed to cold or water.

It is also an important consideration when treating burns. The total body surface area cannot be calculated from the 'rule of 9s' as in adulthood. Special charts need to be devised to enable the relative surface areas to be considered. A paediatric chart (Fig. 17.1) is used to account for surface area differences in children at different ages.

Name...Ward..Unit number............................Date...............................

Age................................

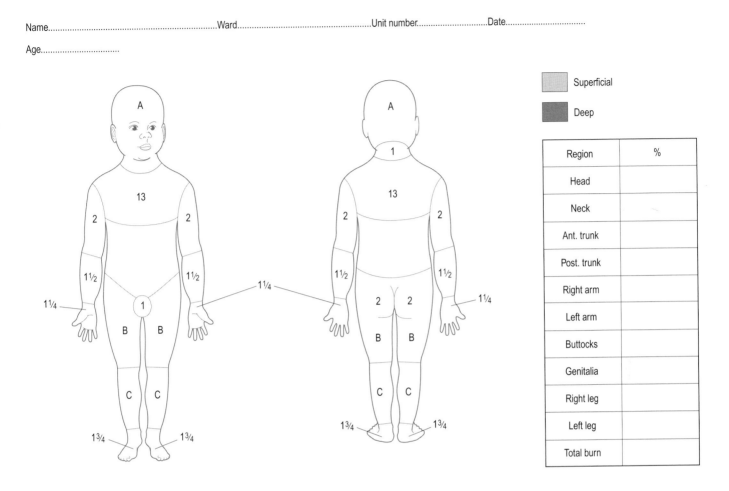

Region	%
Head	
Neck	
Ant. trunk	
Post. trunk	
Right arm	
Left arm	
Buttocks	
Genitalia	
Right leg	
Left leg	
Total burn	

Relative percentages affected by growth

Area	Age 0	1	5	10	15	Adult
A = ½ of head	9 ½	8 ½	6 ½	5 ½	4 ½	3 ½
B = ½ of one thigh	2 ¾	3 ¼	4	4 ½	4 ½	4 ¾
C = ½ of one leg	2 ½	2 ½	2 ¾	3 ¼	3 ¼	3 ½

Fig. 17.1 • A paediatric burns chart (Lund and Browder chart).

Once they reach adolescence it is appropriate to use the 'rule of 9s'. If no chart is available, as may occur in the prehospital phase, the palm of the child's hand can also be used, the surface area corresponding to about 1% of the body.

OTHER DIFFERENCES

A child's bone structure is also different from that in adulthood. The presence of epiphyseal plates is an important factor. Children seldom sprain ligaments. Injuries that in adults can cause a sprained ligament very often result in fractures around the epiphysis, which can be classified using the Salter–Harris classification. Salter–Harris type I fractures are associated with a normal X-ray appearance and are characterized by pain over the distal or proximal end of the involved bone. Fractures in children also heal much more quickly than in adults. Fractures can also remodel providing they are in the plane of movement of the joint, they are close to the epiphyseal plate and there is still substantial growth left. Bones in the hand and face are particularly unforgiving and, if non-alignment is not corrected early, disfigurement will arise.

Wound healing is also rapid in children and it is important therefore that wounds are repaired early if cosmetic defects are to be avoided. It is important that wound closure is done as accurately as possible if long-term disfigurement and scarring is to be obviated.

PHYSIOLOGICAL DIFFERENCES

Physiological differences between infants, children and adults are found in respiratory rates, heart rates, blood pressure and blood volume. Typical values by age are found in Tables 17.3–17.5. There is wide variation and overlap between the age groups and this in turn means that any single value is usually meaningless. One usually has to look for trends in change to gain useful data.

The weight of a child changes with age and varies proportionately with the length of the child in most cases. This means that one can assess therapeutic needs in terms either of the age, length or weight of the child. Consequently, if one knows one of these parameters then it is possible to determine what the others are. This has important consequences for treatment. Most drugs are administered on a weight-for-weight basis. Endotracheal tubes, however, are determined on an age basis. In some circumstances one may not know either the weight of the child nor the age of the child, making length an important parameter.

These parameters have led to the formulation of two distinct methods of estimating drug therapy and resuscitation equipment in the critically ill child. The Oakley chart (Oakley 1988, Fig. 17.2) and the Broselow tape (Luten et al 1992; Fig. 17.3) are both variations on the same theme. Each has its merits and active proponents.

In the prehospital environment the tape measure is probably the most appropriate, particularly if the associated colour-coded packs are similarly provided. In the prehospital phase the stress of having to calculate drugs or endotracheal tube lengths should be avoided if at all possible.

In an emergency an approximate weight of a child can be determined by the following formula:

$$\text{Weight (in kg)} = 2 \times (\text{Age} + 4).$$

Table 17.3 Respiratory rates in children	
Age (breaths min^{-1})	Mean respiratory rate
Birth–3 months	35
3 months–1 year	30
1–5 years	25
5–10 years	20
>10 years	14

Table 17.4 Blood pressures	
Age	Mean blood pressure (mmHg)
Birth	60/40
1 year	95/65
5 years	100/65
Puberty	120/75

Table 17.5 Mean heart rates	
Pulse	Mean heart rate (beats min^{-1})
Birth	125
1 year	125
5 years	100
Puberty	75

Neurological and emotional development

At birth children have a number of primitive reflexes, which should disappear by the age of 6 months. These include the rooting and Moro reflexes. Failure of these to disappear indicates that there is some significant underlying problem with development, often neurological.

By 4 weeks a child should watch its mother and startle at sounds. By 4–6 weeks the child should be smiling and following mother with its eyes. By 3 months the child should be smiling and gurgling. By 5 months head control should be obtained and by 6 months the child should be sitting with support from hands. Most children should be walking by 15 months of age and by 18 months able to climb stairs. A 4-year-old child should be able to dress him/herself, go to the toilet and speak in long sentences. When assessing a child in a critical situation it may not be possible to physically examine these parameters but some idea of the child's development should be obtained. Of particular importance are changes that have occurred in the preceding days, as these may give some idea as to the duration of the child's illness or underlying disorder.

History in the critically ill child

A history should only be obtained once a full assessment of the child's airway, breathing and circulation has been made

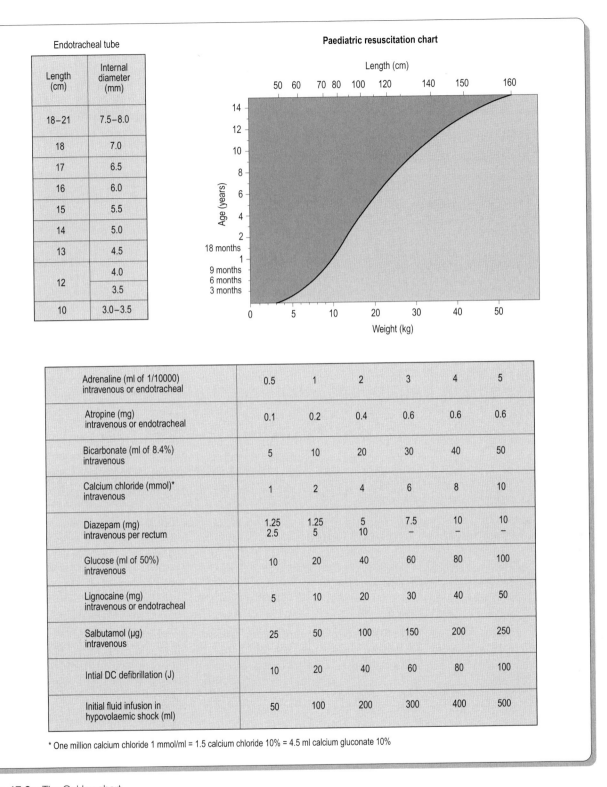

Endotracheal tube

Length (cm)	Internal diameter (mm)
18–21	7.5–8.0
18	7.0
17	6.5
16	6.0
15	5.5
14	5.0
13	4.5
12	4.0
	3.5
10	3.0–3.5

Paediatric resuscitation chart

Adrenaline (ml of 1/10000) intravenous or endotracheal	0.5	1	2	3	4	5
Atropine (mg) intravenous or endotracheal	0.1	0.2	0.4	0.6	0.6	0.6
Bicarbonate (ml of 8.4%) intravenous	5	10	20	30	40	50
Calcium chloride (mmol)* intravenous	1	2	4	6	8	10
Diazepam (mg) intravenous per rectum	1.25 2.5	1.25 5	5 10	7.5 –	10 –	10 –
Glucose (ml of 50%) intravenous	10	20	40	60	80	100
Lignocaine (mg) intravenous or endotracheal	5	10	20	30	40	50
Salbutamol (µg) intravenous	25	50	100	150	200	250
Intial DC defibrillation (J)	10	20	40	60	80	100
Initial fluid infusion in hypovolaemic shock (ml)	50	100	200	300	400	500

* One million calcium chloride 1 mmol/ml = 1.5 calcium chloride 10% = 4.5 ml calcium gluconate 10%

Fig. 17.2 • The Oakley chart.

and one is satisfied that these are secure. The history should be systematic and pertinent to the appropriate problems. Typically, children will be critically ill because there is an underlying either respiratory or circulatory cause. Both of these combine, if left untreated, to merge as cardiopulmonary failure, which in turn will lead to cardiac arrest (Fig. 17.4).

A small percentage of children have underlying long-term illness that makes them more prone to certain types

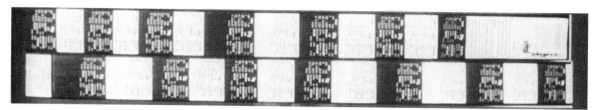

Fig. 17.3 • The Broselow tape.

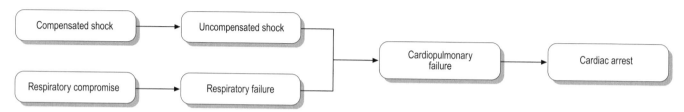

Fig. 17.4 • Progress from circulatory and respiratory problems to critical illness in children.

of illness. If the child has been attended in the prehospital phase by his or her own general practitioner then these predisposing illnesses may be known. However, this is not always the case and certain conditions should be sought.

The history of prematurity is important. A child who has spent time in the neonatal intensive care unit and who has been on a ventilator may well have bronchopulmonary dysplasia. This child may normally be in borderline respiratory failure. Anything that decreases this child's respiratory function will increase the chance of complete respiratory failure. These children will get respiratory infections just like any other child. Bronchiolitis is particularly worrying and most will need inpatient treatment. Children with cystic fibrosis are similarly at risk, as are children with progressive neuromuscular disease.

Children with neurological disease or cerebral palsy may be prone to seizure activity. They may have associated hydrocephalus. Children with hydrocephalus usually have a shunt in place, which can become blocked, leading to atypical neurological symptoms.

Children with underlying cardiac disease may well be living with borderline cardiac function, and they may be tipped into full cardiac failure by the onset of relatively minor infections or intercurrent illness. Antibiotics effective against bacterial endocarditis should be considered in those children with valve disease or who have septal defects and are thought to be at risk by their cardiologist.

Children with proven renal tract abnormalities may be more prone to urinary tract infections. These infections may cause failure to thrive. Apart from giving rise to pyrexia, acute infections may be associated with nausea, vomiting or abdominal pain.

Underlying endocrine disease is also important. Diabetic children are more prone to infection than normal children and infection will, of course, worsen diabetic control. Children who take oral medication for their adrenogenital failure and who start to vomit may well end up with complex metabolic problems with electrolyte disturbance. Again, these children can present in coma and a knowledge of the underlying illness is important to ensure that appropriate treatment is administered.

Children with spina bifida or other neurological problems can develop fractures and skin problems in the limbs distal to the neurological abnormality. These can become infected and may cause septicaemia. These children may present very late because of the absence of pain as a warning sign that something is wrong.

In all of these children with underlying congenital or pre-existing disease, special care needs to be taken and it is probably better for these children to be discussed with their usual attending physician should there be any cause for concern. Often, parents or regular carers will have greater experience of these conditions than health-care professionals, and their advice and experience can be helpful to the prehospital team.

Symptoms of respiratory disease in childhood

Respiratory disease can be associated with increased work of breathing (respiratory distress) or decreased respiratory effort (respiratory depression).

RESPIRATORY DISTRESS

Respiratory distress is common in childhood. Of most concern in the prehospital setting is that of acute onset, or acute onset against a background of respiratory illness (acute on chronic). Sudden onset of respiratory distress may be associated with foreign body inhalation or acute exposure to allergen. Croup (laryngotracheobronchitis) typically has a gradual onset with preceding coryzal illness and cough. Epiglottitis, on the other hand, will have a reasonably acute onset. Often the child will be well going to bed but waken some hours later with the illness.

Wheeze versus stridor

Wheeze can be defined as high-pitched, expiratory noises produced by air moving through the narrowed lower airways. Stridor is a much louder, harsher noise present on inspiration and is associated with obstruction in the upper airways. For either to be present, there must be air entry through the relevant anatomical structures. A history of a child who has noisy breathing that is subsequently getting quieter without treatment can be an extremely ominous sign.

Feeding

A child will preferentially breath rather than feed. In order to maintain a respiratory rate in excess of 50 breaths per minute, as may occur in bronchiolitis or asthma, a child is unable to stop breathing long enough to take any nourishment. This is a particularly worrying sign and is an indication to admit the child to hospital.

Heart failure may present as a child who gets breathless on feeding, who feeds slowly or who sweats during feeding. There may or may not be associated episodes of cyanosis. Differentiating between this and chest infection can be a very difficult clinical decision.

Apnoea

Apnoea can be associated with many conditions in childhood. Most commonly, however, it is associated with bronchiolitis and respiratory disease. The parents should be questioned as to whether the child stopped breathing, for how long and what were the associated signs, e.g. cyanosis. Apnoeic attacks associated with bronchiolitis are an indication to admit the child to hospital.

Apnoea can follow head injury, especially in infants. It is associated with quite significant brain trauma. If present, non-accidental injury, especially by shaking, should be excluded.

RESPIRATORY DEPRESSION

Respiratory depression is typically due to problems outside the respiratory system. Head injury, intracranial infection, epilepsy and poisoning are the commonest causes. A history pertinent to any of these conditions should be obtained and, if time permits, a search should be made of the vicinity for evidence of drug ingestion or alcohol abuse. In the periadolescent child glue sniffing may also have been a feature in the development of respiratory depression.

Symptoms associated with circulatory problems

Circulatory problems are usually due to fluid loss (e.g. haemorrhage, diarrhoea, vomiting or renal loss) or through redistribution (e.g. heart failure, septic shock, anaphylactic shock and neurogenic shock). Of these haemorrhage, diarrhoea, vomiting, renal loss (e.g. diabetes) and septic shock are probably the most common.

HAEMORRHAGE AND BLOOD LOSS

Overt blood loss is rare in the paediatric population. If present it can be associated with many conditions. It is not unusual, however, for infants to have some vomiting associated with blood streaking, particularly due to oesophagitis and hiatus hernia. This, however, is seldom enough to cause hypovolaemia. Blood may be passed per rectum in Henoch–Schönlein purpura, intussusception and Meckel's diverticulum. Blood may be altered (melaena) or fresh in any of these situations. Blood per rectum in intussusception is a late sign.

Bloody diarrhoea may be associated with infective gastroenteritis such as *Salmonella*, *Shigella* and *Campylobacter*. More recently haemolytic–uraemic syndrome, presenting with bloody diarrhoea, caused by infection with *E. coli* O157 has become a public health issue. Evidence of contact with other sufferers should always be sought. Occasionally continued blood loss following minor surgery, e.g. dental extraction, may indicate the presence of a clotting disorder. Many of these are familial and a history of this may give a clue to the diagnosis.

Fluid loss following trauma will usually be intra-abdominal, although obvious fluid loss from an external wound may also be present. A history of trauma therefore should be sought in all children who are apparently hypovolaemic.

VOMITING AND DIARRHOEA

Vomiting is quite a common symptom in childhood. Commonly associated with gastrointestinal infection, it also follows head injury and may be associated with urinary infection and meningitis. One should enquire into the amount and frequency of the vomiting and the presence or absence of bile or blood. Projectile vomiting may be a feature in babies less than 3 months old. If present, pyloric stenosis should be considered. If diarrhoea is present, frequency of stool, consistency and the presence or absence of blood are all important (see above).

It is worth mentioning the diarrhoea of intussusception. Children with intussusception often have one diarrhoeal stool and then develop the classic signs and symptoms of intussusception subsequent to this. These children will be unwell out of all proportion to the volume lost from any associated vomiting or a single episode of diarrhoea.

Polyuria and/or polydipsia may be associated with vomiting and abdominal pain. This combination should alert one to the diagnosis of diabetic ketoacidosis, another cause for fluid loss.

FLUID MALDISTRIBUTION

Fluid maldistribution can occur in cardiac failure, septicaemia, anaphylaxis or neurogenic shock. Of these heart failure and septicaemia are the commonest. The symptoms of heart failure include breathlessness during feeding, weight gain, cyanotic episodes and failure to thrive.

If septic shock is suspected the history may well be one of preceding 'flu'-like illness, which may be of relatively short duration. Parents should be asked about the presence or absence of a rash and how long it has been there. Typically, the rash will be purpuric rather than macular.

Neurogenic shock can be associated with trauma-induced spinal injury, while anaphylactic shock may be associated with contact with a known allergen. Any previous history of allergy should be documented in the child.

Examination of the critically ill child

Recognition skills are vitally important in prehospital management of the critically ill infant. The sequence of assessment follows that of any resuscitation programme, namely the assessment of airway, breathing and circulation (the ABC of resuscitation).

While it is convenient to describe the sequence of resuscitation in this fashion, in reality airway and breathing are assessed together. It is impossible to determine whether the airway is open without looking for breathing; concomitantly breathing will only be present through an open airway. Bearing this in mind, it is easier to progress stepwise through the standard sequence.

ASSESSMENT OF AIRWAY

The airway should first of all be assessed and categorized as being open, partially obstructed or fully obstructed. A fully open airway will allow uninterrupted air entry. The chest wall will be seen to rise symmetrically and there will be no audible stridor or wheeze.

A partially obstructed airway will result in noisy breathing with incomplete lung expansion. Noisy breathing can be characterized as follows:

- gurgling indicating liquid matter in the airway – typically this is vomit, secretions or blood
- stridor indicating upper airway obstruction – foreign body, croup or epiglottitis should be suspected
- wheeze indicating lower airway obstruction.

In a totally obstructed airway there will be no air movement. In the early stages of acute airway obstruction the child may be making vigorous efforts to breath but, unless the airway is rapidly cleared or opened, the child will lapse into coma with subsequent bradycardia and asystolic arrest.

The normal airway will usually need no further treatment except possibly the addition of supplemental oxygen. The partially obstructed airway should be cleared by whatever means possible. As a first stage the chin lift or jaw thrust manoeuvres should be performed, and the head tilted back. In a traumatized child, head tilt will be dangerous and only the chin lift or jaw thrust should be performed. Failure to clear upper airway obstruction with this manoeuvre should lead one to consider suction if gurgling noises are present, or to consider back blows/chest thrusts if a foreign body is suspected. Other causes may require intubation as a matter of urgency. In this situation, or in that of a totally obstructed airway, one should be prepared to perform a needle cricothyroidotomy as a matter or urgency.

ASSESSMENT OF BREATHING

When examining for breathing one should look initially at the respiratory rate and the effort required to breath. Normal respiratory rates for children are given in Table 17.3. A slow, shallow breathing rate may indicate head injury, poisoning, postictal state or raised intracranial pressure. A fast rate may indicate airway disease, pyrexia, pain or hypovolaemia. Of particular concern is a respiratory rate of above 50 breaths min^{-1} in children under 1 year of age and above 40 breaths min^{-1} in older children. This indicates severe respiratory distress. If allowed to continue the child will gradually become exhausted and will eventually progress into respiratory arrest.

Grunting is particularly important. This is a form of physiological positive end-expiratory pressure (PEEP) designed to maximize alveolar gas exchange. If present, it indicates significant respiratory distress.

Chest expansion should be observed and should be symmetrical. Movement of one side more than the other may indicate collapse and/or pneumothorax. In addition, in an intubated child it may indicate intubation of one or other of the main bronchi. Similarly, auscultation may reveal differences in air entry compatible with these same diagnoses.

Ill children may be pale, mottled or cyanosed. Children become cyanosed very late. To wait for cyanosis is to wait too long. Should a child present with cyanosis then he or she is in impending respiratory failure.

Cyanosis is a late sign in children.

Having assessed the breathing one should take measures appropriate to the clinical condition. At the very least supplemental oxygen should be provided via a Venturi mask, or Hudson-type mask with an attached reservoir bag. This will give a percentage of inspired oxygen received by the patient (F_iO_2) of 40–60% with a Venturi mask or to up to 90% with a Hudson mask and reservoir. Failure to improve with this should lead one to provide assisted ventilation using appropriate bag–valve–mask devices.

ASSESSMENT OF CIRCULATION

It is important at this stage to emphasize what one is actually looking for in assessing the circulation. Blood pressure is relatively unimportant in children compared to the adult population. The immense ability of children to compensate for considerable fluid loss means that blood pressure can remain normal until late in the disease process and then drop dramatically. By this stage the child is in uncompensated shock and if untreated this will progress to irreversible shock.

Up to 40% of the circulating volume can be lost before a measurable drop in blood pressure occurs.

Up to 40% of the circulating volume can be lost before a measurable drop in blood pressure occurs (Schwaitzberg et al 1988). This ability to compensate is carried through into early adult life and is one that cannot be overestimated. For this reason it is preferable to talk in terms of end organ perfusion rather than blood pressure. In particular one looks for perfusion in the skin, the brain and the kidneys.

When looking for signs of fluid loss or shock one therefore looks at the physical signs that indicate poor perfusion.

It is important to determine, where a pulse is palpable, the rate and the quality of the pulse. First, peripheral pulses in the normal child can be palpated at the radial or brachial artery in the upper limb, or at the posterior tibial or dorsalis pedis area in the lower limb. If these are weak or absent one should next attempt to feel a femoral pulse. If this is absent one should attempt to feel a carotid pulse. The position of the strongest pulse gives a good rapid assessment of perfusion. Good strong peripheral pulses suggest good peripheral perfusion; weak central pulses indicate significant hypoperfusion.

A rising pulse rate followed by a slowing pulse (without treatment) is an ominous sign. It indicates that the child has impending cardiopulmonary failure and treatment is therefore very urgent.

A high or rising pulse rate may be associated with pain, fear, pyrexia or fluid loss. The rate should be assessed in the context of the clinical picture.

In the normal child capillary refill should be less than 2 s. In a child in a very cold environment up to 4 s may be normal. However, this should be the exception rather than the rule. Anything over 2 s should be considered abnormal and is an indication of circulatory compromise. The higher this is above 2 s the greater the degree of circulatory compromise.

As a child compensates for hypovolaemia by diverting blood to vital areas, the peripheries cool down. This can be assessed by running a hand along the limb. There may be a transition zone where a change from warm to cool can be detected. The closer this transition occurs to the groin in the lower limb or the axilla in the upper limb the more severe the problem. Measurement of urinary output is not practical in the prehospital phase.

Some clue as to the degree of peripheral shutdown and the time that this has taken to occur may be obtained from the frequency with which the child wets a nappy. Mothers are usually quite accurate on how dry and how heavy the nappies are compared to normal. Fathers are less so! This can at best be a guide and cannot be taken as an absolute rule. This can be difficult if diarrhoea is also present.

As detailed above, blood pressure is only useful when it is abnormal. However, *to wait for blood pressure to become abnormal before treatment is to wait too long.* A normal blood pressure with no signs of shock is reassuring; a normal blood pressure with signs as detailed above indicates that a child is in compensated shock. An abnormally low blood pressure with other signs of shock indicates uncompensated or irreversible shock.

The presence of a petechial rash associated with a child who is unwell is a particularly sinister feature. Of most concern is the fact that the child may have meningococcal septicaemia, which can be rapidly life-threatening. A petechial rash should be sought in any child who is unwell with evidence of circulatory failure and an altered level of consciousness. The rash may be minuscule and barely visible but can develop rapidly. *To wait for this to happen before giving oxygen, fluids or penicillin is to wait too long.*

Box 17.2

AVPU scale

- **A** *A*lert
- **V** Responds to **V**erbal stimuli
- **P** responds to **P**ainful stimuli
- **U** *U*nconscious

LEVEL OF CONSCIOUSNESS

Level of consciousness is an important indicator of the state of wellbeing of the child. Children who are hypoxic or hypovolaemic very readily develop an altered level of consciousness. Any child who is comatose or who has altered level of consciousness should have hypoxia and/or hypovolaemia sought and treated as a matter of urgency.

Only when these have been treated can coma be attributed to an intracranial cause.

Measuring level of consciousness is difficult to do reliably in infants and young children. A rapid assessment may be made using the 'AVPU' scale (Box 17.2).

The Adelaide coma scale or the Glasgow paediatric scale can be cumbersome in the field and confer no benefit over the AVPU assessment. Children scoring 'P' or 'U' are at risk of airway obstruction secondary to *either* (a) the tongue falling back to obstruct the oropharynx *or* (b) the loss of gag reflex predisposing to aspiration. Hypoventilation may also ensue, aggravating gas exchange.

Agitation, if present, is a good marker of hypoxia. The agitated or irritable child who will not tolerate an oxygen mask is often the very child who needs oxygen.

PUPILLARY SIGNS

Pupillary changes accompany many disease states. Asymmetrical pupils can be normal (Holmes–Adie pupils). However, this is rare. Children with respiratory distress or depression may have been poisoned. Dilated pupils may be associated with cholinergic-related drugs (atropine, tricyclics) or sympathomimetics (ephedrine, salbutamol).

Pupillary constriction may be associated with opiate poisoning. Intracranial pathology will cause pupillary asymmetry or cycloplegia. Of importance are the changes associated with an acute unilateral expanding intracranial haematoma.

Further assessment and management

Much of the assessment of the sick child relies on a very rapid 'eyes, ears, hands' assessment. An experienced practitioner will get all the above information during clinical examination in the space of approximately 30s. One can then place the child into one of five categories:

1. *Stable* – the child may have some signs but these will not be severe. The child will be in no acute distress.
2. *Respiratory distress* – symptoms and signs of respiratory distress or depression will be present.
3. *Circulatory distress* – signs of shock will be present but the blood pressure will be normal.
4. *Impending cardiopulmonary failure* – the child will have maximally compensated for either a respiratory or circulatory cause and cardiopulmonary failure is imminent.
5. *Cardiopulmonary failure* – the respiratory pattern will be abnormal with totally ineffective ventilation of the lungs. The heart rate will be slow or slowing and uncompensated shock will be present. If untreated, cardiac arrest will ensue within a very short space of time.

Cardiac arrest will be recognized as an unconscious child who exhibits no cardiorespiratory effort. Management of cardiac arrest in children is dealt with in Chapter 19.

When one encounters children in categories 1, 2 or 3 above, there will usually be a history or physical findings compatible with an underlying disease process (Ch. 18). For children who are stable, treatment at home is usually appropriate unless home or social circumstances demand otherwise. Parents or guardians should be advised as to potential ominous signs and given appropriate instructions as to how to proceed to further care if there is concern. Telephone consultation is particularly useful. Children with rare or underlying disease processes should be discussed with the relevant paediatrician, even if only by telephone.

Children with respiratory or circulatory distress will almost invariably require some form of inpatient management. The concept of ambulatory paediatrics within the hospital setting, which will maximize communication between community and the hospital service, would seem to be appropriate for this situation. Ideally, children could be admitted to a short-stay treatment area adjacent to the emergency department from where they can be discharged readily into the community once the situation has stabilized or admitted for longer term inpatient care if not progressing. Further care could then continue in a less acute setting, such as an ambulatory clinic in hospital or GP surgery.

Children in category 4 with impending cardiopulmonary failure will require extensive investigation and resuscitation together with observation. It is appropriate to begin resuscitation in the community and the child should be transferred for inpatient care as a matter of urgency.

Children in category 5 require urgent resuscitation. Often in these situations the simpler the action, the better. It is imperative that the airway is open and the child is ventilated with 100% oxygen. It is not necessary to actually intubate the child in this situation provided that adequate bag–valve–mask technique is being used. Chest compressions may well be needed, particularly if the child is under the age of 1 year and the heart rate is less than 60 beats min^{-1}.

The decision to transfer children with minimal intervention or to 'stay and play' is very difficult to resolve. Hospital-based resuscitation or retrieval teams also enter the equation. These issues should be resolved before they actually arise.

Factors that will influence the various decisions include: geography, availability of local resources and the availability of the expertise in the prehospital setting. No single set of rules will be suitable for all areas but a broad application of general principles is to be advocated, particularly as the incidence of acute life-threatening illness in childhood in many areas is relatively low.

Assessment of the unwell child

Many children present who do not fit neatly into any one of the above categories and the underlying disease is not immediately apparent. These children will not have obvious circulatory or respiratory distress but may just be unwell. Typically the child will have a viral illness with inflamed mucous membranes. Single mucous membrane involvement will usually be bacterial in origin. It is important to have a list of rarer diagnoses that are possible in the back of one's mind. Paramount among these is meningitis, which can present in many ways. Classic patterns of pyrexia, bulging fontanelle and stiff neck are not always present. This is particularly so in the neonatal period, when the child can be simply off feeds and be fussy. The child may be twitchy or jerky in addition. Older children develop more traditional symptoms but occasionally vomiting, lethargy and loss of appetite may be all that is present. A pyrexial child without obvious inflammation of the mucous membranes in the throat or ears or chest should be considered to have an occult focus of infection. This may simply be a viraemia or bacteraemia without a single focus. In addition, however, one should consider appendicitis and osteomyelitis, as well as urinary tract infection.

Children with intussusception can often present without the classic triad of abdominal pain, passage of blood per rectum (redcurrant stool) and palpable mass. In a recent study only 10% of children presented with these signs, although subsequently most children were found to have them as time progressed and the diagnosis was made (Macdonald & Beattie 1995). A child with intussusception may well present simply with screaming and drawing his/her knees into his/her chest, followed by going very pale and quiet. After 6–12 h the child will pass a bloody stool. By this stage the child is usually very unwell.

These diagnoses can be difficult in hospital, let alone in the prehospital phase. There should be a low threshold for referral in these situations, while still adhering to the principles of assessment and care described above.

Non-accidental injury

Non-accidental injury is always a worry when children present for urgent care. However, it is in these children that one must be careful. Four categories of child abuse exist:

- physical abuse
- sexual abuse
- emotional neglect and deprivation
- Munchausen's syndrome by proxy.

The true incidence of each is unknown and many cases certainly go unnoticed or undiagnosed. The first three can occur in combination.

PHYSICAL ABUSE

Physical abuse takes several forms. Usually the child will be beaten, normally with a hand or fist but occasionally with an object such as a stick or belt. Kicking can also occur. It is particularly easy to pick up small babies and infants. For this reason they are prone to shaking or being swung around. The physical signs of this injury are often difficult to detect. Care should be taken with any child who presents with a history of apnoea, breath-holding or prolonged coma. The possibility that the child has been shaken and has sustained significant brain injury must be considered. If shaking is suspected grip marks to the lower limb or chest should be sought and documented.

Thermal injury is also important; parents or guardians have been known to chastise children by placing a hand or other parts of the body on a hot surface or in hot water.

Very few parents or guardians will give a history of actually abusing a child. Often they will fabricate a plausible excuse for the injuries.

Features in the history that suggest that a child has been abused include:

- delay in presentation for medical care
- changing the story
- siblings on the At-risk Register
- time spent separated from parents (especially in the neonatal period)
- previous history of abuse.

Features on examination that are indicative of non-accidental injury include:

- retinal haemorrhages
- bruising of different ages
- marks suggestive of being hit with a stick or a cane
- burns to the buttocks, perineum, feet or back of the hand.

SEXUAL ABUSE

This rarely presents as an emergency. When it does, acute bleeding from perineal injury may be present. Often this is associated with other blunt trauma, which can include attempted strangulation or suffocation. More typically, there will be other features that lead one to think that child sexual abuse is present. Change in behaviour, enuresis (especially if the child has previously been dry), school phobia and change of personality can all be associated with sexual abuse. However, other organic causes must be sought first.

In peripubertal children, truanting, parasuicide and antisocial behaviour are all associated with sexual abuse. Physical signs will include obvious bruising to the perineum or anus, pregnancy or proven sexually transmitted disease.

More often a child will confide in a trusted person, who may be a health-care professional in the prehospital setting. In these situations it is important that the local guidelines are followed, and to this end it is important that all pre-hospital care providers are familiar with the guidelines in their area.

EMOTIONAL NEGLECT AND DEPRIVATION

Emotional neglect and deprivation are difficult to determine. Many children are unkempt and dirty but this does not mean that they are neglected or deprived. Features that may suggest that the child is being neglected include failure to thrive or to achieve milestones. Of particular concern are speech and communication skills, especially if these are seen to regress.

MUNCHAUSEN'S SYNDROME BY PROXY

This is a complex entity in which the child is perfectly well but the parent or guardian is responsible for the child's illness. Factitious presentations such as haematuria or skin ulcers may be features of the problem. It is particularly important to bear in mind that children who present with more than one poisoning episode may be the victim of

Munchausen's by proxy. A high index of suspicion is therefore required. These concerns should be communicated to a local paediatrician or social work department who can instigate further treatment.

MANAGEMENT OF NON-ACCIDENTAL INJURY IN THE PREHOSPITAL PHASE

Abused children are no different from any other child presenting for emergency care. Initially one must ensure that the airway, breathing and circulation are intact. If not they should be treated as described above.

Documentation of all historical issues and facts, together with details of resuscitation events, must be complete. These will be needed as part of any subsequent legal enquiry, which can take months and years to complete. Good contemporaneous notes and diagrams are invaluable and add credibility to the witness.

Each prehospital-care practitioner should be aware of local guidelines on managing child abuse and these should be adhered to in all cases. This will ensure they do all they can to ensure subsequent safety of the abused child.

References

General Register Office for Scotland Childhood Death Statistics 2004

Luten RC, Wears R, Broselow J et al 1992 Length-based endotracheal tube and emergency equipment in paediatrics. Annals of Emergency Medicine 21: 900–904

Macdonald IAR, Beattie TF 1995 Intussusception presenting to a paediatric accident and emergency department. Journal of Accident and Emergency Medicine 12: 182–186

Oakley P 1988 Inaccuracy and delay in decision making in paediatric resuscitation and proposed reference chart to reduce error. British Medical Journal 297: 817–819

Philips GW, Zideman DA 1986 Relation of infant heart to sternum: its significance in cardiopulmonary resuscitation. Lancet 1: 1024–1025

Schwaitzberg SD, Bergman KS, Harris BH 1988 A paediatric trauma model of continuous haemorrhage. Journal of Pediatric Surgery 23: 605–609

Further reading

American Heart Association 1995 Paediatric advanced life support. American Heart Association, Dallas, TX

Luten RC (ed) 1988 Problems in pediatric emergency medicine. Churchill Livingstone, New York

Paediatric emergencies

18

Introduction   209

Airway obstruction   209

Acute asthma in children   211

Pneumonia   214

Inhaled (aspirated) foreign body   214

Epilepsy   215

Metabolic emergencies   215

Management of the comatose child   216

Vomiting and diarrhoea   216

Meningitis   217

Meningococcal septicaemia   218

The pyrexial child   218

Conclusion   219

References   219

Further reading   219

Introduction

Acute life-threatening paediatric emergencies are relatively infrequent in developed countries. However, medical causes still account for large numbers of deaths in the paediatric population in developing countries or in areas affected by war and strife. In these countries diarrhoeal disease is probably the leading problem, although other infections do play a significant part. Respiratory emergencies account for the greatest numbers of problems in the Western world. This chapter describes common paediatric emergencies and provides a guide to their early treatment by prehospital care providers.

Airway obstruction

Acute airway conditions are common in children. During the winter months respiratory disease is the commonest reason for children to be admitted to hospital in the UK. Infective airway obstruction (croup and bronchiolitis) and asthma are probably the most common reasons for admission within this category.

CROUP

Croup (laryngotracheobronchitis) is a disease of viral origin caused by many different viruses. Typically there will be a prodrome with a history of coryza, mild pyrexia and general malaise for a few days prior to the onset of the croup. The croup itself will often be intermittent and is often associated with a harsh, barking cough. Mild cases can be treated at home with steam inhalations and general supportive measures. Evidence that all is not well and that the child is developing problems will be manifest by the presence of signs and symptoms of respiratory distress (see Ch. 17). These will include the use of accessory muscles, increasing respiratory rate, retractions or recession, nasal flaring and an altered level of consciousness. In these situations it is worth trying nebulized adrenaline (epinephrine). There is increasing evidence that steroids decrease the need for intubation and airway intervention (Geelhoed 1996). Oral prednisolone, dexamethasone and nebulized budesonide have all been reported as being useful (Table 18.1). If a child is thought to need such medication, hospital admission should be arranged.

Occasionally children present as if they have epiglottitis but the history is that of croup (Table 18.2). In these situations there is often a secondary bacterial infection with either *Staphylococcus* or the pneumococcus. These children have tracheitis and they can be exceptionally unwell. Because they can have signs and symptoms that mimic epiglottitis they should be treated as such (see below). Direct bronchoscopy will reveal thick inspissated pus over the entire length of the trachea, often blocking the carina, which is the cause of the respiratory obstruction. These children may need to be ventilated and to be on intravenous antibiotics for several days. These children should be treated as for epiglottitis and referred to hospital in the same manner as discussed below.

Table 18.1 Use of steroids in croup

Prednisolone	$2\,\text{mg kg}^{-1}$ orally
Dexamethasone	$0.15\,\text{mg kg}^{-1}$ orally
Budesonide	2 mg via a nebulizer

Table 18.2 Clinical features that can help distinguish viral croup from epiglottitis

	Croup	Epiglottitis
Typical age	< 3 years	2–8 years
Cause	Viral (many different)	Bacterial (*H. influenzae*)
Onset	Slow	Rapid
Prodrome	Usual	Unusual
Toxicity	Apyrexial	Pyrexia
Feeding	Good	Poor
Cough	Barking, harsh	None

EPIGLOTTITIS

Epiglottitis is decreasing in incidence with the introduction of *Haemophilus influenzae* b (Hib) vaccination. However, it still exists and can occur in older children and adolescents who have not had the benefit of immunization. It is characterized by sudden onset of fever, associated with stridor. The child will be extremely toxic, unwell and very quiet. In severe cases the head will be extended and the child will have an altered level of consciousness. This latter in particular indicates that there is an element of hypoxia present. Drooling is not universal. Signs of increased respiratory effort will be present.

If epiglottitis is suspected no effort should be made to examine the child in any great detail. The child should be kept as comfortable as possible, even if this means keeping him or her on his/her mother's knee. In the prehospital phase it is extremely important that this child is accompanied to hospital by practitioners capable of managing all aspects of a paediatric airway. As long as the child maintains his or her own airway there is no need for active intervention.

However, if the child collapses this will almost certainly be due to airway obstruction. The safest and most effective way to deal with this is to perform an emergency needle cricothyroidotomy. The child can then be oxygenated until such time as formal tracheostomy can be secured or the child can be intubated, whichever is easiest in the given situation. While preparing for this procedure the child should be ventilated using a bag–valve–mask device. It may be necessary to depress the 'pop-off' valve (if present) if sufficient pressure is to be generated to ensure that oxygen passes the obstruction. Once the airway is secure intravenous access can be obtained and appropriate antibiotics can be given.

Haemophilus influenzae b is the usual causative organism, and this is increasingly resistant to ampicillin and erythromycin. One of the newer antibiotics such as azithromycin, clarithromycin or a third-generation cephalosporin may be indicated in this situation. It is important that prehospital practitioners know, and keep abreast of, the local antibiotic sensitivities of such important bacteria.

BRONCHIOLITIS

Bronchiolitis is a common respiratory condition typically caused by the respiratory syncytial virus (RSV). Other viruses, however, have been implicated. Typically it occurs during the winter months and is a worldwide phenomenon. At particular risk are those children who are premature, have spent time in a neonatal unit or have underlying cardiac or respiratory disease (e.g. cystic fibrosis or congential heart disease). These children may well have underlying lung problems and reduced respiratory or cardiac reserve, which render the effects of the infection more severe.

A diagnosis of bronchiolitis is made on clinical grounds. It is characterized by:

- increased respiratory rate
- intercostal recession
- wheeze
- widespread crepitations
- hyperinflation of the chest.

This last phenomenon pushes the liver down so that it is invariably palpable about 1 cm below the costal margin. The child may experience difficulty feeding and indeed it is very often this which alerts the mother to the problem. Often there will be an associated dry, hacking cough.

Indications that all is not well with a child with bronchiolitis include failure to feed normally, respiratory rate greater than 50 breaths min^{-1} and apnoeic attacks. In any of these situations the child should be referred for inpatient care.

Care may be given at home in the first instance if these danger symptoms are not present. One method of treatment is to nurse the child upright in a child safety seat. This increases the lung volume and makes it easier for the child to breath. Nebulized ipratropium bromide 125 μg may be helpful in drying secretions. Salbutamol is of little use, although it has been advocated if wheeze predominates (Schuh et al 1990). There is little evidence, however, that it is useful in the long term. Feeds should be offered regularly. While individual feeds may be less than normal, small volumes offered regularly may help keep the child nourished.

Children in whom symptoms are severe, if the mother (or carer) is not coping or where there is concern about apnoeic attacks or underlying disease, should all be referred for inpatient treatment. Children should be given oxygen en route if there is any cause for concern.

If these children do have a respiratory arrest at home there may well be increased difficulty with artificial ventilation due to the narrowed airway increasing airway pressures. It may be necessary to depress the 'pop-off' valve during ventilation with a bag–valve–mask device, although this increase in pressure may cause barotrauma to the lungs with resulting pneumothorax. Associated gastric dilation may also cause respiratory compromise.

Antibiotics are of no proven value in the treatment of bronchiolitis and may be counterproductive. Antibiotic-related vomiting and/or diarrhoea may develop, as may candidal infection.

Acute asthma in children

Asthma is one of the commoner medical emergencies in childhood. Typically there will be a history of atopy (dry skin eczema) or wheeze in infancy. There may also be a family history of wheeze or asthma. A diagnosis of asthma is difficult to make in infants under 18 months of age. There is no doubt that many children in this age group will wheeze but the wheeze is often poorly responsive to standard beta-2-agonist therapy. A firm diagnosis of asthma therefore can really only be made for those children over 2 years of age and the following discussion will relate to these children only.

CLASSIFICATION OF ASTHMA

Asthma may be classified as mild, moderate or severe: in some cases life-threatening features are present, which indicate the need for urgent airway and ventilatory support in addition to standard therapy. The assessment of severity of asthma is primarily by clinical examination. Peak expiratory flow rate and pulse oximetry may be of some use.

Peak expiratory flow rate measurement in children

Peak expiratory flow rate (PEFR) measurement is usually inappropriate for children under the age of 5 years. They are unable to use the machine adequately and may not be sufficiently able to comply with instructions. Over the age of 5 years, however, PEFR should be routinely recorded. This has the benefit of determining the pattern of asthma and response to treatment in the past. Children and carers should be advised to take this information with them wherever they go so that information is available for any potential carer if acute asthma occurs.

Pulse oximetry in children

Pulse oximetry has a place to play in the management of asthma in childhood. It is probably more important for children than adults in the prehospital phase. However, there are certain constraints to its use in children. First only appropriate probes must be used. Smaller children may benefit from using the neonatal-type probes, which are held on with tape. Older children's fingers or toes may be appropriate for the finger clips. Ear clips are not advisable in children. They may be too tight and this will occlude the circulation, thereby making the plethysmographic effect difficult to assess and readings inaccurate. Second, an effort should be made to correlate the heart rate on the pulse oximeter with the heart rate either clinically or on an electrocardiogram (ECG) machine. This will ensure that the plethysmographic function is adequate and that each pulsation is being recorded by the machine. Another check is to ensure that the waveform is of adequate amplitude, be it a linear or sine waveform. If a good waveform is absent, or there is poor correlation between the heart rate on the pulse oximeter and cardiographs, the pulse oximeter reading should be ignored. This indicates that there is poor perfusion to the area being monitored and the pulse oximeter results cannot be relied upon in this situation. All saturation readings should be interpreted in the light of inspired fraction of oxygen (F_iO_2). Ideally, initial readings should be taken while the child is breathing room air.

MILD ASTHMA

Children with mild asthma usually have minimal signs. Typically there will be little in the way of respiratory distress and wheeze will only be audible by auscultation. The child may exhibit a dry cough, particularly at night or after exercise. The child who becomes excessively breathless during exercise should have exercise-induced asthma excluded. The heart rate and respiratory rate will not be unduly raised and the PEFR, if done, will be above 75% of best or predicted value. Oxygen saturations will be above 95% if saturation monitoring is used.

MODERATE ASTHMA

Features of moderate asthma include an audible wheeze, PEFR between 50% and 75% of best or predicted and a mild increase in both respiratory and heart rate. The child may not be able to complete long sentences. Examination of the chest will reveal a mild degree of intercostal recession and there may be a slight degree of accessory muscle use. The child will be fully alert. If available, the oxygen saturation will be above 92%.

SEVERE ASTHMA

A child with severe asthma will be characterized by the presence of an audible wheeze, an inability to talk and a respiratory rate greater than 50 breaths min^{-1} (2–5 years of age) or 30 breaths min^{-1} (>5 years of age) (Box 18.1). There will be marked intercostal recession, sternal recession and accessory muscle use. The child will quite often be agitated, which is a sign of hypoxia. Heart rate will be greater than 130 beats min^{-1} (2–5 years of age) or 120 beats min^{-1} (>5 years of age) and oxygen saturations will often be less than 92% using a saturation monitor, if available. It is often impossible to record PEFR in these children but if recorded, and there is confidence that the recording is accurate, the PEFR will be between 33% and 50% of best or predicted.

LIFE-THREATENING ASTHMA

In addition to the features of severe asthma, life-threatening asthma may be recognized by the development of some

Box 18.1

Severe asthma

- Audible wheeze
- Inability to talk
- Respiratory rate:
  - >50 breaths min^{-1} (2–5 years)
  - >30 breaths min^{-1} (>5 years)
- Intercostal and sternal recession
- Use of accessory muscles
- Agitation
- Heart rate:
  - >130 beats min^{-1} (2–5 years)
  - >120 beats min^{-1} (>5 years)
- Oxygen saturation <92%
- PEFR 33–50% predicted

very sinister signs. The wheeze will become inaudible and there will be genuine inability to talk. The child will often have a significant alteration in level of consciousness. The development of central cyanosis and/or bradycardia are particularly worrying and indicate that the child is heading for cardiopulmonary arrest. The PEFR will be less than 33% of predicted or best, but this is almost certainly a reflection of the inability of the child to cooperate. Consequently it is not useful in this situation. Oxygen saturation readings may be unreliable in these situations because of the development of cardiopulmonary failure and generally poor perfusion, which is associated with this level of illness.

MANAGEMENT OF ASTHMA IN CHILDREN

A stepped plan of action is advocated with treatment being offered according to assessed severity (British Thoracic Society 2008).

Mild asthma

It should be possible to manage children with mild asthma in the community. It is appropriate for parents to be advised to give the child two puffs from a metered dose inhaler of the child's usual beta-2-agonist, with a spacer device if necessary. If the child does not respond to this a further dose of beta-2-agonist can be given after 30 min: steroids should be started at this stage (prednisolone 2 mg kg^{-1} to maximum of 40 mg). If the child does not settle with this, more intensive treatment is required. If this is the first attack in a child who has previously been well, a chest radiograph is advisable. This could be arranged through an open-access X-ray clinic at a time convenient to the clinician, the family and the hospitals involved. This chest radiography will not alter treatment but will help exclude other causes of wheeze.

Table 18.3 Convenient dosage regime for prednisolone when used for asthma in children

Age (years)	Dose (mg)
2–5	20
5–10	30
10+	40

Moderate asthma

Children with moderate asthma will be mildly hypoxic. These children should be given high-flow oxygen therapy pending further treatment. A beta-2-agonist should be given initially 4–10 puffs via a spacer device. Subsequently administration through a nebulizer driven by oxygen may be necessary. Oral steroids should be given to all children with moderate asthma (prednisolone $2\,mg\,kg^{-1}$ to a maximum of 40 mg).

These children need to be assessed 30 min after the beta-2-agonist has been given. If symptoms have improved the child may well be maintained using a beta-2-agonist metered-dose inhaler with a spacer device. If the child has not improved further beta-2-agonist should be given and the child should be transferred for inpatient treatment. Ipratropium bromide may be a helpful adjunct, via a nebulizer.

Transport may be delayed from rural or remote areas, especially if the weather is poor. In this situation the GP, or whoever is providing care, should be prepared to offer this child continuing beta-2-agonist on a regular basis until such times as the steroids have had a chance to work. This may take up to 4–6 h.

Severe asthma

Children with severe asthma should be treated as an emergency and will almost certainly require inpatient care for a prolonged period. In the first instance they should be given high-flow oxygen and this should be followed as soon as possible by nebulized beta-2-agonist driven by 100% oxygen. There is no place for these children to be treated on air. This can be difficult because children in this situation may be agitated, but it should be remembered that the agitation is due to hypoxia in most cases and not to the child being non-compliant. The child should be monitored clinically and, if at all possible, by using either a pulse oximeter, an ECG monitor or both (see above). Steroids (as above) should be given orally if the child can cooperate and is not vomiting (Table 18.3). If this is not possible, intravenous access should be obtained if possible and the child given a dose of intravenous hydrocortisone ($2\,mg\,kg^{-1}$).

Nebulized ipratropium bromide should be added after the beta-2-agonist. The child should be reassessed every 5 min during transfer to hospital. It is desirable that the child is accompanied to hospital by people capable of making appropriate assessments of the clinical condition and also capable of instituting further care in transit to hospital.

Life-threatening features

If life-threatening features such as cyanosis, quiet chest or bradycardia are present the child needs to be treated with extreme urgency. Oxygen therapy should be delivered in as high a concentration as possible. The child should receive a beta-2-agonist via nebulizer and ipratropium bromide should be added. In some situations the child may not be able to breathe deeply enough to gain any benefit from these. In these situations adrenaline (epinephrine) given subcutaneously or salbutamol given intravenously may be required ($15\,mcg\,kg^{-1}$ of $200\,mcg\,ml^{-1}$ solution over 10 min). Aminophylline may also have a role (see above). Almost certainly these children will be unable to swallow and therefore steroids should be given in the form of hydrocortisone $2\,mg\,kg^{-1}$ intravenously.

If the child does not improve with these measures advanced airway care will almost certainly be necessary.

It is extremely difficult to ventilate these children using a bag–valve–mask device. The increased airway pressures make expansion of the lungs almost impossible for ventilation. Pressures can be increased by depressing the 'pop-off' valve if it is present, but this in turn leads to excessive pressures, which can predispose to barotrauma with subsequent development of surgical emphysema, with or without pneumothorax. In addition, the high pressures will force air down the oesophagus and lead to gastric dilation, which will further aggravate the airway compromise.

Intubation will often be needed in these situations and this again is fraught with danger. It should only be contemplated by those with training and experience in managing difficult airways in children. Despite possible drawbacks ketamine is the induction agent of choice and should be used in a rapid sequence induction together with succinyl choline. Ketamine has bronchodilator properties, which may benefit the underlying disease process. A short-acting paralysing agent such as succinyl choline is preferable in case intubation cannot be carried out. Even after intubation, ventilation can be difficult; great care needs to be taken to try and reduce any barotrauma.

Post-emergency treatment of asthma

Children with severe or life-threatening asthma should be transferred to hospital for further care. Children with moderate asthma who respond to an initial diagnosis may be considered for home treatment but should be reviewed early, while those with mild asthma can usually be followed up with general advice via the telephone. In all children who remain at home and who are not followed up in hospital, great care must be taken with the instructions given.

First of all, carers and children should be trained in the use of the devices with which the asthma is being treated. They should be instructed on how to use metered-dose inhalers with or without spacer devices for both beta-2-agonist and steroid. Not every child is able to use this type of therapy and carers (if they are being asked to look after these children) should be given very clear instructions as to when to seek further advice, when to call the GP out and when to take the child to an inpatient facility. If medication has been prescribed the child should have adequate supplies of medication to continue the treatment. This is particularly so for steroids; 3–5 days' supply (depending on local policy) should be provided, and parents should be instructed as to how often and when these should be given. There is no justification for leaving children at home with asthma unless these facilities are available.

Pneumonia

Pneumonia is a common respiratory problem in the paediatric age group. Typical organisms include *Streptococcus pneumonia* and *Haemophilus influenza*. In children under 2 years of age *Staphylococcus aureus* is a rare but important cause of pneumonia. Coliforms and enteric bacteria may infect neonates. *Mycoplasma* infection occurs on a 3–5-year cycle.

Typically, children present with a history of pyrexia, cough and general malaise. Often they will have poor feeding. Physical signs are similar to those in the adult population and include tachycardia, tachypnoea, dullness over the infection and occasionally crepitations in the infected area. These signs can be difficult to detect in small children, particularly if they are crying and uncooperative. If suspected clinically, it is appropriate to treat non-toxic children aged over 2 years with an antibiotic that is effective against the organisms detailed above. As *Mycoplasma* is a rarer organism than the others, treatment with antibiotics such as co-amoxiclav, or erythromycin for those allergic to penicillin, is appropriate.

Failure of the child to settle on this medication would suggest that an atypical pneumonia is present. These children should be referred to hospital for further evaluation.

Children who are toxic, and especially children in the younger age groups, may benefit from intravenous therapy in the first instance, possibly for no more than 12–24 h. If this is deemed necessary it is probably better to transfer these children to hospital for inpatient therapy.

Inhaled (aspirated) foreign body

Inhaled foreign body in the paediatric population is relatively rare. If a child inhales a foreign body the first site it is likely to wedge is at the level of the cricoid cartilage, which is the narrowest point of the paediatric airway. In this situation complete airway obstruction will be present and the child will exhibit signs of acute respiratory distress. Unless dealt with as an emergency the child will rapidly progress into coma, and then cardiac arrest and death. If the child is small enough he/she should be upended and slapped on the back. If this does not work he/she should be placed flat on his/her back and attempts to ventilate him/her should be made. After five breaths have been given, the rescuer should actively compress the sternum five times (as for cardiac arrest) and then check the mouth to ensure that the foreign body has been expelled. If this is not the case the child should be further upended and five back blows given. This cycle of back blows and chest compression alternating with respiratory assistance should be continued until the foreign body has been removed or a needle cricothyrotomy can be performed, following which the child should be rapidly transferred to hospital.

It is very difficult to upend an older child effectively. A Heimlich manoeuvre should be attempted if the child is not comatose. If the child has lost consciousness back blows and chest thrusts as above, interspersed with abdominal thrusts, may be indicated. Again, one should continue until such time as the child is either obviously dead or a foreign body has been removed.

The Heimlich manoeuvre and abdominal thrusts are not advised in infants and small children, when damage can occur to the relatively vulnerable abdominal organs, both solid and hollow.

If the foreign body passes the cricoid it will usually pass to the right main bronchus. The child may be seen to choke briefly followed by a period of coughing and spluttering. If the foreign body is retained and not expelled by coughing the blocked lobe will collapse and infection will supervene. Wheezing may or may not be present. It is important to ask about possible foreign body ingestion in all children with pneumonia, especially if right-sided, if it fails to resolve with standard therapy or is associated with wheeze.

Much more common is the situation where the child aspirates a foreign body that wedges in the upper oesophagus. This may manifest with some of the signs of airway obstruction in that the child may have some stridor and will often be drooling. However, the child will be well. If the child is old enough he/she may complain of something obstructing the upper airway and localize it to the level of the cricoid. This is not amenable to removal by upending or backslapping. The child should be kept upright and transferred to hospital in this situation. Arrangements can then be made for retrieval of this foreign body.

Epilepsy

Epilepsy is quite a common emergency in childhood. While the vast majority of events are either secondary to a febrile illness or idiopathic in nature, a small number will occur associated with other disease or illness. Typically this will include poisoning, head injury, hypoxia or rarely intracranial infection. Most such seizure disorder is grand mal in nature but occasionally focal or unilateral seizures can occur.

It is important to remember that a child can be undergoing seizure disorder that is not manifest by motor activity. Petit mal seizures tend to be characterized by periods of absence when the child appears to stare into space. This usually occurs in children aged 4–6 years and requires no acute treatment. Some children who have had a grand mal seizure may cease having clonic, tonic movements. However, these children may still be fitting, manifest by deviated eyes, flickering eyelids and increase in tone. These children will usually exhibit very poor or minimal respiratory effort. They should be classed as having seizure activity and will usually respond to anticonvulsive therapy. Certainly respiratory effort will improve, with consequent improvement in oxygenation.

On being presented with a child who is fitting it is important to establish a clear airway, to administer oxygen and to assess the circulation. Intravenous access should be established as soon as possible. Intravenous lorazepam $0.1\,mg\,kg^{-1}$ should be given as a bolus. This should be flushed through with a bolus of saline.

If intravenous access cannot be established quickly, rectal diazepam should be administered at $0.5\,mg\,kg^{-1}$ (generally speaking, 5 mg for children <5 years of age, 10 mg >5 years of age). An alternative is to establish intraosseous access and give lorazepam $0.1\,mg\,kg^{-1}$ in a bolus, followed by a bolus of saline. If possible and practical, blood glucose should be tested using a 'stick test'.

If the blood glucose is normal or high (it is rarely low) no further action is needed. If the blood sugar is noted to be low, a bolus of $5\,ml\,kg^{-1}$ 10% dextrose should be administered. If possible, urine should be obtained from small children and saved for analysis for inborn errors of metabolism. This may be the only chance to do this analysis until the next time the child 'goes off' (see the section on 'Metabolic emergencies').

Most children will respond to one dose of either intravenous lorazepam or rectal diazepam (Cock and Schapira 2002). Intravenous lorazepam may be repeated after 10 min if the child is still fitting. *If this is unsuccessful further treatment is usually with paraldehyde or phenytoin, and this should be given in hospital.* If circumstances dictate further treatment at home, paraldehyde 1 ml for each year of age may be administered. Half this dose should be given in each buttock. An alternative is to give paraldehyde 1 ml per year of age rectally diluted 1:1 with arachis oil. In some parts of the world paraldehyde is not freely available and in this situation

one should go straight to phenytoin $18\,mg\,kg^{-1}$, infused, if possible, through an infusion device over 20 min and under electrocardiographic control. It should be recognized that phenytoin is cardiotoxic and this will be aggravated by underlying hypoxia, which is often present in the fitting child. If paraldehyde is chosen as the second-level drug and fails to act then phenytoin will be required. Any child who has failed to stop fitting at this stage will need sedation and paralysis with intensive care treatment. Phenobarbital $15\,mg\,kg^{-1}$ is an alternative second-line drug to paraldehyde.

Metabolic emergencies

Metabolic emergencies are reasonably common in children primarily related to a diagnosis of diabetes. However, in small children (less than 6 months of age) inborn errors of metabolism may present as a comatose or fitting child particularly associated with hypoglycaemia.

HYPOGLYCAEMIA

Most cases of hypoglycaemia are due to an excess of insulin. This will usually be iatrogenic but occasionally (especially in adolescents) will be an overdose or cry for help. As mentioned above, inborn errors of metabolism in small babies may present this way.

Suspected hypoglycaemia should be confirmed by a bedside stick test. If hypoglycaemia is confirmed in a known diabetic, treatment will depend on the level of consciousness of the child. Those children with a reasonably good level of consciousness but acting in a bizarre manner may respond to a small dose of oral glucose. This should not be administered to children who have an inability to protect their airway. Intramuscular glucagon may be an alternative in this situation, at a dose of 0.5–1.0 mg.

If intravenous access can be established easily, 10% dextrose at a rate of $5\,ml\,kg^{-1}$ should be given intravenously. The child may take some time to recover fully. If he or she has not recovered within 30 min blood sugar should be checked again and further therapy given as appropriate.

Hypoglycaemia in a small baby is an indication to consider inborn errors of metabolism. Ideally the child should be taken to hospital as a matter of urgency. If possible a urine sample and blood sample should be saved and the hypoglycaemia treated as appropriate. It is important to try to obtain laboratory tests before treatment if at all possible and in particular if the child is not endangered by delaying treatment.

HYPERGLYCAEMIA

Hyperglycaemia without ketoacidosis is rare in childhood but does occur. More commonly, hyperglycaemia is associated with ketoacidosis. The child may present de novo with a variety of signs and symptoms. Typically there will be a history of thirst, polyuria, polydipsia and general malaise. Occasionally the child will present with abdominal pain and vomiting. In these situations a urine test will show positive for both glucose and ketones. A bedside stick test for sugar will reveal marked hyperglycaemia. Some test sticks may show ketones present as well.

In this situation intravenous access should be established and intravenous treatment started, depending on the severity of the dehydration in the child. If the child is in shock $20\,ml\,kg^{-1}$ of normal saline should be infused over 45–60 min. Insulin should be given at a rate of 0.05 units kg^{-1} intramuscularly. The child should be transferred to hospital as soon as possible where further treatment can be commenced.

In both compensated and decompensated shock blood should be taken if possible for formal blood glucose, urea and electrolytes, and a full blood count. These samples should accompany the child for further analysis at hospital. However, treatment should not be delayed while these samples are obtained. If time permits full physical examination can be performed looking for any underlying cause for ketoacidosis in a known diabetic. Typically, underlying infection, stress or trauma may be the cause.

Caution!

Children with diabetic ketoacidosis should be rehydrated slowly. There is usually no urgency with rehydration. Too rapid rehydration, particularly in the absence of adequate insulin control, may lead to cerebral oedema, which is often intractable.

Management of the comatose child

Coma is rare in childhood but an underlying diagnosis is usually present. Typically one should consider underlying illness such as poisoning with alcohol or other drugs, postictal state, hypoxia or hypoglycaemia. Intracranial problems rarely present as an altered level of consciousness, although children with hydrocephalus may present this way if their shunt becomes blocked. Paramount in the management of these children is the need to secure an airway, to ventilate as needed and to secure intravenous access. Underlying treatable diseases such as hypoglycaemia or hyperglycaemia, seizure disorder or sepsis (see 'Meningococcal septicaemia') should be treated as appropriate. Gastric decontamination with full airway protection may be necessary in poisoned children following admission to hospital.

Table 18.4 Signs of dehydration by severity			
Level of dehydration			
Mild	**Moderate**	**Severe (shock)**	
Level of consciousness	Normal	Irritable	Lethargic (coma)
Eyes	Normal	Sunken	Very sunken
Skin pinch	Normal	Slow return	Very slow return
Mucous membrane	Moist	Dry	Very dry
Drinking	Normal	Thirsty	Drinks poorly

Vomiting and diarrhoea

Gastroenteritis is one of the leading causes of paediatric illness world-wide, and diarrhoeal illness is one of the leading causes of death in small babies.

While vomiting might be a symptom of gastroenteritis, other causes should be sought. These include pyloric stenosis (particularly in males under 3 months), intussusception, intestinal obstruction (associated with volvulus, obstructed hernia), urinary tract infection or meningitis.

If other illnesses can be excluded confidently the child should be treated according to its level of dehydration (see below).

Diarrhoeal disease can be life-threatening, with copious amounts of fluid being lost. Again, treatment will depend on the level of dehydration and shock present (Table 18.4).

TREATMENT

Mild (<5%) dehydration

Most children with less than 5% dehydration can be managed with oral rehydration solution (ORS). This is a balanced salt and glucose solution that replaces lost electrolytes. It can be made at home with 18 g of household sugar, 3 g of table salt and 1 litre of *boiled* water. This solution is given orally in small doses, typically off a teaspoon, until the child has stopped vomiting. Children with diarrhoeal disease should have normal feed on top of this. Breast-fed infants should continue on breast milk, if possible. ORS should be given at a rate of $75\,ml\,kg^{-1}$ over 4–6 h. Maintenance therapy should be continued depending on the volume of the stool and vomit lost. In hot climates these volumes may need to be increased to account for insensible losses. Alternatively, a commercial solution such as Dioralyte® can be used.

Older children may be treated with salty snacks such as salted potato crisps in order to stimulate drinking.

Table 18.5 Approximate amount of oral rehydration solution (ORS) per hour for moderate dehydration

Weight (kg)	<5	5–10	10–15	15–40
Approximate age	<4 months	4–12 months	1–4 years	4–14 years
Amount of ORS (ml h^{-1})	<50–100	100–200	200–300	300–800

Moderate (5–10%) dehydration

Oral rehydration therapy may be tried initially (Table 18.5) but if unsuccessful will need to be augmented by intravenous therapy. Initially the child should be offered repeated doses of ORS from a teaspoon or cup. Vomiting may occur, especially if children gulp the fluid. It is worth persevering for about 1 h, by which time vomiting will have settled and oral rehydration can continue. If unsuccessful, 20 ml kg^{-1} normal saline or Ringer's lactate given over 1 h may speed tolerance of oral fluid. This is in addition to normal daily requirements.

Severe (>10%) dehydration (shock)

Children who have severe dehydration or who are shocked should have intravenous therapy started with an initial bolus of crystalloid 20 ml kg^{-1} given over 30 min (1 h in infants), followed by 70 ml kg^{-1} over the subsequent 3 h (5 h in infants). There is no evidence that colloid is any more effective than crystalloid in these situations. These children should be transferred to a paediatric infectious disease unit for further care.

Meningitis

Meningitis is one of the most feared but actually one of the rarer paediatric emergencies. Three distinct patterns of presentation occur:

- presentation in children under 3 months
- presentation in children aged 3–36 months
- presentation aged over 36 months.

CHILDREN UNDER 3 MONTHS OF AGE

Meningitis in this age group is a difficult diagnosis to make. Signs and symptoms can be as elusive as simply not feeding or being 'off form'. Classic signs of bulging fontanelle and neck stiffness may be absent. There may well be associated illness such as vomiting or diarrhoea. A high index of suspicion is therefore necessary.

Organisms that are commonly present in this age group include *Escherichia coli*, *Streptococcus pneumoniae*, *Haemophilus influenza* and *Neisseria meningitidis*. Viral infection is less common than in the older age group. In developing countries atypical meningitis in the form of tuberculous meningitis has to be considered. Rarely, *Listeria monocytogenes* will be cultured.

CHILDREN AGED 3–36 MONTHS

In this age group symptoms become slightly more reliable. Children at the younger end of this age band may still have open fontanelles, which may be full or bulging. Neck stiffness becomes a much more reliable sign, as does vomiting. Pyrexia is again more likely to be present in this age group than in the 0–3-month-old age group. The same organisms are involved except that *E. coli* is much rarer in this age group.

CHILDREN OVER 36 MONTHS

Meningitis is quite a rare illness in this age group. However, symptoms and signs approach the more classic teaching of stiff neck and headache. Vomiting is also an important feature. Photophobia may also be easier to determine in this age group. The organisms are the same as above. Again, *E. coli* is much rarer than in young infants.

TREATMENT

If meningitis is suspected the level of consciousness should be carefully assessed. If there is any evidence that an altered level of consciousness is present, a lumbar puncture is contraindicated. These children should receive intravenous antibiotics in hospital as directed by local sensitivities and policies. In the 0–3-month-old child treatment should be effective against all the organisms detailed above. If there is to be a delay in getting the child to hospital, penicillin and cefotaxime are suitable drugs. Ceftriaxone alone may be appropriate.

The diagnosis of atypical meningitis is only made if there is no response to other treatment or the results of lumbar puncture indicate otherwise. There is probably no place for this condition to be treated in the prehospital phase. A diagnosis will usually be made somewhere down the line.

Meningococcal septicaemia

The difference between meningococcal meningitis and meningococcal septicaemia must be clearly understood. It is possible to get meningococcal meningitis without any systemic signs. Similarly, it is possible to get meningococcal septicaemia without intracranial involvement. The management of meningitis has been dealt with above.

Typically the child with meningococcal septicaemia will present with a reasonably sudden onset of malaise. It is easy to dismiss the problem at this stage as a flu-like illness. However, there will be no involvement of the mucous membranes in the ears, throat or chest. A urine examination will also reveal no abnormality. Even if a petechial rash is present at this stage it can be very difficult to detect as often the petechiae are of pinpoint size. However, the child will usually be unwell out of all proportion to the signs present. In this situation a strong presumptive diagnosis of meningococcal septicaemia could be made and the child treated appropriately. In the prehospital phase large doses of penicillin are appropriate. For those children allergic to penicillin, chloramphenicol is appropriate. The recommended dose of penicillin is 1200 mg for children aged 10+ years, 600 mg for children aged 1–9 years and 300 mg for children under 1 year of age. Ideally this should be given intravenously but intramuscular administration is acceptable if a vein cannot readily be found. The drug may not be absorbed effectively by the intramuscular route if the child is shocked. For those children allergic to penicillin chloramphenicol 25 mg kg^{-1} to a maximum of 1.2 g is appropriate.

The child should be transferred to hospital for further investigation and treatment to be carried out.

If the child shows any evidence of peripheral shut down s/he should be given high-flow oxygen. Intravenous access should be obtained only if this will not delay transfer to hospital. An intravenous cannula or intraosseous needle can be inserted en route to hospital. If intravenous access is easily and readily obtained 20 ml kg^{-1} normal saline should be infused over 20–30 min.

The pyrexial child

Infectious disease in childhood typically presents with pyrexia. Only in the neonatal period can children be septic without having a pyrexia, although this is still quite rare. It is important to take a history from the parents and/or child if possible. This will include details of contact with other infectious diseases, past history of infectious disease and any underlying symptoms.

A full physical examination should then be performed. The level of the temperature may be of use in determining the urgency of treatment but is usually not all that helpful

otherwise. One should look for evidence of upper respiratory tract infection manifest by checking for inflammation of the mucous membranes. This will include red ears, red eyes, red throat and the possibility of discharge from the nose.

If more than one mucous membrane is involved then a viral aetiology is likely. A single mucous membrane involvement, e.g. pharynx or a single ear, will be more in keeping with a bacterial infection.

Evidence of pneumonia can be difficult to detect, particularly in crying or irritable children.

If these are normal, likely causes will include urinary tract infection, meningitis or orthopaedic infection. Appendicitis is rare but should be considered, particularly in small babies, where signs can be difficult to detect.

In the first instance the temperature should be reduced by paracetamol orally or rectally (15 mg kg^{-1} is a suitable dose to begin with). Viral infections should be treated symptomatically with temperature control and oral fluids.

Aspirin is contraindicated in children because of the risk of Reye's syndrome.

The decision to treat otitis media is a personal one. There is growing evidence that many will settle without antibiotic treatment. However, a child who presents with severe pain, who has a discharge from the ear or in whom symptoms persist for 2–3 days may warrant antibiotics. Amoxicillin or erythromycin are usually effective. The incidence of *H. influenzae* that is resistant to both of these drugs is increasing. It may be that a newer macrolide such as azithromycin or clarithromycin may be preferable in these situations.

If pharyngitis is present, a swab should be taken. Penicillin V may be started orally if symptoms are acute but stopped if the throat swab shows no evidence of bacterial growth. If *Streptococcus* is confirmed then treatment should continue for 10 days.

Children who are toxic with pneumonia or urinary tract infections should probably receive parenteral therapy. It is preferable to observe these children in hospital for 6–12 h or certainly until their toxicity has settled. Once the bacteraemia/septicaemia is under control then outpatient therapy may be contemplated. There is no place for treating meningitis, orthopaedic infections or appendicitis in the community and if diagnosed or suspected these children must be referred for immediate specialist care.

It should be borne in mind that injudicious use of antibiotics in the prehospital phase makes the work of inpatient teams exceedingly difficult. Partial treatment of underlying bacterial disease is made more difficult and outcomes may be hindered by such use of antibiotics. Only if it is impossible to get throat swabs or urine cultures should empiric treatment be started and continued.

Conclusion

True life-threatening paediatric emergencies are rare. Many more children, however, will present for treatment and it is important that the prehospital practitioner is familiar with the differences between paediatric and adult disease presentation.

References

Bone RC 1996 Goals in asthma management: a step care approach. Chest 109: 1056–1065

Cock HR, Schapira AH 2002 A comparison of lorazepam and diazepam as initial therapy in convulsive status epilepticus. Quarterly Journal of Medicine 95: 225–231

Geelhoed GC 1996 Sixteen years of croup in a western Australian teaching hospital. Annals of Emergency Medicine 28: 621–626

Littenborg B 1988 Aminophylline treatment in severe acute asthma. Journal of the American Medical Association 259: 1678–1684

Schuh S, Canny G, Relsman JJ et al 1990 Nebulised albuterol (Salbutamol) in acute bronchiolitis. Journal of Paediatrics 117: 633–637

Further reading

British Thoracic Society Scottish Intercollegiate Guidelines Network 2008 British guideline on the management of asthma. Thorax 63(Suppl 4): 1–121

Paediatric life support

19

Introduction   220

Prevention   221

Paediatric life support   221

Treatment algorithms   225

Complications of resuscitation   227

References   227

Introduction

The resuscitation of infants and children is different from adult resuscitation. Although many of the methodologies are similar there is a fundamental difference in aetiology, which provides a different emphasis. In contrast to adults, children rarely suffer a primary cardiac arrest. The aetiology of paediatric sudden death is usually related to an airway or breathing problem resulting in hypoxia and leading to a severe bradycardic or asystolic collapse. By the time the final collapse has occurred the child's major organs will have suffered a severe prolonged hypoxic insult. Therefore it is not surprising that children who have progressed to a full cardiac arrest are severely physiologically damaged and that the outcome from paediatric cardiac arrest is poor.

Paediatric life support is a difficult and traumatic process, both physically and psychologically. To be successful, paediatric life support requires a level of knowledge and practical skill that can only be achieved by organized training and clinical practice. Paediatric sudden death is a relatively infrequent occurrence and it is therefore difficult, especially in the prehospital setting, to maintain an adequate level of experience. In the prehospital situation the psychological effects can be even more devastating. The progression of the event may not have been noticed or recognized by the carers of the child. The practitioner may have to deal not only with his or her own feelings but also with the supposed 'guilt' of the carers.

The most common cause of death in children under the age of 1 year remains sudden infant death syndrome (SIDS). This is despite the recent campaigns encouraging mothers to put their babies to sleep on their backs and not to wrap their babies in too many blankets resulting in the child overheating. SIDS is particularly distressing as it occurs without warning. Examination at the time of the incident and the detailed post-mortem examination carried out later usually find no specific cause of death. In older children, and in the first four decades of life, the most common cause of death is trauma.

Both SIDS and trauma occur in the prehospital environment and therefore it is extremely important to develop an effective prehospital resuscitation procedure.

In an effort to unify and standardize international guidelines for paediatric resuscitation, the International Liaison Committee on Rescuscitation (ILCOR) published its initial statement in 1997, with updates from its member organizations since then. ILCOR sponsored the 2005 International Consensus on Cardiopulmonary Resuscitation and Emergency Cardiovascular Care Science with Treatment Recommendations (COSTR), which also contains guidelines for paediatric and neonatal resuscitation. The statements not only recommend evidence-based practice but also lists the unresolved issues in an effort to guide research. In the absence of specific data, recommendations were made on the basis of common sense or ease of teaching and skill retention. The European Resuscitation Council has now revised its guidelines to conform with ILCOR and its own requirements (Paediatric Life Support Working Group of the European Resuscitation Council 2005).

Survival from paediatric life support has remained low. Kuisma et al (1995) reported an overall survival rate of 9.6%. This improved to 14.7% when resuscitation had been attempted but fell to 0% when resuscitation followed a witnessed event of cardiac origin. Kuisma's study reported on 79 consecutive paediatric prehospital events collected over 10 years (1985–94). Two-thirds of the events were as a result of SIDS or trauma and, if airway problems and near-drowning were included, together they accounted for nine out of 10 arrests. The most common presenting rhythm was asystole (78.9%); ventricular fibrillation only occurred in 3.8%.

Asystole is the most common arrhythmia in paediatric cardiac arrest.

O'Rourke (1986) reported on 34 children admitted to paediatric intensive care following prehospital cardiac arrest and resuscitation in the casualty department. The aetiological causes were respiratory 8%, SIDS 29% and trauma 50%. O'Rourke's reported survival rate was 21% but all his survivors were neurologically impaired.

Two other recent studies, Losek et al (1987) and Thompson et al (1990), reported on 114 and 70 patients respectively. Their low survival rates of 8% and 4% were further tempered by reports that six out of nine and three out of three survivors, respectively, had neurological impairment. Quan et al (1990) reported on 38 victims of submersion. Although Quan had an initial resuscitation success rate of 69%, survival rates fell to only 12 out of 38, of which four children were found to be neurologically impaired. Quan and her colleagues were able to postulate that the 'downtime' and the length of cardiopulmonary resuscitation were important indicators of outcome in childhood drowning. In an analysis of a further 29 events, Quan & Kinder (1992) reported a return of spontaneous circulation in 13 children, of whom six survived but four were neurologically impaired. The authors were able to predict that submersion for more than 10 min or cardiopulmonary resuscitation for more than 25 min were predictors of death (six of six) or severe neurological deficit (17 of 17) in children.

It is therefore sad to reflect that the outcome results of hospital paediatric resuscitation remain poor, despite advances in methodology and technology. Nonetheless, it can only be by continued striving to improve these results that further advances will be made and the chances of survival from cardiac arrest will be improved.

Prevention

There can be no doubt that it is vitally important to recognize the pre-arrest phase and to treat it appropriately. The child must not, at any cost, be allowed to proceed to the arrest phase. Prevention of the cause, whether medical or traumatic, is in itself also very important. Furthermore the adverse effects of the potential cause of arrest must be minimized by the immediate recognition of the seriousness of the situation and the application of effective first aid. Training is essential and this should be offered not only to health-care providers but to parents and all carers of children so that they fully understand the importance of prevention, can make a rapid and accurate assessment of the situation and can provide appropriate life-saving skills while awaiting the arrival of professional help.

Of all the causes of paediatric arrest, SIDS remains the unresolved dilemma. The recent government guidelines for infant sleeping position and temperature regulation have reduced the number of SIDS cases but there still remains a core group. It is probably the unpredictability of SIDS that makes it so distressing and in this sense it must compare with ventricular fibrillation in adult resuscitation. Unfortunately, the results of resuscitation from SIDS remain extremely poor, unlike the results from adult ventricular fibrillation resuscitation attempts.

Paediatric life support

The advanced techniques of prehospital paediatric life support require a vast array of equipment and technical skills. The size of the victim can vary from the newborn (approximately 3 kg) to a young adolescent 20 times this size. The infrequency of paediatric events can take a heavy toll on both equipment and technical skills. Lack of familiarity with the equipment and the need to perform difficult technical skills in less than ideal surroundings leads to hesitation, restriction of practice and often failure. If the establishment of advanced techniques is not successful then the resuscitator must return to fundamentals before struggling to achieve an 'advanced technique' procedural goal. To delay the circulation of oxygenated blood to the brain and other vital organs could be considered negligent, especially if this were the result of trying to use an advanced procedure rather than a simple, basic but effective technique. Therefore the provision of prehospital paediatric life support still follows the same principles of any resuscitation protocol of establishing an airway, providing efficient ventilation of the lungs and oxygenation of the blood and the re-establishment of a circulation until they can be maintained spontaneously.

The starting point for this description is an unconscious, apnoeic, pulseless child. Although the aetiology of the event may play a part later in the resuscitation sequence it usually has little bearing on the initial resuscitation attempt.

AIRWAY

Tracheal intubation is the gold standard for airway management. The technique of tracheal intubation requires practical skills and technical competence which can only be achieved by supervised training and repeated practice. Therefore despite it being the gold standard it is often not achieved until later in the resuscitation event when the appropriate personnel and equipment are present.

It is of primary importance to establish an airway early in the resuscitation sequence, especially when the loss of the airway has been the underlying cause of the collapse. The simplest method of achieving an airway is by head tilt and chin lift and/or jaw thrust. In infants and small children overextension of the neck can cause airway obstruction as the trachea is soft and may kink. Even the simple management of the airway by these basic manoeuvres is difficult, requiring flexibility of technique and constant monitoring of performance to achieve an effective result.

Airway adjuncts can be effective if properly selected and used. A correctly sized Guedel oropharyngeal airway, when carefully inserted, can overcome the obstruction caused by the tongue. A Guedel airway is sized by comparing the selected airway's length against the distance from the centre of the mouth to the angle of the jaw when the airway is laid along the child's face. If the airway is too small then it will cause obstruction and if too large it can cause trauma to the pharynx on insertion. The airway can be inserted with the aid of a tongue depressor or, in the older child, by inserting it concave side up (upside down) until the tip reaches the soft palate and then gently rotating it through 180° and then sliding it back over the tongue into position.

In children who are semiconscious the oropharyngeal airway may not be tolerated and yet careful airway management will still be required. In this situation a nasopharyngeal airway may be tolerated. A suitable diameter of nasopharyngeal airway is one that just fits into the nostril and a suitable length can be estimated by measuring the distance from the tip of the nose to the tragus of the ear. For small children a shortened tracheal tube can be used. The nasopharyngeal airway should be carefully inserted into the nostril and directed posteriorly over the floor of the nose. Gentle partial rotation of the tube will guide it past the turbinates. The tube should never be forced into position as this will cause damage to the friable nasal mucosa and result in significant haemorrhage. Nasopharyngeal airways are contraindicated in fractures of the base of the skull unless a child has trismus and there is no other alternative.

In 1996 the European Resuscitation Council Working Group on the Management of the Airway and Ventilation During Resuscitation, in its statement on advanced airway management, advocated the laryngeal mask airway (LMA) for use in resuscitation. Grantham et al (1994) described successful use of the LMA in adult prehospital care but it has yet to be evaluated in the out-of-hospital paediatric environment.

Tracheal intubation

Tracheal intubation is the ultimate goal of advanced airway management during resuscitation. Tracheal intubation requires formal training and supervised practice. It should never be regarded as an easy procedure that can be undertaken by those inexperienced in the technique. In such cases, and especially in children, it is better not to attempt intubation but to maintain the airway using the simpler basic techniques already described.

It is recommended that the child's airway is intubated using a straight-blade laryngoscope. This is because the larynx is more cephalad and anterior than in adults and the epiglottis is relatively larger. The straight blade is designed to lift the epiglottis under the tip of the blade. There are a wide variety of design of straight blades; the Seward, Magill, Robertshaw and Oxford are popular designs.

To complicate matters further, the blades are also sized as 0, 1 or 2 and an appropriate length must also be selected (Fig. 19.1). A curved Mackintosh blade can be used for children over the age of 5 years. The technique with a curved blade is to rest the end of the blade in the vallecula. In experienced hands, infants and children can be intubated using an adult curved blade. As in the hospital environment more than one laryngoscope (blade and handle) should be available together with spare batteries and bulbs.

Careful selection of the size (the internal diameter) of the tracheal tube is essential for a successful intubation. If the age of the child is known the formula is:

$$\text{Internal diameter (mm)} = \frac{\text{age}}{4} + 4.$$

Neonates will require a size 3.0 or 3.5 mm tracheal tube. It is recommended that a size above and a size below is also prepared prior to intubation. Straight-sided uncuffed tracheal tubes are used up to size 6 mm (age 8); cuffed tubes can

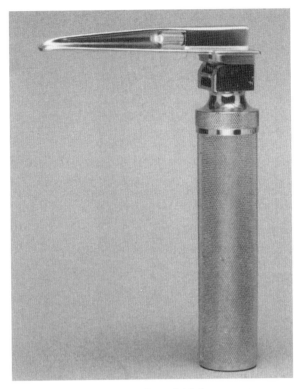

Fig. 19.1 • A straight-bladed paediatric laryngoscope.

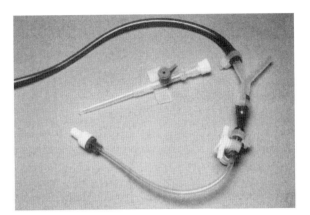

Fig. 19.2 • Equipment for jet insufflation.

be used thereafter. The length of the tube is also important, especially in the small baby where the length of the trachea may only be 2–3 cm. The length of the tracheal tube can be estimated by using one of the following formulae:

length of the tube (cm) = internal diameter (mm) × 3

or

$$\text{length of the tube (cm)} = \frac{\text{age}}{2} + 12.$$

Although tracheal tubes can be cut prior to intubation, most prehospital practitioners carry their paediatric tubes uncut, since in trauma to the larynx or trachea a smaller-sized tube than expected may be required to secure intubation. If all the small-size tubes have been pre-cut then intubation may not be possible, as the appropriate tracheal tube may be too short.

Before any attempt at intubation, the child should be preoxygenated. The technique of tracheal intubation is to hold the laryngoscope in the left hand and to insert the blade carefully into the right side of the child's mouth. The tongue is displaced to the left and the larynx is brought into view by carefully lifting upwards and forwards. Gentle cricoid pressure will help to bring the larynx into view. The selected tracheal tube is inserted between the vocal cords

so that the tip lies 2–4 cm below the cords (until the intubation marker on the tube is at the level of the vocal cords). The laryngoscope can then be removed and the position of the tube checked by auscultating over the apices of both lungs, in both axillae and over the epigastrium. If unequal air entry is detected then the tube should be slowly withdrawn until there is equal air entry into both lungs. The tracheal tube should then be meticulously fixed in position and a note made of the length of the tube at the lips. The correct size of tube is that which allows a slight air leak during ventilation. Should the attempt at intubation take longer than 30 s or fail, the child must then be reoxygenated using a basic airway technique before another attempt is made.

Surgical airway

When all else fails and a patent airway cannot be established then a surgical airway should be considered. The technique, although simple in concept, requires prompt and decisive action. In children under the age of 12 years needle cricothyroidotomy is recommended. A 14 or 16G venous cannula can be directly inserted into the trachea through the cricothyroid membrane. Ventilation is achieved either by using a Y-connector and an oxygen flow of 5–10 l min^{-1} (Fig. 19.2).

By occluding the limb of the Y-connector the gas flow is directed into the lungs and the chest rises. The occlusion is released to allow passive expiration. Alternatively, a self-inflating resuscitation bag can be used to provide slow inspirations. The major problem with the needle cricothyroidotomy technique is that, although it will provide adequate oxygenation, it will not allow adequate removal of expired carbon dioxide, especially when the upper airway is totally occluded. In children over the age of 12 years a formal surgical cricothyroidotomy can be performed using a small vertical incision in the skin followed by a horizontal incision through the cricothyroid membrane. The incision can then be spread and a suitable-sized endotracheal or tracheostomy tube inserted. Performing a surgical airway requires technical

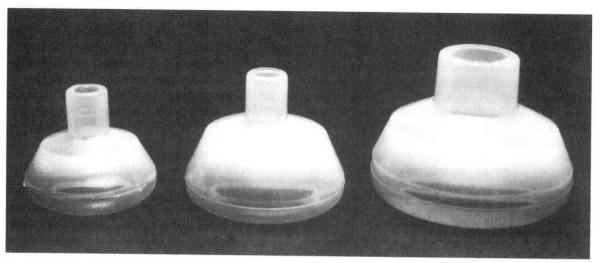

Fig. 19.3 • Infant face masks.

BREATHING

If the child is breathing spontaneously oxygen should be supplied via a facemask with an oxygen reservoir at an oxygen flow rate of 10–15 l min^{-1} (Fig. 19.3). Nasal prongs may be better tolerated in the younger active child.

Where spontaneous respiration is absent or inadequate, assisted ventilation must be provided. Progression of the event may well be prevented by early oxygenation and efficient ventilation. Mouth-to-mouth ventilation in children (mouth-to-mouth and nose in infants) is the simplest way of providing ventilation where no additional equipment is available. An adult pocket mask rotated 180°, so that the nose of the mask is placed over the chin of the child, can also act as a simple breathing adjunct.

Ventilation is best achieved using a self-inflating bag valve mask with an oxygen reservoir attached. There are three sizes of self-inflating resuscitation bag (adult – 1600 ml, child – 500 ml, infant – 240 ml). The paediatric and infant resuscitation bags are fitted with a pressure limiting valve set at 30–40 cmH$_2$O. This is to protect the child's lungs from high airway pressure and thus prevent trauma to the lower airways. In the prehospital scenario where the child may have high airway resistance (asthma) or low lung compliance (drowning), high inspiratory pressures may be required to achieve ventilation. In these cases the valve can be over-ridden by pressing on the top of the pressure relief valve or the metal clip can be slid over the valve to prevent it functioning. Supplemental oxygen must be added to the bag as this will raise the inspired oxygen concentration to approximately 50% without the oxygen reservoir or to as high as 90% with it. The final oxygen concentration will depend on the tidal volume, the frequency of ventilation and the rate oxygen is supplied.

In the initial stages of resuscitation, prior to intubation of the trachea, the resuscitation bag should be fitted with an appropriately sized face mask. In the infant or small child these may be the Rendell–Baker–Suchet design, a mask shaped specifically for an infant's face. Circular design face masks with a soft rim have been found to be more effectively used especially by the inexperienced rescuer (Fig. 19.3).

Following intubation the 22 mm outlet for the resuscitation bag will fit directly onto the 15 mm connector of the tracheal tube.

Portable automatic ventilators are not recommended for use in the prehospital paediatric resuscitation situation. They require expert knowledge, constant observation and continuous monitoring. Portable automated ventilators should only be used by those who have been specifically trained in their use.

CIRCULATION

There are few procedures more fraught with difficulty than establishing venous access in an infant or small child during resuscitation. Brunette & Fischer (1988) and Kanter and colleagues (1986) both demonstrated the importance of establishing circulatory access in successful resuscitation. Direct venous access or intraosseous access are the preferred options. In selecting a route for direct venous access a number of points must be considered. Dalsey et al (1984) demonstrated that vascular access via the superior vena cava by either peripheral or central access routes is preferable during resuscitation. Emerman and colleagues (1988) confirmed this finding and also showed that drugs given via the inferior vena cava take longer to reach the heart. Finally, Barsan et al (1981), Hedges et al (1981) and Kuhn et al (1981) all demonstrated that drugs administered centrally do act more rapidly than those administered via the peripheral route. Viewing the selection from a purely practical viewpoint, central access above the diaphragm is difficult and probably beyond the expertise of most pre-hospital practitioners. Internal jugular vein cannulation in infants and children requires expertise which is rarely gained outside hospital paediatric practice. Subclavian vein puncture usually requires stopping chest compressions while the procedure is carried out and carries a risk of pneumothorax. The external jugular vein can only be cannulated if visible and even then it can be difficult to feed the cannula. Central access below the diaphragm, via the femoral veins, may be attempted but is often difficult. Peripheral access, especially via the brachial vein in the arm or long saphenous vein of the lower limb, is usually simpler, especially during resuscitation. A venous cutdown at these sites will often ensure access. In the infant the brachial vein can be found one fingerbreadth lateral to the medial epicondyle of the humerus; the saphenous vein is half a finger breadth superior and anterior to the medial malleolus. If peripheral venous access is established Emerman and colleagues (1990) recommend that drug administration be followed by a flush of fluid to move the drug more rapidly into the central circulation.

Prehospital practitioners are in an extremely difficult situation when trying to establish direct venous access. The conditions are often not ideal, the lighting is poor and the child is usually peripherally vasoconstricted. Circulatory access can be undertaken on any visible vein but the attempt should be made using a cannula size that will ensure access rather than a size that may be considered ambitious and fail. It cannot be emphasized sufficiently that it is the venous access that is important, providing the ability to administer drugs and fluids, rather than the size of access line.

Intraosseous access (Fig. 19.4) should be regarded as standard practice for sick children who are difficult to cannulate. It is a relatively simple technique and regarded as generally safe. Orlowski et al (1990a), Rossetti et al (1985) and Valdes (1977) have all confirmed that resuscitation drugs and fluids administered by this route reach the heart in a time comparable to direct venous access. Glaeser et al (1993), reporting on a 5-year experience of intraosseous access, found the method suitable for all age groups, including adults. Access by the intraosseous route is classically described as placing the intraosseous cannula through the anterior surface of the tibia, 2–3 cm below the tibial tuberosity or alternatively on the anterolateral surface of the femur 3 cm above the lateral condyle. The criteria for successful entry into the marrow are: a loss of resistance

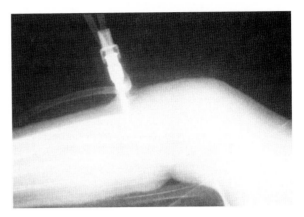

Fig. 19.4 • Intraosseous access.

as the marrow cavity is entered, the needle should remain upright without support, bone marrow can be aspirated with a syringe, and there is a free flow of drugs and fluids without subcutaneous infiltration around the entry point (Berg 1984, Fiser 1990, Spivey 1987). Ummenhofer and colleagues (1992) described how marrow aspirates can be used for estimation of haemoglobin, sodium, potassium, chloride and glucose as well as crossmatching. Almost all drugs and fluids can be administered via the intraosseous route. Complications of intraosseous cannulation have been described as skin necrosis by Christensen et al (1991) and Rimar et al (1988), compartment syndrome by Galpin et al (1991), tibial fractures by LaFleche et al (1989) and subcutaneous extravasation by Simmons et al (1994).

The tracheal route of drug administration should only be used where there has been or is likely to be a significant delay in establishing either direct venous or intraosseous access. It could therefore be argued that in small infants, where access could be difficult, the first dose of adrenaline (epinephrine) should be given via the tracheal tube. There has been little research into the efficacy of drugs administered via the tracheal route. The optimal dose of drug, its volume and concentration as used in children have yet to be formally established. At present a dose of adrenaline ten times that given intravenously is recommended. Orlowski et al (1990b) found tracheal administration of adrenaline to be unreliable. Hornchen et al (1992) reported a depot storage effect of adrenaline in lungs leading to hypertension and tachycardia, neither of which are optimal in the post-arrest myocardium. Bleyaert et al (1980) suggested that severe postresuscitation hypertension could be responsible for a poor cerebral outcome.

Treatment algorithms

In 1997, the International Liaison Committee on Resuscitation published its recommendations for paediatric life

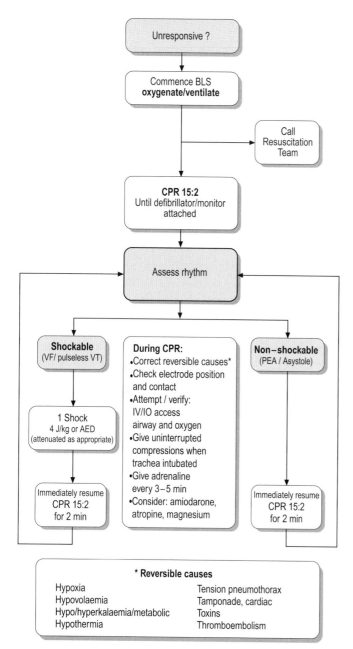

Fig. 19.5 • Paediatric advanced life support algorithm. (Courtesy of the European Resuscitation Council.)

count the pulse. Connick & Berg (1994) have questioned the use of the pulse check during resuscitation, especially in an unresponsive apnoeic child. In advanced life support it is considered reasonable that a health-care provider should spend no more than 10 s determining pulselessness.

The algorithm then divides into two pathways, according to the underlying cardiac rhythm:

- non-ventricular fibrillation or tachycardia (asystole, pulseless electrical activity)
- ventricular fibrillation or pulseless ventricular tachycardia (VF/pulseless VT).

NON-VENTRICULAR FIBRILLATION OR TACHYCARDIA (ASYSTOLE, PULSELESS ELECTRICAL ACTIVITY)

The most common rhythm associated with circulatory collapse in infants and children is asystole or a profound bradycardia. A profound bradycardia, defined as a heart rate of less than 60 beats min^{-1}, does not in itself produce a cardiac output sufficient to sustain life and in many cases precedes an asystolic arrest. Therefore a profound bradycardia must be treated in the same way as asystole. The mainstay of treatment of asystole or pulseless electrical activity is adrenaline (epinephrine). Otto et al (1981) has reported the importance of the administration of adrenaline during resuscitation as, by its alpha-adrenergic activity, it raises the aortic diastolic filling pressure and thereby improves coronary perfusion. The initial dose of adrenaline is 10 μg kg^{-1} given by the intravenous or intraosseous route (10 μg kg^{-1} equals 0.01 mg kg^{-1} or 0.1 ml kg^{-1} of a 1:10000 solution). Ten times this dose (100 μg kg^{-1}) is recommended for administration via the tracheal tube.

The initial intravenous dose of adrenaline (epinephrine) is 10 μg kg^{-1}.

support. This was adopted as the core algorithm for the European Resuscitation Council (2001) (Fig. 19.5).

The algorithm starts by emphasizing the need for basic life support with proper ventilation and oxygenation. The rhythm is then assessed by attaching a cardiac monitor (or defibrillator) and, at the same time, the pulse can be checked. Mather & O'Kelly (1996) and Brearley and colleagues (1992) have documented the inability of lay rescuers and health-care providers to reliably locate or

Administration of adrenaline (epinephrine) is followed by 3 min of ventilation and chest compressions (one ventilation to five compressions at a rate of 100 compressions per minute). A second dose of adrenaline should then be administered. There is little evidence that a higher dose (100 μg kg^{-1}, or 0.1 ml kg^{-1} of 1:1000 solution) has any beneficial effect, but it is recommended in cases where cardiac arrest is thought to be secondary to circulatory collapse. After this, the cycle of 3 min of basic life support followed by another dose of adrenaline should be repeated. Studies by Dieckmann & Vardis (1995), Schindler et al (1996) and Zaritsky et al (1987) have shown that, if a child does not respond to this higher dose of adrenaline, the eventual outcome is likely to be poor. In reviewing the results of these studies, no child survived to discharge who received more than two doses of adrenaline. It is therefore reasonable to surmise that the algorithm, as presented, is self-limiting, but currently there is not enough evidence to suggest a limitation to the time course of resuscitation from asystole.

During resuscitation it is necessary to attempt tracheal intubation and to verify the position of the tracheal tube. Vascular access must be achieved either directly or by the intraosseous route. The monitor electrode position and contacts must be checked to ensure proper electrical connection.

Where there is an electrical cardiac rhythm but no detectable pulse a diagnosis of pulseless electrical activity can be made. In such cases it is necessary to treat any underlying reversible cause. The correctable causes are:

Four 'H's	Four 'T's
• Hypoxia	• Tension pneumothorax
• Hypovolaemia	• Tamponade
• Hyper- or hypokalaemia	• Toxic or therapeutic disturbances
• Hypothermia	• Thromboembolism

In some cases where there is prolonged cardiac arrest or proven metabolic acidosis, sodium bicarbonate can be administered. Sodium bicarbonate should only be given to patients who are ventilated or who have adequate spontaneous respiration. There is probably very little indication to give sodium bicarbonate to the prehospital cardiac arrest except where there has been a prolonged delay in basic resuscitation and the child remains unresponsive to adrenaline (epinephrine). If the arrest has resulted from circulatory collapse, a standard bolus of $20 \, \mathrm{ml \, kg^{-1}}$ of crystalloid should also be given following the first dose of adrenaline.

VENTRICULAR FIBRILLATION OR PULSELESS VENTRICULAR TACHYCARDIA

Although Friesen et al (1982) reported a 23% incidence of ventricular fibrillation in their study, most other investigations, including Eisenberg et al (1983), Fiser & Wrape (1987), Nichols et al (1986) and Torphy et al (1984), report a much lower incidence of less than 10%. Losek et al (1989) and Mogayzel et al (1995) confirmed this low incidence

even when the victim was evaluated within 6 min of alerting the emergency medical services. Nonetheless, the physician must always be aware of the recommended treatment of ventricular fibrillation in children. The second path of the algorithm shows defibrillation as the basis of treatment for ventricular fibrillation. The recommended sequence is to give two rapid defibrillatory shocks of $2 \, \mathrm{J \, kg^{-1}}$, followed by a single shock at $4 \, \mathrm{J \, kg^{-1}}$. All further defibrillation attempts should then be made at $4 \, \mathrm{J \, kg^{-1}}$ in a rapid repeated series of three shocks. Following the first cycle of three defibrillation attempts adrenaline (epinephrine) $10 \, \mathrm{\mu g \, kg^{-1}}$ should be given and basic life support initiated for 1 min. In accordance with previous explanations, further doses of $10 \, \mathrm{\mu g \, kg^{-1}}$ should be given following subsequent cycles of three shocks. When ventricular fibrillation occurs in children there is often an underlying cause and the correction of hypothermia, drug overdose (tricyclic antidepressant overdosage) and electrolyte imbalance (hyperkalaemia) should be considered.

Automated external defibrillators (AED) have not yet been developed for children. The reliable detection of ventricular fibrillation by the machine and the energy levels required to defibrillate a child with an AED have yet to be determined.

Complications of resuscitation

Bush and colleagues (1996) have reported a 3% incidence of medically significant complications. This study examined the documented complications in prolonged paediatric resuscitation carried out by rescuers with a wide variation of skill levels. Other studies (Nagel et al 1981, Powner et al 1984, Spevak et al 1994) confirm this relatively low incidence of complications and support the view that resuscitation should always be attempted in infants and children. Rib fractures, pneumothorax and haemorrhage are rarely seen when appropriately applied resuscitation techniques are used.

References

Barsan WG, Levy RC, Weir H 1981 Lidocaine levels during CPR: differences after peripheral venous, central venous, and intracardiac injections. Annals of Emergency Medicine 10: 73–78

Berg RA 1984 Emergency infusion of catecholamines into bone marrow. American Journal of Diseases in Children 138: 810–811

Biarent D, Bingham R, Richmond S et al 2005 European resuscitation council guidelines for resuscitation. Section 6. Paediatric life support. Resuscitation 67(Suppl): S1, S97–S133

Bleyaert AL, Sands PA, Safar P et al 1980 Augmentation of post-ischemic brain damage by severe intermittent hypertension. Critical Care Medicine 8: 41–45

Brearley S, Simms MH, Shearman CP 1992 Peripheral pulse palpation: an unreliable sign. Annals of the Royal College of Surgeons of England 74: 169–172

Brunette DD, Fischer R 1988 Intravascular access in pediatric cardiac arrest. American Journal of Emergency Medicine 6: 577–579

Bush CM, Jones JS, Cohle S, Johnson H 1996 Paediatric injuries from cardiopulmonary resuscitation. Annals of Emergency Medicine 28: 40–44

Christensen DW, Vernon DD, Banner WJ, Dean JM 1991 Skin necrosis complicating intraosseous infusion. Pediatric Emergency Care 7: 289–290

Connick M, Berg RA 1994 Femoral venous pulsations during open heart cardiac massage. Annals of Emergency Medicine 24: 1176–1179

Dalsey WC, Barsan WG, Joyce SM 1984 Comparison of superior vena caval access using a radioisotope technique during normal perfusion and cardiopulmonary resuscitation. American Journal of Emergency Medicine 13: 881–884

Dieckmann RA, Vardis R 1995 High-dose epinephrine in paediatric out-of-hospital cardiopulmonary arrest. Paediatrics 95: 9019–13

Eisenberg M, Bergner L, Hallstrom A 1983 Epidemiology of cardiac arrest and resuscitation in children. Annals of Emergency Medicine 12: 672–674

Emerman CL, Pinchak AC, Hancock D, Hagen JF 1988 Effect of injection site on circulation times during cardiac arrest. Critical Care Medicine 16: 1138–1141

Emerman CL, Pinchak AC, Hancock D, Hagen JF 1990 The effect of bolus injection on circulation times during cardiac arrest. American Journal of Emergency Medicine 8: 190–193

Fiser DH 1990 Intraosseous infusion. New England Journal of Medicine 322: 1579–1581

Fiser DH, Wrape V 1987 Outcome of cardiopulmonary resuscitation in children. Pediatric Emergency Care 3: 235–237

Friesen RM, Duncan P, Tweed WA, Bristow G 1982 Appraisal of paediatric cardiopulmonary resuscitation. Canadian Medical Association Journal 126: 1055–1058

Galpin RD, Kronick JB, Willis RB, Frewen TC 1991 Bilateral lower extremity compartment syndromes secondary to intraosseous fluid resuscitation. Journal of Pediatric Orthopedics 11: 773–776

Glaeser PW, Hellmich TR, Szewczuga D et al 1993 Five-year experience in pre-hospital intraosseous infusions in children and adults. Annals of Emergency Medicine 22: 1119–1124

Grantham H, Phillips G, Gilligan JE 1994 The laryngeal mask in pre-hospital emergency care. Emergency Medicine 6: 193–197

Hedges JR, Barsan WB, Doan LA 1981 Central versus peripheral intravenous routes in cardiopulmonary resuscitation. American Journal of Emergency Medicine 10: 417–419

Hornchen U, Schuttler J, Stoekle H 1992 Influence of the pulmonary citation on adrenaline pharmacokinetics during cardio-pulmonary resuscitation. European Journal of Anaesthesiology 9: 85–91

International Liaison Committee on Resuscitation 2005 International Consensus on cardiopulmonary resuscitation and emergency cardiovascular care science and treatment recommendations. Resuscitation 67: 157–341

Kanter RK, Zimmerman JJ, Strauss RH 1986 Pediatric emergency intravenous access: evaluation of a protocol. American Journal of Disease in Children 140: 132–134

Kuhn GJ, White BC, Swetman RE 1981 Peripheral versus central circulation time during CPR: a pilot study. Annals of Emergency Medicine 10: 417–419

Kuisma M, Suominen P, Korpela R 1995 Paediatric out-of-hospital cardiac arrests – epidemiology and outcome. Resuscitation 30: 141–150

LaFleche FR, Slepin MJ, Vargas J, Milzman DP 1989 Iatrogenic bilateral tibial fractures after intraosseous infusion attempts in a 3-month-old infant. Annals of Emergency Medicine 18: 1099–1101

Losek JD, Hennes H, Glaeser PW et al 1987 Pre-hospital care of the pulseless, nonbreathing pediatric patient. American Journal of Emergency Medicine 5: 370–374

Losek JD, Hennes H, Glaeser PW et al 1989 Pre-hospital countershock treatment of paediatric asystole. American Journal of Emergency Medicine 7: 571–575

Mather C, O'Kelly S 1996 The palpation of pulses. Anaesthesia 51: 189–191

Mogayzel C, Quan L, Graves JR et al 1995 Out-of-hospital ventricular fibrillation in children and adolescents: causes and outcomes. Annals of Emergency Medicine 25: 484–491

Nagel E, Fine E, Krischer J, Davis J 1981 Complications of CPR. Critical Care Medicine 9: 424

Nichols DG, Kettrick RG, Swedlow DB et al 1986 Factors influencing outcome of cardiopulmonary resuscitation in children. Pediatric Emergency Care 2: 1–5

Orlowski JP, Porembka DT, Gallagher JM et al 1990a: Comparison study of intraosseous, central intravenous and peripheral intravenous infusions of emergency drugs. American Journal of Diseases in Children 144: 112–117

Orlowski JP, Gallagher JM, Porembka DT 1990b: Endotracheal epinephrine is unreliable. Resuscitation 19: 103–113

O'Rourke PP 1986 Outcome of children who are apneic and pulseless in the emergency room. Critical Care Medicine 14: 466–468

Otto CW, Yakaitis RW, Blitt CD 1981 Mechanism of action of epinephrine in resuscitation from cardiac arrest. Critical Care Medicine 9: 321–324

Powner D, Holcombe P, Mello L 1984 Cardiopulmonary resuscitation-related injuries. Critical Care Medicine 12: 54–55

Quan L, Wentz KR, Gore EJ 1990 Outcome and predictors of outcome in pediatric submersion victims receiving pre-hospital care in King County, Washington. Pediatrics 86: 586–593

Quan L, Kinder DR 1992 Pediatric submersions: prehospital predictors of outcome. Pediatrics 90: 909–913

Rimar S, Westry J, Rodriguez R 1988 Compartment syndrome in an infant following emergency intraosseous infusion. Clinics in Pediatrics 27: 259–260

Rossetti VA, Thompson BM, Miller J et al 1985 An alternative route of pediatric vascular access. Annals of Emergency Medicine 14: 885–888

Schindler MB, Bohn D, Cox P et al 1996 Outcome of out-of-hospital cardiac or respiratory arrest in children. New England Journal of Medicine 335: 1473–1479

Simmons CM, Johnson NE, Perkin RM, Van Stralen D 1994 Intraosseous extravasation complication reports. Annals of Emergency Medicine 23: 363–366

Spevak M, Kleinman P, Belanger P, Primack C 1994 Cardiopulmonary resuscitation and rib fractures in infants: a postmortem radiologic-pathologic study. Journal of the American Medical Association 272: 617–618

Spivey WH 1987 Intraosseous infusions. Journal of Pediatrics 111: 639–643

Thompson JE, Bonner B, Lower GM 1990 Paediatric cardiopulmonary arrests in rural populations. Paediatrics 86: 302–306

Torphy DE, Minter MG, Thompson BM 1984 Cardiorespiratory arrest and resuscitation of children. American Journal of Diseases in Children 138: 1099–1102

Ummenhofer W, Frei F, Urwyler A, Drewe J 1992 Emergency laboratory studies in pediatric patients (abstract). Resuscitation 24: 185

Valdes MM 1977 Intraosseous fluid administration in emergencies. Lancet 1: 1235–1236

Zaritsky A, Nadkarni V, Getson P, Kuehl K 1987 CPR in children. Annals of Emergency Medicine 16: 1107–1111

The injured child

20

Introduction   230

Immediate action on arrival   230

Primary survey and resuscitation   232

Triage   237

Secondary survey and definitive care   238

Analgesia   239

Transportation   239

Non-accidental injury   240

Reference   240

Further reading   241

Introduction

Injury remains the commonest cause of death among children. 700 children die every year in the UK because of accidents, half of these road traffic accidents and one third accidents in the home. Many of these deaths are preventable, often by simple prehospital measures. Most of these deaths result from head injury.

Fortunately, individual practitioners will rarely see major paediatric trauma; unfortunately this means that they are unlikely to be familiar with it and at ease in managing it. This may lead to errors in assessment and action,

with adverse outcomes. For this reason everyone who may have to treat children must be certain that they have an excellent theoretical knowledge. They must also practise regularly in moulage-type scenarios to ensure that performance remains optimal. Regular attendance at hospitals to maintain practical and assessment skills is even more vital in paediatric trauma than in adult trauma.

Children have patterns of injuries that are different from those of adults. The response to injury is also different. They compensate well for the physiological effects of trauma but may then rapidly and dramatically decompensate. In addition, many people fear paediatric trauma because of the variations in children's size resulting in the need for different equipment, doses and techniques.

Immediate action on arrival

As with all cases of trauma the first action must be an assessment of the safety of the scene, self and casualty.

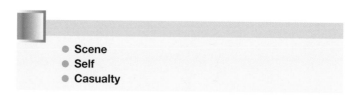

- Scene
- Self
- Casualty

A full assessment of the scene will allow a request for appropriate resources for medical care and for the other emergency services. Every year cases of missed child casualties occur because children are small and are easily thrown from the scene.

It is important, therefore, to ensure that the presence of a child is not overlooked.

- Assess for evidence of a child – a child seat, a teddy bear or toy.
- Look for unexplained details – the broken window on the unoccupied side of a vehicle, the saddled horse with no rider.
- Search the area – this can be done either on foot or from the air. At night the use of thermal imaging cameras can assist.

If the child cannot be found, a search should continue while enquiries are made to see if the child is at home or in another place of safety. The survey of the scene for casualties is also an opportunity to determine the mechanism of injury.

MECHANISM OF INJURY

The child presents a smaller target for trauma. This means that a blow from the same object is likely to cause damage to more body areas in the child than in the adult. The smaller amount of body fat in the child and the increased elasticity of structural components result in less energy absorption by non-vital structures. Hence, internal organ damage is more common and more severe. This is made worse by the close proximity of all the vital organs. Hence, major multiorgan damage is more common in the child. In addition, the skeleton is not fully calcified and therefore the bones may bend rather than break, preventing the absorption of energy in the production of a fracture. For these reasons, external signs of damage and bruising may be small but the internal damage great. External examination in the field may therefore be deceptively normal.

Road traffic accidents remain the commonest cause of death. Inadequate restraint in the vehicle is still a major cause of preventable childhood death. The chance of ejection from a vehicle increases with failure to use seat belts and results in a sixfold increase in mortality. Car design has been greatly improved in order to reduce injuries but is primarily aimed at adult passengers. Airbags will help adult and child passengers, except for infants in rear-facing safety seats. However, some concern is now being expressed following a series of severe or fatal injuries in children resulting from the inflation of airbags. The front of the car is low and curved. This design is not only for aerodynamics but also so that any pedestrian struck by the vehicle is scooped up by a blow below the knee and carried along rather than being knocked to the ground and run over. If the victim is a child, the bumper may hit above the knee. This may have one of two results: the child will either be thrown to the ground and run over or alternatively thrown into the air, suffering a second impact on striking the ground or roadside furniture.

ANATOMICAL AND PHYSIOLOGICAL

The unique anatomical characteristics of the child and significant variations in physiology cause anxiety to carers. These differences, although important, are relatively few. Fear of the differences may cause greater concern and operator error than the difference themselves. The size of equipment and doses of drugs are highly variable in actual amount and in dose per kilogram. A profusion of formulae for different equipment and drugs exist. Correction factors between infant, child and adolescent add to the complexity. The prehospital carer cannot be expected to recall all of these.

It is important that the carer has a rapid source of this information in a comprehensible form. A list of formulae is of no use in an emergency as miscalculations will be common. The Broselow tape is ideal for allowing rapid identification of child's size, the size of equipment and the dose of emergency drugs (Herzenburg et al 1989).

The differences are dealt with in more detail in individual sections of this chapter.

FUTURE GROWTH AND DEVELOPMENT

Any injury may result in impairment of future growth of the child. Injury to a growth centre may require surgical correction to prevent ongoing deformity of an injured limb. The sequelae of brain injury are more severe. Delay in resuscitation may increase the disability produced by injury. Behavioural changes, educational delay and disability can all result from inadequate early treatment, as well as from the initial injury.

Even apparently minor injury can result in dramatic growth abnormality. Compression of a growth plate may have the same clinical appearance as a sprain but can cause cessation of growth at the growth centre.

PSYCHOLOGICAL

An accident upsets anyone. It is essential to be as reassuring as possible. It is important, however, never to lie to a child or trust will be lost. Conversation is the best distraction and the best reliever of anxiety. Silence is the breeding ground of imagination and fear. Studies have shown that up to 60% of children suffering major injury have residual personality changes. Careful handling and reassurance will help the injured by decreasing anxiety and perception of pain. In children this is even more important than in adults. It will be more difficult for them to understand that what you are doing is helping them. They know that in the short term you may be going to inflict pain but do not appreciate why. Careful explanation and a calm nature will often resolve this. The effects of being upset are not only emotional. A crying child decreases his/her ventilation, raising intrathoracic pressure, decreasing cardiac return and raising intracranial pressure.

The presence of a parent is likely to be reassuring and they should be encouraged to stay. Parents as well as children require reassurance and an explanation of what is going on. Carers' anxiety will inevitably be transmitted to the child and make them more upset. The accident has an effect not only on the child victim but also on others within the family unit. Parents and siblings may suffer personality problems and family dynamics may be altered.

Primary survey and resuscitation

The priorities of primary survey and resuscitation are the same as for the adult – ABCDE. The standard principles and procedures are therefore the same whatever the age group.

AIRWAY

Airway is the priority on arrival at the child casualty. In the small baby the cranium is proportionally much larger than the face. The head therefore tends to tilt forwards, resulting in buckling of the immature pharynx and airway obstruction. All trauma cases should have the airway secured, paying appropriate attention to the cervical spine. The neutral spinal position in the child is also the optimal airway position. Hence, the conflict in the adult does not occur. Care must be taken to maintain this position, as the large cranium tends to extend the neck to a position of airway obstruction. The techniques of chin lift and jaw thrust are identical to those in the adult.

The oral airway remains an important airway adjunct, although children are more liable to vomit in the semicomatose state. The nasopharyngeal airway is generally not used until adolescence because of increased vascularity of the nasal passages in younger children.

Endotracheal intubation remains the gold standard of definitive airway control. The larynx of a child is located more anteriorly and caudal than in the adult (Table 20.1). The cords can be brought posteriorly by use of cricoid pressure during intubation. The view is made more difficult

---

Table 20.1 Airway differences in infants and children

- Large cranium
- Compressible soft tissues
- Large tongue
- Anterior larynx
- Floppy epiglottis
- Narrowest part of the airway at the cricoid

---

by the large tongue and the longer, floppier epiglottis. The narrowest point of the airway is at the level of the cricoid, where the structure is circular (rather than the larynx of the adult). Therefore, in infants and toddlers an uncuffed tube can be used, provided that an adequate leak is heard during inspiration as the flow around the tube protects against contamination of the airway from above. For sizing of endotracheal tubes in children see Chapter 19.

Visualize the cords and see the tip of the tube pass through up to the black line on the tube. It is easy in the excitement of successful intubation to intubate the right main bronchus. Once the endotracheal tube is in position, before securing it, listen to both sides of the chest and the epigastrium. Presume that a difference between the sides is due to bronchial intubation and adjust the tube. Remember the possibility of pneumothorax or haemothorax.

Once intubated, the tube must be secured. Small amounts of movement may cause dislodgement. Note the length of the tube at the incisors and tape the tube in position. At this stage apply a semirigid collar. Slight movement of the neck is the commonest cause of tube dislodgement. The position of the tube should be regularly checked.

Nasal intubation is not recommended in children.

If oral intubation is not possible or has failed then it is best to continue with bag–valve–mask ventilation with 100% oxygenation. It is unusual not to be able to achieve adequate ventilation by this method. It does not, however, protect the airway. Because of the paediatric anatomy, insufflation of the stomach during bag–valve–mask ventilation is more common than in adults. This in turn leads to an increased risk of vomiting. Stomach insufflation can be reduced by a second operator applying cricoid pressure. If bag–valve–mask ventilation is not achieving adequate ventilation then needle cricothyrotomy should be undertaken, and the child should be rapidly evacuated to a centre where definitive airway control can be undertaken on arrival.

Surgical cricothyrotomy is contraindicated in infants and children.

If a child's airway cannot be definitively controlled at the scene then immediate evacuation is essential. Other procedures can be continued en route. Delay in establishing adequate airway control is a major cause of death among injured children.

SPINE CONTROL

The mechanism of injury is the main determinant of need for spinal immobilization. Any history or injuries suggesting violent motion of the head indicate the need for immobilization. The presence of neurological signs is an important indicator but may be difficult to elucidate in the distressed child. Unconsciousness precludes assessment and therefore necessitates precautions being taken to protect the neck. The relatively large size of the head gives it greater momentum and more force is therefore exerted on the spine on deceleration.

As with adults, the neck is only adequately protected by one of two methods:

- manual immobilization of head and shoulders
- semirigid collar in association with side supports and strapping.

Both methods must be undertaken in the neutral position. If an infant is laid down on a spinal board in a 'natural position' this does not result in neutral spinal positioning. The large size of the head means that the neck is flexed (Herzenburg et al 1989). It is therefore necessary to place padding under the shoulders to achieve a neutral position. The collar must be the correct size. Most commercially available collars only have one or two sizes for children. There is, therefore, a significant risk that collars will not fit accurately. Too large a collar, causing cervical traction, or too small a collar, allowing movement, are equally dangerous.

Standard spinal boards are designed for adults. Although paediatric boards are produced, they are not yet widely used in the UK. An adult board will allow lateral movement of the child unless padding is put alongside the child between his/her body and the securing straps. Similarly, most extrication devices are designed for adults. The strap positions are not appropriate for children and therefore they should be avoided in paediatric injuries. In infants, a box splint can be used as a spinal board (Herzenburg et al 1989; Fig. 20.1).

Vacuum mattresses have the great advantage that their shape can be individually moulded to the child's requirements. The child's head can be held in the appropriate position while the mattress is adjusted. Similarly, the width and length can be adjusted. The main disadvantage of the vacuum mattress is that it cannot be used as an extrication device. For the small child or infant, who would be swamped in a vacuum mattress, a limb vacuum splint can be used.

Optimum management is probably to use a scoop to lift the child off the ground while manually supporting the neck, following which they can be transferred to a vacuum mattress. Smaller children may be best removed from a vehicle by gentle manual lifting while spinal immobilization is maintained. If a child is trapped, a spinal board can be

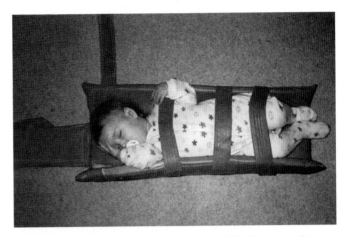

Fig. 20.1 • Using a box splint for spinal immobilization in a child (in a case of suspected spinal injury the 'head' strap would also be applied with appropriate padding to prevent neck movement). (From Herzenburg et al 1989. Reproduced with permission of Rockwater Inc.)

used for extrication and the child can then be transferred on to a vacuum mattress by log rolling prior to transport. If an infant is already in a car safety seat, it may be most appropriate to transport him/her in this seat. The head can be secured by a blanket roll and tape and the child can be tipped to a convenient angle for management of other injuries.

Children will inevitably become frightened if attempts are made to hold them forcibly in one position and to apply an uncomfortable collar. This is made worse if they then cannot see what is happening around them. Further painful procedures such as intravenous cannulation or splintage are also likely to make a difficult situation worse and to cause the child to sit up and look around. The prehospital carer therefore has to use all his/her calming and persuasive powers in this situation.

Children must always be able to see someone who is talking to them and reassuring them. Therefore immobilization is best undertaken from the front. Manual immobilization is generally most effective in the conscious child (particularly in view of the collar sizing problem). Spinal immobilization may require the constant effort of two people. It is therefore not uncommon to need to request additional personnel for paediatric trauma cases. In the unconscious child a collar, side supports and tape can be used. Remember that children in pain or distress often express this by vomiting. Whenever the spine is immobilized it is essential to have a plan of operation in case of vomiting that will prevent aspiration.

When undertaking interhospital transfers, remember that many spinal cord injuries occur in association with normal X-rays; therefore X-rays alone cannot determine that it is safe to remove the semirigid collar and immobilizers (Herzenburg et al 1989).

Table 20.2 Signs of respiratory distress

- Increased respiratory rate
- Use of accessory muscles
- Intercostal and subcostal recession
- Nostril flaring and recession
- Grunting
- Head bobbing

Table 20.3 Causes of immediately life-threatening ventilatory failure in children

- Tension pneumothorax
- Massive haemothorax
- Open pneumothorax
- Flail chest

BREATHING

Children have flexible ribcages with pliable ribs; this means that rib fracture is rare. If rib fractures are present, it suggests major energy dissipation and therefore predicts significant underlying injury. Contusion and injury to internal structures without fracture is more common. Injury to the major airways and rupture of the diaphragm are more common than vascular injuries. Whenever a major organ is found to be injured, a careful search should be undertaken to exclude injury to adjacent organs, as multiorgan damage is common. Once again, a knowledge of mechanism of injury is of vital importance in raising suspicion of an intrathoracic injury.

All trauma patients should receive a high concentration of oxygen. However, the application of an oxygen mask is often frightening for children. Careful explanation is therefore required: saying it is like those that spacemen wear, and similar techniques, may be useful. If the mask upsets the child then it should be removed. A crying child decreases his/her ventilation and oxygenation. It may therefore be better to blow oxygen over the child's face.

In a child with respiratory distress the compensatory mechanisms are different from those of adults (Table 20.2). The respiratory rate increases and the accessory muscles are used. The pressure changes become markedly increased. This causes obvious movement of the nostrils and indrawing of the intercostal and subcostal muscles, and rapidly exhausts the child. This rapidly progresses to respiratory failure and cessation of breathing. Cyanosis is a late sign. Mental state reflects the degree of hypoxia. Restless or combative children who have been injured may simply be upset but it should be presumed that they hypoxic until proven otherwise.

Children with respiratory distress are not only suffering from an oxygenation problem. They are invariably suffering a ventilatory problem, so they are not only hypoxic but also hypercarbic. They need assisted ventilation as well as a high inspired oxygen concentration. Assisted ventilation with a bag–valve–mask is the first action to be taken to improve the child's condition. A high respiratory rate is an indication for assisted ventilation because the depth of respiration will be inadequate (Table 20.3). A search should then be made for the cause of the ventilatory difficulty.

It is important to remember that internal injury with lack of external marking is more common in children than in adults.

Tension pneumothorax is relatively common in children.

In the intubated child it is relatively easy to apply excessive ventilatory pressure and cause a tension pneumothorax. This is most likely when there is lung injury present. Therefore, it is important to ensure that ventilation pressures are not high, that release valves are set to paediatric levels and that constant vigilance is maintained. If there is a sudden increase in ventilatory pressures or deterioration in oxygenation in a ventilated child, the possibility of tension pneumothorax should always be considered.

If tension pneumothorax is suspected then immediate needle thoracocentesis is indicated, using the same technique as for adults. Because of the difficulties with insertion of a chest drain at the scene in a child, this should not usually be undertaken. Rapid transfer to hospital is usually more appropriate unless there is likely to be a significant delay in transfer or aeromedical evacuation is to be employed.

Massive haemothorax is often associated with severe lung injury, including laceration. If a chest tube is inserted exsanguination can rapidly occur. Intravenous access should therefore be established before a chest tube is inserted. Again, the latter may be best done at a specialist centre rather than in the field unless the child is in extremis.

Open pneumothorax is usually associated with impalement injuries. A three-sided dressing or specialized dressing with a one-way valve should be applied. Observation is needed for development of a tension pneumothorax because of the high incidence of underlying lung injury. Flail chest is relatively rare in young children because of the pliability of the ribs, and is treated along the same lines as in an adult. The underlying lung injury is likely to be the fatal injury. Cardiac tamponade needs urgent cardiothoracic surgery and therefore, as in adults, rapid transfer to an appropriate hospital is the best treatment. Cardiac contusion is more common and it is therefore important to remember to monitor the electrocardiogram (ECG) of children with blunt chest trauma.

Most severe chest injuries cannot be adequately treated at the scene. The prehospital carer therefore needs to undertake rapid first-aid measures, ensure adequate oxygenation and ventilation, and transfer the patient as rapidly as possible to a centre that can carry out definitive care. Once a life-threatening ventilatory problem is detected there is no excuse for further treatment of the non-trapped victim at the scene. Circulatory and other problems should be addressed en route to hospital.

CIRCULATION

Children compensate very well for blood loss. The classical signs of hypovolaemia therefore occur late.

The conscious level and general appearance are important in assessment of hypovolaemia. Similarly, the mechanism of injury is important in predicting potential internal haemorrhage. Clinical signs are more difficult to interpret in the child. Fluid loss externally is usually apparent and should be stopped by pressure. The loss from scalp wounds can occasionally be sufficient to cause hypovolaemia.

If external blood loss is not apparent then it is most likely that shock is due to intra-abdominal bleeding, although thoracic or pelvic injuries might be responsible. The presence of intra-abdominal bleeding is extremely difficult to detect clinically in the early stages following trauma. In hospital, ultrasound or computed tomography (CT) scanning are used. The diagnosis will therefore rarely be made with any certainty in the prehospital situation. The mechanism of injury and the presence of hypovolaemia are sufficient for the suspicion to be raised and acted upon. The only way to stop intra-abdominal bleeding is by surgery or angioembolization. Hypovolaemic children therefore need to be delivered to the hospital as rapidly as possible.

Should blood loss be corrected at the scene? The simple answer is no. Establishing intravenous access in a child is difficult in the best of environments, let alone in the usual prehospital care surroundings. Considerable delays in delivery to the hospital may therefore result. If a person is bleeding, some capillary bleeding will stop as the blood pressure falls; elevating the blood pressure may cause this to restart. Because blood is not usually available in the field only one component of perfusion, the perfusion pressure, can be improved and not the oxygen-carrying capability.

The ideal is to transfer the patient rapidly and commence an intravenous infusion en route to hospital. The aim of the infusion is to raise the blood pressure to approximately two-thirds of the normal level – a level at which brain and kidneys will receive adequate perfusion.

Studies in adults show that intravenous access en route is as successful as at the roadside. Success rates in children are lower. The only children needing infusion before hospital are those with significant hypovolaemia. In these cases

intraosseous infusion may be appropriate. This has a high success rate in the ambulance – the marrow of the tibia is a large target. It is therefore recommended that, if infusion is required in the under-6-years age group, intraosseous infusion in the ambulance is the appropriate technique. In trauma it is important to consider the contraindication to intraosseous infusion caused by the injuries present: intraosseous infusion is contraindicated into a fractured bone and into a limb containing a fractured bone. Cutdown to the long saphenous vein at the ankle may also be appropriate in the trapped patient or when transit time will be extremely prolonged. It cannot, however, be performed in a moving ambulance. Alternative cutdown sites are the median cephalic vein at the elbow or main cephalic vein in the upper arm. The external jugular can be used as a peripheral venous access, although this can be difficult while immobilizing the spine.

Initial fluid bolus = 20 ml kg^{-1} of crystalloid solution.

When established, an initial bolus of 20 ml kg^{-1} of crystalloid solution should be given. This should then be administered a second time if there is no satisfactory response. The aim of infusion is to maintain a palpable radial pulse as an indicator of a blood pressure adequate to maintain essential organ perfusion. If this second bolus fails to correct the situation, the child must have critical bleeding. This child needs blood transfusion and probably surgery as a matter of urgency.

One of the most difficult situations in prehospital paediatric trauma care is evolving hypovolaemia. This is usually suspected because of the mechanism of injury. The early signs are easily confused with the reaction to pain or fright. Subtle changes in conscious level are usually the most important early indicators. This is the reason why any child involved in a high-risk accident should be carefully observed and continually reassessed while not delaying transfer to hospital.

Fluid replacement also has dangers. It is simplistic to say that healthy children simply pass more urine if too much fluid is given. It was previously mentioned that pulmonary contusion is common. Excessive fluid replacement will cause pulmonary oedema and decreasing oxygenation. Similarly, it will encourage cerebral oedema, which is a major cause of death.

External haemorrhage in a child can be rapidly life-threatening. Effective compression must be applied. Bleeding from a scalp wound is rarely stopped by a dressing and will need continued manual pressure. Care must be taken when applying dressings. If too large a dressing is applied to a small child it will not apply localized pressure. Hence, the bleeding will continue under or into the dressing. A significant proportion of the child's blood volume may therefore be hidden within the dressing. Applying further dressings over the top will not staunch the flow but may lead to a false sense of security.

DISABILITY AND HEAD INJURY

Head injury remains the commonest cause of death in children.

The AVPU scale can be used initially to assess the conscious level but needs to be done in association with pupillary reaction, mental status and motor response. More accurate assessment can be achieved by the Glasgow coma scale. This does, however, need to be amended for use in children and a suggested adaptation of the speech component is given in Table 20.4.

The use of the Glasgow coma scale is, however, limited in children, as the possibility of changes being due to inter-observer error are greater than in adults. Therefore, the prehospital neurological score of choice remains the AVPU scale. It is important to remember that changes in the Glasgow coma scale may well be due to changes in ABC rather than to changes in neurological status. The two are, of course, interrelated.

The prehospital carer can do nothing about the primary brain injury. Secondary brain injury starts occurring from the time of the accident. No one knows how much this secondary brain injury contributes to morbidity and mortality, as it is impossible to say how much the pathological changes on the initial CT scan were due to primary injury and how much to secondary injury. It has, however, been proved that aggressive early prehospital intervention improves survival and neurological outcome.

We know that the obtunded head-injured child benefits from early intubation and ventilation. Unfortunately, many of the potential survivors of head injury need paralysis before intubation can be attempted. It is therefore vital that the child receives the attention of someone trained in anaesthetic techniques as early as possible, and in the majority of situations this should be on arrival in hospital. The child with a Glasgow coma scale of 10 or less should therefore be rapidly transported to an appropriate centre if the skills are not available on-scene.

It is important to remember that oxygenation can still be achieved without intubation. Using a bag–valve–mask and high concentration of oxygen will buy time pending definitive care. Assisted ventilation may need to be undertaken in the spontaneously breathing patient with decreased conscious level.

The use of mannitol is controversial even in hospital practice. Although it causes a diuresis with lowering of intracranial pressure it can have adverse effects. Lowering intracranial pressure is aimed at improving brain perfusion by increasing perfusion pressure.

Perfusion pressure = mean blood pressure – mean intracranial pressure.

As previously mentioned, hypovolaemia can be difficult to spot. If mannitol is given to a child who is hypovolaemic this will cause a worsening of brain perfusion. Mannitol also causes a delayed rebound increase in intracranial pressure. Its use is therefore best left for two situations:

- the rapidly deteriorating child who is developing a Cushing's response (bradycardia and hypertension) and who has been adequately fluid-resuscitated
- the interhospital transfer, to buy time pending scanning or surgery.

The dose of mannitol is $0.5\,\mathrm{mg\,kg^{-1}}$ by intravenous infusion. The commencement of mannitol in the prehospital environment cannot be recommended except in the most exceptional circumstances, and only then after discussion with the receiving neurosurgeon.

The role of steroids is controversial in head injuries and is currently not recommended.

EXPOSURE AND ENVIRONMENTAL CONTROL

The proportion of surface area to body weight in the child is higher than in the adult. In addition, children have thinner skin and relatively less fatty tissue for insulation. As a consequence, the problem of heat loss is greatly increased. The loss of heat becomes a particularly important problem in the small child. It can combine with the other stresses of major trauma to produce refractory shock, abnormal clotting and depression of neural function, which may combine

Table 20.4 The speech component of the Glasgow coma scale in children

	Paediatric Glasgow coma scale
Smiles, watches, attentive	5
Cries, upset, but consolable	4
Persistently irritable, not consolable	3
Restless, agitated	2
None	1

to produce fatal injuries. In thermal injury the loss of fluid is relatively higher as a percentage of body fluid volume.

Heat loss must be minimized. Although it is important to assess the child, the quest for minor injuries is inappropriate in a cold environment. Whatever the situation, examination must always be followed by covering the child with an insulating layer. Between one-third and one-half of the body heat of a vasoconstricted child is lost through the head. This is because scalp veins do not vasoconstrict. A hat is therefore an important piece of equipment in any child resuscitation. The most effective action is to move the child to a warm environment. The ambulance should be kept warm, and entry and egress minimized in order to reduce heat loss.

Children often have very small reserves of glycogen. They will therefore have difficulty in producing heat. It is insufficient to insulate them from the cold, particularly if they are already cold. Space blankets are popular but a body only warms inside a space blanket if there is a heat source. Warmth must therefore be provided to the injured child. Warm intravenous fluids may help to some degree, and, in addition, warm bags of intravenous fluid can be used as hot water bottles and wrapped inside the blankets around the child.

Triage

Triage in the field is complicated in children. The normal sieve system relies on the person who is walking being triaged out as a low category (see Ch. 48). It is accepted that this initial sieve has pitfalls (e.g. the burns patient or the patient with progressive hypovolaemia). These problems are compounded in the child. The child may not be able to walk yet. When assessing breathing and circulation, the sieve uses adult parameters to determine categorization.

If this is changed to a system of variation from the normal level it becomes more accurate but more difficult to recall and use in an emergency. Many accept that children will be overtriaged.

At the sort phase, the usual policy is to use the Triage Revised Trauma Score. As already mentioned, the Glasgow coma scale has to be modified for children. Because of the variation in physiological parameters with age the Triage Revised Trauma Score is not reliable with children. For this reason the Paediatric Trauma Score has been developed (Table 20.5).

Thus, a maximum score of 10 can be achieved by scoring 2 on each of the five parameters listed in the Paediatric Trauma Score (Table 20.5).

A score of 8 or less indicates critical trauma.

This provides a reliable and reproducible scoring system of triage. It can be used prospectively for triage decision-making. It is different from the Triage Revised Trauma Score in that it does not use physiological parameters alone. By using anatomical scoring as well it predicts change. The age component reflects the increased mortality in younger age groups. The use of palpable pulses rather than blood pressure avoids delay, and acknowledges that a variety of cuff sizes may not be available. The Paediatric Trauma Score can also be used retrospectively as a predictor of outcome. In the multicasualty situation, there may be both adult and child casualties. Clinical judgement must then be used to compare adults assessed by the Triage Revised Trauma Score and children assessed by the Paediatric Trauma Score.

Table 20.5 Paediatric Trauma Score			
	+2	**+1**	**−1**
Size	>20 kg	11–20 kg	<10 kg
Airway	Normal	Assisted, mask	Intubated, cricothyrotomy, obstruction
Conscious level	Awake	Decreased	Unresponsive
Systolic blood pressure	>90 mmHg	51–90 mmHg	<50 mmHg or only central pulses palpable
Fracture	None known	Single closed	Open or multiple
Skin	Normal	Contusion, abrasion, cut <7 cm not through fascia	Tissue loss, gun/knife wound

Certain mechanisms of injury must always be presumed to be associated with hidden major injury:

- ejection from a vehicle
- death of other vehicle occupant
- deformity of seat occupied by the child
- fall of greater than three times the child's height
- damage to protective helmet.

Secondary survey and definitive care

If any life-threatening injury has been identified or the Paediatric Trauma Score is 8 or less, then the patient should be moved to the ambulance and transport should be started before the secondary survey is commenced. Often it will not be possible to undertake the secondary survey before arrival at hospital. The work of initial resuscitation will be more than enough to occupy the carers in the ambulance on the way to hospital. It is more important to deliver the child with the primary survey undertaken and high-quality resuscitation in progress than to have a detailed secondary survey. The secondary survey rarely, if ever, alters the prehospital management of the critically injured child. Splinting and dressing of wounds is only undertaken if it is required as part of 'C' to control haemorrhage.

If the child is stable a different approach can be taken. But delays must still be minimized, as this 'well' child could be a child who is about to decompensate. The findings of the rapid secondary survey of a conscious, stable child may be important in determining treatment en route or destination. Informing the hospital ahead of important findings will also enable the hospital team to optimize their response. Often the secondary survey is undertaken in the ambulance because there is no time delay if the vehicle is already en route and it is warmer.

The secondary survey should take no more than 5 min.

HEAD INJURY

The management of severe head injury has already been discussed. Minor head injuries do, however, form a larger proportion of emergency care. A careful history and baseline set of observations are vital in assessment. Vomiting is common after head injury and usually occurs because of fright or pain. However, persistent vomiting requires investigation. Fits also occur commonly soon after a minor head injury. Providing they are self-resolving in a short time they are usually not of sinister aetiology. The child will need supportive treatment and assessment in hospital. If, however, the fits continue for more than a few minutes then lorazepam should be given intravenously or diazepam rectally. It is important that the dose is carefully titrated and is given slowly. Too large a dose will cause respiratory depression with hypercarbia, the effects of this being to raise intracranial pressure in the head-injured child. Table 20.6 lists the indications for a child who has hit his/her head and is being taken to hospital for assessment and observation.

Any child not taken to hospital must be adequately supervised by a responsible adult. This person must be told to contact medical help immediately if there is any deterioration in the child's state or if any of the above symptoms develop. Paracetamol can be given for the headache.

ABDOMINAL INJURY

In prehospital care the important feature of abdominal trauma is the difficulty in its detection. External markings are often not apparent. Fear and anxiety mean that abdominal examination is more difficult. Distension of the abdomen is frequent and is invariably due to swallowed air. This gastric distension can, on occasions, be sufficient to cause respiratory compromise. In prolonged transfers a nasogastric tube should be used to decompress the stomach. In infants (obligate nasal breathers) and those with facial or head injuries

Table 20.6 Indications for hospital assessment

History

- High-energy mechanism of injury
- Localized trauma, e.g. golf ball injury
- Loss of consciousness
- Lethargy
- Drowsiness
- Amnesia
- Vomiting
- Fitting

Examination

- Associated scalp wound
- Significant scalp haematoma
- Any abnormal neurological signs

Other

- Parental anxiety
- Suspicion of non-accidental injury

an orogastric tube is preferred. Most often abdominal injury is suspected because of the mechanism of injury rather than the clinical findings. Only repeated examination or scanning in hospital can verify or exclude it.

PELVIC AND FEMORAL INJURIES

The blood loss from these injuries can be life-threatening in children as well as in adults. Early effective splintage is vital to decrease blood loss.

The fractured pelvis can account for massive blood loss if unstable. The pelvic component of an extrication device can be used to support the pelvis, as can a strap wrapped around the bony pelvis. It is important that this is firmly applied to decrease bleeding. Manual compression is unlikely to be effective because of the inability to maintain constant force.

The blood loss from a fractured femur can be decreased by traction splintage. By returning the thigh to its normal cylindrical shape from the fractured, shortened, more spherical shape, the volume of the thigh is decreased. Hence, haemorrhage is tamponaded. Tamponade can also be achieved by clothing. A pair of tight jeans or trousers is as effective as a PASG. The temptation to cut the trousers must be resisted; it makes no difference to the prehospital management. If the wound is compound the clothing can have a small window cut in it and a dressing can be applied. If traction splints are not available then the leg should be splinted against its neighbour and manual traction applied.

EXTREMITY INJURY

Clinical diagnosis of fractures in children can be difficult. The pliable bones of the child make certain specific types of injuries more likely. Incomplete greenstick fractures are common, so-called because of the similarity with breaking a green branch, which only breaks on one side. These fractures can only angulate within the constraints of the intact surface. The torus fracture has angulation with impaction, although it is still incomplete. Because there is still a bridge of bone these fractures are usually stable. They are characterized by well-localized bony pain but may have an extraordinarily good range of active and passive movement.

Any child with tenderness above the elbow must be presumed to have a supracondylar fracture. This is associated with injury to the brachial artery. It is important to check pulses and capillary refill. Splinting is best undertaken in the position of comfort. If the elbow is flexed in order to put the arm in a sling the circulation must be checked again once the sling is in place. Flexing of the elbow can cause entrapment of the brachial artery in the fracture fragments.

Analgesia

Children require analgesia just as adults do. In the critically injured, non-trapped patient the delay required to achieve adequate analgesia may be unjustified.

Entonox can be used provided that there is no head or chest injury and the child is capable of self-administration. In practice, this means that it is only used on isolated limb fractures in older children.

Local anaesthesia is rarely practicable in the prehospital setting in children. However, femoral nerve blocks are often useful for fractures of the mid-shaft of the femur. They allow the extrication of the child and the application of a traction splint. They also allow a much more comfortable journey to hospital.

Intravenous opiates are the gold standard of analgesia in trauma care. The intramuscular route is unreliable in the trauma victim, who may be vasoconstricted. The narcotic should be diluted with water and then the dose carefully titrated against effect. Clinical monitoring and pulse oximetry should be continued during and after analgesic administration. Ketamine can also be used for either analgesia or anaesthesia. The incidence of emergence hallucinations is much lower in children. Ketamine can be used as an intramuscular preparation. It may be useful for the extremely restless child in severe pain when an intravenous line cannot be sited. Because there is a risk that the restlessness is due to hypoxia or decreased cerebral perfusion, this technique should only be used by those expert in its use.

Transportation

Care of paediatric trauma needs expertise and experience. The long-term care of these children is often best undertaken in specialist centres.

Extreme airway and breathing problems should be taken to the nearest emergency department for initial treatment.

Children should be taken initially to the unit that can give the best early resuscitation by the most experienced and skilled staff. It may then be appropriate to transfer them for definitive care, if necessary, when immediately life-threatening conditions have been treated.

Informing the hospital of full details of the child's condition will allow an appropriate response to be arranged.

Non-accidental injury

Those involved in prehospital care have a vital role in the detection of non-accidental injury. They are usually the first to be given details by the parents. Careful attention needs to be paid to the history. As soon as any suspicion is raised the exact details *as told* should be written down. A key element in detection of non-accidental injury is the inconsistency in the story given to different health-care providers. When taking the history consider whether it provides a reasonable explanation for the physical findings. Could a child that age have done that? Look around the location for supporting evidence or reasons why the related events could not have happened. The parents' attitude will change when they arrive at hospital. How do they behave in their own home? Does the home suggest a caring environment or one where child safety is neglected? Many accidents are due not to child abuse but to failure to realize risk ('poor parenting'). Prehospital carers have a duty to report means of improving safety in the home. By relaying this to the hospital they can arrange for a health visitor to call who may be able to arrange the loan of safety equipment.

This information about the home environment can only come from the people attending the scene. It is vital that it is noted, passed on to the hospital and written on the patient information sheet.

Examination should also look for the features shown in Table 20.7. Any sign of other injury should be noted. It may be better not to enquire too deeply about these but simply to alert hospital staff to their presence. Care must always be taken not to jump to false conclusions. The child may be suffering from a medical condition that leads to the appearance of violent injury after minimal everyday trauma, e.g. osteogenesis imperfecta or clotting disorders, including leukaemia.

Although some families are at higher risk of committing child abuse, it is important to remember that child abuse affects all socioeconomic groups, all races and all types of family. It may just be that some are more capable than others of avoiding discovery. The role of the health carer is to listen and offer help. It is important not to assume that your suspicions are proved: that is for the courts to decide. All those in health care must be aware of local policy regarding non-accidental injury. The appropriate authority must be informed without delay. This will usually be the local social services. Occasionally, the prehospital carer may refer to an accident and emergency consultant or senior paediatrician.

Table 20.7 Features of non-accidental injury

History

- Delay in presentation without adequate explanation
- Change in story with time or between individuals
- Mechanism of injury not compatible with child's age
- Known history of abuse
- Abnormal parental behaviour, lack of concern
- Frequent injuries or medical attendances

Examination

- Findings not consistent with history
- Injuries of varying ages
- Long bone fracture in child not yet walking
- Signs of neglect
- Injuries
  - Bites
  - Blunt abdominal trauma
  - Oral frenulum tear
  - Pattern burns
  - Pattern/fingermark bruises
  - Perineal injuries
  - Petechial haemorrhage in upper body
  - Retinal haemorrhage
- Skull fracture
- Multiple injuries of varying age
- Unexplained injuries

If you suspect non-accidental injury and the offer to take the child to hospital is refused, immediate action is required. The emergency social worker should be contacted immediately. If danger to the child is imminent then the police should also be summoned.

Whatever the case, careful documentation is of vital importance in the initial assessment, and also in any subsequent action.

Many cases of non-accidental injury will only become apparent after investigation in hospital. The prehospital team may then be contacted by the hospital, police or social services. The importance of careful notes in all cases of paediatric trauma then becomes apparent.

Reference

Herzenburg JE, Hensinger RN, Dendrick DK et al 1989 Emergency transport and positioning of young children who have an injury to the cervical spine. Journal of Bone and Joint Surgery 71A: 15–22

Further reading

Advanced Life Support Group 2005 Advanced Paediatric Life Support: a practical approach, 4th edn. BMJ Publishing, London

Harris BH, Schwaitzberg SD, Seman TM et al 1989 The hidden mortality of paediatric trauma. Journal of Paediatric Surgery 24: 103–106

National Association of Emergency Medical Technicians 1994 Prehospital advanced trauma life support. CV Mosby, St Louis, MO

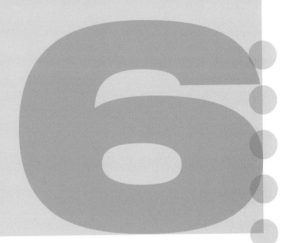

Part Six

21 Scene approach, assessment and safety 245

22 Assessment and management of the trauma patient – the primary and secondary survey 251

23 Head and neck injuries 260

24 Maxillofacial injuries 272

25 Chest injuries 277

26 Spinal injuries 290

27 Abdominal and genitourinary trauma 298

28 The prehospital care of bone and joint injuries 305

29 Prehospital care of soft tissue injuries 315

30 Gunshot wounds and blast injury 322

31 Thermal injury 332

Scene approach, assessment and safety

21

Introduction 245

Approaching the scene 245

Leaving for the scene 246

Driving to the scene 246

Driving techniques 246

Arrival at the scene 249

Conclusion 250

Further reading 250

Introduction

The approach to the scene of a medical emergency starts well before leaving the house, surgery or hospital. Correct preparation, training and equipment are essential for the doctor to ensure his/her own safety and not compromise the safety of others, to be able to interact appropriately with other emergency services and to provide appropriate care for the patient in the prehospital environment.

Prior planning and preparation prevents poor performance.

Approaching the scene

There are several areas that need to be considered even prior to leaving for the scene of the incident.

TRAINING

The level of personal training must be adequate for the types of incident likely to be encountered. While many doctors are competent at dealing with medical emergencies and trauma in a well-equipped hospital, fewer are familiar with providing emergency care in the home or in the street. Fewer still have experience of dealing with chemical injuries or with coordinating medical resources in a mass casualty scenario. On-going training is essential, the aim being to identify areas of personal weakness and to address these areas in a structured way over a period of time. Teaching others is an excellent way of continually refreshing one's own knowledge, of learning new skills and of gaining from others' experiences. Many courses are now available (Table 21.1).

Table 21.1 Emergency care courses

- Pre-hospital Emergency Care (PHEC)
- Pre-hospital Trauma Life Support (PHTLS)
- Basic Trauma Life Support (BTLS)
- Advanced Trauma Life Support (ATLS)
- Advanced Life Support (ALS)
- Paediatric Advanced Life Support (PALS)
- Major Incident Medical Management and Support (MIMMS)

EQUIPMENT

Personal safety equipment and medical equipment must be packed and ready for immediate use. Such equipment should be standardized so that there is no incompatibility with the equipment carried by the emergency services. More details of equipment and clothing are given in Chapter 68. Equipment should not be stored in the vehicle, unless secured in a garage and suitably insured.

The vehicle should be reliable and clearly identifiable as a medical vehicle (removable magnetic labels and lights are ideal, as permanently fitted markings can make the vehicle an attractive target for a thief). Any registered medical practitioner in the course of his/her work may use green flashing lights. Daily checks on the vehicle should include ensuring that the fuel tank and windscreen washer fluid reservoir are full, checking that all lights work and checking the oil and water levels. Monthly checks should include tyre pressure and treads, shock absorbers and brakes. The vehicle should contain maps of the local area, both large- and small-scale, torches and warning triangles. Ideally, the vehicle should be fitted with a hands-free communications system, either mobile phone or radio.

Check your vehicle and equipment regularly.

Leaving for the scene

Before leaving for the scene of an incident, protective clothing should be donned before getting into the vehicle, and controlled drugs, money, identification and a credit card should be collected. Details of the route and destination should be left with a responsible adult. It is better to visit the lavatory in the comfort of home than to improvise at the scene.

Driving to the scene

There is little point in risking becoming a road traffic accident victim on the way to the incident scene. The precise location and nature of the incident and the best route should be clearly established before setting off. Predetermining a place to stop near the final destination in an unfamiliar area will allow the precise location of an incident to be identified. Alternatively, ambulance control or an assistant at home or in the surgery can provide on-going directions using a hands-free mobile phone system. Liaison with ambulance control about any diversions or road blocks that may have been set up as a result of the incident will save a great deal of time and frustration.

Check the route before you set off.

Green flashing lights and two-tone sirens do not give an automatic right of way over other road users, nor do they allow flaunting of the highway code. The aim should be to drive steadily and surely towards the incident, making good progress, so as to arrive calm and unflustered. Attention during the journey should be focused on driving, rather than on anticipating what is happening at the scene and planning management. A good driver will maintain a high level of observation and will accurately match the vehicle's speed and direction to the road conditions while identifying hazards. This takes both training and practice. Useful books are available, as are courses run by local police forces and ambulance services, by the British Association of Immediate Care Schemes (BASICS), by the Institute of Advanced Motorists and by the Royal Society for the Prevention of Accidents.

ESCORTS

The police may occasionally offer an escort to the incident scene, or from the scene to the hospital. This has advantages and disadvantages. An escort allows someone else to concentrate on route-finding and blue lights are better than green ones in clearing a path through busy traffic. On the other hand, the average car may have difficulty keeping up with a powerful police vehicle and particularly with motorcycles. Other road users may pull back into the road in front of the medical vehicle after the police vehicle has passed, not realizing that there is a second emergency vehicle. If the immediate-care doctor is travelling behind an ambulance in the doctor's own vehicle, the same problem may occur. The use of lights and 'two tones' (if carried) may help to avoid this.

A better method is for a number of police motorcyclists to ensure that the road is clear ahead by 'leap-frogging' each other to block side roads and junctions, allowing the medical vehicle a clear route.

Driving techniques

STOPPING SAFELY

The guiding principle is always to be able to stop on your side of the road within the distance that is seen to be clear in front. The distance needed to bring the vehicle to a safe standstill is a combination of the thinking distance and the braking distance.

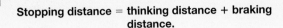

Stopping distance = thinking distance + braking distance.

For example, the average time for a driver to react to a hazard is 0.7 s, at 40 mph the vehicle will cover 12 m in this time. This is the thinking distance. The braking distance will depend on the speed, the type of vehicle and the road surface. At 40 mph the shortest braking distance is 24 m, but this will increase dramatically for a heavy vehicle with old tyres driven downhill on a wet road. The shortest stopping distance at 40 mph is thus 36 m. In order to allow sufficient distance to be able to stop safely, it is best to keep a gap of at least 2 s between oneself and the vehicle in front, doubling this in wet or icy conditions. To estimate this, note when the vehicle in front passes a landmark, such as a lamp post or side street. As it does, say aloud 'Only a fool breaks the 2-second rule'. This will take about 2 s. If you have passed the landmark before finishing the sentence then you are too close to the vehicle in front.

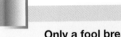

Only a fool breaks the 2s rule.

CADENCE BRAKING

Applying and releasing the brakes in a rhythmic fashion, allowing the wheels to almost lock and then to rotate freely, best effects emergency braking. The vehicle may be steered only while the wheels are rotating. By repeating this sequence regularly speed can be reduced rapidly and control of the vehicle maintained. This is known as cadence braking and antilock braking systems (ABS) replicate this automatically.

CORNERING SAFELY

Correct technique while negotiating bends in the road allows momentum to be maintained and the corner to be completed safely (Fig. 21.1). A vehicle will tend to continue in a straight line unless forces are applied to it. While cornering, it is the grip of the tyres, directed by the steering mechanism, that transmits the forces allowing the vehicle to turn. Tyre grip is reduced by braking and by acceleration. It is therefore of advantage to maintain constant speed around a bend. To do this, the power from the engine will need to be increased to counter the natural tendency of the vehicle to slow down as it changes direction.

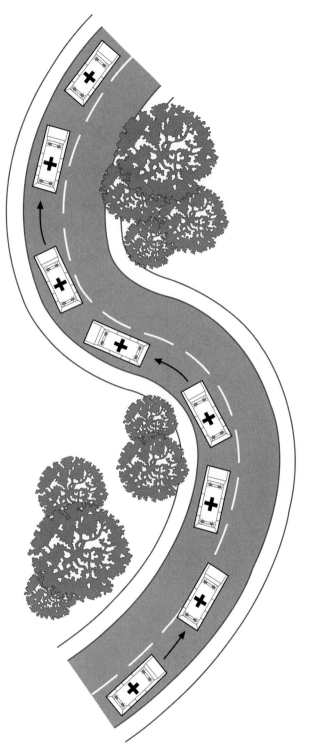

Fig. 21.1 • Safe cornering.

The accelerator should be depressed while cornering in order to maintain a constant speed, not to increase it. A useful way of determining the correct speed while cornering is the *limit point technique* (Fig. 21.2).

a)

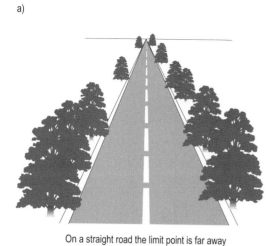

On a straight road the limit point is far away

b)

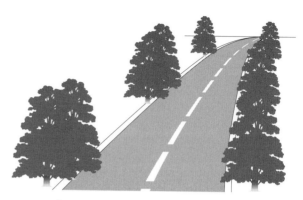

As a corner approaches the limit point moves nearer. Slow down so the vehicle can stop before the limit point

c)

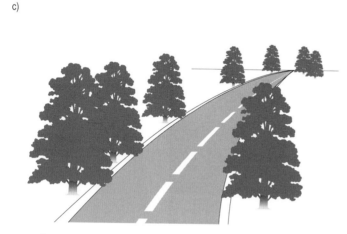

On the corner keep the limit point at a constant distance

d)

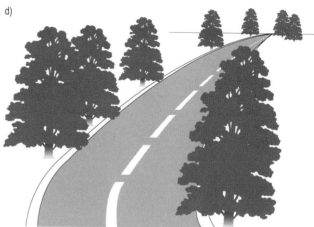

As the corner is left behind the limit point moves away. Increase speed to the maximum that is safe

Fig. 21.2 • Limit point technique.

Use the limit point technique to corner safely.

The limit point is the furthest point along the road that the road surface can clearly be seen. As the bend is approached the limit point appears to remain at the same point on the road, and therefore to come nearer to the vehicle. Speed should be adjusted so that the vehicle can stop before the limit point is reached. As the corner is entered the limit point appears to move round the bend. Speed should now be maintained so that the limit point appears to stay at a constant distance in front of the vehicle. This is the correct speed for the bend. As the corner straightens out the limit point starts to move quickly away. The vehicle should now be accelerated towards this point until reaching the correct speed for the road, allowing for speed limits, traffic and road conditions (Fig. 21.2).

OVERTAKING

Overtaking allows an emergency vehicle to pass slower road users and reach the destination more quickly. It is a dangerous manoeuvre as it may encroach on the path of oncoming vehicles. As a vehicle or other hazard is approached the road ahead should be scanned for information about more hazards such as junctions, other vehicles, bends, signs, road markings and so on. It may be appropriate to alert the vehicle ahead of the intention to overtake by flashing the headlights, activating the siren or green beacon but this must not be relied on. It is important not to antagonize the other driver and to express thanks if action has been taken to allow easy passage. This will make the driver's cooperation next time much more likely. Do not get too close to the vehicle ahead as this will obscure the view forward. Safe overtaking is achieved by checking the mirrors, signalling right and manoeuvring past the vehicle ahead as swiftly as is safe. Once past, the road to the left is assessed for hazards, such as motorcyclists, indicate left and the vehicle can return to the normal carriageway.

Arrival at the scene

PARKING

On arriving at an accident scene the doctor should quickly assess the situation and establish communication with other emergency services. The priorities are safety, scene control and communication. The police will, in general, direct parking and are responsible for overall control of the area around the incident.

If the police have not yet arrived, the vehicle should be parked in a position to protect both the casualty and rescuers. The car is parked in the fend-off position with beacons and/or hazards flashing. In this situation it is permissible to leave the engine running while the vehicle is unattended, to prevent the battery going flat (Fig. 21.3). Ideally, the car should be left unlocked with the keys in the ignition so that the police can move it if necessary. Depending on the area in which the accident occurs, this may represent an unacceptable security risk. In this situation (especially if the doctor is accompanying a patient to hospital in the ambulance), the keys should be handed to a named police officer. Ideally, two sets of car keys should be carried, which will allow the engine to be left running and the car to be locked.

If the incident has taken place off the carriageway, park out of the line of traffic and turn both beacons and engine off. At a motorway accident the doctor's vehicle should be parked beyond the crash, just beyond the ambulance. In this situation the hazard lights should be turned off and the keys should be left in the ignition in case the police have to move the vehicle for reasons of safety or because the doctor has to accompany the casualty to hospital. The comments made above regarding safety still apply.

SAFETY

Having parked the vehicle, the next priority is scene assessment. Here the emphasis is on safety. Common hazards are moving vehicles, fire, electricity, falling masonry and chemicals. The fire service has primacy at an incident scene where hazardous materials are involved, and medical staff should not approach the scene until asked to do so by the senior fire officer present. The police force establishes cordons around the area and controls entry into the incident area.

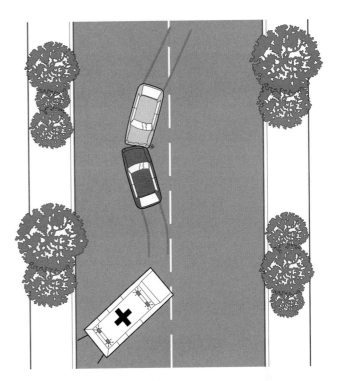

Fig. 21.3 • The 'fend-off' position.

> **Assume that hazards are present until proved otherwise.**

Vehicle hazard

The commonest danger to doctors in the prehospital environment is from road traffic. Personnel working at the scene of road accidents must be constantly alert to danger. The area must be secured with warning signs, cones or the physical barrier of a car or other vehicle. Wearing a reflective jacket and using high-visibility hazard lights is also advised.

Fire hazard

The fire service will deal with any threat from fire but the doctor must be aware of the threat. Car batteries should be disconnected and spilt fuel covered with sand, soil or foam, or washed away with water. Care must also be taken to reduce the risks of sparks from cutting equipment or hobnailed boots, and obviously smoking is prohibited.

Electricity hazard

Any electric cables involved with the incident must be assumed to be live until proved otherwise. Remember that, as bird strikes on electric power cables are so common, the electricity is routinely turned back on 20 min after a disruption without a visual check. Electricity can arc several feet from high-voltage cables. The power company should be alerted to the problem and the electricity turned off and kept off. Power in railway lines may also be restored without warning, and diesel trains can still run even when the power is turned off! If the victim is still in contact with the power cables they should not be touched until it is clear that there is no current flowing, or an insulated pole should be used to separate victim and cable.

Chemical hazard

Huge quantities of chemicals are moved by road in this country, and road traffic accidents involving such vehicles are not uncommon. Doctors may also be called to the scene of an accident at a chemical plant. Information about the load is found on the 'hazard warning' plate on the vehicle. More detailed information may be obtained by ringing the telephone number at the bottom of the warning plate or by using the computer link in the cab of fire rescue tenders. Medical information about poisons is available from regional poisons centres. Fire tenders also carry sealed breathing apparatus and protective clothing that can be used if there is any perceived threat from chemicals or fumes. There is also a risk of the chemical hazard being carried back down the evacuation chain and affecting medical personnel many miles from the incident site. Casualties must be decontaminated and suitable precautions taken by all concerned in the treatment and transport of such patients.

ASSESSMENT

Once safety is assured, assessment of the scene and of the casualties may proceed. The accident should be mentally reconstructed, envisaging the forces involved and the movement of the vehicles. This is known as *reading the wreckage*. From this, patterns of likely injuries can be deduced.

It is worth taking a short time to go through this process before rushing to the nearest casualty, as it will give clues as to the treatment priorities. This approach will also reduce the risk of casualties being missed if they have been ejected some distance from the vehicle, or trapped deep within the wreckage. This is a particular problem with small children, who may easily be overlooked. Conscious casualties must always be asked how many people were in the vehicle and a search of the area around the vehicles must be made for occupants who may have been ejected.

Take care not to overlook casualties.

LIAISON WITH OTHER EMERGENCY SERVICES

Teamwork between all three emergency services is vital at the scene of a major accident. This involves training and practice, and doctors should attend a recognized course, such as the Major Incident Medical Management and Support course (MIMMS). They should also participate in the regular training days organized by the regional emergency services.

At the incident scene the doctor should report to the incident control point (ICP) and identify him/herself to other emergency services. Proof of status as a medical practitioner may be required as there have been instances where bogus doctors have attempted to render assistance at accident scenes. BASICS issues a credit-card-type identity card to members. It is important to recognize and respect the skills that different organizations bring to prehospital emergency care and to use these to the best advantage of the patient by employing a team approach.

SAFETY EQUIPMENT

By their nature accident scenes are hazardous places: wreckage, spilt fuel, chemicals, electricity and the occasional homicidal maniac all present different hazards to the doctor. Early recognition and avoidance of the danger is vital and so is personal protective equipment. More details on protective equipment are found in Chapter 68.

Conclusion

Responding to a medical emergency outside the hospital environment is fraught with potential hazards. There are many things that can go wrong before the doctor has a chance to lay a hand on the casualty. Problems can be minimized by appropriate and on-going training, by meticulous preparation and by making safety the first priority. Once at the scene, an initial brief assessment and a willingness to work closely with the other emergency services will result in more effective administration of care to the patient.

Further reading

Calland V 2001 Safety at scene. Mosby, London

Carley S, Mackway-Jones K 2002 Major incident medical management and support, the practical approach, 2nd edn. Advanced Life Support Group. BMJ Publishing, London

Coyne P 1997 Roadcraft: the essential police driver's handbook. The Stationery Office, London

The Highway Code 1999 The Stationery Office, Norwich

Assessment and management of the trauma patient – the primary and secondary survey

22

Introduction 251

Arriving at the scene 251

Patient assessment and treatment 251

Primary survey – principles 252

Secondary survey 258

Summary 259

Further reading 259

Introduction

The assessment of the trauma patient starts with the initial call to the incident. With experience, details of the likely patterns of injury can often be deduced from a knowledge of the prevailing conditions, the type and location of the incident, especially if it is a so-called 'accident blackspot'. However, because of the urgency of the situation and panic on the part of bystanders the initial details are often confused. Those working in immediate care must have a calm, structured approach but at the same time be able to think flexibly and laterally when there are unusual problems.

To achieve a systematic and structured approach and carry out proper assessment the individual must be properly trained. This is the advantage of the various courses available, such as Pre-hospital Emergency Care (PHEC),

Pre-hospital Trauma Life Support (PHTLS) or Advanced Trauma Life Support (ATLS), which teach a clear, easily applicable method of patient assessment and treatment.

Arriving at the scene

On arrival at the scene of a road traffic accident, a slow approach for the last few moments is essential. During this time the incident can be visually assessed and the correct location for parking the vehicle established. If equipment is to be left in the vehicle it is essential that it is not parked too far away from the accident. If the trauma is not related to a road traffic accident, a similar brief scene assessment, as well as identifying any potential hazards, will still provide vital information about the cause and nature of any injuries.

Frequently the immediate-care worker will be the first on scene at an incident. Recognition of any problems within the first few seconds and appropriate communication with emergency services control is essential for the optimal management of the incident.

Patient assessment and treatment

The assessment and treatment of the injured patient is divided into the following stages:

- primary survey
- resuscitation
- secondary survey
- definitive care.

The *primary survey* is a rapid structured assessment of the patient, searching for injuries that are immediately life-threatening. It is divided into separate phases based on the ABC system (see below). Any immediately life-threatening injury that is identified is immediately treated – *resuscitation*. It cannot therefore be overemphasized that the primary survey and resuscitation phases of the treatment of the trauma victim *take place simultaneously*.

The *secondary survey* is a detailed head-to-toe examination for all other injuries, some of which may be potentially life-threatening. Unless hospital transfer times are likely to be prolonged, the secondary survey should usually be performed following arrival in hospital in order to prevent any unnecessary delay in the patient receiving *definitive care*.

It must never be forgotten that the role of the immediate-care doctor is to deliver the patient to appropriate definitive care as rapidly as possible and in the best possible condition. The separate components of trauma resuscitation are discussed in detail below (Table 22.1).

Primary survey – principles

The primary survey, which can also be applied to the management of medical emergencies, is based on the <C>ABC approach. First, exsanguinating external haemorrhage, if present, is identified and controlled. Then the approach follows the sequence:

- **A**irway with cervical spine control
- **B**reathing
- **C**irculation.

This system is based on the principle that those with obstructed airways will be brain-dead within 3 min. Breathing problems will kill within 6 min on average, and haemorrhage in 9 min. Therefore the aim should be to treat these different systems within a time-specific framework. When there are multiple casualties they can be sorted, or triaged, using the ABC concepts according to the priority with which they must be treated.

The primary survey continues (Table 22.2):

- **D**isability
- **E**xposure and **e**nvironment.

AIRWAY WITH CERVICAL SPINE CONTROL

The first airway step is to assess whether there is a patent airway. The very first approach to the patient will provide valuable information. A patient who is able to answer questions has a functioning brain, a patent airway and reasonable respiratory function. If there is any evidence of any degree of airway compromise, a more formal assessment must be undertaken. The most important signs of airway obstruction are noisy breathing (which may or may not be rapid) and cyanosis. Occasionally, airway obstruction may

Table 22.1 The approach to the trauma patient

- Primary survey
- Resuscitation
- Secondary survey
- Definitive care.

Table 22.2 The primary survey

- **A**irway – with cervical spine control in the injured patient
- **B**reathing
- **C**irculation
- **D**isability
- **E**xposure and environment.

be complete, with no apparent evidence of respiration or disorganized respiratory effort. Potential causes of airway obstruction include:

- the tongue
- foreign bodies
- vomit
- facial injuries
- upper airways haemorrhage.

If there is any evidence of obstruction, or the airway is thought to be at risk because of the patient's position, conscious level or any other factor (e.g. alcohol), steps must be taken to ensure an adequately protected airway. The most common cause of upper airway obstruction is the tongue falling backwards in the unconscious or obtunded patient. The methods involved will range from simple airway manoeuvres to surgical airways; this is known as stepped airway care.

Stepped airway care:
- **Simple manoeuvres – chin lift, jaw thrust**
- **Basic airways – oral and nasal airway**
- **Tracheal intubation**
- **Surgical airways.**

Stepped airway care is discussed in detail in Chapter 4. Occasionally, circumstances may be such that it is essential to turn a patient on to his/her side in order to maintain a patent airway. Patients with facial injuries may be able to maintain a patent airway while sitting forward (which causes a fractured mandible and soft tissue to fall away from the airway) while attempts to lie them supine may result in rapid airway obstruction.

Suction should always be available, and it is important to remember that there is a risk of vomiting in all unconscious patients. The appropriate equipment should be readily available. To achieve this many immediate-care workers carry a first-response bag with them. A reliable suction unit is essential. To guarantee reliability hand- or foot-operated units are ideal for immediate use, particularly when away from a vehicle.

Only when a safe secure patent airway is established, is it possible to move on to the next component of the primary survey.

Part of the management of the airway is to give the patient oxygen. This should be done using a high-flow rate, ideally 10–15 l min^{-1}, via a Hudson (reservoir) mask or a bag and mask device if respiratory support is necessary.

Always give high-flow oxygen.

The most difficult airway situation in trauma is the unconscious and restless head injury. These patients are often blue, struggling and hypoxic, and present a major problem. Proper establishment of a protected airway may only be possible with anaesthesia and intubation, or a surgical airway.

To protect the spinal cord and prevent neurological deterioration, in any traumatic situation the patient's head, neck and shoulders should be kept in alignment as near to the anatomical position as normal. If the head is not in the neutral position, optimal further management is best achieved by bringing the head and neck carefully into the neutral position, facilitating airway management and ongoing cervical spine immobilization.

In certain situations it may not be possible to bring the head to the neutral and anatomical position because of a fracture–dislocation of the facet joints in the neck. In the conscious patient there will be pain in the neck, which is usually severe, and the head will be held slightly rotated and twisted to one side. Under no circumstances should it be forced back to the neutral.

With this exception, once the head is put in the neutral position, this should be maintained by midline manual immobilization without traction. Manual immobilization is an extremely effective method of preventing movement of the cervical spine. Full immobilization requires a semi-rigid collar, sand bags and tape, or foam blocks and straps. Restless, aggressive, struggling patients cannot be satisfactorily immobilized by being strapped down to a spinal board as this makes them likely to rotate their body around the fixed head and neck, thus causing cord damage.

The removal of motorcycle and other helmets is a skill that needs to be learned. It is best performed as a two-person procedure (Fig. 22.1). One of the most common errors is failure to undo the chin strap. One worker needs to support the neck from the front and progressively move their hands up the back of the neck while the eggshell-shaped helmet is tipped forwards and backwards in the vertical plane to clear the occiput and then the nose. While the helmet is being removed, it should be carefully expanded laterally. At each stage the person supporting the neck must have absolute control and should ask the other operator to stop if there are problems.

Occasionally, circumstances demand that a motorcycle helmet is safely removed by one operator (Fig. 22.2). The rescuer kneels above the patient's head, the chin strap is undone and the helmet is carefully expanded laterally and gently tilted forwards until the occiput is cleared, following which the helmet is tipped backwards to release the chin from the chin bar. The rescuer then maintains in-line immobilization by placing his/her hands on the sides of the patient's head and face, and uses his/her forearms to complete the removal of the helmet.

If there is a limited number of trained people and the airway is clear, there is little urgency in removing the helmet as an emergency procedure. This only needs to be done if the patient has an obstructed airway.

BREATHING

The role of the next component of the primary survey is to identify immediately life-threatening chest conditions so that they can be treated appropriately before passing onto the next component of the assessment. These conditions are listed in Table 22.3 and discussed in detail in Chapter 25.

If this part of the examination is done in a cursory manner, critical information will be missed. It needs to be done systematically and carefully to identify potentially life-threatening conditions. The general principles of clinical examination by inspection, palpation, percussion and auscultation (look, feel, tap and listen) are all part of the breathing assessment. Frequently, this examination is skipped and people move on from airway to circulation because the chest remains covered. It should be remembered that every patient has a top, bottom, front, back, right and left. One in four trauma deaths are due to chest injury.

The general inspection should include the patient's general condition, colour and rate of respiration, noting whether it is noisy or quiet. Rapid respiration is indicative of hypoxia or shock, or both. Any respiratory rate above 24 breaths min^{-1} is a sign that the patient is distressed.

Always check the respiratory rate.

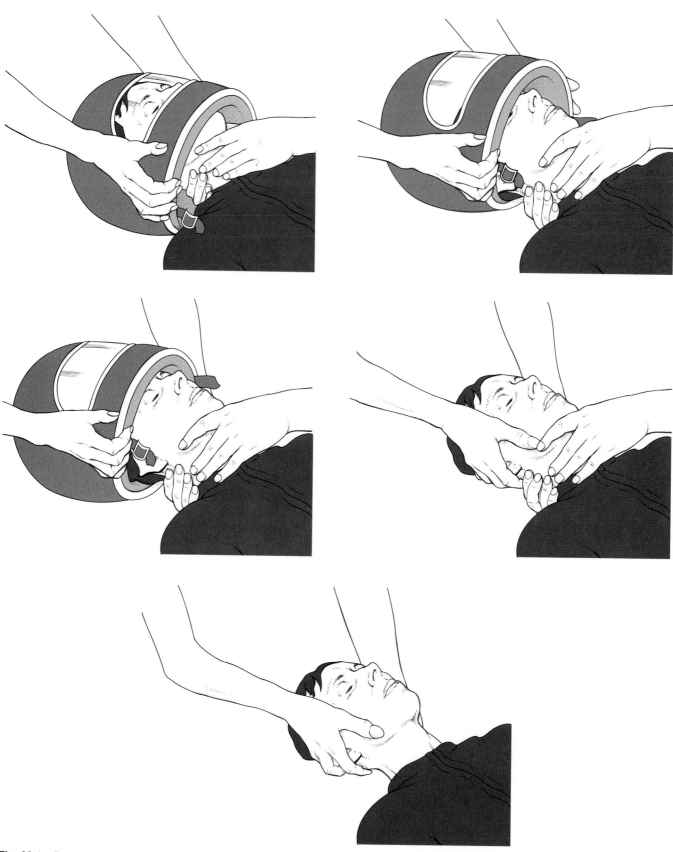

Fig. 22.1 • Removing a motorcycle helmet (two-rescuer approach).

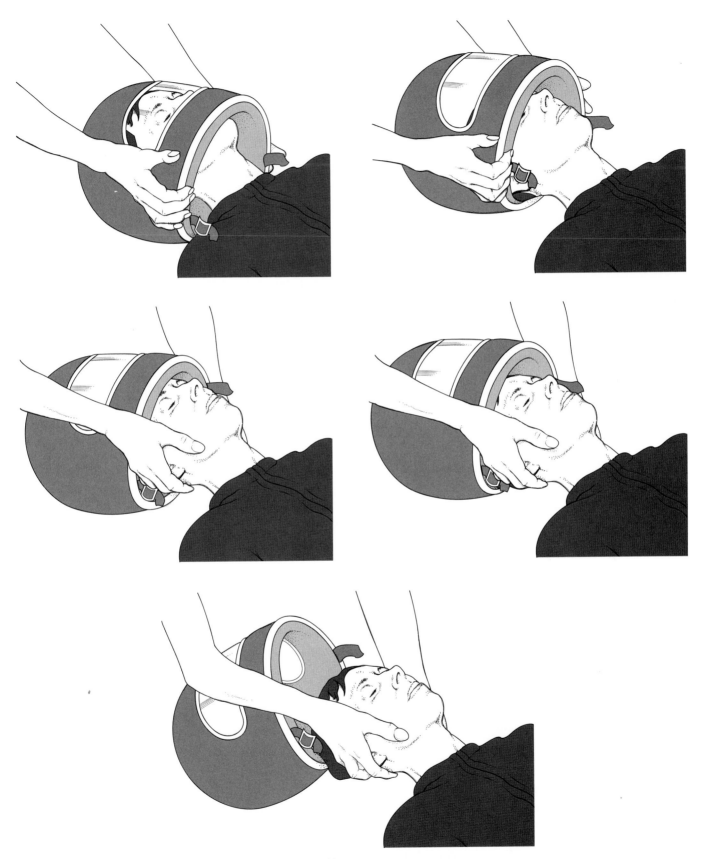

Fig. 22.2 • Removing a motorcycle helmet (one-rescuer approach).

Table 22.3 Immediately life-threatening chest injuries

- Airway obstruction
- Tension pneumothorax
- Massive haemothorax
- Open ('sucking') chest wound
- Cardiac tamponade
- Flail chest.

Table 22.4 Examination of the neck

- Trachea
- Neck veins
- Penetrating trauma
- Soft tissue swelling
- Surgical emphysema.

Table 22.5 Components of the chest examination

- *General inspection*: abrasions, wounds, bruising and pattern bruising, movement (symmetry, paradox)
- *Respiratory rate*
- *Palpation*: asymmetry of movement, bony crepitus, surgical emphysema, tenderness, posterior wounds, flail segments
- *Percussion*: dullness (fluid), resonance (pneumothorax, tension pneumothorax)
- *Auscultation*: air entry, added sounds.

Examination should begin with an assessment of the position of the trachea in the sternal notch and the state of the neck veins as the examiner passes from the head (airway) to the chest. Examination of the neck will also elicit the presence of penetrating trauma, soft tissue swelling and surgical emphysema (Table 22.4).

As part of the inspection the chest needs to be exposed. It can be covered after the examination. Inspection of the chest should include looking for abrasions, wounds, bruising and pattern bruising (Table 22.5). Pattern bruising is important because it is an imprint of an external structure on the skin. This indicates significant force. The inspection must look for open wounds. By careful inspection around the sides and palpation (by running the hands down the sides and the back of the patient and looking for blood on the gloved hand – care is required if there is any possibility of broken glass) penetrating wounds such as a stab or gunshot wound will be identified.

A visual assessment of the chest for any abnormality of movement, including paradoxical movement due to a flail chest, is essential.

Palpation should test for asymmetry of movement. This can be done by placing both hands on the front of the chest and watching to see if both hands move up and down equally. Rib fractures can be identified by fingertip pain over the bone.

A flail chest is identified by paradoxical breathing, so called because when the patient breaths in and the chest expands a negative pressure is created. If a flail segment is present the negative pressure sucks the loose segment inwards so that, instead of the chest wall moving out, it moves in. When the patient breaths out the segment moves outwards. Quite frequently the flail segment is not apparent at the initial stages because the ends of the fractured ribs have not become detached. This occurs some time later.

The purpose of percussion or tapping the chest over a finger is to reveal whether there is a resonant or dull sound. Air trapped inside the chest (but outside the lung) is a feature of pneumothorax or tension pneumothorax and is resonant. Fluid in the chest (in trauma this means blood) is identified by a dull percussion note.

Listening to the chest (auscultation) and comparing the breath sounds is important. This should be done in all areas on both sides to make sure there is equal air entry. Listening to the chest is essential after endotracheal intubation. If the tube is inserted too far it may pass into the right bronchus. Air entry will be heard only on the right side. If there are absent breath sounds on the left after intubation the endotracheal tube cuff will need to be deflated and the tube drawn back.

The findings on examination of the chest in the presence of immediately life-threatening injuries are summarized in Table 22.6. The variability of the signs is due to the underlying injuries associated with some of the conditions described. For example, an open chest wound may be associated with underlying pneumothorax, tension pneumothorax or haemothorax.

CIRCULATION

Once all immediately life-threatening respiratory conditions have been identified and where possible treated, the assessment of the patient can move on to C – *circulation with external haemorrhage control*. It is possible that some chest conditions will simply require immediate transfer to hospital, in which case the remainder of the primary survey is probably best completed during transit. A careful, methodical assessment of the patient's circulatory state, along with the identification of sites and sources of bleeding, is essential.

The pulse should be regularly and repeatedly monitored, and a baseline blood pressure is helpful, although this is often difficult in the prehospital environment. The presence or absence of peripheral pulses provides a useful guide, in that the presence of a radial pulse implies a systolic blood pressure sufficient to maintain vital organ perfusion.

The presence and degree of any tachycardia and pulse volume should be noted. Very occasionally, hypotension occurs as a result of neurogenic shock, resulting from loss of sympathetic tone as a result of a high spinal cord injury. In this situation, although hypotensive, the patient may appear warm and there is no tachycardia. It is usually safer to assume, however, that any patient who has suffered an injury sufficient to cause a spinal fracture has also suffered other injuries resulting in shock due to bleeding. Athletes, patients with pacemakers and elderly patients on beta-blocking drugs may also fail to mount a tachycardia in response to blood loss. It should be remembered that tachypnoea occurs with shock as well as with respiratory problems.

The general examination may reveal the classic signs of shock: pallor, sweating and agitation.

Shock may be classified into four stages depending on the degree of blood loss; this classification is given in Table 22.7 (simplified for use in the prehospital environment).

The stages of shock are most easily remembered by comparing the indicated blood loss in each stage with the scores in a tennis match, Love:15, 15:30, etc.

As part of the C component of the primary survey, any obvious external haemorrhage should be controlled by direct pressure. At the same time a brief assessment of the possible sites of significant haemorrhage should be completed. There are five possible locations for traumatic haemorrhage:

- on the floor – external haemorrhage
- in the chest
- in the abdomen
- in the pelvis
- in the long bones (multiple or open fractures).

Blood on the floor and four more.

A rapid search will indicate the source of the bleeding in the vast majority of patients: blood in the chest should already have been identified under B, palpation of the abdomen may reveal tenderness and guarding, and careful examination of the pelvis may reveal pain or crepitus.

It should be remembered that springing the pelvis may provoke bleeding in unstable pelvic fractures (it is also painful in the conscious patient with a pelvic injury) and it should not routinely be performed.

Any patient who is found to have suffered or to be at risk of haemorrhage will require the insertion of intravenous access. In many situations, if transfer times are short, the most appropriate action will be immediate hospital transfer so that this can be achieved in optimal conditions and surgical referral can be expedited.

Although shock in trauma is most commonly due to bleeding, it may be associated with a number of other conditions:

- tension pneumothorax
- cardiac tamponade
- spinal cord injury (neurogenic shock)
- cardiac contusion.

Shock due to cardiac tamponade or direct cardiac trauma leading to myocardial contusion is suggested by external evidence of local trauma, whether blunt or penetrating. In the presence of cardiac tamponade the neck veins may be elevated. Beck's triad (elevated neck veins, muffled heart sounds and hypotension) is almost impossible to elicit in the prehospital environment. It should be remembered that, in the presence of significant haemorrhage, there may not be enough circulating volume to produce elevated neck veins, even in the presence of tamponade. Shock due solely to myocardial contusion is extremely rare and has a very poor prognosis.

Tension pneumothorax as a cause of shock should already have been identified and treated as one of the immediately life-threatening conditions under B. Signs include reduced breath sounds and a hyper-resonant percussion note on the side of the pneumothorax, tachypnoea, a deviated trachea, hypotension and elevated neck veins.

DISABILITY

Once the life-threatening injuries above have been identified and treated, the next stage is to go on to assess the neurological situation. By continuing the alphabetic code this is 'Disability' (neurological Dysfunction). The basic components of D are an assessment of the level of consciousness and pupillary assessment.

The best initial method of assessment of the conscious level is AVPU:

- Is the patient **A**lert?
- Does he respond to **V**erbal stimuli?
- Does he respond only to **P**ainful stimuli?
- Is s/he **U**nresponsive?

The second component of D is an assessment of pupil size and reactivity. In the absence of obvious local trauma to the eyes, unequal pupils are a sign of a focal intracranial mass lesion. It should be remembered that the pupil first dilates *on the side of the lesion*. Subsequent progression of the rise

Table 22.6 Findings on chest examination

Condition	Neck	Movement	Percussion note	Breath sounds
Tension pneumothorax	Elevated central venous pressure (CVP)	Decreased	Hyperresonant	Reduced or absent
Massive haemothorax	Normal or empty veins	Decreased	Dull	Reduced or absent
Open chest wound	Normal	Varies	Varies	Reduced or absent
Cardiac tamponade	Elevated CVP	Normal	Normal	Normal
Flail chest	Normal	Paradoxical	Varies	Normal or reduced

The findings described are those on the side of (ipsilateral to) the pathology

Table 22.7 Signs and symptoms of shock

	Class I	Class II	Class III	Class IV
Blood loss (ml)	<750	750–1500	1500–2000	>2000
Blood loss (% blood volume)	<15	15–30	30–40	>40
Pulse rate (beats min^{-1})	<100	>100	>120	<140
Blood pressure	Normal	Normal	Decreased	Decreased
Pulse pressure	Normal or increased	Decreased	Decreased	Decreased
Respiratory rate (breaths min^{-1})	14–20	20–30	30–40	>40

in intracranial pressure will produce a dilated pupil on the opposite side as the other third cranial nerve is compressed against the tentorium.

An alternative to the AVPU system is an assessment of the Glasgow coma scale (Table 22.8).

EXPOSURE

The final component of the primary survey is E for exposure. By this stage the patient's chest and abdomen will have been exposed and the further removal of clothing will depend on the environment and clinical necessity. Complete removal of a patient's clothes in the prehospital environment is rarely necessary. It is important to prevent hypothermia and to save the patient embarrassment although, where necessary, clinical priorities will dictate the appropriate actions.

The aim of the E component is to ensure that significant major injuries have not been missed. It is followed by the secondary survey (see below), which is a head-to-toe examination of the patient, searching for any injury whatsoever.

By the time E is reached, any life-threatening injury of the chest will have been identified and hopefully treated; a brief assessment of the abdomen, pelvis and femurs is part

of C. It should be noted that an assessment of the femurs designed to rule out fractures can usually be achieved through trousers. In particular, motorcycle leathers should not be removed as they may provide some splinting action in the shocked patient.

The E component of the primary survey must not delay hospital transfer.

Secondary survey

The secondary survey is the third component of the initial assessment and management of the trauma victim. It consists of a detailed, methodical, head-to-toe examination of the patient and is designed to identify all injuries, however trivial. An essential component of the secondary survey is the completion of a careful record of all the patient's injuries. It is perhaps not surprising, therefore, that a properly performed secondary survey is a relatively time-consuming procedure.

It is absolutely essential that performing the secondary survey does not delay the patient's access to definitive

Table 22.8 The Glasgow coma scale

Component	Response	Score
Best motor response	Obeys command	6
	Localizes to pain*	5
	Withdraws from pain[†]	4
	Flexor response to pain[‡]	3
	Extensor response to pain[§]	2
	No motor response to pain	1
Best verbal response	Oriented	5
	Confused conversation[¶]	4
	Inappropriate speech[‖]	3
	Incomprehensible speech**	2
	No speech	1
Eye opening	Spontaneous	4
	In response to speech	3
	In response to pain	2
	No eye opening	1

* *Moves hand towards pain.*
[†] *Moves away from pain.*
[‡] *Bends arm at elbow and wrist in response to a painful stimulus.*
[§] *Straightens at elbow and knee in response to a painful stimulus.*
[¶] *Disorientated in time and space.*
[‖] *Inappropriate response to question.*
** *Moans and groans.*

Table 22.9 The secondary survey

- Abrasions
- Bruises
- Soft tissue swelling
- Localized tenderness
- Wounds
- Surgical emphysema
- Bony deformity
- Bleeding from body orifices
- Neurological (motor and sensory) deficit.

care. As a result, unless the patient is trapped or transfer is likely to be delayed, or transfer times are expected to be excessively long, the secondary survey will only very rarely be performed in the prehospital situation. It should be remembered that it was designed to be performed in a warm, well-lit emergency department. In addition, particularly in unstable patients, the time to hospital will be more than taken up with a careful primary survey and resuscitation. When a secondary survey is performed it must include a log roll and will therefore require a minimum of four people.

The secondary survey begins at the top of the patient and works down:

- head: scalp and face
- neck
- chest
- upper limb
- abdomen and perineum
- lower limb.

The examination assesses the patient comprehensively, front and back. A thorough examination is made for a complete range of injuries, and the secondary survey is the time to assess in more detail injuries observed during the

primary survey that did not require any further action at that time. A more detailed assessment of any suspected neurological deficit should be completed at this time. A list of findings identified during the secondary survey is given in Table 22.9.

In hospital practice many of the findings above will indicate the need for appropriate investigations; in the prehospital situation they are simply recorded or drawn to the attention of receiving hospital staff.

Summary

The initial approach to the assessment of the injured patient follows the protocol:

- primary survey
- resuscitation
- secondary survey
- definitive care.

The primary survey, which is designed to identify immediately life-threatening injuries, is performed using the <C>ABCDE priority system and takes place simultaneously with the resuscitation phase.

In the majority of cases the prehospital practitioner will progress no further than the primary survey and resuscitation, and in no circumstances should performance of unnecessary assessment be allowed to delay the transfer of the patient with potentially fatal injuries to hospital and definitive care.

Further reading

American College of Surgeons Committee on Trauma 2004 Advanced trauma life support for doctors, Student course manual, 7th edn. American College of Surgeons, Chicago, IL

Driscoll P, Gwinnutt C, Jimmerson CL, Goodall O (eds) 1993 Trauma resuscitation: the team approach. Macmillan, Basingstoke

Greaves I, Hodgetts T, Porter K (eds) 1997 Emergency care: a textbook for paramedics. WB Saunders, London

Head and neck injuries

23

Introduction   260

The pathophysiology of brain injury   261

Preventing secondary brain damage   262

Assessment and examination of the head-injured
patient   263

Open and penetrating brain injuries   265

Planning and carrying out transfer to hospital   266

Managing early deterioration after a head injury   267

Soft tissue injuries of the neck   269

Cervical spine injuries   269

Summary   270

References   270

Introduction

Head injuries are common throughout the world, and their epidemiology has attracted some attention (Kraus 1987, Goldstein 1990). In 1981 Jennett estimated that each year in the UK 1 million people attend hospital emergency departments after a head injury, and that 150 000 of them are admitted to hospital (Jennett & McMillan 1981).

However, probably no more than 10 000 are transferred to a neurosurgical unit.

Neck injuries are also common and range widely in seriousness, from 'whiplash' injuries and superficial neck lacerations to injuries that threaten life by causing major damage to the cervical cord, upper airway, carotid and jugular vessels, or other major structures in the neck.

Injuries of the head and neck have acquired some notoriety, as without skilful assessment and care potentially serious complications can follow. Outcome is best when care is of high quality from the outset, and it is especially important to identify early on those patients who are at risk of complications and to know how to manage them safely before they reach hospital.

For the sake of clarity, injuries to the head and neck will be considered separately in this chapter, but it is important to remember that they can coexist in the same patient. A head injury – especially with altered consciousness – substantially increases the statistical risk of a cervical spine injury (Williams et al 1992, Hills & Deane 1993). Indeed, a high proportion of patients with serious head or spinal cord trauma also have major injuries elsewhere (Gentleman et al 1986, Chesnut et al 1993). It is well established that these can be easy to miss or underestimate when conscious level is impaired, or if attention is focused entirely on the neurological injury (Garland & Bailey 1981, McLaren et al 1983, Ryan et al 1993). Failing to identify and treat them is likely to make the consequences of the neurological injury much worse (Gentleman & Jennett 1990, Lambert & Willett 1993).

Geography and health-care systems vary widely throughout the world and obviously these considerations influence prehospital care. For the purposes of this chapter, it is assumed that the patient has been injured at a location within relatively easy reach of the facilities of a hospital and is being tended at the scene and en route to hospital by a trained health worker: paramedic, doctor or nurse. The organization and delivery of patient care may have to be modified when these assumptions do not apply.

The pathophysiology of brain injury

It is conceptually and clinically useful to think of two types of brain injury: primary and secondary. Primary injury reflects mechanical events in the brain at the moment of injury. Secondary injury occurs later, either because of a chain reaction triggered by the primary injury or as the result of other clinical events.

The central nervous system has only a limited ability to repair itself after injury (Bower 1990, Gentleman 1994), and this underlines the importance of preventing brain damage whenever possible. Primary damage can *only* be reduced by preventative measures – engineering, education and enforcement – as once it has occurred it is not amenable to even the best medical treatment. By contrast, secondary brain injury can be averted or lessened by appropriate treatment, and that knowledge underpins the modern clinical management of head-injured patients (Miller & Becker 1982, Teasdale et al 1982, Gentleman 1992, Chesnut et al 1993).

PRIMARY BRAIN INJURY

Mechanical forces applied to the brain at the moment of injury transfer energy to it. This damages or even destroys neurones and small blood vessels in the brain, with some areas being especially vulnerable. The least severe injuries cause only minor damage and temporary loss of function, which is reflected in the clinical syndrome of concussion: brief loss of consciousness followed by a period of post-traumatic amnesia before an apparently complete recovery. At the other end of the spectrum, the most severe primary brain injuries cause widespread devastation and rapid death, no matter what is done for the patient. In between lie many cases where the transfer of energy kills some neurones but only damages others, with the potential for recovery under the right conditions.

SECONDARY BRAIN INJURY

The injured brain can be further damaged by *secondary insults* minutes, hours, days or even weeks after the head injury itself (Reilly et al 1975, Miller & Becker 1982, Chesnut et al 1993). A common factor with these insults (Table 23.1) is that they cause a mismatch between oxygen demand and supply in the brain. An important goal of

Table 23.1 Causes of secondary brain damage

Intracranial

- Haematoma
- Contusion
- Diffuse brain swelling
- Epileptic seizures
- Intracranial infection
- Neurochemical damage

Extracranial

- Hypoxia
- Hypo- or hypercarbia
- Hypo- or hyperglycaemia
- Systemic shock

managing any head-injured patient is therefore to minimize this secondary damage, which has a profound influence on outcome.

A large body of work now exists to show the harm caused when seriously head-injured patients become hypoxic or hypotensive, even briefly. Studies of severely head-injured patients in Glasgow during the 1980s showed that the proportion of patients who had a favourable outcome was reduced by more than half in those who had been hypoxic or hypotensive during transfer to the neurosurgical unit (Gentleman & Jennett 1990, Gentleman 1992). Such insults can occur even during short transfers within a hospital (Andrews et al 1990) or within a specialist neurosurgical intensive care unit (Jones et al 1994), and action to prevent secondary brain injury must begin at the scene of the accident and continue throughout all stages of care. This is not about complex specialist care but about applying simple principles to support the injured brain (Gentleman 1995).

OXYGEN AND THE INJURED BRAIN

Neurones damaged by mechanical trauma are exquisitely sensitive to changes in their immediate environment and especially to a lack of the oxygen that fuels their metabolic needs (Ishige et al 1987).

Brain cells cannot store oxygen and depend absolutely on a continuous supply of well-oxygenated blood. If this stops completely, consciousness starts to fall after 10–15 s and irreversible brain damage begins after 4 min. The aim is to restore a more normal environment by supplying the oxygen that neurones need.

The oxygen supply can rapidly become compromised by an obstructed airway, hypovolaemia or raised intracranial pressure (ICP). This starves the injured neurones of what they need to repair structural damage and to maintain key cell functions such as ionic gradients across cell membranes. Matters can be made worse if the metabolic demand for oxygen is increased inappropriately by an electrochemical storm of unnecessary action potentials. This occurs when areas of damaged brain trigger epileptic seizure activity or because high concentrations of 'excitotoxic' neurotransmitters released from dead and damaged neurones into the extracellular fluid repeatedly depolarize the cell membrane, wasting neuronal energy stores that would be better used to maintain normal function, repair the cell and inactivate dangerous molecules and ions such as free radicals (Faden et al 1989).

CEREBRAL PERFUSION AND OXYGENATION

Cerebral perfusion must be maintained after a serious head injury. Normal mean intracranial pressure (MICP) is 5–10 mmHg, mean arterial pressure (MAP) is 80–90 mmHg and the difference between them is the cerebral perfusion pressure (CPP) – the 'head of steam' that drives blood through the brain and delivers oxygen to the brain.

> **Cerebral perfusion pressure = mean arterial pressure – mean intracranial pressure**
>
> or
>
> **CPP = MAP – MICP.**

In health, cerebral blood flow (CBF) and oxygen supply are kept constant by reflex dilatation of the cerebral arterioles if CPP falls for any reason, but this 'autoregulation' is impaired after a head injury (Cold & Jensen 1978). Cranial blood flow and cerebral oxygen delivery then become critically dependent on cranial perfusion pressure and vulnerable if it falls (Changaris et al 1987). Cranial perfusion pressure is likely to fall if intracranial pressure rises (e.g. because of a haematoma) or if mean arterial pressure falls (e.g. because of systemic blood loss).

RAISED INTRACRANIAL PRESSURE

High pressure inside the rigid skull damages normal and injured brain tissue alike. Rising intracranial volume from a haematoma or brain swelling causes little change in ICP until a critical point is reached when no more venous blood or cerebrospinal fluid (CSF) can be squeezed out of the cranial cavity (Fig. 23.1). Beyond this point ICP increases steeply if intracranial volume continues to rise, and then CPP, CBF and cerebral oxygen delivery all fall. If the rise in ICP is not corrected, more and more neurones die from the secondary damage caused by an inadequate oxygen supply.

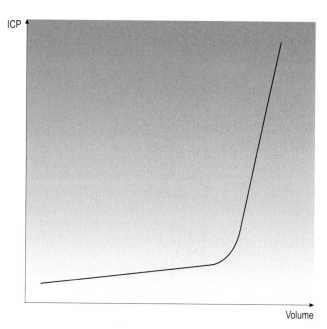

Fig. 23.1 • The relationship between intracranial volume and intracranial pressure.

Preventing secondary brain damage

A knowledge of the disordered pathophysiology of the injured brain allows a rational approach to minimizing further damage after the initial injury. This approach is of critical importance to achieving the best possible outcome, and must begin as soon as possible after injury and be continued through all stages of treatment (Gentleman 1990).

HYPOXIA AND HYPERCARBIA

It is now well recognized that hypoxia and hypercarbia (hypercapnia) are the earliest causes of secondary brain damage. They remain a real threat to the head-injured patient at all times and often develop insidiously. Anything which hinders effective gas exchange in the lungs or which reduces cerebral blood flow at the tissue level can cause hypoxia and hypercarbia.

Hypoxia causes swelling of neurones and glial cells. Hypercarbia leads to unwanted engorgement of the cerebral vessels that is independent of the cranial perfusion pressure. These complications together raise the intracranial pressure, reduce the cranial perfusion pressure and further damage the injured brain.

Preventing and treating hypoxia and hypercarbia depend upon ensuring a clear airway and adequate pulmonary ventilation, and giving high-flow oxygen as soon as possible. These matters are discussed fully in Chapter 4.

SHOCK

Another potent cause of secondary brain damage after head injury is shock, which is defined as inadequate tissue perfusion. Shock impairs cerebral perfusion and oxygenation and in the vast majority of head-injured patients is due to hypovolaemia caused by haemorrhage.

Very rarely an isolated head injury causes shock because of prolonged bleeding from a major scalp injury. Far more often shock is due instead to blood loss from associated extracranial injuries, and these must be identified promptly and the haemorrhage stopped. Fluid replacement is by an initial crystalloid bolus, followed by transfusion of blood or blood substitutes to maintain the oxygen-carrying capacity of the circulation.

INTRACRANIAL HAEMATOMA

The best-known intracranial cause of secondary brain damage is delay in recognizing and treating haematomas. Much attention has therefore been paid to ways of identifying patients who already have a haematoma or may develop one, and getting them to neurosurgical facilities before they deteriorate (Teasdale et al 1982, 1990, Briggs et al 1984).

An expanding haematoma compresses and distorts the brain within the skull and raises the intracranial pressure, producing characteristic clinical features. Large areas of brain contusion have the same effect. If a large haematoma or contusion is not evacuated promptly, intracranial pressure rises and cerebral perfusion pressure falls, lowering cerebral blood flow and cerebral oxygen delivery below critical levels and causing progressive brain damage. A small haematoma may not do this at first but start to do so later if it enlarges, or if other factors like brain swelling come into play.

BRAIN SWELLING

Brain swelling can be focal or general. It results from mechanical or hypoxic damage to the blood–brain barrier and to cell membranes, which allows water to accumulate in the cerebral interstitial space and to enter cells down ionic gradients. This further impairs oxygen delivery at the intracellular level and damages cell metabolism. The intracranial pressure also rises, and this accelerates the chain of adverse events. Established brain swelling is refractory to treatment and it is much better to prevent or limit it by correcting hypoxia and hypercarbia and by surgically removing large areas of contused brain without delay.

FITS

Epileptic fits reflect disordered electrochemical function in the cerebral cortex, whatever the cause. They can occur at any time after a head injury and have two major harmful effects on the injured brain. First, by reducing conscious level and inducing laryngospasm they threaten the airway. Second, they increase the brain's oxygen requirements at a time when oxygen delivery may already be at critical levels because of brain swelling or other complications. Seizures can therefore be devastating to the head-injured patient. The management of seizures before the patient reaches hospital is discussed later.

INTRACRANIAL INFECTION

Certain types of head injury are associated with a risk of secondary damage from delayed intracranial infection. Bacteria can reach the cranial cavity through penetrating wounds (e.g. compound depressed skull vault fractures) or fractures of the skull base. Treatment is based on applying sound surgical principles to wound management and the judicious use of prophylactic antibiotics.

Assessment and examination of the head-injured patient

HISTORY

The paramedic or doctor arriving at the scene of an accident must try to find out as much as possible about the circumstances of the injury. Less seriously head-injured patients can often describe what happened, but with more substantial trauma the patient may be amnesic, confused or even unconscious. It is then necessary to rely upon the testimony of witnesses and one's own observations.

For example, the patient may be lying on the ground near a wrecked vehicle, suggesting ejection and therefore a high risk of multisystem injury. The damage to the vehicle can suggest the force of the impact. Alternatively, there may be circumstantial evidence that the patient fell from a height, or was struck a blow with a weapon. Information about whether the victim had been drinking heavily before the accident is useful for assessment and management. If a friend or relative is present the past medical history can be obtained, including regular medication and allergies.

All too often, little or no useful history is obtained at this stage, and the details only emerge later in dribs and drabs as relatives arrive at hospital or the police make their enquiries. However, this lack of information must never be allowed to delay the provision of effective treatment for the head-injured patient.

PRIORITIES IN EXAMINATION

Under all circumstances, the initial assessment and management of an injured person at the scene begins with a search for life-threatening complications, in the same order as they would threaten life. Vital organs like the brain need adequate quantities of oxygen to function, so attention to the airway, breathing and circulation always takes priority over an assessment of the head injury itself – however obvious that head injury may be. No further harm must be done to the patient and in particular the cervical spine must be protected at all times.

The principles of initial assessment and resuscitation of an ill or injured person at the scene are dealt with in detail in Chapter 22 of this book, and only a summary is given here. A primary survey is conducted in the standard order of catastrophic external haemorrhage airway (with cervical spine control), breathing (with oxygen), circulation (with haemorrhage control), disability and exposure (with environment control) <C>ABCDE. The top priority is to ensure that the patient has a clear airway – whatever it takes to achieve that – as a blocked airway is one of the first things which will kill a patient (Yates 1977). High-flow oxygen is given, ideally through a trauma mask. If conscious level is impaired an airway adjunct such as an oral airway or an endotracheal tube may be required. Throughout all airway manoeuvres the safety of the cervical spine must be guaranteed by assuming that it is injured and taking appropriate precautions to immobilize it. Breathing is assessed clinically and appropriate measures taken if it is compromised (e.g. decompression of a tension pneumothorax). Blood loss is one of the main causes of avoidable early death after injury (Anderson et al 1988) and the circulation is assessed by simple clinical means and supported by intravenous fluids until the patient reaches hospital.

A balance must always be struck between adequate assessment and resuscitation at the scene and avoiding undue delay in getting the patient to hospital. Unless the patient is trapped or the journey is long, the desirable on-scene time is no more than 10 min (Smith et al 1985). Assessment and resuscitation must of course continue during the journey to hospital. Special points about the transfer of head-injured patients are considered below.

NEUROLOGICAL ASSESSMENT DURING THE PRIMARY SURVEY

Only after these first steps have been completed should an initial assessment be made of 'D for disability', i.e. the patient's neurological condition. During the primary survey this is limited to a brief assessment of conscious level and of pupil equality and reaction to light. At this stage the AVPU system (Table 23.2) is a useful (if crude) tool for measuring conscious level and should be combined with an assessment of pupillary size and reactions.

THE SECONDARY SURVEY: THE NEUROLOGICAL ASSESSMENT

After completing the primary survey and dealing with life-threatening injuries, a secondary survey is conducted systematically from head to toe to look for other injuries. Nearly always, this is completed only after arrival at hospital. A detailed neurological examination forms an important part of the secondary survey. It has three components: assessment of conscious level (Glasgow coma scale); the pupil size and response to light; and a neurological assessment of all four limbs. It is rare for other neurological signs to help in the early management of head injury.

The Glasgow coma scale (GCS) is shown in Table 23.3 (Teasdale & Jennett 1974). It is a sensitive and universally used gold standard for assessing disturbances in conscious level in a standardized way, whatever the cause.

Assessing the conscious level by the GCS provides the earliest warning of neurological deterioration after injury. It measures three independent aspects of conscious level: the eye opening response, the best motor response (in the upper limbs) and the verbal response. Each is stratified and

Table 23.2 The AVPU system for measuring conscious level

A: Alert
V: responds to **V**oice
P: responds to **P**ain
U: Unresponsive

Table 23.3 The Glasgow coma scale

Eye opening response

Spontaneous	4
To speech	3
To pain	2
None	1

Best motor response (in the upper limbs)

Obeys commands	6
Localization to painful stimuli	5
Normal flexion to painful stimuli	4
Spastic flexion to painful stimuli	3
Extension to painful stimuli	2
None	1

Verbal response

Orientated	5
Confused	4
Inappropriate words	3
Incomprehensible sounds	2
None	1

described in words that are carefully chosen so as to be unambiguous. Despite relatively low sensitivity at its upper end, the GCS has undoubted value as a practical and user-friendly scale that reliably detects clinically important changes in conscious level. How to use the GCS is described below.

Pupil size and reaction, and limb responses to commands (in the conscious patient) or painful stimuli (in the unconscious patient), are assessed to detect asymmetry between the right and left sides. Such a finding suggests that there is a focal lesion within the brain such as an expanding haematoma.

USING THE GLASGOW COMA SCALE

There are only four possible eye opening responses. The eyes may already be open spontaneously. If not, they may open to (loud and repeated) requests. If not, they may open to a painful stimulus applied to the ear lobe or supraorbital ridge. Finally, they may not open at all.

Testing the motor response in a conscious patient begins by testing the ability to obey commands: 'Lift your hand up', 'Stick out your tongue', 'Squeeze my fingers'. Beware of misinterpreting a grasp reflex as a positive squeeze of the hand in response to command. If the patient does not obey commands, a painful stimulus is applied to the supraorbital ridge or ear lobe to see whether he can 'localize' to the stimulus by raising an upper limb above the level of the clavicles in the direction of the stimulus. Rubbing the sternum produces an ambiguous motor response and unsightly bruising, and should be avoided. If the patient does not localize, a painful stimulus is applied to a fingernail by pressing a pen or pencil down on to it and assessing the response at the elbow: a rapid and coordinated withdrawal; or a slow and spastic flexion; or extension (the decerebrate response). Finally, there may be no motor response to stimulation at all. It is important to emphasize that the motor response is assessed in the *upper* limbs and that it is the patient's *best* motor response that is recorded.

The verbal response is assessed in a conscious patient by testing orientation: 'Where are you?', 'What is this place?', 'What happened to you?' Asking for a name and address is not an adequate test of orientation. It is important to identify a disorientated or confused patient as soon as possible, as the risk of intracranial complications is statistically much higher than in an orientated patient. Sometimes a patient only says inappropriate words at random (often Anglo-Saxon monosyllables!) or only makes incomprehensible sounds such as groans or screams. Finally, there may be no verbal response at all. In a very young child, a modified system of assessing verbal response has to be used, such as the paediatric coma scale (Simpson & Reilly 1982).

In an individual patient accuracy of recording and clarity of communication demand that conscious level is described in words, using these standardized terms. The conscious level should be described in terms of each component of the GCS, not simply a sum of the constituent parts.

The trend in the patient's conscious level over time is at least as important as the measurement of conscious level at any particular time. Therefore it is essential in a head-injured patient to measure conscious level at frequent intervals, using the GCS, and to record the measurements on a neurological observation chart designed for the purpose. For the first 1–2 h after injury, assessments are made at least every 10 min to establish the trend. If conscious level is deteriorating (or failing to improve from an abnormal level) the cause of this must be sought and corrected. If this is not done the patient is likely to suffer secondary brain damage and have a poorer outcome.

THE SECONDARY SURVEY: LOOKING AT THE INJURIES

A boggy scalp haematoma can reflect an underlying skull fracture. Scalp abrasions and minor lacerations need little attention at the scene but larger lacerations can cause profuse external bleeding and are controlled by external pressure with a gauze dressing (which also helps to keep them clean). Scalp bleeding only rarely causes hypovolaemic shock and it is essential to look for other explanations if the patient is in shock. It is wise to be cautious with scalp wounds, as inspection may not reveal whether the skull has been penetrated or the brain exposed. The wound will be thoroughly cleaned in hospital but should be left undisturbed at the scene in case of further bleeding or damage. An impacted foreign body (e.g. a knife or a building strut) should not be disturbed before the patient reaches hospital. This requirement can pose a challenge to emergency services when they need to cut the patient free and get him/her into the ambulance.

Open and penetrating brain injuries

Most head injuries are 'closed' to the outside world, but some involve skull base fractures or open wounds of the skull vault, through which bacteria can reach the cranial cavity to cause meningitis or a brain abscess. Open wounds are seen more often in war or civil unrest than in normal civilian practice.

Knowing the exact mechanism of injury helps in judging whether the skull (and therefore the brain) is likely to have been penetrated, and this information is particularly important when a weapon may have been used.

SKULL-BASE FRACTURES

A fractured skull base implies that considerable force was applied to the head at the time of injury. The dura and

Table 23.4 Clinical signs of skull-base fracture

- Periorbital bruising and swelling
- Subconjunctival haematoma
- Haemotympanum
- Bruising over the mastoid process (Battle's sign)
- Cerebrospinal fluid leak (often bloodstained) from the nose or ear

the mucosa of adjacent cavities (air sinuses, nasopharynx, middle ear) are likely to be torn. This allows bacteria (usually pneumococci or Gram-negative bacilli) to pass into the cranial cavity and cause meningitis or a brain abscess, often days or weeks after injury.

Table 23.4 illustrates the clinical signs of a skull-base fracture, some of which appear only after a few days. Blood-stained cerebrospinal fluid leaking from the ear is shown in Figure 23.2. No specific action needs to be taken before hospital but if evacuation to hospital is delayed for any reason an appropriate antibiotic may be given as prophylaxis against intracranial infection.

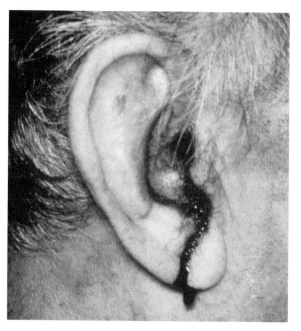

Fig. 23.2 • Blood-stained cerebrospinal fluid leaking from the ear in a base of skull fracture.

DEPRESSED SKULL-VAULT FRACTURE

When the head is struck with a blunt weapon or strikes a protruding object, a piece of the skull vault can break off and be displaced inwards. The dura is often torn and the underlying brain focally contused or lacerated by fragments as they are driven inwards. The overlying scalp wound can be contaminated by hair, dirt or weapon fragments and becomes a portal of entry through which bacteria can penetrate the cranial cavity and (if the dura is torn) the brain itself.

Inspection may reveal bone fragments or even brain tissue in the wound but the wound should not be probed or otherwise disturbed. Treatment before hospital is simply to stop persistent scalp bleeding and to minimize bacterial contamination, and both can be achieved by covering the wound with a dry dressing. If evacuation to hospital is delayed or if there has been heavy wound contamination (e.g. by soil), a broad spectrum antibiotic (e.g. a cephalosporin) should be started. The patient's protection against tetanus is checked at the first opportunity.

A patient with a depressed fracture often has little diffuse brain injury and is conscious but because of focal brain damage may have marked focal neurological signs (e.g. dysphasia, hemiparesis). This type of fracture increases the risk of post-traumatic seizures, which may occur before hospital, and the management of these is discussed below.

STAB WOUNDS OF THE BRAIN

A stab wound of the brain with a knife or other sharp weapon causes a 'slot' fracture of the skull. The overlying wound is easy to underestimate and difficulties in obtaining an accurate history from reluctant witnesses often add to the delay in diagnosis. Whatever the patient's neurological state, an emergency neurosurgical opinion is mandatory if a stab wound of the brain is suspected, as it can be complicated by delayed intracranial haemorrhage from a traumatic false aneurysm as well as by infection (du Trevou et al 1991).

GUNSHOT AND OTHER MISSILE WOUNDS OF THE BRAIN

Low- and high-energy transfer wounds are associated with different patterns of injury. Both lacerate and crush tissue but high-energy transfer wounds also damage tissue extensively by generating shock waves, causing temporary cavitation and sucking contaminated debris into the wound. Bomb and grenade fragments cause high-velocity injuries.

High-energy transfer injuries of the brain carry a high mortality and morbidity (Aldrich et al 1992). Management before hospital is directed at optimizing cardiorespiratory function and monitoring the neurological state by means of the AVPU system and assessment of pupiliary size and reaction described above. The entry and exit wounds (the latter usually much bigger) should be covered and kept clean.

Planning and carrying out transfer to hospital

The principles of transporting injured patients to hospital are described in Chapters 55 and 56. Most of the literature on the hazards of ambulance transfer after a serious head injury relates to journeys between and within hospitals, and from this we know that even short journeys can be potentially hazardous (Gentleman & Jennett 1981, Andrews et al 1990). Taking straightforward precautions can reduce complications and improve outcome (Gentleman & Jennett 1990). There is growing interest in the UK in setting standards to improve the safety of interhospital transfer (Gentleman et al 1993, Munro & Laycock 1993, Joint Working Party on Head Injury Transfer 1996) and very similar principles apply when transporting such patients to hospital from the scene of the accident.

The priority is always to ensure the patient's safety en route as far as possible and this requires that life-threatening injuries are identified and stabilized at the earliest opportunity. In order not to produce unnecessary delays in reaching definitive treatment, although the airway and breathing must always be assessed and stabilized at the scene, support of the circulation can be started en route to hospital if the patient is not trapped and the transport time is not likely to be prolonged.

Throughout the journey to hospital priority must be given to maintaining a clear airway, giving high-flow oxygen, protecting the cervical spine and ensuring adequate breathing and circulation. Experience from interhospital transfer suggests that the risk of secondary brain damage from hypoxia and hypercarbia may be reduced if appropriately trained personnel at the scene can safely intubate and ventilate an unconscious patient (Gentleman 1991). Achieving a stable circulation en route to hospital depends on being able to give enough intravenous fluid to replace blood loss. The patient should have at least one and preferably two reliable, large-bore intravenous lines for crystalloid administration. In a young child, intraosseous infusion is an alternative to the intravenous route. Simple pressure on large external bleeders and splintage of pelvic or limb fractures are important measures but major haemorrhage into the chest or abdomen will inevitably continue until surgically stopped at hospital.

PERSONNEL

Every seriously head-injured patient should be accompanied en route to hospital either by a paramedic or by a doctor called to the scene. In some countries a doctor with intensive care training routinely attends the scene of every major accident and accompanies the patient to hospital but, whoever the escort, that person is professionally responsible for the patient's care during transfer and for ensuring a proper handover to the hospital team.

All paramedics and doctors likely to be involved in transferring seriously head-injured patients to hospital should

have specific training in this area. They should understand the principles of assessing and managing seriously head-injured patients, and the adverse physiological changes associated with moving patients. They also need to know about safe loading and unloading, the practical aspects of working in an ambulance or a helicopter, and the equipment used in transfer.

EQUIPMENT

This is fully dealt with in Chapters 55 and 68. Pulse oximetry at the roadside and en route to hospital gives early warning of desaturation (Finfer & Wishaw 1987, Silverston 1989) but no information about respiration, and can mislead when peripheral perfusion is poor. In a ventilated patient, monitoring end-tidal CO_2 helps to avoid extreme hyper- or hypoventilation, which both reduce cerebral oxygenation. Ideally, blood pressure should be regularly monitored, as palpating the pulse rate and volume is a crude way to monitor the circulation.

INFORMATION TO SEND AT THE TIME OF TRANSFER TO HOSPITAL

The best advice is to send all available information to hospital with the patient, preferably in writing (including any neurological observation chart). Unnecessary delays should not be allowed to result from time spent in the completion of records. The doctor or paramedic should be able to clarify or supplement this and must not leave the emergency department until the doctors and nurses there have been fully briefed. Breakdowns in communication can and do lead to clinical errors.

The staff at hospital need information about patient identification, a succinct mechanism of the injury (including its time), injuries sustained, vital signs and how these have changed over time, what treatment has been given (including drugs), and whether any critical events have occurred at the scene or en route to hospital.

Managing early deterioration after a head injury

Nothing is more frightening at an accident scene or in an ambulance than a head-injured patient whose conscious level is deteriorating in front of one's eyes. Fortunately, halting and reversing this decline is often a straightforward matter. A falling conscious level usually reflects inadequate oxygen delivery to the brain, and each possible reason (Table 23.5) should be considered in turn. If simple measures do not solve the problem, there may be an expanding

Table 23.5 Checklist for action if conscious level deteriorates after a head injury

- Has the oxygen mask slipped?
- Has the airway become obstructed?
- Has the endotracheal tube moved out of position?
- Is there an enlarging pneumothorax?
- Is the patient clinically in shock?
- Is the patient fitting?
- If none of these, consider the possibility of rising intracranial pressure from an intracranial haematoma

intracranial haematoma needing rapid assessment and intervention at hospital. The results of the large CRASH trial have now been published (Roberts et al 2004) clarifying that steroids should have no role in the emergency management of head injuries.

EARLY SEIZURES

A seizure results from a disordered pattern of electro-chemical discharges by damaged or dysfunctional neurones in the cerebral hemispheres. Trauma to the brain increases the risk of fits, especially if there is a haematoma, a penetrating injury or cerebral hypoxia.

Generalized (grand mal) fits are the most common after injury. The loss of consciousness threatens patient safety and airway patency. The limbs jerk convulsively, the tongue may be bitten and swell up, urine is voided and the patient becomes cyanosed with stertorous breathing because of laryngeal spasm. Vomiting and aspiration may also occur.

Managing a convulsing patient goes back to first principles: ensure his/her safety, clear the airway and give high-flow oxygen. Most fits stop spontaneously after 1–2 min. Intravenous lorazepam or diazepam (given either intravenously as Diazemuls, or rectally) should be used only to abort fits that last longer than this, as it can induce respiratory depression. If diazepam is given, the attending doctor or paramedic should be prepared to intervene to support respiration. Phenytoin (unlike diazepam) prevents further fits but is unsuitable for prehospital care, as a loading dose has to be given by very slow intravenous injection under electrocardiogram control (because of cardiotoxicity).

Focal (partial) seizures reflect focal brain pathology (e.g. a haematoma). They cause jerking movements on one side of the body – upper and lower limbs, a single limb or part of a limb. Consciousness may be preserved and the threat to life and function is less than with generalized fits. However, what begins as a focal fit can rapidly become generalized and require the management detailed above.

ANALGESIA AFTER HEAD INJURY

Head-injured patients are often in pain, and this should be alleviated whenever possible. The belief that a head-injured patient should not be given analgesic drugs before assessment at hospital is old-fashioned but dies hard. Good pain relief is far better than leaving untreated pain to raise intracranial pressure and aggravate shock. Anxiety and restlessness are often seen after head injury but it is far better to treat the underlying problem (pain or hypoxia) than to rely upon anxiolytic drugs.

Many head-injured patients have major pelvic or limb fractures and remain conscious. Splinting the fractures can greatly reduce the patient's pain and distress. When an analgesic drug is used, three principles must be followed. First, the dose given should be titrated carefully against the patient's need for analgesia (short-acting drugs have a clear advantage). Second, the dose, timing and route of administration must be clearly recorded, so that those who treat the patient later know what has been given and can interpret the neurological condition accordingly. Third, care must be taken to ensure adequate oxygenation and to support respiratory function, if necessary by intubation and ventilation.

- **Titrate the dose**
- **Record dose, time and route**
- **Ensure oxygenation; support respiration**

Morphine and diamorphine are the drugs of choice when the power of an opioid is required and have the advantage that they are familiar to doctors in primary care. Their euphoric action can also be helpful in a distressed patient. For an adult, the usual starting dose is 5 mg of morphine (or 2.5 mg of diamorphine), given as an intravenous bolus and topped up until the desired analgesic response has been achieved. The synthetic opioid nalbuphine has similar efficacy to morphine but causes less nausea and vomiting. Given in an adult dose of up to 30 mg, it is now used as a standard analgesic in the field by the paramedics of many ambulance services. The most serious complication of all opioids is respiratory depression and it is very important to titrate the dose against the patient's response.

Entonox (an equal mixture of oxygen and nitrous oxide) is carried in many ambulances but is impractical for administration in seriously head-injured patients and can cause enlargement of a pneumothorax or pneumocephalus. It should not be used in head injury except if advised by the hospital.

Soft tissue injuries of the neck

Blunt or penetrating trauma to the neck can injure major structures such as the larynx and trachea, pharynx and oesophagus, carotid and jugular vessels and their branches, vertebral column, cervical spinal cord and nerve roots, and thyroid and lymphoid glands. The airway can be compromised directly or by external compression due to swelling of the traumatized soft tissues or to bleeding into the soft tissues of the neck. Blood loss can be significant enough to cause clinical shock, especially if it is external.

The management of these injuries before hospital is based on the care of the airway and the control of haemorrhage (American College of Surgeons Committee on Trauma 2004).

BLUNT TRAUMA TO THE UPPER AIRWAY

Blunt trauma to the larynx or trachea can threaten the patency of the airway. Laryngeal fractures can cause hoarseness, stridor, tachypnoea and subcutaneous emphysema. Endotracheal intubation should be considered at an early stage in order to protect the airway but if it fails or is not possible a surgical airway may be needed. Before hospital the emphasis is on oxygenation and the preservation as far as possible of a patent airway. Skilled assessment by an anaesthetist at an early stage is essential, then intervention by a head and neck surgeon.

PENETRATING TRAUMA TO THE NECK

Many structures can be damaged by a stab or missile wound of the neck. The extent of the damage may not be immediately obvious when assessing the patient. The wound itself should be left undisturbed before hospital, as should any embedded weapon.

External bleeders should be controlled by pressure, as blood loss can be brisk enough to cause shock. Haemorrhage into the soft tissues of the neck can threaten the airway, and early intubation or a surgical airway may be necessary.

Cervical spine injuries

Other chapters describe the diagnosis and management of injuries to the face (Ch. 24) and cervical spine (Ch. 26), both of which frequently occur in association with head injury. However, it is appropriate in this chapter to consider the prehospital management of suspected or actual injuries to the cervical spine. These are not rare in head-injured patients, they can easily be overlooked when the conscious level is reduced, and the patient's well-being may depend critically upon their safe early management.

The mobility of the cervical spine makes it especially vulnerable to trauma. The thoracic spine is splinted by the ribcage and so is relatively fixed, and cervical spine movement around the fulcrum formed by the cervicothoracic junction commonly causes injury at that level. It is important to remember this point when judging the adequacy or otherwise of cervical spine films.

THE GENERAL APPROACH TO POSSIBLE INJURIES OF THE CERVICAL SPINE

It is vital to have a high index of suspicion for injuries of the cervical spine (American College of Surgeons Committee on Trauma 1997). A useful aphorism is that in patients who have suffered major trauma the neck must be regarded as damaged and unstable until it can be authoritatively shown that it is not. Inevitably the accusation of 'overkill' is levelled against those who advocate this cautious approach, as in the great majority of cases the neck is subsequently shown to be intact and uninjured. However, it is never possible to be sure about this in the early stages of managing a seriously injured person, and once the spinal cord is damaged this is irreversible. No-one who has seen a patient become quadriplegic in hospital because of injudicious neck movement can doubt the wisdom of a policy that errs on the side of caution.

Clearly, there must be sensible limits to this. A patient who has bruised his/her head by stumbling against the corner of a door in his/her own home and who is otherwise well does not need to have the cervical spine immobilized when travelling to hospital. However, it is possible to define three categories of patient who have been shown to have a particularly high risk of cervical spine injury. The first and most obvious is the patient who has symptoms or signs in the neck (pain, stiffness or deformity) or in the limbs (paralysis, weakness, numbness or paraesthesiae). The second is the patient with a significantly altered conscious level, who can be presumed to have sustained a serious head injury and is in no condition to report pain or loss of function. The third is the patient who has suffered trauma involving high-energy transfer (e.g. a high-speed collision or a fall from a height), irrespective of the conscious level or neurological symptoms. Obviously there is a considerable overlap between these three categories.

CLINICAL ASSESSMENT OF THE POTENTIALLY INJURED CERVICAL SPINE

The conscious patient is asked about pain in or around the neck and about neurological symptoms in any part of the upper or lower limbs. In the unconscious patient useful clues to spinal cord injury include limb flaccidity, absence of spontaneous limb movement, loss of anal tone and (occasionally) priapism. If deficits are reported or discovered, they must be fully assessed and documented. A full assessment of motor and sensory function forms part of the secondary survey of every seriously injured patient but this is deferred until after admission to hospital.

If the neck is rotated or laterally flexed, a conscious patient can be asked to move it into the anatomical position but if this cannot be done easily and without pain the position should be accepted, as there may be a unilateral facet joint dislocation between adjacent vertebrae, which will need to be reduced by traction or operation. For the same reason, any attempts to move the neck into the anatomical position in an unconscious patient should be made with caution. Even in skilled hands, the reduction of cervical spine dislocations can be followed by neurological complications (Mahale et al 1993).

Inspection and careful palpation of the back of the neck can elicit soft tissue swelling or bruising (possibly reflecting a haematoma from a bony or ligamentous injury), tenderness over a spinous process or in the paraspinal muscles or a deformity in the alignment of the spinous processes. Occasionally a penetrating wound is found at the back of the neck, raising the question of a penetrating cord injury. Evidence in favour of this includes a complete or partial neurological deficit below the level of the injury or the leakage of CSF from the wound (Peacock et al 1977, Gentleman & Harrington 1984).

IMMOBILIZING THE CERVICAL SPINE

The goal is to prevent movement of the cervical spine until its status can be definitively determined at hospital. One way to immobilize it is to ask someone to place his/her hands on either side of the head and hold it firmly (and without traction) but this is tiring for that person and wasteful of their skills. It is much more practical to immobilize the cervical spine with the combination of a semirigid collar, two sandbags (or equivalent) to wedge the head and broad tape across the forehead and under the chin. Nowadays patients are usually evacuated to hospital on a long spine board with head restraints to substitute for sandbags and straps to replace the need for tape.

The occasional patient is so restless and beyond reason that trying to fix the head and neck to a board is not only impossible but actually dangerous to the cervicothoracic junction. The 'thrasher' may, of course, be hypoxic or in pain and correcting these may solve matters. If not, a possible compromise between safety and practicality is to fit a semirigid collar alone, without sandbags or tape.

Summary

Injuries of the head and neck are common and potentially life-threatening. The first doctor or paramedic on the scene can do much to minimize the danger of further neurological damage. This requires an understanding of the basic physiology of the injured central nervous system, as well as a knowledge of priorities in assessment and treatment and what to do if the patient gets worse before reaching hospital. Equally important, of course, is an awareness of what not to do.

References

Aldrich EF, Eisenberg HM, Saydjari C et al 1992 Predictors of mortality in severely head-injured patients with civilian gunshot wounds: a report from the NIH Traumatic Coma Data Bank. Surgical Neurology 38: 418

American College of Surgeons Committee on Trauma 2004 Advanced trauma life support student manual, 7th edn. American College of Surgeons, Chicago, IL

Anderson ID, Woodford M, de Dombal FT, Irving M 1988 Retrospective study of 1000 deaths from injury in England and Wales. British Medical Journal 296: 1305

Andrews PJD, Piper IR, Dearden M, Miller JD 1990 Secondary insults during intrahospital transfer of head injured patients. Lancet 1: 327

Bower AJ 1990 Plasticity in the adult and neonatal central nervous system. British Journal of Neurosurgery 4: 253

Briggs M, Clarke P, Crockard A et al 1984 Guidelines for initial management after head injury in adults: suggestions from a group of neurosurgeons. British Medical Journal 288: 983

Changaris DG, McGraw CP, Richardson JD et al 1987 Correlation of cerebral perfusion pressure and Glasgow Coma Scale with outcome. Journal of Trauma 27: 1007

Chesnut RM, Marshall LF, Klauber MR et al 1993 The role of secondary brain injury in determining outcome from severe head injury. Journal of Trauma 34: 216

Cold GE, Jensen FT 1978 Cerebral autoregulation in unconscious patients with brain injury. Acta Anaesthesiologica Scandinavica 22: 270

Du Trevou M, Bullock R, Teasdale E, Quin RO 1991 False aneurysms of the carotid tree due to unsuspected penetrating injury of the head and neck. Injury 22: 237

Faden AI, Demediuk P, Panter SS, Vink R 1989 The role of excitatory amino-acids and NMDA receptors in traumatic brain injury. Science 244: 798

Finfer S, Wishaw KJ 1987 Oximetry during transport. Anaesthesia 42: 900

Garland DE, Bailey S 1981 Undetected injuries in head-injured adults. Clinical Orthopaedics and Related Research 155: 162

Gentleman D 1990 Preventing secondary brain damage after head injury: a multidisciplinary challenge. Injury 21: 305

Gentleman D 1991 Transfer-associated hypoxia after severe head injury: the protective role of intubation and ventilation. Injury 22: 250

Gentleman D 1992 Causes and effects of systemic complications among severely head-injured patients transferred to a neurosurgical unit. International Surgery 77: 297

Gentleman D 1994 Growth and repair after injury of the central nervous system: yesterday, today, and tomorrow. Injury 25: 571

Gentleman D 1995 Immediate care after a serious head injury. Journal of the British Association for Immediate Care 18: 14

Gentleman D, Harrington M 1984 Penetrating injury of the spinal cord. Injury 16: 7

Gentleman D, Jennett B 1981 Hazards of inter-hospital transfer of comatose head-injured patients. Lancet 2: 853

Gentleman D, Jennett B 1990 Audit of the transfer of unconscious head-injured patients to a neurosurgical unit. Lancet 335: 330

Gentleman D, Teasdale G, Murray L 1986 Cause of severe head injury and risk of complications. British Medical Journal 292: 449

Gentleman D, Dearden M, Midgley S, Maclean D 1993 Guidelines for resuscitation and transfer of patients with serious head injury. British Medical Journal 307: 547

Goldstein M 1990 Traumatic brain injury: a silent epidemic. Annals of Neurology 27: 327

Hills MW, Deane SA 1993 Head injury and facial injury: is there an increased risk of cervical spine injury? Journal of Trauma 34: 549

Ishige N, Pitts LH, Hashimoto T et al 1987 Effect of hypoxia on traumatic brain injury in rats. Neurosurgery 20: 848

Jennett B, McMillan R 1981 Epidemiology of head injury. British Medical Journal 282: 101

Joint Working Party on Head Injury Transfer 1996 Recommendations for the transfer of emergency head-injured patients to neurosurgical centres. Association of Anaesthetists of Great Britain and Ireland, London

Jones PA, Andrews PJ, Midgley S et al 1994 Measuring the burden of secondary insults in head-injured patients during intensive care. Journal of Neurosurgical Anesthesiology 6: 4

Kraus JF 1987 Epidemiology of head injury. In: Cooper PR (ed) Head injury, 2nd edn. Williams & Wilkins, Baltimore, MD, pp 1–19

Lambert SM, Willett K 1993 Transfer of multiply injured patients for neurosurgical opinion: a study of the adequacy of assessment and resuscitation. Injury 24: 333

McLaren CAN, Robertson C, Little K 1983 Missed orthopaedic injuries in the resuscitation room. Journal of the Royal College of Surgeons of Edinburgh 28: 399

Mahale YJ, Silver JR, Henderson NJ 1993 Neurological complications of the reduction of cervical spine dislocations. Journal of Bone and Joint Surgery 75B: 403

Miller JD, Becker DP 1982 Secondary insults to the injured brain. Journal of the Royal College of Surgeons of Edinburgh 27: 292

Munro HM, Laycock JRD 1993 Inter-hospital transfer: standards for ventilated neurosurgical emergencies. British Journal of Intensive Care 3: 210

Peacock WJ, Shrosbree RD, Key AG 1977 A review of 450 stab wounds of the spinal cord. South African Medical Journal 51: 961

Reilly PL, Adams JH, Graham DI, Jennett B 1975 Patients with head injury who talk and die. Lancet 2: 375

Roberts I, Yates D, Sandercock P et al, CRASH trial collaborators 2004 Effect of intravenous corticosteroids on death within 14 days in 10008 adults with clinically significant head injury (MRC CRASH trial): randomised placebo-controlled trial. Lancet 364: 1321–1328

Ryan M, Klein S, Bongard F 1993 Missed injuries associated with spinal cord trauma. American Surgeon 59: 371

Silverston PP 1989 Pulse oximetry at the roadside: a study of pulse oximetry in immediate care. British Medical Journal 299: 711

Simpson D, Reilly P 1982 Paediatric coma scale. Lancet 2: 450

Smith JP, Bodai BI, Siefkin AD et al 1985 Pre-hospital stabilisation of critically injured patients: a failed concept. Journal of Trauma 25: 65

Teasdale G, Jennett B 1974 Assessment of coma and impaired consciousness. Lancet 2: 81

Teasdale G, Murray G, Anderson E et al 1990 Risks of acute traumatic intracranial haematoma in children and adults: implications for managing head injuries. British Medical Journal 300: 363

Teasdale G, Galbraith S, Murray L 1982 Management of traumatic intracranial haematomas. British Medical Journal 285: 1695

Williams J, Jehle D, Cottington E, Schufflebarger C 1992 Head, facial and clavicular trauma as a predictor of cervical spine injury. Annals of Emergency Medicine 21: 719

Yates DW 1977 Airway patency in fatal accidents. British Medical Journal 297: 1419

Maxillofacial injuries

24

Introduction 272

Mechanism of injury 272

Classification of injury 273

Dental injuries 274

Eye injuries 274

Immediate management of airway and
haemorrhage 274

Airway management 274

Trismus and dislocation of the lower jaw 276

References 276

Further reading 276

Introduction

Maxillofacial injuries are usually considered during the secondary survey, when a detailed examination of the head and neck region is an integral part of the management of the patient. Although not always life-threatening these injuries may be serious if they cause airway obstruction or haemorrhage and should then be managed as part of the primary survey. Cannell et al (1996) suggested that there is underscoring of the contribution of maxillofacial injuries in total injury assessments.

Haemorrhage in the maxillofacial region may be sufficiently severe to result in hypovolaemic shock. It may also be responsible for airway obstruction and should be managed under A of the primary survey.

The prehospital management of maxillofacial injuries may therefore be considered in two groups:

- life-threatening injuries producing airway obstruction and severe haemorrhage
- injuries requiring no specific prehospital care that are treated by the maxillofacial surgeon after arrival in hospital.

Mechanism of injury

An essential part of the immediate management of the trauma patient is an accurate history of events. This includes details of the injury-producing mechanism. Injury to the facial region may be caused by the same mechanisms as injury elsewhere. The most common are:

- blunt trauma
- penetrating trauma
- burns.

Telfer et al (1991) published a survey of trends in the aetiology of maxillofacial fractures in the UK. The survey showed an increase in the overall numbers of patients with maxillofacial injuries although the numbers with severe injuries were decreasing. The main causes in all countries are road traffic accidents, assaults, falls and sports injuries. Although road traffic accidents remain a significant cause of facial injury in the UK, legislation affecting drink-driving and the compulsory wearing of seat belts has produced a decrease in facial injuries. Perkins & Layton (1988) demonstrated a fall in the number of front-seat occupants with maxillofacial trauma from 21% prior to seat-belt legislation to 6% after legislation.

Telfer et al (1991) suggest that two factors are implicated in the increase in facial fractures due to interpersonnel assault – alcohol and unemployment – and showed an increase of 47% in patients injured this way. This contrasted with a fall of 34% in the number of patients injured in road traffic accidents.

Maxillofacial injuries may occur in isolation or as one of a number of injuries. A number of familiar patterns of injury can be identified according to the direction of impact. In particular, an isolated zygomatic (malar) bone fracture is commonly seen on the left side because the majority of assailants are right-handed. Drivers of vehicles are likely to sustain facial injuries in conjunction with one of the common injury patterns.

Classification of injury

Maxillofacial injuries may be divided into those involving the soft tissue and those affecting the hard tissues (teeth and bone). Injuries to the eye will be considered separately.

SOFT-TISSUE INJURY

The face and scalp are well perfused with significant crossover of the arterial supply, with the result that soft-tissue injuries may bleed profusely. The main vessel supplying the face is the facial artery, which is a branch of the external carotid artery. The scalp is supplied by branches of the internal and external carotid arteries. Injuries include superficial cuts and abrasions, lacerations and penetrating wounds. There may also be significant tissue loss. When examining the facial region the mouth should always be examined for injury to the soft tissues. Even a small cut to the oral mucosa can cause severe bleeding and lead to airway obstruction. Degloving injuries may occur (e.g. in the lower labial sulcus when the skin over the chin is forcibly pushed backwards).

HARD-TISSUE INJURY

1. Mandible:
   a. Condyle
   b. Coronoid
   c. Ramus
   d. Angle
   e. Body
   f. Parasymphysis
   g. Symphysis
   h. Dento-alveolar (Fig. 24.1).

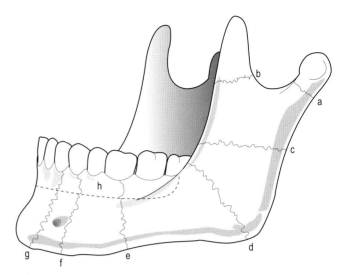

Fig. 24.1 • Mandibular fractures: (a) condyle; (b) coronoid; (c) ramus; (d) angle; (e) body; (f) parasymphysis; (g) symphysis; and (h) dento-alveolar.

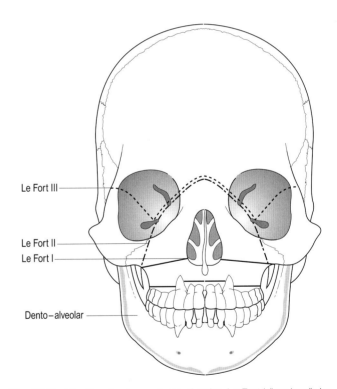

Fig. 24.2 • Maxillary fractures: dento-alveolar; Le Fort I (low level); Le Fort II (pyramidal); and Le Fort III (high level).

2. Maxilla:
   a. Dento-alveolar
   b. Le Fort I (low level)
   c. Le Fort II (pyramidal)
   d. Le Fort III (high level) (Fig. 24.2).
3. Nasal complex.

4. Zygomatico-orbital.

5. Frontal:
   a. Isolated
   b. Associated fractures.

Dental injuries

- Avulsion
- Subluxation
- Fracture.

Subluxed or avulsed teeth can be inhaled and cause airway obstruction or lung collapse. Dentures that have fractured or are poorly fitting can also be inhaled, especially in patients with a decreased level of consciousness.

During the primary survey it is therefore essential to examine the mouth and if necessary perform a finger sweep to remove foreign bodies. Suction using a wide-bore sucker (Yankauer) is useful. Well-fitting dentures may be left in situ as they may aid ventilation using a facemask.

In a patient without a head injury, a completely avulsed tooth (usually a front tooth in a child) can be reinserted immediately. The patient can be asked to hold the tooth in place until definitive splinting can be achieved. Alternatively, the tooth can be placed into a container of milk and taken with the patient to hospital.

Patients with a head injury are at particular risk from inhalation of a foreign body and it may be advisable to reinsert the tooth in hospital where immediate fixation is possible. In the past it has been suggested that the tooth could be transported in the patient's buccal sulcus but this is absolutely contraindicated in a patient with a decreased level of consciousness.

If the tooth is fractured all the pieces should be found and taken with the patient to hospital. A chest radiograph is essential if there is any suspicion of a missing fragment.

Eye injuries

Ocular injuries commonly occur in patients with facial fractures. Al-Qurainy et al (1991), in a prospective study of 363 patients who had sustained midfacial trauma sufficient to lead to a fracture, studied the characteristics of the eye injuries in relation to the aetiology and type of fracture. 90% of patients sustained ocular injuries of various severities. 63% of patients had minor or transient ocular injuries, 16% suffered moderately severe ocular injury and 12% sustained severe eye damage. Road traffic accidents were associated with the highest incidence of severe ocular disorder, while assaults had the second highest incidence at 11%. Decrease in visual acuity was the main clinical finding accompanying the majority of significant eye injuries.

In the prehospital environment patients with significant eye injuries should simply be transferred as rapidly as possible to hospital. Any penetrating foreign body should be left in place.

Immediate management of airway and haemorrhage

Profuse bleeding from facial and scalp wounds should be arrested during the primary survey. Pressure applied directly to the wound using a gauze swab is usually sufficient. Failing this, insertion of large stitches across the bleeding area or inversion of the bleeding scalp edge may be effective. Penetrating wounds should not be explored, and neck wounds should be covered and managed definitively in hospital, where arteriography may be necessary. Foreign bodies should be left in place unless they involve the cheek. These may be removed to allow haemorrhage to be controlled by direct pressure from inside and outside the mouth. During the secondary survey a thorough examination of the face and scalp should be made and all wounds recorded. These may be cleaned with chlorhexidine gluconate 0.05% and covered with a gauze dressing.

Airway management

Maxillofacial injuries may compromise the airway in a number of ways and it is essential that these are considered during the primary survey.

INHALATION OF FOREIGN BODIES

A full intraoral examination of the mouth may reveal loose fragments of teeth or bone. The patient may vomit or there may be a broken denture. Finger sweep of the mouth and thorough suction using a wide-bore sucker is necessary to clear the airway.

HAEMORRHAGE

The tissues of the mouth bleed profusely even with just a small cut of the mucosa. Once again, a full mouth examination and careful suction will relieve airway obstruction from inhaled blood. If the patient is sufficiently conscious, intraoral bleeding from a tooth socket can be controlled by rolling up a piece of gauze, placing it over the bleeding point and asking the patient to bite firmly down. Most other areas of bleeding can be controlled by direct pressure.

Profuse haemorrhage can result from damage to the terminal branches of the maxillary artery associated with a

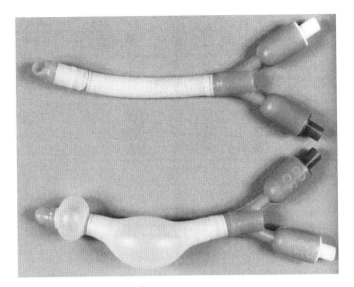

Fig. 24.3 • Nasal Epistats®.

maxillary fracture, as well as from the anterior and posterior ethmoidal arteries. Bleeding can be so massive as to produce not only respiratory obstruction but also significant hypovolaemia. Nasal Epistats® (Fig. 24.3) are particularly easy to use and effective in the control of haemorrhage from the nose.

Cannell et al (1993) have described the use of Nasal Epistats® and have demonstrated their effectiveness in controlling maxillofacial bleeding. Other techniques include anterior and posterior nasal packing using ribbon gauze soaked in a vasoconstrictor and an inflated Foley catheter. In the absence of a maxillary fracture, nasal bleeding can be controlled with expanding Merocel foam packs or tampons inserted into the nostrils.

Ultimately, in the presence of severe nasal or oral haemorrhage, the only guaranteed method of achieving a secure protected airway is endotracheal intubation. If this is not practical, nursing the patient face down in order to allow drainage of blood away from the airway may be life-saving. Patients with severe facial injuries who are sitting upright and forwards should never be compelled to lie down, as this may result in fatal airway obstruction.

INTRAORAL SWELLING

Oral tissues can swell rapidly following injury and cause airway obstruction. Insertion of an oropharyngeal airway, nasopharyngeal airway or endotracheal tube in the unconscious patient may be necessary.

LOSS OF TONGUE CONTROL IN A FRACTURED MANDIBLE

Fractures of the mandible may be either unilateral or bilateral, and occur in recognizable patterns. A blow to the left side of the jaw may produce a left-angle fracture and a right-condylar neck fracture. Similarly, a fall on to the chin may cause a midline fracture and bilateral condylar neck fractures ('guardsman's fracture').

In a patient who is able to maintain his/her own airway, fractures of the mandible are not usually life-threatening. Problems can arise, however, in head-injured patients or those who are intoxicated and are unable to maintain their own airway. Severe comminution of the mandible or bilateral fractures producing an unstable mandible are of particular concern. The muscles of the tongue are attached to the genial tubercles in the midline of the jaw on the lingual aspect. Any mandibular fracture leaving this segment free may allow the tongue to fall backwards, impinging on the posterior wall of the pharynx and causing obstruction. Immediate management should be to pull the tongue forward, either manually or by passing a large suture (0 gauge black silk) transversely through the dorsum of the tongue. A large safety pin may be used and a thread attached to it. The tongue should be pulled into an unobstructed position and the suture taped to the side of the face.

POSTERIOR IMPACTION OF THE FRACTURED MAXILLA

The maxilla articulates with the base of the skull along an inclined plane directed downwards and backwards. Trauma to the midface of sufficient force to produce a Le Fort fracture (at any level) may move the maxilla along the inclined plane and result in airway obstruction as the soft palate impinges on the posterior wall of the pharynx. Immediate management of this potentially life-threatening situation involves inserting the index and middle fingers of a gloved hand into the mouth and hooking them behind the soft palate. The maxilla is then pulled forward to disimpact it.

DIRECT TRAUMA TO THE LARYNX

Any injury involving the neck must be examined carefully and any bruising or stiffness, particularly with pain, must be taken seriously. Laryngeal or tracheal injury may be suspected if the patient has a hoarse voice, dyspnoea or neck swelling. Airway obstruction can occur if there is swelling and displacement of the vocal cords or epiglottis. Unless airway obstruction is complete or rapidly progressive, the majority of these patients should be transferred rapidly to hospital for definitive management. In the unconscious patient who requires intervention, intubation may be attempted. This may not be possible, especially if complete transection has occurred. If intubation cannot be achieved a surgical airway is the only other option.

Trismus and dislocation of the lower jaw

The word trismus is derived from the Greek *trismos* meaning gnashing. It is defined as a prolonged, tetanic spasm of the jaw muscles resulting in restricted jaw opening (locked jaw). Normal adult mouth opening is in the range 35–50 mm, measured between the incisor teeth. Patients presenting with trismus may complain of an inability to open their mouth or difficulty with speech and eating. Management of a patient complaining of difficulty in opening the mouth starts with a full history to determine how long the trismus has been present. There may be a clear event such as trauma to the jaw or the onset may be more chronic.

Examination of the patient to determine the degree of opening between the upper central and lower central incisors will indicate the severity of the trismus. The temporomandibular joint should be palpated to elicit any tenderness or swelling (particularly in the pre-auricular region). If there has been a history of trauma to the face a full maxillofacial examination will be essential in order to exclude any mandibular fractures. Traumatic (acute) causes of trismus following mandibular injuries may be due to a fracture in the condylar region resulting in mechanical obstruction or fractures elsewhere leading to guarding by the patient. Fractures of the zygomaticomaxillary complex may produce restricted jaw opening by direct impingement on the coronoid process. Haematomas in the muscles of mastication (perhaps following a recent local anaesthetic infiltration) can produce trismus and postsurgical causes (after third molar extraction) are common.

Dislocation of the condylar head from the fossa may occur following trauma or simply after yawning widely. The patient may present with his/her mouth fixed open, unable to speak, in some considerable pain and drooling saliva. Reduction of the dislocation, which may be unilateral or bilateral, depends on how relaxed the patient can be made and the length of time following the dislocation.

If sedation is required, reduction should take place in hospital. Reduction is achieved by seating the patient in a low chair with the clinician standing in front. Both thumbs are placed on the posterior lower teeth (or bony ridges in an edentulous patient) and pressure is applied in a downward and backward direction. A successful manoeuvre produces instant relief for the patient and the clinician can readily feel the jaw go back into its correct position.

Inability to open the mouth due to muscle spasm is a relatively common finding in head-injured patients. It may settle following oxygenation with a mask and a nasopharyngeal airway. Concern regarding intracranial placement of a nasal airway in the presence of a risk of basal skull fracture should not be allowed to prevent the insertion of such an airway in these patients. The only other options are rapid transfer to hospital, rapid sequence induction of anaesthesia or a surgical airway.

Inability to open the mouth due to muscle spasm is a relatively common finding in head-injured patients.

References

Al-Qurainy A, Strassen LFA, Dutton GN et al 1991 The characteristics of mid-facial fractures and the association with ocular injury: a prospective study. British Journal of Oral and Maxillofacial Surgery 29: 291–301

Cannell H, Paterson A, Loukota R 1996 Maxillofacial injuries in multiply injured patients. British Journal of Oral and Maxillofacial Surgery 34: 303–308

Cannell H, Silvester KC, O'Regan MB 1993 Early management of multiply injured patients with maxillofacial injuries transferred to hospital by helicopter. British Journal of Oral and Maxillofacial Surgery 31: 207–212

Perkins CS, Layton SA 1988 The aetiology of maxillofacial injuries and the seat belt law. British Journal of Oral and Maxillofacial Surgery 26: 353

Telfer MR, Jones GM, Shepherd JP 1991 Trends in the aetiology of maxillofacial fractures in the United Kingdom (1977–1987). British Journal of Oral and Maxillofacial Surgery 29: 250–255

Further reading

American College of Surgeons Committee on Trauma 2004 Advanced trauma life support for doctors. Student course manual, 7th edn. American College of Surgeons, Chicago, IL

Association for the Advancement of Automotive Medicine 1990 Abbreviated injury scale booklet, (AIS 90 revision). Association for the Advancement of Automotive Medicine, Des Plaines, IL

Chable injuries

25

Introduction   277

Anatomy   277

Respiratory pathophysiology   278

Mechanism of injury   279

Examination   280

Examination of the chest   280

Other injuries   283

Practical procedures   285

Analgesia   288

References   289

Introduction

Injuries to the thorax are responsible for 25% of all trauma deaths, usually as a result of acute tissue hypoxia or hypovolaemia. However, only 15% require operative intervention by a thoracic surgeon (McSwain 1992). Most of the rest can be managed by maintaining adequate oxygenation and perfusion. As a result, it is extremely important that thoracic injuries are recognized and managed, with early assessment and treatment of the problems that require expert help.

Anatomy

The trachea commences below the cricoid cartilage and continues to the carina, at the level of the sternal angle (second rib), where it divides to form the right and left main bronchi. The trachea is a tube measuring 2.5 cm in diameter, made of fibrocartilage strengthened by incomplete cartilaginous rings and lined by mucous membrane. As the right main bronchus lies more vertical than the left, foreign bodies are more likely to enter the right-hand side. The bronchial tree continues to divide into smaller and smaller branches until the respiratory bronchioles are formed.

The respiratory bronchioles, as well as the alveoli and ducts they give rise to, are known as the respiratory portion of the lung. This is the only part of the lungs where oxygen is taken up from the inspired air and carbon dioxide released from the blood. Gas exchange by diffusion is facilitated by the extremely thin and closely applied walls of the airway and blood vessels and the extremely large surface area.

The lungs and chest wall are both lined by pleura. The potential cavity between these layers is known as the intrapleural space. Both the lung and chest wall contain elastic tissues, which pull in opposite directions. Consequently, the chest wall is continually trying to open out, whereas the lungs are trying to collapse. The interface between these two opposing forces results in a negative pressure in the intrapleural space. This stretches the lungs so that their outer surfaces are closely applied to the chest wall.

During inspiration the intercostal muscles contract, causing the ribs to move upward and outward. Simultaneously the diaphragm contracts and moves downwards. This increases the intrathoracic volume and hence the intrapleural pressure falls further. As a result the lungs are further stretched and air is drawn into them. The opposite process occurs in expiration.

If there is an opening in the lung or chest wall, air is sucked into the intrapleural space, causing a pneumothorax. The lung elasticity will now be unopposed and the lung will collapse. In this situation gas exchange is markedly impaired because of the decrease in the surface area of the respiratory portion of the lung and a fall in perfusion of this area.

As the pleural cavity and lung projects above the clavicle, and below the 12th rib, penetrating injuries to the neck or lower back may result in a pneumothorax. During expiration the diaphragm is elevated and the lower seven ribs lie over the abdominal cavity. Consequently a penetrating wound between the nipple line (fifth rib in males) and the costal margin can result in both abdominal and chest injury.

The trachea, oesophagus, heart and major blood vessels lie in close proximity in the centre of the chest and are collectively known as the mediastinum. The heart is covered by the pericardium, which is a tough inelastic fibrous sac.

Respiratory pathophysiology

The main function of the lungs is oxygen uptake and carbon dioxide elimination. To achieve this, oxygen must flow into the alveoli (ventilation), blood must flow to the pulmonary capillaries (perfusion), and oxygen (O_2) and carbon dioxide (CO_2) must diffuse between the alveoli and the pulmonary capillaries. The balance between ventilation and perfusion must also be correct. Impairment of any of these processes will lead to a low level of oxygen in the blood (hypoxia) and a high level of carbon dioxide in the blood (hypercapnia).

VENTILATION

The tidal volume is the amount of air taken into the chest with each breath. It is normally equal to $7-8\,ml\,kg^{-1}$ (or 500 ml in a 70 kg patient at rest). The minute volume is the volume of air inspired each minute, and can be calculated by multiplying the tidal volume by the respiratory rate. Normally this is approximately $5\,l\,min^{-1}$ for a 70 kg patient at rest.

Only 70% (350 ml) of each tidal volume reaches a point distal to the terminal bronchioles where gas exchange occurs. The remaining 150 ml fills the airway proximal to this point and therefore is not involved in gas transfer. This is known as the *anatomical dead space*. Failure of gas transfer also occurs in the areas of the lung that are ventilated but not perfused with blood. When these areas are added to the anatomical dead space, a volume known as the *physiological dead space* is produced. In healthy individuals

the anatomical and physiological dead spaces are approximately equal, as ventilation and perfusion are well matched.

PULMONARY PERFUSION

The cardiac output of the right ventricle passes through the pulmonary circulation. As the pressures in the pulmonary circulation are much lower than in the systemic circulation, there are differences in blood flow between the apex and base of the lung. Apical alveoli are relatively poorly perfused, giving rise to dead space, whereas basal alveoli are over perfused. Discrepancy between ventilation and perfusion leads to some blood not having the chance to eliminate its CO_2 and take up O_2. This blood is termed 'shunted' blood. In the healthy patient this effect is minimized by hypoxic pulmonary vasoconstriction, which diverts blood from poorly ventilated (hypoxic) areas to alveoli that are better ventilated.

DIFFUSION

Gas exchange between the alveoli and blood across the pulmonary or respiratory membrane occurs as a result of passive diffusion (Table 25.1).

Gases move from areas of high to low partial pressure. Blood entering the pulmonary capillaries has a partial pressure of oxygen (Po_2) of 40 mmHg. In contrast, the partial pressure (Po_2) in the alveoli is 100 mmHg. Consequently, oxygen rapidly diffuses from the alveoli into the blood. If the gradient is reduced (e.g. by breathing a hypoxic mixture) the partial pressure of oxygen falls and diffusion is reduced.

The partial pressure of CO_2 in the pulmonary capillary blood is 45 mmHg and in the alveoli is 40 mmHg. This is much smaller than the gradient for oxygen but the rate of diffusion is made up for by the fact that CO_2 is 20 times more soluble than O_2. In the healthy state it takes approximately the same time for O_2 and CO_2 exchange to occur.

The lung is ideally suited for diffusion as the surface area of the pulmonary membrane is large but extremely thin. Reduction in the surface area (e.g. from a pneumothorax) or an increase in thickness (e.g. from fluid in the alveoli) will reduce gas exchange. The rate of diffusion will also fall if the concentration of oxygen (or, more accurately, the Po_2) in the alveoli falls, either as a result of decreased ventilation or a lowering in the inspired oxygen concentration.

Table 25.1 Factors affecting gas exchange between alveoli and blood

- Partial pressure gradient of the gas
- Solubility
- Barrier surface area
- Barrier thickness

In the trauma situation abnormalities are seen in ventilation, perfusion and diffusion in conditions such as pulmonary contusion. The permeability of the small pulmonary capillaries increases, leading to oedema in the alveoli and surrounding tissues. This increased permeability is worsened by an associated hypoxia. As the lungs become stiffer, the effort required to inflate the lungs increases and the tidal volume decreases. The respiratory rate initially increases in an attempt to maintain alveolar ventilation. As the patient becomes exhausted, the respiratory rate falls and ventilation is reduced, leading to progressive hypoxia. Mismatch in ventilation and perfusion of the lung also makes a major contribution to hypoxia (for a further explanation of this, see West 1990).

Mechanism of injury

Optimal care of the trauma patient is dependent on early identification of all injuries, so that treatment can be started before deterioration occurs. However, even with good assessment many injuries may be missed if the index of suspicion is not high. An accurate history, correctly interpreted, allows for the prediction of more than 90% of the patient's potential injuries (McSwain 1992), even before a hand has been laid on the patient. The history should be thought of in three phases (National Association of Emergency Medical Technicians 2003):

- pre-incident
- incident
- postincident.

Important factors in the pre-incident phase include ingestion of alcohol, pre-existing medical conditions and the mental state of the patient. The most important information obtained is that regarding the incident itself. This process of assessing the accident scene and mechanism of injury in order to predict injuries is known as 'reading the wreckage'. For instance, by inspection of a road traffic accident it is possible to assess who hit what and where, and to estimate, with the help of any witnesses, what speed the vehicles were travelling at and the stopping time. Inspection of the vehicle will indicate whether the patient was restrained by a seat belt and whether an airbag was activated. The damage caused to the vehicle will also help in

the prediction of the exact injuries to the patient (Fox et al 1991). The postincident phase starts from the moment of impact, as events during this period will influence the prognosis for the patient (Table 25.2).

BLUNT TRAUMA TO THE CHEST

The two forces commonly involved are shear (due to the change in speed) and compression. In a road traffic accident the driver of the car often suffers a blunt chest injury as the chest impacts the steering column. On impact the sternum will stop moving but the intrathoracic organs and the posterior thoracic wall will continue to move forward. The descending aorta is fixed to the posterior thoracic wall, whereas the heart and ascending aorta are relatively free to move. The resulting difference in rate of deceleration causes a shearing force, which may lead to tearing at the junction between the arch and the descending aorta. Similar shearing forces can occur between the relatively fixed trachea and the more mobile main bronchi and lungs. Compression of the chest wall is common in frontal and lateral impacts and may produce rib fractures or even a flail chest. In frontal impacts the front of the car often bends and is compressed as it stops suddenly (Fig. 25.1). The rear of the car may continue to move forward, forcing the driver into the steering column. Pulmonary and cardiac contusions can also result from this mechanism, as may injuries to intra-abdominal organs.

Rotational impact collisions tend to result in injuries that are a combination of those seen in frontal and lateral impacts. In the case of the roll-over of a vehicle, it is very difficult to predict injuries. Patients ejected from a vehicle sustain two impacts; the initial one and a second with the ground or other object outside the vehicle.

Ejected patients are six times more likely to sustain fatal injuries than non-ejected patients.

Table 25.2 Scene assessment
- Talk to witnesses
- Position of vehicles
- Speed and direction of impact
- Damage to vehicles
- Seat belt, head rest, airbag

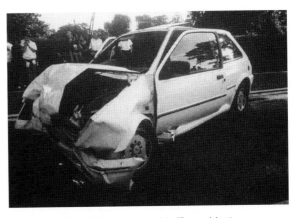

Fig. 25.1 • A frontal impact road traffic accident.

Pedestrians struck by a car may sustain severe chest and abdominal injuries. The bumper usually strikes the lower legs, which are driven out from under the pelvis and torso, so that the chest and abdomen impact with the bonnet.

Victims of falls commonly suffer multiple injuries, the nature of which is dependent on which part of the body hits the ground first. The severity of injury depends on the height of the fall and the type of surface the victim landed on. Falls from more than three times the height of the victim generally result in serious injuries.

BLAST INJURIES

Blast injuries to the respiratory system are discussed in detail in Chapter 30. In general, the primary effects of blast on the lung include alveolar haemorrhage with consolidation, acute pulmonary oedema, pneumothorax, haemopneumothorax and pneumomediastinum. Secondary effects due to the impact of fragments are associated with penetrating injuries, and tertiary injuries result from displacement of the body.

PENETRATING INJURIES

Damage caused by a penetrating injury is dependent on the energy of the weapon or object. Low-energy weapons, including knives and other sharp instruments, cause damage by the sharp edge of the instrument, with little secondary trauma. The significance of the injury will depend on the structures involved. Injuries can be predicted from the path of the instrument through the body. If the weapon is still in place, it should not be removed. If the instrument has been removed, attempts should be made to find out its nature in order to assist with the prediction of possible injuries. It should always be remembered that such weapons are of forensic significance and are best handled by the police.

It must be remembered that the knife may have been moved around inside the victim and therefore any structures within reach of the knife may have been damaged. It must also be remembered that the diaphragm reaches the level of the nipples on deep inspiration; therefore a stab wound to the lower chest will involve both intra-abdominal and intrathoracic organs in 75% of cases. Similarly, a stab wound to the upper abdomen may have damaged intrathoracic organs. Central wounds, defined as lying between the midclavicular lines and the clavicles and sternal notch superiorly and the costal margin inferiorly, both front and back, tend to inflict severe injuries often requiring surgical intervention. This is because of the vital organs situated in this region. Organs particularly at risk include the heart and great vessels, trachea and mainstem bronchi, oesophagus and spinal cord, and intra-abdominal organs such as

the liver, spleen, pancreas and stomach, and major vascular structures. All patients with penetrating chest injuries should be rapidly transported to hospital. Intravenous access and fluid administration should take place en route to hospital.

If you find one stab wound, look for another!

Gunshot wounds to the chest are fortunately still rare in the UK. The majority (85%) of thoracic bullet wounds will not require operative intervention. Wounds to the lungs are often through-and-through injuries and may involve relatively little tissue damage even with high-energy missiles. Clearly, any missile striking bone or parts of the mediastinum will be associated with greater destruction. Thus, a major predictor of the severity of a missile injury is the distribution of organs involved. In the prehospital environment, management is restricted to careful attention to the primary survey priorities and, in particular, the insertion of intercostal drains if any life-threatening chest injury is present or ventilation is to be carried out. The small number of patients who will clearly require urgent thoracotomy should be transferred to hospital without delay.

Examination

The primary survey is a rapid assessment of <C>ABCDE to detect and correct any immediately life-threatening conditions (Ch. 22).

The airway must be assessed, cleared and secured while maintaining cervical in-line stabilization (Ch. 4). All patients with chest injuries have an increased oxygen demand and therefore require a high inspired oxygen concentration.

Examination of the neck can be difficult once the cervical collar is fitted. It is therefore advisable that those factors indicative of chest trauma are detected before the collar is applied.

Examination of the chest

The chest should be inspected for bruising, penetrating wounds, intercostal or supraclavicular indrawing and abnormal chest movements. This requires clothing to be removed, even though this may prove difficult in certain trapped patients. The breathing rate and volume should be noted, as rapid shallow ventilation occurs in chest injury as

Table 25.3 Examination of the chest

- Look
- Feel
- Percuss
- Listen
- Check back

Table 25.4 Immediately life-threatening conditions of the chest

- Tension pneumothorax
- Open pneumothorax
- Flail chest
- Cardiac tamponade
- Massive haemothorax

Table 25.5 Signs of a tension pneumothorax

- Tachypnoea
- Shock
- Hyperresonant hemithorax
- Decreased air entry to hemithorax
- Tracheal deviation (late)
- Raised jugular venous pressure (JVP) (if no hypovolaemia)
- Cyanosis (late)

well as developing hypoxia. The chest should then be palpated for tenderness, crepitus and surgical emphysema, and assessed for equality of chest movement. Auscultation and percussion are often extremely difficult in the prehospital environment because of noise levels. When possible, they help to determine whether pneumothorax (resonance and decreased air entry) or haemothorax (dullness and decreased air entry), or a combination of the two, is present. Although access may be difficult, it is important to check the patient's back, particularly in the case of penetrating trauma, as life-threatening wounds may otherwise be undetected (Table 25.3).

A rapid assessment of the patient's colour and capillary refill time, as well as the presence of carotid, femoral and radial pulses, needs to be carried out. At least one intravenous peripheral line (14–16G) should be sited, with fluid started depending on the mechanism of injury and the patient's clinical state. In many cases intravenous access is best sited in the back of the ambulance en route to hospital. Blood taken at this stage can often be sent ahead of the patient to the hospital for investigations and cross matching.

There are five immediately life-threatening conditions of the chest; these are shown in Table 25.4.

TENSION PNEUMOTHORAX

This type of pneumothorax arises when a one-way valve is created, allowing air to enter but not to leave the pleural space. It can be a consequence of direct trauma to the lung or the rupture of an emphysematous bulla. This condition is also associated with the insertion of subclavian or internal jugular lines, or when manual or mechanical ventilation is commenced in a patient with chest trauma. The patient rapidly becomes shocked as cardiac output falls, and ventilation becomes progressively more difficult as the

intrapleural pressure increases. If the trauma victim is being ventilated an increase in resistance to manual inflation, or raised inflation pressures on the ventilator, may be noticed (Table 25.5).

The classical signs of a tension pneumothorax are tachypnoea and tachycardia with hyperresonance of the hemithorax on the affected side and with decreased chest movement and air entry also on this side. If the patient is not hypovolaemic a raised jugular venous pressure may be noted. As tracheal deviation to the contralateral side is a late sign, treatment should not be delayed until this is present. Cyanosis is a premorbid sign which only occurs when more than 5g of deoxygenated haemoglobin is in the circulation.

A high index of suspicion is required when dealing with all trauma patients as tension pneumothorax can develop at any time and is easily missed. This is particularly true in the prehospital environment where clinical assessment is more difficult. Therefore, if the patient's condition deteriorates it is necessary to recheck for signs of a tension pneumothorax.

As patients can die within minutes from this condition, appropriate treatment must be started as soon as the diagnosis is made. The emergency management is needle thoracocentesis to decompress the chest (see the section on 'Practical procedures'). The subsequent insertion of a prehospital chest drain is controversial. Barton et al (1995) retrospectively reviewed the use of needle thoracocentesis and chest drains in 207 trauma patients who underwent one or both of these procedures in the field. Improvement of clinical status and overall mortality was similar with both procedures but average on-scene time was greater in the patients who had a chest drain inserted. It was concluded that needle thoracocentesis is a relatively rapid intervention in the treatment of suspected tension pneumothorax in the prehospital setting. Nevertheless, chest drainage is an effective adjunct for definitive care without increasing morbidity or mortality. Consequently chest drainage is appropriate in the prehospital setting if transfer is delayed, the patient is deteriorating or helicopter transfer is used. With needle decompression, the needle is prone to being displaced from the chest wall with respiration and also to blockage (especially if there is blood in the pleural space).

Regular and careful observation for signs of re-accumulation of the tension pneumothorax is therefore essential.

OPEN CHEST WOUND

These are often the result of knife or gunshot wounds but can also occur from impalement, road traffic accidents and falls. An open chest wound will cause a pneumothorax on the ipsilateral side. If the wound is more than two-thirds of the diameter of the trachea, air preferentially enters the chest through this hole during inspiration. This leads to a failure of ventilation of the lung, which eventually collapses. A 'sucking chest wound' occurs when air is heard to enter the pleural cavity through the wound. Conversion of such a wound into a tension pneumothorax may occur if the wound is fully sealed in the presence of an associated lung lesion.

Management of an open chest wound with a dressing sealed on three sides is often suggested. The rationale is that air can escape during expiration but not enter the defect during inspiration. However, this type of dressing can be associated with the development of a tension pneumothorax due to misapplication (see above). An alternative is to manage these patients in the prehospital environment with immediate insertion of a chest drain through a different site to drain the pneumothorax. The wound can then be covered completely with a dressing. Alternatively, an Aschermann® dressing specifically designed for this situation can be used (Fig. 25.2); the Bolin® seal is an alternative. If a tension pneumothorax develops any occlusive dressing must immediately be removed, thereby opening the wound and allowing air to escape.

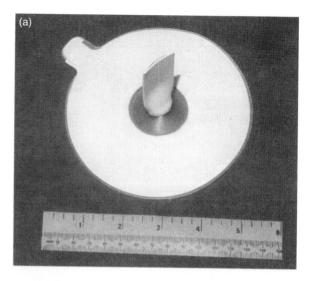

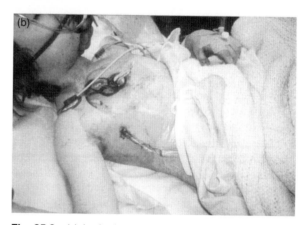

Fig. 25.2 • (a) An Aschermann chest seal, and (b) the seal in use.

FLAIL CHEST

In this condition at least two adjacent ribs are each fractured at more than one site. Alternatively, the first rib and clavicle can be fractured in two places. The three main problems associated with this injury are paradoxical movement, pain and pulmonary contusion. Paradoxical movement of the chest occurs when the affected segment moves inward on inspiration. Immediately after the injury there is significant muscle spasm in an attempt to reduce the pain of the rib fracture; hence paradoxical movement is seldom apparent at this stage. However, it does occur with a central flail, a massive flail or an elderly patient with weak intercostal muscles. Later, usually after the patient has been admitted to hospital and given analgesia, paradoxical movement may be seen. This has the effect of decreasing pulmonary ventilation because of the reduction in the amount of intrathoracic negative pressure possible during inspiration. Pulmonary contusion is usually a greater problem than paradoxical movement (McSwain 1992) and has the effect of increasing the effort of breathing and increasing the chance of hypoxia. Manual

stabilization of the flail segment relieves pain and may improve the mechanics of respiration sufficiently to delay further deterioration during the prehospital phase.

Patients with a flail chest present with tachypnoea, dyspnoea and pain. If hypoxic, they may also be agitated. Examination can reveal bruising, crepitus, subcutaneous emphysema and paradoxical movement. Management is by administration of high-flow oxygen. Analgesia should be given in the form of intravenous opioids, titrated to effect. If there is any delay in transportation to hospital, or the patient develops signs of respiratory distress, a chest drain should be inserted. Some patients will require intubation and ventilation to correct hypoxia and this may be required in the prehospital phase (Table 25.6). Pulse oximetry is extremely useful in detecting these patients (Silverston 1989).

CARDIAC TAMPONADE

This injury can result from blunt or penetrating trauma but those due to penetrating trauma (e.g. stab wounds) are

Table 25.6 Patients with flail chest requiring ventilation

- Falling oxygen saturation
- Exhaustion
- Respiratory rate >30 breaths min^{-1}
- Significant associated abdominal or head injury

Table 25.7 Signs of cardiac tamponade

- Beck's triad – shocked, raised jugular venous pressure (JVP), decreased heart sounds
- Pulsus paradoxus >10 mmHg
- Kussmaul's sign – raised JVP on inspiration

Table 25.8 Signs of a massive haemothorax

- Decreased air entry to hemithorax
- Dull percussion note over hemithorax
- Shock
- Raised jugular venous pressure

most likely to survive owing to the arrival of medical assistance. A stab wound at any site in the chest, upper abdomen or neck can reach the heart provided that the knife is long enough. The closer the wound to the lower part of the sternum, the greater the probability of this.

Cardiac tamponade occurs when blood, fluid or air fills the pericardium. This leads to a decrease in the diastolic filling of the heart and hence the stroke volume. The normal pericardium can admit 80–100 ml of fluid without an increase in pressure, but addition of a further 20–40 ml will lead to a doubling of the pressure in the pericardial sac (Anderson 1993). Consequently, in trauma the onset of cardiac tamponade is usually rapid. Aspiration of a similar volume of fluid from the pericardial sac in this situation will lead to a rapid increase in cardiac output and an improvement in the patient's clinical condition.

The classical presentation of Beck's triad (hypotension, a raised jugular venous pulse and muffled heart sounds), pulsus paradoxus and Kussmaul's sign is only seen in one-third of patients with cardiac tamponade (Table 25.7); in addition, such signs are often difficult to elicit in the prehospital environment. However, 90% of patients are shocked due to impaired left-ventricular filling. The jugular venous pressure (JVP) can be elevated as a result of poor venous return to the right ventricle but this will not be seen in patients with coexisting hypovolaemia.

Temporary relief from the symptoms of cardiac tamponade can be gained by optimizing venous return (e.g. by raising the legs or by increasing the rate of intravenous infusion) and by aspirating the pericardial sac (see the subsection on 'Pericardiocentesis'). This can be falsely negative in at least 25% of cases, usually because the blood in the pericardial sac has clotted. The procedure also has the potential for significant morbidity because of the risk of laceration to a coronary artery. If blood is aspirated, the cannula should be left in the pericardial space and allowed to drain freely. This will delay the development of any recollection, but in all cases thoracotomy will be required for definitive care.

MASSIVE HAEMOTHORAX

This is defined as a collection of more than 1.5 litres of blood in the pleural cavity or drainage of more than 200 ml h^{-1} of blood for 4 h. A patient with a massive haemothorax will therefore have the signs of hypovolaemic shock (Table 25.8). It usually results from a laceration of either an intercostal vessel or the internal mammary artery. It can also occur if the hilum is torn. Bleeding from the lung parenchyma usually stops once the lung has re-expanded because of the low pulmonary perfusion pressure. However, if the source is a blood vessel then an emergency thoracotomy will be required.

Management of a haemothorax requires high-flow oxygen, fluid resuscitation and the insertion of a chest drain (see the section on 'Practical procedures'). In civilian practice in the UK, prehospital thoracotomy is almost always inappropriate, and the patient should be resuscitated and transferred to hospital without delay. Intravenous access must be obtained prior to insertion of the chest drain. This is because it may be difficult after the drain has reduced the tamponade effect and precipitated further haemorrhage.

Other injuries

MAJOR TRACHEOBRONCHIAL INJURIES

These injuries are rare, accounting for less than 1% of chest injuries following blunt trauma. They can occur at different levels.

Larynx

Injuries in this area result from impacts with dashboards, steering wheels, clothes lines, fists or feet. On examination three classical signs may be present: hoarseness, crepitus and surgical emphysema. There may also be tenderness and bruising around the larynx, reduced prominence of the thyroid notch and dyspnoea.

Initial management is to ensure airway patency. Orotracheal intubation may be technically impossible and some of these patients will require a surgical airway, especially if complete disruption of the larynx has occurred. Needle cricothyrotomy may allow sufficient time to transfer the patient to hospital for a more definitive procedure.

Once the airway has been secured, the patient will require resuscitation and immediate transfer to hospital for definitive care from the ENT surgeon.

Trachea

This can be damaged by a direct impact, decelerative force, compressive force or penetrating trauma. During deceleration a shearing force develops, which may act at the cricotracheal junction. A compression injury may cause a sudden increase in airway pressure against a closed glottis, resulting in a longitudinal tear in the membranous part of the trachea or major bronchi. Ruptures of the smaller airways are intrapleural and may cause a pneumothorax or persistent air leak. Penetrating trauma can occur at any level but most commonly occurs in the neck where it is frequently associated with injuries to other vital structures, such as the carotid artery, jugular veins, oesophagus and laryngeal and phrenic nerves.

If the lumen of the trachea is exposed by penetrating injury, blood, spray and bubbles are often seen in the wound. The priority is to clear and secure the airway, and it is sometimes possible to insert an endotracheal tube directly into the trachea through the wound. In complete airway obstruction the patient will show signs of respiratory distress, and there may be vigorous movement of the chest and diaphragm even though no air is passing through the trachea. If the defect in the trachea is small, basic airway management may be all that is required until the trachea can be properly examined in hospital.

Bronchi

As the trachea and proximal bronchi are relatively fixed in comparison to the distal structures, shearing forces can develop distal to the carina following rapid deceleration (Anderson 1993). Consequently, 80% of tears in the bronchi occur less than 2.5 cm from the carina. These can be partial or complete. The high mortality of 30% is due to the associated injuries that occur with this type of injury.

On examination there may be haemoptysis, surgical emphysema, a pneumothorax and overt signs of chest injury. If the insertion of an intercostal drain does not relieve a pneumothorax and bubbles are produced with each expiration, suspicion of bronchial rupture should be raised. Definitive management of these patients is by a cardiothoracic surgeon, with bronchoscopy and either conservative or surgical management.

Vascular disruption

Blunt injury to major vessels may result from deceleration, compression or shearing forces. These may cause rupture of the aorta or avulsion of a major artery or vein. Aortic rupture is a frequent cause of death from road traffic accidents, accounting for 10–15% of all deaths (Anderson, 1993). The mechanism of injury is thought to be shearing due to the difference in rate of deceleration between the relatively fixed descending aorta and the relatively mobile arch of the aorta. Other contributory stresses are bending and torsion, and the water–hammer stress due to a sudden increase in intra-aortic pressure, which results from increased intra-abdominal pressure in compression injuries to the abdomen. 90% of patients with aortic injury will die at the scene of the incident and little can be done to save them. In the remaining 10%, the adventitial layer provides a tamponade effect and only about 500 ml of blood will be lost from the systemic circulation. If there are no other associated injuries, the patient will not demonstrate the classical signs of shock. It is important to remember, however, that physical examination in patients with aortic disruption can be misleading and up to 50% may have no external signs of chest trauma.

Treatment at the scene consists of rapid primary survey and stabilization with speedy transfer to hospital with appropriate facilities. Subsequent chest X-rays may assist diagnosis but the definitive investigation is either by angiography or computed tomography (CT) scan. Survival depends on surgical repair of the aorta before the adventitial layer ruptures.

SIMPLE CHEST INJURIES

Simple pneumothorax

A trauma patient may have a simple rather than a tension pneumothorax. This is not immediately life-threatening and may be difficult to detect clinically at the scene of an accident. Treatment is not usually required in the pre-hospital environment. However, it must be remembered that a tension pneumothorax can develop from a simple pneumothorax at any time, particularly when manual or mechanical ventilation is used.

Insertion of a formal chest drain may be necessary if the patient is trapped, journey times are likely to be prolonged, or intermittent positive pressure ventilation is in progress or is being considered.

Small penetrating wounds can also produce a pneumothorax. This is due to injury to the underlying lung tissue rather than continuous air leak from the outside.

Simple rib fractures

This is the most common chest injury, occurring in 36% of patients with non-penetrating chest injuries (Anderson 1993). The fracture occurs most commonly at the site of impact or at the lateral aspect of the ribs. Young children less commonly sustain fractured ribs as their bones are more pliable. In children, considerable forces may cause significant internal chest injuries without overlying rib fracture.

Fractures may be single or multiple and may cause damage to underlying tissues. Associated injuries depend on the site, force and direction of the impact. Fractures of the upper three ribs require great force, are usually associated with severe intrathoracic pathology and have a mortality of 50%. The presence of these life-threatening conditions must be suspected at an early stage. The fourth to ninth ribs may be fractured by a direct blow or as the result of an anterior–posterior compressive force. Fractures of these ribs may be associated with pneumothoraces or lung contusion. The intercostal neurovascular bundle is closely related to each rib and, if damaged, will cause bleeding into the chest cavity. The lower ribs also cover the abdominal cavity and, when fractured, may be associated with intra-abdominal visceral injuries.

Considerable forces may cause significant internal chest injury in children without overlying rib fractures.

Patients with rib fractures present with pain which is worse on deep inspiration. Palpation may elicit localized tenderness and crepitus over the site of the fracture. There may also be signs of pneumothorax, haemothorax or damage to solid viscera.

Management of rib fractures involves anticipation of potential problems such as pneumothorax and hypovolaemia, and identification and management of associated life-threatening injuries. High-flow oxygen and analgesia should be administered. Strapping of the chest used to be popular but is now considered inappropriate as it decreases ventilation and increases lung collapse. Symptomatic relief of pain in the period immediately following injury can be achieved by encouraging the patient to use his/her hands to 'splint' the rib fractures. The patient should be transferred to hospital for further clinical and radiological assessment.

Pulmonary contusion

This may result from deceleration, compressive, explosive, blunt or penetrating injury. The most common cause is road traffic accidents, followed by falls, explosions and crush injuries. The mortality from pulmonary contusion is 16% but mortality for a patient with pulmonary contusion associated with a flail chest is 42%.

Within 1–2 h of injury, alveolar and interstitial haemorrhage develops, with oedema forming over a 24 h period. This leads to a reduction in pulmonary compliance and an increase in work of breathing with increasing hypoxia.

25% of patients with pulmonary contusion will have no external evidence of chest injury.

Patients may complain of shortness of breath, chest pain or haemoptysis. They may be dyspnoeic and tachypnoeic, and in severe cases may be cyanosed. On examination there may be chest tenderness, bruising or evidence of rib fracture or flail chest. There could also be absent breath sounds over the affected area, with additional local or widespread crepitations and wheeze. However, at the scene of the incident there may only be the mechanism of injury and the presence of associated injuries to suggest the possibility of a pulmonary contusion.

Practical procedures

NEEDLE THORACOSTOMY

Indications for needle thoracocentesis are given in Table 25.9. This is an emergency procedure to rapidly decompress the chest in a patient with a tension pneumothorax by converting it into a simple pneumothorax. A 16G cannula connected to a 10 ml syringe is inserted into the second intercostal space in the midclavicular line. A rapid release of air confirms the diagnosis, following which the cannula is slid over the needle into the pleural cavity. The syringe and needle are then removed, leaving the cannula in place (Fig. 25.3). As with all patients with chest trauma, pulse oximetry is extremely useful in these cases.

If, on insertion of the cannula, there is no release or only a slow release of air and froth, the diagnosis of tension pneumothorax is unlikely. In this situation, the cannula should be left in place, first to prevent progression to tension pneumothorax and second to identify that the procedure has been carried out, as a formal chest drain may be needed on arrival in hospital. An alternative is to remove the needle, with close and continuing observation for deterioration. In this situation it is essential that the hospital is informed that needle thoracocentesis has been performed.

If the patient's condition deteriorates again after needle thoracocentesis, it is possible that the cannula has become kinked, or has slipped out of the pleural space, and the

Table 25.9 Indications for needle thoracocentesis

- Tension pneumothorax
- Deteriorating trauma patient with decreased air entry
- Electromechanical dissociation with chest trauma

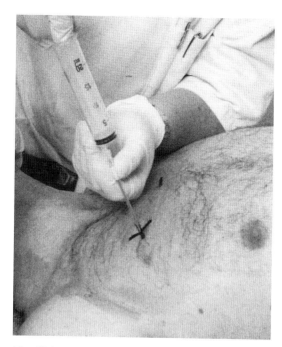

Fig. 25.3 • Needle thoracocentesis.

patient has redeveloped a tension pneumothorax. The patient must be reassessed (starting with the airway) and another needle thoracostomy carried out with a new cannula if this is suspected.

INSERTION OF A CHEST DRAIN

In the majority of cases, insertion of a formal intercostal drain should be delayed until arrival in hospital. Indications for the prehospital insertion of a drain include:

- chest trauma with intermittent positive pressure ventilation where pneumothorax is suspected, following needle thoracocentesis and where hospital transfer is likely to be delayed
- massive haemothorax where transfer is likely to be delayed or prolonged, or the patient is trapped or deteriorating, and following insertion of intravenous cannula
- simple pneumothorax with respiratory compromise, where transfer is likely to be delayed or prolonged, or the patient is trapped.

A chest drain should be inserted into the fifth intercostal space, just anterior to the midaxillary line.

Equipment

- Skin preparation solution
- Swabs
- Sterile gloves
- 1% lidocaine 10 ml
- Syringe and needle
- Scalpel and blade
- Suture, at least 0 in thickness, scissors
- 36G Silastic chest drain with trocar removed
- Portex chest drainage bag
- Two large clamps.

Procedure

The patient's arm is abducted and the fifth intercostal space is palpated (usually at the level of the nipple in males). If there is a rib fracture at this level, an intercostal space immediately above is chosen.

Using aseptic technique, the patient's chest is cleaned. Local anaesthetic is injected into the fifth intercostal space anterior to the midaxillary line. The needle is then directed down on to the fifth rib and local anaesthetic is injected on to the periosteum and over the superior surface of the rib into the underlying pleura. This approach is necessary as the intercostal vessels lie under the inferior surface of the ribs. It is important to aspirate regularly while injecting to ensure that the needle has not entered a blood vessel.

A 3 cm transverse incision is then made through the anaesthetized area down to the fifth rib. Using a clamp, a track is formed and the pleura above the rib is breached. The operator must then insert a finger through the incision and sweep around the intrapleural space to detect the presence of a ruptured diaphragm or lung adhesions. If adhesions prevent the passage of a finger, a fresh incision should be made in the fourth intercostal space just anterior to the mid-axillary line. The end of the chest drain is then clamped and the other clamp is used to guide the tip of the drain through the incision (Fig. 25.4). If the drain is correctly placed in the pleural cavity, condensation of water vapour will cause fogging of the tube. The trocar should never be used, as inappropriate placement can cause injury to lung, mediastinum and abdominal viscera.

The drain is then connected to the Portex chest drainage bag and the clamp is removed. The incision must be closed using sutures and the chest drain must then be firmly secured using both sutures and adhesive tape. A firm gauze dressing is then applied. After insertion of the chest drain, the chest must be re-examined to ensure that the lung is now ventilating. On admission to hospital, a chest X-ray will be required to check the position of the drain and exclude other lung pathology.

The operator needs to be experienced in the technique as several complications may occur (Table 25.10).

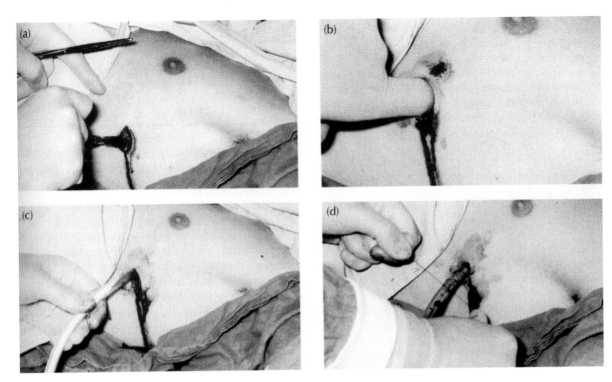

Fig. 25.4 • Insertion of an intercostal drain.

Table 25.10 Complications of intercostal drainage

- Bleeding
- Damage to intercostal vessels and nerves
- Lung and mediastinal injury
- Damage to abdominal viscera and vessels
- Infection

Table 25.11 Indications for pericardiocentesis

- Penetrating wound in danger area
  plus either
- electromechanical dissociation
  or
- hypovolaemic shock and no response to fluid challenge

Kinking, blockage with blood clot or displacement of the chest drain may cause a recurrence of the original problem.

Table 25.12 Complications of pericardiocentesis

- Pneumothorax
- Damage to coronary vessels
- Damage to myocardium
- Damage to other mediastinal structures
- Infection of skin, mediastinum or peritoneum

PERICARDIOCENTESIS

Pericardiocentesis may be life-saving in well-defined situations but is also associated with significant morbidity and mortality (Tables 25.11 and 25.12).

Equipment

- Skin preparation solution
- Swabs
- Sterile gloves
- A long 16 or 18G cannula connected to a 10ml syringe
- Electrocardiogram (ECG) monitor.

Procedure

If there is time, aseptic precautions are taken and the xiphoid area is cleaned. The skin is then punctured 1–2 cm inferior to the left of the xiphochondral junction. While continually aspirating, the needle is advanced at an angle of 45° towards the tip of the left scapula. The ECG must be constantly observed for injury patterns (ST elevation or depression) and dysrhythmias (ventricular ectopics). These would suggest that the needle had advanced too far and was touching the myocardium. In this situation the needle should be slowly withdrawn until a normal ECG is obtained. However, the needle can penetrate the heart without causing ECG changes.

Once the needle enters the pericardium, as much blood as possible should be aspirated. As the cardiac tamponade is drained, ventricular filling will increase and the myocardium will move towards the needle, and ECG changes may occur. Slow withdrawal of the needle in this case should result in return to a normal ECG. The tap and cannula are then secured in place with gauze and tape and allowed to drain freely.

THORACOTOMY

There has been much controversy over the years regarding the indications for emergency thoracotomy in the resuscitation room in the case of trauma patients. A considerable amount of research has been done to identify a group of patients in which this procedure is worthwhile (Bodai et al 1982, Cogbill et al 1983, Adkins et al 1985, Pons et al 1985, Feliciano et al 1986, Krome & Dalbec 1986, Boyd et al 1992).

Survival rates for emergency department thoracotomy quoted in studies are variable. The group of patients most likely to survive the procedure are those with an isolated penetrating injury to the chest (Bodai et al 1982, Karrel et al 1982, Feliciano et al 1986, Schwab et al 1986, Boyd et al 1992). Those with stab wounds have a higher survival rate than those with gunshot wounds (Bodai et al 1982, Durham et al 1992). Those who deteriorate and arrest in the department have a better prognosis than those who require prehospital cardiopulmonary resuscitation (CPR) (Cogbill et al 1983).

Many studies (Tavares et al 1984, Adkins et al 1985, Schwab et al 1986) have stressed the importance of rapid transfer to hospital of all patients with isolated penetrating cardiac stab wounds. Studies have shown no survivors from emergency department thoracotomy in patients with no signs of life at the scene (Cogbill et al 1983), and also in those requiring CPR prior to transport to hospital. Endotracheal intubation was the only prehospital intervention which was shown to improve survival in chest-injured patients (Durham et al 1992). Hence, it has been recommended that on-scene time should only be extended for intubation and all other interventions should take place en route to hospital, unless they can be undertaken without prolonging on-scene time. Pneumatic antishock garments (PASG) have been shown to be of no benefit in patients with penetrating chest trauma and short transfer times (Mattox et al 1986) and can actually have a deleterious effect on victims of isolated penetrating chest trauma, possibly by interfering with ventilation. The presence of pupillary reactions and spontaneous respiratory effort have been shown to be reliable indicators of successful outcome in patients undergoing emergency department thoracotomy (Lorenz et al 1992).

In contrast to penetrating cardiac injury, many studies have shown extremely poor outcome from emergency department thoracotomy in patients with blunt thoracic trauma (Bodai et al 1982, Krome & Dalbec 1986), the vast majority showing no survivors (Flynn et al 1982, Cogbill et al 1983, Schwab et al 1986, Boyd et al 1992, Durham et al 1992). Hence, it is considered inappropriate to perform this procedure in this group of patients. Similarly, patients with penetrating wounds below the diaphragm who present in cardiorespiratory arrest refractory to usual methods of resuscitation have a dismal prognosis.

PREHOSPITAL THORACOTOMY

Apart from anecdotal case reports (Wall et al 1994), there has been little research into thoracotomy in the prehospital environment. Although there may be situations where this may be considered useful, in civilian practice in the UK prehospital thoracotomy is not generally appropriate. In certain circumstances where the appropriate expertise is available, thoracotomy may be performed in patients with penetrating trauma who have shown witnessed and recent signs of life. Patients with penetrating chest wounds should be intubated if necessary (Durham et al 1992) and then rapidly transported to hospital without delay. The hospital should be alerted to the imminent arrival of such a patient so that an appropriate surgical team can be waiting in the emergency department. Intravenous lines and fluid resuscitation should be initiated en route. The factors most affecting survival are the time between trauma and emergency department thoracotomy, and the presence or absence of signs of life at the scene (Bodai et al 1982, Cogbill et al 1983, Feliciano et al 1986, Schwab et al 1986, Boyd et al 1992).

Analgesia

There is no ideal analgesic for chest injury in the prehospital environment. Consequently, each situation must be assessed and the most appropriate analgesic used. The doctor or paramedic administering the drug should always be familiar with its use and take into account the age and previous medical history of the patient (if available) and the effects of any coexisting drugs that may have been taken. The subject of analgesia is covered in detail in Chapter 14.

The management of chest injuries is summarized in Table 25.13.

Table 25.13 Chest injuries, summary
● Consider mechanism of injury
● Primary survey and initial resuscitation
● Secondary survey only if patient is stable
● Analgesia
● Rapid transfer to appropriate hospital

References

Adkins RB, Whiteneck JM, Woltering EA 1985 Penetrating chest wall and thoracic injuries. American Surgeon 51: 140–148

Anderson DR 1993 The diagnosis and management of non-penetrating cardiothoracic trauma. British Journal of Clinical Practice 47: 97–103

Barton ED, Epperson M, Hoyt DB et al 1995 Pre-hospital needle aspiration and tube thoracostomy in trauma victims: a six-year experience with aeromedical crews. Journal of Emergency Medicine 13: 155–163

Bodai BI, Smith JP, Blaisdell FW 1982 The role of emergency thoracotomy in blunt trauma. Journal of Trauma 22: 487–491

Boyd M, Vanek VW, Bourgeut CC 1992 Emergency room resuscitative thoracotomy: when is it indicated? Journal of Trauma 33: 714–721

Cogbill TH, Moore EE, Millikan JS, Cleveland HC 1983 Rationale for selective application of Emergency Department thoracotomy in trauma. Journal of Trauma 23: 453–460

Durham LA, Richardson RJ, Wall MJ et al 1992 Emergency centre thoracotomy: impact of pre-hospital resuscitation. Journal of Trauma 32: 775–779

Feliciano DV, Bitondo CG, Cruse PA et al 1986 Liberal use of emergency centre thoracotomy. American Journal of Surgery 152: 654–659

Flynn TC, Ward RE, Miller PW 1982 Emergency department thoracotomy. Annals of Emergency Medicine 11: 413–416

Fox MA, Fabian TC, Croce MA et al 1991 Anatomy of the accident scene: a prospective study of injury and mortality. American Surgeon 57: 394–397

Karrel R, Haffer MA, Franaszec JB 1982 Emergency diagnosis, resuscitation and treatment of acute penetrating cardiac trauma. Annals of Emergency Medicine 11: 504–517

Krome RL, Dalbec DL 1986 Emergency thoracotomy. Emergency Medicine Clinics of North America 4: 459–465

Lorenz HP, Steinmetz P, Lieberman J et al 1992 Emergency thoracotomy: survival correlates with physiological status. Journal of Trauma 32: 780–785

McSwain NE 1992 Blunt and penetrating chest injuries. World Journal of Surgery 16: 924–929

Mattox KL, Bickell WH, Pepe PE, Mangelsdorff AD 1986 Prospective randomised evaluation of antishock MAST in post-traumatic hypotension. Journal of Trauma 26: 779–786

National Association of Emergency Medical Technicians 2003 PHTLS. Basic and advanced pre-hospital trauma life support, 5th edn. Mosby Lifeline, London

Pons PT, Honigman B, Moore EE et al 1985 Pre-hospital advanced trauma life support for critical penetrating wounds to the thorax and abdomen. Journal of Trauma 25: 828–832

Schwab CW, Adcock OT, Max MH 1986 Emergency department thoracotomy. A 26-month experience using 'agonal' protocol. American Surgeon 52: 20–29

Silverston P 1989 Pulse oximetry at the roadside: a study of pulse oximetry in immediate care. British Medical Journal 298: 711–713

Tavares S, Hankins JR, Moulton AL et al 1984 Management of penetrating cardiac injuries: the role of emergency room thoracotomy. Annals of Thoracic Surgery 38: 183–187

Wall MJ, Pepe PE, Mattox KL 1994 Successful roadside resuscitative thoracotomy: case report and literature review. Journal of Trauma 36: 131–134

West JB 1990 Respiratory physiology – the essentials. Williams & Wilkins, Baltimore, MD

Spinal injuries

26

Introduction	290
Recognition	291
Immediate management	292
Immobilization	294
Transport of spinal injuries	295
References	296

Introduction

The incidence of spinal cord injury within the UK is about 10–15 cases per million of the population per year (Swain & Grundy 1993). Spinal injury occurs in between 2% and 12% of trauma victims according to published reports (Cohn et al 1991, Davis et al 1993). Traffic accidents account for about 55% of admissions to spinal injury units (with motorcycle accidents constituting 31% of the total), 22% result from falls, 5% from criminal assault and, disturbingly, the remainder of 18% from sporting events (Peach & Grundy 1991). Spinal injuries do not always occur in isolation – in fact up to 50% of patients with spinal injuries will have other injuries also.

The number of injuries affecting the cervical spine has increased in recent years and now more injuries affect this part of the spinal column (55%) than elsewhere (dorsal spine 35%; lumbosacral spine 10%) (Swain & Grundy 1993). In 5% of cases injuries coexist in more than one part of the spine (Calenoff et al 1978, Korres et al 1981). Injuries involving the upper cervical spine are more likely

to be fatal (Alker et al 1975, Bucholz et al 1979). 14% of spinal injuries implicate the cord (Riggins & Kraus 1977).

In 5% of cases spinal injuries will occur at more than one level.

The concern of rescue workers in the field is the development of secondary injuries to the spinal cord from improper handling and immobilization, and this is claimed to have occurred in up to 17% of such cases reviewed in the USA (Macdonald et al 1990, Gerrelts et al 1991, Davis et al 1993). Such occurrences are, of course, extremely difficult to prove retrospectively and spinal cord injury specialists believe that most cord damage occurs as a primary event, the problem being that very frequently this is not recognized and either the extent of the cord damage may increase or the injury may be aggravated by secondary complications (e.g. respiratory difficulties or pressure sores, etc.). Up to 30% of patients with delayed diagnoses may suffer deterioration (Reid et al 1987) but in one spinal injury unit it has been claimed that as many as 50% of admitted patients have suffered neurological deterioration at the receiving district hospital (Toscano 1988). It is difficult to distinguish between complete and incomplete cord injuries without careful specialist evaluation and it may take up to 24 h for the full extent of the neurological lesion to develop.

The emphasis of prehospital care must be upon establishing that a patient has, or is at risk of, a spinal injury rather than attempting a precise neurological diagnosis of complete or partial lesions.

Thus, there is an onus on the field worker both to have a high index of suspicion of spinal injury cases and to provide good quality spinal column immobilization and general care when that suspicion is raised.

Recognition

BLUNT INJURY

In common with all trauma at the scene of an accident, the emphasis should be on determining the mechanism of injury. This is particularly true in spinal trauma when the initial injury is a skeletal one resulting from the application of forces to the spine (Table 26.1). The direction or type of force applied will determine the type and extent of injury.

The most common forces are those of flexion and extension, and the relevance of this can be seen if the spine is considered as one long bone with joints at either end but with the head acting as a weighted lever and exerting a moment of force particularly upon the neck. The most vulnerable parts of the spinal column are the faceted joints. Thus, combinations of flexion or extension with rotation are most likely to cause damage particularly in the areas of maximum curve or lordosis (e.g. C5–C6) or where the spine changes direction (e.g. cervicothoracic or thoracolumbar junctions), the latter being the most difficult areas to determine clinically (Riggins & Kraus 1977, Green et al 1981).

A number of accident situations are classically associated with blunt spinal column injury:

- Deceleration in vehicular accidents, especially when there are additional lateral forces – combinations of flexion and rotation resulting in fracture dislocations of the cervical spine are important injuries as they are frequently associated with spinal cord trauma.
- Ejection from a motor car or motorcycle – one study revealed that serious neck injury occurred in one in 14 casualties ejected from a motor vehicle compared with one in 483 who remained within the damaged vehicle (Huelke et al 1981).
- Falls from a horse.
- Collapse of a scrum in sport – a particularly dangerous aetiology that can result in flexion, rotation and compressive forces.

Table 26.1 Forces involved in the mechanism of spinal column injuries

- Flexion
- Extension
- Rotation
- Lateral flexion
- Axial loading (compression)
- Distraction

- Falls from a height, especially if more than 6 m.
- Blows to the head resulting in extension injury – there is stated to be a 5–10% incidence of unstable cervical injury in patients with significant head trauma (Irving & Irving 1967, Evans 1971).
- Head-first dives (especially into a shallow pool) resulting in an extension injury – diving is an activity carrying a high risk of spinal injury (Peach & Grundy 1991) and immersion casualties should always be suspected of having a spinal injury (Morgan & Winter 1986).
- Objects falling onto the (flexed) spine – once a common injury in mine workers. This results in hyperextension.

PENETRATING INJURY

The penetrative causes of spinal injury (e.g. knife and bullet wounds) are often overlooked but are increasing in frequency. It is important to remember that the site of spinal cord/column damage may be at some distance from the entry wound. Again, a high index of suspicion is required.

Why do some spinal injuries get overlooked?

Notwithstanding our knowledge and awareness of the causes of spinal injury and its clinical presentation, the diagnosis of spinal injury is often missed (Bohlman 1979, Ravichandran & Silver 1984, Ravichandran 1989). A number of conditions explain why this may be so:

- Major trauma may be associated with the *acute stress reaction* causing the 'fight or flight' phenomenon associated with the outpouring of the sympathetic catecholamines. One of the effects of this stress reaction is 'pain masking' caused by natural hormones (endorphins) with narcotic-like properties. There is some degree of acute stress reaction present with all types of violent injury, making the patient and the examination somewhat unreliable. Any case with a positive mechanism of injury, especially in the presence of an acute stress reaction, must be treated as a spinal injury.
- *Distracting injuries* – frequently the pain or spasm from a spinal column injury is not appreciated because of the urgency and intensity of injuries elsewhere in the body.
- *Brain injury* – as there is a significant association between spinal cord and brain injury, it follows that many spinal injuries will be found in patients with a depressed level of consciousness. Aggressive and uncooperative behaviour may be an indicator of brain damage and may mask the diagnosis of the spinal injury.
- *Intoxication* – many accidents responsible for spinal cord injury are associated with the consumption of alcohol (Peach & Grundy 1991) or the use of drugs, and the effects of intoxication on the level of responsiveness may mask spinal symptoms.

- *Abnormal mental status* – spine injury assessment is unreliable in patients with psychosis or other forms of severe mental illness.
- *Communication difficulties* – these are seen in the elderly, the young, the histrionic and patients in whom there is a language barrier. Beware the patient thought to be feigning or hysterical.

Immediate management

When discussing the management of spinal injuries, appropriate emphasis is placed on injuries to the cervical spine. It must not be forgotten, however, that adequate immobilization of all levels of the spine is equally important.

POSITIONING

When a diagnosis of spinal injury is suspected, it is important to immobilize the spine as soon as possible. Initially this will be by applying manual in-line stabilization (MILS) – *not traction* – to the head according to the method formally taught on the Advanced Trauma Life Support (ATLS) and Pre-hospital Trauma Life Support (PHTLS) courses (Fig. 26.1).

When the head is not lying in a neutral (midline) position future interventions, including immobilization, are greatly facilitated by bringing it gently into the midline position without traction. This manoeuvre may also take pressure off a compromised spinal cord. In some cases an attempt to return the head and neck to neutral will result in resistance to movement such that the midline position can not be achieved without force. In this situation the neck must be immobilized in the position at which resistance is found, as the patient may have a unilateral facet joint when dislocation and reduction will be impossible.

It is desirable to place the patient supine in the anatomical position by gently correcting any flexion, extension or rotational posture of the spine; this aids immobilization and facilitates assessment and resuscitation.

Unconscious casualties are at risk of passive gastric regurgitation, vomiting and aspiration when lying on their back. Suction must therefore be available at all times. If the patient is on a long spine board, this can be tilted in the event of vomiting. If the patient is not on a long spine board, careful observation with suction and log rolling in the event of vomiting is most appropriate. At the scene, if the patient is likely to be left unattended, he should be placed in the lateral position by log rolling. A correctly performed log roll will require at least four people acting in a coordinated manner.

The lateral position shown in Fig. 26.2 is an acceptable position for when a spinal-injured patient has to be left unattended – the upper shoulder is tilted slightly forward and the head is supported in neutral on the underlying arm. A modification to this position has been proposed (Gunn et al 1995) in which the lower arm is raised above the head in full abduction and used to support the patient's head. Abducting the lower arm carries a small risk of brachial plexus traction damage and impairment of the upper limb venous return, so an anatomical side stable position might be the best compromise. However, this requires physical support from at least one rescuer at all times.

PRIMARY SURVEY AND RESUSCITATION

The prevention of hypoxia and hypotension is just as important in spinal trauma as it is in cranial trauma (Sonntag & Douglas 1992) and thus meticulous attention to the airway, breathing and circulation is essential.

Airway

Opening, clearing and maintaining a patent airway is the first priority in all patients suspected of having sustained injury to the cervical spine. With the head supported by a hand on each side, the airway can be opened with a jaw thrust (Fig. 26.3). This position can be maintained until

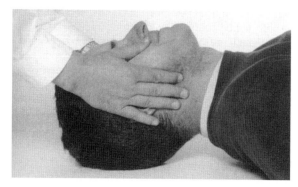

Fig. 26.1 • In-line spinal stabilization.

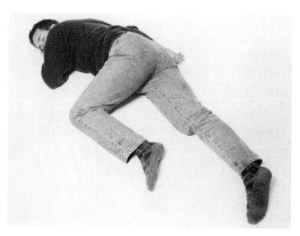

Fig. 26.2 • The lateral position.

the head can be properly immobilized (see below) or the airway secured.

It has been suggested that in skilled hands tracheal intubation in spinal injury is best performed by the nasotracheal route without moving the neck (Aprahamian et al 1984). However, most practitioners in the UK are more familiar with orotracheal intubation. Studies have shown that, provided movement of the neck is minimized by an assistant providing MILS, there is no evidence of any risk in employing intubation by the oral route (Majernick et al 1986, Bivins et al 1988, Rhee et al 1996).

Overaggressive pharyngeal suction should be avoided in the presence of a high spinal cord lesion because unopposed vagal stimulation can precipitate cardiac arrest (Frankel et al 1975). Accordingly, some authorities would advocate the use of atropine 0.5 mg when performing an upper airway manoeuvre in the presence of a high cervical cord lesion.

Breathing

Respiratory impairment is common in patients with spinal cord injury. There may be concomitant injuries to the thorax (rib fractures, pulmonary contusion, haemopneumothorax) which (if combined with intercostal muscle paralysis from thoracic or cervical spinal cord trauma or diaphragmatic paralysis from a phrenic nerve injury) may impair the cough reflex or produce a ventilation–perfusion mismatch.

The effect of the resulting hypoxia is to aggravate oedema within the spinal cord, which may develop over the next 24 h and result in respiratory failure. Spinal cord injury victims should be treated with a high concentration of oxygen given through a well fitting facemask with oxygen reservoir. The tissue oxygen saturation level can be monitored by pulse oximetry and a low threshold for assisted ventilation should be adopted.

Circulation

Monitoring of the pulse and respiratory rate, capillary refill and blood pressure may reveal clinical shock. When

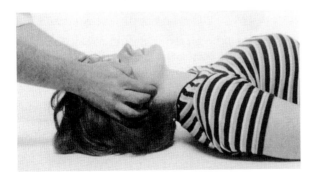

Fig. 26.3 • The jaw thrust and in-line stabilization.

hypotension is discovered this nearly always implies hypovolaemia with blood or tissue fluids lost from other or associated injuries; the correction of volume deficit, in the usual manner, is a top priority. It should be remembered that trauma sufficient to cause spinal injury is also likely to have caused injuries elsewhere, which might result in bleeding. A careful assessment is therefore required before hypotension is considered to be due to neurogenic shock.

With a cord injury above the level of T5 *neurogenic* shock may be a cause of the hypotension (Burt 1988, Sonntag & Douglas 1992). When the thoracolumbar sympathetic outflow (T1–L2) is interrupted, vagal tone is unopposed; the blood pressure will fall and the heart rate slow. This effect can be seen in some paraplegics as well as with tetraplegia. In neurogenic shock the patient is hypotensive but, in contrast to hypovolaemic shock, is bradycardic and vasodilated (rather than tachycardic and peripherally shut down).

It must be remembered that *spinal shock* is a syndrome of *neurological* signs that might be considered to be akin to 'concussion' of the spinal cord. It does not in itself have cardiovascular consequences and it is not relevant to the prehospital management of the patient with spinal injuries. Despite the confusing terminology, it must not be confused with neurogenic shock.

Although restoration of fluid volume is essential, overinfusion of fluids may be deleterious in such patients (Meyer et al 1971). Atropine in small increments should be given if the heart rate falls below 50 beats min^{-1} but large doses of atropine may be toxic in spinal-injury patients (Baker & Silver 1984). Elevating the patient's legs may also be valuable.

Disability

Assessment of pupillary reaction and AVPU ('mini neurological examination') is an important component of the primary survey and it must be remembered that in an unconscious patient any painful stimulus should be applied *above the neck* in order to avoid an inappropriate lack of reaction in the patient with a spinal injury, which might occur if finger pressure was used.

Exposure

Appropriate exposure may reveal obvious external evidence of localized spinal injury as well as priapism, differential movements of the upper and lower limbs, and vasodilatation. It should be remembered that patients with neurogenic shock are at particular risk of hypothermia.

SECONDARY SURVEY

In the prehospital care of suspected spinal-injury patients time should not be wasted on a detailed secondary survey particularly aimed at identifying the exact level of the cord lesion. The emphasis should be on adequate immobilization of the spine and transport to definitive care.

However, a brief neurological assessment may be useful in confirming the presence of spinal cord injury or conversely, when used in conjunction with the mechanism of injury and the absence of symptoms, ruling out spinal injury cases. But it should be remembered that patients with spinal injuries do not always complain of neck or back pain (Maull & Satchatello 1977, Bresler & Rich 1982). A spine-injured patient, even in the absence of spine pain and tenderness, may have some abnormality of motor or sensory function. Goth (1995) describes tests of motor function that can be carried out reliably and rapidly at the accident scene, and these are:

- *Finger abduction/adduction* (T1 nerve root) – ask the patient to spread the fingers of both hands and keep them spread while you attempt to squeeze the index and ring fingers together. You should experience a spring-like resistance felt equally in both hands.
- *Finger/hand extension* (C7 nerve root) – ask the patient to keep the hands and fingers spread straight out while you attempt to push them down. (With your other hand support the patient's hand at the wrist.) Normal resistance should be felt.
- *Foot plantar flexion* (S1–S2 nerve root) – place your hands on the undersides of both feet and ask the patient to push against them as if pushing down on an accelerator pedal. Both sides should feel strong and equal.
- *Big toe dorsiflexion* (L5 nerve root) – holding the top of the foot across the toes ask the patient to pull back on the big toe, keeping the foot still. Both sides should feel strong and equal.
- *Knee extension* – holding the knee, place the hand on the anterior calf and ask the patient to push against the resistance.

As well as tests of motor function, sensation – to upper and lower limbs – can be assessed quickly by checking light touch and *light* pinprick. One side of the body should be compared with the other.

It may be useful to remember MSC × 4:

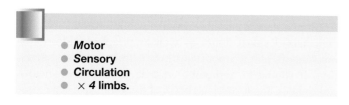

- **Motor**
- **Sensory**
- **Circulation**
- **× 4 limbs.**

Immobilization

Any patient in whom spinal injury is suspected or, from the mechanism of injury, is possible and cannot be excluded must have full spinal immobilization applied. The only safe form during rescue is a correctly applied semirigid collar, lateral immobilization to the head and strapping to secure the body firmly to a rigid board (Chandler et al 1992, Prinsen et al 1995). The use of a collar alone or improperly applied immobilization may be worse than no immobilization at all.

COLLARS

The only acceptable collars are those with a semirigid reinforcement and a chin cup. Simple foam collars are unsuitable (Johnson et al 1981, Podolsky et al 1983).

It is important that the collar is correctly sized using the manufacturer's guidelines. Universal adjustable one-piece semirigid collars are now available. The collar must be applied direct to skin and not over clothing.

Although there have been studies demonstrating a rise in intracranial pressure associated with the prolonged wearing of collars (Raphael & Chotai 1994), this complication is a lesser risk in prehospital care than inadequate immobilization (Craig & Neilsen 1991). However, in cases of severe head injury a collar applied in the field should be removed as soon as feasible in hospital.

LONG SPINAL BOARDS

The long spinal board used with a collar and head blocks is an excellent device permitting immobilization of the spinal column during extrication and transport. Most of the experience with the long spinal board is from the USA and is anecdotal – as there have been no randomized controlled trials. Nevertheless, spinal boards make the handling of patients very much easier and their slippery surface facilitates extrication. The spinal board is primarily a tool for general rescue but is particularly useful in aiding extrication in road traffic accidents. In the latter case they may be used in conjunction with specialist extrication splints, e.g. the Kendrick extrication device (KED) or the Russell extrication device (RED) (Cline et al 1983, Graziano et al 1987, Howell et al 1989).

All patients should be placed in a cervical collar. Unless used with a specialist extrication splint, the spinal board must further be augmented by a cervical immobilization device (e.g. head blocks, rolled blankets and tape, or a single-use corrugated board device) to prevent lateral movement of the head. The disposable cervical immobilization device appears to be more effective at restricting lateral neck movement than the reusable foam block, is easier to store and is marginally quicker to apply (Manix et al 1995).

The steps to be followed in the application of a spinal board, e.g. in the case of a casualty seated in a motor vehicle, are given below.

- In-line immobilization should be applied and maintained at all times.
- A correctly sized semirigid collar is applied.
- The board should be slid down behind the seated patient from the head end or under the patient from the side through an open door.
- Blocks and straps are used with the board to secure the head and torso.
- Straps should be applied to the chest, abdomen and thighs, and the head restraint is then applied. They should be applied transversely only and must not be crossed over the chest (Bauer & Kowalski 1988, Mazeloweski & Manix 1994).
- Rolls of blanket can be applied at the sides to support smaller patients.
- The spinal board must be secured to the trolley cot.

When faced with a standing patient with possible spinal injury the 'take down' technique may be employed whereby the spinal board is placed behind the patient and the patient and the board are moved backwards into the horizontal position.

Spinal boards are not ideal if the patient is already supine because a log roll to turn the patient requires a number of trained people and is not a technique free from risk (McGuire et al 1987). An orthopaedic ('scoop') stretcher is preferred for lifting a suspected spinal-injury patient who is already on the ground. However, an alternative to the log roll may be considered, which entails sliding the board under the patient during a 'spinal' lift using at least four people. This method can be associated with unacceptable degrees of movement when arms are placed under the casualty prior to the lift.

EXTRICATION

Techniques for extrication are described elsewhere in this book. However, in the context of suspected spinal injury it should be recalled that the standard method of extrication is by the rear route through a hatchback tailgate or the car's rear window, or vertically through the roof after it has been removed. Routine immobilization of a spinal-injury patient should be an unhurried team effort, often involving medical supervision and employing a specialist extrication device. When extrication is required urgently but access is limited the use of a KED or RED could be dispensed with. The side route for extrication should be used in emergencies only when there is a major risk to life (e.g. vehicle fire or serious airway or breathing problems) and ambulance crews have to be prepared to take risks with the spine in order to preserve life.

SPINAL IMMOBILIZATION IN CHILDREN

In children no method has yet been demonstrated that reliably achieves a neutral neck position (Curran et al 1995). A collar alone is insufficient and a padded board and straps are usually required (Huerta et al 1987).

Transport of spinal injuries

There has been a lot of concern expressed about how long a person can safely lie on a spinal board and when and where they should be taken off. It is accepted that, in patients who have had injury to the spinal cord, pressure sores can develop in as little as 45 min after placement on the board (Chan et al 1994, Cordell et al 1995). There have been suggestions that spinal boards could be padded (Walton et al 1995) but the advantage of comfort and protection from skin damage is outweighed by the disadvantage of loss of efficiency as a rescue tool. For transportation of a spinal-injury patient, especially over a long distance, a vacuum mattress is preferred (Johnson et al 1996).

Patients can tolerate a 30-min journey on a long spinal board. The receiving emergency department staff should be alerted immediately as to how long the patient has been on the board so that they can make an appropriate judgement on the timing of its removal. The duration of time on the spinal board should be recorded on the ambulance's patient report form.

If a journey time of more than 30 min is anticipated, the patient should be transferred from the spinal board on to a vacuum mattress using a scoop stretcher. Wide-bodied vacuum mattresses are of great value for the transportation of spinal-injury cases. They cannot, however, be used for extrication. Vacuum mattresses are vulnerable to damage, particularly from glass at the scene of a road accident, and it may be difficult to stow them in a front-line ambulance vehicle. Thus, there may be merit in retaining a vacuum mattress in reserve to be used electively or brought out specifically to the scene of a suspected spinal injury. If there is clear paralysing injury to the spinal cord, on-line medical advice should be sought with regard to the use of the spinal board, the benefits of which may be limited while the risk of pressure sores may be very high. In such circumstances the use of a vacuum mattress may be preferred. However, the use of a vacuum mattress requires specific training and, as half the cases of spinal injuries have other serious injuries also, unnecessary delay at the scene or in transit should be avoided.

The most important feature in the mode of transport of spinal-injured patients is that it should be smooth. If the patient is adequately protected with a vacuum mattress then there is no requirement for a dead crawl pace (traditionally associated with spinal care journeys) – often a high-speed escorted journey is best, provided that roundabouts and intersections are guarded to prevent excessive acceleration and breaking. For long journeys consideration should be given to the use of air ambulance helicopters, where, because of the excessive vibration experienced, the use of a vacuum mattress is mandatory.

If cervical immobilization has been attempted by the insertion of skull calipers at the primary centre then the maintenance of steady skull traction during a secondary transfer to a spinal injury unit may be considered. In practice this is difficult, although the Povey frame developed by the RAF overcomes this problem by incorporating a constant tension device linked by cable to the skull calipers. Traction, however, is not a prerequisite for the secondary transfer of patients with unstable cervical fractures. What is most important is that effective splintage is applied, and this can be achieved by the use of the vacuum mattress described above (Burney et al 1989).

In long journeys the need for thermal insulation must also be appreciated. Because the sympathetic nervous system is paralysed in tetraplegia, the normal vasomotor responses to temperature changes are impaired. The patient is said to be poikilothermic – and hypothermia may become a real risk. Thermally insulating blankets may be required.

In the UK the care of patients with spinal cord injury is best provided in a spinal injury unit. Advice should be sought from the specialist staff of the nearest unit as soon as the diagnosis is made, in order that appropriate care can be recommended and secondary complications prevented.

References

Alker GJ, Young SO, Leslie EV et al 1975 Postmortem radiology of head and neck injuries in fatal traffic accidents. Radiology 114: 611–617

Aprahamian C, Thompson BM, Finger WA, Darin JC 1984 Experimental cervical spine injury model: evaluation of airway management and splinting techniques. Annals of Emergency Medicine 13: 21–24

Baker JHE, Silver JR 1984 Atropine toxicity in acute cervical spine injury. Paraplegia 22: 379–382

Bauer D, Kowalski R 1988 Effect of spinal immobilisation devices on pulmonary function in the healthy, non- smoking man. Annals of Emergency Medicine 17: 915–918

Bivins HG, Ford S, Bezmanilovic Z et al 1988 The effect of axial traction during orotracheal intubation of the trauma victim with an unstable cervical spine. Annals of Emergency Medicine 17: 25–29

Bohlman AH 1979 Acute fractures and dislocations of the cervical spine. Journal of Bone and Joint Surgery 61A: 1119–1141

Bresler NJ, Rich GH 1982 Occult cervical spine fracture in an ambulatory patient. Annals of Emergency Medicine 11: 440–442

Bucholz RW, Burkagad WZ, Graham W, Petty C 1979 Occult cervical spine injuries in fatal traffic accidents. Journal of Trauma 19: 768–771

Burney RE, Waggoner R, Maynard FM 1989 Stabilisation of spinal injury for early transfer. Journal of Trauma 29: 1497–1499

Burt AA 1988 Thoracolumbar spinal injuries: clinical assessment of the spinal cord injured patient. Current Orthopaedics 2: 210–213

Calenoff L, Chessare JW, Rogers LF 1978 Multiple level spinal injuries: importance of early recognition. American Journal of Roentgenology 130: 665–669

Chan D, Goldberg B, Tascone A et al 1994 The effect of spinal immobilisation on healthy volunteers. Annals of Emergency Medicine 23: 148–151

Chandler DR, Nemeja C, Adkins RH, Waters AL 1992 Emergency cervical spine immobilisation. Annals of Emergency Medicine 21: 1185–1188

Cline JR, Scheidel E, Rigsky FF 1983 A comparison of methods of cervical immobilisation used in patient extrication and transport. Journal of Trauma 25: 649–653

Cohn SM, Lyle WG, Linden CH, Lancey RA 1991 Exclusion of cervical spine injury: a prospective study. Journal of Trauma 31: 570–574

Cordell WH, Hollingsworth JC, Ulinger ML et al 1995 Pain and tissue interface pressures during spine board immobilisation. Annals of Emergency Medicine 26: 31–36

Craig GR, Neilsen MS 1991 Rigid cervical collars and intracranial pressure. Intensive Care Medicine 17: 504–505

Curran C, Dietrich AM, Bowman MJ et al 1995 Paediatric cervical spine immobilisation: achieving neutral position? Journal of Trauma 39: 729–732

Davis JW, Dhreaner DL, Hoyt DB, Mackeisie RC 1993 The etiology of missed cervical spine injuries. Journal of Trauma 4: 342–346

Evans JP 1971 The International Symposium on Head Injuries. Journal of Neurosurgery 35: 367–370

Frankel HL, Mathias CJ, Spalding MR 1975 Mechanism of reflex cardiac arrest in tetraplegic patients. Lancet 2: 1183–1185

Gerrelts BD, Petersen EU, Mabry J, Petersen SR 1991 Delayed diagnosis of cervical spine injuries. Journal of Trauma 31: 1622–1628

Goth P 1995 Spine injury: clinical criteria for assessment and management. Medical Care Developments, Augusta, ME

Graziano AF, Scheidel EA, Cline JR 1987 A radiographic comparison of pre-hospital cervical immobilisation methods. Annals of Emergency Medicine 16: 1127–1131

Green BA, Callahan RA, Klose KJ, de la Torre J 1981 Acute spinal cord injury: current concepts. Clinical Orthopaedics 154: 125–135

Gunn BD, Eizenberg N, Silberstein M, Gutteridge GA 1995 How should an unconscious person with a suspected neck injury be positioned? Prehospital and Disaster Medicine 10: 239–244

Howell JM, Burrow R, Dumontior C, Hillyaro A 1989 A practical radiographic comparison of short board technique and Kendrick Extrication Device. Annals of Emergency Medicine 18: 943–946

Huelke DF, O'Day J, Mendelsohn RA 1981 Cervical injuries suffered in automobile crashes. Journal of Neurosurgery 54: 316–321

Huerta C, Griffith R, Joyce SM 1987 Cervical spine stabilisation in paediatric patients: evaluation of current technique. Annals of Emergency Medicine 16: 1121–1126

Irving MH, Irving PM 1967 Associated injuries in head-injured patients. Journal of Trauma 7: 500–511

Johnson RM, Owen JR, Hart DL et al 1981 Cervical orthoses. Clinical Orthopaedics 154: 34–43

Johnson DR, Hauswald M, Stockhoff C 1996 Comparison of a vacuum splint device to a rigid backboard for spinal immobilisation. American Journal of Emergency Medicine 14: 369–373

Korres DJ, Katsaro SA, Pantazopoulos T, Hartofilakios-Garofalios T 1981 Double or multiple level fractures of the spine. Injury 13: 147–152

Macdonald RL, Schwartz ML, Mirich D, Sharkey PW, Nelson WR 1990 Diagnosis of cervical spine injury in motor vehicle crash victims: how many X-rays are enough? Journal of Trauma 30: 392–397

McGuire RA, Neville S, Green BA, Watts C 1987 Spinal instability and the log-rolling maneuver. Journal of Trauma 27: 525–531

Majernick TG, Bienek R, Houston JB, Hughes HG 1986 Cervical spine movement during orotracheal intubation. Annals of Emergency Medicine 15: 59–62

Manix TH, Gunderson MR, Garth GC 1995 Comparison of pre-hospital cervical immobilisation devices using video and electromyography. Prehospital and Disaster Medicine 10: 232–238

Maull KI, Satchatello CR 1977 Avoiding a pitfall in resuscitation: the painless cervical fracture. Southern Medical Journal 70: 477–478

Mazeloweski P, Manix TH 1994 The effectiveness of strapping techniques in spinal immobilisation. Annals of Emergency Medicine 23: 1290–1295

Meyer GA, Berman IR, Dotty DB 1971 Haemodynamic responses to acute quadriplegia with or without chest trauma. Journal of Neurosurgery 34: 168–177

Morgan GAR, Winter NJ 1986 Drowning and near drowning. British Medical Journal 293: 395

Peach F, Grundy D 1991 How preventable are spinal cord injuries? Health Trends 23: 62–66

Podolsky S, Baraff LJ, Simon RA et al 1983 Efficacy of cervical spine immobilisation methods. Journal of Trauma 23: 461–464

Prinsen RK, Syrotuik DG, Reid DC 1995 Position of the cervical vertebrae during helmet removal and cervical collar application in football and hockey. Clinical Journal of Sport Medicine 5: 155–161

Raphael JH, Chotai R 1994 Effects of the cervical collar on cerebro-spinal fluid pressure. Anaesthesia 49: 437–439

Ravichandran G 1989 Errors and omissions in the acute management of spinal cord injury. Report of the Medical Defence: 14–16

Ravichandran G, Silver JR 1984 Recognition of spinal cord injury. Hospital Update January: 77–86

Reid DC, Henderson R, Saboe L, Miller JDR 1987 Etiology and clinical course of missed spine fractures. Journal of Trauma 27: 980–987

Rhee KJ, Green W, Holdcroft JW 1996 Oral intubation in the multiply injured patient: the risk of exacerbating spinal cord damage. Annals of Emergency Medicine 19: 511–514

Riggins RS, Kraus JF 1977 The risk of neurological damage with fractures of the vertebrae. Journal of Trauma 17: 126–133

Sonntag VKH, Douglas RA 1992 Management of cervical spinal cord trauma. Journal of Neurotrauma 9: 5385–5394

Swain AH, Grundy D 1993 In: At the accident. ABC of spinal cord injury. BMJ Publications, London, p 1

Toscano J 1988 Prevention of neurological deterioration before admission to a spinal cord injury unit. Paraplegia 26: 143–150

Walton R, Besalvo JF, Ernst AA, Shahane A 1995 Padded vs unpadded spine board for cervical spine immobilisation. Academic Emergency Medicine 2: 725–728

Abdominal and genitourinary trauma

27

Introduction	298
Anatomy	298
Mechanisms of injury	299
Examination and physical signs	300
Treatment	301
Genitourinary trauma	302
Genital injuries	303
References	304

Introduction

Abdominal injuries resulting from trauma are common. They can range from life-threatening conditions that require immediate resuscitation and emergency laparotomy to those that require more conservative management. Unfortunately, these emergencies can be difficult to assess and correctly diagnose. Consequently, emphasis has to be put on assessing the severity of the patient's condition and managing it appropriately. In particular, it is important to recognize those patients who require immediate resuscitation and urgent transfer to hospital.

Anatomy

In considering the mechanisms of abdominal trauma, it is necessary to be familiar with the relevant anatomy.

The abdomen is a cavity bounded by bone and muscle. The anterior abdominal wall lies between the anterior axillary lines, the posterior abdominal wall lies between the posterior axillary lines, whereas the flanks lie between the anterior and posterior axillary lines. The posterior wall is semirigid, comprising the spine and paraspinal muscles. The anterior wall and flanks are musculotendinous, extending from the costal margins of the thorax to the pelvic girdle. The diaphragm divides the upper abdomen from the thoracic cavity. As the diaphragm moves downwards with inspiration, the liver, spleen and stomach are pushed down below the partial protection of the lower ribs and costal margins. The lower border of the abdomen is formed by the pelvic floor muscles.

The internal aspect of the abdominal cavity is lined with a thick double layer of peritoneum. This divides the organs that are intraperitoneal from those that are retroperitoneal. As the outer layer of peritoneum is supplied by nerves, which also supply the skin overlying that area, accurate localization of injury is often possible. This is not possible with the inner layer because it has a different nerve supply. The layers of peritoneum carry the vascular and nervous supply to the abdominal organs.

Retroperitoneal structures lie on the semirigid posterior abdominal wall (Table 27.1). They include the aorta, inferior vena cava, ascending and descending colon, duodenum, pancreas, kidneys and ureters. These structures have limited mobility and therefore cannot move out of the way during injury. Hence, they are more likely to be damaged in this situation than the more mobile intraperitoneal small bowel and transverse colon.

In the case of blunt trauma, the blood supply of intraperitoneal structures, such as the small bowel, may be disrupted if mobile vessels are sheared from the immobile

Table 27.1 Retroperitoneal structures

- Aorta
- Inferior vena cava
- Ascending and descending colon
- Duodenum
- Pancreas
- Kidneys
- Ureters

Table 27.2 Major vessels which can cause life-threatening haemorrhage

- Aorta
- Inferior vena cava
- Coeliac axis
- Superior mesenteric vessels
- Iliac vessels
- Renal vessels
- Hepatic artery
- Portal vein

aorta as well as from the caval and portal venous systems. Similarly, shearing forces can result in vascular disruption to the liver and spleen where mobile vessels join more fixed ones. These organs are very vascular and blunt traumatic forces can cause shearing of their solid tissue. The duodenum lies coiled around the pancreas high in the retroperitoneal space and significant blunt or penetrating injury may damage both together. The mobility of the kidneys and ureters is closely related to the movement of the diaphragm during respiration. They are generally well protected by the lower ribs and lumbar musculature but are prone to direct blunt trauma and shearing forces acting through their vascular connection with the aorta.

Mechanisms of injury

Assessment and appropriate management of the trauma patient depends on the identification of actual and potential injuries. An accurate history and assessment of the scene will greatly help in this process. In countries where civil violence is still relatively rare, the ratio of penetrating to blunt abdominal injury is approximately 1:10. In contrast, places with a high level of violence and crime, such as the USA, have a ratio of at least 1:1 (Rignault 1992).

BLUNT ABDOMINAL INJURIES

Blunt abdominal injuries most commonly occur as the result of road traffic accidents (American College of Surgeons' Advanced Trauma Life Support). During a collision, the forward motion of the body stops but the organ continues to move forward, causing tears at the point of attachment of the organ to the abdominal wall. If the organ is attached by a pedicle, a tear can occur to this. During deceleration injury the liver may be lacerated on impact with the ligamentum teres, which is attached to the anterior abdominal wall and the left lobe of the liver.

Pelvic fractures may cause injury to the bladder or to the pelvic blood vessels. Approximately 10% of patients with a pelvic fracture have a genitourinary injury (Spirnak 1988).

During frontal impact, organs may rupture as they are pressed against the vertebral column. This type of injury frequently involves the liver, spleen, pancreas and kidneys. An increase in intra-abdominal pressure, e.g. on impact with the steering column, may occasionally lead to rupture of the diaphragm. An increase in intra-abdominal pressure can also rarely cause retrograde blood flow, leading to rupture of the aortic valve.

In blunt abdominal trauma, the organs most frequently involved are the spleen, liver, retroperitoneal vasculature, kidney and small bowel.

PENETRATING ABDOMINAL INJURY

In cases of stabbing the most commonly injured organ is the liver (Lacqua & Sahdev 1993), because of its large size and high position. Other commonly injured organs include the colon, small bowel and stomach. 10% of abdominal stab wounds cause vascular injuries (Rignault 1992). When a major vessel is involved, the victim's life is immediately at risk (Table 27.2).

Rapid transportation with adequate resuscitation and prompt surgery are essential if the patient is to survive. Stab wounds have a lower potential for injury than gunshot wounds as they are much less likely to cause injury to multiple organs and are not associated with cavitation. In victims of stabbing, the site of entry of the weapon has a marked influence on the likelihood of intra-abdominal injury. In one study (Sirinek 1990) intra-abdominal injury was found at laparotomy in 66% of patients with anterior stab wounds, 51% of patients with flank stab wounds and 35% of those with back stab wounds.

In gunshot patients hollow viscera are commonly involved, most frequently the small bowel (Rignault 1992). However, other structures may be involved, including the mesentery and omentum, liver, colon and diaphragm. In gunshot wounds, the likelihood of intra-abdominal injury is dependent more on the type of weapon used than the entry site of the bullet. High-energy weapons cause more severe injury than medium-energy weapons (Ch. 30).

Shotgun injuries can range from minor pellet wounds to devastating soft tissue and visceral injuries. At close range, shotgun wounds produce similar injuries to high-velocity weapons. In contrast, at longer range each pellet becomes a low-energy missile, as the pellets spread before reaching the target. It has been shown that 80% of all abdominal gunshot wounds penetrate the peritoneum and 95% of these cause significant intra-abdominal injury (Lacqua & Sahdev 1993).

THE PATIENT WITH A CHEST AND PELVIC INJURY

The patient with a chest and pelvic injury is likely also to have an abdominal injury. This is because of the close anatomical relationship between the chest and the abdomen and between the abdomen and the pelvis.

Chest injury + pelvic injury = abdominal injury.

The upper abdomen is protected anteriorly by the lower ribs and posteriorly by the vertebral column. The liver, spleen, diaphragm and stomach all lie in this region and any may be injured as a result of injury to the sternum or lower ribs. The liver and spleen are most commonly injured by the same forces that cause fractures to the lower ribs. The lower abdomen gains some protection from the bony pelvis. However, pelvic fracture may be associated with injuries to the pelvic organs, intra-abdominal viscera and retroperitoneal and pelvic vascular structures. Fractured pelvic bones are themselves associated with significant haemorrhage and, as a consequence, hypotension in such a patient may be due to many causes.

When making an initial assessment of a patient with chest and pelvic injuries, it is essential to maintain a high index of suspicion that an abdominal injury is also present even if this is not clinically obvious. The patient should be treated as if such an injury is present until this can be confirmed or excluded by further investigations in hospital.

Diaphragmatic rupture is usually due to upper abdominal trauma, typically resulting from road traffic accidents. It is commonly associated with other chest and abdominal injuries and is often initially overlooked. Severe compression to the abdomen may cause the intra-abdominal pressure to rise enough to rupture the diaphragm. This will allow the abdominal organs such as the colon, small intestine and spleen to enter the thoracic cavity. This restricts lung expansion and reduces ventilation. Consequently, the conscious patient may complain of shortness of breath.

PATIENTS WITH ASSOCIATED PENETRATING CHEST INJURIES

Patients who have penetrating wounds to the lower part of the chest may also have abdominal injuries. During maximal expiration the diaphragm ascends to the fourth intercostal space anteriorly, the sixth intercostal space laterally and the eighth intercostal space posteriorly. Hence, a stab wound at or below this level may pass through the diaphragm and cause damage to intra-abdominal viscera. Organs particularly at risk in this situation are the spleen, liver, stomach, pancreas and major vascular structures (see Ch. 25 on chest injuries). In the case of gunshot wounds, the bullet may be deflected on hitting bone and hence it is often not possible to determine clinically the exact path of the bullet, particularly if there is no visible exit wound. In this situation it is safer to assume that any missile entering the thorax may have crossed the diaphragm and caused intra-abdominal injury.

Examination and physical signs

Unrecognized abdominal injuries remain a frequent cause of death from trauma because signs and symptoms of abdominal injury are subtle and often unreliable. They may be masked by unconsciousness, head injury, spinal injury, alcohol or drugs. In the UK 40% of patients with intra-abdominal haemorrhage have benign abdominal signs when first assessed in the emergency department. With all the difficulties faced in the prehospital environment, this figure is likely to be much higher for assessment at the scene. The peritoneal cavity is also a potential reservoir for massive blood loss. Hence, it is essential to have a high index of suspicion of abdominal injury in trauma patients, based on the mechanism of injury.

Initial assessment of the patient with abdominal or genitourinary trauma should follow the Advanced Trauma Life Support (ATLS) guidelines instituted by the American College of Surgeons. Safety of the scene must be ensured before approaching the patient. A rapid assessment can then be made of the mechanism of injury, hence enabling prediction of likely injuries. On reaching the patient, a primary survey and resuscitation should be commenced in the usual manner. The patient with abdominal trauma may show signs of shock. Indeed, the most reliable indicator of intra-abdominal bleeding is the presence of shock from an unexplained cause.

The conscious patient may complain of pain, although this may be masked as stated previously. On inspection of the abdomen, bruising and abrasions may be visible. There may be obvious external haemorrhage, penetrating wounds, impaled objects or evisceration (Fig. 27.1).

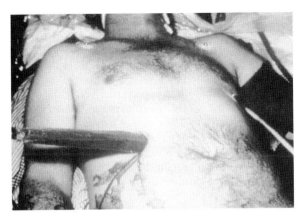

Fig. 27.1 • Penetrating abdominal trauma.

Palpation of the abdomen may reveal tenderness, guarding, rigidity and rebound tenderness, all of which suggest underlying abdominal injury. Pelvic injury may be elicited by careful examination of the pelvis. Fractures associated with instability are usually also associated with significant haemorrhage. Consequently, if careful examination suggests pelvic injury, a pelvic splint should be applied.

Auscultation of the abdomen is difficult at the scene and does not alter patient management; therefore is not recommended. Examination of the chest is essential in patients with abdominal injuries as coexisting chest injuries are common. The secondary survey should not delay the transfer of an unstable patient to hospital.

Treatment

This should follow the Advanced Trauma Life Support (ATLS) approach; therefore it starts with initial resuscitation during the primary survey, and management of the airway and cervical spine, breathing and circulation (ABC). As stated previously, the most reliable indicator of intra-abdominal bleeding is the presence of hypovolaemic shock from an unexplained cause. Similarly, if a patient's level of hypovolaemic shock is greater than can be explained by other injuries, this should also raise suspicion of intra-abdominal haemorrhage.

The definitive treatment for intra-abdominal bleeding is laparotomy to stop the bleeding process. Hence, the patient must be transferred without delay to the nearest hospital with the facilities to perform emergency surgery. All trauma patients with abdominal injuries should be given high-flow oxygen and kept warm. Time should not be wasted at the scene in attempt to determine the exact nature of the injury, as this will often not be apparent until laparotomy has been performed.

PREHOSPITAL FLUID

The value of intravenous fluid administration in the prehospital phase remains controversial because of associated delays in transport and the inadequate fluid volumes that are usually infused. Given that the definitive life-saving treatment for patients with abdominal bleeding is laparotomy, any delay in transportation may lead to the death of a salvageable patient and is therefore unacceptable. In many cases, particularly in urban areas, transport time to hospital has been shown to be less than the time taken to establish an intravenous line (Pollack 1993). The small volumes of fluid infused in transit have little influence on the final outcome as many prehospital personnel are reluctant to infuse fluids at rates necessary to produce any benefit (O'Gorman et al 1989).

It has been shown that intravenous access can be gained en route to the hospital in the majority of patients, and with equal success rates to those at the scene (O'Gorman et al 1989, Slovis et al 1990). Hence, ideally, intravenous access should only be initiated en route in a moving ambulance. There has also been controversy as to whether the resuscitation of hypovolaemic trauma patients with intravenous fluids before surgery to stop haemorrhage is of any benefit. The rationale behind this treatment is to give fluid in order to maintain perfusion to vital organs. However, in giving intravenous fluid in order to increase organ perfusion, the blood pressure is also increased, and this may increase haemorrhage from an abdominal injury (Martin et al 1992). It has been suggested that elevation of blood pressure before haemorrhage has been surgically controlled may be detrimental to the survival of the patient. This appears to be supported by research showing a better outcome in patients in whom fluid resuscitation was delayed until surgical haemostasis was achieved (Kaweski et al 1990, Martin et al 1992, Bickell et al 1994). However, much of this research has been done on young trauma patients with penetrating injuries and short prehospital times, and extrapolation to older patients, blunt injuries and rural areas may not be appropriate.

Until further research determines the true benefits of prehospital fluid resuscitation in major trauma, it is recommended that intravenous therapy in the field is initiated in a way that ensures that patient transport to definitive care is not compromised. Hence, intravenous line establishment in the hypotensive patient who is not trapped should occur in a moving ambulance, and not at the scene.

IMPALED OBJECTS

Removal of impaled objects at the accident scene may cause further abdominal trauma, and increase bleeding. They should be left in place until the patient has been assessed in hospital and transferred to the operating theatre. If the object is fixed, or large enough to prevent patient transfer, the involvement of the fire brigade may be necessary in order to facilitate rescue. This will enable the patient to be transferred without complete removal of the object.

An impaled object should be immobilized and supported to prevent further movement during transportation. External bleeding should be stopped using direct pressure, and the patient should be transferred without delay to a hospital with the facilities for immediate surgery.

EVISCERATION

This is the protrusion of part of the intestine or other organ outside the abdominal cavity through an open wound. No attempt should be made to push the protruding organ back into the abdomen. It is essential to keep the protruding organ moist by covering it with sterile pads soaked in saline as, when the tissues become dry, necrosis will occur.

PELVIC FRACTURES

These usually result from severe blunt trauma and have a mortality of 5–20% (Spirnak 1988). They are frequently associated with other severe visceral injuries, most commonly the bladder and urethra. The pelvis is a rigid ring of bone, joined by tough fibrous tissue at the pubic symphysis and sacroiliac joints. It provides considerable protection to the bladder, prostate and part of the male urethra. As it is a ring structure, fracture at one point in the ring without fracture, diastasis or dislocation elsewhere in the ring is uncommon. The bladder is predominantly an abdominal organ during early childhood and takes up its position beneath the symphysis pubis at approximately 6 years of age, thus becoming a pelvic organ.

Most pelvic fractures result from road traffic accidents, especially amongst pedestrians and motorcyclists. However, they may also result from falls, crush injuries and sports accidents. Urethral injuries occur in up to 11% of patients with pelvic fractures (Spirnak 1988), although rarely in females, as the urethra is short, mobile and not attached to the pubis. Bladder rupture occurs in 5–10% of patients with pelvic fracture (Hanno & Wein 1984, Spirnak 1988). Combined urethral and bladder injuries occur in 1% of patients with pelvic fracture (Spirnak 1988).

Consequently, all patients considered to have a pelvic fracture should also be suspected of having a urethral or bladder injury. Macroscopic haematuria and blood at the external urethral meatus indicate this type of injury. Inability to void urine may indicate a urethral or bladder injury or may simply be due to an empty bladder or to severe pain from the pelvic fracture.

Genitourinary trauma

In the patient with severe multiple trauma, injuries to the genitourinary tract are often of secondary importance. Nevertheless, when initial assessment and stabilization has been achieved, it is essential that these injuries are not overlooked. Any suspicion of genitourinary injury should simply be communicated to the receiving medical staff on arrival at hospital. Urinary tract injuries are usually associated with other injuries, typically pelvic fractures and abdominal injuries.

URETHRAL INJURIES

The membranous and bulbous parts of the urethra are most susceptible to trauma because of their lack of mobility. Injury to the bulbous urethra is frequently associated with straddle-type falls, whereas injury to the membranous urethra is most frequently associated with pelvic fractures. Suspicion of urethral injury should be raised by any direct trauma to the perineum.

Retrograde urethrography in the emergency department will aid diagnosis. Urethral injuries may be treated surgically or conservatively. Prehospital management of patients with urethral injuries should be directed at treatment of life-threatening injuries and transportation to a hospital with appropriate facilities.

BLADDER INJURIES

The bladder may be injured by blunt or penetrating trauma. After a direct blow the intravesical pressure may rise rapidly to a level high enough to cause rupture of the bladder wall. In the case of a pelvic fracture the bladder may be injured directly from a bony fragment. If both pubic rami are fractured on both sides, the incidence of bladder rupture is increased to 20% (Hanno & Wein 1984). Penetrating injuries to the abdomen may also involve the bladder. This type of injury should therefore be suspected in a patient with pelvic fractures, lower abdominal injuries or suprapubic pain following trauma. Classical signs are gross haematuria and inability to pass urine. If the rupture is intraperitoneal, signs of peritonitis may develop but these often occur very late. Between 5% and 10% of patients with a fractured pelvis will have an associated bladder rupture (Hanno & Wein 1984, Spirnak 1988).

Penetrating trauma to the bladder is relatively uncommon. Frequently associated injured organs include the rectum and sigmoid colon, often with devastating results, the small intestine and the iliac vessels. Treatment of penetrating bladder injuries is by surgical exploration.

URETERIC INJURIES

Trauma to the ureters is relatively uncommon as they lie in a well-protected position. Other more life-threatening injuries take priority in initial management. However, ureteral trauma should be considered if there is a penetrating injury in the area of the ureter or if the course of a penetrating object crosses the path of the ureter (Hanno & Wein 1984). Deceleration injury with hyperextension of the spine is associated with ureteropelvic junction disruption. Haematuria, or the presence of a flank mass, should also raise the suspicion of a ureteric injury. Ureteral injuries require a high index of suspicion for diagnosis and confirmation of the injury is by intravenous pyelogram after more serious injuries have been excluded or managed.

RENAL INJURIES

The kidneys lie in the retroperitoneal space, anterior to the lower ribs, inferior to the liver, spleen and diaphragm, and hence are relatively well protected from trauma. They are relatively mobile organs, fixed by their attachments to the ureters and their vascular attachments to the aorta and inferior vena cava. They are surrounded by a tough renal capsule, which requires great force to tear it. The kidney is also surrounded by fascia, which has a tamponade effect on renal haemorrhage. If this fascia is damaged, massive bleeding into the retroperitoneal space may occur.

Blunt renal injury

This is most commonly associated with road traffic accidents, when sudden deceleration forces occur (Hanno and Wein 1984, Guerriero 1988). Direct blows during football and other contact sports are also common causes. The mobile kidney may move on its pedicle, colliding with the ribs to cause renal contusions. When the trauma causes rib fractures, renal lacerations may also occur (Table 27.3).

Haematuria is not always present in renal injury (Hanno & Wein 1984, Guerriero 1988) and there is poor correlation between the amount of haematuria and the severity of the renal injury (Hanno & Wein 1984).

Initial management of these patients is by primary survey and resuscitation, followed by rapid transfer to a hospital with the facilities to perform appropriate investigations and prompt surgery when required, although the majority of patients with blunt renal injury can be managed conservatively.

Penetrating renal injury

80% of patients with penetrating renal trauma will have an associated intra-abdominal injury requiring laparotomy (Guerriero 1988). This is almost universal in the case of penetrating gunshot wounds, whereas stab wounds, particularly those to the flank, are less likely to cause serious associated injury (Guerriero 1988). The abdominal injury often poses a greater threat to life than the renal injury, although renal haemorrhage can be massive when the tamponade effect of the renal fascia is lost. Immediate management of the patient with penetrating renal trauma is therefore similar to treatment for patients with penetrating abdominal trauma. Consequently, the patient requires a primary survey, resuscitation and rapid transfer to a unit with appropriate facilities. Definitive management entails evaluation with intravenous urography, and may often require laparotomy.

Genital injuries

These can be classified into penetrating injuries, blunt injuries and avulsion injuries.

PENETRATING INJURIES

Immediate management at the scene is similar to that for penetrating abdominal injuries (see earlier in text). If urethral damage is suspected, retrograde urethrography will be necessary. Otherwise hospital management includes wound irrigation and debridement, removal of foreign bodies, surgical exploration and repair as appropriate.

BLUNT INJURIES

Direct blows to the penis or scrotum are associated with marked pain and swelling. Cold packs, rest and elevation will usually be adequate. If there is persistent bleeding, surgical haemostasis and drainage may be necessary. If rupture of the testis or corporal tissue is suspected, immediate exploration and surgical repair will be necessary.

Table 27.3 Factors suggestive of renal injury

- Mechanism suggestive
- Deceleration injury
- Direct blow to the flank
- Fractures of lower ribs or upper lumbar vertebrae
- Flank pain or tenderness
- Swelling in flank
- Haematuria
- Hypovolaemic shock

Table 27.4 Summary – management of abdominal and genitourinary trauma

- Consider mechanism of injury
- Primary survey and immediate resuscitation
- Consider intravenous fluids
- Rapid secondary survey (if the patient is stable)
- Transfer without delay to appropriate hospital

AVULSION INJURIES

Accidents involving machinery may lead to the avulsion of penile or scrotal skin. Immediate management at the scene consists of analgesia, wrapping the injured part in sterile saline-soaked dressings and transportation to a hospital with appropriate facilities. Definitive care includes broad-spectrum antibiotics, tetanus prophylaxis and surgical debridement with skin grafting. If the testes cannot be covered with skin, they may be implanted beneath the skin in the thighs.

References

Bickell W, Wall M, Pepe P et al 1994 Immediate versus delayed fluid resuscitation for hypotensive patients with penetrating injuries. New England Journal of Medicine 331: 1105–1109

Guerriero WG 1988 Etiology, classification and management of renal trauma. Surgical Clinics of North America 68: 1071–1084

Hanno PM, Wein AJ 1984 Urological trauma. Emergency Medical Clinics of North America 2: 823–840

Kaweski SM, Sise MJ, Virgilio RW 1990 The effect of pre-hospital fluids on survival in trauma patients. Journal of Trauma 30: 1215–1218

Lacqua MJ, Sahdev P 1993 Effective management of penetrating abdominal trauma. Hospital Practice 4 June: 31–38

Martin RR, Bickell WH, Pepe PE et al 1992 Prospective evaluation of pre-hospital fluid resuscitation in hypotensive patients with penetrating truncal injury: a preliminary report. Journal of Trauma 33: 354–361

O'Gorman M, Trabulsy P, Pilcher DB 1989 Zero time pre-hospital IV. Journal of Trauma 29: 84–86

Pollack CV 1993 Pre-hospital fluid resuscitation of the trauma patient – an update on the controversies. Emergency Medicine Clinics of North America 11: 61–70

Rignault DP 1992 Abdominal trauma in war. World Journal of Surgery 16: 940–946

Sirinek KR 1990 Is exploratory celiotomy necessary for all patients with trunkal stab wounds? Archives of Surgery 125: 844

Slovis CM, Herr EW, Londorf D et al 1990 Success rates for initiation of intravenous therapy en route by pre-hospital care providers. American Journal of Emergency Medicine 8: 305–307

Spirnak JP 1988 Pelvic fracture and injury to the lower urinary tract. Surgical Clinics of North America 68: 1057–1062

The prehospital care of bone and joint injuries

28

Introduction   305

Mechanisms of injury   305

Classification   306

Diagnosis and assessment   308

Principles of management   308

Local injuries   309

Further reading   314

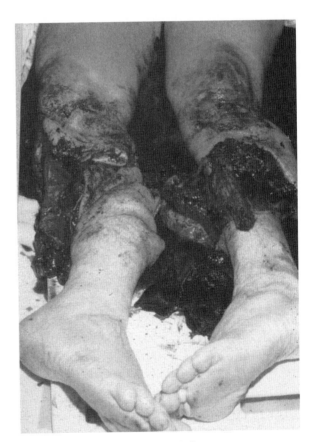

Fig. 28.1 • Life-threatening limb injuries.

Introduction

Limb trauma and fractures are the commonest injuries that a prehospital care practitioner will encounter. These injuries are rarely life-threatening, and it must be remembered that the care of the airway, breathing and circulation must take precedence over fracture management – however spectacular the sight of the limb trauma may appear. Exceptions occur if a fracture in some way influences the care of the above, e.g. causing external blood loss that requires haemorrhage control (Fig. 28.1). Although unlikely to be life-threatening, fractures may pose multiple problems to prehospital care personnel particularly with regard to immobilization, appropriate pain relief and subsequent safe, painless extrication.

Mechanisms of injury

Bone is strongest under compressive load-bearing forces and weakest if distracted and twisted. Fractures of the ankle involving twisting forces to the tibia and fibula where the foot is fixed are classic examples. Bone may also fracture as a result of direct force. Examples include fracture of the tibia from a kick in football and fracture of the ulna in assuming a defensive position during an assault where direct forces far exceed the strength of the bone. The type of force, direction and degree of tension or compression determine the type of fractures that may occur.

Classification

FRACTURE

A fracture is a loss of continuity of the cortex of a bone. It occurs as a result of forces being applied to a bone that exceed its strength. The results may range from a small hairline fracture, such as a march (stress) fracture, to a more major disruption of the bone, such as occurs in high-speed road traffic accidents.

Fractures can be broadly divided in a number of ways. The majority of classifications are irrelevant to the prehospital carer as they are based on X-ray appearance but give valuable information to the hospital practitioner as to the degree and nature of the violence to which the bone has been subjected. On X-ray appearance the fracture may be divided as to the pattern or direction of the break (e.g. a transverse fracture, spiral fracture, oblique fracture.) The *comminuted* fracture contains multiple small fragments of bone that may well represent a measure of the amount of force that has been applied to cause the fracture. A simple classification of fractures is given in Fig. 28.2.

A *complicated* fracture is defined as one where there is associated damage to vessels or nerves.

When the shaft of a long bone fractures it may do so in a straightforward transverse manner; introduction of a rotational component to the fracturing force may result in an *oblique* or *spiral* fracture. If a fragment of bone separates from the shaft this is a *butterfly* fragment. Flat bones, such as those found in the skull, usually suffer linear fractures, although if a segment of bone becomes detached a *depressed* fracture may occur as it is displaced inwards by the force of the causative blow.

SIMPLE AND COMPOUND (CLOSED AND OPEN)

Simple (closed) fractures are those where there is no overlying wound communicating with the fracture site. Although described as simple, this in no way reflects their complexity or the potential problems that such fractures may cause. For example, a simple fracture that extends into a joint may cause far more significant pain, stiffness and post-treatment disability than an open injury of the shaft

of the bone. In open fractures there is an overlying wound that communicates with the fracture.

One of the most important aspects of prehospital fracture management is preventing simple fractures from becoming compound as a result of inappropriate handling.

The open fracture can be subdivided according to whether the wound has been caused by the bone exiting the skin (from within outwards) or by an object entering the body through the skin (from without inwards). Although this information may be of use to the hospital practitioner, it is of little value in the field.

All open wounds need protecting from further contamination, dressing with a moist sterile dressing and then immobilizing. If an iodine dressing, such as Betadine or a similar substance, is available this should be poured over the inner aspect of the dressing, but if not saline is a good alternative.

Once a wound over an open fracture has been dressed, the wound should be left undisturbed in order to reduce the risk of further contamination. The gold standard of care is to carry a Polaroid camera and photograph the injury prior to the application of a dressing. The photograph should accompany the patient report form to hospital.

Open wounds may lose more than twice the volume of blood that a closed fracture of the same bone would be expected to lose, and it may be necessary to apply some form of compression dressing to limit external haemorrhage. In this situation, treatment of the open wound may be part of the primary survey.

PATHOLOGICAL FRACTURES

Bone may fracture through abnormal areas where sites of bony weakness exist. Abnormal bone is typically seen where a malignancy has spread to bone with the formation of secondary deposits, or where there is intrinsic bone malignancy such as a sarcoma. Other potential causes of pathological fracture include benign tumours of bone, sites of bony infection or metabolic conditions of bone. Owing to the structural weakening of the bone, the forces required to produce a fracture may be minimal.

There may be a history compatible with pain in the bone leading up to the fracture in a patient with a known history of malignancy. In general, the fractures seen in the elderly where bone has been weakened by osteoporosis (a disease characteristically affecting elderly patients where there is loss of bone strength and fractures occur with very little force) are not regarded as pathological. The commonest fractures resulting from osteoporosis are vertebral

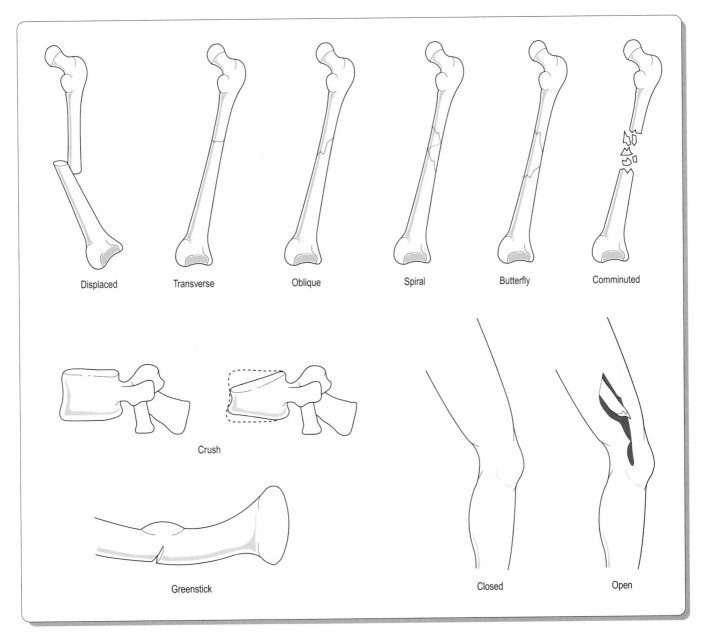

Fig. 28.2 • A classification of fractures.

compression fractures, fractures of the neck of the femur and humerus, and the Colles fracture of the wrist.

FRACTURES IN CHILDREN

Fractures in children need special consideration. The areas of active bone growth at the epiphyses are weak and at increased risk of fracture. If these fractures are not correctly managed, abnormalities of subsequent growth may occur.

Because bone in childhood is softer than in adulthood, children's bones may bend in response to trauma. This produces two characteristic appearances on an X-ray: the torus fracture, where one cortex is buckled (hence the alternative term 'buckle' fracture), and the greenstick fracture, where one cortex and medullary bone is fractured but the other cortex is buckled but intact.

DISLOCATIONS

A dislocation is the complete disturbance of the congruity of a joint such that the joint surfaces are no longer in contact. Some dislocations are complicated by a fracture of a bony part of the joint (fracture dislocations). Posterior dislocation of the hip following a road traffic accident, where the knee strikes the dashboard and the hip is driven backwards fracturing the posterior lip of the acetabulum, is an example of such an injury.

The principle of treatment of any dislocation is rapid reduction. Some dislocations should, if possible, be immediately relocated at the scene (e.g. a dislocation of the knee, especially if associated with vascular complications). Subluxation is a partial loss of normal congruity of joint surfaces; a common example is subluxation of the acromio-clavicular joint due to a fall on the point of the shoulder.

Diagnosis and assessment

The diagnosis of a fracture, like any other injury, is based on the history and examination. The hospital practitioner has the benefit of special investigations, such as X-rays. A knowledge of the mechanism of injury and the forces involved is of the greatest value in determining the possibility of fracture. The patient may complain of pain at the fracture site but there may be circumstances (such as a head injury) that make interpretation of pain and other symptoms difficult or make it difficult for a patient to complain.

On examination of the affected part there may be obvious signs of swelling, bruising, deformity and angulation (Table 28.1). There may be pattern bruising (e.g. car tyre tracks) across the limb. Any form of movement may elicit the sound and feel of crepitus – the grating of broken bone on broken bone. As a sign this should not be elicited in the conscious patient but may be detected as a deformed limb is straightened.

There may be obvious signs of an open wound. Abnormal movement of the limb at sites that would normally not be expected to move may be revealed on examination. It is imperative to check sensation, capillary refill and pulses distal to the fracture but in the prehospital environment the appropriate amount of exposure required should be just enough to ascertain these are normal or abnormal and no more.

Tight jeans or motorcycle leathers may provide valuable splintage and tamponade of bleeding, and removing such garments may be detrimental as it may increase blood loss and limb swelling if proper traction and immobilization is not possible.

If the limb is grossly deformed it should be straightened. This manoeuvre should be performed with gentle traction and appropriate analgesia. Both before and after correction of the deformity it is mandatory to check that there has been no change in vascular or neurological status. If on initial examination there is an absence of pulses with a distorted limb then the limb should be immediately straightened and the pulses reassessed. Suspicion of vascular injury is heightened if the limb appears cooler than its opposite number and has diminished pulses. Many sources state that there may be diminished oxygen saturation in the injured limb when measured by pulse oximetry but there are many variables that may affect this. Peripheral vasoconstriction due to cold (especially if the limb has been exposed to check the pulses and to arrange immobilization), as well as hypoxia due to other general injuries, may alter the saturation of oxygen in the blood. A vascular injury also has to be very severe before a drop in saturation occurs, particularly if the patient is breathing 100% oxygen.

Principles of management

The initial priorities in the management of a patient with a fracture are:

- Safety
- Control of exsanguinatory external haemorrhage
- Airway and cervical spine control
- Breathing with high flow oxygen
- Circulation with haemorrhage control
- Disability
- Exposure.

The essential components of fracture management are reduction and immobilization. How these are best achieved will depend on the nature of individual fractures and the clinical state of the patient.

CLOSED FRACTURES

Wherever possible, gross deformity should be reduced by whatever method is thought appropriate at the scene. The limb is returned to its natural alignment by traction on the limb, lengthening any shortening caused by the fracture

---

Table 28.1 Features of fractures

- Pain
- Swelling
- Tenderness
- Deformity
- Crepitus
- Loss of function

---

and associated muscle spasm. Reduction and splintage may be painful procedures and adequate analgesia should always be given. Definitive splintage, especially of the lower limbs, may only be possible once the patient has been extricated from a vehicle. A properly reduced and splinted limb is usually much more comfortable during evacuation and transport to a facility for definitive treatment.

Correct reduction of a fracture will result in lower blood loss into the surrounding tissues (in the case of a fractured femur, the shortening of the thigh allows the swelling thigh to approach the shape of a sphere rather than that of a cylinder: the volume of blood that a sphere can contain is much greater than that of a cylinder for a given surface area). Following reduction the limb should be immobilized; this may be achieved in a number of ways (Ch. 54).

OPEN FRACTURES

These differ from simple closed injuries only in that the wound needs dressing with a sterile dressing and appropriate measures need to be applied to control haemorrhage. Reduction of the fracture may be accompanied by the replacement of exposed bone back under the skin; this is not a problem as the correct treatment of any open fracture once in hospital is a thorough debridement and exploration of the wound. Apart from dressing the wound the treatment of an open fracture differs in no way from that of a closed fracture. Exactly the same methods of immobilization are used but may be even more important in the case of an open wound as the blood loss may be at least double that of its closed equivalent.

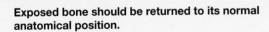

Exposed bone should be returned to its normal anatomical position.

DISLOCATIONS

The priority of treatment in these injuries is to reduce the dislocation so that the normal congruence of the joint surfaces is restored. The treatment of dislocations will vary from case to case. For example, for the patient with a simple dislocation of a shoulder the provision of simple support, analgesia and transfer to hospital for reduction is usually most appropriate. However, in a patient with a complex fracture dislocation of an ankle with no distal pulses, an immediate attempt should be made to reduce the dislocation under appropriate analgesia in order to reduce the risk of irreversible skin necrosis and neurovascular damage. It must be remembered that the optimal management of a dislocation may be effected by the presence of an unrecognized associated fracture. Prehospital care practitioners, therefore, are best advised only

to reduce dislocations where the limb is threatened or the possibility of an associated fracture can effectively be excluded (examples include lateral patellar dislocations or recurrent shoulder dislocations).

Local injuries

UPPER LIMB INJURIES

These injuries are common in all age groups. Mechanisms of injury vary greatly from complex fractures resulting from high-speed road traffic accidents to distal radial fractures occurring in the frail elderly as a consequence of simple falls. They are common in children, and particularly in boys, who are generally more adventurous than girls.

Finger and hand fractures

These injuries usually occur as a result of direct violence, including crush injury and during fist fights. They may be accompanied by cuts or teeth marks over the fracture where an attempt to punch an antagonist has resulted in contact with his/her teeth. In these cases there is a high risk of infection and antibiotic therapy will be required. The commonest hand fracture is a fracture of the fifth metacarpal (boxer's fracture). Hand injuries need to be taken extremely seriously, as the potential for loss of function due to bony deformity or damage to tendons and nerves is high; it is mandatory, therefore, for such injuries to be seen in a hospital emergency department no matter how trivial they may appear.

Dislocations and fractures of fingers occur in a variety of situations, including sports, and the dislocations are often reduced by the patients themselves or by bystanders. Many of these injuries can simply be treated with some form of neighbour strapping provided that there is no major deformity of the fingers (swelling excluded) or malrotation of the fingers when flexing to form a fist (Fig. 28.3).

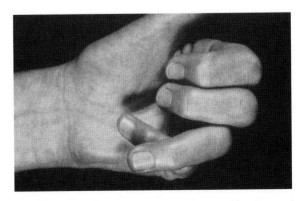

Fig. 28.3 • Malrotation of the little finger secondary to a metacarpal fracture.

If malalignment occurs with rotational injuries the ability to form a fist may be seriously hampered by underriding of the fingers. As an associated fracture cannot be excluded on clinical grounds, hospital attendance for X-ray assessment is essential. Prehospital care is usually limited to analgesia and the application of a broad arm sling.

Rings must be removed from every injured hand.

Wrist fractures

Fractures involving the carpus itself are quite uncommon, although they may occur after falls with forceful flexion or extension. The most common is a scaphoid fracture, which normally occurs as a result of a fall on an outstretched hand. If a scaphoid fracture is suspected the patient should be referred to an emergency department for assessment and careful follow-up. Features include pain in the wrist, characteristically at the base of the thumb, and tenderness in the anatomical snuffbox and over the dorsum of the scaphoid with pain on axial compression of the thumb.

Distal radial and ulnar fractures such as the Colles fracture are more common. These are particularly common in the osteoporotic elderly following a fall, usually on to an outstretched hand. The injured arm should be placed in a broad arm sling and then transported to hospital for further investigation and reduction if required. A rolled-up tabloid newspaper can be used as an improvised splint.

A fall on flexed wrist may produce a reversed Colles or Smith's fracture. The prehospital management is identical to that for a Colles fracture.

Any child complaining of pain in the wrist following a fall should be suspected of having a greenstick fracture and referred to hospital for an X-ray. A broad arm sling is appropriate for initial immobilization.

Forearm fractures

These fractures are more common in active young men. They may be caused by a fall on to an outstretched hand or by a direct blow. The latter may result in the so-called 'night-stick' injury to the ulna (an isolated fracture of the ulnar following a direct blow with a stick or pickaxe handle or similar implement where the patient, in an attempt to ward off the blow, raises his/her forearm.). The majority of forearm fractures in the adult will require open reduction and fixation; therefore they should be splinted in a support such as a broad arm sling or a box splint and transferred to hospital. Angulation should be corrected if it is very marked or there is neurovascular compromise; otherwise the fracture should be splinted unreduced for transfer to hospital.

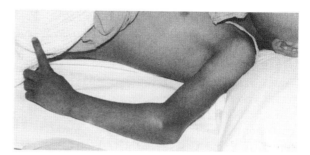

Fig. 28.4 • A displaced supracondylar fracture.

Injuries of the elbow

These may take the form of dislocations or injuries to any of the bones around the elbow. Supracondylar fractures are particularly common in children, and varying degrees of deformity are found. Severe deformity may be associated with vascular compromise due to kinking of the brachial artery, detected by the absence of a radial pulse and the presence of an ischaemic white hand with increased capillary refill time. In the prehospital environment, manipulation of the fracture in an attempt to regain the vascular supply may be difficult but circulation usually returns as the elbow is extended. If there is deformity with no loss of vascular supply the elbow should not have its position changed as the process of manipulation can itself result in loss of vascular supply. The arm should be splinted and transfer to hospital arranged. As well as vascular compromise, neurological compromise, especially of the median nerve, may occur.

Proximal ulnar (olecranon) fractures usually result from a fall directly on to the point of the elbow. Rarely they can result from resisted elbow extension because of the pull of triceps. Radial head and radial neck fractures commonly occur as a result of a fall on the outstretched hand and result in painful limitation of all elbow movements, especially rotation. Marked tenderness may be elicited on compression of the proximal radius anteriorly and laterally.

Dislocations of the elbow may occur following falls on to an outstretched hand, and rapid transfer to hospital for reduction is appropriate. A neurovascular assessment is essential and analgesia should be given.

Displaced supracondylar fractures (Fig. 28.4) and dislocated elbows are best immobilized in a vacuum splint in the position in which they are found or the position that restores optimal circulation. Alternatively, a padded box splint may be used. Undisplaced supracondylar fractures, olecranon fractures and fractures of the head or neck of radius may be immobilized in a broad arm sling.

Humeral fractures

Fractures of the middle third of the humerus may be associated with radial nerve damage, which is characterized by a wrist drop or weakness in extending the wrist. Classically, this is a transient problem, as the radial nerve is only bruised. In high-velocity injuries there is a greater chance of the radial nerve being torn and requiring operative intervention. Immediate treatment is either with a pad between the arm and the chest wall and two narrow triangular bandages above and below the fracture in combination with a broad arm sling, or alternatively padding and triangular bandages with the arm by the patient's side. A vacuum splint may also be used.

Fractures of the neck of the humerus most commonly occur in the elderly in association with osteoporosis. The mechanism is usually a fall either on to an outstretched hand or directly on to the upper arm. The patient usually supports the arm at the elbow and all movements are painful. Marked swelling is usually present. The arm should be placed initially in a broad arm sling, A collar and cuff is used after confirmation of the fracture in the emergency department.

SHOULDER INJURIES

Shoulder injuries usually follow a fall on to an outstretched hand or direct trauma. (Posterior dislocation of the shoulder may follow an epileptic fit or electric shock.) In the young person with no history of previous dislocations, a dislocation of the shoulder generally requires significant force. The majority of dislocations are anterior and many will show a characteristic abnormality of shoulder contour (Fig. 28.5). If previous dislocations have occurred resulting in instability then unguarded movement alone may be enough to cause dislocation. In both the young and the elderly, dislocations may be associated with a variety of fractures around and involving the humeral head.

In the elderly, fracture at the level of the surgical neck of the humerus is a common injury and may be complicated by a variety of fracture patterns that pass through the humeral head.

Uncomplicated dislocations of the shoulder are best left in a position of comfort during transfer. This is usually with the patient sitting up and supporting his/her own arm, often on a pillow across his/her knees. Although it is sometimes appropriate at sporting events for an experienced medical practitioner to perform an immediate reduction under analgesia, in most cases transfer to hospital for reduction following the exclusion of any associated fracture is more appropriate.

The prehospital management of posterior dislocation is the same as that of anterior dislocation.

CLAVICULAR FRACTURES

Clavicular fractures result either from direct trauma or transmission of forces along the upper limb in a fall on to

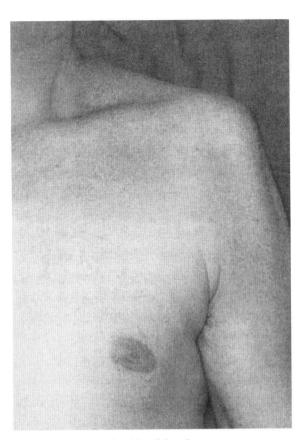

Fig. 28.5 • Anterior shoulder dislocation.

an outstretched hand. They are most common in sportsmen and children. In the prehospital setting, they require support in a broad arm sling, neurovascular assessment and transfer to hospital for confirmation of the diagnosis. Sometimes the clavicle may dislocate at the acromioclavicular joint, leading to a significant, but relatively harmless, deformity and marked point tenderness over the acromioclavicular joint. Treatment out of hospital does not differ from that of a clavicular fracture.

An unusual complication of a clavicular injury is damage to the subclavian artery as it passes from the chest to the arms, or damage to the brachial plexus. These complications tend to occur following very displaced fractures of the clavicle but may also occur when the sternoclavicular joint dislocates. This rare dislocation results from high-energy injuries that force the clavicle posteriorly or anteriorly. If posterior, the proximal end of the clavicle digs into the root of the neck, where it may compress the major vessels and/or the trachea, resulting in airway compromise. This injury is potentially life-threatening and should be reduced as soon as possible. The safest manoeuvre is to pull the clavicle forward by placing the fingers behind it at the same time as traction is applied to the arm.

SCAPULAR INJURIES

These injuries result from direct trauma to the scapula either in the form of a blow or as a result of an impact resulting from a high-velocity road traffic accident, such as a motorcyclist thrown from his/her bike. There may be an associated brachial plexus injury, particularly if there has been a forced rupture of the supporting shoulder musculature. In the worst scenario, complete dissociation of the shoulder girdle from the thoracic wall may occur, resulting in a useless limb. Support of the limb in a broad arm sling is the treatment of choice out of hospital in isolated scapular injury.

PELVIC FRACTURES

Although minor pelvic fractures (usually of the pubic rami) can occur in the elderly as a result of minimal trauma, they are more often found as a component of multisystem injury in the victims of high-energy accidents, such as road traffic accidents or falls from a height. Pelvic fractures may dramatically influence the findings of the primary survey as they may be associated with extremely high blood loss. Unexplained blood loss can often be attributed to bleeding into the pelvis. Accompanying injuries include abdominal and genitourinary injuries, femoral shaft fractures and damage to surrounding structures, including the lumbar spine, nerve roots and nerves (typically the sciatic nerve) as well as vascular structures (normally the venous plexuses around the sacrum).

If the mechanism of injury suggests a pelvic fracture or the patient complains of pelvic pain or there is pelvic deformity, the pelvis should not be examined. A pelvic splint should be applied.

Pelvic fractures may be difficult to detect, although classically there may be pain on careful examination of the pelvis. Unstable pelvic fractures effectively result in an expanded diameter of the pelvis and thus a bigger potential space for fracture haematoma. Thus, closing of the fracture pattern (i.e. reducing the diameter of the pelvis) should result in decreasing the blood loss. Pelvic fractures can be stabilized by a vacuum mattress, extrication device such as the Russell extrication device (RED), the Kendrick extrication device (KED) or the ED 2000 turned upside down with the extrication 'wings' strapped around the pelvis (Fig. 28.6).

LOWER LIMB FRACTURES

Fractures around the hip

The commonest of these is the fractured neck of femur commonly seen in the elderly patient following minor trauma. Although it is classically described as leaving the leg with the appearance of shortening and external rotation, this

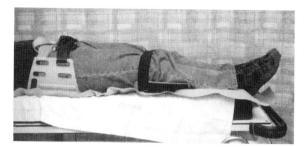

Fig. 28.6 • Using an extrication device for pelvic stabilization.

is by no means universal as the fracture may be undisplaced. An inability to straight leg raise may be useful in suggesting the presence of a bony injury. Any patient in whom there is any suspicion of a fracture of the proximal femur requires assessment in hospital. Appropriate analgesia should be given.

Femoral neck fracture in the younger patient is invariably the result of a high-velocity injury, such as a road traffic accident. In the adolescent, a traumatic acute slipped upper femoral epiphysis may present with the same features as a femoral neck fracture. Patients with a suspected fractured neck of the femur should be immobilized in a traction splint or the injured leg can be splinted to the intact limb during transport.

The commonest hip dislocation is that of a hip prosthesis, which is inevitably posterior and may occur with little provocation such as simply rising from a chair. Posterior dislocations following accidents present with shortening and internal rotation, adduction and flexion of the leg. They are normally a result of a force driving the femur backwards while the patient is in a sitting position, and are associated with road traffic accidents where the patient is sitting in an upright position and is thrown forwards, striking his/her knee on the dashboard. The limb should be splinted to the good leg using padding and triangular bandages with a pillow or rolled blanket supporting the knees. Alternatively, a vacuum mattress may be contoured to support the limb. Attempts to straighten the leg should be avoided. Neurovascular assessment is mandatory. Sciatic nerve injury is indicated by the presence of a foot drop. Urgent reduction is necessary following prompt transfer to hospital.

If the patient sustains a hyperextension injury to the hip, such as occurs in motorcycle accidents, an anterior dislocation may be found. This dislocation is associated with a high incidence of injuries to the femoral artery vein and nerve. The limb is splinted, and urgent reduction in hospital is necessary.

Femoral shaft fractures

Femoral shaft fractures are frequently associated with high-velocity road traffic accidents and are common in young men. These fractures may be associated with significant blood loss (anywhere between 2 litres in a closed injury and 4 litres in an open injury), and damage to the femoral artery and sciatic or femoral nerves. Fractures around the knee are associated with specific problems, which are discussed below. If the patient is wearing tight trousers these should be left on as to some extent they may tamponade blood loss within the thigh. The most appropriate form of immobilization is a traction splint. Analgesia for these injuries can be achieved with a femoral nerve block or titrated intravenous opiate analgesia.

Supracondylar fractures of the knee

These are often seen in the elderly, and again are related to osteoporosis. Vascular damage may occur, either at the site of the fracture or due to angulation of the fragments into the popliteal fossa. Fractures in the elderly may occur just above or involving a total knee replacement as a periprosthetic fracture. Immobilization is best achieved with a vacuum splint or box splint.

Use of a traction splint is relatively contraindicated because it may allow more angulation at the fracture site due to unopposed action of gastrocnemius on the distal femoral fragment. Care should be taken while examining this region as after a high-velocity injury the presence of a knee dislocation may be misinterpreted as a supracondylar fracture; in general a knee dislocation merits emergency reduction. This is achieved by pulling forwards on the tibia while applying longitudinal traction. Adequate analgesia is necessary.

Patellar fractures

Patellar fractures usually result from a fall on to the knee and are more common in the elderly. They may also result from sudden contraction of the quadriceps muscle in resisted extension, e.g. when the foot becomes trapped in a pothole. These injuries can be immobilized by positioning the knee in a box splint, avoiding pressure from the straps on the knee. Patella fractures may be diagnosed by palpating a gap in the patella or by local swelling and bony tenderness. Complete transection of the patella is associated with loss of active straight leg raising. Some fractures may be undisplaced, with the quadriceps tendon, patellar tendon and the surrounding reticular fibres of the patella intact, and thus straight leg raising may be preserved.

Patellar dislocations (Fig. 28.7) are invariably lateral and may occur in any age group but are common in young active females. There may be a history of recurrent dislocations and the patient may be used to reducing his/her own patella. If possible, the dislocated patella should be relocated as soon as possible by straightening the knee and applying medial force to the patella. Patellar dislocation

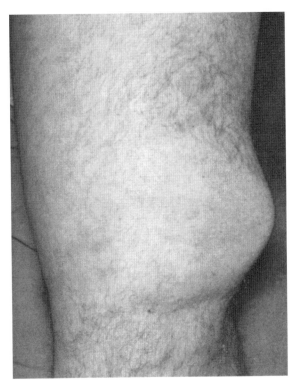

Fig. 28.7 • Patellar dislocation.

is extremely painful and parenteral analgesia may be necessary. Even if the patella reduces immediately, it is wise to seek hospital review. Immobilization of the leg once reduced is best achieved using a box splint. If the patella cannot be reduced, padding and triangular bandages with a blanket under the knee will provide support. A contoured vacuum mattress is an alternative.

Fractures of the knee

Fractures of the knee take three forms: tibial plateau fractures, usually due to varus or valgus compression; avulsion fractures of the insertions of the ligaments of the knee; and intra-articular fractures due to direct trauma. In each case precise diagnosis is likely to be difficult because of pain, swelling and loss of movement. Therefore, in all cases where there is a possibility of a significant knee injury, the leg should be immobilized in a box splint and the patient transferred to hospital for assessment and follow-up.

Tibial fractures

The mechanism of injury in tibial fractures varies from direct trauma during sport or a road traffic accident to a stress fracture following excessive physical activity. Tibial fractures run a particular risk of being open as the medial border is subcutaneous and free of muscle covering. Marked

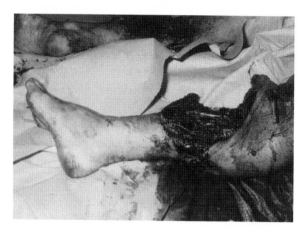

Fig. 28.8 • An open tibia and fibula fracture.

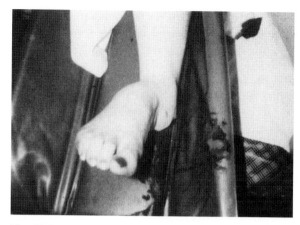

Fig. 28.9 • A complex ankle fracture requiring urgent reduction.

angulation is common. Any open wound should be treated as outlined above (Fig. 28.8). Immobilization is best achieved using a box splint, although a vacuum splint or traction splint can be used. Careful neurovascular assessment is necessary before and after application of any form of splintage. Tibial fractures may be associated with the development of compartment syndrome.

Fibular fractures

Isolated fractures of the shaft of the fibula are usually the result of direct trauma, e.g. a kick in football. Prehospital management is confined to immobilization in a box splint and appropriate analgesia. Occasionally, a fibular shaft fracture occurs as a result of the rotational forces that have also resulted in an ankle fracture.

Ankle fractures

These injuries are common in all ages and are the commonest lower limb fractures. Suspicion of an ankle fracture is suggested by a history of inversion or eversion of the ankle with or without associated rotation with the foot fixed. Common clinical features include swelling, pain, tenderness over the malleoli or fifth metatarsal and an inability to bear any weight. Support can be provided using a box splint, typically with a right-angled foot piece.

Fracture dislocations are normally recognized by the considerable displacement or distortion of the ankle (Fig. 28.9). Often there may be threat to the foot because of ischaemia due to kinking of the arterial vessels, there may also be tenting of the skin over the fracture site and the skin may

appear threatened. Reduction can be achieved by steady traction on the joint pulling the leg out to length and correcting the deformity. Very unstable ankle dislocations may redislocate within the splint and therefore considerable care should be taken once reduction is achieved to try to achieve good splintage of the ankle prior to transfer to hospital.

Foot fractures

These are relatively rare injuries, although occasionally fractures of the hind- and midfoot may occur following falls from a height (e.g. fractured calcanei) or from forced dorsiflexion during a road traffic accident where the foot is forced against one of the foot pedals (resulting in fractures of the navicular or talus). Other potential injuries include fracture of the fifth metatarsal following inversion injuries of the ankle, where the tendon of peroneus brevis is attached to the proximal and lateral portion and avulses it. Crush injuries to the foot after direct trauma may result in a number of forms of fracture dislocations or straightforward fractures. All foot fractures require simple immobilization in a box splint and transfer to hospital.

Further reading

Court-Brown CM, McQueen MM, Quaba A (eds) 1996 Management of open fractures. Mosby-Year Book, Chicago, IL

Greaves I, Porter KP 2007 Oxford handbook of prehospital care. Oxford University Press, Oxford

McRae R, Esser M 2008 Practical fracture treatment, 4th edn. Churchill Livingstone, Edinburgh

Prehospital care of soft tissue injuries

29

Introduction 315

Definitions 315

History, examination and management 316

Injuries to specific tissues 317

Compartment syndrome 319

Amputated parts 320

Tetanus prophylaxis 320

Antibiotic cover 321

Further reading 321

Introduction

Soft tissue injuries are common in prehospital care and, although generally minor, may occasionally be life- or limb-threatening. These injuries may be divided anatomically according to the structures involved:

- Skin
- Tendon
- Nerve
- Vessel
- Muscle
- Complex injuries.

Soft tissue injury patterns vary dramatically depending on the anatomical area of the injury, the type of object involved (blunt or sharp), the direction and degree of the force applied, and often the place of injury (injuries on the football field will be different from those in an industrial setting).

In the prehospital arena, unless a soft tissue injury is clearly uncomplicated and trivial, referral to an emergency department for exclusion of associated bone, nerve or tendon damage will usually be required. Although soft tissue injuries are often a low priority in the immediate resuscitation of the injured person, avoidable excess morbidity undoubtedly results from inadequate assessment and poor rehabilitation and follow-up.

Definitions

LIGAMENT

Ligaments are tough fibrous tissues linking bones at joints and range from flat bands to thick cords. They are responsible for much of the stability of joints and forces insufficient to result in bony fracture may produce ligamentous damage. Combinations of ligament and bony injury can also occur.

TENDON

Tendons are tough collagenous structures that join muscle to bone and transmit the contraction of a muscle to allow movement of a joint. Like ligaments, they may be damaged by direct trauma, although forced muscular contraction may also result in injury to an involved tendon (rupture of

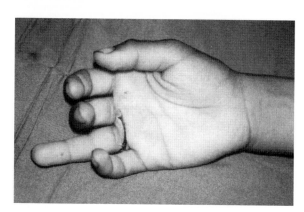

Fig. 29.1 • Complete rupture of the flexor tendon demonstrated on flexion of the fingers ('pointing finger' sign).

the quadriceps tendon may occur when a patient mistimes his/her step and falls, resulting in a sudden and excessive contraction of the quadriceps muscle). Tendon injuries are, however, most commonly due to lacerations involving glass and other sharp objects.

STRAIN

Strains are soft tissue injuries resulting in damage to muscle or tendon. They are characterized by pain on attempting to move the muscle.

SPRAIN

A sprain is a soft tissue injury to a joint ligament or capsule characterized by pain on both passive or active stressing of the structure concerned.

RUPTURE

A rupture is a complete discontinuity in the normal structure of a soft tissue – normally a muscle, tendon, ligament or joint capsule (Fig. 29.1).

History, examination and management

HISTORY

The mechanism of the injury should be clearly established. Pointers to the extent and nature of the injury include:

- Mechanism of injury
- Magnitude of applied force
- Anatomical location

- Open or closed injury
- Loss of function
- Associated bony injury.

EXAMINATION

The examination of any injury can be divided into three components:

- Look
- Feel
- Move.

In hospital practice, the information acquired from the examination is supplemented by radiological investigation.

Look

If an injury is closed (i.e. there is no break in the continuity of the skin) then the skin over the particular area should be carefully inspected and any signs of deformity, swelling, discoloration or bruising noted. Particular attention should be paid to underlying anatomical structures. Previous scars should also be noted. The position in which the limb is held may also give some diagnostic clues.

Feel

Deformity and swelling should be carefully palpated before the function of a limb is examined. Local and anatomically well-defined areas of swelling may help in determining the underlying pathology. The sensation and vascular status distal to any wound should be assessed and recorded.

Open wounds may be extremely difficult to examine because of accompanying bleeding or contamination. If this is the case, a sterile dressing should be applied and the wound suitably immobilized. It is not in the remit of the prehospital carer to attempt a detailed formal assessment of an open wound, as this may lead to extension of contamination and damage to vital structures, and more importantly is unlikely to reveal any useful information. It is acceptable to wash off gross contamination with a sterile fluid and, if the wound is contaminated with chemicals, this forms an important part of the first-aid process.

Move

If appropriate, active and passive movement should be assessed and the findings recorded. This may not always be possible and attempts should not be made in the presence of severe pain. The function of the limb distal to a wound should be assessed in order to determine the presence of any nerve or tendon injury. If indicated, the various ligaments around a joint should also be tested for pain on stressing and laxity indicating a sprain or possible rupture.

It may be difficult to determine with great precision whether deficiencies in function are due to the pain of the wound or to structural damage, and it is particularly difficult to exclude a partial tendon injury. Therefore any laceration that overlies, or is close to, a tendon should be referred to an emergency department for assessment.

MANAGEMENT

Many soft tissue injuries require some form of first aid. During sporting events initial first aid may be rendered by physiotherapists or trainers. This will almost inevitably consist of commencing a combination of:

- **R**est to the limb
- **I**ce
- **C**ompression
- **E**levation
- Analgesia.

This is a good philosophy to adopt for the majority of soft tissue injuries. Dirty wounds will need to be cleaned (see below) and dressed, while wounds where there may be fractures or joint instability will need immobilization in a splint.

Injuries to specific tissues

SKIN INJURIES

These may be worse than they initially appear, particularly if the mechanism of injury is crushing. All crush injuries require hospital assessment and radiological investigation. Simple, clean cuts to the skin may be sutured or Steri-Stripped. Few prehospital carers carry suturing equipment and it is probably not an appropriate activity to be performing in the community unless the wound is clean and simple, relevant clinical examination does not suggest any neurovascular or tendon injury, and a trip to the nearest hospital unit for suturing is likely to be unacceptably inconvenient. Simple cuts can be glued using sterile tissue adhesive. Dirty wounds require cleaning; this may be best achieved by mechanical methods (wiping with a gauze swab) or by irrigation with sterile water or saline. Extremely contaminated wounds may require vigorous surgical cleaning under general or regional anaesthesia.

Avulsed skin should never be discarded as it may subsequently be used to obtain cover of any defect; this also applies to avulsed body parts that appear to be unsuitable for reimplantation. However tenuous its connection, skin should be laid carefully over the defect and a sterile dressing

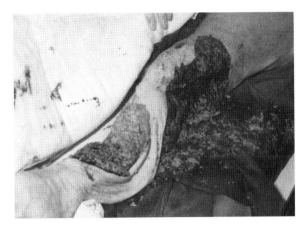

Fig. 29.2 • A degloving injury.

applied prior to transfer to hospital. Care should be taken that there are no twists in any skin pedicle as this may further threaten the viability of the tissue. Contaminated abrasions resulting from the skin being scraped across a gravel surface should be carefully examined for evidence of embedded gravel. If not removed, gravel will cause permanent tattooing of the skin. Vigorous cleaning of these wounds, often including scrubbing, is usually required.

Degloving injuries, in which the skin is avulsed by shearing forces from its fascial attachment, commonly occur in road traffic and industrial accidents. In the domestic setting, they may result from a patient catching a ring on a fixed point, resulting in finger degloving. These injuries are often dramatic. Quite commonly however, the true extent of the tissue damage may only become apparent on formal hospital assessment. The prehospital management is restricted to the application of a sterile dressing and urgent referral to a hospital with appropriate facilities (Fig. 29.2).

Subcutaneous haematomas, while not appearing to be severe at the scene, may continue to expand and provide a threat to the overlying skin. Large haematomas should always be referred to hospital for assessment and, if necessary, appropriate drainage. At the scene these can be treated with gentle compression from a wool and crepe bandage or a simple crepe bandage. If there is going to be any delay in evacuation to hospital, an ice pack and elevation can be used to help reduce swelling. Bandaging should not be so tight as to reduce blood flow to the limb distally, and any wounds under the bandage should be dressed before application of the bandage.

Local bleeding from a skin wound can almost always be stopped by applying a pressure dressing and elevating the limb.

VASCULAR INJURIES

Vascular injuries may complicate open lacerations, closed soft tissue injuries and either closed or open bony injuries.

The treatment of these injuries in the prehospital environment is limited. Recognition of the presence of these injuries is vital and viability of tissues distal to the injury must be assessed. The completely ischaemic limb is recognized by the presence of the five 'Ps':

- Pain
- Pallor
- Pulselessness
- Perishing with cold
- Paraesthesia.

Optimal management of limb ischaemia is time-dependent as the patient has a maximum of 6h of 'warm ischaemia' time (ischaemia at body temperature) before irreparable damage is done. There is no current evidence to support prehospital cooling of a limb in an attempt to prolong this period.

If associated with profuse arterial haemorrhage, open injuries may require a tight compression bandage and elevation to prevent further blood loss. Occasionally the use of pressure points and tourniquets may be necessary.

MUSCULAR INJURIES

Unless part of a complex injury involving other soft tissues (such as a laceration), these are often a result of inappropriate muscular contraction or of overexertion. They rarely need active treatment in the prehospital environment except simple measures such as 'RICE' (see above) and analgesia. Many muscular strains will require little further treatment other than good physiotherapy and rehabilitation. However, unless the prehospital carer is experienced in the care of these injuries, they should be referred on to hospital for appropriate review and follow up.

TENDON INJURIES

Tendon injuries usually result either from a direct laceration or from forcible muscular contraction. All lacerations to the hand require careful assessment. Only if complete or partial tendon injury can be absolutely excluded is hospital referral not required for further assessment. In partial tendon injury, loss of function may not occur and the injury may only be discovered on formal wound exploration. It must be remembered that the extent of the skin wound may not give an accurate guide to the extent of internal injury. Any laceration, therefore, which is in close proximity to any tendon requires exploration under general or local anaesthesia in optimal conditions before such an injury can be excluded.

Injury to the Achilles tendon deserves special mention as it is the most commonly missed closed tendon injury.

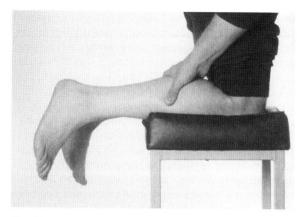

Fig. 29.3 • Thompson's or Simmonds' test.

The patient often complains of a sensation like being kicked in the back of the heel. Following an Achilles tendon injury, weight-bearing is difficult and plantar flexion against resistance is reduced or absent. Examination reveals swelling over the distal tendon, and a clear gap in the tendon may be felt. Simmond's test (squeezing the muscles of the proximal calf with the patient prone or kneeling) reveals normal plantar flexion on the unaffected side and absent plantar flexion on the side of the tendon rupture (Fig. 29.3).

If rupture of the Achilles tendon is suspected or confirmed, transfer to hospital for further management should be arranged. Suitable splintage may be provided for pain relief.

Tenosynovitis or tendonitis present with pain on a specific movement due to inflammation of a tendon or its sheath, usually caused by vigorous repetition of that movement. Swelling, tenderness and crepitus are found at the site of the inflammation. The most common example is tenosynovitis of the wrist, which is often seen in keyboard operators. If a fracture can be excluded, and the history and physical findings are appropriate, tenosynovitis and tendonitis are treated with rest, immobilization and anti-inflammatory analgesia.

NEUROLOGICAL INJURIES

Nerve function in any limb requires a careful and thorough evaluation, particularly in areas that have a complex nerve supply such as the hand. Any patient who has a cut over the site of a major nerve or whose wound may extend deep enough to involve a nerve should have a careful history taken particularly relating to any subjective loss of sensation, any pins and needles (paraesthesia), or any odd sensations such as feeling as if the limb or digit is covered in cotton wool. This should be followed by a careful physical examination.

Nerve assessment will include the ability to distinguish light touch and painful stimuli as well as, in the hand, the ability to discriminate between two closely approximated points (two-point discrimination). The latter test in the hand is said to be the most sensitive clinical discriminator of nerve function, and may be performed by using a bent paperclip set with the tips 5 mm apart (in the hand the normal range is about 5 mm). Motor function distal to a laceration should always be carefully assessed.

Any patient in whom a nerve injury is suspected or cannot be excluded should be referred to hospital.

LIGAMENTOUS INJURIES

Ligamentous injuries are usually the result of excessive strain on a joint – typical injuries are a sprained ankle or a knee ligament sprain; occasionally they may result from penetrating trauma.

There may be a good history of an excessively violent injury to the joint, such as in the case of a rugby or football player who has taken a forceful tackle where there is an acute valgus or varus strain on the knee. After the injury, if the sprain is of any significance, there will be a considerable loss of function of the joint. Typically, in lower limb injuries there will be inability to weight-bear. In the case of ligamentous injuries to the knee, there may be a range of differing signs and symptoms.

If there are sprains of either the medial or lateral collateral ligaments, the patient will complain of pain around the area of the ligament on weight-bearing, or the examiner may reproduce symptoms by stressing the affected ligament. If the ligament is completely ruptured then there may be little pain but a considerable degree of instability when attempting to walk. If injury to the anterior or posterior cruciate ligaments has occurred, a rapidly forming haemarthrosis will be found, with very reduced movements because of pain.

In the prehospital environment, the practitioner will frequently be exposed to the acute stage of the ligamentous injuries (when rapid formation of an effusion, soft tissue swelling or haemarthrosis is occurring). In general, a haemarthrosis occurs immediately after the injury, whereas an effusion or soft tissue swelling takes some time to develop. Haemarthrosis is invariably a hallmark of significant internal derangement of the knee (Fig. 29.4). The fundamentals of prehospital management are ice, support bandaging and arrangement of appropriate hospital referral or follow-up. If the injury is extremely painful then immobilization, as for a fracture, is appropriate.

In the case of ankle injuries, swelling pain and disability may make it difficult to distinguish a sprain from a fracture. Absence of tenderness over the malleoli and fifth metatarsal, combined with swelling, bruising and tenderness

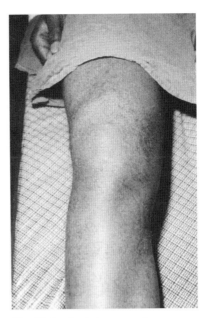

Fig. 29.4 • Acute knee swelling.

over the anterolateral aspect of the ankle, are suggestive of a simple sprain. If any doubt exists then the injury should be completely immobilized as for a fracture and transfer to hospital arranged.

Compartment syndrome

A compartment syndrome occurs when swelling or bleeding into a group of muscles following trauma raises the pressure within a closed fascial space, such that the microvascular blood supply is significantly reduced. This can result in ischaemic injury and muscle infarction if it is not recognized in time. Normally, compartment syndrome takes several hours to develop and in the conscious patient is characterized by unremitting pain that is worse on passive movement of the muscles affected by the process. Even opiate analgesia may not relieve the pain. In the unconscious patient a high index of suspicion must be maintained in any limb where there has been a significantly comminuted injury or significant crush injury. Essentially, any of the limb compartments may be affected, from the upper arm to the fingers and from the thigh to the small muscles of the foot. The diagnosis is generally made in hospital as its onset is sufficiently delayed for the patient to reach hospital before it occurs. Compartment syndrome may present late; it may also occur in intravenous drug abusers. The presence of distal pulses is no indication that a compartment syndrome is not developing. In the prehospital environment, if a patient has been trapped with significant crush to a limb for several hours the presence of compartment syndrome must be considered if there appears to be unremitting pain. Little can be done at the roadside (elevation of the limb may help an early compartment syndrome but may paradoxically worsen a rapidly developing one) as the mainstay of treatment is surgical release of the affected compartment. The recognition of the problem should hasten the urgency with which someone is transported to hospital.

Amputated parts

Digits or limbs that have been avulsed with shredding of the amputation site are unlikely to be suitable for reimplantation, particularly if the amputated part has been crushed. However, the amputated part may provide skin and bone for reconstruction, and should be sent with the patient to hospital. The part should be wrapped in a sterile dressing dampened in saline and placed in a waterproof plastic bag or container. This should then be further surrounded by a bag or container containing a mixture of ice and water, such that there is no way that the limb or digit can rest for any length of time in direct contact with a piece of ice and sustain thermal injury.

Decisions regarding the suitability of body parts for reimplantation should not normally be made in the prehospital situation. In general, however, clean guillotine amputations are more likely to be suitable than ragged avulsive amputations, especially if the latter involve crush injuries (Figs 29.5 and 29.6). The severity of a patient's associated injuries will determine treatment priorities and may mean that a reimplantation procedure is not appropriate.

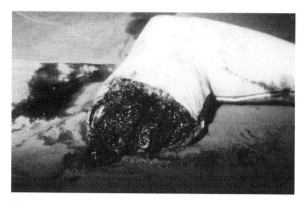

Fig. 29.5 • A guillotine amputation.

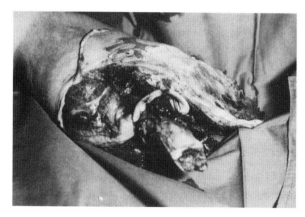

Fig. 29.6 • An avulsive amputation.

Tetanus prophylaxis

Although a rare disease, tetanus has a significant mortality and morbidity. Tetanus spores may be found in the soil and many cases of full-blown tetanus occur following minor abrasions or a 'trivial' wound in patients who are not adequately immunized. The causative organism is *Clostridium tetani*, which is anaerobic and thrives in an environment containing dead tissue. Prehospital care workers should be aware of the risks both to themselves and to their patients. The treatment of any wound that is thought to pose a risk of tetanus is thorough cleaning with debridement, if necessary.

For the prehospital practitioner the most important thing is to recognize the risk of a contaminated wound and ask the patient about his/her immunization status. In the case of a heavily contaminated wound (or a contaminated wound containing devitalized and crushed tissue) and an individual who is not immunized, passive immunity should be gained by giving tetanus immunoglobulin, obtainable from the blood transfusion service but normally stocked by any hospital emergency department. Candidates who should

be considered for immunoglobulin treatment also include those who have never received active immunization and those who have a wound that is more than 6 h old before treatment is started. They require a dose of 250–500 units of tetanus human immunoglobulin (TIG). Administration of immunoglobulin is only part of the treatment, which must include good wound toilet, in addition to starting the tetanus vaccination regime (0.5 ml tetanus toxoid by intramuscular injection using a different syringe and into a different limb) in order to develop active immunity. In wounds where there is little risk of contamination but the patient has never received or completed a course of tetanus immunization, immunization should be started, with a second dose being given at 4 weeks and the third dose at 4 months postinjury. Maintenance doses of tetanus toxoid should be given at 10-year intervals to maintain an effective level of immunization. In patients who are fully immune and have a wound that is unlikely to be contaminated, no vaccine is necessary; however, if significant contamination is likely then a booster dose of adsorbed vaccine should be given.

Antibiotic cover

In the prehospital environment there are few indications for starting antibiotic therapy in the *injured* patient. If there is to be a significant delay between the patient's injury and admission to hospital, e.g. in more remote areas, it may well be worth commencing antibiotics. In this case, a broad-spectrum antibiotic such as cefuroxime intravenously (starting with a loading dose of 1.5 g) is appropriate. If the wound might be contaminated with anaerobic organisms, then a suitable regime will include metronidazole (500 mg intravenously) as well. In a case of penicillin allergy then erythromycin would be a sensible alternative to a cephalosporin.

Further reading

British Medical Association 2008 British national formulary 56. British Medical Association, London

Driscoll P, Skinner D, Earlam R (eds) 1999 ABC of major trauma. BMJ Publishing, London

Greaves I, Porter KP 2007 Oxford handbook of prehospital care. Oxford University Press, Oxford

Gunshot wounds and blast injury

30

Gunshot wounds: prevalence and epidemiology   322

Wound ballistics   323

Patterns of injury   325

Safety, immediate assessment and resuscitation   326

Blast injury   327

Blast mechanisms   327

Patterns of injury   328

Summary   330

References   331

Gunshot wounds: prevalence and epidemiology

Injury following exposure to bomb blast and from penetrating ballistic missiles has tested the expertise of physicians since the arrival of firearms on the battlefields of Europe in the middle of the 14th century. Once confined to war and the wards and operating theatres of military field hospitals, these injuries now equally concern both civil and military medical practitioners. The latter half of the 20th century saw a significant shift in the epidemiology of these injuries, so that by the 1990s the great majority of patients were managed in the peacetime environment, including the prehospital setting.

In the USA, where trauma has reached epidemic proportions, deaths from gunshot wounds comprise 22% of total (deliberate and accidental) deaths (Pre-hospital Trauma Life Support 1994). Even in the most AIDS-prevalent age group of 25–34-year olds, deaths from gunshot wounds equal or exceed AIDS-related causes. More than 60% of murders in the USA are associated with the use of firearms.

Even in countries where blunt trauma following road traffic and industrial accidents greatly exceeds penetrating injury, worrying trends towards multiple shootings and terrorist incidents are recorded. In the UK in recent years there have been numerous incidents resulting in large numbers of dead and wounded, most notably at Hungerford with 32 people killed or wounded, and at Dunblane where one man shot dead 16 children and their teacher using a variety of modern handguns. Similar trends are observed in most developed parts of the world, including Europe, South Africa and Australia (Chapman 1995).

Terrorist incidents are now endemic in most developed societies and pose unique problems. Most result in large numbers of wounded presenting with complex, multisystem injury threatening to overwhelm medical facilities, and are particularly testing for prehospital medical personnel.

Although this chapter is concerned with management following injury, some comment must be made on prevention. Following the Dunblane incident, the UK government introduced swingeing legislation to control the availability of handguns. Apart from .22-calibre pistols, which must be kept secure in gun clubs, all other weapons are banned. In North America, the increasing availability and ease of access to handguns has been associated with an alarming rise in the use of these weapons. A study of Canadian and USA cities where legislation has been relaxed in recent years has shown a sevenfold increase in gun-related murders

(Sloan et al 1988). A further study showed a rise of over 60% in gun-related murders by under 18-year olds between 1980 and 1991 (Shepherd & Farrington 1995). Effective legislation, therefore, appears to be mandatory if current trends are to be reversed.

Wound ballistics

Wound ballistics is the study of wound production by missiles, irrespective of their origin. In this section the emphasis is on wounds caused by bullets. In a later section injury caused by blast-energized fragments will be discussed.

Following penetration, bullets interact with tissues by performing work and transferring energy, which is manifested as cutting, laceration and crushing of tissues and structures directly in their path. They may also cause additional injury to structures remote from the visible, permanent wound track (Fig. 30.1).

The extent of injury caused by bullets is variable and is the cause of much debate and often needless controversy (Ryan et al 1997). Bullets vary greatly in their range and penetrating power and are usually classified as high- or low-energy. Low-energy bullets tend to be short and squat and are generally propelled from handguns, whereas high-energy bullets are long and thin and propelled from rifles (Fig. 30.2).

This is a broad generalization and the distinction is increasingly blurred, with modern automatic pistols capable of propelling small, high-energy rounds. This classification is useful for ballisticians but has little relevance for medical personnel and may actually be misleading as impact velocity is merely one of the variables concerned with injury

potential. Equally, the commonly quoted kinetic formula for a missile may mislead. The formula

$$KE = \frac{1}{2}MV^2$$

defines the available kinetic energy and therefore its capacity to perform work. Units of energy are joules (J) when M is mass in kilograms (kg) and V is velocity in metres per second (m s^{-1}). The available kinetic energy (KE) should not be equated with the energy transferred to a given wound. The amount of energy actually transferred is governed by the extent to which the bullet is retarded by the tissues and this, in turn, is related to numerous and variable factors. These include bullet and tissue characteristics (Tables 30.1 and 30.2).

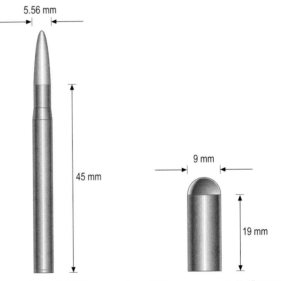

Fig. 30.2 • A 5.56 mm modern, high-energy assault rifle round is shown on the left. Note its slender, elongated shape and sharp, pointed nose. On the right is a short, squat, blunt-nosed 9 mm low-energy handgun round.

Table 30.1 Bullet characteristics
• Velocity at impact and within tissue
• Bullet mass (weight)
• Presented area at impact and along the wound track – 'nose on' or yaw/tumble
• Missile construction – jacketed or unjacketed

Table 30.2 Tissue (wound) characteristics
• Wound track density and elasticity
• Wound track length

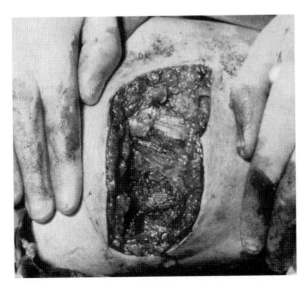

Fig. 30.1 • A clinical photograph of a typical gunshot wound showing contusion and laceration of soft tissue in the track of the bullet. These are the features of a low energy transfer wound (see text).

It should now be obvious that attempts to classify wound severity prior to detailed surgical assessment is spurious and should be avoided. Most clinicians now defer description of wound severity until surgical exploration and then use the 'energy transfer' classification rather than one based on presumed missile velocity. From the standpoint of the prehospital personnel caring for victims these debates are largely irrelevant. They are outlined here to inform the reader and to avoid confusion (Cooper & Ryan 1990). The clinical approach to be adopted in the prehospital setting is one based on the ABCDE method used by most modern life-support systems.

INTERACTION OF BULLETS WITH TISSUES

The events that follow bullet penetration are varied and largely unpredictable; consequently injury severity ranges from modest to life-threatening. The following may occur and affect injury severity:

- Temporary cavitation
- Yaw and changes in presented area
- Bullet fragmentation and deformation
- Wound contamination.

Temporary cavitation

Bullets of high available energy because of size, muzzle velocity or tendency to fragment exert considerable retardation forces within wound tracks, which may lead to the formation of a significant temporary cavity. The maximum size of a cavity is related to energy transfer, and it is noteworthy that even low-energy bullets will cause some degree of cavitation. Cavities vary in size, shape and clinical consequences. Very elastic tissues such as lung and muscle stretch readily and, although bruised, remain viable. More dense, inelastic tissues such as liver, loaded colon and bone are more susceptible, leading to serious clinical consequences.

The position of the maximum cavity size tends to be deeply placed with long wound tracks, typically with chest or abdominal wounds. In limbs, where impact upon bone is a feature, maximum cavity size may be evident as a large and ragged wound.

The formation of a significant temporary cavity is important but it is not the only factor in the production of a high-energy wound. Other factors are listed and discussed below.

Yaw and changes in presented area

Most bullets are inherently unstable. This instability is largely, but not fully, overcome by imparting a spin to the bullet during flight. The remaining instability is manifested as yawing. This is a minute altering deviation along the bullet's long axis (Fig. 30.3). This *relative* stability is achieved by rifling the barrel of the weapon. However, it is lost as soon as a bullet penetrates any target, including human tissue – the angle of yaw then increases and, if the wound track is long enough, the bullet may begin to tumble end over end, altering its presented area in so doing. The clinical significance of this is greater retardation, a wavering wound track, and a more severe and unpredictable wound. This phenomenon also enhances any tendency towards temporary cavitation.

Bullet fragmentation – deformation

If a penetrating bullet breaks up or deforms within a wound track, the result may be devastating. Military bullets are fully jacketed to prevent break-up, and this is required by the Hague and Geneva Conventions. However, these rules do not apply to sporting or police bullets and are certainly not observed by criminals and terrorists. Non-military bullets may be scored, have soft noses or hollow points, and may be partially jacketed. These are designed to fragment, deform or shed their lead cores. The object is to ensure retention of the bullet within the body and maximum 'energy dump' (energy transfer). For the police, this effect is desired in order to prevent accidental injuries to innocent bystanders in urban firefights. For sportsmen, the effect increases the likelihood of a kill, thus preventing a wounded animal from fleeing into the bush to suffer a slow and painful death.

Notable fragmenting or deforming bullets include the British 'dumdum', the Glaser® safety slug and the Black Talon® round. The Glaser® has a hollow point filled with shot. The Black Talon® round has a copper-alloy nose with a central hollow cavity and a steel insert in the base – it is referred to as a 'barbed round' because of the manner in which it deforms within tissue.

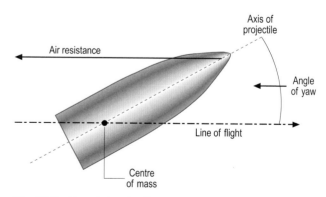

Fig. 30.3 • Yaw during the flight of a rifle bullet in air. The axis of the bullet deviates from the line of its trajectory. The angle (φ) between the trajectory and the axis is the angle of yaw.

Clinical presentation is variable following gunshot injury. A bullet that deforms or sheds part of its lead core is retarded significantly and is likely to remain within a target, thus giving up ('dumping') all its available energy. Cavities are typically large and may be complex or multiple. Susceptible tissues fare badly, and morbidity and mortality are increased. There may be little to guide prehospital medical personnel other than clinical evidence of severe hypovolaemic shock. In the hospital setting, preoperative radiology showing a trail of radio-opaque material should heighten suspicion. Fragmenting bullets may be even more devastating. Multiple diverging wound tracks may arise with the involvement of multiple body cavities and systems, yet a single wound of entry may be the only external evidence of injury. In some ways these patients have features in common with terrorist victims who present with multiple wounds from fragments.

Wound contamination

Wound contamination is a particular feature of terrorist fragment injury and will be discussed later. Contamination following bullet wounding, while less extensive, is still significant and should not be ignored. Bullets are usually pointed and will transfer little material directly into wounds. However, penetrating and perforating bullets associated with temporary cavities tend to draw in tiny fragments of clothing and other materials from the environment because of the negative pressure generated by cavity formation. It is sensible to consider all penetrating missile wounds to be heavily contaminated and at risk of developing systemic sepsis, irrespective of the wounding agent. The most effective means of dealing with such contamination is by early and adequate surgical excision. Antibiotics should be seen as adjuncts to this despite some claims to the contrary in the ballistic literature (Bowyer et al 1998).

In concluding this section it should be recognized that wound severity is unpredictable and the worst should be assumed. From a biophysical and physiological point of view, wounds will fall into two broad classes:

- low energy transfer wounds
- high energy transfer wounds.

LOW ENERGY TRANSFER

These are characterized by injury confined to the wound track and due to laceration and crushing. Injury severity will be determined by the structures in the wound track. Low energy wounds are the typical consequence of wounding by low-energy handgun bullets, high-energy bullets that perforate a short, soft-tissue wound track, modern military antipersonnel fragments and knives.

> If the track involves a vital structure such as the heart or brain, injury may be lethal and debates concerning high- or low energy transfer become irrelevant.

HIGH ENERGY TRANSFER

High energy transfer wounds are characterized by cutting and contusion in the missile path and also by remote injury radial to the wound track produced by temporary cavitation with or without bullet fragmentation. Such injury may be lethal. Temporary cavitation involving the liver, brain or heart is associated with very high mortality. High-energy wounds are associated with injury caused by many high-velocity bullets and fragments, large low-energy fragments, shotgun injury at close range, and 'designer bullets' such as Glaser® and Black Talon®.

Patterns of injury

Bullet wounds in the peacetime setting tend to result in single wounds or small numbers of wounds to individuals or small groups. This is in contradistinction to war and terrorism, which are associated with multiple casualties presenting with multiple injuries. Rare exceptions include the multiple shootings at Hungerford and Dunblane.

In most instances the presence of a wound will be obvious and may have been reported by the police or other agency.

Bullets tend to penetrate deeply and are no respecters of body cavities or anatomical regions. The position of the body at the time of wounding (which is often not known) is an important determinant of possible injuries. It is vital therefore not to make any predictions concerning injury severity based on presumed entry or exit wound sites. Neither should predictions be made concerning structures encountered. However, one should be particularly suspicious concerning bullet wounds close to the shoulders and thighs – these may well involve the adjacent body cavities of chest and abdomen, producing significant injuries even in the apparently fit and stable patient. Many victims are young adults capable of an excellent physiological response, who may lose up to 30% of their blood volume and suffer considerable faecal spillage without overt clinical evidence in the first hour (American College of Surgeons Committee on Trauma 1997). In the prehospital setting, undressing a casualty may be neither possible nor appropriate. Heavy, multilayered clothing may readily disguise small entry wounds, particularly those to the back. The clinician should always take heed of the history and be guided by the clinical condition of the patient. Equally, witnesses should not be disbelieved because a wound is not immediately evident. Some gunshot wounds may be tiny and external bleeding may be minimal or even absent. If it is safe and appropriate, *and will not delay transfer to hospital*, a search may be made for an exit or second entrance wound. The principal risk to a gunshot wound patient is exsanguination. Signs of this should be sought, treatment commenced (usually en route to hospital – inappropriate delays should not be introduced while infusions are commenced) and the search for wounds left to hospital personnel after transfer.

Forensic texts oversimplify identification of entry and exit wounds. In the field setting it may be impossible to reach a decision – time should not be wasted on a fruitless exercise. If a gun is fired at point-blank range there will be tattooing and burns around the entrance wound from the propellant and there may be further evidence on overlying clothing. This finding should be recorded and care taken with clothing cut away by prehospital personnel. Clothing should not be cut through gunshot holes. Clothing and other objects should be placed in a bag, labelled, sealed and handed to the police.

Preserve clothing for forensic purposes.

SHOTGUNS AND AIRGUNS

Shotguns have a smooth bore and are designed to fire multiple pellets. Shot size is defined by a number: the higher the number the smaller the shot. The range is from 12, which is the smallest, referred to as birdshot, to 00, the largest, called buckshot.

Clinical effects are determined by the size of shot and the range. Birdshot fired from more than 10 m will produce multiple, superficial, very low energy wounds. At a range between 5 and 10 m pellets may penetrate deep fascia but the wounds will still be low-energy in nature. At a range of less than 5 m the multiple pellets behave as a single mass with a wide presented area and may result in a lethal, localized, high-energy wound. Close-range shotgun wounds are heavily contaminated with skin, clothing and the wadding from the shotgun cartridge. There is a significant risk of wound infection among survivors.

Airgun pellets produce single low-energy wounds but may have lethal consequences in small children or if the eye is perforated with intracranial involvement. The wounding power of airguns should not be underestimated.

Safety, immediate assessment and resuscitation

The first priority for medical personnel at the scene of a shooting is safety. The site is often still a place of danger

and will usually be under the control of the police or other security service. Their instructions must be followed and no approach to a patient made until clearance to do so is given. On approaching a victim a check should be made for weapons. No attempt should be made to pick up or make safe any weapon found.

The first priority at a shooting is safety – be guided by the police.

It should not be forgotten that a wounded, hypoxic, hypovolaemic victim may be frightened or disorientated and may attempt to shoot anyone who approaches. This is particularly true if the victim is a terrorist or criminal. Once the scene is declared safe the clinical approach is the same as for injury following a road accident. As a rule critical decision-making is easier in penetrating injury, particularly when caused by a gun. All patients require prompt hospital transfer with a view to surgical exploration.

The assessment and treatment priorities are control of exsanguinating external haemorrhage airway, breathing, circulation and disability (central nervous system) and exposure. This process has been outlined in earlier chapters (<C>ABCDE).

The following additional points are important when dealing with gunshot wound victims.

- In the UK, surgical intervention is considered mandatory for all gunshot wounds. Therefore, there should be no delay even with stable patients.

Do not 'stay and play'.

- Many gunshot wound victims bleed profusely, often from multiple sites. If the bleeding is external it should be controlled by direct pressure. Artery forceps and tourniquets should be avoided wherever possible.
- When faced with a shocked patient with bleeding into the chest or abdomen it is important to be particularly careful with intravenous resuscitation. The key to survival for such patients is prompt surgical intervention in a facility equipped for the task.

Delay caused by attempts at vascular access or surgical intervention at the roadside may be fatal. The concept of hypotensive resuscitation for victims of penetrating injury to chest and abdomen is now generally accepted. Bickell and others working in Houston, Texas (Martin et al 1992, Bickell et al 1994) have shown the benefit of withholding intravenous fluids until the patient is at first surgery. Their view is that 'scoop and run' for patients who are hypovolaemic following penetrating torso injury is safer than a policy of roadside fluid resuscitation. This appears sensible, as giving large fluid volumes to patients bleeding into body cavities does nothing to prevent ongoing bleeding and may, by inappropriately raising blood pressure to normal or hypertensive levels, exacerbate further bleeding. An important caveat is time. The hypotensive approach demands early (30–60 min) access not just to hospital but to an operating theatre, and implies that an agreed system, including prehospital to hospital communication, must be in place. If intravenous fluid resuscitation is considered mandatory, sufficient should be given to ensure the presence of a palpable radial pulse in order to avoid precipitating clot displacement and further bleeding.

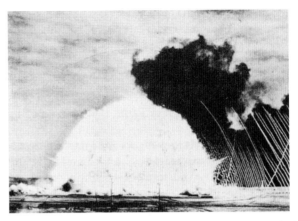

Fig. 30.4 • A photograph following detonation of high explosive. The shock front can be seen on the left of the picture as a hemisphere preceding the mass movement of air (With permission from Department of Military Surgery, Royal Defence Medical College, Gosport, Hampshire, UK).

Blast injury

Injury resulting from the effects of blast poses unique problems in the prehospital setting. Medical personnel are usually faced with multiple casualties suffering multisystem injury of mixed aetiology and may have to function in a climate of continuing danger. Blast injury may arise in a number of settings:

- Terrorism
- Conventional war
- Domestic
- Industrial.

This section is concerned with injury resulting from acts of terrorism but the principles hold true irrespective of aetiology. The objectives of terrorist bomb attacks are to provoke fear and panic in the target population by indiscriminate maiming and killing of groups of people. In a detailed analysis of over 200 bombing incidents over a 25-year period, Frykberg & Tepas (1988) found that all involved multiple casualties with a mean of 15. Just over 12% died immediately, the majority of survivors presented for medical attention but a relatively small number, only 30%, required hospital admission. This low admission rate, however, masks a significant group who suffer long-term disability from diverse conditions such as post-traumatic syndromes and hearing loss.

Blast mechanisms

The physical and chemical events surrounding a bomb explosion are complex and are still the subject of continuing debate: attending medical personnel need not be overconcerned with them (Cooper et al 1983, 1997).

The terrorist bomb typically contains high explosive (which requires a detonator but will explode without confinement) surrounded by some form of casing, which may vary from a milk churn down to a small, chocolate-box-sized container for use under vehicles – the 'car bomb'. Modern terrorist bomb materials are odourless, malleable and difficult to detect – Semtex is a typical example. These substances require chemical decomposition to cause detonation and the use of a percussion cap is typical. Following detonation, the explosive substance is rapidly converted into a large volume of gas, which results in the formation of a *blast shock wave* (Fig. 30.4).

Behind the shock front and moving more slowly is a body of displaced air – this is called the 'mass movement of air' or *blast wind*. Within the area affected by the shock front and air displacement there is the potential for fragmentation of the environment. Finally, there is the additional flash phenomenon and the risk of igniting the environment, resulting in fires of variable intensity. In a closed or contained environment, such as a pub or motor vehicle, the effects may be devastating, with additional injury resulting from structural collapse and disintegration of the environment (see below).

BLAST SHOCK WAVE

The blast wave is a rapidly expanding front of overpressure in the shape of a sphere, arising instantaneously and moving away from the point of detonation at a velocity greater than the speed of sound in the affected environment (air or water) – in other words, supersonic in the affected medium. The magnitude of the wave decays rapidly as the distance from the source increases. The effect is accentuated within an enclosed environment, where reflection of the incoming incident wave from walls and other surfaces is a particular feature. The overpressures at reflecting surfaces, where the incidence wave meets the reflected wave, may be of an order of magnitude many times that of the approaching incident wave. In addition, the incident or approaching wave will flow over and around barriers such as walls or screens and may injure those taking cover behind.

The effects of the front are very variable and are determined in the main by the magnitude and duration of the associated overpressure. This in turn is determined by the type of explosive employed. A conventional high explosive such as Semtex results in overpressures of milliseconds duration; a thermonuclear device may result in overpressures lasting seconds.

BLAST WIND

The blast wind is the mass movement of the air surrounding the blast environment, which is displaced by the expanding gas from the explosion. Moving more slowly than the shock wave, it follows behind it and may be of sufficient intensity to disrupt the environment. For example, if a pane of glass is exposed to a bomb blast, the shock wave or front will break the glass, and the following mass movement of air will take the broken shards and widely disperse them. The same holds true for masonry, metal, wood and any other materials encompassed by the explosion, including body parts. The mass movement of air is also referred to as the *dynamic* pressure from the blast and has obvious potential to cause severe injury.

FRAGMENTATION

Most military explosive munitions are contained within carefully engineered shells or casings, which may be manufactured to fragment in particular patterns (Ryan et al 1991). This is the basis of most modern hand grenades, mortars and artillery shells. Most terrorist devices use the same principle but depend on the affected environment as sources of fragments, or include 'fragments' such as nails within the bomb. Terrorist bombs inside buildings or vehicles are common examples. Fragments generated from the bomb casing or contained within the bomb are commonly referred to as *primary fragments*, those generated within the environment are *secondary fragments*. Primary fragments are usually metal and range from millimetres to centimetres in size – potential depths of tissue penetration are very variable. Secondary fragments include glass, masonry, metal, wood or vehicle parts. They may also include human tissue, including bone from victims. The impact on victims of such body parts may result in the transmission of infective disease, especially hepatitis.

Table 30.3 Effects of blast

- Primary injury (effects of the shock wave – ears, lungs, abdomen)
- Secondary injury (fragment injury)
- Tertiary injury (effects of the blast wind – impact injury and amputations)
- Crush injury
- Burns
- Psychological

FLASH AND CONFLAGRATION

An explosion is an exothermic event. Intense heat is generated and a thermal pulse or flash is produced that may be of sufficient magnitude and duration to cause superficial burns to exposed skin. The pulse may also cause the environment to ignite. This is particularly a feature of terrorist explosions inside buildings.

Patterns of injury

The clinical consequences of exposure to blast may be classified under six broad headings. These are listed in Table 30.3 and are discussed below.

PRIMARY INJURY

Primary injuries are caused by exposure of the body to the blast shock wave. Fortunately, the human body is remarkably resistant to primary injury. Solid and fluid structures such as the liver and spleen are rarely damaged by the shock wave – they may of course be damaged by other effects of the explosion. Structures most at risk are those that have solid–fluid and air components interfacing. Most notable are the lung, ear and bowel.

The most important primary effect upon the body is contusion injury within the lung. This results in a haemorrhagic contamination of the alveoli due to damage to the alveolar septa and stripping of the bronchial epithelium. The exact mechanisms are still the subject of controversy (Maynard et al 1989). Two phenomena are implicated: low-frequency shear waves result from inward distortion of the chest wall by the shock wave but, in addition, high-frequency stress waves (compression waves) are coupled into the chest wall (Cooper & Taylor 1989, Cooper et al 1991). It is the stress waves that have the greatest capacity to cause injury at fluid–air interfaces. The clinical picture is of acute lung injury, similar to blunt lung contusion. A syndrome similar to adult respiratory distress syndrome (ARDS) may supervene.

Injury to the auditory system has long been recognized. The tympanic membrane is particularly vulnerable to blast. A wide spectrum of injury is seen from bruising to disruption of the ossicular chain. The likelihood of injury is related to blast intensity and orientation of the external ear canal to the approaching incident wave. Rupture of the tympanic membrane may occur with an incident wave of less than 15 kPa if the ear drum is diseased. With overpressures of 100 kPa, ear drum injury may be expected in over 50% of cases (Cooper et al 1997). In practice, a large number of surviving victims will have deafness to a variable degree that may make communication difficult.

> **The absence of deafness does not indicate that the patient has not been exposed to a significant blast loading.**

Clinically significant injury to bowel is uncommon following exposure to blast shock wave in air. It is a notable feature following underwater exposure, where a 'water ram' effect results. Reported injuries vary from simple bowel wall contusions to acute perforation with faecal peritonitis. In practice, isolated gut injury among survivors is rarely a feature of exposure to air blast.

A small percentage of victims will die with little sign of external or internal injury. These deaths are probably due to dysrhythmias or coronary artery air embolization (Fig. 30.5).

SECONDARY INJURY

The blast shock wave and dynamic pressure (blast wind) working in concert will disrupt the casing of the explosive

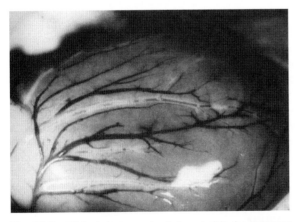

Fig. 30.5 • Clinical photograph of air emboli in the coronary arteries following exposure to blast shock wave (With permission from Department of Military Surgery, Royal Defence Medical College, Gosport, Hampshire, UK).

device and parts of the exposed environment, and then disperse the resulting fragments. Close in to the explosion these fragments will travel at very high velocity. Victims penetrated will usually die from a combination of primary blast and secondary penetrating injury. The vast majority of survivors will have multiple injuries caused by fragments of lower velocity and by blast-wind energized debris (Mellor & Cooper 1989). Injury will be both penetrating and blunt. In practice, casualties will usually be found to have multiple, shallow, penetrating wounds, abrasions and contusions. All wounds will be grossly contaminated, with a significant risk of subsequent sepsis.

TERTIARY INJURY

The forces exerted by the dynamic pressure (blast winds) are considerable and, while less than the blast shock wave, are of longer duration. Their effects are destruction of the environment and displacement of individuals within it. The clinical sequelae include traumatic amputation, whole body disruption and crush injury. Lesser injuries include skeletal fractures, lacerations and contusions resulting from impact with walls and other surfaces.

CRUSH INJURY

Entrapment following blast within buildings is common and will result in danger to both victims and rescuers alike. Most casualties will have multiple injuries of the types already described. If rescue is delayed and victims are exposed to continuing pressure, crush injury leading to crush syndrome may ensue. Crush syndrome occurs when a large muscle bulk is involved and a delay of hours or longer occurs before release. Rhabdomyolysis follows muscle injury, and there is a leakage of protein-rich fluid into the intravascular space, producing oedema, which may be of sufficient extent to result in hypovolaemic shock. On release of the affected limb reperfusion occurs leading to more severe hypovolaemia and hyperkalaemia. Myoglobin and free radicals from the injured muscle compound the insult, leading to acute renal failure. Good management demands anticipation, vigorous intravenous fluid resuscitation with potassium-free fluids (although, where possible, this should not be allowed to delay transfer to hospital, if there are multiple casualties, resuscitation may be commenced on-scene) and rapid transfer to a critical care environment. In a climate of war or disaster early management may require the application of a tourniquet before release, followed by prompt amputation. Such a drastic approach is rarely necessary in a peacetime environment where early release, on-site resuscitation and rapid transfer to hospital should be possible.

BURN INJURY

Flash burns to exposed areas such as the face, hands and arms are a feature of exposure to a thermal pulse or flash within a closed environment. Most will be superficial in depth but inhalation injury should be suspected in all cases. Overt signs of inhalation injury may not be present in the early hours following exposure. In addition, if the environment ignites, flame burn injury may ensue and should be managed along standard lines.

PSYCHOLOGICAL INJURY

Various syndromes will be seen extending from immediate panic reaction to late-onset post-traumatic stress disorder (PTSD). PTSD is unlikely to present a problem to prehospital personnel involved in the early hours of management. However, they may have to cope with panic and disorientation among injured and uninjured survivors. Survivors may also feel guilt at having survived. Many will be tearful and need reassurance. Anger and rage may also pose problems and should be handled with tact and calmness. Assistance from the police or security services may be required.

Longer term problems such as PTSD and related syndromes may affect victims and medical personnel alike. Arranging follow-up for victims will be a task for GPs and hospital personnel. Medical personnel helping in the field should be offered psychological debriefing and regular follow-up. The initial debrief for the entire rescue team should take place as soon as possible after 'stand down' and is a team leader responsibility (Advanced Life Support Group 2002).

MANAGEMENT

Terrorist bomb blasts are associated with large numbers of casualties and this is part of the terrorist's intention. The vast majority of the fatalities occur immediately or very soon after detonation. These are deaths in the first peak of the trimodal distribution of deaths described by Trunkey (American College of Surgeons Committee on Trauma 1997). Many others will have no physical injury but will be distressed and disorientated. Those injured by the explosion need to be identified and separated from other groups. This requires skilled and prompt triage.

TRIAGE

Triage is the process of sorting or sieving casualties on the basis of medical need. The concept and methodology is covered comprehensively by Hodgetts and Mackway-Jones (Advanced Life Support Group 2002) and in Chapter 21 of this book. Failure to perform a proper triage sieve followed by a triage sort will result in chaos, with large numbers of uninjured and lightly injured patients being transferred to first-line hospitals, which may then be overwhelmed and unable to accept the small number of seriously injured urgently in need of resuscitation and surgery.

INITIAL ASSESSMENT AND EARLY MANAGEMENT

The triage sieve process should identify those in most urgent need. These victims should be moved to a place of safety for immediate assessment and resuscitation. The approach is precisely as described for any other victim of trauma. The <C>ABCDE – primary and secondary survey approach will identify those with life-threatening injury. Where appropriate a 'treat on the spot' or 'scoop and run' policy can then be initiated.

The following points are particularly relevant to a terrorist bomb setting:

- In making a judgement concerning transfer to hospital, weight must be given to the circumstances and mechanisms of injury.
- When dealing with victims following an explosion inside a building, a high index of suspicion is required for inhalation injury and impending acute lung injury. If in doubt, the patient should be transferred to hospital, where a further triage process will be performed.
- Early administration of supplemental oxygen in high concentration using masks with reservoir bags is mandatory if any form of lung injury is suspected. Pulse oximetry is particularly helpful.
- Careful assessment for signs of abdominal injury is needed. In the early period following injury there may be few unequivocal physical signs – it is important to remember the importance of the mechanism of injury.
- Most victims will complain of deafness. Most recover in a few hours. Tympanic membrane assessment is not easily performed in the prehospital setting. Therefore, the history should be recorded and a note made of the need for later auditory assessment.
- The vast majority of the surviving injured will have been struck by primary or secondary fragments. Casualties with penetrating injuries *must* be transferred to hospital irrespective of the victim's general condition.
- Burn victims are managed along standard lines but evidence of airway injury in those exposed to the flash should be sought.
- Psychological injury to victims and medical attendants should not be forgotten.

Summary

Gunshot and blast victims have much in common. The majority will present with penetrating ballistic injury and management will be guided by standard advanced trauma life support protocols and guidelines. There are, however, notable differences between the groups and these must be recognized. Gunshot victims usually present singly or in small numbers and are readily managed without resort to major incident procedures. Victims resulting from blast exposure are almost always multiple, with multisystem complex injury, and require special efforts by carers. Most bomb blast incidents require a major incident response with clear communication between prehospital and receiving-hospital personnel. In the prehospital setting, the security services take the lead role and this may affect the pace and intensity of the medical response. Medical personnel require knowledge and training, and must be prepared to work within a multidisciplinary team and within pre-agreed guidelines. Triage holds the key to early success. Early clinical assessment and interventions for individuals are the same as for single patients and an agreed trauma life support system must be followed.

References

Advanced Life Support Group 2002 In: Hodgetts TJ, Mackway-Jones K (eds) Major incident medical management and support, 2nd ed. BMJ Publishing Group, London

American College of Surgeons Committee on Trauma 1997 Advanced trauma life support student manual, 6th edn. American College of Surgeons, Chicago, IL

Bickell WH, Wall MJ, Pepe PE et al 1994 Immediate versus delayed fluid resuscitation for hypotensive patients with penetrating torso injury. New England Journal of Medicine 331: 1105–1109

Bowyer G, Ryan JM, Kaufmann CR 1997 General principles of wound management. In: Ryan JM et al (eds) Ballistic trauma – clinical relevance in peace and war. Arnold, London

Chapman S 1995 Gun control. British Medical Journal 310: 284

Cooper GJ, Ryan JM 1990 Interaction of penetrating missiles: some common misapprehensions and implications for wound management. British Journal of Surgery 77: 606–610

Cooper GJ, Taylor DEM 1989 Biophysics of impact injury to the chest and abdomen. Journal of the Royal Army Medical Corps 135: 58–67

Cooper GJ, Maynard RL, Cross NL, Hill JF 1983 Casualties from terrorist bombings. Journal of Trauma 23: 955–967

Cooper GJ, Townend DJ, Cater SR, Pearce BP 1991 The role of stress waves in thoracic visceral injury from blast loading – modifications of stress transmission by foams and high-density materials. Journal of Biomechanics 24: 273–285

Cooper GJ, Mellor SG, Dodd KT, Harmon JW 1997 Ballistic and other implications of blast. In: Ryan JM et al (eds) Ballistic trauma – clinical relevance in peace and war. Arnold, London

Frykberg ER, Tepas JJ 1988 Terrorist bombings. Lessons learnt from Belfast to Beirut. Annals of Surgery 208: 569–576

Martin RR, Bickell WH, Pepe PE et al 1992 Prospective evaluation of pre-operative fluid resuscitation in hypotensive patients with penetrating truncal injury. Journal of Trauma 33: 354–362

Maynard RL, Cooper GJ, Scott R 1989 Mechanisms of injury in bomb blasts and explosions. In: Westaby S (ed) Trauma – pathogenesis and treatment. Heinemann Medical Books, Oxford, pp 30–42

Mellor SG, Cooper GJ 1989 Analysis of 828 servicemen killed or injured by explosions in Northern Ireland 1970–1984. British Journal of Surgery 76: 1006–1010

Ryan JM, Cooper GJ, Haywood IR, Milner S 1991 Field surgery on a future conventional battlefield: strategy and wound management. Annals of the Royal College of Surgeons of England 73: 13–20

Ryan JM, Rich NR, Burris DG, Oshsher MG 1997 Biophysics and pathophysiology of penetrating injury. In: Ryan JM et al (eds) Ballistic trauma – clinical relevance in peace and war. Arnold, London

Shepherd JP, Farrington DP 1995 Preventing crime and violence. British Medical Journal 310: 271–272

Sloan JH, Kellerman AL, Reay DT et al 1988 Handgun regulations, assaults and homicide. New England Journal of Medicine 319: 1256–1262

Thermal injury

31

Introduction   332

Pathophysiology of thermal injury   333

Causes of thermal injury   334

Classification of thermal injuries   340

Wound assessment and fluid resuscitation   340

Specific considerations at a major incident involving burns   342

Summary   343

References   343

Further reading   344

Introduction

The term 'thermal injury' is preferred to 'burns' because it encompasses chemical, cold and electrical injury as well as flame burns and scalds. Most injuries are trivial. Many are self-treated, sometimes with bizarre remedies – butter, bicarbonate of soda or toothpaste. Others are managed by GPs or emergency department staff as outpatients.

Deeper or larger burns should be treated at hospital, and many are managed as day or short-stay cases. The goal is to ensure that the patient receives prompt, appropriate surgical management to minimize disfigurement or disability.

Life is seldom at risk in burns covering less than 10% of the body surface.

On the other hand, a small number of thermally injured patients each year suffer a massive or complicated life-threatening burn (Fig. 31.1). These are devastating, with the prospect of prolonged treatment in hospital, multiple operations, painful rehabilitation, long-term disability and lifelong social isolation if they survive.

Between these extremes is a significant number of moderate injuries. These are serious enough to become complicated or lethal if inadequately assessed or treated. Referral to an appropriate burn care facility, where all aspects of the injury can be managed by experienced staff, is essential for all but minor burns.

It is therefore pertinent to start this chapter with a brief description of the pathophysiology common to all burns (Dziewulski 1992), then to look in more detail at

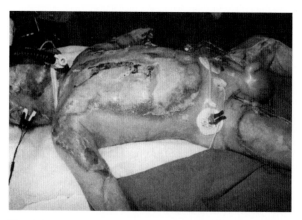

Fig. 31.1 • A child with 70% body surface burns and smoke inhalation. Severe facial burns complicate this injury.

individual causes and complications, specifying the relevant immediate care principles.

Pathophysiology of thermal injury

Injured tissue triggers an inflammatory reaction, which, in thermal injury, is proportional to the area of skin destroyed. It is non-specific and common to all tissue damage whether from trauma, sepsis or surgical intervention. Designed to initiate healing, the inflammatory response is a normal physiological process that nevertheless itself causes damage if the injury is large. It is well described in standard texts and is summarized in Figure 31.2. It produces an immediate effect on the burn itself but in large burns also affects the whole patient, particularly if complicated by respiratory injury.

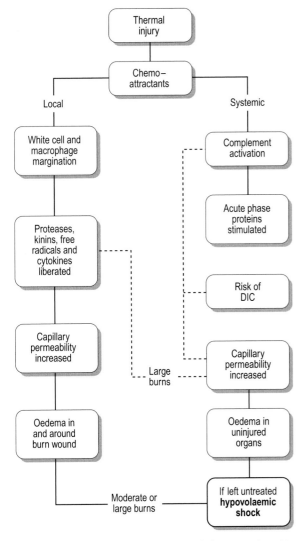

Fig. 31.2 • The inflammatory response in burns and scalds (simplified).

THE BURN WOUND

The immediate consequence of thermal injury is a thin layer of dead or dying tissue over a proportion of the body surface area. In response to chemoattractants derived from the injured tissue, there is margination and microaggregation of white cells and macrophages in capillaries. This gives rise to a 'zone of stasis' in the area under the wound. Capillary flow may be renewed when the inflammatory response subsides but, if not, this zone becomes an addition to the original depth of the burn. Inadequate intravenous resuscitation makes this more likely by decreased perfusion in the zone of stasis. On the other hand, over-zealous resuscitation increases oedema.

Inflammatory mediators are released by the white cells (Fig. 31.2). These cause an increase in capillary permeability, allowing extravasation of a fluid similar to plasma. Oedema develops in and around the burned tissue, made up of water, electrolytes and plasma proteins. In superficial burns in which the eschar (dead skin) is thin, blisters form. In larger burns, the fluid loss gives rise to hypovolaemic shock endangering the function of vital organs, especially the kidney.

Enough inflammatory mediators are produced in response to a large burn to cause oedema in unburned tissues as part of a generalized response, the systemic inflammatory response syndrome (SIRS), which is more commonly associated with massive sepsis. Some authors describe a burn toxin or myocardial depressant factor as well, although others suggest these are merely the inflammatory mediators described by their clinical effects.

Heat coagulation of blood in the subcutaneous capillary beds accompanies full thickness burns, causing red cell destruction proportional to burn size. This does not contribute to the hypovolaemic shock of thermal injury however, as that is caused by the body's reaction to the burn as described above. Burn shock is slower in onset than hypovolaemic shock due to haemorrhage, so that commencing intravenous fluid resuscitation should not delay the patient being taken to hospital provided this can be achieved within 1 h or so.

Do not delay transfer to hospital in order to achieve intravenous access unless transfer times are long.

HEAT LOSS AND THERMOREGULATION

The metabolic response to thermal injury causes thermoregulation to be reset upwards. A steady pyrexia (37.5°C in adults, up to 38.5°C in children) is seen within hours of injury, especially in children (Childs 1995).

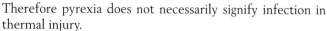

Therefore pyrexia does not necessarily signify infection in thermal injury.

On the other hand, some patients with major or complex burns seem unable to restore their body temperature after cooling (Platt et al 1997). Failure of heat generation may be to blame, or heat may be lost by evaporation from an extensive wound, or a combination of both may be responsible. Keeping burned patients warm is therefore a vital part of immediate care for these patients.

All body tissues have a high water content and therefore a high specific heat of vaporization/condensation – i.e. they retain heat energy for several minutes after thermal injury and continue to burn until tissue temperature falls below 52°C. The temperature threshold for pain is lower, at 42°C. Consequently, an important first-aid measure is to cool the burn quickly to remove heat energy, and the best agent readily available is cold tap water. The cooling process may take 15 min to be effective.

Clearly, there is a need to balance first aid for the burn against the risk of hypothermia. The need for warmth may override the need for first-aid cooling in large burns. However, cooling with running cold water should be applied unless conditions overwhelmingly dictate otherwise. Cooling should be confined to the wound as far as possible and then measures to actively ensure warmth for the patient should be instituted. Once in the emergency department it is often too late for cooling to be effective and maintaining body temperature has priority.

Always balance the risk of hypothermia with the need for burn cooling.

Many fire and ambulance services now routinely carry the newly developed water-gel coverings (e.g. Burnshield®). These have a remarkable capacity for absorbing heat to cool the wound but maintain a warm covering for the patient. Benefit from cooling falls dramatically the longer it is delayed so water cooling must still be applied until the fire service arrives, unless these materials become more widely available.

Some guidelines for general immediate care are given in Box 31.1.

Causes of thermal injury

A high proportion of burned patients are either children or the elderly. Scalds are common in children, whereas adults are more often injured by flame. Electrical, chemical and similar injuries are usually the result of industrial or domestic accidents. The main causes of thermal injury are listed in Box 31.2.

Box 31.1

Guidelines for general immediate care of thermal injury

- *Ensure the environment is free from avoidable risk to the carer.*
- **Remove the patient from the heat source and extinguish flames if necessary.**
- **Give specific first aid for *Airway* and *Breathing* as needed.**
- **Give specific first aid for the cause of injury, as described below.**
- *Cool* the wound (up to 15 min) – use water, or water-gel dressings.
- **Wrap the wound in sterile dressings, laundry-clean towels or polythene food wrap (e.g. ClingFilm) (this material is excellent for this purpose: the wound can be inspected through it; plasticizers in the wrap inhibit bacteria).**
- *Warm* the patient. Wrap well in clean blankets, duvet, anything to ensure body heat is retained. Remove to a warm environment if possible.
- **Assess for the likelihood of other injuries.**
- **Make (brief but accurate) notes about the circumstances and times of the injury.**
- **Remove to hospital. Ensure the ambulance is well heated.**
- **If transfer to hospital is delayed more than 30 min, attend to the *Circulation* – carry out wound area assessment and start intravenous fluid resuscitation.**

Box 31.2

Causes of thermal injury

- **Scalds**
- **Flame burns**
- **Explosions**
- **Contact burns**
- **Chemical burns**
- **Electrical injury**
- **Ionizing radiation**
- **Non-accidental injury**

SCALDS

Between 40% and 50% of all burn unit admissions are children, and 85% of these are scalds in children under 3 years of age (Smith & O'Neill 1984). Domestic hot water is often set at a high temperature, commonly 65–100°C. It has a high specific heat so can cause serious injury. Kettles, saucepans, cups and mugs are easily upset, and prevention is better than cure. Every health-care worker must therefore accept a responsibility to increase public awareness of simple safety precautions in using hot water (Box 31.3). Practical application of these common-sense precautions in every home would prevent most scalds.

Box 31.3

Precautions to avoid domestic scald injury

- Handle hot drinks with care, especially when children are around.
- Never pass a hot drink to someone else across a child.
- Treat kettles and saucepans as potentially very dangerous.
- Turn saucepan handles inwards towards the wall.
- Keep children out of the kitchen when cooking.
- Use safety devices such as short or coiled kettle flexes, cooker guards, etc.
- When filling a bath start with cold water and add hot to achieve the desired temperature.
- Never leave young children unattended by an adult when a bath is being run.

Box 31.4

Guidelines for specific immediate care of scald injury

- Immediately cool the wound with running cold water for up to 10 min.
- Warm the patient to prevent hypothermia during transfer to hospital.
- Cover the wound using sterile, or at least laundry-clean, towels or polythene food wrap (e.g. ClingFilm).
- Most scalds occur in children – comfort the patient; reassure the parents.
- Transfer to hospital, well wrapped up, in a well-heated ambulance.

Very rarely, even a simple scald can be dangerous. Sporadic case reports have appeared in the literature of respiratory obstruction due to swelling, not always caused by swallowing or inhaling the hot liquid but simply in association with a scald of the neck. Toxic shock syndrome (Childs et al 1994) is occasionally seen in small children with scalds colonized by *Staphylococcus aureus*. If treatment is delayed, this may prove fatal. A minor scald is therefore not always a safe scald.

The elderly are also vulnerable to scalds. They spill hot liquids more readily than younger adults. If they climb into a bath that is too hot they are unable to get out quickly. Because of infirmity or dementia, they may react too slowly to high temperatures. Installation of thermostatic mixers on bath taps would go a long way to prevent this kind of accident, yet too few nursing homes have taken this elementary precaution. Bath handles will assist escape if something does go wrong.

Scalds at any age may be caused by disability, epileptic fits, myocardial infarction, diabetic crisis, hypoglycaemia, cerebrovascular accident or other medical emergencies. Both alcohol and drugs make accidents more likely.

Burns due to other hot liquids

Chip pans and deep fat fryers are a hazard in the kitchen. Fat usually causes deep injuries, as do tar and molten metal. Treatment is the same as for other burns but they can be serious. Some guidelines for specific immediate care are given in Box 31.4.

FLAME BURNS

Flame burns are commonly associated with house fires. Fire may also occur in a road traffic accident, or clothes may catch light in the home. In children, playing with matches or cigarette lighters is a common cause. Petrol or other accelerants may sometimes be a factor in an accident or a suicide attempt, or as a means of assault. Barbecue and bonfire accidents are increasingly frequent in the summer. Smoking in bed is an avoidable hazard, to which the elderly are again vulnerable. Drugs, alcohol, sudden illness or pre-existing disability make accidents due to flame more likely and will impede ability to escape.

Flame burns are often complicated by smoke inhalation. Additionally there may be other injuries, e.g. following a road traffic accident or an explosion. A history from the rescuers is important: has there been a roof collapse, for example, or has the patient escaped by jumping?

Do not forget the possibility of associated injury.

Guidelines for specific immediate care are given in Box 31.5.

EXPLOSIONS

Explosions occur in house fires more often than is commonly realized because flammable materials may vaporize at very high temperatures, forming an explosive mixture with air. Explosions due to liquid petroleum gas (LPG, butane, propane) are not uncommon in boats, caravans and some residences. Natural gas leaks, due to carelessness or poor maintenance, cause injury by explosion.

Carbon monoxide poisoning is likely in victims of domestic gas explosions. A gas leak may have gone unnoticed for some time by an intoxicated or sleeping person, or a suicide attempt may have gone wrong. Direct blast trauma may have occurred in addition to burns. Blast injury to the

Box 31.5

Guidelines for specific immediate care of flame burn injury

- **Extinguish the flames and ensure the safety of rescuers and carers.**
- **Cool the wound with water or water-gel dressings.**
- **Assess and support the *Airway* and maintain *Breathing*, especially if smoke inhalation is suspected. See the section on 'Respiratory tract injury'.**
- ***Circulation*: if the burn is large, assess the burn size, calculate fluid requirements and set up an intravenous infusion of Hartmann's or 0.9% saline solution (large cannula).**
- ***Disability*: assess the conscious level – this may help the hospital decide the likelihood of hypoxia at time of injury, or concussion from explosion.**
- ***External* examination of the patient may reveal other injuries.**
- **Measures *C*, *D* and *E* should not cause delay in transfer to hospital.**
- **Ensure an accurate, timed history is written down: Was the patient resuscitated by firemen? Did the patient jump from an upper floor? Was the patient unconscious at any time? Get as much detail as possible from bystanders and rescuers about the situation from which the patient was rescued.**
- **Transfer to hospital, well wrapped up, in a well-heated ambulance.**

Box 31.6

Guidelines for specific immediate care of explosion injury

- **As for flame burns.**
- **Remember: this group is very likely to have other injuries.**

Box 31.7

Guidelines for specific immediate care of contact burn injury

- **Full ABC assessment, bearing in mind that the burn may be less serious than the illness or injury that caused it.**
- **Hot source injury: immediately cool the wound with running cold water.**
- **Cool heat source (e.g. radiator): cooling is unlikely to be of benefit.**
- ***Priority*: the precipitating cause of the contact injury may be a stroke, drugs or alcohol, any of which may have impaired temperature regulation. Significant hypothermia may therefore be present. Re-warm the patient.**
- **Set up a good intravenous infusion, if time.**
- **Transfer to hospital, well wrapped up, in a well-heated ambulance.**

lung, concussive brain damage and shrapnel injuries must be expected and may be difficult to distinguish from the effects of hypoxia caused by smoke inhalation. Some guidelines for specific immediate care are given in Box 31.6.

CONTACT BURNS

Contact burns occur when part of the body comes in contact with a hot object. The burn may be small or large, depending on the nature and temperature of the heat source and the duration of contact. A child touching a cooker ring momentarily will sustain a deep injury, as will an ill elderly person lying against a domestic heating radiator for several hours. Some guidelines for specific immediate care are given in Box 31.7.

CHEMICAL BURNS

Industrial accidents, domestic violence or deliberate assault can cause chemical burns, giving rise to skin damage indistinguishable from a burn. They are fortunately rare.

Four modes of chemical injury need special mention (Box 31.8).

- *Phosphorus burns*: phosphorus ignites spontaneously and burns fiercely, even in the presence of water, causing scattered, small, deep burns often amounting to a substantial total area. They can be difficult to assess accurately.

- *Phenol burns* (Horch et al 1994): phenol is absorbed through the skin and may cause renal failure. Paradoxically, the burn itself is often mild.

- *Hydrofluoric acid burns* (Kirkpatrick & Burd 1995, Kirkpatrick et al 1995): hydrofluoric acid causes intensely painful, deep burns. It is absorbed systemically, leading to depletion of ionized calcium. It is widely used in glass manufacture, in electronics and for cleaning purposes in industry, where safety measures should be explicit and rigidly applied. Even small (less than 2.5% body surface area burned) injuries can be fatal.

- *Cement burns*: cement is a weak alkali that may cause a burn on prolonged contact. It is an important cause of full-thickness burns to the lower leg in building-site labourers.

Guidelines for specific immediate care are given in Box 31.8.

Box 31.8

Guidelines for specific immediate care in chemical burn injury

General

- Always protect yourself – wear rubber gloves and other appropriate protection.
- *Except as indicated below*, first aid starts with copious irrigation using running water. All industries using chemicals should have conveniently placed showers.
- Antidotes – sodium bicarbonate for acids and weak vinegar for alkalis – are less useful than you would imagine because they may cause an exothermic reaction; they should not therefore be used.
- Phosphate buffer solution is safer but water is most readily available.

Phosphorus

- The phosphorus particles must be picked out with forceps, which is helped by turning them black using 1% copper sulphate solution – *but beware*: this can cause systemic copper toxicity if used on a large area. Water irrigation does not stop the burning while phosphorus remains in the wound.

Phenol

- Water or saline soaks on the wound are *absolutely contraindicated* as they may enhance absorption of the phenol through the skin, although irrigation with copious running water can help. Polyethylene glycol soaks may be of benefit. Ingestion should be treated using activated charcoal. *Drinking water enhances absorption by dilution, so is contraindicated if phenol is swallowed.*

Hydrofluoric acid

- Immediate irrigation with cold water.
- Removal of finger or toe nails if the acid has penetrated beneath.
- Calcium gluconate gel rubbed in continuously until pain is relieved – very large quantities may be needed.
- *Avoid secondary injury* by making sure all care personnel are protected from contact with the acid on the patient.
- In hospital:
  - Intra-arterial injection of calcium gluconate 10% to relieve pain and preserve the part if the injury is distal to the area supplied by the artery, e.g. radial artery injection for a hand injury.
  - Infiltration of 10% calcium gluconate under the wound is advocated, but is often ineffective.
  - Serum calcium levels must be measured frequently.
  - Immediate excision of the wound may be the only way to remove the hydrofluoric acid once it has penetrated the superficial layers of the skin.

Box 31.9

Guidelines for specific immediate care of electrical burn injury

- Ensure the environment is safe and there is no danger to rescuers.
- ABC assessment to exclude immediate danger to the patient's life.
- Immediate cooling of the wound is much less useful than in other circumstances because of the extreme depth of the injury.
- Set up an intravenous infusion (high-tension injuries).
- Urgent transfer to hospital is vital, and the ECG, pulse rate and blood pressure should be monitored during transfer.
- Treat shock aggressively.

ELECTRICAL BURNS

Electrical injuries (Haberal 1986) may be caused by low- or high-tension current sources, and the two result in different kinds of damage. Small, deep burns at each entry and exit point characterize low-tension injuries. Depending on the path of the current and the time for which it flows, cardiac dysrhythmias may occur. It is wise to monitor the electrocardiogram (ECG) for dysrhythmias during transfer to hospital, where a 12-lead ECG or a history of cardiac arrest at the time of the accident will show whether routine ECG monitoring is necessary.

High-tension electricity may arc, causing a flash burn. Entry and exit burns may be small but are often large. Microvascular capillary coagulation inflicts extensive ischaemic damage on soft tissues, which may be dead while retaining intact peripheral pulses. Paralysis from spinal cord and other nerve damage is possible. Muscle spasm induced by the high-tension current may have caused fractures, or there may be other fractures, including the spine, associated with a fall from an overhead high-tension source. In hospital, myoglobin and other products from damaged tissue may cause renal failure. Disseminated intravascular coagulation is not uncommon. *Hypovolaemic shock is usual and cannot be predicted by burn surface area.* Guidelines for specific immediate care are given in Box 31.9.

IONIZING RADIATION

Radiation accidents are fortunately extremely rare (Ch. 50). They should be suspected whenever victims are rescued from fire in a nuclear installation, although the suspicion is usually groundless.

Burns due to radiation (Oughterson & Warren 1956) are initially caused by flash or flame. The burn seems at first to heal well, then disorders of formation of granulation tissue,

> ### Box 31.10
>
> **Guidelines for specific immediate care of ionizing radiation injury**
>
> - Rescuers must take appropriate precautions against contamination.
> - Remove the patient from the source of radiation.
> - *ABC* assessment and support.
> - Copious water irrigation using soap or detergent.
> - Transfer to hospital for appropriate management of the injury and of ARS.

infection, thrombocytopenia and agranulocytosis become apparent. There is ongoing damage due to the effects of the radiation itself, mediated by free radicals such as the hydroxyl radical. The full acute radiation syndrome (ARS) may develop, with haemopoietic (bone marrow), gastrointestinal and neurovascular manifestations.

An occasional cause of minor radiation burns is therapeutic radiotherapy. These injuries heal slowly and, if grafted, take of the skin graft is poor. Some guidelines for specific immediate care are given in Box 31.10.

NON-ACCIDENTAL INJURY

Non-accidental injury (NAI) by burning is a particularly vicious form of NAI because it frequently demonstrates premeditation or cruelty. NAI is most often seen in children in the UK but it can occur in adults (abuse of a spouse or elderly relative due to exasperation).

Cigarette burns, pattern burns due to holding a child on a hot grill, buttock and foot pad sparing and absence of splash injury in bath scalds, for example, are very clearly due to abuse. Scalds of non-accidental origin are often deeper than accidental ones. In other cases, inconsistency in the history triggers suspicion of NAI and is confirmed by careful investigation, which may reveal, for instance, old, healed fractures.

Poor social circumstances, momentary carelessness and ignorance of risk are common factors contributing to all scald injuries in children. In some, inadequate or neglectful parenting exacerbates the risk. The full child protection machinery (the UK Children Act 1989) must be applied in these latter circumstances but they are outside the strict definition of the label 'non-accidental injury'. Telling the difference between neglect and NAI can be very difficult and requires multidisciplinary investigation by experienced people, led by a paediatrician. The prehospital environment is emphatically *not* the setting in which NAI can be confidently diagnosed, but any suspicion, if present, must be passed on to the emergency department doctors. Some guidelines for specific immediate care are given in Box 31.11.

> ### Box 31.11
>
> **Guidelines for specific immediate care of non-accidental injury (NAI)**
>
> - The patient has priority – full ABC assessment.
> - NAI needs careful investigation by the proper authorities and must not precede or prejudice appropriate immediate care of the patient's injury.
> - A non-judgemental approach must be adopted, even when abuse seems the most likely cause of injury.
> - The natural rights of parents or relatives in relation to the child must be respected unless there is continuing danger to patient or carers.

RESPIRATORY TRACT INJURY

There are two ways in which the respiratory tract may be damaged (Kinsella 1988):

- Heat injures the upper airway causing *oedema of the pharynx and larynx*, leading to respiratory obstruction. Once oedema has started to form, the loose glottic tissues swell easily and rapidly occlude the airway. Early signs or symptoms of respiratory obstruction therefore require urgent intervention (Fig. 31.3). The prognosis is good if obstruction is relieved quickly. The mucosae absorb heat so that thermal damage below the larynx is unusual.

- Smoke is inhaled into the bronchial tree and causes *smoke inhalation injury*.

No two fires are the same in respect of the *products of combustion* (Prien & Traber 1988). These depend on the temperature, the materials burned and the availability of oxygen. Carbon dioxide, carbon monoxide and cyanide are usually present, and oxygen is likely to have been exhausted in order to support combustion so that patients may be asphyxiated. Aromatic compounds, oxides of sulphur and nitrogen, hydrochloric acid and other strong acids, and many more compounds, have been identified in smoke.

Carbon dioxide (CO_2) is an anaesthetic at 30% inhaled concentration. Normally, we breathe out 5% CO_2. At the concentrations found in smoke, often in excess of 12%, it dulls the mind. The victim therefore is often unable to gather his/her wits in order to escape. It also stimulates respiration. Initially, the glottis closes in response to smoke. Lack of oxygen then stimulates a deep breath, which causes smoke and more carbon dioxide to be inhaled. Hypercarbia causes hyperventilation, so the amount of smoke inhaled increases as time passes.

Carbon monoxide (CO) binds more firmly to haemoglobin than does oxygen, with a half-life of about 4 h in air and 40 min in 100% oxygen. The oxygen dissociation curve

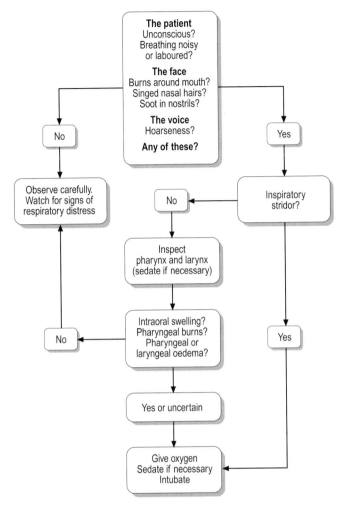

Fig. 31.3 • Decision guide for intubation in burns patients.

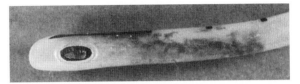

Fig. 31.4 • Mucus, soot and cellular debris in a child's tracheal tube.

inflammatory response (Fig. 31.2) but the consequences of this for the lungs are very different from those for the skin (Traber et al 1988):

- Interstitial pulmonary oedema develops, increasing the diffusion gradient for gas exchange. The alveolar–arteriolar oxygen gradient increases as a result.
- The mass (weight) of the lung tissue is increased by the oedema. This weighs heavily on the lower, dependent parts of the lung, so that small airway closure occurs earlier in the respiratory cycle, or throughout it for some lung components.
- Atelectasis is inevitable, causing consolidation, adding to the weight of lung tissue. A vicious circle develops that can lead inexorably to respiratory distress syndrome.
- In the larger airways, mucus production increases and it commonly becomes viscid. These secretions, mixed with soot and debris (migrant leukocytes, fibrin and damaged mucosal cells), have the consistency of thick, black glue. The mucosal wall of the major airways may be killed and may separate. These components combine to form 'casts', which can block the airway (Fig. 31.4).
- Inflammatory mediators, in particular arachidonic acid precursors, such as thromboxane A_2, which are potent smooth muscle constrictors, cause bronchospasm.

The patient has almost certainly been asphyxiated in the fire. In addition, he is now at risk of upper airway obstruction, bronchial narrowing due to oedema and secretions, bronchospasm and lung damage. Gas exchange is inhibited, oxygen delivery to the tissues is reduced and oxygen uptake and utilization by tissues is diminished. Inhalation injury thus affects the whole patient, not just the lungs.

As if to add insult to injury, inflammatory mediators released from the injured lung add to the effect of those derived from the skin burn. Mortality in burns is therefore greatly increased when complicated by respiratory injury, exceeding 50% in most published series. On the other hand, smoke inhalation is only occasionally fatal unless accompanied by a skin burn. It is the combination of the two that worsens the prognosis. Some guidelines for specific immediate care are given in Box 31.12.

is shifted to the left, which reduces the ability of haemoglobin to give up its oxygen in tissues. At the cellular level it attaches to myoglobin, having a half-life of about 24 h at this level. Lastly, it inhibits cytochrome oxidase.

Cyanide also poisons the mitochondria and inhibits cytochrome oxidase, exacerbating the effects of CO. Carbon monoxide and cyanide together therefore cause three deleterious effects:

- reduced oxygen carriage by the blood
- reduced oxygen transfer to the tissues
- impaired use of oxygen in the energy production cycle.

The end result is significant tissue hypoxia.

The mechanism of lung injury

Other components of smoke cause chemical injury to the tracheobronchial tree. This, like the skin burn, sets up an

Box 31.12

Guidelines for specific immediate care of respiratory tract injury

- **Extinguish any flames and ensure safety for rescuers.**
- **An adequate *Airway* must be assured. Tracheal intubation may be needed (see Fig. 31.3).**
- **Oxygen, via a Hudson mask, at high concentration (60%+), or 100% if intubated.**
- ***Assisted breathing (ventilation) may be needed.***
- **Unconsciousness at the scene may signify carbon monoxide inhalation and/or severe hypoxia. Such patients benefit from immediate intubation, and ventilation with 100% oxygen.**
- ***Circulation: these patients benefit if intravenous resuscitation is started early. Use 1 litre of Hartmann's solution or 0.9% saline solution. However, do not significantly delay despatch to hospital in order to set up an infusion.***
- **Transfer to hospital, well wrapped up, in a well-heated ambulance.**

Classification of thermal injuries

It is helpful to subdivide thermal injury into four main groups:

- *Small injuries*: these seldom threaten life. Oedema forms only locally so the physiological upset is minimal. Immediate cooling with tap water minimizes the depth of the injury, and may reduce the need for surgery. Early surgical treatment, when needed, can make a difference to the likelihood of future disability or disfigurement.
- *Moderate injuries*: these are less than 30% body surface area burned (bsab) and more than 15% bsab (10% bsab in children and the elderly, who are more vulnerable). Except perhaps in the very young or the elderly, they are rarely life threatening. Hypovolaemic shock can occur if they are not properly treated, so intravenous resuscitation is always necessary.
- *Large injuries*: in major burns, the inflammatory response causes oedema to be formed in unburned tissues (Fig. 31.2). Fluid loss causes a drop in cardiac index, which may further be depressed by inflammatory mediators. Cardiac index may, on the other hand, be increased by catecholamines released in response to injury. Disseminated intravascular coagulation or respiratory distress syndrome, or both, can occur, even in the absence of smoke inhalation, starting a decline into multisystem organ failure. Early excision of the burn wound gives the best hope of survival.
- *Complex injuries*: include patients with airway obstruction and/or smoke inhalation, high-tension electrical burns, which often feature extensive soft tissue damage, and patients with significant comorbidity or other injuries. These all behave more like larger burns, even when the total percentage bsab is small or moderate.

An alternative method of crudely assessing the severity of injury is to calculate the sum of the percentage of body surface area burned (% bsab) and the patient's age. If this sum exceeds 100, the prognosis is grave. A burn score between 75 and 100 indicates a major injury, as age and area of burn are the two main determinants of prognosis.

Wound assessment and fluid resuscitation

Appropriate fluid replacement depends on an accurate assessment of burn surface area. However, such an assessment should not be allowed to delay transfer of the patient to hospital by ambulance. Knowledge of assessment and resuscitation is therefore essential at a major incident (see below), when longer times may elapse before evacuation is possible.

Wound area assessment is best done using a Lund & Browder chart (Fig. 31.5). The wound area is drawn on the chart and the proportion of each chart area affected is estimated. The total of these estimated areas is then added together. The accuracy of this method is surprisingly good, even in inexperienced hands, provided it is done with great care.

Lund & Browder charts may not be available in the prehospital environment, in which case the Rule of Nines (Fig. 31.6) will suffice. For this method of assessment, the body of an *adult* patient can be roughly subdivided into areas in multiples of 9, the burned area estimated as a proportion of each 9% or multiple, and the total added up. Unlike the Lund & Browder chart, the Rule of Nines makes no allowance for the different proportionalities in children compared to adults. It is therefore a second-best assessment most suited to field work as in a major disaster, when paperwork is unavailable and a crude but useful assessment is better than nothing.

A further guide is the *patient's* hand, which equates to approximately 1% of body surface. Lastly, a simple check of accuracy is possible by assessing the *un*burned area also, subtracting this figure from 100%, and comparing with the first calculation.

Fluid requirements should be calculated *from the time of injury*, and initial therapy given according to one of the formulae in Box 31.13. In the immediate care situation the simplest effective solution is Hartmann's or 0.9% saline solution. The appropriate formula is given in Box 31.13. Once in hospital, the emphasis is on careful clinical monitoring which quickly takes over from the formula as the means of achieving the desired goal.

It is common to over- or underestimate the wound size by inclusion of erythema or exclusion of superficial injury mistaken for erythema. In practice, in the prehospital setting this is unlikely to result in harm to the patient.

Chart for estimating severity of burn wound

Name..Date..................................

Age.. Admission weight...............................kg

Ignore simple erythema

Partial thickness lost (PTL)

Full thickness loss (FTL)

Lund and Browder charts

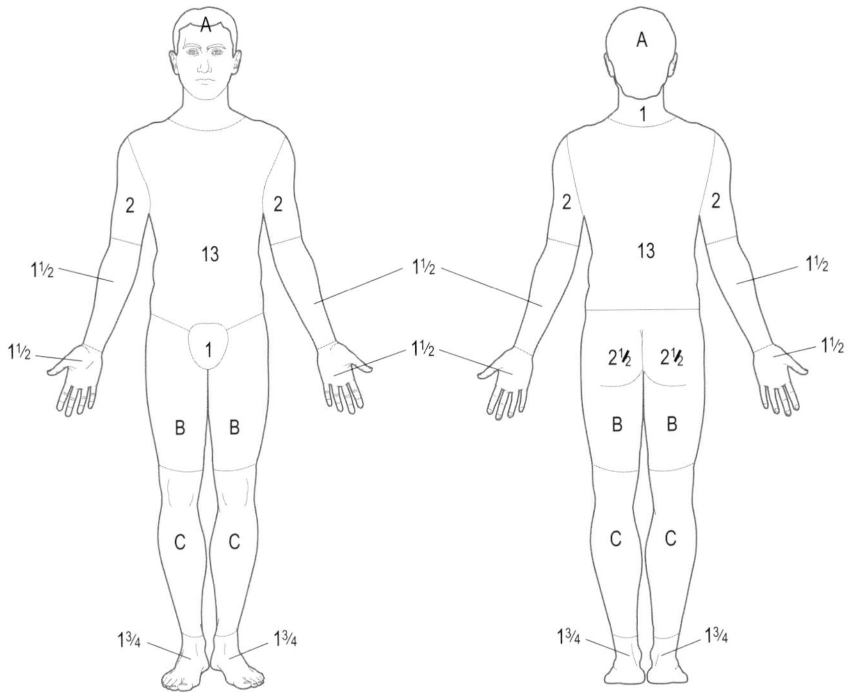

Region	%	
	PTL	FTL
Head		
Neck		
Ant. trunk		
Post. trunk		
Right arm		
Left arm		
Buttocks		
Genitalia		
Right leg		
Left leg		
Total burn		

Relative percentages of body surface area affected by growth

Area	Age 0	1	5	10	15	Adult
A = ½ of head	9½	8½	6½	5½	4½	3½
B = ½ of one thigh	2¾	3¼	4	4½	4½	4¾
C = ½ of one leg	2½	2½	2¾	3¼	3¼	3½

Fig. 31.5 • Lund & Browder burn area assessment chart.

THE BURN WOUND

It is important to keep the wound covered when it is not being assessed. This can be achieved using sterile dressings if available, or laundry-clean towels, or polythene food wrap (e.g. ClingFilm). This latter material is excellent for the purpose: the wound can be inspected through it, and plasticizers in the wrap inhibit bacteria. Circumferential ClingFilm dressings should not be applied in view of the risk of circulatory compromise due to developing swelling.

PAIN RELIEF

It is very easy to be so engrossed in the priorities described above that the patient's pain is forgotten (Laterjet & Choinière 1995). A major, full-thickness burn may be surprisingly free of severe physical pain but the patient is usually very distressed by the horror of what has happened and needs support, of which analgesia is an important component.

Although the nerve endings in a full-thickness burn are damaged, the wound edges are still innervated and even

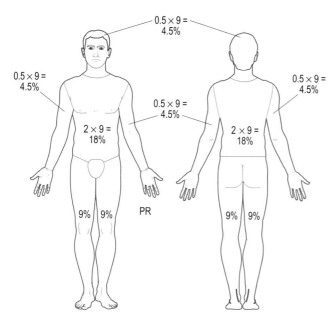

Fig. 31.6 • Wallace's Rule of Nines for burn wound area assessment. Each body area is deemed to be a multiple or submultiple of 9%; an estimate is made of the proportion of each 9% involved in the burn, and the estimates are then totalled.

Box 31.13

Fluid resuscitation formulae

Baxter (Parkland) Formula (using crystalloid)

● Lactated Ringer's (Hartmann's) solution 4 ml kg^{-1}% bsab^{-1} in the first 24 h
 – half to be given in the first 8 h from time of injury
 – or, to simplify, 0.25 ml kg^{-1}% bsab^{-1} per hour from time of injury.
● Children will need additional metabolic water as dextrose 5%
 – 1–3 ml kg^{-1} h^{-1} depending on age.

---

subcutaneous tissues carry pain fibres. In contrast, partial-thickness and especially superficial burns can be very painful. Attention should therefore be given as soon as possible to high-quality analgesia and relief of distress in all patients with a thermal injury.

Entonox is very helpful initially and is available on most ambulances. In major burns intramuscular injections are unreliable and pain relief must be immediate. If a doctor is present, or the ambulance paramedics have the required certification, intravenous analgesia may be given using small increments of diluted morphine, diamorphine or nalbuphine, titrated until comfort is achieved. Non-steroidal anti-inflammatory drugs (NSAIDs), such as ibuprofen, enhance the analgesic benefit of opiates synergistically and

are thought by some to blunt the inflammatory response. There is therefore nothing to be lost and possibly much to be gained, by adding NSAIDs to the analgesia regimen from the start.

Relief of distress needs the humane approach of calm, reassuring professionals who keep the patient informed, answer questions and respond to anxieties expressed.

Specific considerations at a major incident involving burns

Burn injuries do not account for a large proportion of the victims of major incidents, but when a major fire occurs it hits the headlines. Facilities in the UK for treating major burns are, however, limited. Specific planning for the management of large numbers of burned victims is therefore a necessary part of a major accident and disaster plan.

Most of the fire disasters occurring in recent years have been written up in the literature. The collective findings are well summarized by Mackie & Koning (1990) in a paper originally produced as evidence to the Dutch Department of Health. The main points emphasized by this paper are as follows:

● Owing to the greater potential for escape, more immediate survivors requiring urgent triage are to be expected from outdoor than from indoor disasters. Some of these will inevitably be lethal injuries, however, with no prospect of survival because of massive or complex injury. Burned patients are often surprisingly well, conscious and lucid for hours after a lethal injury because of the relative slowness of the pathological response compared to that caused by blunt trauma.

● A higher number of inevitably lethal injuries (more than 70% bsab, especially if complicated by smoke inhalation) can be expected following outdoor incidents than from indoor. These patients will initially present alive and must be identified in order to:
 — avoid inappropriate diversion of resources from those more likely to benefit
 — enable them to receive appropriate comfort care.

● Common to both types of disaster, injuries of an intermediate severity – 30–70% bsab, with or without respiratory injury – are comparatively few in number. This group will benefit most from early intervention.

● The vast majority of survivors will have significant but not life-threatening injuries, less than 30% bsab. It should be remembered that such injuries *may* threaten life in small children or the elderly.

The first priority therefore is to perform early, effective triage (Box 31.14). The second priority must be to estimate burn surface area as accurately as possible and to institute appropriate intravenous fluid therapy according

Box 31.14

Triage of burns patients at a major incident

All major accident plans should address the issue of how large numbers of burned casualties are to be managed.

The following points regarding the care of burns are considered essential components in a major accident plan.

A. Identification in the plan (by name or role) of a burns care specialist from the Burn Centre who should be called to the designated receiving hospital(s) (or accident site, see below) to direct burns triage. This will usually be a surgeon, as the intensive care team will be needed at base to receive the complex major injuries.

B. Prompt removal of patients to the designated receiving hospital where effective triage can take place. If prompt evacuation is not possible the triage team (*including* the burns specialist) must be taken to the accident scene.

C. Triage as follows:
- Application of standard immediate trauma care principles, particularly <C>*ABC*.
- Prompt commencement, after <C>*ABC* and *simultaneously* with triage, of burn size assessment (Wallace's Rule of Nines) and intravenous fluid therapy for all burns > 15% bsab (children and the elderly: > 10% bsab). Other injuries must also be identified and appropriately treated.
- Triage should achieve a five-way separation of burns victims as:
  a. minor
  b. intermediate needing fluid resuscitation
  c. major (>30%) or complex including respiratory injury and/or other injuries
  d. lethal burns
  e. respiratory injuries without cutaneous burns.
- Identification of burns likely to benefit from onward referral to a Burns Centre (mostly triage group c, above).
- Identification of any patients with smoke inhalation or airway injury in the *absence* of a significant skin burn (triage group e, above). These patients may need *active ITU care* but need not necessarily go to a Burns Centre.
- Identification of lethally injured patients for whom comfort care is appropriate (triage group d, above).
- Organization of care, under the direction of a consultant plastic surgeon, for the remaining burns (<30% bsab, uncomplicated – triage groups a and b, above).

to protocol. If removal from the site is slow, triage must be undertaken at the disaster scene to prioritize evacuation, under guidance from a burns specialist. The *goal* in all cases, irrespective of the detail of the disaster situation, is to achieve early ABC assessment and management of airway difficulties, followed by early commencement of intravenous resuscitation.

The objectives of triage in a burn disaster are given in Box 31.14.

A designated person should be identified to handle media enquiries. Burn disasters are always emotive, and careful choice must be made of the person to fulfil this role.

Summary

Major burns make up just a small proportion of all thermal injuries, but can be frightening for the inexperienced. Changes occur more slowly and more predictably than in other trauma, so the goal is to transfer the patient quickly to hospital for referral, if need be, to a specialized Burn Centre.

Assessment of burn surface area and intravenous fluid administration according to formulae are necessary if removal to hospital could be delayed, as in a major incident.

Minor injuries also require accurate assessment and often the expertise of a plastic surgeon, and should not be lightly dismissed although they usually pose no threat to life.

The main objectives for immediate care can be summarized as:

- *Cool* the burn
- *Warm* the patient
- Resuscitate (<C>ABC) appropriately
- Transfer to hospital.

References

Childs C 1995 Temperature regulation in burned patients. British Journal of Intensive Care 4: 129–134

Childs C, Edwards-Jones V, Heathcote DM et al 1994 Patterns of *Staphylococcus aureus* colonization, toxin production, immunity and illness in burned children. Burns 20: 514–521

Dziewulski P 1992 Burn wound healing: James Elsworth Laing Memorial Essay for 1991. Burns 18: 466–478

Haberal M 1986 Electrical burns: a five-year experience – 1985 Evans Lecture. Journal of Trauma 26: 103–109

Horch R, Spilker G, Stark GB 1994 Phenol burns and intoxications. Burns 20: 45–50

Kinsella J 1988 Smoke inhalation. Burns 14: 269–279

Kirkpatrick JJR, Burd DAR 1995 An algorithmic approach to the treatment of hydrofluoric acid burns. Burns 21: 495–499

Kirkpatrick JJR, Enion DS, Burd DAR 1995 Hydrofluoric acid burns: a review. Burns 21: 483–493

Laterjet J, Choinière M 1995 Pain in burn patients. Burns 21: 344–348

Mackie DP, Koning HM 1990 Fate of mass burn casualties: implications for disaster planning. Burns 16: 203–206

Oughterson AW, Warren S 1956 Medical effects of the atomic bomb in Japan. McGraw-Hill, New York

Platt AJ, Aslam S, Judkins KC et al 1997 Temperature profiles during resuscitation predict survival following burns complicated by smoke inhalation injury. Burns 23: 250–255

Prien T, Traber DL 1988 Toxic smoke compounds and inhalation injury – a review. Burns 14: 451–460

Smith RW, O'Neill TJ 1984 An analysis into childhood burns. Burns 11: 117–124

Traber DL, Linares HA, Herndon DN 1988 The pathophysiology of inhalation injury – a review. Burns 14: 357–364

Further reading

Clarke JA 1992 A colour atlas of burn injuries. Chapman & Hall, London

Driscoll PA, Gwinnutt CL, Jimmerson CL, Goodall O (eds) 1993 In: Burns. Trauma resuscitation – the team approach. Macmillan, London, ch 12

Herndon DN (ed) 1996 Total burn care. WB Saunders, London

Martyn JAJ (ed) 1990 Acute management of the burned patient. WB Saunders, London

Settle JAD (ed) 1996 Principles and practice of burn management. Churchill Livingstone, Edinburgh

Part Seven

32   The elderly patient 347

The elderly patient

Introduction   347

Assessment of the elderly patient   347

Major clinical problems in old age   348

References   357

Further reading   358

Introduction

An account of the elderly patient in the context of a book about prehospital medicine would seem to exclude consideration of issues of frailty and disabling chronic disease. Such an exclusion is wrong, as the distinctive nature of clinical emergencies in frail old people is inextricably linked with chronic disease and the precarious health of an elderly person perhaps living alone and already dependent on support from others. Age is only a rough proxy for such frailty, and we all know people in their late 80s who seem younger as well as those in their 50s and 60s who seem old. Nevertheless, over the age of 75 years the prevalence of disabling diseases, the number of people living alone, perhaps recently bereaved, and the occurrence of multiple pathology, as well as visual and hearing difficulties rises sharply and therefore it is reasonable to focus on this age group.

Assessment of the elderly patient

THE NATURE OF ACUTE ILLNESS IN OLD AGE

Some generalizations can be made.

- Acute illnesses in old people often fail to present with convenient and 'classical' symptoms or physical signs:
    - A myocardial infarct may present without crushing central chest pain and rather with a fall, acute onset of mental confusion or simply breathlessness.
    - Acute infections may fail to mount the response of an immune reaction (raised white cell count) or a raised body temperature.
- Acute illnesses in old people arise in the context of a general background of failing health such as:
    - *memory loss and impairment of intellect* – the elderly brain is especially susceptible to the toxic effects of any acute illness so that acute onset of mental confusion may be a presenting symptom that resolves provided that the underlying cause is treated
    - *failing eyesight or hearing*
    - *increase in postural sway* so that acute illnesses may present as falls
    - *impaired central control of bladder function* so that acute illnesses may present with urinary incontinence
    - perhaps most importantly *an accumulation of other diseases* so that a fairly trivial acute illness may arise in a person already compromised by heart failure and further limited by impaired mobility following an operation for a fractured neck of femur.

- Acute illnesses in old people often arise in a situation of precarious social circumstances in which the support network for the individual is already stretched.
- Acute illnesses in old people are often partly or wholly related to drug therapy.

Therefore, an apparently minor illness in an old person can have very different consequences from the same illness in a young person.

HISTORY AND EXAMINATION – GETTING THE INFORMATION

Communicating with old people

Problems such as impaired hearing, anxiety, neurological problems (stroke, dementia, depression) and the effects of social isolation may cause problems in communicating with old people. Simple measures such as ensuring that a hearing aid is switched on and that dentures are worn may make a huge difference. In people with impaired hearing, ensuring good lighting and that the patient can see your face clearly may assist with lip reading, at which many old people are extremely adept.

The home environment: clues to aid diagnosis and management

The paramedic, doctor or district nurse may be in a unique position when called to an emergency in the home of an old person. The major illnesses of old age often leave environmental clues to give assistance to the hospital or primary care team. This investigative role of the medical, paramedical or nursing visitor is especially crucial when the patient is a recluse, perhaps not well known to neighbours, or to the primary care team. If reluctant to go to hospital, the patient may play down or deny that problems exist.

Major clinical problems in old age

THE 'GIANTS' OF GERIATRIC MEDICINE: INTRODUCTION

The effects of ageing and acute or chronic illnesses often manifest as conditions best described as in 'functional failure'. These are described in this section. Professor Bernard Isaacs, one of the first generation of academic geriatricians, characterized these common manifestations of illness in old age as 'the giants of geriatric medicine': *intellectual disorder* (dementias and acute confusional states), *immobility*, *incontinence* and *instability* (a tendency to fall). Add to these the social ill of isolation often worsened by the common handicap of *visual and hearing impairment* (described in the second section of this chapter). Another common

problem, often undetected or untreated, is *depression*. Multiple ailments, so common in old people, often result in multiple drug therapy. Approximately 10% of acute admissions to geriatric wards are as a result of *adverse drug reactions* (ADR) (Williamson & Chopin 1980). All these aspects will be described later.

INTELLECTUAL IMPAIRMENT (ACUTE CONFUSIONAL STATES AND DEMENTIAS)

Some impairment of memory and concentration is so common in later life as to be considered normal and not indicative or predictive of dementia. This thought is a great relief to its victims but is occasionally responsible for a delay in diagnosis of genuine dementia. This type is seldom in any way disabling. In simple terms, intellectual impairment is of two types: due to disease outside the brain (extrinsic) and due to intrinsic brain disease (dementia).

Extrinsic causes (acute or toxic confusional states)

These are a common cause of acute illness and are properly treated as a medical emergency. They may arise in a patient apparently mentally normal before the event but more commonly arise in a person with underlying dementia.

The causes of acute confusional states are indicated in Table 32.1.

The intellectual dysfunction associated with these extrinsic causes is usually short-lived, unless there is coexisting intrinsic brain disease.

Intrinsic causes (dementia)

Dementia is a pathological state characterized by diffuse loss of brain tissue. When brain tumour and other focal conditions have been excluded the usual causes are Alzheimer's disease, multifocal vascular disease and a mixture of these. Dementia also occurs in Parkinson's disease, Huntington's chorea and other rarer brain diseases.

Alzheimer's disease is characterized pathologically by plaques and neurofibrillary tangles in the brain substance, and biochemically by loss of cholinergic and other neurotransmitters. It is a slowly progressive disease with a 10-year course on average. While some cases can present in the fifth and sixth decades, most appear in the eighth and ninth decades.

Vascular brain disease, also called multi-infarct dementia, occurs often in hypertensive patients, who suffer progressive loss of brain tissue, with or without focal neurological signs. The course of this disease is more rapid than that of Alzheimer's disease, and many patients die from cardiac disease or stroke.

Patients may give a very misleading history of the illness, as they are unable to assess their current state, but may be

Table 32.1 Causes of toxic confusional states

Causes	Clinical examples
Drugs	Psychoactive drugs, diuretics, sedatives, alcohol intoxication or withdrawal
Infections	Pneumonia, urinary tract infection, acute viral illness, shingles
Hypoxia	In cardiac or respiratory failure
Dehydration	In hot weather, due to drugs or failure of access to oral fluids
Electrolyte disorders	For example hyponatraemia (diuretics)
Disturbances of carbohydrate metabolism	For example hyperglycaemia, often due to newly diagnosed or poorly controlled maturity-onset diabetes mellitus; hypoglycaemia due to starvation, illness or overtreatment in known diabetic
Renal and hepatic failure	Characteristic 'metabolic' flapping tremor may be absent
Thyroid disorders	Hypo- or hyperthyroidism
Vitamin B_{12} and folate deficiency (rare cause)	More often presents with features of spinal cord degeneration
Head injury with or without intracranial haemorrhage	Any fall followed by a toxic confusional state must alert the clinician to possibility of head injury, CT head scan to exclude subdural or extradural haematoma
Acute stroke	May present as toxic confusional state that precedes localized neurological signs

Table 32.2 The history in dementia

- An increased use of the telephone, especially in the middle of the night
- Frequent losses of key, pension books, money, jewellery
- Accusations that others have stolen these
- Burning out kettles
- Leaving the gas on unlit
- Resistance to bathing and changing clothes
- Changes in sleep–wake patterns
- Soiling of clothes and neglect of personal appearance
- Leaving the house and getting lost
- Repeatedly asking the same question
- Misidentifying or failing to identify near relatives
- Speaking of the past as if it were the present, and of dead people, e.g. parents, as if they were still alive

Box 32.1

Confusional states as a medical emergency

Two cardinal features distinguish acute confusional states from dementia:

- **Acute onset (and usually rapid resolution)**
- **Disturbed or fluctuating conscious level may be a feature. Consciousness may be impaired (drowsy) or the patient may be agitated and hypervigilant but without true engagement with other people or surroundings.**

In dementia, the problems may place an intolerable strain on carers, neighbours and statutory services. Eventually a crisis occurs that carers can no longer accept and the resulting breakdown of domestic support may masquerade as a medical emergency. Problems or disruption at night are common precipitants for a demented person to be considered for residential or nursing home care. However, the clinician has the responsibility for considering and excluding a superimposed toxic confusional state. A sudden change in behaviour in a demented person should lead to a search for a toxic cause, but disruptive behaviour is often due to the natural progression of a dementing illness.

able to talk convincingly and positively of their past life. Patients have considerable skills of deception. Be very wary of patients who make even the slightest lapse from consistency or accuracy in answering questions, and seek information from relatives who have watched them over a period of time. The tell-tale signs of dementia are indicated in Table 32.2.

An alternative approach to admission for a badly demented individual is innovative flexibility in domestic supervision encompassing night times and weekends, as well as considering intermittent respite care in a residential setting to allow willing but worn-out relatives to 'recharge their batteries'.

IMMOBILITY

What are the barriers to maintaining mobility in old age?

Physical barriers

Unfortunately, old age brings with it an increasing prevalence of a number of diseases, often more than one at a time:

- Joint problems, especially osteoarthritis of knees and hips
- Neurological deficit: impaired balance, stroke, Parkinson's disease

- Previous falls
- Sensory deprivation: deafness, impaired vision
- Cardiovascular and respiratory diseases.

Mental barriers

- Reduced expectations of an 'active life'
- Loss of adaptability and creativity
- Introversion with reduced social contact
- Anxiety and fear of going out (or of allowing others to).

Social barriers

- Retirement brings with it dangers of reduced social contact, and a drop in income. The retired person may regard a motor car as an unnecessary expense. Many regret having got rid of their car.
- Living alone: an epidemic problem in ageing women.
- Nowhere to go: insufficient outside interests or activities.

What are the consequences of immobility?

- *Loss of choice* – any of the following choices may be lost to us:
  - Being able to get to where we want to be and thus able to do what we want to do
  - Being alone or with others
  - Having the television on or off (look around any hospital ward)
- *Loss of capability*:
  - Getting to the toilet in time/answering the door/getting upstairs
  - Social responsiveness
  - Worsening physical dependency.

An old person's world may thus contract, and after becoming housebound he (or more often she) then becomes restricted to the lower half of the house and eventually to what the geriatricians sometimes call a 'triangular' existence – from bed to chair to commode.

INCONTINENCE

Prevalence and effects – urinary incontinence

Because of the social stigma and personal embarrassment unfairly associated with this problem, estimates of prevalence are almost certainly a gross underestimate. Data from a number of sources (Royal College of Physicians of London 1995) indicate that it is a problem throughout adult life but that its prevalence rises with age and is much more common in women over 65 years (10–20%) than in men aged over 65 (7–10%).

Box 32.2

Immobility as a medical emergency

People with severe immobility at home, especially if alone, live on a knife-edge of critical dependency on others and at risk of social breakdown if:

- withdrawal of carer support occurs
- intercurrent illness renders them unmanageable, bedbound or chairbound.

In these circumstances, the individual will be unable to access food, fluid or toilet, which justifies emergency support at home or admission to hospital. If denied such access, the situation will worsen, with the risk of falls and incontinence.

The effects on the individual may be devastating. Old people may be ostracized or even institutionalized. In adult women with urinary incontinence, 60% avoid leaving their home, 50% feel inferior to others, 45% avoid public transport and 50% avoid sexual activity. There is also significant psychiatric disturbance, principally depression.

The cost of managing (in contrast to diagnosing and treating) the problem is enormous. Components include loss of earnings, costs of nursing and provision of incontinence aids. In the USA it was estimated to cost 2% of the health budget. This estimate would translate into a cost of approximately £1.4 billion per annum.

Prevalence and effects – faecal incontinence

Although less common than urinary incontinence in older people, faecal incontinence is a significant problem, especially in institutions. In their own homes about 3–5% of people over 65 years of age and 15% over 85 years suffer from this problem. Institutions have a higher prevalence (residential homes – 10%; nursing homes – 30%; NHS care elderly medical and psychiatric – 60%). At home the effects on carers, who may have to clean up faecal incontinence, not infrequently precipitate a crisis of care and may lead to emergency hospital admission.

Causes in elderly people

Table 32.3 indicates the main causes of urinary and faecal incontinence.

Additional factors in frail people

Anyone can become incontinent if not able or not allowed to have access to proper toilet facilities. The elderly are more vulnerable because of poor mobility, and frequency

Table 32.3 Causes of urinary and faecal incontinence in older people

Urinary incontinence

Women	Men
Stress incontinence (sphincter weakness)	Outflow obstruction (enlarged prostate)
Detrusor instability (constitutional)	Detrusor instability
Neurogenic bladder (associated with stroke, dementia, Parkinson's disease)	Underactive (atonic) bladder
Overflow incontinence due to urine retention	Neurogenic bladder (associated with stroke, dementia, Parkinson's disease)
Urine infection	Faecal impaction
Faecal impaction	Drugs
Confusional states	
Drugs, e.g. diuretics	

Faecal incontinence

Colorectal conditions:
  diarrhoea
  overflow – impaction
  cancer (especially rectal)
Chronic straining at stool
Neurological problems:
  autonomic neuropathy (e.g. diabetes mellitus)
  spinal cord disease (e.g. multiple sclerosis)
  dementia and acute confusional states
Drugs, e.g. laxatives and antibiotics

and urgency of micturition. As indicated above, *any acute illness* is likely to be associated with deterioration in continence but usually this is transient. Likewise, any *change of environment* such as admission to hospital may also lead to a temporary period of incontinence.

Management

Diagnosis of the cause of incontinence is crucial. Most patients will present a diagnosis after careful history and examination.

In addition to management of specific problems, the approach must be one of optimism as, in the absence of severe dementia, approximately 30% overall will be cured, 30% improved and in the remainder much can be done to reduce the social and psychological handicap with the use of toileting regimes and equipment such as pads (many quite acceptable cosmetically), penile sheaths and various bed pads. Urinary catheters, often considered a last resort, can occasionally relieve the discomfort of constant incontinence associated with excoriation of the skin and poor mobility or inability to manipulate underclothes and pads.

Box 32.3

Incontinence as a medical emergency

The social stress on carers of coping with severe incontinence, often unassessed and hidden, may result in a crisis that results in emergency admission to hospital or rapid and usually inappropriate transit to a nursing home. Genuine medical emergencies include:

- urinary incontinence as the presentation of urine retention secondary to prostate disease or faecal impaction
- urinary incontinence associated with urine infection and septicaemia
- faecal incontinence due to acute diarrhoea (infection or inflammatory bowel disease) or a distal colonic or rectal cancer
- occasionally, melaena secondary to a brisk upper gastrointestinal bleed may present with faecal incontinence.

INSTABILITY AND FALLS

Instability

Balance

Balance is a set of biological strategies designed to maintain the body in the erect posture. Mechanisms involved include ocular, vestibular and proprioceptive receptors found in the neck and elsewhere, especially in the weight-bearing joints and in the tendons and ligaments of the trunk. Under normal circumstances, the body undergoes oscillations around a fixed point known as the sway path. The amplitude of the sway path reaches a minimum during adolescence and is maintained at this level until the late 40s, when the amplitude of sway begins to increase. Women display greater amplitude of sway at any given age.

Balance mechanisms deteriorate in old age
The centre of mass of the human body lies somewhere in the region of the second sacral vertebra. Any shift of weight away from the region of this vertebra is under vigilant surveillance of the nervous system in order to prevent overbalancing.

- *Ocular mechanisms*: Under normal circumstances, visual cues are constantly used to correct minor deviation from the fixed point. In old people visual acuity is frequently reduced, as is the threshold for light stimulation.
- *Vestibular mechanisms*: The vestibule is mainly involved with rotatory movements of the head and neck, whereas the otolith organ is involved with acceleration/deceleration. With advancing age, these mechanisms are relatively inefficient, although this component of balance declines in importance with ascent of the evolutionary scale. Vestibular mechanisms may be implicated in walking over uneven

ground, or have some part to play in instability during rising from a chair.

- *Proprioceptive mechanisms*: Position sense is important for maintaining balance. Sensory information from propriocep-tors in the central spine and major weight-bearing joints may be impaired with ageing and arthritis or after joint replacement.

In summary, imbalance in old age is due to a combination of ageing of the various balance mechanisms leading to an increased likelihood of falls.

Falls

About 20% of elderly men and 40% of elderly women will give a history of a recent fall, and the liability to fall rises with age: the probability going up from a 30% chance of falling at the age of 65 years to 50% at the age of 85. Of course, the majority of falls are not reported *and only about 3% sustain an injury that requires medical atten-tion*. Nevertheless, in an average size Health District of 250 000 people, with about 37 000 people over 65 years of age, between 16 and 20 beds will be occupied by patients admitted as a direct result of a fall. It is one of the com-monest causes of emergency admission to an acute geriat-ric ward, often after a prolonged period lying on the floor unable to get up.

Consequences

Falls are the sixth leading cause of death in old people. Serious soft tissue injuries occur in 5% and fractures in a further 5% (Tinetti et al 1988). They account for a quarter of elderly medical admissions. Apart from the morbidity associated with serious injury, falls result in loss of confi-dence, immobility and increasing dependency on others.

Risk factors

A number of prospective studies have examined the fac-tors associated with an increased risk of falling. Tinetti et al (1988) examined 336 free-living individuals aged over 75 years, identified risk factors and recorded the incidence of falls within 1 year of assessment. 32% fell within 1 year, and a quarter of the fallers had serious injuries, including six with fractures. They showed the dramatic deleteri-ous effect of sedative drugs and of other risk factors such as cognitive impairment and multiple risk factors. These results are displayed in Table 32.4. Interestingly, the dem-onstration of significant postural hypotension, often quoted as a risk factor, did not figure in this study.

Where and when do falls occur?

Most occur indoors or very close to the house, in daytime. If on stairs they are more likely when descending.

Table 32.4 Risk factors for falls in elderly people

Risk factor	Odds ratio
Sedative use	38.3
Cognitive impairment	5.0
Disability of lower extremities	3.0
Impaired gait and balance	1.9
Foot problems	1.8

Risk of falling increases with multiple risk factors	
Number of factors	**Fall rate within 1 year (%)**
0	8
1	19
2	32
3	60
4 or more	78

Source: Reprinted with permission from Tinetti ME, Speechley M, Ginter SF 1988 Risk factors for falls among elderly persons living in the community. New England Journal of Medicine 319: 1701–1707. Copyright © 1988 Massachusetts Medical Society. All rights reserved.

What are the clinical features?

They fall into two broad categories:

- *Extrinsic*, in which an external factor is responsible: tripping or accident. These falls typically occur in younger, fitter people and the vast majority are unreported and cause no serious injury. The consequences are slight, with no restriction in activities or loss of confidence.
- *Intrinsic*, in which the dominant cause is failure of balance for the reasons described above and in which one or more precipitating factors (described below) may play a part. In this case the patient is older and more frail, and typically the consequences are much more serious regardless of physical injury: loss of confidence, restriction of activity and a loss of mobility, typically fear of going out of doors unaccompanied.

Precipitating causes

- *Change of posture* – getting out of a chair, an unstable situation requiring strength and coordination in antigrav-ity muscles. (Not usually due to postural hypotension, an uncommon cause of falls but much loved by medical students and doctors.)
- *Extended movement* – in which the person reaches out or up, puts his/her centre of gravity outside his/her ground-base but because of a slowing of postural reflex move-ments is unable to compensate by moving his/her feet quickly enough to prevent a fall.

Box 32.4

Falls as a medical emergency

From the foregoing discussion, it is clear that all falls in old people must be taken seriously. Falls that do not reach medical attention occur frequently. The patient may not wish to make a fuss nor to be admitted to hospital. When called to see such a patient after a fall at home, a full history (giddy turns? recurrent falls? precipitating event?) and examination (in pain? off feet? sign of fracture or soft tissue injury? environmental hazards? neurological deficit? joint disease?) must be completed.

- It is usually safe to leave such a patient at home in the following circumstances:
  - up and about and confident
  - normal or safe gait
  - able to get up off the floor unassisted
  - no injury or pain
  - cognitively intact
  - no serious coexisting disease (acute illness, cardiac failure, severe arthritis)
  - a companion available for at least 24 h.
- Urgent admission to hospital should be considered if:
  - giddy, impaired gait, history of recurrent falls
  - off feet or in pain or suspicion of a fracture
  - unable to get up off floor
  - living alone
  - environmental hazards (e.g. unavoidable stairs)
  - unable to perform simple activities of daily living (ADL).

- *Illnesses* – any acute illnesses, such as cardiac disease or arrhythmias, poor vision.
- *Drugs* – especially diuretics, hypnotics and drugs for hypertension.

What is the prognosis?
Falls in the very old often indicate serious underlying disease and have a gloomy outlook. About a quarter will die within 1 year of their index fall. If they have lain for more than 1 h, half will be dead in 6 months (Overstall et al 1977).

DEPRESSION

Depression is both a subjective mood state and an objective psychiatric illness. It is important to distinguish one from the other.

The psychiatric illness of depression is characterized by *low mood, unaffected by external circumstances*, feelings of unworthiness and helplessness. Suicidal ideas may be present. The future looks bleak. There is appetite disturbance, usually leading to weight loss. Sleep disturbance, characteristically early morning wakening, occurs. Concentration is poor and there is a decrease in normal interests, even in family and friends. In a severe illness, psychotic phenomena may be present such as delusions and hallucinations. Delusions are usually of poverty or nihilistic, thinking things have disappeared, never to exist again. Hallucinations are usually second-person and are derogatory statements, for example 'you are dirty', 'you should be dead'. In elderly patients with depression *hypochondriacal ideas* are more often present (e.g. worries about heart disease, cancer, etc.). This is often in the setting of real illness, which is then exaggerated by fears and worries.

Masked depression

Hypochondria or anxiety symptoms are predominant and there is no complaint of depression, although symptoms are there if questioned. It should be noted that new onset of anxiety, phobic, obsessional or hysterical illnesses are exceedingly rare over the age of 65 years. If a previous stable premorbid personality 'changes', a depressive illness should be sought.

'Pseudodementia'

Pseudodementia is the term given to a syndrome that presents with poor self-care and poor cognitive ability. This change in function is brought about by a retarded depression. All the features mentioned above will be present, lack of interest will result in poor self-care and cognitive function. These patients will often answer 'don't know' to questions rather than confabulate. The history of onset of the illness is weeks or months rather than years as in a true dementia. There may be a family or previous history of affective disorder.

Prevalence of depression

A study of prevalence of depression in a community survey amongst elderly people (UK and USA in 1976) showed:

- 22% possibly depressed
- 13% minor depressive disorder
- 1.6% major depressive disorder.

Factors predisposing to depression

Old age is a time of losses. Giving up work, the death of relatives or friends, physical illness or a constricted lifestyle all set the scene for a depressive illness. Diseases common in old age and associated with depression include Parkinson's disease, stroke and disabling arthritis.

Box 32.5

Depression as a medical emergency

Patients exhibiting delusional ideas, or who are failing to thrive with loss of interest in eating or drinking, require urgent attention. If medication is ineffective or not taken, it may be necessary to invoke the Mental Health Acts to arrange compulsory admission to hospital. In this circumstance, close liaison between psychiatric and medical services is essential because medical as well as psychiatric treatment may be required.

STROKE (ACUTE CEREBROVASCULAR DISEASE IN OLD AGE)

Definitions

Cerebrovascular disease has three ways of presenting acutely: as subarachnoid haemorrhage (SAH: acute bleeding, usually from an arterial aneurysm into the subarachnoid space); transient ischaemic attack (TIA: acute neurological deficit resolving within 24 h); and stroke (the acute neurological deficit does not resolve within 24 h).

Epidemiology

Subarachnoid haemorrhage is the least common presentation and stroke the most common. Only stroke will be further considered. Because two thirds of stroke sufferers survive, and half of the survivors are left with some degree of disability, the burden of stroke is more closely related to the prevalence. As a rough guide, the prevalence of stroke in Western countries lies between 400 and 600 cases per 100 000 of the population.

For a description of the clinical features, treatment and complications, the reader is referred to other accounts (Wade et al 1985, Main 1995). In the context of this book, further discussion will be confined to stroke as a medical emergency in the community and the continuing burden of stroke at home or after discharge from hospital.

Hospital or home?

Various surveys have reported that between 40% and 70% of patients were admitted to hospital after an acute stroke. In the Oxfordshire Community Stroke Project (OCSP; Bamford et al 1986) and in earlier studies, patients were more likely to be admitted to hospital if they:

- lived alone
- were unconscious
- had a severe neurological deficit overwhelming the capacity of a carer or community-based services to cope.

Patients more likely to stay at home were those with mild or quickly resolving strokes.

Should more patients be admitted to hospital?

Hitherto, the decision about whether to admit a patient with an acute stroke to hospital has not depended upon any perception that specific hospital-based intervention would be helpful. However, recent evidence (Langhorne et al 1993) has suggested that coordinated stroke care by a multidisciplinary team or in a stroke unit reduces mortality when compared with 'ordinary' stroke care. In addition, thrombolysis for acute stroke is becoming a standard part of emergency stroke management in a sub-group of patients, and therefore assessment in hospital as soon as possible after the onset of stroke symptoms is mandatory. Thus, in the future, efficient organization of acute stroke services might alter the pattern of referral to hospital. In an editorial accompanying the results of Langhorne et al's work, it was pointed out that it is very hard to discern which aspects of therapy are successful. It seems likely that better nursing and medical care, as well as perhaps greater use of anticoagulants to prevent vascular complications, are responsible. In view of the evidence discussed above, acute hospital services need to be organized in a way to allow good and consistent quality of medical and nursing care, access to computed tomography (CT) scanning, standard application of treatment regimes (in or out of clinical trials), and smooth transition from high-dependency nursing and medical care to coordinated rehabilitation and multidisciplinary discharge planning. There can be little reason now for patients with strokes being scattered throughout acute medical wards. Clinical indication for referral to a stroke unit will depend on whether the unit is for high-dependency early management or for rehabilitation. In the former case, patients most suitable would be those with severe strokes, those being considered for acute drug intervention or those who require expert nursing to prevent the early complications.

FITS AND FAINTS

Making a diagnosis: was it a fall, faint or fit?

If the episode was witnessed, the diagnosis should be fairly easy. If a fit was seen, careful questioning may determine also the type of fit and even the underlying cause. If not witnessed the diagnosis includes simple falls and syncope (transient loss of consciousness due to interruption of cerebral blood flow). If the patient has no recall of a period of unconsciousness and therefore reports a fall, suspicion of an epileptic fit or syncope should arise if there is no obvious environmental or intrinsic physical cause for falls, or if an exact description of the events surrounding the fall is hard to extract. Distinguishing between a fit and syncope from the history in these circumstances can be difficult. In a known diabetic, hypoglycaemia should be considered, especially if the episode occurred at night or if there is doubt about drug or dietary compliance. Of course, prolonged hypoglycaemia per se may cause a fit.

Faints (syncope)

As described above, unless witnessed a faint may be difficult to distinguish from a fit or from transient cerebral ischaemia resulting in a short-lived focal neurological deficit. A true faint may be precipitated by coughing, micturition or defecation. It may occur as a result of failure of postural reflexes on standing or at night it can occur when rising from a warm bed into a cold bedroom. Compromise of the postural reflexes may be caused by drugs or carotid sinus disease.

Fits (epilepsy)

In an established epileptic patient, attention is likely to be centred on the adequacy of drug treatment, the patient's compliance with therapy and complicating factors such as alcohol (or alcohol withdrawal).

What type of seizure?

A simple clinical classification of generalized convulsions (Tallis 1992) is helpful:

- Tonic
- Absence
- Myoclonic
- Other clonic
- Partial
- Simple (consciousness retained)
- Complex (consciousness impaired)
- Evolving to generalized fits.

In patients referred to a specialist centre, generalized fits account for about one-fifth, of which tonic–clonic fits are the most common. Much more common are partial fits, of which over half are complex (associated with impaired consciousness). In elderly patients, generalized fits predominate.

Interpretation of investigations of fits in elderly patients

As cerebrovascular disease is the most common cause, the urgent search for a tumour may receive less emphasis. Initially, the search for a remediable metabolic cause should receive urgent consideration (Fig. 32.1). An electrocardiogram (ECG) may detect an arrhythmia associated

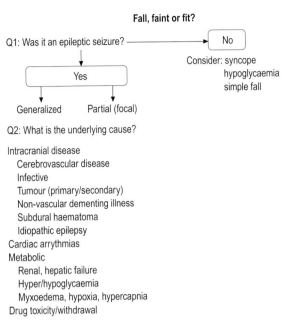

Fig. 32.1 • Fall, faint or fit? – an algorithm.

with syncope and, along with a blood glucose estimation, is likely to be the only investigation available prehospital. A positive electroencephalogram (EEG) will support a diagnosis of epilepsy and may indicate a focal abnormality suggesting a local neurological cause, such as ischaemia or a tumour. However, a normal EEG does not rule out the diagnosis of epilepsy. CT is indicated if a focal abnormality is suspected clinically or on EEG. Although cerebrovascular disease may be strongly suspected on clinical grounds, a negative CT scan will be reassuring to a patient worried about cancer because there is a very low false-negative rate.

Principles of management

Initial management in the prehospital environment will concentrate on the maintenance of a clear protected airway and an adequate circulation.

Much fear surrounds this condition and there is a certain perceived stigma attached to the diagnosis. Reassurance and demystification about the condition is required early on. There should be avoidance of dangerous activities without over-restriction. Advice on freedom of activities will only be possible when the pattern and frequency of fits is established and when optimal control is achieved with drug treatment. Unfortunately, even a single fit necessitates cessation of driving. Current practice is that a single fit is not usually treated. The drugs usually used in maintenance treatment are phenytoin, valproate and carbamazepine. Further discussion will be restricted to the management of status epilepticus.

Box 32.6

Steps in treatment of status epilepticus

1. Rapid control of fits: – Diazemuls 10 mg in 2 ml over 3–5 min intravenously.
2. High-flow oxygen by mask and reservoir bag.
3. Search for and exclude hypoglycaemia or poisoning (Fig. 32.1).
4. Failure of control with above regime will require hospital admission; in unusual circumstances the following may need to be considered:
   a. diazepam infusion up to 40 mg h^{-1}
   b. phenytoin intravenously.
5. If status is prolonged, or respiratory failure results from diazepam use, assisted ventilation may be required.

Status epilepticus is a medical emergency. It occurs when seizures are prolonged or when there is no recovery between frequent attacks. The steps in treatment are given in Box 32.6.

ACCIDENTS AND FRACTURES

Introduction

Accidents are a major cause of mortality and morbidity in old age. The majority of accidental deaths are related to falls, usually within the home, but burns and road traffic accidents are also significant causes.

Fractures

Fractures in elderly people are the inevitable outcome when the dangerous combination of the tendency to fall is added to a substantial reduction in bone strength, due mainly to osteoporosis. The most serious fracture in terms of cost and human misery is proximal femoral fracture but fractures of the humerus, wrist and pubic ramus are also significant.

The numbers of hip fractures in the UK have been growing steadily and this rise can confidently be expected to continue because of the increasing numbers of elderly people as well as an increase in the age-specific incidence.

The current costs in the UK of managing these fractures is probably in excess of £200 million per annum and this represents only the direct cost of hospital care.

Road traffic accidents

Road traffic accidents are an important cause of morbidity and mortality in old age and are second only to falls as an important cause of accidental death, particularly in people over 75 years of age.

The two most significant groups of elderly road users are drivers of private cars and pedestrians. In relation to elderly drivers, there is little doubt that the rate of crashes rises steeply with advancing age. The reasons are much the same as those discussed for burns but include especially increased reaction time and poor vision. Furthermore, in elderly patients with dementia the rate of crashes is substantially increased, possibly as much as fivefold over age-matched controls.

Despite these rather alarming figures, the number of accidents involving elderly drivers remains relatively small and it seems likely that this is because elderly drivers cover fewer miles and avoid potentially dangerous situations (particularly driving at night). Accidents to elderly pedestrians are an important problem and again one that is likely to grow. For many elderly people, walking remains their major mode of transport and an accident can have devastating consequences. The reason for the high level of pedestrian accidents amongst the elderly clearly has much to do with the sort of factors already discussed, but vision and hearing are likely to be important, as is walking speed. Steps have been taken to make streets safer for elderly pedestrians but clearly much more needs to be done. The creation of pedestrian precincts, measures to calm traffic speed and the provision of audible crossing signals are well established, and are also popular with the wider community.

ADVERSE DRUG REACTIONS

For the reasons described above, an old person is especially vulnerable to the toxic effects of drugs. In addition to the increased susceptibility of target organs, such as the brain and kidney, additional problems of compliance with medication result from mental impairment, impaired manual dexterity and poor vision. In addition, old people are prescribed far more medication than younger people and are often poorly monitored by their doctors (Cartwright & Smith 1988).

Table 32.5 indicates the commonest culprits in causing problems in old people. The doctor or paramedic called to see an old person should (with permission) search for all medication (prescribed and 'over-the-counter') and bring them with the patient to hospital. They may be crucial in assisting diagnosis, especially when the patient is unable to give an accurate history.

PHYSICAL ABUSE

Recently there has been increasing interest and concern in this important topic. Abuse may be physical, sexual, financial or due to neglect by relatives, carers or (it could be argued) by the State, which leaves many old people on very low incomes or insufficiently supported in their

Table 32.5 Drugs that may cause problems in elderly patients

Drug group		Symptoms and signs
Diuretics		Falls, confusion, dry mouth, dehydration, postural fall in blood pressure, urinary incontinence
Compound analgesics		Drowsiness, confusion, falls, constipation
Tricyclic antidepressants		Greater risk of anticholinergic effects: urine retention, constipation, dry mouth, postural hypotension and confusion
Digoxin		Reduced renal excretion. Increased risk of side effects such as sickness, diarrhoea and slow pulse rate and other heart rhythm disorders causing dizziness, fainting or falls
Beta-blockers		Falls, confusion, heart failure, slow pulse, postural hypotension, asthma attacks, cold limbs
Hypnotics		Increased and prolonged effects. Confusion, drowsiness, staggering and falls (especially at night)
Major tranquillizers		Symptoms of Parkinson's disease such as shake (tremor), stiffness and general slowing-up
Non-steroidal anti-inflammatory drugs		Fluid retention and renal failure more likely to occur. Gastrointestinal bleeding
Antibiotics	Tetracycline	Reduced renal clearance may cause renal failure
	Co-trimoxazole	Renal failure
	Corticosteroids	Increased risk of osteoporotic fractures and poorly healing skin abrasions

own homes. Paramedics and doctors should be trained in the signs of non-accidental injury. Much attention has been paid to this topic in children and adults in violent households, but only recently has the problem in old people been addressed. Injuries such as finger mark bruising (especially on the upper arms), cigarette burns (which may not be self-inflicted), bruising around the head and neck and on non-extensor surfaces may be due to assaults and should be carefully documented. Usually, they are blamed on falls and, in direct confrontation, the old person will often deny abuse, which is often from a stressed carer on whom the old person depends. Physical abuse most often occurs within a caring relationship, in which a stressed carer, often inadequately supported, is dealing day and night with a person who is mentally or physically very dependent. Management of the situation demands great sensitivity, with care and treatment not only for the abused person, but for his or her carer.

ACCESS OF EMERGENCY ADMISSIONS TO ACUTE CARE

The reasons for an observed steady rise in the demand for emergency admissions to hospital in the UK is alarming. The reasons are not entirely clear but include:

- a rise in the proportion of elderly people in the population and among admissions
- fear among GPs of litigation for negligence of sick patients managed at home
- increased use by GPs of deputizing emergency services
- increased expectations of the general public.

The result is a downward pressure on length of hospital stay, seen by many managers as a symbol of success. For the frail patient it can be a disaster for the following reasons:

- premature discharge, before adequate recovery has occurred, may result in readmission
- insufficient time to plan a safe discharge
- inappropriate placement of patients from acute wards in residential or nursing home care
- increased pressure on relatives and district nursing services.

The solutions are difficult, although improved funding and organization of primary care and social support services may in the future prevent crisis admissions due to inadequate support at home. Proper funding and supply of acute beds to match demand is desirable but difficult to achieve efficiently in the face of budget restraints and wide fluctuations in the demand for emergency admissions. Proper organization of elective medical and surgical procedures with an emphasis on day cases frees up hospital beds but inevitably puts extra strain on community nursing services.

References

Bamford J, Sandercock P, Warlow C, Gray M 1986 Why are patients with acute stroke admitted to hospital? British Medical Journal 292: 1369–1372

Cartwright A, Smith C 1988 Elderly people, their medicines and their doctors. Routledge, London

Langhorne P, Williams BD, Gilchrist W 1993 Do stroke units save lives? Lancet 342: 395–398

Main A 1995 Acute stroke and other neurological disorders. In: Sinclair AJ, Woodhouse KW (eds) Acute medical illness in old age. Chapman & Hall, London

Overstall PW, Exton-Smith AN, Imms FJ, Johnson AL 1977 Falls in the elderly related to postural imbalance. British Medical Journal 1: 261–264

Royal College of Physicians of London 1995 Incontinence. Causes, management and provision of services – a report. RCPL, London

Tallis R 1992 Epilepsy. In: Evans JG, Williams TF (eds) Oxford textbook of geriatric medicine. Oxford University Press, Oxford, ch 18.11

Tinetti ME, Speechley M, Ginter SF 1988 Risk factors for falls among elderly persons living in the community. New England Journal of Medicine 319: 1701–1707

Wade DT, Langton Hewer R, Skilbeck CE, David RM 1985 Stroke – a critical approach to diagnosis, treatment and management. Chapman & Hall, London

Williamson J, Chopin JM 1980 Adverse reactions to prescribed drugs in the elderly: a multicentre investigation. Age and Ageing 9: 73–80

Further reading

Audit Commission 1995 United they stand. Co-ordinating care for elderly patients with hip fracture. National report. UK Audit Commission, London

Bennett GJ, Ebrahim S 1992 Health care of the elderly. Edward Arnold, London

British Geriatrics Society 1995 Guidelines, policy statements, and statements of good practice. British Geriatrics Society, London

Coni N, Davison W, Webster S 1984 Ageing: the facts. Oxford University Press, Oxford

Cullinan T 1986 Visual disability in the elderly. Croom Helm, London

Isaacs B, Livingstone M, Neville Y 1972 Survival of the unfittest. Routledge & Kegan Paul, London

NHS Health Advisory Service 1997 Eldercare towards 2000. The multidisciplinary assessment of elderly people and the delivery of high quality continuing care. A thematic review. Stationery Office, London

Pitt B 1982 Psychogeriatrics – an introduction to the psychiatry of old age, 2nd edn. Churchill Livingstone, Edinburgh

Timiras PS (ed) 1988 Physiological basis of ageing and geriatrics. Macmillan, London

Wolfson LI 1992 Gait and mobility. In: Evans JG, Williams TF (eds) Oxford textbook of geriatric medicine. Oxford University Press, Oxford, ch 18.15

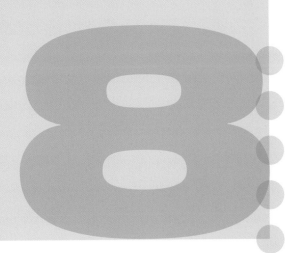

Part Eight

33 Hypothermia 361

34 Rescue from remote places 376

35 Near drowning 383

36 Heat illness 389

37 Acute diving emergencies 398

38 Electrocution injury 405

39 Risk of infection in prehospital care 410

Hypothermia

33

Introduction   361

Hypothermia   362

Methods of rewarming   367

Late effects   372

Practical management   372

Finally   373

References   374

Introduction

Cold can kill. Humans have known this since prehistory but appear to have forgotten with the development of modern civilization. Unfortunately, misunderstandings and dogmas bedevil hypothermia and its management (Lloyd 1986).

COLD RISK

In the timber industry, and on building sites and farms, workers are exposed to all weathers. Because of cold, fishing is a particularly hazardous occupation, the accident rate being five times greater than the most dangerous land-based transport industry. For divers the water temperature below 100 m depth is a constant 4°C dropping to −2°C in the Arctic.

Deep-freeze stores are installed in large depots, individual shops (e.g. butchers), refrigerated lorries and medical facilities (e.g. blood transfusion) and workers are exposed to temperatures of −20 to −40°C, sometimes with an additional fan producing wind-chill. People can also be exposed to potentially dangerous levels of cold at home in poor-quality housing, during travel and following an accident.

Exposure to cold also occurs during sport and recreation. Any person in the hills, whether as a climber, skier, or recreation walker, is at risk, especially if s/he is injured or there is a sudden change in the weather. On the Scottish hills, between 1967 and 1977, 15% of surviving casualties were hypothermic, 10% of the fatalities were attributed to hypothermia and the effects of cold exposure probably contributed to many of the deaths due to physical injury.

Water-sports participants experience cold (e.g. scuba divers, where hypothermia has been implicated in 20% of diving fatalities). Swimmers are immersed in cold water, and sailors suffer wind-chill and wetting from spray and unexpected immersion. Drowning is the commonest cause of death in water and may follow loss of consciousness due to hypothermia. Cavers may also be immersed in cold water. The effects of cold exposure are listed in Table 33.1.

Hypothermia is a risk of trauma and in trauma has a deleterious effect on survival, with 40% mortality if the core temperature is below 34°C compared with 7% if the core temperature is above 34°C. Hypothermia also contributes to the coagulopathy that accompanies massive transfusion (Nolan 1993).

REGULATION OF BODY TEMPERATURE

Body temperature is controlled through a central mechanism in the hypothalamus that is activated by changes in

Table 33.1 Effects of cold exposure

Muscular

- Muscle and tendon tears
- Shivering

Cardiovascular

- Angina on decreased exertion
- Rise in blood pressure – increased risk of:
  - Stroke
  - Myocardial infarction
  - Heart failure

Respiratory

- Asthma
- Rhinorrhoea on return to warm room

Peripheral nervous system

- Loss of manual dexterity
- Loss of sensitivity

Central nervous system

- Coordination impaired
- Visual acuity reduced
- Alertness reduced
- Reflexes slowed
- Increased mistakes
- Visual and auditory sensory input misinterpreted
- Hallucinations

Other

- Increased risk of 'bends'

the temperature of the blood and by peripheral receptors, mainly in the skin. Spinal thermostatic reflexes alone are insufficient to control body temperature. The thermostat regulates the body temperature by adjusting heat production and heat loss but the setting of the thermostat itself may be altered (Maclean & Emslie-Smith 1977).

The body, being warmer than the surrounding environment, loses heat through radiation, conduction, convection and evaporation. These mechanisms are discussed in detail in Chapter 36.

The rate of heat loss (cold stress) is not solely related to temperature. Air movement (wind or draughts) and moisture (humidity, rain or damp) cause a marked increase in the rate of heat loss, and a body is losing less heat at −10°C in still air than at +10°C with a 20 mph wind (Lloyd 1986). Both convective and evaporative heat losses are increased in windy conditions – the 'wind-chill' (Table 33.2).

The body responds to cold by constriction of the peripheral vessels, which, while very effective in reducing heat loss by reducing the temperature differential between the skin and the environment, increases the risk of local cold injury. The head has minimal vasoconstrictor activity, and the rate of heat loss through the head increases in a linear manner between +32°C and −20°C. At rest in −4°C the heat loss from the head may equal half the total heat production (Lloyd 1986).

Heat production falls in hypothermia and rises through increased muscle metabolism and tone, leading to shivering, or by deliberate activity. Activity and shivering need an increased blood supply to the muscles, which increases heat loss. Only 48% of the extra heat generated is retained in the body.

Increased heat production is always accompanied by a rise in oxygen consumption. To maintain normothermia for any level of exercise the oxygen consumption is higher in a cold environment than in a warm one (Horvath 1981), as seen clinically when angina develops during a particular level of activity in the cold but not at normal temperatures. If hypoxia is present, as at high altitude, there will be a decrease in the total possible heat production, and shivering may be inhibited (Alexander 1979). With very vigorous exercise in very severe cold the oxygen demand may exceed the maximal oxygen uptake, and unexpected and unsuspected hypothermia may develop. Finally. in exhaustion or malnutrition, heat production cannot be increased because of the lack of substrate (fuel) for metabolism (Lloyd 1986).

There are racial variations in the response to cold, and at the extremes of age there is an increased risk of hypothermia. Many medical disorders predispose to hypothermia (Maclean & Emslie-Smith 1977) and a range of drugs, including anaesthetics, increase the risk through impairing vasoconstriction or depressing metabolism. Mental stress, even of as mild a degree as mental arithmetic, increases heat loss, as do nausea, vomiting, fainting, trauma and haemorrhage (Lloyd 1986).

During sleep the cerebral thermostat is reset to a new low level, vasoconstriction is reduced with an immediate rise in skin temperature and the metabolic rate is reduced (Lloyd 1986). Although alcohol produces a number of effects that increase the risk of hypothermia, the greatest danger occurs because it decreases the awareness of cold and increases bravado while impairing the ability to assess risks (Lloyd 1986). Improving fitness results in an increase in the maximum oxygen uptake, and fit people work and sleep better and are more comfortable in the cold (Horvath 1981).

Hypothermia

DEFINITION AND CLASSIFICATION

When a person is exposed to cold, the temperature of the superficial (shell) tissues falls before there is any drop in core

Table 33.2 Wind-chill chart showing the effect of wind on increasing the degree of cooling

Wind speed (mph)	Equivalent chill temperature (°C)									
0	4	−1	−7	−12	−18	−23	−29	−34	−40	−46
5	2	−4	−9	−15	−21	−26	−32	−37	−43	−48
10	−1	−9	−15	−23	−29	−37	−44	−51	−57	−62
15	−4	−12	−21	−29	−34	−43	−51	−57	−65	−73
20	−7	−15	−23	−32	−37	−46	−54	−62	−71	−79
25	−9	−18	−26	−34	−43	−51	−59	−68	−76	−84
30	−12	−18	−29	−34	−46	−54	−62	−71	−79	−87
35	−12	−21	−29	−37	−46	−54	−62	−73	−82	−90
40	−12	−21	−29	−37	−48	−57	−65	−73	−82	−90
	Little danger			Increasing danger Flesh may freeze within 1 min			Great danger Flesh may freeze within 30 s			

temperature: there is a fall in total body heat. *Hypothermia* is present if the core temperature is below 35°C (selected to allow for the maximal diurnal variation) (Royal College of Physicians 1966). This very artificial definition may lead to the attitude that 35.5°C is safe while at 34.5°C the patient is in danger. This is obviously ridiculous and takes no account of total body heat. In fact, there are many non-hypothermic cold-related illnesses that result in more deaths than occur as a result of hypothermia (Lloyd 1986, 1991b).

Unfortunately hypothermia is often considered as a single entity, and the single measurement of core temperature is used to produce a classification of hypothermia into mild, moderate and severe (Moss 1986, Danzl & Pozos 1987, American Heart Association 1992, Weinberg 1993). Frequently the recommended treatment depends on the severity level of the hypothermia. This is akin to classifying and deciding the treatment of anaemia purely on the measurement of the haemoglobin level, and is made even less logical by the fact that there is disagreement over the temperature ranges of the different grades; e.g. mild 36–34°C and severe <30°C (Danzl & Pozos 1987, American Heart Association 1992, Weinberg 1993), or mild 35–32°C and severe <28°C (Moss 1986).

Among the many physiological effects of exposure to cold there are three which are of particular relevance to the safe management of cases of hypothermia (Lloyd, 1986, 1992).

Energy reserves

The body responds to cold by increasing heat output, which depletes the energy reserves, the final level depending on the length of time the increased output of heat lasts.

Fluid balance

Cold-induced vasoconstriction shunts blood from the peripheral vasculature into the deep capacitance veins. The body counteracts this relative central overload by means of a diuresis, and the body suffers a net loss of fluid (Popovic & Popovic 1974, Moss 1986). Water immersion, even thermoneutral, also causes a marked increase in diuresis (Hayward 1983).

Cold air is dry, evaporation is rapid and even $1–2\,l\,d^{-1}$ sweat loss may be unnoticed. Respiratory moisture loss is increased by exercise, especially in cold dry air (e.g. in the polar regions and at high altitude).

During exposure to cold there is also a shift of fluid from the intravascular space into the extracellular and then intracellular space (Hamlet 1983) where it is no longer immediately available to the circulation. This shift reverses during rewarming, and the circulating volume can rise to 130% above the normothermic volume (Popovic & Popovic 1974) depending on the potential volume of fluid available, which in turn is related to the duration of cold exposure and the rate of rewarming. Even with total body dehydration, exercise also reverses the fluid shifts (Tappan et al 1984) and this may contribute to further diuresis.

An individual will lose a varying proportion of total fluid loss through each of the above mechanisms.

Vascular responses

During cooling vasoconstriction reduces the volume of the vascular bed in active use. On removal from the cold the continuous stimulus of cold on the skin stops. The vasoconstriction therefore relaxes, thus increasing the active vascular bed. This is further increased by active surface warmth.

Immersion in water produces a hydrostatic squeeze with effects similar to vasoconstriction. Removal from water removes this hydrostatic squeeze (Golden et al 1991).

TYPES OF HYPOTHERMIA

Using these parameters, it is possible to describe different types of hypothermia (Lloyd 1986).

Acute ('immersion') hypothermia

The cold stress is so great that the heat production is overwhelmed and the body cools before the energy reserves are exhausted. There has also been very little time for any diuresis or shifts of body fluid to have occurred. The victim will therefore rewarm spontaneously and inevitably once removed from the cold stress.

The commonest cause of this type is falling into cold water. Someone on dry land who becomes hypothermic while drunk also falls into this category.

Subacute ('exhaustion') hypothermia

The cold is less severe, and cooling only occurs when the energy reserves are exhausted. Therefore rewarming spontaneously is less certain and cooling may continue even with very little continuing heat loss. In this type, therefore, every potential route for heat loss must be stopped and even minimal additional heat may be vital.

There will also have been a net loss of circulating fluid volume from diuresis and intercompartmental shifts. Removal from the cold will result in an increase in the active vascular bed with no increase in the circulating fluid volume. This will produce a relative hypovolaemia and a drop in blood pressure, sometimes severe, a phenomenon often seen soon after a patient is admitted to hospital (Burton & Edholm 1955, Lloyd 1973).

This is most commonly found in mountaineers, hill walkers or in other endurance activities, and may occur during the activity or after stopping.

Subchronic ('urban') hypothermia

The cold, while relatively mild, has been prolonged. The core temperature remains normal (35°C or above) possibly for weeks, before drifting or being precipitated into hypothermia, e.g. by a fall. Vasoconstriction may not have occurred because the cold was relatively mild or because the physiological mechanisms are impaired. There may, therefore, have been no cold-induced diuresis. However, time has allowed vast intercompartmental fluid shifts, and any

intravascular loss has been replaced through fluid intake. If the rate of return of the sequestered fluid during rewarming exceeds the ability of the kidneys to remove it, fluid overload will occur, leading to cerebral and/or pulmonary oedema and death. The energy reserves will be very variable.

Active rewarming of this group results in 100% mortality unless treated in an intensive care unit (Lloyd 1986), where intermittent positive pressure ventilation (IPPV) can be used if required to counteract the oedema. Even spontaneous rewarming must be kept below 0.5°C h^{-1} to avoid the risk of triggering cerebral or pulmonary oedema (Bloch 1965, Lloyd 1990).

This type is most common in the elderly living in poor housing or in those with malnutrition.

Superacute ('submersion') hypothermia (Lloyd 1986, Moss 1986)

There are now a considerable number of reports of cases where patients have been known to have been without oxygen for up to 60 min and yet have been successfully resuscitated without brain damage. A common factor has been that all were totally submerged in ice-cold water. The younger the victim the better the chance of survival. Children have a larger surface area to body mass ratio and will therefore cool faster than adults. In addition, the head is an important route for heat loss, with very poor vasoconstrictor activity, and the younger the child the larger the head in proportion to the rest of the body. Very rapid cooling could therefore be expected if the body is totally submerged, and this has been demonstrated in cases where time of submersion and rescue, as well as rescue temperatures, are known, with rates of temperature drop of up to 36°C h^{-1} being recorded (Lloyd 1986). This phenomenon used to be called the *diving reflex*.

- **Acute ('immersion') hypothermia**
- **Subacute ('exhaustion') hypothermia**
- **Subchronic ('urban') hypothermia**
- **Superacute ('submersion') hypothermia**

The different types are best illustrated by case histories.

- A climber in a snowstorm disabled by a broken leg will probably cool as rapidly as if immersed, through the shock of the injury increasing the rate of heat loss, and the secondary factor of the fracture preventing the person generating heat to his full capacity and therefore preventing exhaustion.

- Deep diving (below 150 m) with the use of oxyhelium gas breathing mixtures may cause 'immersion' hypothermia, even in a 'dry' chamber, because of the tremendous respiratory heat loss from the heat transfer capacity of the compressed gas.

- A swimmer lost overboard in relatively warm water is a candidate for 'exhaustion' hypothermia.
- A child with severe malnutrition is likely to develop 'urban' hypothermia, whereas a fit 70-year-old out walking in the hills probably has 'exhaustion' hypothermia.

It is important to make the correct diagnosis because inappropriate treatment may result in death during rewarming. Collapse is almost unknown during rewarming from 'immersion' hypothermia whereas it is common with 'exhaustion' hypothermia. Survival in 'submersion' hypothermia depends on the institution of resuscitation immediately on rescue.

DIAGNOSIS

One of the earliest signs of hypothermia is a change in personality or behaviour, but unfortunately not only can similar changes be due to other factors, such as hypoglycaemia, exhaustion or heat stroke, but the person involved is likely to be the last person to notice the change. A variety of signs and symptoms have been described (Table 33.3) in an attempt to give a clinical guide to the level of hypothermia, but these can only be a very general guide as they were described mainly as a result of immersion, and individuals show a great range of responses; e.g. loss of consciousness may occur at temperatures as high as 33°C, but in one case consciousness was still present at a rectal temperature of 24.3°C and there are many other causes of loss of consciousness even at normothermia. Similarly, shivering is considered to cease at 30°C but has been recorded at a core temperature of 24°C. At the other extreme, some experimental subjects can cool without shivering and many mountain rescue cases never shiver (Lloyd 1986). Even the presence of a J wave (Fig. 33.1) on the electrocardiogram (ECG) is not diagnostic, being present in only 80% of hypothermia patients and also being present in sepsis and with central nervous system (CNS) lesions (Weinberg 1993).

The ideal diagnosis is by recording the core temperature using a low-reading thermometer. The *rectum* is the usual site but rectal temperature may not reflect cardiac temperature if the body is rewarming. Also, measurement may be difficult because of clothing or an uncooperative casualty (Handley et al 1992). The inner ear or *tympanic membrane* is accurate but requires special equipment. The *oesophagus* is accurate and sensitive but there is the remote risk of triggering ventricular fibrillation (VF), and inserting the probe may be difficult if the jaw is clenched with the cold. The *mouth* temperature has the same problem with teeth, is inaccurate but will not be higher than the core (Lloyd 1986). In the situations where casualties occur, low-reading

Table 33.3 Signs and symptoms at different levels of hypothermia

Core temperature (°C)	Signs and symptoms
37.6	'Normal' rectal temperature
37	'Normal' oral temperature
36	Increased metabolic rate to attempt to balance heat loss. Respiratory and pulse rate increase
35	Shivering maximum at this temperature. Hyperreflexia, dysarthria, delayed cerebration
34	Patients usually responsive and with normal blood pressure; lower limit compatible with continued exercise
33–31	Retrograde amnesia, consciousness clouded, blood pressure difficult to obtain, pupils dilated, most shivering ceases
30–28	Progressive loss of consciousness, increased muscular rigidity, slow pulse and respiration, cardiac arrhythmia develops, ventricular fibrillation may develop if heart irritated
27	Voluntary motion lost along with pupillary light reflex, deep tendon and skin reflexes. Appear dead
26	Victims seldom conscious
25	Ventricular fibrillation may appear spontaneously
24–21	Pulmonary oedema develops: 100% mortality in shipwreck victims in Second World War
20	Heart standstill
18	Lowest adult *accidental* hypothermic patient with recovery
17	*Iso-electric EEG*
15.2	Lowest infant *accidental* hypothermic patient with recovery
9	Lowest artificially cooled hypothermic patient with recovery
4	Monkeys revived successfully
1–7	Rats and hamsters revived successfully

thermometers are unlikely to be available. For practical purposes, therefore, a casualty should be treated as a 'cold casualty' if the body *feels* 'as cold as marble' and, in particular, if the armpit is profoundly cold (Handley et al 1992). Probably the most important factor in making the diagnosis is that the medical attendant must *suspect* that hypothermia may be present (Table 33.3).

In hypothermia other diagnoses are difficult because the clinical features are masked by the effects of cold (Lloyd 1986). In hypothermia the reflexes are affected and there is a general increase in rigidity that makes accurate neurological diagnosis impossible. Slurred speech, ataxia and the development of incoordination or a change in personality may be due to hypothermia and not neurological damage. The changes in the electrical and mechanical functions of the heart cause problems for cardiologists. Gastrointestinal motility slows and may cease during cooling, and as a result gastric dilatation and decreased or absent bowel sounds are common in hypothermia. Lungs may show clinical and X-ray features similar to pneumonia (Fig. 33.2), although these clear on rewarming. It is therefore important that the patient should be normothermic before any diagnosis is made or any irrevocable treatment started.

DEATH IN HYPOTHERMIA

The clinical picture in profound accidental hypothermia is very difficult to distinguish from death, with a pulse that is very slow and undetectable because of vasoconstriction and such profound respiratory depression that the patient appears apnoeic. Temperature is no guide to potential

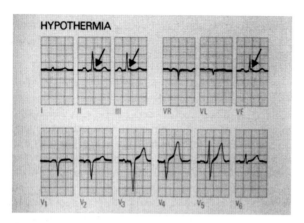

Fig. 33.1 • 'J' waves. (Courtesy of Dr WJ Mills Jr, of Anchorage, AL, USA.)

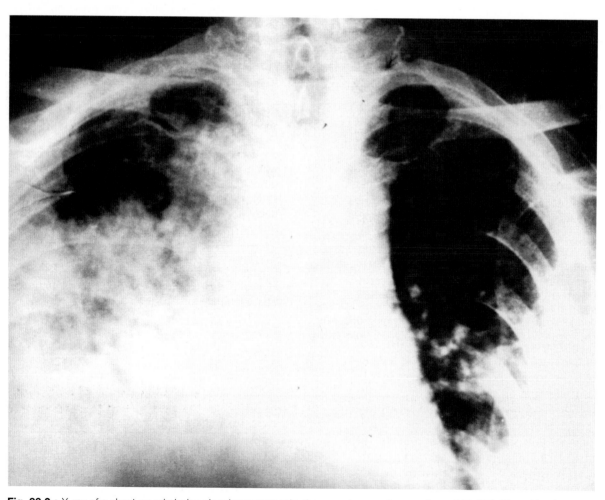

Fig. 33.2 • X-ray of a chest on admission showing pneumonic changes at a core temperature of 32.5°C. (From Lloyd 1986. With permission of Evan Lloyd.)

survival, with recovery recorded from a temperature of 9°C from induced hypothermia (Niazi & Lewis 1958) and in accidental hypothermia from 16°C (Wood 1977), 14.4°C (Lexow, personal communication) and 15.2°C (a 23-day-old infant revived with no sequelae; Nozaki et al 1986). Neither the total absence of cardiorespiratory activity nor a flat EEG is a certain indicator of death in hypothermia.

The only certain diagnosis of death in hypothermia is failure to recover on rewarming.

This statement has to be tempered with common sense for the rescuers, as the victim can be accepted as dead if the core temperature is equal to or lower than the air temperature, or if the mouth and nose are filled with snow or ice. There may also be the situation in the field where rewarming is impossible or when rewarming attempts may jeopardize the survival of the rescuers.

Sudden entry into very cold water produces marked responses that may cause death or unconsciousness or incapacity, and therefore drowning (Fig. 33.3).

CAUSE OF DEATH AFTER RESCUE

Despite the belief that once a person has been removed from the cold stress situation they are safe, deaths still occur after rescue (Lloyd 1986, 1992). Death following rescue may be due to the following:

- An imbalance between the active vascular capacity and the effective circulating fluid volume. As discussed earlier, the different types of hypothermia have different physiological changes and inappropriate rewarming may result in death if either the vascular bed becomes too large for the actual circulating blood volume (relative hypovolaemic shock) or the reversal of the fluid shifts is too great, overloading the circulation and resulting in cerebral and/or pulmonary oedema. This matches clinical and experimental observations and is the commonest cause occurring during rewarming.
- Ventricular fibrillation (VF). The risk rises as the core temperature falls but, if left undisturbed, the cooling heart usually stops in asystole. VF is frequently probably the result of treatment. VF may be triggered by mechanical irritation, sometimes as mild as the heart having its position changed by rolling a patient for bed-making. Other triggers are hypoxia of the heart muscle and rapid changes in temperature gradients within the heart muscle, or in pH or electrolytes in the blood (Lloyd & Mitchell 1974, Lloyd 1996). (Rewarming is the primary treatment for biochemical abnormalities in hypothermia (Weinberg 1993).) Occasional case reports have implicated endotracheal intubation in hypothermia as being the event that has triggered VF. However, in several large series (Ledingham & Mone 1980, Miller et al

1980, Hall & Seyverud 1990, Lloyd 1990) endotracheal intubation was performed on many patients (lowest core temperature 24.3°C (Lloyd 1973)) and no cases of VF were recorded. All patients were preoxygenated before intubation.

- Continued cooling.
- Hypoxia, in association with serious illness or injury, may contribute to some deaths.

Methods of rewarming

The main aim of management is to produce a warm, live patient. There is a widespread feeling that the patient should be rewarmed as fast as possible because hypothermia may cause death. However, there is no evidence that faster rewarming is better than slow (Moss 1986) and Golden (1979) examined all the reasons given for using active rewarming and concluded that none were valid. Rewarming methods currently available are given below.

SPONTANEOUS REWARMING

Preventing further heat loss to the environment and allowing the body to rewarm without supplying any additional heat.

ACTIVE REWARMING

Supplying additional heat, which may be through two main routes:

- Surface heating – this includes immersion in a hot bath, hot water circulating through plumbed garments, heating pads and hot-water bottles, hot blankets, hot air blowers, heat cradles and in front of a fire
- Central rewarming – the methods that have been used to date are:

  — Extracorporeal blood warming, e.g. cardiopulmonary bypass and haemodialysis

  — Irrigation of body cavities, e.g. mediastinal irrigation, pleural irrigation and peritoneal dialysis

  — Other methods, e.g. intragastric, intra-oesophageal and intracolonic balloons, intravenous infusion and diathermy
- Airway warming.

COMBINATION TREATMENT: TREATMENT USING A NUMBER OF DIFFERENT METHODS

The effectiveness of these methods should be assessed on the following criteria (Lloyd 1986).

- Heat gain, not only in terms of absolute quantities of heat added and heat loss prevented, but also where the heat gain occurs.

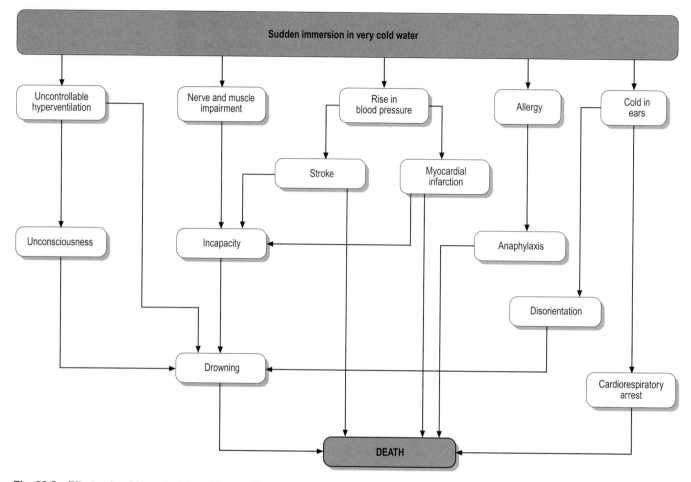

Fig. 33.3 • Effects of sudden entry into cold water. (Redrawn with permission from McLatchie et al 1995.)

- Other effects on the body. These may be beneficial or adverse, and should include consideration of cardiovascular, cerebral, respiratory and renal function.
- Where the method can be used (practical potential). Each method has to be evaluated as to its safety and utility through the whole medical sequence from discovery of the victim through first-aid treatment, transport, treatment at base or hospital to final recovery.
- Mortality rates rather than warming rates should ultimately dictate the choice of therapy. It is important to remember that people die slowly in the cold but inappropriate aggressive treatment can kill in a hurry.

Patients who are young and/or suffering from immersion or exhaustion hypothermia have a very low mortality, whereas urban hypothermic patients tend to have a high mortality. However, where the treatment has been carried out in an intensive care unit (i.e. a unit with intensive monitoring of physiological and biochemical changes and the facilities to make rapid corrections of any abnormality that may occur) there is a very low mortality in all types of hypothermia, with any deaths being due to medical conditions that were either pre-existing or developed after rewarming. It is probably true that if a patient with hypothermia is in an intensive care unit any method of rewarming can be done safely.

Rubbing the skin of the victim is absolutely contraindicated because it provides a sense of warmth to the skin without providing heat. This suppresses shivering and increases the risk of hypotensive collapse. It may also damage the cold skin.

Physical exercise produces increased heat and has been recommended as a last resort in mountain hypothermia (Kaufman 1983), but exercise is only safe if the core temperature is greater than 35°C (Moss 1986). In a hostile environment continued forced exercise is frequently lethal, whereas 'going to ground', i.e. taking shelter, has saved many lives (Lloyd 1986).

SPONTANEOUS REWARMING

This is used automatically by the rescue services as soon as the victim is found. Insulating the body surface usually reduces the heat loss sufficiently to allow the patient to rewarm spontaneously from endogenous heat production. Any available material can be used but the 'space blanket' made of metallized plastic sheeting, which is often recommended as part of the insulating package, was shown on theoretical grounds and in experiments to be no better than a similar thickness of polythene, which is much cheaper (Lloyd 1986). The insulation must include the head as up to 70% of total heat production can be lost by this route (Lloyd 1986). Adequate insulation between the casualty and the ground must be ensured. The hands and feet should be kept cool, i.e. the hands should be down the side of the patient and not on the abdomen. Warm hands and feet reduce the stimulus for heat production and allow reduction of vasoconstrictor tone, thus increasing heat loss and increasing the risk of vasomotor collapse.

In the field, part of the insulation is to provide shelter from the wind (e.g. a hut, lifeboat cabin, survival bag, in a snow hole or behind a large boulder). However, if the environmental cold is very severe, if the insulation is poor or incomplete, or if the metabolism is depressed through drugs or low body temperature, the heat production may be insufficient to compensate for the continued heat loss and the patient may then fail to rewarm, or may continue to cool.

Even in hospital the rate of rewarming is very variable, depending on the metabolic rate. In urban hypothermia, if the rate exceeds 0.5°C per hour, covers should be removed to slow rewarming to reduce the risk of pulmonary/cerebral oedema.

If the person is shivering, rewarming will be fairly rapid. However, shivering may be dangerous, especially in the presence of hypovolaemia (e.g. following trauma) because it requires an increase in peripheral blood flow with the risk of hypotension. In addition, shivering requires an increase in oxygen consumption (up to 400%), which is dangerous during the rewarming period for critically ill patients (Rodriguez et al 1983), those with trauma or hypovolaemia (Nolan 1993) or those with pre-existing myocardial or pulmonary disease (Lloyd 1986). The shift to the left in the oxyhaemoglobin dissociation curve in hypothermia will impair oxygen delivery, possibly leading to lactic acidosis and increasing cardiac irritability. Shivering will therefore compound the lactic acidosis and decreased hepatic metabolic clearance of lactic acid that typically accompany hypovolaemia (Nolan 1993). Warmth on the skin depresses shivering and reduces oxygen consumption, but at the expense of reduced heat production. Shivering is also inhibited by airway warming but, despite the decreased oxygen consumption, rewarming is not slowed (Conn 1979).

SURFACE HEATING

This is often used because the rescuers feel that they must do something active. However, the warmed superficial tissues have an increased oxygen demand (10°C rise in tissue temperature gives a 100% increase in O_2 demand (Maclean & Emslie-Smith 1977)). As described above, in cold blood less oxygen is available for the tissues. In addition, superficial perfusion is impaired in hypothermia. The combination of warm tissues and impaired perfusion with cold blood may produce hypoxia of the superficial tissues and be the cause of the acidosis seen during surface warming (Paton 1983). Surface warming also reduces vasoconstriction and has been associated with rewarming collapse (Lloyd 1986). However, radiant heat applied to the blush area of the head and neck will inhibit shivering without markedly impairing vasoconstriction (Sharkey et al 1993). If there is no circulation (or very little) through the skin, as may be the case with cardiac depression or arrest, surface warming is ineffective and may cause burning even at 'baby bath' temperatures (Lloyd 1986).

The hot bath is the fastest method of rewarming a person and it became standard therapy following early experiments (Alexander 1945), although survival rates were not quoted and, in some, the hot bath used was boiling water (Berger 1990). The hot bath technique has many disadvantages and limitations. The main benefit only occurs within the first 20 min of removal from the cold, cardiopulmonary resuscitation (CPR) cannot be used (Lloyd 1986) and it should only be used for casualties who are conscious, shivering and uninjured and can get into the bath with minimal assistance (Handley et al 1992). The temperature of the bath should approximate but not exceed 40°C, i.e. elbow comfort temperature. This temperature should be maintained by constantly stirring and adding hot water as necessary. This technique requires large quantities of hot water, too much for the ordinary domestic hot-water supply, even supposing the hot-water system is active when the rescue team reaches the nearest house. Heavy outer clothing should be gently removed before the casualty is immersed to the neck. Assistance should be given with removing the rest of the clothing once the casualty is comfortably settled in the bath. Almost immediately on immersion, shivering will stop but this is not an indication for removing the casualty. When the casualty feels comfortably warm, he should be helped out of the bath, dried, covered with blankets and kept lying flat. He should not be allowed to stay in the bath if he complains of feeling hot or starts sweating.

Radiant heat in the form of an open fire is very dangerous and often lethal. During the retreat from Moscow in 1812, Napoleon's doctor Baron Larrey noticed that hypothermic soldiers died if they were close to the camp fires.

Heating pads and hot-water bottles placed at the neck, axilla and groin can be used. Plumbed garments, which circulate warm fluids, are effective but are rare, expensive and restrict access to the patient.

One method reputedly used by mountain rescue teams is body to body contact inside a sleeping bag. Unless three people can provide simultaneous body heat the method is potentially dangerous (Collis et al 1977) and in practice the standard sleeping bag will only just admit one body – the victim.

CENTRAL REWARMING

The heat is supplied to the 'core' first, and rewarming proceeds from core to periphery. The core organs, 8% of the total body weight, contribute 56% of the heat production in basal metabolism at normothermia and a higher percentage in hypothermia because the muscles and superficial tissues have cooled more than the core and are therefore producing a lower percentage of the total body heat production. As the temperature of a tissue rises, the heat generated also rises rapidly. Therefore, by concentrating the heat gain in the core, the thermal benefits will be significantly greater than calculations alone would suggest (Lloyd 1986).

Airway warming (Lloyd 1986, 1990)

Airway warming is similar to spontaneous rewarming in that the main thermal input comes from the body's own metabolic heat production. Even with perfect surface insulation, the patient is still losing heat and moisture through breathing. Airway warming stops this heat loss, with a possible small heat input to the vital core. In the only clinical study which has compared airway warming with spontaneous rewarming during the same episode of hypothermia, airway warming produced a significant increase in the rate of rewarming (Lloyd 1990) and this finding was repeated in animal experiments (Lloyd et al 1976a). It is therefore only of value as an addition when insulation of the rest of the body is already being used. It is now widely recommended in the management of accidental hypothermia (American Heart Association 1992, American College of Surgeons Committee on Trauma 1997, Handley & Swain 1994).

Airway warming produces a marked improvement in cardiovascular function (Lloyd et al 1976b, Lloyd, 1990) (a feature shared with peritoneal dialysis), cerebral function, conscious level and cardiorespiratory control. With both airway warming and peritoneal dialysis there have been case reports of VF reverting spontaneously to sinus rhythm at a core temperature about 28°C. Even using air as the inspired gas, airway warming produced an improvement in blood gases (Roberts et al 1983).

In young patients suffering from immersion or exhaustion hypothermia, airway warming has a lower mortality than spontaneous rewarming or hot bath rewarming (Miller et al 1980). However, in urban hypothermia, airway warming should not be used without intensive care facilities because the accelerated rate of rewarming may precipitate cerebral and/or pulmonary oedema.

There are a variety of equipment designs (Lloyd 1991a) that can produce warm, moist air or oxygen, which should not be above 45°C to avoid thermal burns to the face and pharynx. Many designs are sufficiently portable to be used in the prehospital situation (Fig. 33.4). These include electrically operated hospital humidifiers (not nebulizers), gas-powered heaters, a system that utilizes the chemical reaction between soda lime and carbon dioxide (the portable version weighs 3 kg – Fig. 33.5) and a condenser humidifier attached to a facemask (Fig. 33.6). Although the condenser humidifier is the least efficient, it is simple, light and cheap and could be carried as part of a first-aid kit.

Airway warming has the advantage that it can be started in the field and continued to, and in, hospital. It is non-invasive and can be combined with other rewarming methods.

Intravenous fluids

All fluids, including blood, should be warmed during resuscitation in hypothermia. A level 1 fluid warmer warms all fluids from 10°C to 35°C at flow rates of 350–500 ml min^{-1} (Nolan 1993). In the field, heat packs or body warming can reduce the risk of cold fluid. Battery driven fluid warmers

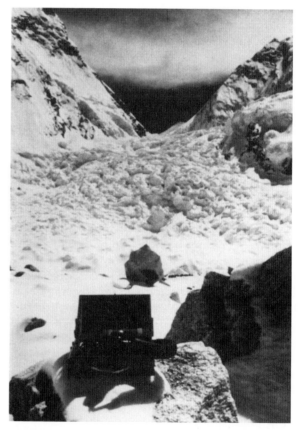

Fig. 33.4 • 'Lloyd' airway warming equipment on Mt Everest: the Khumbu ice-fall is in the background. (From Lloyd 1986. Reproduced with permission of Evan Lloyd.)

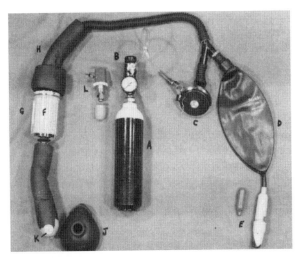

Fig. 33.5 • Lightweight 'Lloyd' portable airway warming equipment. (A) Oxygen cylinder. (B) First-stage reducing valve and gauge. (C) Demand reducing valve with manual override to allow a 2 litre reservoir bag (D) to be filled if ventilation needs to be assisted. The demand valve may be replaced by a button valve. (E) Corkette® (Sparklet Corkmaster®) with the distal portion of the needle removed and inserted into the tail of the reservoir bag. Spare Sparklet cylinder alongside. (F) Soda lime. (G) Paediatric waters canister. (H) Insulation, neoprene foam tubing. (J) Facemask. (K) Thermometer registering mean air temperature at mask inflow. (L) Adapter for refilling the small oxygen cylinder from a large cylinder. *Instructions for use*: empty one Sparklet cylinder into the system by using the Corkette® (E). Open the valve (B) on the oxygen cylinder (A). Apply the facemask (J) to the patient. If appropriate, the facemask may be replaced by an endotracheal tube. The reservoir bag (D) should be inflated by depressing the centre of the demand valve (C) or the alternative button valve. Thereafter the system will work on demand or by intermittent refilling of the reservoir bag. The thermometer (K) should be observed. This will rise steadily into the working range and when the temperature again drops to 35°C, place a new Sparklet cylinder in the Corkette® (E) and depress the lever to allow CO_2 to flow for 3 s. This should be repeated whenever the airflow temperature falls to 35°C. Where possible the waters canister (G) should be vertical rather than horizontal to reduce the risk of gases channelling along the side of the canister. The gauge on the oxygen cylinder should be checked regularly and the cylinder should be refilled from a large cylinder after use. The soda lime (F) should be replaced in the waters canister after use, ensuring, by tapping and shaking, that the canister is completely full to reduce the risk of gases channelling along the side if the canister is horizontal. The equipment, which weighs 3 kg (7 lb), can be carried in any convenient container. The device should provide warmed moist oxygen for 2 h before the soda lime needs to be replaced. (With permission from Lloyd & Croxton 1981.)

such as enFlow® (Zoll) are also available. The addition of saline warmed to 70°C to an equal volume of cold-packed (4°C) red cells results in a diluted unit of blood at 37°C with no adverse effect on red-cell survival (Nolan 1993).

Unfortunately, the risk of fluid overload and cardiac arrhythmias reduces the value of this method in pure hypothermia.

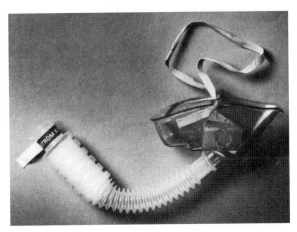

Fig. 33.6 • Condenser humidifier with facemask attached. This can be used in the emergency treatment of accidental hypothermia. The end of the humidifier should be under the clothing next to the skin and the whole device, including mask, covered with a scarf. (From Lloyd 1991a. © 1991 Wilderness Medical Society. From *Journal of Wilderness Medicine*. Reprinted by permission of Alliance Communications Group, a division of Allen Press, Inc.)

Extracorporeal warming

Cardiopulmonary bypass may be considered to be the ideal method of rewarming as the vital organs in the core are rewarmed first with well oxygenated fluid and the circulation is artificially supported. It is only available once definitive medical care has been reached. Although it has been suggested that cardiopulmonary bypass is the only effective treatment for a hypothermic patient in VF or asystole (Althaus et al 1982), it is not always successful (Jui et al 1988). In addition, a patient with induced hypothermia was successfully rewarmed from 9°C in asystole (Niazi & Lewis 1958), another patient with accidental hypothermia in VF at 25°C was successfully rewarmed, using airway warming and cardiac lavage, and cardioverted (Osborne et al 1984), and a patient in asystole at 23.2°C was rewarmed using peritoneal lavage, warm intravenous fluid, a hot-water bottle and blankets, with spontaneous return of sinus rhythm at 28°C (Lexow 1991). Because of its heating pattern, bypass rewarms no faster than peritoneal dialysis (Moss 1986), and there have been incidents of recooling and problems with cardiovascular stability, respiratory problems and renal failure (Lloyd 1986). Cardiopulmonary bypass requires an experienced team, is only available in a few large hospitals and may be in use for its primary purpose (i.e. open heart surgery). In practice, it is usually adopted after other methods have been started.

All the methods of rewarming mentioned above have been used successfully but all have disadvantages and problems (Lloyd 1986). Some require expertise or equipment only available in a few large hospitals, and some that have been advocated for use by the emergency services (e.g. diathermy or peritoneal dialysis) should only be used with medical supervision because of inherent dangers or risks (Lloyd 1986). There are many reports of successful rewarming using many different methods, singly or in combination. However, most are of individual cases managed in an intensive care unit, and in this environment all methods of rewarming are effective and safe (Lloyd 1986, Moss 1986). The best method therefore depends on the environment and what is available.

OTHER TREATMENT

The cold myocardium is unresponsive to pacing and cardioactive drugs, and relatively insensitive to DC shock defibrillation (American Heart Association 1992, Handley & Swain 1994).

Contrary to earlier belief, oxygen is not dangerous and should be given to hypothermic patients (Lloyd 1986, Moss 1986, American Heart Association 1992, Weinberg 1993). However, if the oxygen is too cold, e.g. because the cylinder has been lying in the snow, changing from warm expired air resuscitation may cause cardiac arrest, either through cold inhalation or through the vagal stimulation of cold on the face.

There is no evidence that barbiturates or antibiotics given prophylactically have any benefit (American Heart Association 1992, Handley and Swain 1994). Corticosteroid levels are often above normal in hypothermic patients but these may have fallen from higher, stress-induced levels (Lloyd 1986). While steroids cannot be considered as a routine measure, large intravenous doses given as a last resort in the field have had almost miraculous effects (MacInnes 1971).

Glucose levels fall during rewarming and patients, particularly those with exhaustion hypothermia, may require glucose as a metabolic substrate. Hypothermia can be precipitated by hypoglycaemia and the symptoms of the two conditions are very similar. Glucagon is ineffective in glycogen depletion when glucose is required.

Intensive care is one of the most important measures in the hospital management of hypothermia. All patients should be transferred to intensive care after initial stabilization in the emergency department. With urban hypothermia, if unnecessary deaths are to be avoided, rewarming should only be undertaken with intensive care monitoring.

Late effects

Most patients have no after-effects following rewarming but some patients may develop diffuse intravascular coagulation, which can produce thrombosis and lead to stroke. This is more common following rapid rewarming from severe hypothermia, as also are haemolysis and acute tubular necrosis. Postrewarming pancreatitis also occurs and may be another effect of the coagulopathy, or may have a different mechanism.

Practical management

At all times it is important to ensure the safety of the rescuer as well as the casualty. This is particularly important if the casualty is in a hostile environment such as in the water or on a hillside. As well as being aware of the dangers of falling rocks, unstable snow or unsafe ice, rescuers must ensure that they do not also become hypothermic either through exhaustion or as a result of donating their own clothing to the casualty.

If possible a casualty should be rescued horizontally, especially from water, but it is sometimes more important to get the casualty to safety quickly than to cause delay in order to achieve horizontal rescue (Handley et al 1992). When safe, the casualty should be laid flat, given essential first aid for any injury and resuscitated if necessary. The casualty should be insulated and airway warming, if available, should be performed. Oxygen can be valuable but should not be given if the cylinder is very cold. Intravenous fluids should be prewarmed. The casualty should be carefully moved to shelter.

In a conscious cold casualty, a hot drink provides comfort but alcohol must not be given.

At all times, including during transport, the casualty should be kept lying flat or slightly head down to avoid orthostatic hypotension (Lloyd 1986, American Heart Association 1992, Handley et al 1992, Weinberg 1993). Any unnecessary movement of the unconscious or semiconscious casualty should be avoided because movement may precipitate VF. These points may sometimes have to be ignored during the practical difficulties of a rescue.

To avoid catastrophic heat loss, wet clothing should only be removed when the victim is in a warm shelter out of the wind. If shelter is not available, extra layers of clothing should be added, especially a layer that is impervious to wind and water (Handley et al 1992). If the person is unconscious the wet clothes must be cut off to avoid movement. Even in a warm environment the casualty should be kept insulated to prevent the surface warmth causing a further increase in vascular dilatation and a catastrophic drop in blood pressure.

Maintain close observation. Get help as soon as possible and transport the casualty to hospital.

PRACTICAL REWARMING RECOMMENDATIONS

In the prehospital (field) situation choice of treatment is governed by many factors (e.g. distance, local risk, including weather, number and experience of rescuers and their physical condition, and the availability of equipment) (Mills 1992). The only methods of rewarming that can be considered practical are spontaneous rewarming, airway warming and surface heating, although the last is not first choice (Lloyd 1986, Handley et al 1992).

In an emergency department spontaneous rewarming and airway warming can be used and peritoneal dialysis should also be available. These should be sufficient. Other measures require specialist expertise, which is not always available (Lloyd 1986).

RESUSCITATION IN HYPOTHERMIA

This follows the normal ABC of resuscitation. In hypothermia the heart may still be working, even if clinically undetectable, but the mechanical irritation of chest compression may trigger VF with total loss of cardiac function and the person is then worse off. However, even in hypothermia, cardiac arrest may be due to some other cause. If the heart has stopped through drowning or heart attack, resuscitation with mouth-to-mouth respiration and chest compression must be started at once if there is to be any hope of the person surviving. This dilemma for the rescuers causes controversy but the widest consensus (Lloyd 1986, Steinman 1986, Danzl & Pozos 1987, Handley et al 1992) is as follows:

- If breathing is absent, becomes obstructed or stops, standard airway management should be started, including expired air resuscitation if appropriate.
- Chest compression should be started *only* if indicated (Table 33.4): there is the danger that if the rescuers become exhausted by doing CPR they may themselves become casualties.
- The rates for expired air ventilation and chest compression should be the same as in normothermia (Lloyd 1986, Moss 1986, Handley et al 1992, Handley & Swain 1994) to compensate for the pulmonary restrictions (decreased chest wall elasticity and decreased pulmonary compliance), the altered rheological properties of the blood (Lloyd 1986, Danzl & Pozos 1987) and the heart feeling 'as hard as stone' (Althaus et al 1982). The aims should be to inflate with a volume of air sufficient to cause the chest to rise visibly, and to compress the sternum to a depth of 4–5 cm in an adult (2–3 cm in a child; 1–1.5 cm in an infant).
- If at any time a pulse is detected CPR must stop while it is still present.

In hypothermia, an apparent VF may merely be an electrical artefact or due to shivering. A 'flat ECG' may be due to asystole, a bad electrical conduction through cold skin or problems of adhesion of the electrodes because of the cold damp skin (Weinberg 1993). Sterile hypodermic needles inserted through the gel portion of the electrodes improve

Table 33.4 Indications for starting cardiopulmonary resuscitation in hypothermia

- No carotid pulse is detectable after feeling in the correct place for at least 1 min
  or
- cardiac arrest is observed, i.e. a pulse that was present previously has disappeared
  or
- there is a reasonable chance that a cardiac arrest occurred within the previous 2 h
  and
- there is a reasonable expectation that effective CPR can be provided with only brief periods of interruption for movement until the casualty can be transported to hospital, where full advanced life support can be provided.

adhesion and conduction (American Heart Association 1992, Weinberg 1993). If VF is identified, the normal first three DC shocks should be given immediately. Further shocks should wait until the patient has been rewarmed to 30°C (American Heart Association 1992, Weinberg 1993, Handley & Swain 1994).

Casualties, especially if young, who have been in very cold water can recover even after periods of up to 1 h of known total submersion (Lloyd 1986). A man who was very cold and showed no signs of life was successfully resuscitated on the sea front using external cardiac compression and expired air resuscitation after he had been hauled out of a cold winter sea by the rope which had formed a loop round his neck (Frankland 1983). Similarly, one young woman was revived with expired air resuscitation after being buried for 20 min in a wet-snow avalanche (Gray 1987). Standard CPR has been continued for 2.5 h during a helicopter rescue (Althaus et al 1982), for 4 h during transport in a snow vehicle, ambulance and helicopter (Steinman, personal communication), for 4.5 h during transport and rewarming when cardiac arrest occurred at a rectal temperature of 23°C with the rhythm varying between asystole and VF (Stoneham & Squires 1992), and for 6.5 h including air ambulance transport when asystole occurred at 23.2°C (Lexow 1991), with ultimate survival of the patients.

Finally

It is salutary to remember that physiological responses have limited value in severe cold and behavioural changes such as taking shelter early are the most effective survival mechanisms (Moss 1986).

References

Alexander G 1979 Cold thermogenesis. In: Robertshaw D (ed) Environmental physiology III. University Park Press, Baltimore, MD, pp 43–155

Alexander L 1945 The treatment of shock from prolonged exposure to cold, especially in water. Combined Intelligence Objective Subcommittee, Item No. 24, File No. 26–37

Althaus U, Aeberhard P, Schupbach P et al 1982 Management of profound accidental hypothermia with cardiorespiratory arrest. Annals of Surgery 195: 492–495

American College of Surgeons Committee on Trauma 1997 Advanced trauma life support student manual, 6th edn. American College of Surgeons, Chicago, IL

American Heart Association 1992 Guidelines for cardiopulmonary resuscitation and emergency cardiac care. Part IV: Special resuscitation situations. Journal of the American Medical Association 268: 2244–2246

Berger RL 1990 Nazi science – the Dachau hypothermia experiments. New England Journal of Medicine 322: 1435–1440

Bloch M 1965 Re-warming following prolonged hypothermia in man. MD thesis, University of London

Burton AC, Edholm OG 1955 Man in a cold environment. Edward Arnold, London

Collis ML, Steinman AM, Chaney RM 1977 Accidental hypothermia: an experimental study of practical rewarming methods. Aviation Space and Environmental Medicine 48: 625–632

Conn, ML 1979 Evaluation of inhalation rewarming as a therapy for hypothermia. MSc thesis, Simon Fraser University, Victoria, BC, Canada

Danzl D, Pozos RS 1987 Multicenter hypothermia study. Annals of Emergency Medicine 16: 1042–1055

Frankland JC 1983 The Blackpool tragedy. Journal of the British Association of Immediate Care 6: 34–35

Golden FStC 1979 Why rewarm? In: Matter P, Braun P, de Quervain M, Good W (eds) Skifahren und Sicherheit III. Buchdruckerei Davos, Davos, pp 163–167

Golden FStC, Hervey GR, Tipton MJ 1991 Circum-rescue collapse: collapse, sometimes fatal, associated with rescue of immersion victims. Journal of the Royal Naval Medical Service 77: 139–149

Gray D 1987 Survival after burial in an avalanche. British Medical Journal 1: 611–612

Hall KN, Seyverud SA 1990 Closed thoracic cavity lavage in the treatment of severe hypothermia in human beings. Annals of Emergency Medicine 19: 204–208

Hamlet MP 1983 Fluid shifts in hypothermia. In: Pozos RS, Wittmers LE (eds) The nature and treatment of hypothermia. Croom Helm, London, pp 94–99

Handley AJ, Swain A 1994 Advanced life support manual, 2nd edn. Resuscitation Council (UK). Burr Associates, Slough

Handley AJ, Golden FStC, Keatinge WR et al 1992 Report of the Working Party on Out of Hospital Management of Hypothermia. Medical Commission on Accident Prevention. Royal College of Surgeons of England, London

Hayward JS 1983 The physiology of immersion hypothermia. In: Pozos RS, Wittmers LE (eds) The nature and treatment of hypothermia. Croom Helm, London, pp 3–19

Horvath SM 1981 Exercise in a cold environment. Exercise, Sport and Science Review 9: 221–263

Jui J, Hauty M, Harder R 1988 Hypothermia on Mt Hood. Wilderness Medicine Newsletter 5: 4–7

Kaufman WC 1983 The development and rectification of hiker's hypothermia. In: Pozos RS, Wittmers LE (eds) The nature and treatment of hypothermia. Croom Helm, London, pp 46–57

Ledingham IMcA, Mone JG 1980 Treatment of accidental hypothermia: a prospective clinical study. British Medical Journal 1: 1102–1105

Lexow K 1991 Severe accidental hypothermia: survival after 6 hours 30 minutes of cardiopulmonary resuscitation. Arctic Medical Research 50(Suppl 6): 112–114

Lloyd EL 1973 Accidental hypothermia treated by central rewarming via the airway. British Journal of Anaesthesia 45: 41–48

Lloyd EL 1986 Hypothermia and cold stress. Croom Helm, London

Lloyd EL 1990 Airway warming in the treatment of accidental hypothermia: a review. Journal of Wilderness Medicine 1: 65–78

Lloyd EL 1991a Equipment for airway warming in the treatment of accidental hypothermia. Journal of Wilderness Medicine 2: 330–350

Lloyd EL 1991b The role of cold in ischaemic heart disease: a review. Public Health 105: 205–215

Lloyd EL 1992 The cause of death after rescue. International Journal of Sports Medicine 13: S196–sS199

Lloyd EL 1996 Accidental hypothermia. Resuscitation 32: 111–124

Lloyd EL, Croxton D 1981 Equipment for the provision of airway warming (insulation) in the treatment of accidental hypothermia in patients. Resuscitation 9: 61–65

Lloyd EL, Mitchell B 1974 Factors affecting the onset of ventricular fibrillation in hypothermia: an hypothesis. Lancet 2: 1294–1296

Lloyd EL, Mitchell B, Williams JT 1976a Rewarming from immersion hypothermia. A comparison of three methods. Resuscitation, 5: 5–18

Lloyd EL, Mitchell B, Williams JT 1976b The cardiovascular effects of three methods of rewarming from immersion hypothermia. Resuscitation 5: 229–233

MacInnes C 1971 Steroids in mountain rescue. Lancet 1: 599

McLatchie GM, Harries M, Williams C, King J (eds) 1995 ABC of sports medicine. BMJ Publishing, London

Maclean D, Emslie-Smith D 1977 Accidental hypothermia. Blackwell Scientific Publications, Oxford

Miller JW, Danzl DF, Thomas DM 1980 Urban accidental hypothermia: 135 cases. Annals of Emergency Medicine 9: 456–461

Mills WJ 1992 Field care of the hypothermic patient. International Journal of Sports Medicine 13: S199–sS202

Moss J 1986 Accidental severe hypothermia. Surgery, Gynecology and Obstetrics 162: 501–513

Niazi SA, Lewis FJ 1958 Profound hypothermia in man: report of a case. Annals of Surgery 147: 254–266

Nolan JP 1993 Techniques for rapid fluid infusion. British Journal of Intensive Care 3: 98–105

Nozaki RN, Ishabashi K, Adachi N 1986 Accidental profound hypothermia. New England Journal of Medicine 315: 1680

Osborne L, Kamal El-Din. AS, Smith JE 1984 Survival after prolonged cardiac arrest and accidental hypothermia. British Medical Journal 2: 881–882

Paton BC 1983 Accidental hypothermia. Pharmacology and Therapeutics 22: 331–377

Popovic V, Popovic P 1974 Hypothermia in biology and medicine. Academic Press, London

Roberts DE, Patton JF, Kerr DW 1983 The effect of airway warming on severe hypothermia. In: Pozos RS, Wittmers LE (eds) The nature and treatment of hypothermia. Croom Helm, London, pp 209–220

Rodriguez JL, Weissman C, Damask MCetal 1983 Physiologic requirements during rewarming: suppression of the shivering response. Critical Care Medicine 11: 490–497

Royal College of Physicians 1966 Report on the Committee on Accidental Hypothermia. Royal College of Physicians, London

Sharkey A, Gulden RH, Lipton JM, Giesecke AH 1993 Effect of radiant heat on the metabolic cost of postoperative shivering. British Journal of Anaesthesia 70: 449–450

Steinman AM 1986 Cardiopulmonary resuscitation and hypothermia. Circulation 74(Suppl 4): 29–32

Stoneham MD, Squires SJ 1992 Prolonged resuscitation in acute deep hypothermia. Anaesthesia 47: 784–788

Tappan DV, Jacey MJ, Heyder E, Gray PH 1984 Blood volume responses in partially dehydrated subjects working in the cold. Aviation Space and Environmental Medicine 55: 296–301

Weinberg AD 1993 Hypothermia. Annals of Emergency Medicine 22: 370–377

Wood V 1977 Case of hypothermia. Canadian Medical Association 117: 16–17

Rescue from remote places

34

Introduction   376

Mountain rescue   377

Cave rescue   378

Ski patrolling   380

Lifeboats   380

Search and rescue helicopters   381

Remote industrial sites   381

References   381

Further reading   382

These areas include:

- mountain rescue
- ski patrolling
- cave rescue
- the lifeboat service
- search and rescue helicopters
- remote industrial sites.

This chapter covers the rescue of patients suffering from trauma, medical problems or drowning, all of which can be complicated by hypothermia. Without exception, all the rescue work discussed in this chapter is carried out by individuals who have the specialist training, physical ability and equipment necessary for working in the remote circumstances in which they operate. The main message of this chapter must be that, unless one possesses, or is prepared to acquire and maintain, the knowledge, skills and physical attributes of these individuals, one should under no circumstances attempt to participate in their rescue activities. The only qualification for being a member of such a rescue team should be the ability to perform physically at the same level as other members of the team. If you cannot, other members of the team will be put at risk. Medical skills can only be regarded as a bonus to be provided if one's physical skills are appropriate.

This statement covers all areas discussed in this chapter. This may seem obvious with regard to mountain rescue; an example of a less obvious situation can be seen in the lifeboat service where someone who is not used to travelling in a small boat in rough seas will not physically be able to cope with such circumstances and will be unable to contribute to patient management. This person may even have

Introduction

For most medical practitioners, rescues from remote places are events confined to news bulletins. For doctors and other personnel working in particular areas of the UK, however, they occur relatively frequently and form a significant component of the workload, especially at certain times of the year. It is important to recognize, however, that there is a wide range of situations in which remote area rescues become necessary and an appropriate definition is therefore required.

Remote places may be defined as areas where rescue is likely to be significantly prolonged because of the location and likely to require the use of individuals with specialist training and skills for working in such areas.

to be looked after by a member of the crew, removing this crew member from his/her normal function.

People involved in prehospital care are encouraged not to attempt rescue from these areas without the use of such specialist teams, and should not attempt to provide a service to replace these established rescue services. It is likely, therefore, that providers of prehospital care will be involved in meeting specialist rescue teams at a prearranged rendezvous point and providing the ongoing treatment and transportation of the rescued person or people to an appropriate hospital. The purpose of this chapter is therefore to discuss the relevant rescue services, the degree of medical involvement in such services, the medical rescue equipment used by such services and the particular medical problems that may be encountered.

As with all patients in the prehospital situation, the collection of as much information as possible about the history leading to the need for medical help (and the patient's past medical history) is vital. Of particular note in these situations will be information on:

- treatment already given by the rescue personnel – it should be noted that rescue teams carry drugs, sometimes including injectable morphine
- observations, in particular serial observations that may have been undertaken during a prolonged rescue.

Most rescue teams will have members who have had training in first aid with particular reference to the situations and environment they are likely to encounter. This fact should be kept in mind and as much use made of such experience as possible. It is important to remember when considering situations where trauma is the most common problem that people do still suffer medical problems such as asthma and myocardial infarction and that this may be their only or most significant problem.

Mountain rescue

There are a variety of publications covering first aid for mountaineers, and many mountaineering textbooks contain chapters on first aid. It is therefore possible that people climbing with the patient may have applied first-aid skills at an early stage.

Mountain rescue is undertaken by teams of volunteers. Such teams do not usually include a doctor but most teams will contain members who have advanced first-aid skills. Mountain rescue teams normally have a doctor as their medical adviser. This doctor will be involved in training and may give advice to the team via a radio. It can often be expected, therefore, that the patient will have had advanced first-aid procedures performed before contact is made with the standard emergency services.

Table 34.1 Mountain hypothermia guidelines		
Definitely dead	No respiration No signs of circulation *and* obvious fatal injury *or* airway blocked by blood/snow/vomit or debris *or* temperature more than 32°C (if available)	No action Evacuate as dead
Definitely alive	Conscious	Insulate from heat loss Monitor regularly Evacuate
Definitely alive	Unconscious Respiration and/or pulse present	Insulate from heat loss Maintain airway Evacuate (in modified recovery position if possible)
May be alive	No respiration *and* no carotid pulse *and* airway clear *and* no obvious fatal injury *and* temperature less than 32°C	Ask for radio assistance

In November 1997, a conference was held in Scotland to bring together accident and emergency consultants, surgeons, anaesthetists, mountain rescue team doctors, senior mountain rescue team first-aiders and other relevant personnel in order to produce consensus guidelines on the treatment of patients suffering accidental mountain hypothermia. Table 34.1 summarizes the guidelines produced (Grant et al 1998).

Decision-making support for 'may be alive' casualties is summarized in Table 34.2.

Despite this, the environment and need for transportation of the patient will have limited the procedures that will have been undertaken. It can be expected that initial observations will have been completed, and spinal immobilization with a cervical collar and possibly a vacuum mattress may also have been applied. Injured limbs may have been splinted, dressings applied to open wounds, and warmed oxygen and Entonox given. The patient is likely to have been placed in a rescue stretcher. Two are currently used in this country, the McInnes stretcher and the Bell stretcher (Fig. 34.1).

Ingram (1994) has shown that helicopters are involved in 59% of all mountain rescues and therefore the main purpose of these stretchers is to provide easy transportation of the patient without the risk of the patient falling out of the stretcher, combined with the ability of the stretcher to be

Table 34.2 Decision-making support for 'may be alive' casualties

Better chance	Poor chance
Prognosis	
Recent vital signs	Cardiac arrest more than 2 h ago in the open
Witnessed cardiac arrest	
Burial/snow hole/shelter	Helicopter/ambulance more than 2 h
Easy evacuation	Difficult evacuation
Treatment	
Insulate from heat loss, including respiratory heat loss	Evacuate as dead (death must be certified by a doctor at some point)
Evacuate (in modified recovery position if possible)	
Commence cardiopulmonary resuscitation (CPR) if:	
no carotid pulse for 1 min	
or cardiac arrest observed	
or cardiac arrest within 2 h	
and CPR can continue until hospital is reached	

used for lifting the patient into a helicopter. It can be difficult to get patients out of these stretchers while protecting them against the risk of further damage to an injured spine, and special consideration must be given to this problem. If the team carries a vacuum mattress the patient should be enclosed in this before being put into the mountain rescue stretcher. This makes the removal of patients from such stretchers much easier, and the patient should continue to be transported in this until arrival at hospital.

Puttick & Lawler (1989) have assessed the use of pulse oximeters in mountain rescue and helicopter evacuation. They found them useful to monitor the continued effectiveness of respiration while the patient was being moved.

Arrival at an ambulance will often, however, be the first opportunity to do a full primary survey. Special consideration should be given to the fact that the patient may be hypothermic, and rough handling may induce a cardiac arrhythmia. Clothing should only be removed sufficiently to allow necessary examination, or if damp clothing is liable to cause further hypothermia. It is important to remember that a hypothermic patient cannot usually be certified dead until taken to hospital and rewarmed.

Hypothermia in mountain rescue deserves special consideration as Crocket (1991) showed this to be the cause of 13% of all mountain rescue incidents. It is important to remember that hypothermia can occur in both summer and winter, and that wind and damp clothing can be causes of hypothermia as well as the surrounding air temperature. Snadden (1993) has suggested that, in mountain rescue, where the measuring of the patient's core temperature is

impossible, shivering should be used as a differentiating factor. If the patient is shivering the hypothermia can be considered to be mild and the patient should be passively rewarmed and evacuated. If the patient is hypothermic and not shivering, probably with an altered state of consciousness, then he should be considered to be severely hypothermic, not allowed to walk and not subjected to any more movement than is absolutely necessary. In considering an appropriate hospital for the patient, thought should be given to transporting the patient to a hospital with facilities for rewarming. In remote areas this may be the nearest hospital with dialysis facilities.

As a general rule, most members of mountain rescue teams will carry aspirin, glucose and a non-steroidal anti-inflammatory drug. There will also be a team first-aid pack, which is likely to contain morphine for intramuscular injection, salbutamol and an antihistamine. It is due to the efforts of a Manchester surgeon (Wilson-Hay) some 30 years ago that mountain rescue teams have the facility to give morphine.

An indication of the patterns of injury seen in mountain rescues is given by Ingram (1994) and shows the following statistics:

- lower limb injuries – 46% of injured
- bruising – 19% of injured
- head injuries – 21% of injured.

An analysis of fatal injuries shows the following:

- 38% due to head injuries
- 15% due to multiple trauma
- 18% due to medical conditions.

In view of the high incidence of head injuries, it is worthwhile considering the delivery of a person with advanced airway skills to the scene by helicopter.

Cave rescue

Much of what has been said above about mountain rescue applies to cave rescue. There are, however, some differences as the cave systems that are explored frequently contain tunnels the diameters of which are not much greater than that of the human body. Caves also contain water, and cavers may have been involved in diving activities. Thus, even if skilled medical attention in the form of a doctor or paramedic can be delivered to the location of the injured caver, the only procedures that can be adequately undertaken are basic airway maintenance measures, pain relief, splinting of fractures and monitoring of the patient. It is unlikely that bulkier pieces of equipment will be able to be delivered to the patient or that such equipment can be used on the patient in the cave.

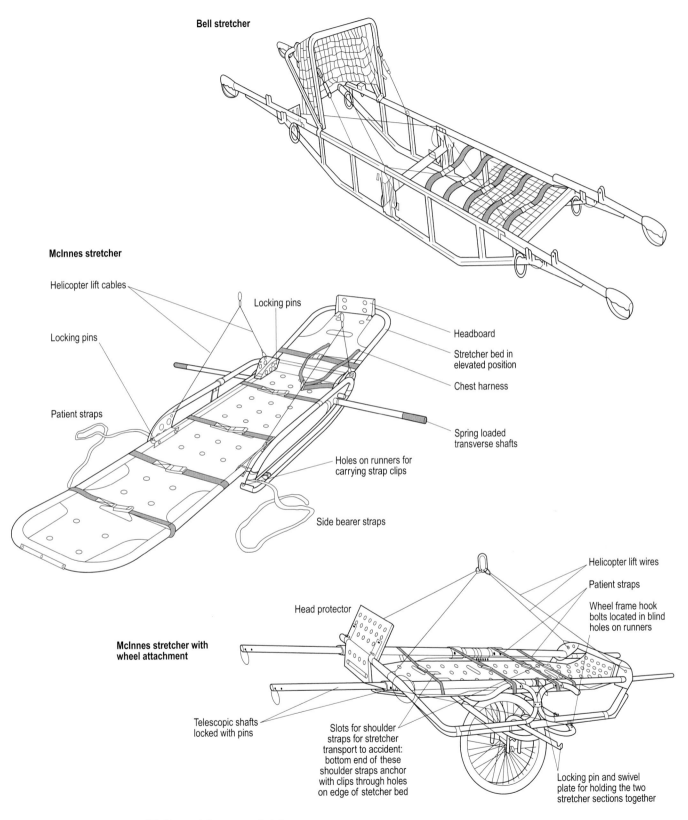

Bell stretcher

McInnes stretcher

Helicopter lift cables

Locking pins

Locking pins

Patient straps

Headboard

Stretcher bed in elevated position

Chest harness

Spring loaded transverse shafts

Holes on runners for carrying strap clips

Side bearer straps

McInnes stretcher with wheel attachment

Head protector

Helicopter lift wires

Patient straps

Wheel frame hook bolts located in blind holes on runners

Telescopic shafts locked with pins

Slots for shoulder straps for stretcher transport to accident: bottom end of these shoulder straps anchor with clips through holes on edge of stetcher bed

Locking pin and swivel plate for holding the two stretcher sections together

Fig. 34.1 • The McInnes and Bell mountain rescue stretchers.

Stokes litter

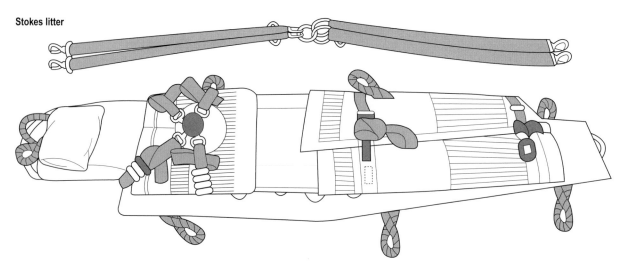

Neil Robertson stretcher

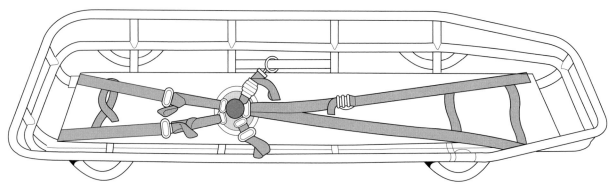

Fig. 34.2 • The Stokes litter and Neil Robertson stretcher.

Morphine can be given by cave rescue teams. The previous advice regarding hypothermic patients applies. The management of such patients will usually be the application of an exposure bag before they are put on to a suitable stretcher, such as a Stokes litter or a Neil Robertson stretcher (Fig. 34.2).

It is important to remember that if the injured person has been diving s/he should not be given Entonox.

Ski patrolling

Apart from members of the general public, the first layer of planned medical provision on ski slopes is provided by ski patrollers. Such persons may well be members of the British Association of Ski Patrollers, an organization that runs courses in advanced first aid and courses to Emergency Medical Technician standard. It is likely that the injured person will be brought to an ambulance rendezvous point by the ski patroller, probably on a sledge. The problems of hypothermia and skeletal injury mentioned previously will again apply, and it is important to remember that areas of

possible frostbite should not be actively rewarmed during the transportation phase.

Langran et al (1996) showed an injury rate of 2.43 per 1000 skier days. American and Australian studies report rates of 3.0–3.8 per 1000 skier days (Sherry 1984, 1985, Sherry & Fenelon 1991). No fatalities were reported. Of the 486 casualties, most injuries were musculoskeletal and 32 required admission to hospital (again, mostly with musculoskeletal problems). Apart from musculoskeletal problems, there were two head injuries, two facial fractures and a cervical spine fracture. Knee injuries made up one-third of all injuries.

This pattern is similar to other studies (Moller-Madsen et al 1990, Johnson & Pope 1991, Sherry & Fenelon 1991, Schydlowsky et al 1993).

Lifeboats

Rescue at sea and around the coasts of Britain and Ireland is efficiently organized by a combined operation between statutory organizations, voluntarily organizations and the armed forces. Major contributors are the Royal National Lifeboat Institution (RNLI), the Coastguard Service, and the Royal Air Force and Royal Navy rescue helicopters.

Each lifeboat station has a lifeboat doctor known as the station honorary medical adviser (SHMA). This doctor has a variety of duties, including advising on the health of the crew and first-aid training. The doctor is also encouraged to attend regular lifeboat exercises and can go to sea with the lifeboat in an emergency if it is felt that the doctor's services may be required. The RNLI estimates that in 10% of its call-outs the rescued will require medical attention, and that in 1% of its call-outs a doctor will go to sea with the lifeboat. Currently, total call-outs for the RNLI are approximately 6000 per year.

Provision is also made for any member of a lifeboat crew who has paramedical skills to have appropriate equipment and to make use of these skills when on a rescue. All crew members are encouraged to attend first-aid courses run specifically for lifeboat crews by the Royal National Lifeboat Institution. As well as covering first aid, these courses also include the use of oxygen and Entonox, and special techniques for airway maintenance and patient immobilization where lack of space may not allow conventional techniques to be employed. Special attention is paid to prolonged care and monitoring of the rescued as it may take some considerable time for such persons to reach hospital.

If the situation warrants it the SHMA can be requested to give medical advice to the lifeboat crew via the radio.

First Aid for Lifeboat Crews (Guild 1993), the RNLI first-aid manual, states that under the Dangerous Drugs Regulations 1985 the Home Office has granted permission for coxswains and mechanics of the institution's lifeboats to be in possession of morphine for certified crew members to administer at sea. This is done after obtaining approval from the SHMA by radio.

Lifeboats usually carry a basket stretcher and a Neil Robertson stretcher. As well as large lifeboats there are, of course, inshore rescue craft. Crew on these are likely to have first-aid training and the equipment is generally carried in a first-aid pouch.

Search and rescue helicopters

This service is provided by the Royal Air Force, the Royal Navy and helicopters supplied by private companies and painted in coastguard livery. Requests for the use of such helicopters are normally made via the police or coastguard.

The crew members who undertake the functions of winchmen and winch-operator will generally have advanced first-aid training. In addition, on some occasions a doctor may accompany the helicopter, depending on availability and whether or not the extra weight would use up critical fuel supplies. These helicopters may also take on board mountain rescue team doctors.

The type of equipment available can be quite extensive and may include a first-aid kit, battery-operated suction apparatus, a pneuPAC ventilator, Entonox, traction splints and pneumatic antishock garments (PASGs).

Remote industrial sites

Certain types of work such as quarrying, oil drilling, fish farming, forestry and estate management may now take place in remote areas, requiring a lengthy journey to hospital. These activities frequently involve the use of a great deal of heavy mechanical equipment and there is always, therefore, a risk of serious injury. Regulation 3 of the Health and Safety (First Aid) Regulations 1981 requires employers to make provision for first aid in the workplace. This involves the provision of equipment, facilities and suitable persons to provide adequate and appropriate first aid to employees who are injured or become ill at work. These regulations are interpreted in different ways by employers in these industries. Some sites will be totally dependent on the emergency services. Others will have appropriate items of equipment for rendering first aid and persons who have undertaken a standard certificate, 4-day first-aid course and may have had further training directed to the particular problems of their working environment. On the better sites, equipment such as survival bags, stretchers, splints, rigid cervical collars, resuscitators, Entonox, oxygen and manual suction equipment may be available. If cyanide is used, a Kelocyanor kit should also be available.

When treating patients at these sites it is important to remember to use appropriate equipment and clothing to ensure the rescuers' own safety. This may require borrowing equipment from site personnel. Patients are, of course, at risk of spinal injury, and protection of the spine and airway while extricating and transporting the patient may be a particular problem.

It may be particularly important to carefully assess the patient's need for urgent transport; if this is not felt necessary it is wise to take time to carefully complete a primary survey before attempting transportation. A thorough knowledge of the extrication devices and stretchers that can be used for lifting purposes is important for working in this area.

References

Crocket KV 1991 Scottish mountain accident statistics. Scottish Mountaineering Club Journal

Grant P, Snadden D, Symem D, Walker T 1998 Freezing to death. Scottish Medical Journal 17: 3

Guild WJ 1993 First aid for lifeboat crews. Training Division, Royal National Lifeboat Institution, Poole, Dorset

Ingram A 1994 Scottish mountain rescue study. Scottish Mountain Rescue Committee, Glasgow

Johnson RJ, Pope MH 1991 Epidemiology and prevention of skiing injuries. Annales Chirurgiae et Gynaecologiae 80: 110–115

Langran M, Jachacy GB, MacNeill A 1996 Ski injuries in Scotland. A review of statistics from Cairngorm ski area Winter 1993/94. Scottish Medical Journal 41: 169–172

Moller-Madsen B, Jakobsen BW, Villadsen I 1990 Skiing injuries: a study from a Danish community. British Journal of Sports Medicine 24: 123–124

Puttick NP, Lawler PGP 1989 Pulse oximetry in mountain rescue and helicopter evacuation. Anaesthesia 44: 867

Schydlowsky P, Halberg G, Galatius-Jensen SP 1993 Skiing injuries: review over the winter of 1990–91 in a clinic in the French Alps [in Danish]. UgeskriftforLaeger 155: 387–390

Sherry E 1984 Skiing injuries in Australia. Medical Journal of Australia 140: 530–531

Sherry E 1985 Medical problems in skiers [Letter]. Medical Journal of Australia 143: 92

Sherry E, Fenelon L 1991 Trends in skiing injury type and rates in Australia. A review of 22,261 injuries over 27 years in the Snowy Mountains. Medical Journal of Australia 155: 513–515

Snadden D 1993 The field management of hypothermic casualties arising from Scottish mountain accidents. Scottish Medical Journal 38: 99–103

Further reading

British Association of Ski Patrollers 2003 Outdoor first-aid and safety manual, 8th edn. British Association of Ski Patrollers, Glencoe, Argyll

McInnes H 1984 International mountain rescue book. Constable, London

Malacrida LC, Anselmi LC, Genoni M et al 1993 Helicopter mountain rescue of patients with head injuries and/or multiple injuries in southern Switzerland 1980–1990. Injury 24: 451–453

Steele P 1992 Medical handbook for mountaineers. Constable, London

Near drowning

35

Incidence   383

Pathophysiology   383

Aspects of rescue   384

Immediate care   385

Treatment of cardiac arrest   386

Transport to hospital   387

Results and prognosis   387

Conclusion   388

References   388

Incidence

Death from drowning is responsible for more than 500 deaths per annum in the UK, and estimates of immersion incidents suggest that near-drowning accidents are 8–10 times more frequent than this. Children aged 1–4 years are particularly vulnerable as they have rarely learnt to swim but have a fascination with water. Death from drowning is the third most common form of accidental death in children in the UK and the second most common in the USA. In teenagers and young adults the male to female ratio is approximately 3:1. With the increased interest in water sports, immersion incidents are liable to increase. There also seems to be an increased interest in swimming among elderly people and this group is particularly prone to cardiovascular and cerebrovascular accidents after entering cold water. Amateur diving is increasingly popular and if divers suffer an immersion accident they will not be afforded the cerebral protection of hypothermia as they are invariably clothed in a very efficient insulation suit.

Pathophysiology

Death from drowning occurs due to one or a combination of the following four factors:

- Unconsciousness
- Inability to swim
- Exhaustion
- Hypothermia.

UNCONSCIOUSNESS

Anyone who suffers trauma to the head and neck that reduces or causes unconsciousness before entering the water will have an unprotected airway, water will replace air in the lungs and the victim will die a rapid death from hypoxia. Other factors that lead to unconsciousness or diminished consciousness include:

- epilepsy
- cerebrovascular accident
- myocardial infarction
- acute hypoglycaemia
- severe alcohol or drug overdosage.

Death by drowning is also a recognized form of suicide.

INABILITY TO SWIM

Anyone who is unable to swim and finds him/herself out of his/her depth of water will make frantic efforts to keep the airway above the water line by beating the water with outstretched arms and keeping the head in an extended position. This will be successful for a variable period of time but usually leads initially to the ingestion of what can be very cold water and inevitably to attempts at inspiration when under the water. It is thought that this leads only to minimal aspiration but precipitates violent bronchospasm, with resulting inability to control respiration and, as a consequence, repeated inspirations under water. This leads to a downward spiral of increasing aspirations leading to increasing hypoxia until eventually unconsciousness occurs.

EXHAUSTION

It used to be thought that drowning from exhaustion only occurred in warm water after an accident resulting in the patient being stranded many hours from rescue or without prospect of rescue. It is now known that an acute exhaustion-like picture can also be precipitated by cold water in a matter of minutes. This has been reported on many occasions and has been the subject of a Royal Navy video film, when world-class swimmers were unable to swim for protracted periods in cold water. The reason this acute exhaustion-like picture occurs is thought to be the steady onset of hypothermia.

HYPOTHERMIA

Being plunged into ice-cold water can occasionally lead to sudden death from cardiac arrest and it is thought that this is largely due to asystole. Most swimmers manage to control the initial involuntary hyperventilation, and then coordinate breathing, arm and leg movements as long as their temperature remains above 35°C. Swimming without protection in cold water will, however, inevitably, lead to a gradual cooling of the body, enhanced by the muscular effort required to maintain normal swimming progress. Below 35°C there is a period of confusion, with an inability to coordinate and ataxic swimming movements that have been likened to a dog paddling motion with no forward propulsion. Victims rescued at this point may be amnesic and deny that they were in any difficulty. If rescue is not achieved at this point further cooling leads to the increasing onset of unconsciousness. The airway then slips below the water and drowning occurs through an unprotected airway. Cold-water swimmers die from drowning but the reason they drown is that they have become unconscious through hypothermia.

Shallow lakes and pools are frequently at freezing point in winter, when death can occur in as little as 10 min. At 5°C (a common winter sea temperature) survival times are estimated as between 30 min and 2 h. Even at a summer sea temperature of 15°C or 16°C swimmers can be lost after 2 h, although there is little doubt that at this temperature acclimatized cold-water swimming can lead to prolonged survival (Barnet 1962).

Hypothermia can be described as the 'Jekyll and Hyde' of the drowning process as although it is undoubtedly the main killer of fit, unprotected swimmers it is also the probable reason why there have been some remarkable cerebrally normal survivors after prolonged submersion. It is thought that cold affects first the skin then the gastrointestinal system and finally the pulmonary vascular bed, leading to a cooling of the venous return and consequently of the blood being pumped to the brain. It is known that respiratory arrest usually occurs before cardiac arrest in drowning, and as long as the heart remains in sinus rhythm then cooled blood will continue to be pumped to the brain leading to relatively quick cooling. In animals cerebral oxygen requirements are reduced by 30% at 30°C and this provides a degree of cerebral protection from hypoxia (Stern & Good 1960). Normal cerebral survival after prolonged submersion has always been accompanied by severe hypothermia. Many of these survivors have been children with a high body surface area to weight ratio, leading to increased superficial cooling.

The common pathophysiological pathway for drowning from any cause is a right–left shunt leading to profound hypoxia. This leads to tissue ischaemia, with resulting metabolic acidosis. Metabolic acidosis is an invariable finding when hypothermia is severe and pH levels below 7.0 are frequently recorded. Vomiting and aspiration of gastric content are a frequent terminal event and are found in 40% of post-mortems in deaths due to drowning.

Much has been made in the past of the importance of the different pathophysiology between salt- and freshwater drowning. Essentially, hypertonic salt-water drowning can be shown in animals to lead to an osmotic movement of water through from the capillary into the lung alveolus. Similarly, freshwater hypotonic drowning can lead to a movement of water into the circulation and subsequent haemolysis. In clinical practice both these events are extremely rare. As far as rescue, resuscitation and outcome go, treatment is identical and it is the temperature rather than the type of water that is important.

Aspects of rescue

It is of fundamental importance to appreciate that every year some near-drowning incidents are turned into fatalities, but with the loss not of the initial victim but of those who attempt rescue. It is self-evident that rescuers should be competent swimmers but it is equally important that they be suitably dressed to withstand the effects of cold and attached by a line to a safe retrieval point, particularly in rescues from ice-covered lakes in winter or from rocky shores in stormy seas. Each year rescuers are lost because they either cannot themselves escape from submersion under ice or cannot get back to safety from a rough sea. The common pattern in the latter event is for the rescuer to suffer a head injury attempting to clamber up rocks. Those who are not adequately insulated will rapidly suffer an acute exhaustion-like state, as has been previously described.

The retrieval of immersion victims from deep water, in particular, can be very difficult and has exercised the minds of professional rescue organizations ever since Golden et al (1991) identified the potential catastrophic drop in cerebral perfusing pressure that can occur when the victim is moved from the horizontal to the vertical position. In the water the victim has a potential benefit of a positive pressure to the body exerted by the surrounding water. This was described by Golden et al as the 'hydrostatic squeeze'. The position that most unconscious victims adopt, especially if wearing a life jacket, is semihorizontal. If they are removed from the water in a vertical position, not only is the hydrostatic squeeze lost but the pressure of blood perfusing the brain is reduced.

This has led to reports of unconsciousness developing in at least three helicopter rescues (Simcock 1986). Attention is now directed towards using a double-strop method of lifting, but this requires careful airway control by the rescuer if the victim is unconscious. Rescue into boats, particularly high-sided boats, presents its own problems but wherever possible winches and lifting devices should be used to avoid a vertical lift. With dinghies, shallow water and swimming pools it may be possible to use a bounce and roll technique to successfully retrieve the victim in a horizontal position (Fig. 35.1).

Immediate care

THE CONSCIOUS PATIENT

The cornerstone of resuscitation is the identification and relief of hypoxia in the shortest possible time. Ideally, this would be started in the water as soon as the accident is discovered but in practice this is only feasible with highly trained personnel and in calm water. The vast majority of rescues should concentrate on the identification of hypoxia as soon as the patient is removed from the water. The time between the initial aspiration and relief of the ensuing hypoxia has been referred to as the 'hypoxic gap' and it is the reduction of this to a minimum that will govern

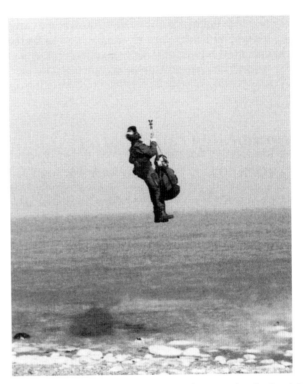

Fig. 35.1 • Removing the victim from the water in a horizontal position.

not only survival but cerebrally normal survival (Simcock 1986). The fundamental questions to ask are:

- Is this patient breathing?
- Is this patient breathing adequately?

Many rescues will result in a patient who has aspirated water but is still conscious and breathing with an apparently normal respiratory rate and depth. Respiration will be accompanied by frequent coughing, retrosternal pain and the expiration of small amounts of grey frothy sputum. Until there is any objective evidence to the contrary, it is wisest to assume that these people are either hypoxic or potentially hypoxic and they should be given high-flow oxygen therapy by mask at the accident site and during transport to hospital. The cardiovascular effects of near-drowning mimic those of hypovolaemia, with poor circulation, low pulse pressure, tachycardia and low blood pressure. It is wise, therefore, to maintain the horizontal position and it may be of benefit to raise the legs. Where personnel and equipment allow, the siting of an intravenous cannula and infusion of $10\,\mathrm{ml\,kg^{-1}}$ of isotonic fluid can only be of benefit. These are simple straightforward measures that require little time and certainly should not delay the speedy transport of the patient to a well-equipped emergency department in a hospital equipped with intensive care facilities. Monitoring of the electrocardiogram (ECG) should begin as soon as possible, together with pulse oximetry, although it must be remembered that peripheral shutdown may render the oximetry results invalid. Communication with the hospital emergency department or intensive care personnel is a wise precaution to avoid any delay in the continuity of treatment on arrival at hospital.

There are undoubtedly a large number of immersion victims who recover rapidly after rescue and immediate care. Some of these may be only briefly unconscious and with careful airway and oxygen management appear to recover completely at the accident site. It is wise to insist that these patients are also taken to hospital, as the late onset of acute respiratory failure or so-called 'secondary drowning' is well documented, although its incidence is only of the order of 2–3%. The onset of tachycardia, tachypnoea, cough with frothy sputum and eventually hypoxia and unconsciousness is potentially lethal and may require urgent ventilation and intensive care management. All patients should therefore be admitted to hospital, where the situation may be reappraised after 6 h. The Resuscitation Council (UK) guidelines (2004) suggest that discharge can be considered 6 h after admission if the patient is clinically normal, the chest X-ray is clear and the partial pressure of oxygen (P_aO_2) is normal when breathing air. Any doubt about these criteria should mean overnight admission and careful observation.

THE UNCONSCIOUS PATIENT

The immediate care management of the unconscious immersion victim who has not suffered cardiac arrest presents one of the most rewarding challenges to immediate care specialists. Priority must be given to airway management, especially as most of these patients will have an airway obstructed with water, foreign matter or even vomitus. The possibility of cervical spinal injury should always be considered but fortunately this is rare in immersion accidents and is largely restricted to those who have dived into unexpectedly shallow water. However, airway clearance is still feasible in these patients with in-line immobilization: finger sweeps are acceptable practice in all except small children but a portable sucker should be used whenever available. In small children of light weight there is still a case to be made for turning into the recovery position and then elevating the pelvis and legs above the head to facilitate simple drainage. Once cleared, the airway must be maintained and supplementary oxygen therapy instituted as soon as possible. Bag and mask ventilation can be used to override the patient's spontaneous effort and, if facilities and training are available for endotracheal intubation this can usually be achieved without resorting to supplementary intravenous drugs. The patient's own spontaneous ventilation is usually restricted to a few gasps

involving purely diaphragmatic movement and the exhalation of small amounts of inhaled water. If endotracheal intubation has been achieved then artificial ventilation should commence with as high an oxygen percentage as is available, wherever possible 100% oxygen via a manual inflating bag with reservoir. Again, the patient's spontaneous respiratory effort is easily overcome without adjuvant drug therapy but ventilation may be accompanied by the necessity for frequent suction of the upper airway. If endotracheal intubation has not been achieved then the risk of vomiting and aspiration should always be borne in mind. With a cuffed oral endotracheal tube in place, the airway is sealed from the danger of regurgitation but aspirated water will often regurgitate up the endotracheal tube on expiration. It is in this situation that the portable sucker with endobronchial catheters is particularly useful.

The circulatory state of the unconscious near-drowned patient is akin to hypovolaemia in that there is invariably poor pulse pressure, poor peripheral circulation and usually tachycardia with hypotension.

Where facilities exist, the siting of an indwelling intravenous cannula should be considered as this can be followed by the rapid infusion of $10 \, ml \, kg^{-1}$ of fluid without any risk of circulatory overload. The peripheral circulation is usually shut down and venous access is not easy. Undue time should not be spent inserting a cannula but it is worth remembering that the external jugular vein is frequently easily visible in this group of patients and can be cannulated rapidly and with minimal morbidity. Those practised in cut-down techniques may find this a quick and easy method of gaining venous access, but again undue time should not be spent as transport to hospital should not be delayed.

Most of these patients will have temperatures below 35°C but it is the restoration of cardiorespiratory normality that is important as long as there is still a cardiac output. However, insulation from further heat loss is a simple and wise precaution. The use of so-called space blankets should probably be abandoned, but covering the patient in warm woollen blankets or dry clothing should prevent further heat loss and is quick and easy to do. The use of steroids and antibiotics has become controversial in the last decade and there is probably little advantage in considering this in the field situation. It is the relief of hypoxia and rapid transfer to hospital that will determine the survival and degree of residual cerebral impairment of this group of patients.

Treatment of cardiac arrest

A decision not to treat a patient after cardiac arrest due to immersion is difficult, and it is unwise to assume that simply because there is no clinical evidence of cardiac output the victim is irretrievable. Certainly in a small percentage of cases an ECG will reveal slow sinus rhythm although there is no palpable peripheral pulse. With vigorous airway and cardiovascular resuscitation these patients are eminently recoverable. Similarly, there have been some remarkable survivors after cardiac arrest following prolonged submersion in cold water. The maximum survivable period in cold-water immersion is probably unknown, but a child of 2 years recovered after submersion for 66 min in water at a temperature of 5°C (Botte et al 1988). Orlowski (1987), reviewing the world literature, found many cerebrally normal survivors after prolonged cardiopulmonary resuscitation extending up to 3 h. Virtually all cases of survival after cardiac arrest due to immersion have occurred in cold water. Certainly the apparently dead should be assessed carefully before assuming they are beyond resuscitation. The key questions to ask are:

- How long was the period of submersion?
- What was the temperature of the water?
- What does the ECG show?

It is not always easy to ascertain the answers to the first two questions with any great accuracy, but periods of immersion of less than 66 min in cold water should certainly be considered suitable for resuscitation. As will be discussed later, the risk of cerebrally damaged survivors after resuscitation is fortunately low. If in doubt it is wise to commence conventional cardiopulmonary resuscitation and continue this until hospital assessment can be made when the patient has been rewarmed. It is now generally accepted that cardiopulmonary resuscitation should follow conventional lines.

Clearance of the airway (remembering that approximately 40% of these patient will vomit and aspirate) is the first priority. Artificial ventilation should commence with as high an oxygen percentage as possible. Ideally, this should be using endotracheal intubation with a cuffed tube and 100% oxygen. However, it is well recognized that both bag ventilation and expired air resuscitation are compatible with normal cerebral recovery. Once commenced, artificial ventilation must be continued during rescue and transport. It is also generally accepted that where there is clinical evidence of cardiac arrest then external cardiac massage should commence along conventional lines.

The ECG is particularly useful in identifying the small group that are still in sinus rhythm. Again, once commenced, external cardiac massage must not be discontinued before the patient is rewarmed. The question of defibrillation is controversial and it is conventionally taught that the myocardium is refractory to drug management and defibrillation in the presence of hypothermia. There have, however, been isolated reports of successful defibrillation in children at temperatures as low as 28°C (Simcock 1986).

It is reasonable to attempt defibrillation if the ECG shows ventricular fibrillation, but repeated attempts should not be continued if there is no initial success as damage to the myocardium itself can be caused.

There are many recorded cases and anecdotes of successful cardiac resuscitation leading to the restoration of circulating blood volume and spontaneous ventilation at the accident site or before the victim reaches hospital. All such patients require admission to intensive care facilities.

If initial measures do not appear successful, cardiopulmonary resuscitation should not be abandoned in the immediate care scenario. Where feasible, intravenous cannulation and volume resuscitation with $10\,ml\,kg^{-1}$ of intravenous fluid should be commenced. This should not, however, be at the detriment of conventional cardiopulmonary resuscitation guidelines. Resuscitation has to continue in the hypothermic cardiac arrest immersion victim until the patient has been rewarmed to at least 32°C. It is only at this point that a reassessment and decision on whether to abandon resuscitation can be made. This can only be done in the intensive care unit or emergency department, where facilities for rewarming and temperature monitoring are available.

Transport to hospital

The importance of trying to maintain rescue in the horizontal position and avoiding the drop in cerebral perfusion pressure with a vertical lift have already been discussed. Once rescue has been achieved, then treatment at the accident site, during movement and transfer to hospital should always be in the horizontal position. Treatment, once commenced, must continue. Wherever possible the receiving hospital should be notified of the patient's condition and should arrange to meet the rescue vehicle on arrival at the emergency department. There is no place for a gap in treatment on arrival at the hospital site and the hospital resuscitation team should be able to perform ventilation with 100% oxygen, perform endobronchial suction, continue external cardiac massage and be able to monitor temperature and ECG as soon as the patient arrives.

It is on arrival in a well equipped emergency department that the secondary survey can be performed. Anyone who is still unconscious or hypoxic should be then moved to an intensive care unit. Careful assessment and monitoring of the cardiac arrest victim should be set up in the emergency department and the patient should then be transported to an intensive care unit for continued rewarming if necessary.

Results and prognosis

The results of treating patients who have suffered an immersion accident without cardiac arrest are excellent.

A paediatric survey in the UK reported 100% normal survival in 125 children who suffered an immersion accident but received resuscitation at the accident site and who had recovered consciousness by the time they were admitted to hospital (Kemp & Sibert 1991). The Cornwall Drowning Study has retrospectively studied survivors for 21 years and is now able to report on 287 survivors out of 291 treated prior to cardiac arrest. All of these survivors were also cerebrally normal.

The question of cerebral damage is essentially concerned with the cardiac arrest group, although a Toronto study found that that those children with blunted consciousness after resuscitation showed 94% full recovery but those who remained comatose had a significant number of brain-damaged survivors (Conn & Barker 1984). The paediatric UK study reported on 61 normal survivors out of 64 children with impaired level of consciousness on admission.

The cardiac arrest group show significantly poorer survival rates but an encouraging number of cerebrally normal survivors compared with other groups of cardiac arrest victims. The Cornwall Drowning Study has 10 survivors out of 45 cardiac arrest victims treated, and seven of these are cerebrally normal. Perhaps what is encouraging is that, if we look at paediatric cardiac arrest as a whole, the figures for survival after hypothermic immersion cardiac arrest are considerably better than for any other cause. Kuisma et al (1995) reported only five survivors out of a survey of 79 out of hospital paediatric cardiac arrests. Only five of the 79 were as a result of immersion accidents, and three out of these five survived. Poor prognostic indicators are: prolonged submersion, delayed on-site resuscitation, asystole, fixed dilated pupils and prolonged resuscitation before first spontaneous gasp.

Conclusion

The case for effective rescue and immediate care of the immersion victim is paramount not only to survival rates but cerebrally normal survival rates. It is the management in the first few minutes after rescue and the reduction or elimination of the hypoxic gap that is the most important factor in determining survival. Even the apparently dead should be assessed carefully before resuscitation is withheld, as the results of treating hypothermic cardiac arrest after near-drowning are better in children than in any other single cardiac arrest group. The future in improving survival, therefore, lies very much at the accident site.

References

Barnet PN 1962 Report from Arctic Aerospace Laboratory. AA TDR 61: 656

Botte RG, Black PG, Bowers RS et al 1988 The use of extracorporeal rewarming in a child submerged for 66 minutes. Journal of the American Medical Association 260: 377–379

Conn A, Barker G 1984 Freshwater drowning and near drowning – an update. Canadian Anaesthetic Society Journal 31: 538–544

Golden FStC, Harvey GR, Tipton MJ 1991 Circum-rescue collapse, sometimes fatal, associated with rescue of immersion victims. Journal of the Royal Naval Medical Service 77: 139–149

Kemp A, Sibert J 1991 Outcome in children who drown, a British Isles study. British Medical Journal 302: 931–933

Kuisma M, Suominuen P, Kopela R 1995 Paediatric out-of-hospital cardiac arrest – epidemiology and outcome. Resuscitation 30: 141–150

Orlowski J 1987 Drowning, near-drowning and ice-water submersion. Pediatric Clinics of North America 30: 75–92

Resuscitation Council (UK) 2004 ALS manual, 4th edn (revised). Resuscitation Council, London, ch 13, p 108

Simcock AD 1986 The treatment of immersion victims – a review of 130 cases. Anaesthesia 41: 643–648

Stern WE, Good RG 1962 Studies on the effect of hypothermia on CSF oxygen tension and carotid blood flow: 1960. Surgery 48: 13–30

Heat illness

36

Introduction 389

Temperature regulation 389

Normal body temperature 390

Acclimatization 390

Risk factors for heat illness 391

The scope of heat illness: minor and major syndromes 392

Assessment 393

Cooling techniques 394

Treatment 394

Complications 394

Prevention 395

References 396

Further reading 397

Introduction

It has long been recognized that exposure to heat can have severe consequences for wellbeing. The ancient Greeks described a condition precipitated by warm weather and resembling stroke, naming it siriasis, after a star that only appears in the summer months. Heat emergencies arise when the body can no longer adequately dissipate heat, so that the core temperature rises. In heat exhaustion this process is usually reversible; however, in heatstroke a complete breakdown of thermoregulation may develop.

Military personnel, industrial workers and athletes often have to perform under conditions of extreme heat stress. Other groups at particular risk include children and the elderly, the chronically ill, those who have to wear encapsulating protective clothing, alcoholics and people taking various prescribed or illicit medications.

This chapter will provide an outline of the physiology of thermoregulation and the pathophysiology of heat illness, followed by an account of its clinical features, treatment and complications.

The International Classification of Diseases classifies heat illness into 10 distinct entities, the most significant being heatstroke because of its significant potential for morbidity and mortality.

The basis of prevention is the education of at-risk groups and exercising precaution, while effective clinical management relies upon vigilance combined with early recognition and intervention.

Temperature regulation

Body temperature is determined by the complex balance of heat production and dispersion, and is controlled by endocrine, behavioural, somatic and autonomic influences. Heat is created by such diverse processes as the basal metabolic rate, muscular exertion and the assimilation of food substrates. This heat gain must be counterbalanced by

Table 36.1 Mechanisms of thermoregulation

Heat production	Heat dispersal
Basal metabolic rate	Evaporation of sweat
Food substrates	Radiation
Skeletal muscle activity	Convection
Brown fat (infants)	Conduction
Radiation, convection and conduction	Respiration, urination and defaecation

dissipation through radiation, evaporation of sweat, convection and conduction (Table 36.1). Humans are homeothermic animals, whose complex biochemistry and enzyme systems will only function within a narrow temperature range. The hypothalamus must therefore maintain body temperature within precise limits, no matter what the prevailing environmental conditions.

Thermoregulation in children is less highly developed: they have a lower sweating capacity and produce more heat per kilogram than adults so, when compared to those of adults, core values commonly show a 0.5°C increment. Consequently, it is inadvisable that they should be exposed to high-intensity exercise during warm weather.

MECHANISMS OF HEAT PRODUCTION

The body acquires heat from exothermic intracellular metabolic reactions and by absorption of heat through conduction, radiation and convection. The basal metabolic rate contributes approximately $100\,kcal\,h^{-1}$ in an average adult; in the absence of cooling mechanisms this would result in a 1.1°C rise in temperature every hour.

In hot weather, radiation from the sun contributes a further $300\,kcal\,h^{-1}$ to the heat load, but the greatest contribution comes from the contraction of skeletal muscle, with strenuous activity producing up to $900\,kcal\,h^{-1}$, i.e. sufficient heat to raise the core temperature by 1°C every 5 min. Heat emergencies occur when the body is unable to adequately dissipate the heat that is produced so that the core temperature begins to rise.

MECHANISMS OF HEAT LOSS

Conduction

This is direct transfer of heat to another object or substance in contact with the source. The amount of heat lost by conduction is related to the thermal gradient between the body and its surroundings. Air is an efficient insulator, so only 2% of body heat is dissipated by this process. In contrast, water conducts heat 32 times more proficiently than air, making immersion an effective method of cooling.

Convection

This is transfer of heat to a circulating liquid or gas. This is largely dependent on wind velocity and the prevailing temperature, generally accounting for about 15% of heat dispersal.

Evaporation

In circumstances where the environmental temperature rises above 35°C virtually all heat is lost through evaporation of sweat; however, at levels of humidity over 75%, the rate of evaporation slows and sweating becomes a less efficient means of heat loss. Hence, it is the combination of humidity and temperature, rather than the absolute temperature alone, that is critical in determining the intensity of the prevailing heat stress.

Radiation

Although a major determinant of heat loss at lower temperatures, the importance of radiation diminishes as warmer conditions are experienced, so that eventually the body gains heat from its surroundings.

Normal body temperature

Human core temperature conforms to a circadian cycle, with fluctuations of 0.5°C between morning and evening readings being commonplace. The normal value is taken as 37°C, but can vary between 36.3°C and 37.1°C. Precise temperature readings will depend upon the site of measurement, and in hot weather the oral and extremity values tend to be 0.5°C and 1°C lower, respectively, than the core. Obviously this has implications when using temperature as a means of diagnosing heatstroke or for measuring the clinical response to cooling interventions.

In contrast, rectal and core temperatures closely approximate and are less affected by, ambient changes. It is the core temperature (rather than the cutaneous temperature receptors) that the anterior hypothalamus scans and responds to, with the cutaneous sensors being more involved in the detection of low temperatures.

Acclimatization

Both hyperthermia and dehydration contribute to the reduction in physical and mental performance seen when individuals work or exercise in hot conditions. Physiological

Table 36.2 Physiological adaptation to heat

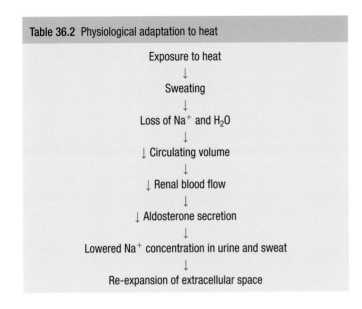

Exposure to heat
↓
Sweating
↓
Loss of Na^+ and H_2O
↓
↓ Circulating volume
↓
↓ Renal blood flow
↓
↓ Aldosterone secretion
↓
Lowered Na^+ concentration in urine and sweat
↓
Re-expansion of extracellular space

Table 36.3 Risk factors for heat illness

Increased heat production	Exercise
	Acute febrile illness
	Drugs: cocaine, phencyclidine hydrochloride (PCP or 'angel dust'), Ecstasy, amphetamines, lysergic acid diethylamide (LSD), tricyclic antidepressants
	Hyperthyroidism
Decreased heat dissipation	Heavy or non-breathable clothing
	Poor fitness levels
	Obesity
	Children
	Old age
	Cardiovascular illness
	Widespread skin disease
	Drugs: antihistamines, phenothiazines
Dehydration	Prolonged exertion: athletics, religious pilgrimages, military training
	Preparation for sports competitions: boxing, body building, etc.
	Diarrhoea and vomiting
	Diabetes mellitus
	Mental retardation
	Drugs: diuretics, alcohol

adaptation to heat involves alterations to the thermoregulatory responses, extending downwards as far as the cellular and molecular levels (Table 36.2). The process of acclimatization is largely complete by 7–12 days but can continue for several weeks. Horowitz (1986) describes acclimatization as being a two-phase process: an initial short-term adaptation lasting 5–7 days, succeeded by a more prolonged state that becomes established after 28 days of exposure to the new climate. Metabolic and cardiovascular changes produce a lowering of the core temperature and a diminution of the threshold for sweating, the key feature being the aldosterone-mediated modification of the sodium and water balance.

Cardiovascular adaptations include an increase in plasma and stroke volume, a diminished rate of rise in the heart rate on exercising, an increase in maximum oxygen uptake ($Vo_{2\,max}$) and a resetting of the vasodilatation threshold for the skin. Cutaneous blood flow can vary from $0.2\,l\,min^{-1}$ in a cold environment to $7–8\,l\,min^{-1}$ in a hot one.

Cardiac output increases to help compensate for the drop in blood pressure caused by the expanded peripheral pooling in the vessels of the skin. Once blood pressure can no longer be maintained, the peripheral vascular resistance increases. Although cutaneous vasoconstriction may help restore blood pressure, it markedly impairs heat loss, so that the core temperature begins to rise.

Tek & Olshaker (1992) point out that the process of acclimatization can be augmented by a graduated exercise programme of 60–90 min sessions; exposing the individual to the heat but avoiding the hottest part of the day.

PATHOGENESIS OF HEAT ILLNESS

Heat illness is most likely to occur when there is disruption or imbalance of the normal thermoregulatory mechanisms caused by either increased heat production or reduced heat dissipation; heat gain may be exogenous (classical heat illness) or endogenous (exertional heat illness). A point is reached where these mechanisms are overwhelmed and core temperature increases. Following failure of the thermoregulatory mechanism, the temperature rises further, resulting in denaturing of proteins, cell necrosis and organ system failure. Hepatocytes, neurones and vascular endothelium are especially at risk.

Risk factors for heat illness

A series of factors often conspire to produce a heat emergency. These include not only the environmental temperature and endogenous heat production but also aspects as diverse as the state of hydration, the wearing of unsuitable multilayered clothing and the presence of predisposing illness and ingestion of various drugs. Risk factors may be classified into three groups (Table 36.3):

- Factors causing increased heat production
- Factors producing decreased heat dispersal
- Factors contributing to dehydration.

INCREASED HEAT PRODUCTION

Heat gain may either be from endogenous or exogenous sources, with the two conspiring to overload the thermoregulatory systems. Increases in endogenous production are seen following physical work, the ingestion of certain drugs, in febrile illness and where the basal metabolic rate has been altered, as in hyperthyroidism.

REDUCED HEAT LOSS

Tight-fitting or heavy clothing reduces heat loss by evaporation and hastens the onset of dehydration. The elderly and the obese cope less well because of lack of cardiovascular fitness, so that they may not be able to increase the cardiac output to the level required to compensate for the reduced venous return induced by cutaneous vasodilation. Alcohol exacerbates any dehydration and can adversely affect behavioural responses, so that an intoxicated individual may not seek cooler surroundings or adjust the amount of clothing worn to a more suitable level.

The scope of heat illness: minor and major syndromes

Rather than relying on strict definitions, the various conditions may be better regarded as lying along a continuum of heat injury. Heat oedema, heat syncope, heat cramps, heat tetany and heat exhaustion comprise minor heat illness. Heatstroke is the most severe form of heat illness and is characterized by hyperthermia with neurological impairment and failure of thermoregulation.

Dickinson (1994) estimates the incidence of exertional heat illness in the more active branches of the Armed Services to be 70 per 100 000, 74% of which are heat exhaustion and 13% heatstroke. While instances are more numerous in the summer months, a significant proportion are seen in the winter, reflecting the relative importance of endogenous heat. Heat-related illness is even more widespread in the USA, where total heat-related deaths in 1980 were 1700, and during a recent heatwave in Philadelphia lasting 8 days the Centers for Disease Control and Prevention (1994) found that 118 deaths were directly attributable to the heat.

MINOR HEAT ILLNESS

Heat syncope

Heat syncope occurs when blood pools in the peripheral circulation, thus reducing venous return. As such it is similar to postural hypotension, with both conditions being due to a relative volume depletion. Clearly, dehydration may also be a contributory factor. Those at increased risk include the unacclimatized, groups standing stationary for long periods (e.g. soldiers on parade) and patients on diuretics, with the latter group fitting Knochel & Reed's (1987) proposal that potassium depletion may have a central role because of its detrimental effect on cardiac reflexes and vasomotor control.

The simple vasovagal faint must be distinguished from the more serious central nervous system (CNS) dysfunction seen with heatstroke, and collapse in a hot environment warrants measurement of rectal temperature to exclude this possibility. On-scene evaluation includes a rapid screening examination for significant cardiovascular, neurological and metabolic disorders that may have precipitated the collapse, along with assessment of any injuries sustained in the resulting fall. Prevention consists of avoidance of contributory circumstances, maintaining adequate hydration and wearing support stockings to prevent venous pooling.

Heat exhaustion

Heat exhaustion is a reversible condition of heat overload, and may be a precursor of heatstroke. By definition, the core temperature is less than 40°C and gross changes in neurological or mental status are absent. The clinical picture is characterized by a combination of imprecise symptoms including weakness, fatigue, light-headedness, headache, palpitations, nausea, vomiting, sweating, cramps, flushing and, paradoxically, piloerection (Table 36.4). Armstrong (1987) provides a description of the signs encountered in more advanced cases, and these include tachycardia, hypotension, tachypnoea and syncope, reflecting the volume depletion that contributes to the collapse.

The features that allow differentiation from heatstroke are a core temperature of less than 40°C and an absence of neurological impairment, although telling the two conditions apart can often be difficult. It is perhaps safer to assume that all heat casualties are victims of heatstroke and to treat accordingly until the true diagnosis can be confidently established. On occasions it may only be when the patient has been observed for some time in the emergency department that the distinction can be made. It should be noted that a core temperature of 37°C does not rule out heat illness.

Heat exhaustion arises either where there has been prolonged exposure of an unacclimatized individual to a heat load over several days, or following shorter bouts of heavy exertion. Cardiovascular strain induced by the body's attempt to maintain a thermal setpoint, in conjunction with dehydration and electrolyte depletion, are the main precipitants. Tek & Olshaker (1992) state that two types of heat exhaustion exist, depending on whether the depletion is primarily one of water or salt; however, pure forms of either type are rare and differentiation is irrelevant in the

Table 36.4 Signs and symptoms of heat illness

Condition	Rectal temperature	Signs and symptoms
Heat exhaustion	Less than 40°C	Feeling weak, light-headedness, dizziness, nausea, headache, cramps. Ataxia, disorientation, profuse sweating, tachycardia, tachypnoea, vomiting, vasodilatation, syncope
Heatstroke	Over 40°C	As above
		Confusion, irritability, coma. Rising rectal temperature

prehospital environment. Were laboratory testing available it would confirm abnormalities of sodium, chloride, magnesium and potassium, the precise nature and magnitude of which would depend on which fluid, if any, had been used for rehydration.

Once heatstroke has been definitively ruled out, treatment consists of removing the patient from the heat to a cooler location and administering fluids. Most will recover with cool oral fluids alone, given at a rate of 1 litre h^{-1} over several hours, but where vital signs are altered intravenous administration of a crystalloid solution should be started promptly. Cooling by evaporation, using a spray of lukewarm water supplemented by a fan to increase the rate of convection, will help to aid recovery. Additional cooling methods are detailed below. All but the most mild cases should be transported immediately to hospital and admitted for a minimum observation period of 24h. This will allow monitoring for developing rhabdomyolysis, renal and cardiovascular complications. Under no circumstances should an apparently recovered individual be permitted to recommence activity.

MAJOR HEAT ILLNESS

Heatstroke

Heatstroke is a potentially fatal disorder and represents the severe end of the heat illness spectrum. It can occur in those working or exercising in high ambient temperatures, or in less extreme conditions where the process of acclimatization is incomplete and the workload has been extreme. The mortality rate is estimated at 10%, although this rises considerably where a temperature of 39°C or more is allowed to persist (Horowitz 1989). Heatstroke may be defined as heat-induced illness exhibiting the combination of acute neurological impairment with hyperthermia.

Heatstroke has been classified into classical and exertional patterns, with the former occurring during heatwaves in children, the infirm and the elderly. It is caused by increased exogenous heat gain combined with reduced heat dispersal. The exertional pattern, by comparison, affects a younger age group and is associated with increased endogenous heat produced by skeletal muscle activity.

History

It is important to ask about the circumstances surrounding the collapse, any alteration of consciousness, prescribed or recreational drug use, and what treatment if any has been given thus far. Knowledge of the past medical history may allow diagnosis of conditions that might otherwise be missed in the initial assessment, e.g. hyperthyroidism. If any significant degree of alteration to the mental status is present, relatives or ambulance personnel may be better placed to provide this information.

Examination

The initial assessment will often reveal tachycardia, hypotension and tachypnoea. The core temperature should be measured rectally and is often found to be in excess of 40°C, although it may be lower if bystanders or medical personnel have instigated cooling. A temperature reading of less than 40°C should not deter one from making the diagnosis of heatstroke.

Unsteadiness is an early expression of CNS problems, and may progress to altered levels of consciousness, confusion, irritability and combative behaviour, with fitting, decorticate posturing and coma in more advanced cases. An AVPU score should be taken as a baseline against which further change can be compared.

Classically, patients with heatstroke have been described as having hot, dry skin as a result of shock causing vasoconstriction. While this may indeed be a feature it is by no means invariable, and the presence of sweating is an unreliable indicator to exclude heatstroke.

The presence of sweating does not exclude a diagnosis of heatstroke.

A short differential diagnosis of heatstroke is given in Table 36.5.

Assessment

It is vital to have an accurate measurement of core temperature and under field conditions a compromise must be reached between accuracy and convenience. It is recommended that rectal measurement is the most suitable for use in the field and problems of modesty should not deter its use. Sheets or clothing can be used to afford some degree of privacy while taking a reading. Serial measurements

Table 36.5 Differential diagnosis of heatstroke

- Heat exhaustion
- Sepsis
- Malaria
- Meningitis/encephalitis
- Brain abscess
- Fits from any cause
- Drug overdose
- Cerebrovascular accident
- Psychosis
- Hyperthyroid storm
- Malignant hyperthermia

of rectal temperature, pulse and blood pressure give a useful guide to the success or otherwise of the treatment. Hypotension is associated with a poor outcome, as it may herald profound circulatory collapse. Where pulse oximetry and electrocardiogram (ECG) monitoring are available, they provide useful corroboration of the clinical findings.

Cooling techniques

There has been extensive debate about the most appropriate and effective method of lowering body temperature, with much of the work being performed on animal models. Outside of hospital, available methods include evaporation and fanning, strategic placing of ice packs and immersion. Evaporation and convection using a fine mist delivered from hand-held sprays (such as are used to water household plants) combined with fanning allows easy access to the patient so that monitoring can continue. Harker & Gibson (1995) reviewed several methods, concluding that evaporative cooling is the most efficient. A highly developed form of this technique has been employed by Weiner & Khagali (1980), who developed the Makkah Body Cooling Unit to provide immediate care to pilgrims adversely affected by the heat. Care must be taken when cooling the body not to *actively* reduce the rectal temperature to below 38°C: Ash et al (1992) have shown an incidence of 33% overcooling because of marked rectal temperature lag during periods of rapid cooling.

Any transport should ideally be air-conditioned or at least well ventilated, and it may be necessary to ensure that the doors of a vehicle or helicopter are held open.

Treatment

The overriding principle in the management of heatstroke is cooling concurrent with resuscitation. This means attending to the usual priorities of airway, breathing and circulation but at the same time ensuring that aggressive measures to normalize the body temperature are commenced. Horowitz (1989) applies the concept of the 'golden hour' to heatstroke, with prognosis being directly related to the duration of the hyperpyrexia.

Many prehospital personnel are unfamiliar with the cooling methods employed and the rate of temperature reduction that should be aimed for, therefore it is important to have protocols or guidelines in place.

RESUSCITATION

The casualty should be removed from the heat to an area of shade, or if available an air-conditioned room, and cooling procedures started immediately. As discussed previously, the standard principles of ABC apply, and supplemental oxygen should be given via a mask with reservoir bag.

One or two large-gauge cannulas are used to gain circulatory access, and fluid resuscitation is commenced with normal saline or Hartmann's solution, as opposed to a colloid preparation. Shapiro & Seidman (1990) advise administrating 2l over the first hour followed by $1\,lh^{-1}$ over the next 3h. Other workers contend that because of the risk of pulmonary oedema a total of only 1–2l should be given. In the author's experience with a military population, young, fit adults generally tolerate the fluid load without difficulty. This does not remove the need for careful monitoring, more so in the case of children and the elderly.

The patient is undressed as far as is practicable, sprayed with a fine mist of water and fanned by whatever means is available in order to increase the evaporative heat loss. Ice-packs, such as are used for sports injuries or in picnic hampers, can be placed at strategic points in the groin, axilla and neck, but should be wrapped in cloth first. These should only be regarded as an adjunct to evaporative techniques because used alone they do not produce a sufficiently high rate of cooling. A rate of temperature reduction of 1°C every 10–15 min is ideal.

Fits must be controlled quickly as they will promote a further rise in temperature. Suitable drugs include intravenous lorazepam, or rectal diazepam if intravenous access cannot be obtained.

Complications

The variety of possible complications following heatstroke is an indication of how widespread the tissue injury can be.

CENTRAL NERVOUS SYSTEM

Brain cell injury is directly related to the duration of the thermal insult and results in cerebral oedema, convulsions and coma. Delaney (1992) observed that coma persisting for more than 3 h is associated with a poor prognosis. Common clinical features include confusion, agitation and delirium, which may then progress to loss of consciousness, decerebrate rigidity, hemiplegia and late parkinsonism. Constricted pupils and loss of rectal tone have also been described. While recovery is usual, hemiparesis, ataxia due to cerebellar atrophy and memory loss may persist.

CARDIOVASCULAR SYSTEM

Hubbard et al (1995) outline the cardiovascular changes seen with thermal stress: sinus tachycardia is almost invariable, with blood pressure being maintained within normal limits up to the point where the rectal temperature exceeds 41°C. After this the diastolic pressure begins to drop, advancing later to hypotension and frank shock. Abnormalities of conduction and disturbance of the ST segment and T wave may be seen on the ECG tracing. While heart failure, cardiovascular collapse and pulmonary oedema can accompany heatstroke in any age group, the elderly are especially prone. Garcia-Rubira et al (1995) give an account of acute myocardial infarction with diffuse myocardial damage in a man aged 33 years.

RESPIRATORY SYSTEM

Aspiration, carpopedal spasm as a result of hyperventilation, and adult respiratory distress syndrome (ARDS) have all been described (El-Kassimi 1986).

LIVER

Cellular damage to the liver may almost be considered a diagnostic feature of heatstroke. Centrilobular necrosis is seen 12–24 h after the initial event and is manifested by increases in aspartate transaminase (AST), alanine aminotransferase (ALT) and bilirubin, although frank jaundice is rare. An estimated 10% proceed to liver failure, with death superseding some 2 weeks later unless a liver transplant is performed. Thus, while hepatic complications are not often encountered in the prehospital setting, the inherent risk alone is a potent reason to admit even seemingly normal cases for a period of observation.

RENAL SYSTEM

Hassanein et al (1992) suggest that acute renal failure is seen in 25% of patients with exertional heatstroke and in 5% of those with the non-exertional variety. Severe rhabdomyolysis and decreased renal blood flow are thought to be the chief precipitants. Rhabdomyolysis is secondary to the release of myoglobin and other cellular contents into the circulation, which follows heat injury to skeletal muscle. Haematuria and proteinuria can be detected on urinalysis at an early stage, whereas the dark urine of myoglobinuria is sometimes a late presenting feature in apparently recovered individuals who give a history of recent severe exertion or exposure to heat.

GASTROINTESTINAL SYSTEM

Constriction of the vascular beds in the gut mesenteries produces areas of mucosal necrosis. This in turn leads to vomiting and diarrhoea, with haematemesis and melaena supervening when disseminated intravascular coagulation has ensued.

HAEMATOLOGICAL

Disseminated intravascular coagulation is a significant cause of mortality that presents approximately 12–36 h after the acute phase. The presence of hypovolaemic shock and rectal temperatures over 41°C increase the likelihood of this complication.

Prevention

EDUCATION AND AWARENESS

The chances of developing heat-related illness can be lessened by acclimatization, maintaining a good level of cardiovascular fitness, adequate hydration and the wearing of appropriate clothing. Athletics coaches, referees and military instructors in charge of recruits need to be familiar with these issues, along with any local guidelines, so that they may advise on suitable levels of exercise for a given degree of thermal stress. Attention must be paid to provision of rest and water breaks, and the activity may be safer if rescheduled to a cooler time of the day. Where an event with numerous participants is being organized, medical packs and equipment should be readily available. This will include intravenous and oral fluids, ice-packs, fans and perhaps a child's paddling pool where immersion can be carried out. Prior arrangements for emergency transportation should be in place and supervising staff should be familiar with these.

IDENTIFICATION OF SUSCEPTIBLE INDIVIDUALS

Some individuals appear to be more susceptible to heat than others but it is unclear whether this represents the expression of a predisposing factor or is due to a residual heat injury. Bourdon & Canini (1995) contend that heatstroke is associated with an inherited abnormality of skeletal muscle that is similar to malignant hyperpyrexia. Epstein (1990) recommends that those subjects who have experienced an episode of heatstroke should have their heat tolerance tested 8–12 weeks later in order to detect any residual impairment to thermoregulation. In the interim they should avoid strenuous activity. Armstrong et al (1990) found that recovery from heatstroke was idiosyncratic, taking up to 1 year, and that it was not uncommon for unusually high levels of creatinine phosphokinase to occur on subsequent exposure to heat.

RECOGNITION OF RISK FACTORS

Endogenous heat is of greater importance than the ambient temperature, although hot conditions render exercise-induced heat harder to dissipate. Any conditions that reduce the ability to sweat, cause excess heat production or dehydration will place an individual at increased risk. These have been outlined in Table 36.3.

Hydration

The subject should commence work or exercise in a well hydrated state, as prior dehydration has a detrimental effect on heat tolerance, even on low-intensity training where sweat loss appears to be minimal. Terrados & Maughan (1995) suggest that when the duration of work is in excess of 40 min there should be a regular fluid intake. This should take place on a fixed time schedule regardless of thirst as ad libitum drinking alone results in significant dehydration.

Guidelines include consuming 500 ml of fluid 2 h prior to exertion, followed by another 500 ml 15 min before starting. This is supplemented by 100–200 ml aliquots every 15 min during exercise. Cool water is the most suitable fluid, although some sources advise a carbohydrate/electrolyte-containing sports drink. White & Ford (1983) found that sports drinks aid hydration because of their enhanced palatability; although in terms of maintaining the plasma volume there is little to choose between them and water. Reluctance to drink tepid, chemically purified water can result in significant dehydration.

Manipulation of environment

The Centers for Disease Control and Prevention (1994) recommends the use of air-conditioning and fans as protective measures and encourage taking advantage of other air-conditioned areas such as shopping malls, etc. Cool baths may also be helpful.

Table 36.6 Heat stress index

Temperature (°C)	Restriction on activity
< 24	Activities may proceed, but remain vigilant for early signs of heat illness
24.0–25.9	Rest periods needed Water stops every 15 min
26–29	No activity for unacclimatized or at-risk individuals. Others need to be carefully monitored
> 29	No unnecessary activities should take place

Appropriate clothing

Clothing should be lightweight and single-layer, with the ability to 'wick' sweat away from the skin. The greater the area of skin exposed the greater the potential for evaporation. This applies particularly to the head, which can account for almost 40% of the evaporative loss. Firefighters and the military may require full encapsulation in protective clothing. Montain et al (1994) have shown that under these conditions exhaustion is reached at a lower core temperature.

Fitness and apposite exercise regimes

Bannister (1989) in a letter to *The Times*, stated 'The notion that courage and esprit de corps can somehow defeat the principles of physiology is not only wrong but dangerously wrong; lives can quite needlessly be lost and survivors be left with permanent brain damage'. Relatively safe levels of exercise can be estimated from the wet bulb globe temperature (WBGT), which is an index of environmental heat stress incorporating measures of the ambient temperature, humidity and solar radiation. Hubbard et al (1995) present a suggestion for activity levels based on the heat stress index or WGBT (Table 36.6). Such recommendations are guidelines at best, and in extreme conditions neither acclimatization nor attention to fluid replacement can entirely eliminate the risk of developing heat illness.

References

Armstrong LE 1987 Signs and symptoms of heat exhaustion during strenuous exercise. Annals of Sports Medicine 3: 182

Armstrong LE, De Luca JP, Hubbard RW 1990 Time course of recovery and heat acclimation of prior exertional heatstroke patients. Medicine and Science in Sports and Exercise 22: 36–48

Ash CJ, Cook JR, McMurray TA, Auner CR 1992 The use of rectal temperature to monitor heat stroke. Missouri Medicine 89: 283–288

Bannister 1989 Letter to The Times

Bourdon L, Canini F 1995 On the nature of the link between malignant hyperthermia and exertional heatstroke. Medical Hypotheses 45: 268–270

Centers for Disease Control and Prevention 1994 Heat-related deaths – Philadelphia and United States, 1993–1994. Journal of the American Medical Association 272: 1

Delaney KA 1992 Heatstroke. Underlying processes and lifesaving management. Postgraduate Medicine 91: 379–388

Dickinson JG 1994 Heat illness in the services. Journal of the Royal Army Medical Corps 140: 7–12

El-Kassimi FA 1986 Adult respiratory distress syndrome and disseminated intravascular coagulation complicating heat stroke. Chest 90: 571

Epstein Y 1990 Heat intolerance: predisposing factor or residual injury? Medicine and Science in Sports and Exercise 22: 29–35

Garcia-Rubira JC, Aguilar J, Romero D 1995 Acute myocardial infarction in a young man after heat exhaustion. International Journal of Cardiology 47: 297–300

Harker J, Gibson P 1995 Heatstroke: a review of rapid cooling techniques. Intensive Critical Care Nursing 11: 198–202

Hassanein T, Razack A, Gavaler JS, van Thiel DH 1992 Heatstroke: its clinical and pathological presentation. American Journal of Gastroenterology 87: 1382–1389

Horowitz M 1986 Heat acclimation: cardiac performances of isolated rat heart. Journal of Applied Physiology 60: 9

Horowitz BZ 1989 The Golden Hour in heatstroke: use of iced peritoneal lavage. American Journal of Emergency Medicine 7: 616–619

Hubbard WH, Gaffin SL, Squire DL 1995 Heat-related illness. In: Auerbach PS (ed) Wilderness medicine. Mosby, St Louis, MO, p 167–212

Knochel JP, Reed G 1987 Disorders of heat regulation. In: Kleeman CR, Maxwell MH, Narin RG (eds) Clinical disorders of fluid and electrolyte metabolism. McGraw-Hill, New York

Montain SJ, Sawka MN, Cadarette BS et al 1994 Physiological tolerance to uncompensatable heat stress: effects of exercise intensity, protective clothing and climate. Journal of Applied Physiology 77: 216–222

Shapiro Y, Seidman OS 1990 Field and clinical observations of exertional heat stroke patients. Medicine and Science in Sports and Exercise 22: 6–14

Tek D, Olshaker JS 1992 Heat illness. Emergency Medicine Clinics of North America 10: 299–310

Terrados N, Maughan RJ 1995 Exercise in the heat: strategies to minimize adverse effects on performance. Journal of Sports Sciences 13: S55–S62

Weiner J, Khagali M 1980 A physiological body-cooling unit for treatment of heat stroke. Lancet 1: 507–509

White J, Ford MA 1983 The hydration and electrolyte maintenance properties of an experimental sports drink. British Journal of Sports Medicine 17: 51–58

Further reading

Froom P, Caine Y, Shochat I, Ribak J 1993 Heat stress and helicopter pilot errors. Journal of Occupational Medicine 37: 720–724

Ganong FG 1995 Review of Medical Physiology. Appleton & Lange, Stamford, CT

Havenith G, Inoue Y, Luttibolt V, Kenney WL 1995 Age predicts cardiovascular, but not thermoregulatory responses to humid heat stress. European Journal of Applied Physiology and Occupational Physiology 70: 88–96

Ohtsuka Y, Yabunaka N, Watanabe I et al 1995 Thermal stress and diabetic complications. International Journal of Biometeorology 38: 57–59

Pascoe DD, Shanley LA, Smith EW 1994 Clothing and exercise: biophysics of heat transfer between the individual, clothing and environment. Sports Medicine 18: 38–54

Acute diving emergencies

37

Introduction   398

Physiology and physics   398

Diving emergencies   399

Acute decompression illness   400

References   404

Introduction

This chapter is designed to be a basic introduction to some of the diving problems that may be encountered by a prehospital care physician, and is not intended to be a definitive diving text (for a definitive diving text see Bennett & Elliott 1993). Little information is given regarding saturation diving problems, as these dives tend to be undertaken under professional conditions where experienced medical cover is usually available.

Diving is an increasingly popular sport within the UK and like any sport it has associated injuries and dangers. It is estimated that there are 50 000 sports divers in the UK (Jagger & Jackson 1997). The British Sub Aqua Club, which is only one of many sports diving associations, reported 16 fatalities in 1997 (British Sub Aqua Club 1997). The Institute of Naval Medicine, which runs an acute decompression illness database, reports an average of more than 100 cases a year (Surgeon Commander Benton, personal communication). The majority of serious accidents require treatment in the prehospital phase but a significant proportion of more minor conditions present directly to emergency departments or general practitioners.

Diving problems can be broadly divided into the following groups:

- Physical injury (unrelated to the diving process)
- Hypothermia
- Near-drowning
- Barotrauma
- Acute decompression illness
- Nitrogen narcosis
- Oxygen toxicity
- Infections.

The first three problems are considered elsewhere in this book and are therefore not covered in this chapter.

Physiology and physics

In order to understand the pathology of diving problems it is essential to understand the physiology and physics that accompany diving.

Air is composed of approximately 21% oxygen, 79% nitrogen and 0.03% carbon dioxide. Each of these gases exerts a partial pressure in proportion to their percentage concentration.

At sea level the air exerts a pressure of 1 atmosphere, which is equal to approximately 100 kPa. Water is considerably more dense than air and consequently a depth of only 10 m of water exerts the same pressure as the entire atmosphere of air at sea level. A diver at a depth of 10 m is thus subject to a pressure of 2 atmospheres; on diving

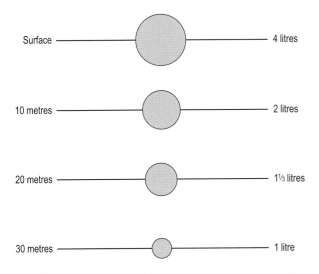

Surface ———————————— 4 litres

10 metres ———————————— 2 litres

20 metres ———————————— 1⅓ litres

30 metres ———————————— 1 litre

Fig. 37.1 • Volume of a bubble of air as it rises to the surface.

deeper to a depth of 20 m the diver is subjected to a pressure of 3 atmospheres.

It is important to appreciate the relationship between volume and pressure of a gas, as expressed in Boyle's law, in which volume (V) is inversely proportional to pressure (P)

$$V \propto 1/P.$$

The practical effect of this pressure and volume relationship is to reduce the volume occupied by a gas on increasing the depth of diving and, conversely, to increase the volume on returning to the surface. If divers take a breath on the surface and then dive to a depth of 10 m, the volume of air in their lungs would be reduced to half its volume on the surface as a result of the pressure having doubled. From Fig. 37.1 it can be appreciated that the largest changes in volume occur within the first 10 m.

Divers breathe air at a pressure equal to that of their depth, the volume of each breath remaining unchanged by the pressure change, this being delivered by a device known as the regulator. Having filled their lungs from this compressed air supply, while at a depth of 10 m, divers will double the volume of air in their lungs on returning to the surface, unless exhalation occurs on ascent.

The fact that the diver is breathing gas at a higher pressure brings into play another of the gas laws, namely Henry's law. This law relates to the solubility of gases in a fluid. The diver will increase the amount of nitrogen dissolved in the blood and tissue fluids as the pressure increases. This will come out of solution on return to the surface as the pressure is decreased.

Diving emergencies

BAROTRAUMA

Barotrauma, or the trauma produced directly by pressure, can occur on either ascent or descent and affects rigid-walled, air-filled body cavities, e.g. the lung, middle ear, facial sinuses and tooth cavities.

Descent

As the diver begins to descend, pressure is exerted by the water on gas-containing spaces, resulting in a 'squeeze' effect. From the physiology discussed above, it will be appreciated that this problem will predominantly occur near the surface, where the greatest changes in volume occur. This squeeze is noted particular in the middle ear, causing pressure on the ear drum. The squeeze can be prevented by equalizing the difference across the drum by 'clearing the ears', which involves either swallowing or performing a Valsalva manoeuvre. Difficulty with this manoeuvre can occur if the eustachian tube is obstructed by mucosal congestion, as occurs with a 'cold'. If equalization is not possible then damage to the tympanic membrane occurs, which may initially be limited to haematoma formation but can eventually result in rupture of the drum. The inpouring of cold water can then cause severe (calorific) vertigo.

Sudden severe pressure changes between the middle and inner ear can result in rupture of the round or oval windows. This results in a sensorineural hearing deficit and vestibular dysfunction. A useful guide to aid diagnosis is a clear history as to the onset of signs and symptoms, namely during descent, on arrival at the bottom, on ascent or following arrival at the surface. This history is particularly relevant, as mechanical damage to the middle and inner ear can mimic true acute decompression illness. A patient presenting with barotrauma to the ear will usually have abandoned the dive on the descent because of his/her symptoms.

Barotrauma on descent, without rupture of the tympanic membrane, will result in erythema and possible haemorrhage into the drum and mucosal oedema. This can be treated with decongestants and avoidance of diving until symptoms have fully resolved, which usually takes some 2 weeks. Antibiotics should be considered if there is a past history of otitis externa or concern that the water was significantly polluted. If tympanic rupture has occurred, antibiotics are required and referral to an ear, nose and throat clinic is appropriate. Damage to either the oval or the round window requires urgent ENT referral.

Barotrauma on descent can occur at other sites such as the nasal sinuses, where mucosal congestion results in air-trapping. In this case the diver may develop a sudden epistaxis and complain of tooth pain.

Another problem that can occur on descent is 'mask squeeze' due to the diver failing to equalize the pressure between the facemask and the outside water pressure. This is normally achieved by periodically exhaling through the nose into the mask. Mask squeeze results in erythema, bruising and petechial haemorrhage to the face and conjunctiva, but is primarily a cosmetic problem and requires no treatment.

Ascent

Barotrauma of ascent is in essence the reverse problem of squeeze: as the diver returns to the surface the volume of gas in the air-containing areas increases. This should not cause a problem if the diver ascends slowly, breathing out on the way. If, however, the diver ascends rapidly and fails to exhale then sudden and dramatic increases in volume can cause a variety of problems.

Expansion in the middle ears does not normally cause a problem as the increased volume is vented through the eustachian tubes, which if obstructed will have caused problems on descent likely to have prevented the dive. Occasionally a problem will occur if the diver has taken a decongestant the effect of which has worn off by the time the diver is ready to ascend. In this case the drum can rupture as a result of expansion of the air in the middle ear.

The rapid expansion of air within the lungs can be associated with pulmonary barotrauma. This condition may be asymptomatic or the individual may develop symptoms very rapidly. This condition is more likely to develop in an individual who suffers from asthma or other conditions in which air-trapping occurs. The patient is likely to develop a cough with the production of frothy red sputum and with signs of surgical emphysema (usually felt in the neck) appearing over a short period of time. A pneumothorax may develop. If this has developed during ascent it may present as a tension pneumothorax on arriving at the surface due to rapid gas expansion in the final stages of ascent. The treatment of this condition is administration of oxygen and drainage of the associated pneumothorax. In the extreme case this may require needle decompression through the second intercostal space. The patient then requires transfer to a suitable facility, as there may be an associated decompression illness problem. It is vital that the patient has a thorough neurological examination to determine the involvement of other systems.

The most dramatic complication of pulmonary barotrauma is the development of an arterial gas embolism affecting the brain. In accidents that involve a cerebral arterial gas embolus, there is evidence that 5% of the divers die on, or shortly after, arrival at the surface, 60% will experience a neurological deficit followed by some spontaneous recovery but are highly likely to relapse and 35% have a sustained or deteriorating neurological deficit (Gorman 1990). Such an event will result in the development of unilateral signs that are the same as a stroke but are usually associated with unconsciousness. The arterial gas embolism can involve other sites and produce cardiopulmonary arrest. The treatment of this extreme condition is identical to that for any electromechanical dissociation arrest together with urgent transfer to a suitable hyperbaric facility.

Acute decompression illness

BACKGROUND

The term acute decompression illness (DCI) tends to cause considerable confusion. This probably relates to the fact that the term was previously divided into a number of separate categories:

● type I or mild, which relates to limb or cutaneous bends where there is no neurological deficit
● type II or serious, where there is neurological, respiratory, gastrointestinal or cardiac signs and symptoms.

This is further compounded by lay terminology such as bends, hits and staggers, which are used by divers themselves to describe their illness. To a large degree it is now accepted that this division is artificial, as any evidence of minor manifestations does not exclude a more significant problem and neurological injury may be 'silent' (Palmer et al 1981, Polkinghorne 1998). On the basis of this concept of acute decompression illness, it is appropriate to refer all suspected cases to a hyperbaric facility.

The majority of patients who present with symptoms of acute decompression illness develop them rapidly, with 50% occurring within 10 min and 85% by 1 h (Francis & Pearson 1988). It is accepted that presentation can be delayed, and we have experience of a presentation at more than 36 h. It should also be appreciated that some divers are initially reluctant to admit symptoms as they feel it reflects badly on their abilities as a diver. This attitude is only slowly changing as education in clubs informs divers that the development of decompression illness does not automatically imply that a 'mistake' has been made. Honesty in relation to the dive profile should be encouraged. Diagnosis should be based on a through clinical examination. The diagnosis cannot be excluded on the grounds that the patient has not deviated from the correct diving practice. The database held at the Institute of Naval Medicine supports the proposition that at least 10% of recorded incidents of DCI are from 'non-provocative' dives.

PREDISPOSING FACTORS

There are a number of factors that are not supported by an evidence-based approach but which, on theoretical grounds and empirical experience, are thought to increase the risk of development of acute decompression illness. Many of these factors result in reduced tissue perfusion and, hence, dissolved gas being able to leave tissues less quickly on ascent.

The following are associated with an increased risk of development of decompression illness:

- Lack of physical fitness – this probably relates to tissue perfusion during exercise
- Low water temperature – because of decreased tissue perfusion and increased solubility of gas at lower temperatures
- Increased physical exertion – this increases uptake of nitrogen by muscles when at depth; on the surface this can result in supersaturation of the blood returning from muscles
- Obesity – fat is a nitrogen-absorbing material
- Females – probably as a result of having a higher proportion of body fat
- Increasing age – this is probably related to poorer tissue perfusion
- Injuries – probably as a result of local changes in blood flow
- Dive profile – the type and depth of the dive and the speed of ascent
- Recurrent dives – repeat dives before the tissues have fully desaturated increases the tissue loading of nitrogen
- Increasing altitude – the higher the altitude the lower the air pressure and, hence, the greater the pressure change on surfacing
- Dehydration – reduced hydration results in reduced tissue perfusion and, hence, the elimination of nitrogen
- Alcohol – acutely affects judgement and causes skin vasodilatation with cooling. The hangover effect causes dehydration.

Of all these factors, recurrent dives appears to be the most significant, and there is some evidence base for this as a cause of acute decompression illness.

PATHOPHYSIOLOGY

When a diver descends the increase in pressure of the inspired air and, hence, the partial pressure of nitrogen causes more nitrogen to be absorbed into the blood from the alveoli (Henry's law). This nitrogen is then taken up by different tissues, at varying rates and to varying degrees, depending on the blood flow to that tissue and its composition. Some tissues take up nitrogen rapidly but are only able to absorb limited amounts. Other tissues take up nitrogen slowly but are able to absorb a greater amount (e.g. fatty tissue). Gas uptake is measured in half-lives relating to *theoretical* tissue compartments representing various tissue such as blood, muscle, fat and bone. In acute decompression illness it is this nitrogen, which has been absorbed into the tissues while under pressure, being released suddenly when the pressure is reduced on rapid ascent that results in the conditions encountered. In simplistic terms, this can be visualized as a shaken bottle of fizzy drink having its cap released suddenly. The gas dissolved in the drink is suddenly forced out of solution by the pressure reduction. Bubbles appear within the drink, causing it to fizz (and froth out of the bottle). Slow release of the bottle cap enables a gradual change of pressure and a slow release of gas from the drink without the frothing.

On a normal ascent, as the pressure reduces, nitrogen is released from the tissues: this process is referred to as *decompression*. The speed of this release, like uptake, depends on the blood flow and the type of tissue. This nitrogen is then released in the lungs. If ascent is slow there is sufficient time for nitrogen to be released without undue problems, although it must be appreciated that nitrogen continues to be released for hours after the dive, hence the problems that can occur with recurrent dives. During this off-loading phase a reduction in atmospheric pressure (e.g. flying) significantly increases the likelihood of clinical decompression illness. There are many recorded incidents of patients presenting to their emergency department on return from a diving holiday with symptoms that have developed in the aircraft on the flight home.

If the rate of ascent is too great for the nitrogen load that has accumulated during the dive, the blood flow is insufficient to remove the nitrogen being released from the tissues. The result is the formation of a gas phase. It should be appreciated that bubbles should not form in the arterial limb of the circulation as the blood has just passed through the lungs and therefore equilibrated with the ambient partial pressure. The arterial pressure also makes the formation of a gas phase highly unlikely (unless horrendously fast depressurization occurs, which will be fatal).

Bubbles develop in the venous limb of the circulation as the tissues release nitrogen. Some degree of bubble formation is thought to occur in all divers but no symptoms are suffered as these bubbles are filtered by the lungs. It is now thought (Wilmshurst 1997) that the development of cerebral decompression illness requires that there must be a right to left shunt. It is recognized that up to 25% of individuals have a minor patent foramen ovale, which under normal circumstances is asymptomatic but is a route for bubble transfer. Of the 25% of the population with a patent foramen ovale, there is good evidence that only 5% have haemodynamically significant communication, thus reducing the percentage population at risk. A small degree of left to right shunting is also thought to occur in the lungs between the pulmonary and systemic supplies (Francis 1990).

Once a bubble has passed into the arterial limb it will act as an embolus, with the potential to block small vessels. The contact of the bubble with the endothelium of the vessel causes damage, resulting in activation of the clotting mechanism and loss of the blood–brain barrier. In patients who are symptomatic with acute decompression illness there is evidence of complement activation. Thus, although the bubble itself may be rapidly reabsorbed, damage will already have been caused. It may be wondered as to how hyperbaric treatment is of benefit in this situation. The answer almost certainly relates to the increased oxygen carriage. At 2.8 atmospheres, sufficient oxygen is carried dissolved in the blood to enable survival in the absence of haemoglobin! Oxygen is able to be delivered to 'hypoxic' areas of the brain by diffusion through tissue fluid due to the greatly increased oxygen gradient and the improved solubility (this also explains some of the other uses for hyperbaric oxygen therapy). At 3 atmospheres, the diffusing distance of oxygen at the arterial end of a capillary is increased fourfold, and at the venous end is increased twofold. Furthermore, oxygen breathing facilitates the wash-out of nitrogen, thereby reducing the potential for microemboli to collide, coalesce and subsequently develop to a clinically significant gas phase.

Nitrogen bubbles can also occur in situ in tissues and are referred to as 'autochthonous' bubbles (although it is accepted that this is controversial (Francis, 1990)), the most hazardous location being the white matter of the spinal cord. The myelin sheath is able to absorb large amounts of nitrogen and hence bubbles can occur at this site on sudden depressurization. As pressure is reduced these bubbles expand and cause pressure in the cord because that there is little room for expansion, the cord being encased in the rigid structure of the spinal column. This pressure results in reduction of blood flow, initially by compressing the venous return. These bubbles reduce in size when repressurization occurs in a hyperbaric facility. It should also be appreciated that damage to the spinal cord can, and almost certainly does, occur from microemboli in the same way as cerebral damage occurs.

Nitrogen bubbles can occur in other tissues, resulting in pain, alterations in blood flow and restriction of lymph drainage. The classical joint pain that is associated with the bends is thought probably to be related to bubble formation in the subperiosteal tissue, ligaments and joint capsule rather than to gas in the joint space (Edmonds et al 1992).

CLINICAL FEATURES

The geographical location and the type of diving may have a functional relationship with the manifestation and outcome of acute decompression illness; as a consequence different textbooks may show a variation in the presentation of the disease. Relevant data are given in Table 37.1.

The most commonly described symptoms are those of general lethargy, weakness and apathy. Symptoms may be more specific, with the development of a specific site of pain or numbness or more severe neurological symptoms.

Musculoskeletal

Pain may be confined to a single joint. This is usually initially ill defined and may be described as numbness.

Table 37.1 Clinical presentation of acute decompression illness

	N	%
Cases	**1422**	
Male	1199	
Female	202	
Unknown	21	
General category – signs and symptoms		
Sensory abnormality	545	
Weakness	266	
Altered level of consciousness	24	
Higher function	139	
Sphincter abnormality	38	
Manifestations		
Neurological	721	78
Limb pain	454	49
Constitutional malaise undue fatigue	248	26.8
Skin	86	9.3
Pulmonary	36	3.9
Lymphatic	8	0.9
Girdle/back pain	23	2.5
Other	3	
Number of manifestations		
Limb pain only	10	
Patient with single manifestation	445	49
Patient with two manifestations	299	32.5
Patient with three manifestations	135	14.8
Patient with four manifestations	33	3.7
Patient with five manifestations	3	0.3

Source: reprinted with permission from the database of the British Hyperbaric Association, run by the Royal Navy Institute of Naval Medicine – data as of 25 September 1997

Over several hours the discomfort progresses to a constant pain. Movement of the joint may become limited. It is not unusual for these symptoms to be attributed to 'sustaining an injury on getting into the boat'.

Cerebral

The signs and symptoms depend on the site of the vascular lesion, which is normally multifocal, hence the disease is often described as being disseminated. Symptoms tend to be similar to a cerebrovascular accident (CVA) but affecting multiple sites. Thus, the patient can have loss of motor or sensory function affecting a single limb or multiple limbs. Other presentations include headaches and confusion.

Cerebellar

If the cerebellum is affected the patient will present with symptoms similar to those of a cerebellar CVA: unsteadiness, loss of coordination, dysarthria and nystagmus.

Spinal

The patient usually complains of spinal or girdle pain initially and then may develop tingling and numbness in the lower limbs before developing more disturbing symptoms of paraplegia. These patients are at significant risk of developing urinary retention, and attention to the treatment of this condition is required early.

Inner ear

This is rare in scuba diving and is usually only seen in relation to helium dives. The symptoms are those of vertigo and hearing deficit, and are therefore easy to misinterpret as barotrauma to the ear.

Peripheral nerves

The patient presents with numbness, tingling and occasionally motor weakness. The distribution can be patchy or glove and stocking. Major nerve plexuses may be involved. It is important to distinguish between peripheral and incomplete spinal lesions, the former having a better prognosis.

Skin

Pruritus and a rash can occur, the rash usually being red and punctate and distributed over the trunk. Red papules, plaques or pale areas with cyanotic mottling also occur. Lymphatic obstruction may cause local swelling.

The chokes

This is the result of nitrogen bubbles forming in the pulmonary capillary beds, interfering with gaseous exchange and leading to areas of reduced perfusion, which in turn lead to pulmonary oedema and reduced lung compliance. An adult respiratory distress (ARDS)-type picture can develop.

Local ischaemia

As in the case of cerebral DCI, bubble formation in the arterial limb of the circulation can cause obstruction to the blood supply to other organs, resulting in damage to the spleen, kidney, gastrointestinal tract or heart. Damage to the myoneural conducting system of the heart can also occur.

TREATMENT

The most important role of the prehospital doctor in the management of acute decompression illness is to suspect the diagnosis. During assessment and treatment the ABCDE approach is followed, as for any acute resuscitation.

- All divers suspected of suffering with symptoms of acute decompression illness should be treated with high-concentration oxygen via a mask with a reservoir bag. It should be noted that symptoms may initially appear to get worse (possibly related to diffusion of oxygen into nitrogen bubbles, increasing their size). Oxygen therapy improves hypoxic areas and aids nitrogen offloading. Although symptoms can improve while breathing atmospheric oxygen, this is not an appropriate treatment and simply reflects the waxing and waning seen in the disease process. Previous suggestions as to the positioning of the patient are now thought to be unhelpful, and the head-down position is contraindicated as it increases intracranial pressure, worsening cerebral hypoxia. Any other resuscitative measures that may be required should also be instigated.

- Fluids should be given intravenously or orally depending on the level of consciousness. It is well recognized that immersion, cold-induced diuresis and the fluid shunting that occurs with hypothermia all contribute to an overall state of volume depletion.

- Analgesia is contraindicated as it masks the development of clinical signs. Entonox is absolutely contraindicated as nitrous oxide has a rapid diffusion rate, diffusing into nitrogen bubbles and increasing their size.

- Any diver who is suspected of suffering from decompression symptoms should be rapidly transferred to a suitable hyperbaric facility, which must be hospital-based and staffed by suitably trained individuals, including medical staff trained in hyperbaric medicine. The requirements for chambers are laid down in a document produced by the Royal College of Physicians (1994). A suitable treatment centre should comply with the standards for a 'level 1 chamber'. Although there are, or have been, non-hospital-based facilities that offer an excellent service there are also chambers that are wholly inadequate for the task. Information as to where to obtain details of suitable chambers is given in Table 37.2.

Table 37.2

If radio or telephone advice is sought for divers while at sea, a history should be taken, with the name of the vessel and its location, and direct them to contact the Coastguard on VHF channel 16. Your information should also be related to the Coastguard.

- Royal Navy – Institute of Naval Medicine Telephone Advice Line
  Telephone: 0831 151523 or 02392 818888
- Scotland Telephone Advice Line – Aberdeen Royal Infirmary
  Telephone: 0845 408 6008 or 01224 681818 (ask for the duty hyperbaric doctor)
- The Coastguard
  Telephone: 999

- The temptation to recompress the diver by a further descent in water should be avoided. The water is a hostile environment and re-immersing an ill patient with equipment that may be faulty is a recipe for disaster.

Divers normally dive with a 'buddy'. If the buddy has followed a similar dive profile to their partner s/he will also be at risk of developing acute decompression illness, even if s/he currently has no symptoms. It is usually appropriate, therefore, for the buddy to accompany his/her ill colleague. It is also important for the diver's equipment, including the dive computer (if one was used), to follow the diver to the treatment centre in order for it to be examined.

Acute decompression illness is unlikely to be related to an isolated organ or system and should *always* be viewed as a multisystem problem.

NITROGEN NARCOSIS

Nitrogen narcosis is not something that will be seen on the surface but may affect a diver during a dive and result in him/her having an accident that will require medical intervention. Nitrogen narcosis is the result of nitrogen acting in a similar manner to anaesthetic gases, although the effects are most marked on intellectual and cognitive function rather than motor activity. There is no specific depth at which narcosis occurs, but it is not usually apparent at depths of less than 30 m and factors such as fatigue and exercise are important. The risk significantly increases with depth, and it is this that limits the depth of air diving to a maximum of 50 m. For deeper dives other gases are used to replace nitrogen, or its partial pressure is reduced by using nitrox (nitrogen and oxygen mixtures). It should be noted that other 'inert' gases cause narcosis at high partial pressure.

Acute oxygen toxicity

Acute oxygen toxicity affects the central nervous system, resulting in convulsions. This is clearly potentially disastrous during diving.

Acute oxygen toxicity is not normally seen in amateur diving as the partial pressure of oxygen required to cause it is usually in excess of 2 atmospheres, although the length of time of exposure and other factors, such as exercise, form part of the equation. In hyperbaric chambers acute oxygen toxicity is not normally seen until pressures reach 3 atmospheres, but toxicity at 2 atmospheres has been witnessed by the authors. With the advent of so-called 'technical diving' using nitrox or oxygen-enriched air mixtures, by increasing the percentage and thus partial pressure of oxygen it is anticipated that oxygen-induced convulsions will occur during diving, with potentially disastrous consequences.

INFECTIONS

Although individual infections will not be discussed in this section, it is important for physicians to appreciate the potential for such problems. It is an unfortunate fact that most waters in which dives are undertaken are polluted by sewage and human waste. Thus, gastroenteritis, hepatitis A and Weil's disease may all occur in divers.

References

Bennett P, Elliott D 1993 The physiology and medicine of diving, 4th edn. WB Saunders, London

British Sub Aqua Club 1997 Diving incidence report. British Sub Aqua Club, Ellesmere Port, Cheshire

Edmonds C, Lowry, Pennefather J 1992 Diving and subaquatic medicine, 3rd edn. Butterworth-Heinemann, Oxford

Francis, J 1990 Pathophysiology of decompression sickness. In: Diving accident management proceedings, the 41 UHMS Workshop. UHMS PVB 78: 38–57

Francis J, Pearson RR 1988 Central nervous system decompression sickness-latency of 1070 human cases. Undersea Biomedical Research 15: 402–411

Gorman, D 1990 Principles of recompression treatment. In: Diving accident management proceedings, the 41 UHMS Workshop. UHMS PVB 78: 57–69

Jagger RG, Jackson SJ, Jagger DC 1997 In at the deep end: an insight into scuba diving and related dental problems for the GDP. British Dental Journal 184: 209

Palmer AC, Calder IM, McCallum RI 1981 Spinal cord degeneration in a case of recovered spinal decompression sickness. British Medical Journal 283: 888

Polkinghorne PJ, Sehmi K, Cross MR et al 1998 Ocular fundus lesions in divers. Lancet 2: 1381–1383

Royal College of Physicians 1994 Code of good working practice for the operation and staffing of hyperbaric chambers for therapeutic purposes. Royal College of Physicians, London

Wilmshurst P 1997 Brain damaged divers. British Medical Journal 314: 689–690

Electrocution injury

38

Introduction   405

Occurrence   405

Relevant electrical principles   406

Pathophysiology of injury   406

Immediate care in electrical injury   407

Conclusion   409

References   409

Introduction

The frequency of accidental death by electrocution is 0.54 per 100 000 population per year in the USA, where it accounts for approximately 1000 deaths annually (Leibovici et al 1995). The precise incidence in the UK is unclear.

Cardiac arrest from electrical shock or lightning strike is associated with significant mortality and requires prompt, aggressive resuscitation. The majority of victims have associated multisystem involvement including neurological complications, cutaneous and internal thermal injury and secondary blunt trauma. Consequently, a combination of advanced cardiac and advanced trauma life support skills is required if the outcome is to be successful.

In the prehospital arena, application of these skills must occur in an environment that has been made safe; a rescuer's awareness of safety in a situation where electrical injury has occurred is paramount.

This chapter discusses the occurrence of electrocution injury, relevant principles of electricity flow, basic pathophysiology and patterns of injury, practical aspects of scene safety and immediate management.

Occurrence

INDUSTRIAL/OCCUPATIONAL INCIDENTS

Electrocution is the fifth leading cause of fatal occupational injuries among men (Centers for Disease Control 1982), with a fatality rate of 1 per 100 000 workers per year. The highest death rates (10 per 100 000 workers per year) occur amongst utility workers (Jones et al 1991). More than half of job-related electrocutions result from power line contact (electric power linemen suffer an average electrocution rate of 33.4 per 100 000 workers per year; Fish 1993) and a further quarter during the use of electrical tools and machines (Jones et al 1991).

DOMESTIC INCIDENTS

The majority of household electrocutions result from failure to earth tools or appliances properly, or from using electrical devices near water (Fontanarosa 1993). 20% of all electrocutions occur in children (Fontanarosa 1993); the incidence of electrocution injury in youth is bimodal, with toddlers at one peak and adolescents at the other (Leibovici et al 1995). Toddlers are prone to electric shocks because they inspect their surroundings and are apt to take various objects into their mouths: biting electrical cords causes typical and specific electrical injury in this population. Adolescents engage in dangerous activities such as climbing electrical poles or playing with electrical sources.

Bathtub incidents comprise 2.5% of all deaths due to electrocution (Patten 1992).

LIGHTNING STRIKE

Lightning strike causes between 150 and 300 fatalities per year in the USA (more than most other natural disasters combined) and causes serious injuries in a further 1000–1500 patients (Duclos & Sanderson 1990).

Between 75% and 85% of all lightning deaths and injuries are to men. 30% of all deaths involve people who work out of doors and 25% involve people participating in recreational activities (Cox 1992). The increasing popularity of outdoor activities (such as golf, sailing and hiking) is likely to result in increasing numbers of lightning injuries.

OTHER INCIDENTS

Other cases of electrocution injury and death include railway-related incidents, injury during electroconvulsive therapy (McKenna et al 1970), deliberately applied electric shocks from stun guns and shock batons (Robinson et al 1990), suicide (Fernando & Liyanage 1990) and homicide-related events (Al-Alousi 1990).

Relevant electrical principles

Patterns of electrical injury are better understood if the basic principles of electricity are considered.

Electric current is defined as a motion of electrical charges. The electrical driving force is called potential difference or voltage. The magnitude of the electrical current is measured in amperes. Current flow through a material (e.g. skin, nerve tissue and muscle) is dependent on the driving voltage and the resistance of the material. This relationship is governed by Ohm's law:

$$I = V/R,$$

where I is the current, V is the voltage and R is the resistance. Current flows preferentially through tissues with least resistance to flow (e.g. nerve tissue) and this is reflected in observed patterns of injury, where nerve tissue is often damaged by electrical shock while other tissues remain relatively intact.

Skin resistance depends on its thickness and humidity, and is lowest on the wet thin skin of moist palms and highest on thick, calloused skin. After thermal injury, skin resistance drops dramatically, greatly reducing its protective effect (Abroute et al 1993).

The amount of thermal energy generated is proportional to the resistance of the material, the time of contact and the square of the current flow; energy release is manifest as thermal injury as current passes through the body, and therefore injury severity is most critically dependent on the magnitude of the current passing through the tissues.

Direct current (DC) refers to an unchanging direction of current flow (e.g. that produced by a battery). Alternating current (AC) refers to an electric source with a changing direction of flow (e.g. domestic UK electricity supply, which is 240 V, 50 Hz AC current). Alternating current is substantially more dangerous than direct current of the same magnitude (Salem et al 1977). Contact with alternating current may cause tetanic skeletal muscle contractions, preventing victims from releasing their hold of the electrical source and leading to prolonged current delivery and hence greater injury. Direct current usually causes a single violent flexion contracture and thrusts the victim away from the source.

The voltage of a lightning strike may be between 20 million and 200 million volts and the current up to 50 000 amperes (Cox 1992). The time exposure of a lightning strike, however, is so small (less than 0.2 s) that the amount of energy discharged into the victim is greatly limited. As discussed above, the pathway of the current defines the damage that is caused, and in lightning incidents there is insufficient time for the current to breach the skin. As a consequence the energy usually pours over the outside of the person, the so-called 'flashover effect' (Craig 1986). As a result deep burns are infrequent; cardiac asystole is possibly caused by the brief but very intense electric and magnetic fields.

Pathophysiology of injury

SKIN

Burns caused by current flowing through tissue are called electrothermal burns, which usually cause most damage at the skin surface, where resistance to flow is high. An electrothermal burn will occur when the magnitude of current flowing through a given skin resistance causes enough heat to be generated. Local electrothermal burns of the skin occur at points of entry and exit of electrical energy to and from the body. Alternating current produces entry and exit wounds of approximately the same size. Direct current produces a small entrance wound and a much larger exit wound. These entrance and exit wounds are local lesions, with a central region appearing charred, a middle zone of whitish coagulation necrosis and an outer area of brighter red, oedematous, damaged tissue.

Electrothermal burns of the mouth and lips occur in children biting or sucking an electrical cord, and are a characteristic injury of the toddler population.

Arc burns are due to the radiation of heat from an electrical current arcing through the air. Thermal burns may be caused by being in the vicinity of an arc (without electricity flow through the body) or may be thermal and electrothermal if the arc is conducted into the body. These burns occur, therefore, with no direct contact between the source of electricity and the victim. Thermal cutaneous burns may also occur from surrounding burning materials such as clothes, or from materials heated by electric currents.

NERVOUS SYSTEM

Injury to the nervous system occurs in 70% of cases of electric shock (Grube et al 1990). Brief loss of consciousness is frequent and benign, but coma persisting for more than 10 min or deteriorating conscious level indicates cerebral oedema or intracranial haemorrhage.

Spinal cord lesions from electric shock may lead to spastic paresis, gait ataxia and bladder dysfunction, and may be progressive after the injury. It should be remembered that clinical signs suggestive of spinal injury in electric shock incidents should alert the caregiver to the possibility of secondary blunt trauma.

Peripheral nerves are directly injured by current passing through them, by local ischaemia or by a polyneuritis distant to the point of contact.

CARDIORESPIRATORY SYSTEM

Cardiac arrest is the primary cause of immediate death due to electrical injury. Alternating current and low-voltage injuries are associated with ventricular fibrillation (VF), whereas high-voltage electrical shocks produce asystole (Browne & Gaash 1992). Electrothermal injury to the skin of the anterior chest wall is associated with significant myocardial injury and a poor prognosis (Chandra et al 1990).

AC shock is usually associated with VF, DC shock with asystole.

Less serious arrhythmias are common among survivors of an electrical shock, the incidence depending on the voltage and the current pathway. The commonest arrhythmias are sinus tachycardia and ventricular ectopic beats, but ventricular tachycardia, atrial fibrillation and complete heart block are all recognized. The commonly occurring arrhythmias present early and tend to be benign and self-limiting in the absence of previous heart disease. Ventricular tachycardia and complete heart block will require close monitoring and appropriate intervention if causing compromise.

Respiratory arrest may be due to prolonged tetanic paralysis of the respiratory muscles and/or damage to the respiratory centre in the brain stem, and may persist from minutes to hours. Cardiac output may spontaneously return shortly after electrical insult due to automatic activity of cardiac pacemaker cells but, in the presence of prolonged respiratory arrest, if attention is not given to ensure adequate ventilation secondary hypoxic cardiac arrest will follow.

Adequate ventilation may prevent secondary hypoxic cardiac arrest.

VASCULAR INJURY

Local vascular injury may be associated with cutaneous burns. Arterial pulses may not be palpable through eschar or subcutaneous oedema. Where major vascular injury has occurred, this is associated with sepsis and subsequent loss of the affected limb. This is usually caused by high-voltage (1000 V or more) electric shock, and morbidity may be increased by an underestimation of the extent of tissue injury and resultant delayed surgical debridement of devascularized non-viable tissues.

LIMB INVOLVEMENT

Joint dislocation and secondary long bone fracture may represent secondary blunt trauma (e.g. falling from a pylon following electric shock). Thermoelectric injury to muscle causes massive necrosis, and muscle distal to major vascular injury will be rendered ischaemic.

A significant electrical injury that has passed through a limb will render it pale, cold and senseless. Compartment syndromes will develop as injured muscle becomes oedematous and swells rapidly. A combination of muscle, nerve and vascular injury may necessitate subsequent limb amputation. In this setting, sepsis must be anticipated.

Massive muscle damage will result in rhabdomyolysis with release of myoglobin systemically, precipitating subsequent renal failure, as well as producing a risk of hyperkalaemia and cardiac arrest.

Immediate care in electrical injury

MAKING THE SCENE SAFE – PRACTICAL CONSIDERATIONS

The therapeutic approach to electric shock victims begins with making the scene safe by discontinuing the electric current or by clearing the victim from the electrical source. Extreme caution must be exercised to prevent injury to the rescuer: despite precautions, injuries to would-be caregivers have been reported (Viener & Barrett 1986).

DOMESTIC AND INDUSTRIAL INCIDENTS

The rescuer must be certain that the current is switched off before attempting to touch the victim or remove the victim from the electrical source. If possible, the current should be switched off at its source. If this cannot be done quickly, precautions must be taken to prevent electric shock to the rescuer (such as using non-conductive material such as dry wood, electrical safety gloves, polypropylene rope, etc.).

In electricity pylon accidents, it will be necessary to telephone the electricity board to prevent them reconnecting an interrupted source, which they do as a matter of routine after 20 min (as the cause of most temporarily interrupted sources is bird strike). Downed wires may physically move when energized if the current is resupplied and it is therefore sensible to secure them with a heavy object.

A victim may be unable to release an alternating current electrical source because tetanic muscle contraction occurs. The only course of action is to disconnect the source of electricity, as separation of the victim from a live source will be impossible.

When a power lineman on an electricity pole is electrocuted, expired air ventilation can often be initiated by rescuers on the pole, with chest compressions started as soon as the victim can be lowered to the ground. Appropriate precautions will be required to prevent rescuers from falling.

RAILWAY INCIDENTS

Railways are a hazardous environment and one should not go on to the track unless absolutely necessary; be aware of warning signs indicating 'Reduced Lineside Clearance' or 'No Refuge'. Always face oncoming traffic and wear a high-visibility tabard.

Electrical lines should always be regarded as live until there is positive assurance to the contrary.

Telephones at crossings and signals provide direct communication with rail network control; using these telephones, or through the ambulance control network, permission should be obtained from rail network before venturing on to the track and an official railway lookout should be requested. Overhead line structures, signal numbers or mile post numbers can be used to identify the exact location.

It has been suggested that, if the victim is over 1 m below the wire it is not essential for the current to be switched off, provided that the rescuer can also be over 1 m below the wire at all times. However, whenever possible, the current should be discontinued.

The current isolation procedure in the UK is as follows:

Using lineside telephones, state: 'Emergency call', your name, your location and why the current needs to be switched off. Then wait for definite assurance that the electricity supply has been discontinued.

If a major incident occurs, a Railtrack incident officer will be appointed.

BASIC LIFE SUPPORT AND CASUALTY TRIAGE

After ensuring scene safety, an immediate assessment of the patient's cardiorespiratory status should follow. In the absence of spontaneous respiration and circulation, assisted ventilation and external cardiac massage should commence immediately using standard basic life support techniques. The airway should be secured and supplemental oxygen administered with assisted ventilation. Blunt trauma must be assumed, particularly in unresponsive victims and in unwitnessed incidents, and appropriate spinal immobilization must be maintained.

This triage priority is different to priorities in non-electrocution cardiac arrest situations because respiratory arrest may be prolonged beyond cardiac arrest, with little actual tissue damage in an individual who probably has no pre-existing cardiac morbidity. Although the victim may appear dead, remarkable recoveries have been reported, and aggressive and prolonged resuscitation efforts should be undertaken (Patten 1992).

Lightning strike victims should receive the same triage priorities as victims of electric shock. 70% of all lightning fatalities involve a single victim, 15% involve groups of two victims and 15% involve three or more victims at once (Cooper 1989). Virtually all victims of lightning strike who do not experience cardiac or respiratory arrest survive; therefore, casualties who appear clinically dead following the strike should be treated before other victims who show signs of life (Fontanarosa 1993). A suitable motto is:

'Treat first those who appear to be dead, for they may live. Those who are alive, although in need of medical aid, can wait, for they will live in spite of treatment delay.' (Leibovici et al 1995)

ADVANCED LIFE SUPPORT

Local burns, swelling and soft tissue injury may prove challenging for airway management manoeuvres but, as with any life support situation, securing a patent airway, by endotracheal intubation if indicated, is the first priority. Cardiac arrhythmias (ventricular fibrillation, asystole, etc.) should be treated along conventional advanced life support (ALS) guidelines, with standard drug doses and direct current (DC) shocks delivered if necessary at conventional energy levels.

Victims with significant electrothermal injury should have an aggressive fluid regime (similar to that for an extensive crush injury) to correct ongoing fluid losses and maintain a diuresis in order to avoid renal failure in the face of myoglobinuria and hypotension; a solution such as Ringer's lactate is suitable. Because of the significant deep tissue and internal injury associated with a large electrothermal insult, despite what may be a small cutaneous burn, fluid requirement will be higher than that calculated from standard formulae based on the cutaneous thermal burn alone. Luce & Gottlieb (1984), for example, reported that adequate fluid resuscitation of patients with electrical trauma required $7\,\mathrm{ml\,kg^{-1}}$ per 1% body surface area burned (compared with the Parkland formula for a thermal burn of $4\,\mathrm{ml\,kg^{-1}}$ per 1% body surface area).

Lightning strike victims, unlike electric shock victims, seldom have significant underlying tissue destruction, and aggressive fluid administration is unnecessary. On return of spontaneous circulation and adequate peripheral perfusion, fluid administration should be restricted in order to prevent any exacerbation of the cerebral oedema that may accompany lightning strike (Cooper 1989).

Conclusion

Electrocution is an uncommon but potentially lethal event. It is essential for immediate care providers to be familiar with the therapeutic approach to the management of electrical injury and the necessary precautions that need to be taken at the incident scene, to offer appropriate assistance and to avoid further injury to themselves. An appreciation of the basic physical principles of electrical energy helps to understand the pathophysiology and patterns of injury consequent upon accidental electrocution and lightning strike. Electrical injuries have a generally favourable outcome if intervention is prompt, adequate and appropriately prioritized. The nature of electrocution injury allows the well prepared immediate care provider to demonstrate skill and knowledge in terms of scene safety and life support.

References

Abroute M, Cohen IL, Lumb PD 1993 Cardiovascular problems in the post-operative trauma patient. In: Grande CM (ed) Textbook of trauma, anaesthesia and critical care. CV Mosby, St Louis, MO, p 773–775

Al-Alousi LM 1990 Homicide by electrocution. Medicine, Science and the Law 30: 239–426

Browne BJ, Gaash WR 1992 Electrical injuries and lightning. Emergency Medicine Clinics of North America 10: 211

Centers for Disease Control 1982 Fatal occupational injuries – Texas. Morbidity and Mortality Weekly Report 34: 130–139

Chandra NC, Sin CO, Munster AM 1990 Clinical predictors of myocardial damage after high voltage electrical injury. Critical Care Medicine 18: 293

Cooper MA 1989 Lightning injuries. In: Auerbach PS, Geehr EC (eds) Management of wilderness and environmental emergencies, 2nd edn. CV Mosby, St Louis, MO, p 173–193

Cox RA 1992 Lightning and electrical injury. Journal of the Royal Society of Medicine 85: 591–593

Craig SR 1986 When lightning strikes. Postgraduate Medicine 79: 109–124

Duclos PJ, Sanderson LM 1990 An epidemiological description of lightning-related deaths in the United States. International Journal of Epidemiology 19: 673–679

Fernando R, Liyanage S 1990 Suicide by electrocution. Medicine, Science and the Law 30: 219–220

Fish R 1993 Electric shock, part 1: Physics and pathophysiology. Journal of Emergency Medicine 11: 309–312

Fontanarosa PB 1993 Electrical shock and lightning strike. Annals of Emergency Medicine 22: 378–387

Grube BJ, Heimbach DM, Engrav LH, Coppas MK 1990 Neurological consequences of electrical burns. Journal of Trauma 30: 254

Jones JE, Armstrong CW, Woolard CD 1991 Fatal occupational electrical injuries in Virginia. Journal of Occupational Medicine 33: 57–62

Leibovici D, Shemer J, Shapira S 1995 Electrical injuries: current concepts. Injury 26: 623–627

Luce ES, Gottlieb SE 1984 'True' high-tension electrical injuries. Annals of Plastic Surgery 12: 321–326

McKenna G, Engle RP, Brookes H, Dalen J 1970 Cardiac arrhythmias during electroshock therapy: significance, prevention and treatment. American Journal of Psychiatry 127: 530–535

Patten BM 1992 Lightning and electrical injuries. Neurologic Clinics 10: 1047

Robinson MN, Brookes CG, Renshaw GD 1990 Electric shock devices and their effects on the human body. Medicine, Science and the Law 30: 285–300

Salem L, Fisher RP, Strate RG 1977 The natural history of electrical injury. Journal of Trauma 7: 487–492

Viener SL, Barrett J 1986 Lightning-related injuries and electrical burns. In: Trauma management for civilians and military physicians. WB Saunders, Philadelphia, PA, p 446–451

Risk of infection in prehospital care

39

Introduction   410

Classification of the infectious diseases   410

Risk to emergency health-care workers from
occupational diseases   411

Immunization of prehospital health-care workers
against infectious diseases   412

Use of personal protective equipment   413

Adoption of safe working practices   413

Procedures for postexposure prophylaxis   415

References   416

Further reading   416

Introduction

Providers of prehospital care should be aware of the risks posed by different types of infectious disease and should know what measures to be followed in reducing those risks. Such measures include:

- an awareness of the disease processes, how infection is transmitted and the risk to health-care workers
- adequate immunization of prehospital health-care providers against the common infectious diseases to which they could be exposed
- the use of appropriate personal protective equipment

- the adoption of safe working practices when dealing with infectious disease cases
- a knowledge of the procedures for postexposure prophylaxis.

Classification of the infectious diseases

Prehospital care providers might wish to adopt the classification of infectious diseases used by ambulance service in the UK. Infectious diseases may be classed as:

- category I – where no precautions are necessary (Table 39.1)
- category II – where simple precautions are required
- category III – where special precautions pertain.

The category II infectious diseases can be further classified according to the mode of spread or portal of entry into the body (Table 39.2).

The highly infectious diseases in category III include those given in Table 39.3.

Some conditions occur in more than one category, their categorization depending on the form and type of illness. For example, human immunodeficiency virus (HIV), hepatitis B virus (HBV) and ophthalmia neonatorum require no special precautions unless there is a risk of spillage of blood or body fluids, in which case they are placed into category II. Methicillin-resistant *Staphylococcus aureus* (MRSA) is usually a category I infection as it poses no risk to healthy, non-immunocompromised health-care workers. However, where there is MRSA contamination of open areas of skin, such as in burns or in infection around external fixators, there is a significant risk to other patients who may be in close contact; in such cases MRSA is better considered as a category II infection.

Risk to emergency health-care workers from occupational diseases

The conditions causing most concern to health-care workers in emergency situations are hepatitis B and HIV. HBV has been shown to be capable of transmission in the following ways.

- Percutaneous transmission with:
  - blood and blood products
  - intravenous drug abuse
  - contaminated needle, syringe and instruments

Table 39.1 Category I infections

- Brucellosis
- Erysipelas
- Glandular fever
- Hepatitis B
- HIV/AIDS
- Intestinal worms
- Legionellosis
- Leprosy
- Leptospirosis
- Listeriosis
- Malaria
- Methicillin-resistant *Staphylococcus aureus* (MRSA)
- Ophthalmia neonatorum
- Q fever
- Scabies
- Tetanus
- Toxoplasmosis
- Whooping cough

Table 39.3 Category III infectious diseases

- Ebola fever
- Lassa fever
- Marburg disease
- Pneumonic plague
- Rabies
- Viral haemorrhagic fever

Table 39.2 Category II infectious diseases

Category II(a) – infections that are transmitted by airborne spread and pass from the air into the respiratory system, e.g. by droplets:

- Encephalitis
- Measles
- Meningitis
- Mumps
- Pneumonias
- Psittacosis
- Rubella
- Scarlet fever
- Streptococcal tonsillitis
- Streptococcal pharyngitis

Category II(b) – the contagious diseases that are transmitted by skin contact:

- Anthrax
- Chicken pox
- Hepatitis B
- Hepatitis C
- Herpes zoster (shingles)
- HIV/AIDS
- Impetigo
- MRSA
- Ophthalmia neonatorum
- Pyrexia of unknown origin

- Puerperal fever
- Tuberculosis (cutaneous with discharge)
- Verminous infestations (lice)

Category II(c) – infections which are transmitted by the faecal/oral route passing into the body as contaminated food or fluid taken by mouth:

- *Campylobacter*
- Cholera
- Diarrhoeal diseases, including diarrhoea in HIV/AIDS
- Dysentery
- Food poisoning
- Gastroenteritis
- Hepatitis A
- Paratyphoid
- Poliomyelitis
- Salmonella
- Typhoid

Category II(d) – infections transmitted from lung to lung via sputum, and so on:

- Anthrax, pulmonary
- Diphtheria
- Tuberculosis, pulmonary

- Other routes of transmission:
  - transfer of body secretions
  - oral transmission
  - intimate (sexual) contact
  - perinatal
- Blood-borne contamination.

BLOOD AND BLOOD PRODUCTS

Blood and blood products may be the sources of infection from HIV, HBV, hepatitis C virus, cytomegalovirus (CMV), trypanosomiasis, malaria, syphilis and brucellosis. Of these, the most frequent is HBV, by which it has been estimated that, in the USA, 12 000 health-care workers are infected every year (Department of Labor Occupational Safety and Health Administration 1989). In 5–10% of these a chronic disease will develop and there are 200 deaths of health-care workers in the USA from hepatitis B each year. It has been estimated that between 7% and 30% of needlestick incidents involving blood from a HBV-positive patient will result in clinical infection in a health-care worker.

HBV is between 30 and 100 times more infectious than HIV. It has been estimated that the risk of the transmission of HIV following percutaneous exposure to blood is as low as 0.3% (Henderson et al 1990, Marcus et al 1993).

In Europe, the rates of seroconversion to HBV following occupational exposure have been reviewed (Peréz et al 1993). Out of 19 cases reported, 18 occurred in nurses and 17 of these were cases involving the recapping of needles (see below).

TRANSMISSION OF HEPATITIS B INFECTION FROM OTHER BODY FLUIDS

Seroconversion of viruses in health-care workers known to have been contaminated with HBV from patients' mucous membranes or patients whose skin has not been broken is extremely rare.

Blood is the only substance from which there has been documented occupational infection. However, HBV and HIV may be found in other body fluids, including amniotic fluid, semen, pleural, pericardial, peritoneal and vaginal fluids. Therefore, transmission is theoretically possible and precautions should be taken. Urine, saliva, sputum, tears and sweat can be considered as non-infectious (Oksenhendler et al 1986).

RISKS OF INFECTION INVOLVING MOUTH-TO-MOUTH RESUSCITATION

It has been shown that direct mouth-to-mouth resuscitation may result in exchange of saliva between patient and rescuer. Fortunately, as HBV and HIV are not infectious in saliva, there has never been a documented case of transmission of either of these agents during mouth-to-mouth resuscitation. Similarly, there is no perceived risk of transmission of HBV from resuscitation manikins in training classes (Glaser & Nadler 1985).

However, there is a risk of the exchange of blood that may contaminate saliva in mouth-to-mouth resuscitation (e.g. if there are wounds to patient or rescuer about the face) and of course there is the confirmed risk of transmission of other infectious agents such as herpes simplex, Neisseria meningitidis and the category II(d) infections – pulmonary anthrax, diphtheria and pulmonary tuberculosis. The spread of tuberculosis by mouth-to-mouth resuscitation poses a significant risk.

For this reason, members of the public are given training in the use of interposition barrier devices or mouth to mask devices during resuscitation training classes, and health-care workers are advised to avoid direct mouth-to-mouth contact.

Immunization of prehospital health-care workers against infectious diseases

In the UK the general guidelines for immunization against infectious diseases are contained in a book of the same name published by the Department of Health (1996). The main conditions against which health-care workers should be immunized are tetanus, poliomyelitis, tuberculosis, hepatitis B and rubella.

Prehospital care workers who may be called upon to work overseas should also consider immunization against the commoner tropical diseases (hepatitis A, typhoid and paratyphoid, and yellow fever) and take prophylaxis against malaria.

IMMUNIZATION AGAINST HEPATITIS B

Hepatitis B immunization should be provided to all health-care workers, including students and trainees, who have direct contact with patients' blood or blood-stained body fluids, or with patients' tissues. Clearly, this applies to all front-line workers in the prehospital environment who may have to deal with victims of accidents or sudden illness.

The basic immunization regime consists of three doses of vaccine, each of 500 IU, with the first and second dose separated by 1 month and the second and third dose separated by 6 months.

Hepatitis B immunoglobulin (HBIG) is available for postexposure prophylaxis, and is normally used in combination with HBV vaccine to confer passive and active immunity after the exposure (see below). If a health-care worker who has not previously been vaccinated against HBV receives a needlestick injury then that, by implication, is a demonstration of risk, and that person should be provided with active and passive immunization postexposure.

IMMUNIZATION AGAINST OTHER CONDITIONS

Influenza

Currently, immunization of all health-care workers against influenza B is not recommended. It has not yet been demonstrated to be cost-effective and, more importantly, supplies of the vaccine should be conserved for selective immunization of those at greater risk. Nevertheless, a number of trials of immunization of health-care workers including general practitioners and ambulance workers are under way and this guidance may change in due course.

Rubella

Rubella is offered as part of the normal vaccination regime for infants and young children. However, there have been cases of rubella infection of maternity patients from health-care workers of both sexes who were not immunized against rubella when they were young. For this reason, all health-care workers should have their rubella antibodies checked at the commencement of their employment and, where deficient, active immunization should be instituted.

Meningococcus

Routine immunization with meningococcal vaccine is not recommended as the overall risk of meningococcal disease is very low. Occasionally, postexposure antibiotic prophylaxis against meningococcus is recommended for health-care workers (see below).

Tetanus

Tetanus is another condition for which routine pre-school immunization is provided. Although the protection afforded by immunization lasts for many years, a booster injection given 10 years after the primary course and again 10 years later will maintain satisfactory levels of protection which will probably be life-long.

Tuberculosis

All health-care staff working in the prehospital field should be considered at risk of tuberculosis and should be provided with testing (reading of the Heaf or Mantoux test) and bacille Calmette–Guèrin (BCG) vaccination as appropriate.

Use of personal protective equipment

Prehospital care workers who are used to performing in dangerous and alien environments will be aware of the necessity for personal protective equipment. Fortunately, with careful selection, some of the items used for personal protective equipment against chemical or radioactive contaminants can also be used for protection against infectious diseases.

The following is a list of personal protective equipment for infectious diseases giving the appropriate British or European Standard and/or levels of infection protection available.

- Protection to the eyes:
  - either wrap-round visor on protective helmet (EN 166); or
  - protective goggles with wrap-round side protection (BS 2092.1/CE 95.0086); or
  - wrap-round visor attached to a facemask (Medical Devices Agency (MDA) Standard).
- Respiratory protection:
  - surgical facemask for the mouth and nose (EN 149 FFP 25) OEL 12 – (providing 12 occupational exposures); or
  - for greater degrees of risk, masks with particulate filters.
- Protective gloves:
  - single-use, disposable PVC or latex gloves (MDA Standard); or
  - hypoallergenic gloves for patients with skin hypersensitivity.
- Protective gowns/overalls:
  - ranging from simple plastic aprons to give protection from blood splashes to
  - full overalls incorporating hood, wrist and ankle protection (EN Type 6 EN 3635) to
  - full one-piece protective suits.

A guide to personal protective equipment used when travelling with known infectious disease cases is given in Table 39.4.

Adoption of safe working practices

UNIVERSAL PRECAUTIONS

All health-care workers, whether working inside or out of hospital, are advised to heed the advice relating to universal precautions published by the Centers for Disease Control of the United States Health Department (Centers for Disease Control 1988):

Since medical history and examination cannot reliably identify patients infected with HIV or other blood-borne pathogens, blood and body fluid precautions should be consistently used for all patients. All patients should be assumed to be infectious for HIV and other blood-borne pathogens. Health-care workers should protect themselves from contact with blood and body fluids from all patients.

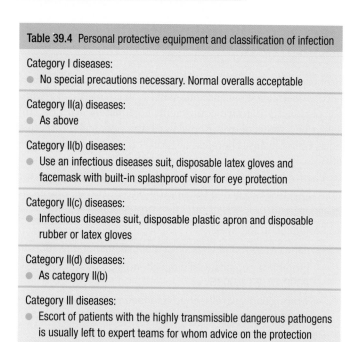

Table 39.4 Personal protective equipment and classification of infection

Category I diseases:
- No special precautions necessary. Normal overalls acceptable

Category II(a) diseases:
- As above

Category II(b) diseases:
- Use an infectious diseases suit, disposable latex gloves and facemask with built-in splashproof visor for eye protection

Category II(c) diseases:
- Infectious diseases suit, disposable plastic apron and disposable rubber or latex gloves

Category II(d) diseases:
- As category II(b)

Category III diseases:
- Escort of patients with the highly transmissible dangerous pathogens is usually left to expert teams for whom advice on the protection required in dealing with conditions, such as viral haemorrhagic fever, has been provided by the Advisory Committee on Dangerous Pathogens (1997)

Table 39.5 Suggested precautions for prehospital procedures

Procedures requiring gloves only	Procedures requiring gloves, eyewear and mask	Procedures requiring gloves, eyewear, mask and gown
Venepuncture	Intubation and airway manipulation when droplet infection is likely	Central vascular procedures
Placing and removing intravenous lines	Oral procedures	Nasogastric intubation
Contact with laboratory specimens		Obstetric procedures
Management of wounds		Chest drainage procedures

In dealing with patients in whom there is a risk of infection from blood or body fluids, therefore, barrier methods should be used and gloves should be worn. Health-care workers are one of several groups that have a higher risk of developing a natural rubber latex allergy (Baumann 1999). Wherever possible, latex-free gloves should be available for health-care workers, and only gloves that conform to European Community (CE) standards must be used. Gloves should be worn for as short a period as possible. Following a procedure gloves should be removed before driving. Any skin wounds (such as simple scratches or abrasions) of the health-care worker should be covered by a waterproof adhesive plaster, and health-care workers with exudative lesions should avoid direct patient care. Masks and goggles or face shields should be used when there is a risk of droplet infection. Gowns or plastic aprons should be used when there is a risk of blood splashing. Mouth-to-mouth resuscitation should be avoided. The hands should be washed immediately after patient contact.

Table 39.5 lists procedures that could well be applied in the prehospital environment when special precautions are necessary.

HAND WASHING

Hand washing is the single most important factor in the prevention and spread of infection. Hand-washing facilities are available in all ambulance stations and hospital departments. Wherever possible the hands should be washed immediately after patient contact. However, few ambulance vehicles have proper hand-washing facilities. Where it is not possible to wash hands, a water-based handwipe followed by an approved alcohol handrub should be used. Alcohol gel will not penetrate through blood or dirt, so hands should be wiped with a moist wipe before gel is applied, unless hands are not soiled, when gel alone can be used. To maximize the effectiveness of hand washing, nails should be kept short and clean and jewellery should be kept to a minimum. Skin cream can help to reduce cracking and dry skin on frequently washed hands, helping to reduce the risk of lesions developing. If a particular soap, antimicrobial handwash or alcohol product causes skin irritation an occupational health team should be consulted.

SAFETY WITH SHARPS

Much work has been done on the cause and prevention of needlestick injuries, of which a staggering 2000 per day are estimated to occur in the USA (Morgan 1990). Although new, inexperienced staff are at the greatest risk (Albertoni et al 1992), the major risk factor is recapping of the needle (Jagger et al 1988) which has been incriminated in one-third of needlestick incidents. Other factors include the use of complex devices and the unsafe disposal of needles or sharps after they have been used.

The following guidelines should be considered in the use of sharps:

- Do not recap needles.
- Do not bend or break needles or remove them from the attached disposable syringe.

- Immediately after use place the sharp in an approved sharps container.
- Never reach into the sharps container.
- Always replace the sharps bin when three-quarters full or at the safety line indicated by the manufacturer.
- Avoid the use of needles for adding drugs or fluids to an intravenous line. Instead make greater use of Luer-Loks, stopcocks or three-way taps.

If unfortunate enough to sustain a needlestick injury, health-care workers should be aware of the local procedures for immediate management and postexposure prophylaxis (see below). In general, the advice is:

- **Wash it**
- **Bleed it**
- **Report it.**

Simple skin punctures should be encouraged to bleed, and should be washed with soap and water. Any wounds should be irrigated with disinfectant. Exposed mucosae can be decontaminated by flushing with clear water. Health-care workers are required to seek early assistance after accidental puncture with a needle or other sharp.

DISPOSAL OF CLINICAL WASTE

There are three main groups of waste materials which apply to prehospital care providers.

- Group A – tissues and dressings – all human tissue including blood, whether infected or not, related swabs and dressings.
- Group B – sharps including discarded syringe needles, cartridges, broken glass and any other contaminated disposable sharp instruments or items.
- Group C – infected materials including items used to dispose of urine, faeces and other body secretions or excreta other than those in Group A.

All waste within these three groups should be disposed of by incineration only. There is no need to segregate wastes further other than by ensuring sharps (Group B items) are put in the appropriate container.

Tissues, dressings and infected materials should be placed in a yellow plastic bag and sealed with special adhesive tape prior to incineration. Disposable items coming into this category include oxygen therapy equipment, suction catheters, disposable pharyngeal airways and examination gloves.

Approved sharps containers should be used by prehospital care providers. Inexpensive, small, portable sharps

containers are available for inclusion within a first-response bag. Full sharps containers should be sealed and prepared for disposal. They should not be placed in a plastic bag, whether yellow or not.

Items for disposal should be handled carefully using the appropriate protective devices (gloves, aprons, etc.). Arrangements should be made for items for incineration, including yellow bags and sharps bins, to be accepted in a designated area at the receiving hospital or to be delivered to an appropriate alternative site as soon as is practicable.

AMBULANCE VEHICLE AND EQUIPMENT CLEANING

It is important to maintain high standards of hygiene within the emergency vehicle to prevent the spread of infection. A suitable cleaning schedule should be developed and maintained for each vehicle. Certain items of equipment used by prehospital care workers are classified as single-use only and must never be re-used. They should be disposed of, as clinical waste, immediately after use and replaced. Reusable equipment should be appropriately decontaminated after each patient, using only the method advised by the manufacturer. It is important to follow local procedures for cleaning and disinfection of equipment and vehicles.

Procedures for postexposure prophylaxis

As discussed previously, the main risk to health-care workers is from blood-borne contamination with HIV or HBV. Recently, in the UK, guidance has been published on the postexposure prophylaxis for health-care workers occupationally exposed to HIV (Department of Health 1997).

Although the risk to health-care workers of HIV from needlestick injuries is small (less than 3 per 1000 injuries), and the risk of acquiring HIV through mucous membrane exposure is less than 1 in 1000, where there is knowledge of exposure to an HIV case this risk can be reduced still further if zidovudine is taken prophylactically as soon as possible after the occupational exposure.

Health-care workers who have sustained blood-borne exposure to a possible contaminant (e.g. through a needlestick injury) should present as soon as possible, and ideally within 1 h, to a centre where a risk assessment can be undertaken and postexposure prophylaxis can be given. Such centres include occupational health departments and, out of hours, emergency departments. Although attendance within 1 h is ideal, there is some evidence that postexposure prophylaxis may be effective even if 1–2 weeks have elapsed since the exposure.

The postexposure management of needlestick cases would involve the following:

- The boosting of active immunization to conditions such as hepatitis B and tetanus
- The provision of passive immunization against HBV by the administration of immunoglobulin
- Blood sampling for initial, and later, titres of HBV and HIV in the health-care worker's blood
- Consideration of the HIV status of the patient (source subject) if known and, when appropriate and with the patient's consent, estimation of the HIV antibody status of the patient
- Following a risk assessment, when appropriate, the administration of zidovudine to the health-care worker
- Occupational follow up with counselling and support.

Emergency and occupational health departments may need to provide postexposure prophylaxis and monitoring for other conditions, e.g. tuberculosis, meningococcus and, rarely, leptospirosis. In the case of meningococcus, recent advice indicates that the routine administration of antibiotics to health-care workers who have dealt with a meningococcal septicaemia case is not required unless there has been intimate personal contact, such as the performance of mouth-to-mouth resuscitation.

References

Advisory Committee on Dangerous Pathogens 1997 Guidance on the management and control of viral haemorrhagic fevers. London, HMSO

Albertoni F, Ippolito G, Petrosillo N et al and the Latium Hepatitis B Prevention Group 1992 Needlestick injury in hospital personnel: a multicenter survey from Central Italy. Infection Control and Hospital Epidemiology 13: 540–544

Baumann NH 1999 Latex allergy: an orthopaedic case presentation and considerations in patient care. Orthop Nurs 18(3): 15–22

Centers for Disease Control 1988 Update: universal precautions for prevention of transmission of human immunodeficiency virus hepatitis B virus and other blood-borne, pathogens in health care settings. Morbidity and Mortality Weekly Report 37: 377–388

Department of Health 1996 Immunisation against infectious disease. HMSO, London

Department of Health 1997 Chief Medical Officer's Expert Advisory Group on AIDS, guidelines on post-exposure prophylaxis for health care workers occupationally exposed to HIV. HMSO, London

Department of Labor Occupational Safety and Health Administration 1989 Occupational exposure to blood-borne pathogens: proposed rule and notice of hearing. Federal Register 54: 23042–23139

Glaser JB, Nadler JP 1985 Hepatitis B virus in a cardiopulmonary resuscitation training course: risk of transmission from a surface antigen-positive participant. Archives of Internal Medicine 145: 1653–1655

Henderson DK, Fahey BJ, Willy M et al 1990 Risk for occupational transmission of human immunodeficiency virus type (HIV 1) associated with clinical exposures. Journal of the American College of Physicians 10: 740–746

Jagger J, Hunt EH, Brand-Elnaggar J, Pearson RD 1988 Rates of needlestick injury caused by various devices in a university hospital. New England Journal of Medicine 319: 284–288

Marcus R, Culver DH, Bell DM et al 1993 Risk of human immunodeficiency virus infection among emergency department workers. American Journal of Medicine 94: 363–370

Morgan DR 1990 HIV and needlestick injuries. Lancet 335: 1280

Oksenhendler E, Harzic M, Le Roux JM et al 1986 HIV infection with seroconversion after a superficial needlestick injury to the finger. New England Journal of Medicine 315: 582

Peréz L, de Andrés R, Fitch K, Najera R, the European Study Group on Accidental Exposure to HIV 1993 HIV seroconversion following occupational exposure in European health care workers. In IXth International Conference on AIDS and the IVth STD World Congress, Berlin. Abstract PO-C18-3040

Further reading

British Medical Association 1987 Report of the Board of Science and Education, immunisation against hepatitis B. London: British Medical Association

Centers for Disease Control 1988 Update: acquired immunodeficiency syndrome and human immunodeficiency virus infection among health care workers. Morbidity and Mortality Weekly Report 37: 229–234

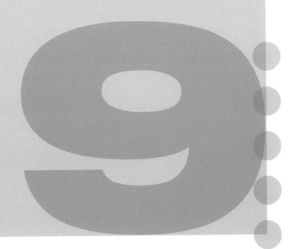

Part Nine

40 Emergencies in pregnancy 419

41 Trauma in pregnancy 433

42 Childbirth 439

43 Neonatal resuscitation and transport 448

Emergencies in pregnancy

40

Introduction 419

Anatomy and physiology of pregnancy relating to emergencies in pregnancy 420

Approach to and management of the severely ill pregnant woman 423

Emergency conditions of pregnancy presenting to the immediate care physician 425

Non-obstetric causes of abdominal pain during pregnancy 430

Other medical problems 431

Summary 431

References 432

Introduction

The management of pregnancy and labour over the past 50 years has changed out of all recognition from the doctor-led approach with GPs and community midwives conducting the majority of deliveries (including instrumental ones) at home, to midwife-led care with the vast majority of deliveries being conducted in a hospital setting with early discharge home, often as early as 6h post-partum and usually within 48h of delivery. The consequence of this change is that GPs have almost completely withdrawn from intrapartum obstetrics. Since 1981 only 1% of all deliveries have involved a GP. This is a major change from 30 years ago when most GPs would have possessed current competencies in all except surgical deliveries. Many GPs at that time would also have been comfortable with instrumental delivery. For a variety of clinical, medicolegal and operational reasons this is no longer the case (Brown 1994). The situation is further compounded by the falling birthrate and increasing numbers of doctors and midwives in training chasing a falling number of opportunities for training and experience in intrapartum skills.

As a result of this there is no longer a large pool of physicians available in the community with current intrapartum care skills. It is, therefore, a core skill of any physician dealing with a pregnant woman to be able to recognize the presence of an emergency and to arrange immediate referral to a specialist obstetrician, just as it is a core skill of any physician to be proficient in resuscitation.

Despite these changes, it is Department of Health policy to encourage more out-of-hospital deliveries. By no means all ambulance services within the UK have commissioned specific training in extended skills for ambulance personnel for obstetric cases. Even in those services that have commissioned such training an individual ambulance paramedic is unlikely to use such skills frequently. Furthermore, skill retention problems coupled with inadequate scope of permitted practice for ambulance personnel may result in underdiagnosis and undertreatment, particularly in obstetric haemorrhage. Although many GPs may not possess current technical skills they do have the clinical knowledge and judgement to decide when not to persist with interventions and when to 'scoop and run'.

Emergencies in pregnancy are a prime example of where access to on-line medical supervision of paramedics may be beneficial. There are still a significant number of locations where transport times to a specialist obstetric and gynae-cological unit are long enough to warrant physician and/or midwife support. It must be remembered that every NHS GP has a terms of service obligation to respond to emergency calls within his or her practice area. As a result of the changes discussed above, there now exists the paradoxical situation of a need for greater immediate care skills in relation to emergencies in pregnancy at a time when the opportunities, particularly for physicians, to remain skilled in this field are fewer than ever before.

Pregnancy is a normal, natural phenomenon and approaches that unnecessarily 'medicalize' the process are to be discouraged. However, when a pregnancy goes wrong it can do so swiftly and with devastating results. It is important to remember that *any* emergency can arise during pregnancy, not simply those related to pregnancy itself. It is axiomatic that the mother rather than the fetus must be resuscitated first.

The Confidential Enquiry into Maternal and Child Health (CEMACH) is a self-governing body that runs confidential enquiries into maternal, perinatal and child health.

Find further information and current statistics for the Confidential Enquiry into Maternal and Child Health at www.cemach.org.uk.

Table 40.1 details the contribution of substandard care to common categories of maternal death.

The following conclusions can be drawn for the pregnant woman:

- Treatment precedes definitive diagnosis
- A high index of suspicion for haemorrhage is essential, especially for concealed haemorrhage
- There must be a low threshold for transportation to a hospital with obstetric facilities
- The patient must be transferred to the *appropriate* hospital in the appropriate timescale using the appropriate mode of transport.

Anatomy and physiology of pregnancy relating to emergencies in pregnancy

The logical management of emergencies in pregnancy must be related to the anatomical and physiological changes in the mother which occur during pregnancy. In the prehospital phase it is unnecessary to have a detailed knowledge of fetal physiology as the approach must be to assess, stabilize and treat the mother first. For a fetus to have any prospect of survival (except close to term under the circumstances

Table 40.1 The contribution of substandard care to common categories of maternal death

Category	Deaths	Substandard care
Hypertensive disorders	20	16 of which had substandard care
Haemorrhage	15	11 of which had substandard care
Thrombosis and thromboembolism	35	12 of which were antenatal deep vein thromboses (DVTs) 13 of which were post-caesarean-section DVTs
Ectopic pregnancy rupture	9	1 of which died of adult respiratory distress syndrome All of the other eight involved substandard care

Source: Department of Health 1996

of a maternal perimortem emergency caesarean section), the mother must be resuscitated first. Thus, the only features that will be discussed are those impinging upon resuscitation management namely:

- airway with cervical spine control
- breathing with high-concentration oxygen supplementation
- circulation with haemorrhage control and attention to maternal posture.

Maternal physiological changes are directed toward accommodation of the enlarging uterus, growth of the fetus and placenta, and preparation for labour and subsequent lactation. The average weight gain of 12.5 kg (range 0–23 kg) places a significant load on the cardiorespiratory system and the metabolic load of pregnancy increases progressively toward term due to the maturing fetus, enlarging uterus and increased maternal efforts in servicing and transporting the average 12.5 kg full-term pregnancy.

AIRWAY AND ANATOMICAL CHANGES

The anatomical changes of pregnancy all affect any resuscitative attempt on the mother (Table 40.2). In the developed world most countries positively encourage dental health and it is now likely that the mother will have a full dentition, which must be protected, particularly during advanced airway manoeuvres. As pregnancy progresses breast tissue engorges and fat is deposited in other tissues, especially around the face and neck. This may lead to some difficulties in sizing and fitting cervical collars; thus in the pregnant trauma victim extra care must be taken to ensure an adequate fit. In addition it may be difficult to intubate using a McIntosh blade.

Table 40.2 Anatomical and physiological changes in pregnancy: airway

- Full dentition
- Facial and airway swelling (consider a smaller endotracheal tube)
- Neck swelling
- Breast engorgement (may lead to difficulty with intubation)
- Increased risk of gastro-oesophageal reflux

Table 40.3 Anatomical and physiological changes in pregnancy: breathing

- Increased minute volume – 50% at term (mainly increased tidal volume)
- Reduced functional residual capacity
- Relative hyperventilation
- Increased tidal volume

Thomson & Cohen (1938) showed that the shape of the chest alters during pregnancy. The lower ribs flare outwards and the diaphragm rises by 4 cm. The increase in the transverse diameter of the chest caused by the flaring of the ribs alters the ratios of the various lung volumes (De Swiet 1991) although the forced expiratory volume in the first second (FEV_1) and peak expiratory flow rate (PEFR) are unaffected in normal pregnancy. Total body water increases during pregnancy, leading to generalized tissue oedema including the supraglottic tissues, necessitating selection of a smaller endotracheal tube.

The uterus progresses from being a thick-walled pelvic organ up to 12 weeks' gestation to an increasingly thin-walled abdominal organ displacing the diaphragm upwards maximally at 34 weeks. This causes the thoracic volume alterations outlined above and the heart to move cephalad, the apex moving laterally and anteriorly and then rotating upon its axis transversely. The change in position of the heart is reflected in electrocardiogram (ECG) changes with large Q waves and T-wave inversion in lead III; this is caused partly by the general cardiac enlargement. Progressive growth of the uterus increasingly splints the diaphragm and as the chest wall splays the ribs are also splinted and the ventilatory mechanical pattern shifts from a predominantly diaphragmatic one to a thoracic cage movement pattern. It is thought that up to one-third of women at term have airway closure during supine tidal respiration, resulting in increased atelectasis and ventilation–perfusion mismatches.

The compressive effects of increasing uterine size upon the stomach, coupled with:

- altered gastro-oesophageal junction mechanics
- progesterone-induced reduced upper oesophageal sphincter pressure
- increased gastric acid secretion
- delayed gastric emptying,

all increase the risk of acid reflux and therefore the potential for airway soiling with gastric contents. Thus, the airway should be secured at an early stage using cricoid pressure (Sellick's manoeuvre) if intubation is performed. The use of antacids or H_2-receptor-blocking drugs is unlikely to be effective in the prehospital environment unless a long transfer is envisaged. The rescuer must be aware that altered chest wall dynamics can make assessment of respiratory excursion difficult.

BREATHING WITH OXYGEN SUPPLEMENTATION

The anatomical factors outlined above together with the physiological effects of pregnancy markedly affect breathing during pregnancy (Table 40.3). The changes are not solely confined to the mechanics of breathing and lung performance but also occur in the higher centres and in biochemical systems. In order for both mother and fetus to prosper during pregnancy there has to be a satisfactory P_{CO_2} gradient from fetal P_aCO_2 (6 kPa) to maternal (4 kPa) to alveolar air. This is achieved by fine tuning of the maternal respiratory centre by progesterones reducing the threshold for stimulation of respiration and by oestrogens increasing the respiratory centre sensitivity to P_aCO_2. Prowse & Gaensler (1965) showed a fourfold increase in the pregnant woman's minute volume from 1.5–6 l min^{-1} for a 1 mmHg rise in CO_2. The increased minute volume is of the order of 50% by term and is achieved by increased tidal volume rather than by increased respiratory rate. Vital capacity is unchanged but the functional residual capacity of the lungs is reduced by around 20%; this means that there is less expired air left in the lungs to be mixed with the fresh inspiratory gases and aids maintenance of a steep P_aCO_2 gradient from fetus to maternal alveolus.

Vital capacity increases by as little as 100–200 ml at term and may actually decrease in the obese mother. Effectively these changes mean that the pregnant woman is hyperventilating to maintain the steep P_{CO_2} gradient and that she operates in a state of chronic compensated respiratory alkalosis with reduced P_aCO_2, reduced bicarbonate and a normal pH. The maternal P_aO_2 is conversely raised by 10 mmHg, thus preserving an oxygen gradient from alveolus via mother to fetus. The overall rise in tidal volume during pregnancy is of the order of 30–40% and rapidly returns to normal by 6–8 weeks postpartum (Gazioglu et al 1970). Minute ventilation values rise in parallel with tidal volume also by 50% from 7.5–10.5 l min^{-1}.

The practical consequences of the respiratory changes during pregnancy are that, coupled with the high oxygen demand of the fetus and the work of the mother (particularly during labour), there is a very high oxygen flux. This, in the environment of a reduced functional residual capacity and a high tidal volume, can result in rapid preoxygenation

Table 40.4 Anatomical and physiological changes in pregnancy: circulation

- Increased cardiac output (heart rate and stroke volume)
- Cardiac muscle hypertrophy
- Cardiac chamber enlargement
- 'Left ventricular strain' on ECG
- Risk of inferior vena caval obstruction
- Increased circulating blood volume (50% at term)
- Relative anaemia

but with less benefit because of reduced oxygen reserve. More rapid gaseous induction with gaseous anaesthetic agents and rapid desaturation of the blood during apnoea also occur. Oxygen must be administered at the highest possible inspired concentration and at a high flow rate. In the spontaneously breathing mother this requires use of a Hudson face mask with reservoir bag. If there are any doubts as to the adequacy of ventilation or any question of airway compromise, early intubation and early intermittent positive pressure ventilation should be considered, although this may require expeditious transfer to hospital.

CIRCULATION AND POSTURE

The most important physiological changes of pregnancy impacting upon the seriously ill or injured mother are those of the cardiovascular system. Both the haemopoietic and the circulatory system are affected (Table 40.4).

During pregnancy cardiac output rises by 40% by the end of the second trimester, with 60% of the rise in cardiac output occurring by 10 weeks' gestation (Robson et al 1989). This is achieved by a 10% increase in stroke volume through increased venous filling and an increase in heart rate of 15 beats min^{-1} from as early as 2 weeks' gestation (Clapp 1985). The increase in stroke volume is partly achieved by hypertrophy of the cardiac muscle and enlargement of the cardiac chambers, which cause unfolding of the heart on the aorta.

On ECG monitoring these changes will show as 'left-ventricular strain' with inverted T waves in V_2 and V_3 leads. The hyperkinetic, hypervolaemic state may uncover a systolic ejection murmur, a third heart sound or an internal mammary artery murmur (Tabatznik 1960), the majority of which have no significance and in prehospital care may not be audible.

During labour cardiac output may rise a further 30%, entirely as a result of increased stroke volume. If venous return is compromised by inferior vena caval obstruction then cardiac output cannot rise proportionately.

In pregnancy the plasma volume increases by 50% (Pirani et al 1973, Whittaker & Lind 1993) in healthy women and

although there is haemodilution the red cell mass increases by between 18–30% depending on whether the mother takes iron supplementation (Hytten & Leitch 1971). Thus, although there is a 50% increase in the circulating blood volume there is no corresponding increase in oxygen-carrying capacity. This is even more important in multiple pregnancy where the plasma volume increase is proportionately greater as is the haemodilution (MacGillivray et al 1971).

As pregnancy proceeds, the systemic blood pressure alters with a slight reduction in systolic pressure and a more marked reduction in diastolic pressure. Thus, the normal physiological response in pregnancy is a widened pulse pressure almost entirely due to reduced peripheral resistance (from a generalized relaxation of smooth muscle tone coupled with, in effect, a low resistance shunt within the circulatory system caused by the uterine circulation). Holmes in 1960 showed the effects of maternal posture on blood pressure and found that 70% of women have a 10% drop in blood pressure and 8% of women a 30–50% drop in the supine position. Several other workers have also demonstrated the effects of pressure from the gravid uterus upon inferior venal caval patency and therefore venous return. Vena caval compression is thought to reduce venous return to the heart by up to 40%. In the face of complete obstruction of the inferior vena cava, some venous return is maintained via the azygos veins, paravertebral veins and ovarian veins.

If the supine hypotension syndrome is allowed to become established, the fall in cardiac output not only induces hypotension but markedly reduces cerebral and uteroplacental perfusion. The catecholamine release caused by the hypotension will further compromise uteroplacental circulation as a result of vasoconstriction.

To prevent fetal distress and achieve the best possible outcome for a mother with trauma or serious illness, it is vital that caval compression is relieved by:

- manually holding the uterus over to the left
- a sandbag pillow or other similar object under the right buttock (beware in lower spinal injury)
- nursing the victim on a long spinal board tilted 25–30° to the left.

This last method is probably the best prehospital, especially now that such equipment is widely available on front-line ambulances. The use of a human wedge in the absence of suitable equipment has been described (Goodwin & Pearce 1992), in which the victim is log-rolled to the left and a rescuer (or two) kneels on the right side of the victim with the knees a few centimetres from the patient's left side. The victim is then gently log-rolled back on the thighs of the rescuer(s) (Fig. 40.1).

It is possible, (although not easy) for a single rescuer to perform external cardiac compression from this position, but not expired air respiration, so at least two skilled rescuers are required. When there is only one rescuer, the

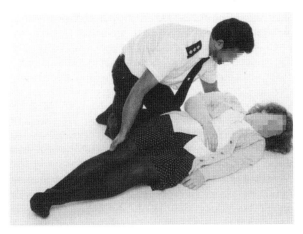

Fig. 40.1 • The human wedge.

most effective and convenient method of relieving caval obstruction is by inserting an appropriate article under the right buttock. The importance of relief of caval compression cannot be overstated. To illustrate the point, competent, effective basic life support gives at very best 30% of normal cardiac output. Caval compression reduces venous return by 40% and therefore Starling's law of the heart would indicate inevitable failure of resuscitation attempts in the face of unrelieved caval compression.

Haemopoietic system changes within pregnancy of significance in prehospital care have already been alluded to, namely the relative haemodilution arising from increased plasma volume and an increase of around 15% in the red cell mass to around $30\,ml\,kg^{-1}$ at term.

The cardiovascular changes described above are all designed to ensure that the 20% increase in oxygen demand in pregnancy and 60% increase during labour can be met. Oxygen delivery is proportional to blood flow through tissues and therefore under normal circumstances proportional to the arterial oxygen content of that blood P_aO_2. Normal oxygen consumption is around $250\,ml\,min^{-1}$ or $140\,ml\,min^{-1}\,m^{-2}$ body area and in the non-pregnant woman there is a factor of 4 margin of excess capacity in oxygen delivery to the tissues, i.e. approximately $1000\,ml\,min^{-1}$. However, where the pregnant woman is concerned, since the delivered oxygen to all intents and purposes remains little altered, the margin of safety falls to threefold and in labour to even less. Further analysis reveals that the only effective way of increasing oxygen delivery is by maintaining or increasing cardiac output, together with attention to maintenance of high F_iO_2 and adequate ventilation.

Successive confidential enquiries into maternal deaths have shown repeatedly that causes of maternal death from haemorrhage arose from:

- failure to identify the high-risk mother
- failure to deal efficiently with haemorrhage when diagnosed, commonly because of underestimation of

losses or undertransfusion and on occasion because of overtransfusion leading to pulmonary oedema
- failure to anticipate, detect or treat coagulation failure.

The first two categories are definitely within the remit of prehospital care. Massive blood loss must be considered to have occurred once the patient has lost 1000–1500 ml blood. Because in many conditions affecting pregnancy there is concealed haemorrhage, with or without a coagulation problem, the practical message is that a very high index of suspicion of significant haemorrhage must be maintained at all times. The normal, fit, healthy pregnant woman is already using some of her compensatory mechanisms simply to cope with her pregnancy and her margins of reserve are reduced when an emergency arises. Signs of haemorrhage may initially be absent because of the marked increase in circulating volume, and it may be only when approximately 33% of her blood volume has been lost that signs appear. This is the rationale behind aggressive fluid therapy and swift transport of the pregnant woman to definitive care in hospital.

Approach to and management of the severely ill pregnant woman

Dealing with the severely ill or traumatized pregnant women is undoubtedly stressful. This is compounded by the fact that any one prehospital-care worker is unlikely to see severely ill or injured pregnant women with any degree of frequency.

There are very few specific prehospital interventions that can be directed at the fetus, except, perhaps, the replacement of a prolapsed umbilical cord. The emphasis is on the principle of assessment, stabilization and treatment of mother first. Restoration of the mother's physiological status gives the best chance of fetal survival with minimal fetal morbidity.

Mother's uterus is the best transport incubator for the fetus.

Many immediate care emergencies involving pregnancy are time critical and several factors will affect the critical decision to 'stay and play' or 'load and go':

- The clinical condition of the patient
- The working and possible diagnoses
- Distance and time to the appropriate hospital
- Availability of consumables such as oxygen and fluids
- Skills available within the team on the day.

If definitive care is less than 15–30 min away, the emphasis should be on attending to airway, breathing with oxygen supplementation, circulatory support with attention to posture, and loading and transferring rapidly. Especially with time-critical haemorrhage and particularly in the pregnant victim, there can be no excuse for delay on scene or in transit to execute or reattempt therapeutic measures purely to stay within protocol if the delays so caused equal or exceed the time remaining to hospital.

If the definitive hospital is a significant distance or time away then consideration should be given to aeromedical evacuation by helicopter. Space constraints and loading configurations in many aircraft preclude the conduct of delivery or prevent access below the umbilicus and, while it might be clinically necessary to gain access by landing the aircraft, it may be operationally impossible.

On long journeys consideration should be given to using a community hospital en route as a staging post or rendezvous where the patient can be re-evaluated under optimum conditions, a midwife or second physician may join the team and further clinical supplies can be obtained.

THE APPROACH

The approach to the pregnant victim is exactly the same as to the non-pregnant victim (Table 40.5).

Special emphasis is given to early oxygen supplementation to obtain as high an F_IO_2 as possible, early intervention to assist ventilation, and appropriate measures to protect the integrity of the airway. It is prudent to cannulate early even in the absence of any signs of haemorrhage and commence intravenous fluids. The supine hypotension syndrome from inferior canal obstruction must be avoided by attention to the pregnant victim's posture.

HISTORY TAKING

If the pregnant victim is conscious and answering questions, in addition to normal history taking, questions should be focused on her gynaecological status, in particular the date of last menstrual period, the usual menstrual cycle length and regularity and the number of weeks of the pregnancy. The patient's maternity cooperation card may contain information such as ultrasound scan results. A previous history of miscarriage, premature labour, antepartum haemorrhage, pelvic/abdominal surgery, assisted conception or

ectopic pregnancy should be noted. It is useful to find out how many pregnancies and live births she may have had.

Contraceptive usage may be relevant as intrauterine contraceptive devices are associated with higher ectopic pregnancy rates, as are the progesterone-only and 'morning after' postcoital contraceptive pills. A recent history of termination of pregnancy may point to bleeding from incomplete removal of products of conception or to sepsis.

A pre-existing ovarian cyst or uterine fibroid may suggest torsion of the cyst pedicle or red degeneration of the fibroid, whereas recent attempts at assisted conception may point to collapse from the associated increased incidence of ectopic pregnancy. More rarely, circulatory collapse from hypotension, embolic phenomena and adult respiratory distress syndrome (ARDS) (Schenker & Weinstein 1978) associated with the ovarian hyperstimulation syndrome may occur. Most assisted conception attempts are conducted in the outpatient setting on a private basis with minimal postoperative surveillance.

Not all women will admit to the possibility of pregnancy, because of either fear, denial or social stigma, and it is important that a woman is given the opportunity to answer questions in as much privacy as possible and to one professional only.

Based upon the answers it should be possible to come to a reasonable working diagnosis. Gynaecological examination should be confined to abdominal palpation to confirm or refute the correlation between calculated gestation and fundal height. The perineum should be *inspected* for blood or fluid loss. There is almost no place for vaginal examination, either bimanually or with a speculum, in the prehospital field, particularly because of the risk of precipitating uncontrollable haemorrhage. In hospital practice vaginal examination may be undertaken with the back-up of immediately available theatre facilities and in general practice a vaginal examination may be performed in conditions of bleeding in early pregnancy to differentiate between a threatened (os closed) and inevitable (os opened) miscarriage, thus preventing needless admission to hospital in the former and allowing admission if required or next day pregnancy viability assessment plus Rhesus status assessment in the latter. How much can be achieved in the field will depend on the facilities available and the professional status of the immediate-care provider. There are two conditions where vaginal examination may be justified – for removal of a retained tampon in toxic shock syndrome and in incomplete miscarriage, where retained products of conception are entrapped in the endocervical canal preventing uterine contraction and thus causing continuing uterine haemorrhage. Under both sets of circumstances vaginal examination may be warranted provided that no undue delay in transportation is caused.

Only when the mother has been assessed and resuscitated should fetal assessment be performed by palpation of the uterus for contractions and for fetal movements.

Table 40.5 Approach to the pregnant patient
• Call for (extra) help if required
• Attend to your own safety
• Attend to scene safety
• Attend to the victim's safety
• Evaluate the victim's ABC

Beyond 22 weeks' gestation it may be possible to auscultate fetal heart sounds; however, time should not be wasted on this in a noisy environment. Fetal heart rates of 120–160 beats min^{-1} are reassuring but a rate below 110 min^{-1} is indicative of fetal distress and mandates rapid transfer with concomitant attention to optimizing maternal resuscitation. The information gleaned from fetal assessment may be of poor value in comparison to the time taken to obtain it. History taking is important, particularly in a call to a woman of reproductive age, and in prehospital care a very high index of suspicion for concealed haemorrhage must be maintained. Any woman of reproductive age with collapse or abdominal pain should be suspected as having a pregnancy-related cause until proven otherwise.

If massive blood loss is a possibility or already present then four questions require to be answered:

- What essential procedures need to be executed on scene and en route in connection with resuscitation?
- Which is the most appropriate hospital, taking into account transit times and the facilities available?
- If transport time is prolonged, what is the appropriate mode of transport?
- What scale of medical/surgical/obstetric/paediatric resuscitation reception should be ready on arrival at hospital?

Swift transport to a hospital offering definitive surgical facilities is mandatory and time must not be wasted on-scene hunting collapsed veins or performing cutdowns if the execution of that clinical task is going to extend the time to hospital by more than a few minutes. The golden hour belongs to the patient and the aim should be to be on scene for no more than 10–15 min in a non-entrapment incident. In many situations the hospital will be less than 30 min away and there is much to be said for securing the airway, supplementing breathing with oxygen, loading the patient and making a single attempt at cannulation within a maximum 3 min time frame before swift transportation with a call to the receiving hospital warning them to be on standby.

If further attempts at cannulation are to be made in a moving ambulance and there is a reasonable chance of success then this is a reasonable course of action, but transportation should not be delayed by repeated attempts, which may in addition destroy all the remaining venepuncture sites.

It is important to recognize that pregnancy itself is not pathological but that as well as emergencies specific to pregnancy any medical emergency such as asthma, diabetes or epilepsy can occur. As far as prehospital emergency care is concerned the treatment of such emergencies in the prehospital setting is little different from the non-pregnant state. The question of drug administration and teratogenicity is, as always, a balanced calculation of risk versus benefit. The problem of respiratory depression in the newborn in the face of maternal opiate or benzodiazepine administration can be predicted and neonatal resuscitation should be within the repertoire of skills of a prehospital care physician.

In a woman of reproductive age with a last menstrual period more than 4 weeks ago the safe option is to assume pregnancy until proven otherwise.

GENERAL RESUSCITATIVE MEASURES

The institution and maintenance of general resuscitative measures require frequent measurement of pulse, blood pressure and respiratory rate with regular assessment of trends. Semi-automatic and automatic monitoring machines are a useful aid but are no substitute for intelligent use of the human senses. Caution should be exercised in the interpretation of pulse oximetry.

Emergency conditions of pregnancy presenting to the immediate care physician

The immediate care physician is likely to be called to a pregnant or potentially pregnant woman because of collapse, abdominal pain or bleeding per vaginam or any combination of these symptoms. It is frequently impossible to make a definitive diagnosis in the field and as always general resuscitation along the lines discussed above is the correct course of action.

Table 40.6 Common emergencies in pregnancy

- Ectopic
- Miscarriage
- Toxic shock syndrome
- Antepartum haemorrhage
  - Placenta praevia
  - Placental abruption
- Hypertensive disorders
  - Eclampsia
  - Pre-eclampsia
- Non-obstetric causes of abdominal pain
- Medical emergencies
  - Asthma
  - Diabetes
  - Epilepsy

ECTOPIC PREGNANCY

A missed ectopic pregnancy can have devastating, if not fatal, results. During the period 2000–02 there were 11 deaths from ectopic pregnancy (CEMACH 2004), some due to substandard care and failure to consider the possible diagnosis.

Comments from the *Confidential Inquiry into Maternal Deaths in the United Kingdom* (1991–93) are still relevant today:

When a woman presents … with unexplained abdominal pain, with or without vaginal bleeding, every means available must be used to exclude ectopic pregnancy…. The management of the collapsed patient bleeding from a ruptured ectopic must be swift and expertly carried out. Teamwork is essential.

Ectopic pregnancy occurs when the conception implants outside the uterine cavity and is associated with:

- previous pelvic inflammatory disease
- intrauterine contraceptive devices and progesterone-only contraception pills
- history of previous tubal surgery
- previous ectopic pregnancy
- assisted conception manoeuvres.

During the period 2000–02 there were an estimated 30 100 ectopic pregnancies (CEMACH 2004), a rate of approximately 1% of all pregnancies. Analysis of predisposing conditions leads to the conclusion that there is a rising incidence of ectopic pregnancy and this is confirmed by Coste et al (1994).

Presenting symptomatology can be variable with pain in 90% of cases, amenorrhoea in 80% and abnormal vaginal bleeding in only 50% of cases. The abdominal pain may be low and to one side and if coupled with a history of amenorrhoea should immediately raise the possibility of ectopic pregnancy. The duration of amenorrhoea will depend upon the site of aberrant implantation, with fallopian tube implantations presenting at approximately 5–7 weeks whereas other sites tend to present at 8–10 weeks. The duration and presenting order of symptoms can be misleading and Clancy & Illingworth (1989) state that symptoms may be present for more than 1 week. The abnormal vaginal bleeding can vary from a 'prune juice' discharge to bright red blood. The classic story of pain preceding bleeding is unreliable and shoulder tip pain occurs in less than 20% of ruptures, requiring diaphragmatic irritation to occur. Any history of fainting should also arouse suspicion of ectopic pregnancy.

The management of ectopic pregnancy is to suspect the diagnosis, resuscitate if necessary and obtain precautionary intravenous access with a large-bore cannula. Routine attention to airway maintenance and oxygen supplementation must be instituted and suction must be to hand in case of vomiting. The patient must be kept warm and be frequently reassessed.

MISCARRIAGE

The old clinical terms threatened, inevitable, missed and septic abortion (Fig. 40.2) are best replaced with the term miscarriage because of the social stigma the term abortion now carries. Whatever the cause, miscarriage is cessation of pregnancy with the consequent death of the conception/fetus before 24 weeks gestation. The viability threshold for a fetus in law within the UK is now 24 weeks gestation. The term 'induced abortion' should be reserved for a deliberate act intended to terminate pregnancy, whether legally or illegally.

Miscarriage falls into the following categories:

- Spontaneous miscarriage
  - Threatened
  - Inevitable
  - Missed
- Induced miscarriage
  - Complete
  - Septic
  - Incomplete.

Three characteristic features of all miscarriages are:

- Abnormal, unexpected vaginal bleeding
- Pain (except in the missed miscarriage, which may present with a feeling of no longer being pregnant)
- The uterus being smaller than the period of amenorrhoea would suggest.

The differential diagnosis between threatened and inevitable miscarriage depends on the additional findings of a closed os in threatened miscarriage, whereas the os is open in an inevitable miscarriage. Speculum examination can also reveal non-pregnancy-related causes of vaginal bleeding. The reality in prehospital emergency care is that abnormal vaginal bleeding constitutes, in the 12–55 age group, a complication of pregnancy until proven otherwise and therefore transport to hospital is mandatory unless a physician member of the team with relevant obstetric/gynaecological skills is able to satisfy himself by appropriate gynaecological examination that the cause is a threatened miscarriage and can therefore be managed conservatively with bedrest and appropriate timely professional follow-up.

The management of miscarriage in the prehospital phase is along standard resuscitative lines. If the patient fails

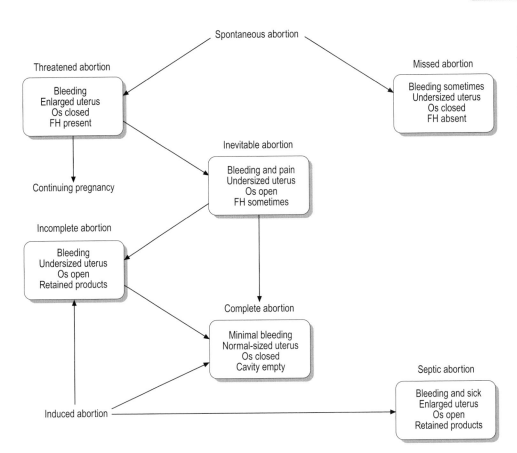

Fig. 40.2 • Classification of abortion. FH, fetal heart. (Redrawn with permission from Chamberlain G (ed) 1995 Gynaecology by ten teachers, 16th edn. Edward Arnold, London.)

to respond it may be due to products of conception lying in the endocervical canal preventing uterine retraction. How this is dealt with will depend upon the qualifications of the prehospital emergency responder. A physician may use a speculum and sponge forceps to remove the tissue and then give Syntometrine (ergometrine 500 μg and oxytocin 5 units ml^{-1}) 1 ml by intramuscular injection. If the transfer to a definitive unit is prolonged then it is worth considering rendezvous with a physician if bleeding cannot be stopped.

Occasionally after incomplete miscarriage or an incomplete termination and frequently following criminal abortion attempts, infection can supervene (septic abortion). Added to the features of miscarriage will be pain and elevated temperature but little bleeding. Sometimes circulatory collapse may supervene as a result of endotoxic Gram-negative shock causing peripheral vasodilation. This is likely to manifest as a tachycardia, a widened pulse pressure with a full bounding pulse, a temperature and pink or cyanosed extremities. These patients are seriously ill and require immediate transport to hospital. If transport is delayed or prolonged it may be necessary to take swabs and blood cultures (most GP surgeries in rural areas carry such items, together with transport media) and antibiotics should be started parenterally.

A cephalosporin and metronidazole should cover most eventualities and it is important to remember to hand in the specimens at the hospital.

TOXIC SHOCK SYNDROME

A small number of women using intravaginal tampons during their menstrual period develop toxic shock syndrome which classically develops on the second to fourth day of menstruation, although Williams (1990) noted many cases not associated with menstruation. It is an aggressive staphylococcal infection caused by the tampon introducing the organisms into the vagina, where they multiply, aided by the decidua-soaked tampon acting as a wick. Classically victims have fever, circulatory collapse, diarrhoea and a macular rash. Inspection of the vagina may reveal a purulent, offensive discharge and the tampon tracer ribbon. General resuscitative measures should be instituted and the patient should be transported immediately to hospital. If it is possible to remove the tampon, this should be done. If transport is delayed, penicillin should be started, having taken swabs and blood cultures. Toxic shock syndrome is rare.

ANTEPARTUM HAEMORRHAGE

Antepartum haemorrhage (APH) is defined as bleeding from the birth canal at any time from the 24th week of gestation until delivery. It is important to note that the gestational threshold for the definition has reduced from 28 to 24 weeks thus paralleling the change in the UK definition of fetal viability. There are three categories of APH:

- Placental abruption
- Placenta praevia
- Other incidental causes such as cervical ectropion, polyp, vas praevia and coagulation defects.

Whatever the origin of APH, the risk of massive haemorrhage is significant and the only appropriate prehospital response is mandatory transport to hospital with general resuscitative measures as necessary. Vaginal examination is expressly forbidden as the risk of provoking life-threatening haemorrhage is great.

Vaginal examination is forbidden in antepartum haemorrhage.

Although the differential diagnosis of the precise aetiology may seem academic to the prehospital care worker, it is important because placental abruption can result in massive, concealed, life-threatening haemorrhage. Estimates of the incidence of APH vary according to maternal age, parity and smoking status but the general consensus is that the incidence of placenta praevia is between 0.4% and 0.8% of all pregnancies and the incidence of placental abruption is 1% of all pregnancies. The confidential inquiry for the 1991–93 triennium reported seven deaths from APH, four from placenta praevia and three from placental abruption, with almost three-quarters of cases involving substandard care.

PLACENTA PRAEVIA

Placenta praevia occurs when placental implantation wholly or partly encroaches on the lower segment of the uterus and may, in extreme cases, lie over the cervical os (Fig. 40.3).

With routine use of ultrasound scanning in antenatal care the incidence of undiagnosed placenta praevia should fall. Because of uterine contraction patterns, haemorrhage is inevitable during labour. Usually placenta praevia gives warning by painless bright red bleeding per vaginam at any time from 24 weeks' gestation. The clinical picture can range from minor blood spotting to maternal collapse from torrential haemorrhage. Other salient clinical findings may

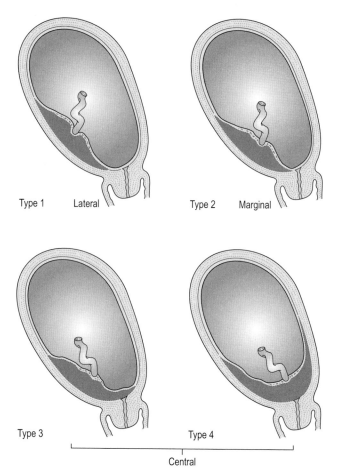

Type 1   Lateral   Type 2   Marginal

Type 3   Type 4

Central

Fig. 40.3 • Placenta praevia.

include an unengaged head or a transverse lie, particularly close to term. From the prehospital viewpoint the actions are resuscitation if necessary and transportation to the obstetric unit, having inserted a precautionary large-bore intravenous cannula and commenced an intravenous infusion. The woman should be transported in the left lateral position. Vaginal examination is contraindicated.

PLACENTAL ABRUPTION

Placental abruption occurs when a normally located placenta separates from the uterine wall, the aetiology being obscure, complex and incompletely elucidated, although abruption is a recognized complication of blunt abdominal trauma. Haemorrhage occurs at the placental/uterine wall interface. Maternal blood flow to the placenta is approximately $600 \, ml \, min^{-1}$. At the site of placental abruption, in addition to the possibility of feto-maternal haemorrhage, thromboplastic substances are released into the maternal circulation, which predisposes to disseminated intravascular coagulation. Maternal blood dissects either under the membranes or under the placenta itself, further stripping

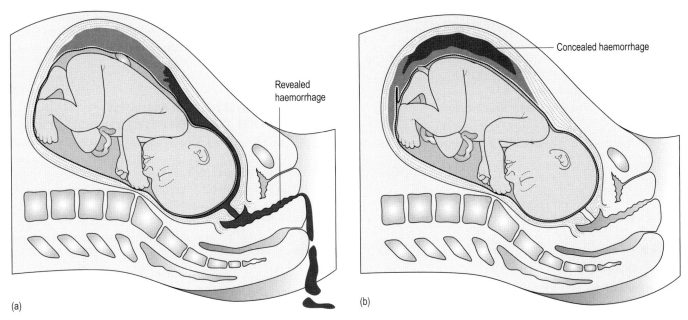

Revealed
haemorrhage

Concealed haemorrhage

(a)

(b)

Fig. 40.4 • Placental abruption: (a) with revealed haemorrhage, (b) with concealed haemorrhage.

the placenta from the uterine wall and further aggravating the abruption. The uterus undergoes tonic contraction, adding to the vicious spiral of rising intrauterine pressure and falling uteroplacental perfusion.

The call to the emergency services is usually for lower abdominal pain of sudden onset, which is initially of a steady, severe nature, although labour pains may supervene. The important feature is that haemorrhage may be concealed (Fig. 40.4). Revealed haemorrhage makes the diagnosis easy but the degree of shock may be out of all proportion to the observed blood loss. Sometimes abruption, if of traumatic origin, may not present for up to 48 h after the insult. As a consequence it is important to enquire about trauma and specifically ask whether mother has noticed reduced or absent fetal movements over the past day.

Vaginal examination is prohibited although perineal inspection may help diagnosis if there is bleeding per vaginam. Abdominal palpation may reveal the tender, hard Couvelaire uterus with a fundal height greater than expected for dates. It helps future assessment by subsequent carers if the initial fundal height is marked on the abdominal wall. The major diagnostic and therapeutic pitfall is to fail to recognize and treat the possible concealed haemorrhage. Diagnostic confusion can arise from other conditions, such as torsion of an ovarian cyst or red degeneration of a fibroid. The major diagnostic difference between placenta praevia and placental abruption is that the former is painless and the latter painful.

In placenta praevia it may only be necessary to insert an intravenous cannula and to frequently re-measure, note and interpret trends in vital signs. More severe degrees of bleeding, particularly in placental abruption, may require

general resuscitative measures. The pain of placental abruption may be relieved by titrated intravenous doses of morphine.

The rarer causes of APH require the same prehospital management pattern as placenta praevia and placental abruption.

HYPERTENSIVE DISORDERS

Hypertensive disorders occur in about 8% of pregnancies. From the immediate care viewpoint the two categories of patient likely to be encountered are:

● the mother who is developing pre-eclampsia
● the mother with impending or actual eclamptic fits.

Proteinuria is also a feature of pre-eclampsia. Often there are other symptoms (Table 40.7). Pre-eclampsia is a spectrum of hypertensive placental originated disease and management is dependent on severity. The definitive treatment is delivery of the fetus and placenta.

The blood pressure reading constituting the boundary between normality and pathology is generally taken as 140 mm/90 mm. However the trend of the blood pressure is also important and a rise in blood pressure of more than 30 mmHg systolic and 15 mmHg diastolic over baseline booking blood pressure readings is taken by many to constitute pregnancy-induced hypertension. It is also important to recognize that progression from normality to pre-eclamptic levels can occur over several hours rather than several weeks as in other types of hypertension.

Table 40.7 Symptoms and signs of pre-eclampsia

- Over 20 weeks' gestation
- BP over 140/90 or rapidly rising BP
- Rising proteinuria
- Excessive rate of weight gain
- Upper abdominal pain from liver capsule stretching
- Headache
- Visual disturbance, flashing lights/jagged lines
- Clonus or hyperreflexia

The common risk factors for pre-eclampsia are:

- Maternal
  - Primigravida
  - Maternal age under 20 or over 25
  - Previous history of eclampsia, migraine, renal disease or hypertension
  - Family history positive

- Fetal
  - Multiple pregnancy
  - Hydatidiform mole
  - Hydrops fetalis.

Any evidence of hypertensive disease alone with no other findings requires review after 6h. If there are any additional symptoms or signs or if review cannot be arranged, the safest course is transportation to the obstetric unit for management review. A woman in the imminent pre-eclamptic phase must be transferred to the obstetric unit. Intravenous magnesium sulphate is the treatment of choice. An initial dose of 4g should be given over 5–10min, and further boluses of 2g can be given to control recurrent seizures.

If an eclamptic fit supervenes the woman must be turned on to her left side (if she is not already in that position), to give protection should she vomit and relieve caval compression. Airway maintenance and ventilatory support with oxygen supplementation must be instituted. If repeated seizures occur despite magnesium, intravenous diazepam (10mg boluses) may be necessary. Where extreme delays in hospital transfer are likely, reduction of severe hypertension is best achieved with hydralazine or labetaol.

Rarely, severe intractable convulsions may require general anaesthesia with thiopental, itself a powerful anticonvulsant. This should only be performed by those trained in general anaesthesia and is a last resort in the prehospital environment. Transport should not be delayed and the use of flashing lights and sirens should be kept to a minimum,

as noise, vibration, movement and flashing lights can provoke further fits. Concerns regarding fetal depression are secondary to the absolute requirement to control maternal fits.

Non-obstetric causes of abdominal pain during pregnancy

Misdiagnosis of abdominal pain in pregnancy can carry significant morbidity and mortality for both mother and fetus. Traditional signs may be altered by the presence of a gravid uterus. From the prehospital perspective hospital investigation will be required to confirm or establish the diagnosis and therefore transportation with general resuscitative measures is necessary.

RED DEGENERATION OF FIBROID

This presents with tenderness, vomiting and a mild fever, usually around 12–18 weeks, and may cause diagnostic confusion with appendicitis.

TORSION OF FALLOPIAN TUBE AND OVARY

This presents with low abdominal pain in early pregnancy and, in view of the need to exclude ectopic pregnancy, is a diagnosis made by exclusion requiring investigation at hospital.

PELVIC LIGAMENT PAIN

Pelvic ligament pain is due to stretching of the ligaments between 16–20 weeks and presents as a form of low abdominal pain. It is a diagnosis made after exclusion of abruption.

OVARIAN CYSTIC TUMOUR PAIN

This produces localized unilateral lower abdominal pain in early pregnancy. Admission to exclude ectopic pregnancy will again make ovarian cystic tumour rupture a diagnosis of exclusion.

PYELONEPHRITIS

Pyelonephritis is common in the second trimester and the patient may have vomiting, fever and loin pain. She is more likely to present to her GP with 'a urinary infection'. However if she presents in the immediate care situation, admission may be necessary, particularly if dehydration is present.

APPENDICITIS

Diagnostic confusion and the changed position of maximal pain intensity can make accurate diagnosis difficult and contributes to the doubling of the perforation rate in the second trimester and a fivefold rise in the third trimester, where a perforation rate of up to 70% has been reported. Weingold (1983) showed that rebound tenderness only occurs in 58% of cases and guarding in 33% and no fever was detected in around half of cases. Compounded by the fact that nausea, vomiting and anorexia may be features of normal pregnancy the possibility of missed diagnosis is high and assessment by the surgeons is necessary. Transportation to hospital is therefore mandatory. Horowitz et al (1985) showed maternal mortality of up to 17% and fetal mortality of up to 43% with perforated appendix.

Other medical problems

ASTHMA

Pregnancy usually has little effect upon asthmatic control. Acute deterioration in asthmatic status is frequently triggered by infection and should be treated along standard guidelines, bearing in mind that the pregnant woman has a reduced margin of safety in oxygen-carrying capacity and that her cellular oxygen demand is 25–30% increased from normal. First principles also demonstrate that the fetus is intolerant of hypoxia. In the prehospital phase every effort must be made to ensure the highest possible F_iO_2 coupled with early intervention and a lowered threshold for instituting intermittent positive pressure ventilation. The mother must be treated first, using standard drug regimes for acute, severe and life-threatening asthma. Rapid evacuation is essential and, if any concerns about respiratory status arise, it may be necessary to radio ahead for a resuscitation team to be on standby.

CARDIAC DISEASE

Occasionally, a pregnant woman with pre-existing cardiac disease decompensates during pregnancy. Treatment is along conventional lines, using general resuscitative measures, opiates and vasodilators.

DIABETES

Because of lowered renal threshold for glucose all estimations must be by finger prick blood glucose testing strips. Diabetic ketoacidosis supervenes at lower blood glucose levels than in non-pregnant women and because of the expanded plasma volume the degree of ketoacidosis may not be matched by the degree of dehydration. A high index of suspicion is required and appropriate fluid resuscitation should be initiated. In the vast majority of prehospital scenarios it is preferable to leave soluble insulin administration until arrival in hospital.

DEEP VEIN THROMBOSIS AND PULMONARY EMBOLUS

Deep vein thrombosis is a recognized complication of 0.3% of pregnancies and 3% of women delivering by caesarean section. From the prehospital viewpoint the major need is to recognize the condition and transport the patient to hospital. 12 patients died antenatally from pulmonary embolism in the 1991–93 period, several of which were missed before admission. In the 2000–02 report, 25 patients died of pulmonary embolus (including the postpartum period). The presenting picture may range from pleuritic chest pain, with or without haemoptysis, via dyspnoea and cyanosis with tachycardia to complete collapse. The prehospital management is general resuscitative measures and swift transportation to hospital. Guidelines regarding thromboprohylaxis have now been issued by the Royal College of Obstetricians and Gynaecologists (2004).

EPILEPSY

There is debate as to the influence of pregnancy on seizure frequency in women. Nash & Price (1997), quoting Montouris et al (1979), state that seizure frequency increases in almost half of epileptic women. Chamberlain (1994) states that for most women the frequency of epileptic seizures is not affected by pregnancy. The advantages and disadvantages of one anticonvulsant over another in pregnancy are outside the scope of prehospital care and the management of the epileptic fit is, as for non-pregnant women, along general resuscitative lines. Intravenous diazepam emulsion is the best drug for control of fits. It is important if possible to estimate blood pressure and, if the patient has become incontinent, test for urinary protein in case the fit is eclamptic rather than epileptic in origin.

Summary

In the prehospital phase of emergency medicine adequate treatment and resuscitation of the mother provides the optimum outcome for both mother and fetus. The mother must always be treated first and considerations of effects on the fetus must not prevent administration of emergency drugs. The risk of haemorrhage, including concealed haemorrhage, is greater in pregnancy, and physical signs present late; it must therefore be anticipated and treated proactively. Maternal and fetal oxygen requirements mandate close attention to airway patency, adequacy of ventilation and high inspired oxygen concentration. It is safer in the field to avoid vaginal examination.

References

Brown DJ 1994 Opinions of general practitioners in Nottinghamshire about provision of intrapartum care. British Medical Journal 309: 777–779

CEMACH 2004 Why mothers die 2000–2002 – The Sixth Report of Confidential Enquiries into Maternal Deaths in the United Kingdom (ed G Lewis). Royal College of Obstetricians and Gynaecologists Press, London

Chamberlain G (ed) 1994 ABC of antenatal care, 2nd edn. BMJ Publishing, London

Chamberlain G (ed) 1995 Gynaecology by ten teachers, 16th edn. Edward Arnold, London

Clancy MJ, Illingworth RN 1989 The diagnosis of ectopic pregnancy in an accident and emergency department. Archives of Emergency Medicine 6: 205–210

Clapp JF III 1985 Maternal heart rate in pregnancy. American Journal of Obstetrics and Gynecology 152: 659–660

Coste J, Job-Spira N, Aublet-Cuvelier B et al 1994 Incidence of ectopic pregnancy. First results of a population-based register in France. Human Reproduction 9: 742–745

Department of Health, Welsh Office, Scottish Home and Health Department, Department of Health and Social Services Northern Ireland 1996 Report on confidential inquiries into maternal deaths in the United Kingdom, 1991–1993. HMSO, London

De Swiet M 1991 The respiratory system. In: Hytten F, Chamberlain G (eds) Clinical physiology in obstetrics, 2nd edn. Blackwell Scientific, Oxford

Gazioglu K, Kaltreider NL, Rosen M, Yu PN 1970 Pulmonary function during pregnancy in normal women and in patients with cardiopulmonary disease. Thorax 25: 445–450

Goodwin APL, Pearce AJ 1992 A manoeuvre to relieve aortocaval compression during resuscitation in late pregnancy. Anaesthesia 47: 433–434

Holmes F 1960 Incidence of supine hypotensive syndrome in late pregnancy. Journal of Obstetrics and Gynaecology of the British Empire 67: 254–258

Horowitz MD, Gomez GA, Santiesbastian R, Burkitt G 1985 Acute appendicitis during pregnancy. Archives of Surgery 120: 1362–1367

Hytten FE, Leitch I 1971 The physiology of human pregnancy, 2nd edn. Blackwell Scientific, Oxford

MacGillivray I, Campbell DM, Duffus GM 1971 Maternal metabolic response to twin pregnancy in primigravidae. Journal of Obstetrics and Gynaecology of the British Commonwealth 78: 530–536

Montouris GD, Fenichel GM, McLain LW 1979 The pregnant epileptic. Archives of Neurology 36: 601–603

Nash P, Price J 1997 Obstetric emergencies. In: Skinner D, Swain A, Peyton R, Robertson C (eds) Cambridge textbook of accident and emergency medicine. Cambridge University Press, Cambridge

Pirani BBK, Campbell DM, MacGillivray I 1973 Plasma volume in normal first pregnancy. Journal of Obstetrics and Gynaecology of the British Commonwealth 80: 884–887

Prowse CM, Gaensler EA 1965 Respiratory and acid base changes during pregnancy. Anaesthesiology 26: 381–392

Robson SC, Hunter S, Boys RJ, Dunlop W 1989 Serial study of factors influencing changes in cardiac output during human pregnancy. American Journal of Physiology 256: H1060–H1065

Royal College of Obstetricians and Gynaecologists 2004 Thromboprophylaxis during pregnancy, labour and after normal vaginal delivery. Guideline No. 37. RCOG, London, Available on line at www.rcog.org.uk

Schenker JG, Weinstein D 1978 Ovarian hyperstimulation syndrome: a current survey. Fertility and Sterility 30: 255–268

Tabatznik B, Randall JW, Hearsch C 1960 The Manumory souffle in pregnancy and lactation. Circulation 22: 1069

Thomson KJ, Cohen ME 1938 Studies on the circulation in pregnancy II. Vital capacity observations in normal pregnant women. Surgery, Gynecology and Obstetrics 66: 591–597

Weingold AB 1983 Appendicitis in pregnancy. Clinics in Obstetrics and Gynaecology 26: 801–810

Whittaker PG, Lind T 1993 The intravascular mass of albumin during human pregnancy: a serial study in normal and diabetic women. British Journal of Obstetrics and Gynaecology 100: 587–592

Williams GR 1990 The toxic shock syndrome. British Medical Journal 300: 960

Trauma in pregnancy

41

Accidental injury – scope of the problem	433
Road traffic accidents	434
Anatomical and physiological change	434
Basic management – primary survey	435
Basic management – secondary survey	435
Major obstetric haemorrhage	436
Blunt trauma and assault	436
Penetrating trauma	437
Burns	437
Brain-stem death in pregnancy	437
Sport, occupational and toxic injury	437
Perimortem and postmortem caesarean section	437
Conclusion	438
References	438

Accidental injury – scope of the problem

Treatment of the acutely injured pregnant woman involves two patients but the Advanced Trauma Life Support (ATLS) principle (American College of Surgeons Committee on Trauma 1997) is that:

Treatment priorities for an injured pregnant patient remain the same as for the non-pregnant patient.

Fetal outcome depends on maternal morbidity and there is no doubt that the mother must be resuscitated before attention is given to the state of the fetus. Thus, the priority in the traumatized pregnant female is assessment and stabilization of the mother when possible.

Assess and stabilize the mother first.

In the 1930s, childbirth was one of the major causes of death in otherwise young, healthy women. Very few women learned to drive until during and after the Second World War. Fortunately, childbirth has become much safer but more young women, at various stages of their pregnancy, are now involved in road traffic accidents.

To give the scale of the problem, in the most recent report on maternal deaths during the period 2000–02, eight were caused by road traffic accidents, and 11 by interpersonal violence (CEMACH 2004).

Vaizey et al (1995) stated that trauma is a major cause of maternal death in pregnancy and should be managed according to the ATLS guidelines. The use of properly fitted and worn seat belts does seem to have reduced the incidence of maternal morbidity and mortality without necessarily improving fetal outcome.

London (1991), however, considers that it is not possible to give confident and authoritative data on the subject because of poor data collection. He found that, in 5 years,

Table 41.1 Deaths during pregnancy – unnatural deaths in the UK 1991–93

Road traffic accident	9
Injecting substance abuse	4
Murder	2
Drowning/suicide open verdict	3
Burning – house fire	2
Alcohol-related	1
Overdose – suicide	1

Source: Departments of Health 1996.

Table 41.2 Mortality rates – approximate annual death rates per million

Non-pregnant women aged 15–44 from trauma	500
Pregnant women from trauma	8
Deaths in pregnancy – causes other than trauma	110

the Birmingham Accident Hospital dealt with 17 injured pregnant patients with 21 injuries. London compared the approximate annual death rates from injury in non-pregnant women aged 15–44 and in pregnant women from causes other than trauma with the death rate from trauma in pregnant women (Table 41.2).

There is very little literature from the UK, in contrast with the extensive list of publications from workers and trauma units in the USA. The extensive review by Griffiths et al (1993) could find no data on the incidence of significant fetal or maternal injury as the result of road traffic accidents in pregnancy. They estimated, however, that there might be about 250 trauma-related fetal deaths per year in the UK.

Other injuries in pregnancy are seldom seen in British practice but the US literature contains many articles on knife and gunshot wounds.

In road traffic accidents, bomb and blast injuries and mass casualty situations, mothers usually suffer extreme mental distress (sometimes without physical damage) and this alone can precipitate labour, which may be accompanied by vaginal bleeding as the cervix dilates. Antepartum haemorrhage can also be triggered by extreme maternal distress.

Road traffic accidents

The injuries sustained by pregnant women may reflect the anatomical changes of pregnancy and differ from those commonly seen in road traffic accidents.

Entrapment is more common with advanced gestation because of the size of the pregnant abdomen and the relative immobility of the patient. It is possible that a heavily pregnant abdomen may have an air-bag effect and actually reduce the severity of chest and facial injury. The uterus, placenta and fetus are particularly vulnerable to deceleration injury (Connor & Curran 1976). The soft tissues of the pelvis and uterus are easily damaged by pelvic fracture. Rib fractures are more likely to cause damage to the abdominal viscera. It can be difficult to diagnose a ruptured spleen or liver because of anatomical displacement or confusion with uterine pain.

Maddox et al (1991) reported a case of ruptured diaphragm in a pregnant woman, pointing out the frequent occurrence of this as a delayed or missed diagnosis.

It is always important to 'read the wreckage', but practitioners should know about the types of injury associated with poorly worn or fitted seat belts. Griffiths et al (1993) addressed this important topic and showed that the compulsory use of seat belts by front seat occupants since 1993 in the UK has reduced the severity of injuries. Griffiths et al (1991) reported a case of fetal death where traumatic bisection of the placenta was caused by a poorly placed high lap strap. In another case, a similarly too highly placed lap belt led to placental abruption and fetal demise. In one case (Cottingham R, Valentine BH 1996, personal communication) a patient suffered a ruptured uterus with abdominal extrusion and death of the fetus in a deceleration injury probably related to poor seat-belt usage. Griffiths et al (1993) also discussed the design of suitable restraints in pregnancy, including purpose-designed belts where the lap strap can be pulled below the pregnant abdomen and advised that all pregnant women should always wear properly fitting seat belts when travelling by car. A special cushion with a comfort strap passing between the legs is available that holds the lap portion of the seat belt securely below the gravid uterus.

Anatomical and physiological change

Pregnancy changes the pattern and presentation of injuries. The severity and degree of hypovolaemia may be masked by the remarkable ability of the pregnant woman to cope with major haemorrhage.

The management of the injured pregnant patient should attempt to restore the physiological values unique to the gravid state. Injury is often complicated and exacerbated by conditions peculiar to pregnancy such as placental abruption (separation of the placenta from the uterine wall) and ruptured uterus (Table 41.3).

The review by Nash & Driscoll (1991) outlines the anatomical changes that are seen in the uterus. Other

Table 41.3 The three most common abdominopelvic injuries during pregnancy

- Placental abruption
- Uterine rupture
- Pelvic fracture

anatomical and physiological changes are discussed in detail in Chapter 40.

Basic management – primary survey

Treatment priorities for an injured pregnant patient remain the same as for the non-pregnant patient. Standard protocols must be followed. The assessment of injuries and resuscitation must take account of the pregnant state. Under no circumstances should a vaginal examination be performed following trauma in pregnancy, as this may precipitate catastrophic haemorrhage.

Do not perform a vaginal examination.

Obvious external exsanguinating trauma must be controlled.

A patent and protected airway should be maintained and the neck stabilized. Intubation may be necessary in the unconscious patient or the patient whose airway is at risk for any other reason. This is fortunately rarely necessary, since most airways can be managed using simpler methods. In the unconscious patient intubation may be straightforward; otherwise induction of anaesthesia or the formation of a needle cricothyrotomy or surgical airway present the only alternatives to immediate transfer to hospital.

Endotracheal intubation may provoke coughing and vomiting in the otherwise reasonably quiet, semiconscious patient and persistent attempts at intubation in the unconscious patient are dangerous and may detract from the more important task of ventilating the lungs with high-flow oxygen. Pregnant patients rapidly become cyanotic if deprived of oxygen.

The chest should be examined for life-threatening injury and high-flow oxygen should be administered through a mask reservoir system (Hudson mask). Assisted ventilation, if indicated, must take account of the increased tidal volume of pregnancy. If the patient regurgitates or vomits, she should be turned into the left lateral position and the airways aspirated. If the patient is on a spinal board, the board can be tilted and elevated at the foot end. Pulse oximetry is useful prior to hospital admission and the maintenance of normal maternal oxygen saturation is a reasonable indicator of fetal oxygenation. It can, however, be unreliable in a severely shocked patient.

In second- and third-trimester patients the right hip should be raised with a sandbag or pillow; alternatively an assistant can be asked to manually displace the uterus to the left or use their knees as a 'human wedge'. If the patient is immobilized on a spinal board and the neck is stabilized with a rigid cervical collar, then the board may be put into a semi-left-lateral tilt.

Large-bore intravenous access should be obtained, although this must not be allowed to delay transfer to hospital. Rapid fluid replacement with crystalloid or colloid is started. It must be remembered that a pregnant patient may easily lose 2 litres of blood with remarkably few clinical signs and that the fetus may be at risk from maternal hypovolaemia even if the mother appears relatively stable.

Cardiac arrest is seldom encountered and carries an appalling prognosis in the injured pregnant woman. Chest compression may be difficult because of the large breasts and abdomen but standard cardiopulmonary resuscitation (CPR) is applied. The principles of arrhythmia management and defibrillation are the same as for the non-pregnant patient.

Dysfunction of the central nervous system is rapidly assessed using the AVPU system, followed by exposure of the patient to aid examination before she is suitably covered. Blood loss or a baby between the patient's legs should always be sought. Rapid delivery may occur after trauma and an unexpected fetus may be found in cases where an injured woman has concealed her pregnancy.

Basic management – secondary survey

The secondary survey should be carried out following arrival in the emergency department. A detailed head to toe examination is not appropriate in the prehospital environment.

ASSESSMENT OF THE UTERUS AND FETUS

It is vital to look for the maternity records, which may be with the patient. The conscious patient may be able to give a history of the pregnancy together with the all-important gestational age, as well as any problems associated with the present or any previous pregnancy.

The fetus may be viable after 24 weeks' gestation but the obstetrician will be reluctant to deliver a baby before 32 weeks of the pregnancy.

Fundal height is assessed and the symphysis pubis to fundus measurement in centimetres corresponds with the weeks of gestation. If the fundus is above the umbilicus then the fetus may well be viable.

The presence of uterine contractions, continuous uterine pain and tenderness are ascertained. A tense, hard uterus suggests a major placental abruption heralding the demise of the baby. The presence and amount of vaginal bleeding or amniotic fluid loss is noted. The degree of vaginal bleeding is a poor guide to volume replacement because of the frequent presence of concealed haemorrhage within the uterus.

Placental abruption can occur up to 48h following trauma and a high index of suspicion for this life-threatening injury is essential (Table 41.4). Placental abruption occurs in as many as 5% of episodes of minor trauma and 50% of cases of major trauma. Although the classic presentation is with increasing fundal height, this may not be apparent in the prehospital environment. A mark applied to the abdomen indicating the fundal height on initial examination may, however, act as a useful baseline for reassessment in hospital. A fundal height that clearly exceeds what is expected must be considered a strong indicator of possible abruption.

If it is easy to feel the fetus in a severely shocked patient, traumatic uterine rupture with extrusion of the baby into the abdomen may have occurred. This is much rarer than placental abruption (Table 41.5). Vaginal bleeding and abdominal pain are not invariably present.

It is almost impossible, even with a Pinard stethoscope, to hear the fetal heart at the accident scene, in the back of an ambulance or in the hubbub of an emergency department. In the presence of a tense, hard uterus and placental abruption, it is often difficult to hear the fetal heart even in the quieter confines of the labour ward. The normal fetal heart rate is 120–160 beats min^{-1} and the presence of fetal heart decelerations or tachycardia or bradycardia suggest severe fetal distress.

Even if the mother's condition is satisfactory after apparently minor trauma, it is essential that she is transported to hospital for examination. Lesser degrees of placental abruption may be difficult to detect but can jeopardize the life of the fetus. Such lesser abruptions may result in the production of maternal antibodies due to the leak of fetal cells into the maternal circulation. This can have catastrophic consequences for future pregnancies and Kleihauer testing and appropriate treatment will be necessary.

Scorpio et al (1992) studied the factors affecting fetal outcome in 51 trauma patients who either delivered successfully or experienced fetal loss and found that fetal demise was related to the severity of maternal injury as characterized by the injury severity score (ISS).

Major obstetric haemorrhage

It may be difficult for the prehospital practitioner to determine whether the shocked obstetric patient is bleeding from obstetric complications, internal trauma or a combination of both. Suffice it to say that the degree and speed of haemorrhage in the pregnant woman can be alarming and the combination of revealed and concealed haemorrhage may lead to underestimates of the blood loss. A high index of suspicion and continuous and careful observation and assessment are therefore essential.

The maternal mortality reports have often demonstrated the problem of substandard care by inexperienced doctors after pregnant women have died from haemorrhage.

Blunt trauma and assault

Most serious blunt trauma in pregnant women in the UK occurs in road traffic accidents but accidental falls and physical assaults occasionally occur. Pelvic fractures are an important cause of maternal morbidity and mortality. In pregnancy the pelvic venous plexuses are engorged and rupture can lead to massive haemorrhage. Urgent transfer to hospital is appropriate, with placement of intravenous lines en route or at the scene if evacuation is delayed or prolonged or the patient is trapped. Pelvic fractures are usually managed conservatively and operative fixation is rarely performed unless there is life-threatening haemorrhage from the pelvic vasculature.

Speer & Peltier (1972) found that 16 of 32 women with pelvic fracture were delivered normally, five required caesarean section and 11 had dead babies.

Roe (1993) reported a prevalence of physical abuse of 17% in urban patients in the USA and that 60% of physically

---

Table 41.4 Signs and symptoms of placental abruption

- History of trauma
- Uterine tenderness
- Lower abdominal pain
- Maternal shock
- Vaginal bleeding
- Fetal distress
- Premature labour
- Increased fundal height

Table 41.5 Signs and symptoms of uterine rupture

- Maternal shock
- Fetal bradycardia or loss of fetal heart sounds
- Palpable fetal parts
- Vaginal bleeding
- Abdominal pain

abused women reported two or more episodes of assault. Abdominal blows do occur but injury was more common to the head, neck and limbs and there was a fourfold increase in the incidence of genital trauma in this group. Ribe et al (1993) reported three cases in which blows to the abdomen of pregnant women in the third trimester resulted in fetal death due to placental abruption. Two cases were domestic assaults while one was a third-party assault. In these cases, the mother had minimal apparent injuries, although one experienced a small degree of vaginal bleeding and another had some contractions. The patients noticed loss of fetal movements shortly after the assault.

Penetrating trauma

Most cases of penetrating trauma to the pregnant abdomen in the UK involve impalement by various parts of a vehicle in road traffic accidents, although most level 1 trauma centres in the USA are very familiar with gunshot and knife wounds.

The pregnant uterus to some extent shields the mother from the full effect of penetrating gunshot wounds. The enlarged uterus is most likely to be injured in gunshot wounds and is, for the mother, perhaps not such a vital organ. The small intestine is displaced into the upper abdomen and can be protected from the destructive path of the bullet. Buchsbaum (1979) found that fetal injuries occurred in 59% of gunshot wounds to the gravid uterus, with a perinatal mortality of 55%.

The prehospital management of gunshot wounds follows the standard trauma guidelines.

The prognosis of stab wounds is far better than that of gunshot wounds (Hammar & Carter 1960). In late pregnancy, a stab wound to the lower abdomen may injure the uterus and fetus but other organs are protected by the large womb. Upper abdominal wounds may cause injury to the displaced small intestine.

Burns

The immediate management of burns in pregnancy follows the usual ABCDE approach. In calculating fluid replacement, the circulatory changes discussed above should be borne in mind. Larger volumes of fluid are usually required. Nash & Driscoll (1991) state that immediate transfer to hospital and delivery is indicated when maternal burns exceed 50% of body surface area in the second or third trimester. The complications that threaten the fetus are hypotension and hypovolaemia, hypoxia, sepsis and electrolyte imbalance. The USA guidelines (Buchsbaum 1979) for the management of the burned pregnant woman stress good routine burn care with particular attention to fluid resuscitation, greater attention to maternal oxygenation and more

prompt correction of any electrolyte imbalance. Jain & Garg (1993) reviewed the treatment of 25 pregnant patients with burns over a period of 6 years. They emphasized that, with proper care, the prognosis of pregnant patients with burns is encouraging and is comparable to any other burns patient. Abortion was common in the first trimester of pregnancy. Septicaemia was the commonest cause of abortion.

Fatovich (1993) studied case reports of electric shock in pregnancy. Information on voltage, gestation, injury-to-delivery interval and outcome was collected. Among the 15 victims, the fetal mortality was 73% and there was only one normal pregnancy following electric shock. The fetus is much less resistant to electric shock than the mother. Any mother who suffers from an electric shock in pregnancy, however minor, requires prompt fetal monitoring and careful obstetric supervision.

Brain-stem death in pregnancy

Intensive care unit physicians and obstetricians are increasingly having to deal with the difficult problem of a brainstem dead patient on a ventilator with an apparently intact fetus. Before 24 weeks a decision has to be made about prolonging ventilation and support for the mother to allow the fetus to develop to a reasonably mature gestation before delivery by caesarean section.

Sport, occupational and toxic injury

Pregnant women are increasingly active during their pregnancy, taking part in such activities as skiing, horse-riding, yoga and aquarobics. Nearly 50% of the workforce is now female and pregnant women occasionally work up to term. They will, therefore, be exposed to the hazards of the workplace. The report by the four UK Departments of Health (Departments of Health 1996) on maternal mortality recorded four deaths from injecting substance abuse compared with nine deaths in road traffic accidents in the period 1991–93. The most recent report cites two deaths from overdose of street drugs (CEMACH 2004).

Perimortem and postmortem caesarean section

Current resuscitation guidelines suggest that, at a gestational age in excess of 28 weeks, caesarean section should be undertaken in the emergency department if there is no maternal response to resuscitation after 5 min. This is a difficult decision and there may be controversy as to whether this action should be authorized by the team leader or by an attending obstetrician.

The 1991–93 maternal mortality report (Departments of Health 1996) discusses this issue. There is a report of a postmortem caesarean section being performed on a woman of 38 weeks gestation who had died instantly from multiple injuries sustained in a RTA 45 min earlier. The baby was resuscitated and survived for 48 h but died of cerebral damage due to intrauterine anoxia. This case highlights the poor success rate for fetal survival for postmortem caesarean sections, which, unless performed immediately following the death of the mother, are almost invariably associated with severe fetal anoxia and consequent cerebral damage.

The report therefore classifies these operations into perimortem and post-mortem caesarean sections. Perimortem caesarean sections are defined as cases in which the mother was close to death at the time of operation, was unconscious, was receiving CPR and failed to regain consciousness after delivery. There were no surviving babies following postmortem caesarean sections, whereas the fetal results for perimortem sections performed under optimal conditions were good.

Conclusion

The prehospital medicine practitioner should treat the injured pregnant patient according to standard guidelines. Extra attention must be paid, however, to adequate oxygenation of the mother and prompt correction of hypovolaemia, which will improve the outcome for both mother and fetus.

In these cases, the emergency department should be forewarned that the trauma patient is pregnant in order that appropriate specialists can be available on arrival.

Fetal damage must be suspected even in the presence of minimal maternal trauma and close obstetric follow-up must be arranged.

References

American College of Surgeons Committee on Trauma 1997 Advanced trauma life support student manual, 6th edn. American College of Surgeons, Chicago, IL

Buchsbaum HJ 1979 Trauma in pregnancy. WB Saunders, Philadelphia, PA

CEMACH 2004 Why mothers die 2000–2002 – The Sixth Report of Confidential Enquiries into Maternal Deaths in the United Kingdom (ed G Lewis). Royal College of Obstetricians and Gynaecologists Press, London

Connor E, Curran J 1976 In utero traumatic deceleration injury to the fetus. American Journal of Obstetrics and Gynecology 125: 567–569

Departments of Health 1994 Report on Confidential Inquiries into Maternal Deaths in the United Kingdom, 1987–1990 (Department of Health, Welsh Office, Scottish Home and Health Department, Department of Health and Social Services Northern Ireland). HMSO, London

Departments of Health 1996 Report on confidential enquiries into maternal deaths in the United Kingdom, 1991–1993 (Department of Health, Welsh Office, Scottish Home and Health Department, Department of Health and Social Services Northern Ireland). HMSO, London

Fatovich DM 1993 Electric shock in pregnancy. Journal of Emergency Medicine 11: 175–177

Griffiths M, Hillman G, Usherwood MMcD 1991 Seat-belt injury in pregnancy resulting in fetal death. British Journal of Obstetrics and Gynaecology 98: 320–321

Griffiths M, Siddall-Allum J, Reginald PW, Usherwood MMcD 1993 Road traffic accidents in pregnancy – the management and prevention of trauma. In: Studd J (ed) Progress in obstetrics and gynaecology 10. Churchill Livingstone, Edinburgh

Hammar B, Carter TD 1960 Intrauterine stab wound of fetus. Central Africa Journal of Medicine 6: 362

Jain ML, Garg AK 1993 Burns with pregnancy. Burns 19: 166–267

London PS 1991 The severely injured pregnant patient. In: Baldwin RWM, Hanson GC (eds) The critically ill obstetric patient. Farrand Press, London

Maddox PR, Mansel RE, Butchart EG 1991 Traumatic rupture of the diaphragm: a difficult diagnosis. Injury 22: 299–302

Nash P, Driscoll P 1991 Trauma in pregnancy. In: Skinner D, Driscoll P, Earlam R (eds) ABC of major trauma. BMJ Publishing, London

Ribe JK, Teggatz JR, Harvey CM 1993 Blows to the maternal abdomen causing fetal demise. Journal of Forensic Sciences 38: 1091–1096

Roe J 1993 Trauma in pregnancy. In: Markovchick VJ, Pons PT, Wolfe RE (eds) Emergency medicine secrets. Hanley & Belfus, Philadelphia, PA

Scorpio RJ, Esposito TJ, Smith LG, Gens DR 1992 Blunt trauma during pregnancy: factors affecting fetal outcome. Journal of Trauma 32: 213–216

Speer DP, Peltier LF 1972 Pelvic fracture and pregnancy. Journal of Trauma 12: 474

Vaizey CJ, Jacobson MJ, Cross FW 1995 Trauma in pregnancy. British Journal of Surgery 82: 279

Childbirth

42

Introduction	439
Emergency childbirth	440
The first stage of labour	440
The second stage of labour	441
The third stage	442
Abnormal deliveries	445
Babies born before arrival	445
Confidential Enquiry into Maternal and Child Health	446
Concealed pregnancy	446
Conclusion	446
References	446
Further reading	446

Introduction

Childbirth is a natural event and will usually occur without any complications but babies may arrive anywhere and at any time and may surprise both the mother and practitioners of prehospital medicine.

It is therefore essential to know how to deliver a baby and to care for the pregnant patient during her labour and the immediate puerperium, as well as to be able to care for the newborn. Obstetrics is one of the most unpredictable branches of medicine. Sometimes, almost without warning, an uncomplicated, low-risk delivery may turn into an extremely acute emergency threatening the lives of mother and baby. The practitioner should also know how to manage the major obstetric emergencies either outside hospital or while the patient is being transported to the obstetric unit.

Confidential Enquiry into Maternal and Child Health (CEMACH) is a self-governing body that runs confidential enquiries into maternal, peri-natal and child health. The major causes of direct deaths remain thromboembolism, hypertensive disorders of pregnancy and haemorrhage.

 www.

Further information about CEMACH and current statistics can be found at
www.cemach.org.uk.

Home childbirth can best be divided into planned, unplanned, unbooked and concealed delivery. The natural childbirth movement emphasizes the importance of women's choice and the number of home births is increasing. At the same time, there has been a reduction in the willingness of GPs to attend home births because they lack the necessary continued experience required to maintain their skills and may fear litigation following suboptimal obstetric outcomes. Obstetric flying squads are fast disappearing and midwives, who have a statutory duty to attend their patients in labour, are likely to call the front-line paramedic ambulance to help in emergencies. In some areas, doctors belonging to immediate care schemes may be called upon to attend the obstetric patient. Some planned home deliveries are conducted by independent midwives and the patient may have hardly seen a medical practitioner during her pregnancy.

Planned childbirth also takes place in better equipped settings such as GP cottage hospitals, midwife-led units, GP beds attached to consultant units and as 'domino' (domiciliary-in-and-out) deliveries by the community midwife in a consultant unit. Paramedics are occasionally called to GP- or midwife-led delivery units, which are usually in small or cottage hospitals, often fairly remote from the nearest specialist unit.

Unplanned delivery can happen anywhere. These births, often known as BBAs (birth before arrival) frequently occur in the back of an ambulance. Such a situation may also occur by chance or through bad planning in the case of an in utero transfer of a mother from a smaller district general hospital to a larger hospital with a special care or intensive care neonatal unit. Delivery occasionally occurs in the emergency department when there is insufficient time to summon a midwife.

Some women, especially the multiparous, will be unbooked for delivery and may attempt to avoid care by both doctors and midwives, even though the close family is fully aware of the situation. Members of certain sects may also only seek the help of lay friends.

Concealed pregnancy is often a tragedy and disaster for the mother, with a very poor perinatal outcome. Practitioners need to be aware of the need to involve the police or the police surgeon, who may wish to collect forensic evidence at the scene of the birth.

Emergency childbirth

Because normal childbirth is a natural event even in the prehospital setting, the practitioner's role may be confined to providing reassurance and support to a worried and frightened mother. A healthy baby will normally adapt well to the extrauterine environment in the arms of its mother.

Labour involves the delivery of the fetus and placenta and starts with the onset of regular painful contractions and progressive dilatation of the cervix. Sudden birth may, however, occur within minutes, especially in multiparous patients, who can have an extremely short first and second stage. Precipitate delivery may lead to the baby being delivered in a cold, unprepared environment.

The first stage of labour

During the first stage of labour, the cervix effaces, then dilates, and there is a 'bloody show' as the plug of blood-stained mucus in the cervical canal is displaced. Once cervical dilatation has reached 10 cm, the first stage of labour

is complete. During this time, the amniotic sac bulges through the cervical os and ruptures, releasing amniotic fluid. During the first stage of labour contractions become increasingly painful and increase from every 20 min to every 3 min. Towards the end of the first stage, the fetal head descends into the pelvis (Fig. 42.1).

The patient, especially if a primigravida, can be reassured that she is in labour. Emotional support is vital. The main job of the attendant is to consider whether s/he will need to deliver the baby him/herself or if there is time to call on more experienced help or to transfer the patient to hospital. It is also necessary to be on guard and ready to undertake the immediate care of any complications.

Assessment involves five components:

- The history
- Vital signs of the mother
- Vital signs of the fetus
- Progress of labour
- Recording of the above.

Trouble can often be predicted and sometimes avoided by taking a history from the mother or her other attendants. The crucial questions are:

- Does the patient have obstetric notes?
- Where is she booked for delivery?
- What is the expected date of delivery (based on last menstrual period and ultrasound examination)?
- Have there been any problems in this pregnancy?
- Have there been any problems in a previous pregnancy?
- How long has the woman had symptoms and signs such as contractions, breaking of waters or bleeding?
- Has anyone been making any maternal or fetal observations?

Specific questions may be necessary, especially with regard to the estimation of blood loss.

The present and past history of the patient will give much information about the present delivery and also as to whether any problems are to be expected.

Vital signs include level of consciousness, colour, blood pressure and pulse measurements. In suspected preeclampsia, it is essential to look for oedema and test the reflexes. At this stage, the nature of maternal pain can be observed.

The condition of the baby is monitored by listening to the fetal heart before, during and after maternal contractions. A cardboard toilet roll is a useful alternative to the Pinard fetal stethoscope. Observation of meconium in the amniotic fluid is also extremely useful.

Progress of labour is best judged by vaginal examination to detect progressive dilatation of the cervix. Vaginal examination is, however, not really necessary in a prehospital

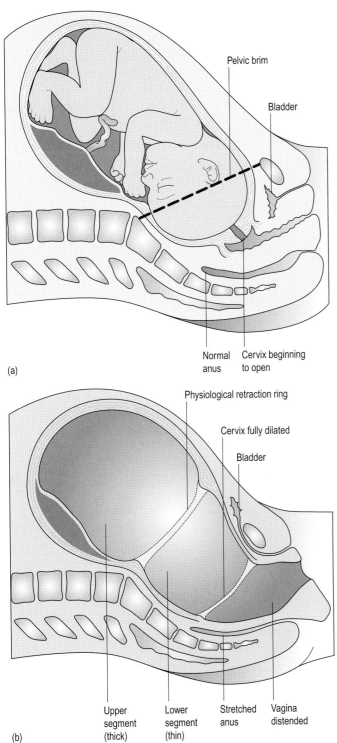

(a)

Pelvic brim

Bladder

Normal anus | Cervix beginning to open

Physiological retraction ring

Cervix fully dilated

Bladder

Upper segment (thick) | Lower segment (thin) | Stretched anus | Vagina distended

(b)

Fig. 42.1 • The birth canal (a) at early first stage and (b) at the beginning of the second stage of labour (the baby is not shown in (b)).

presenting part and its engagement in the pelvis. If the mother wants to open her bowels, care must be taken to ensure that this does not herald the desire to push and imminent delivery. Finally, all the above observations should be recorded in order to aid further management of the patient and, perhaps, an eventual transfer to a hospital unit.

Once management of labour is under way, the options are:

- Preparing for delivery
- Calling for help at the scene
- Transferring the patient to hospital.

The second stage of labour

Preparation of the delivery site should be made. A home delivery kit will be available for planned delivery. In an emergency, however, surprisingly little equipment is needed and the provision of a warm environment for the baby is the most important aim.

The principal symptom of the second stage is the urge to push. The principal signs are bulging of the perineum, anal dilatation and appearance of the baby's head at the vulva.

During the second stage, the baby's head flexes then internally rotates so that the occiput is anterior and the face posterior. The head extends at birth. The occiput delivers first, followed by the vertex, forehead and face (Fig. 42.2).

CROWNING OF THE HEAD

Delivery should be allowed to proceed normally without any restraint. The practice of 'protecting the perineum' with a pad or hand is conventional but has little influence on perineal damage. It is also common to put the other hand on the head to control delivery, but again this should not be necessary with a normal delivery. A midwife or experienced practitioner will, however, control delivery in such a fashion, but her judgement will prevent injudicious use of such manoeuvres.

RESTITUTION

When the head has emerged from the vagina, it will turn to a lateral position to allow the shoulders to negotiate the widest part of the outlet. The midwife may support the head in this position (Fig. 42.3).

THE CORD

The attendant can now check the umbilical cord. If it is wound around the baby's neck, it can be slipped over the

setting when the vital signs of the mother and the fetus are satisfactory. The length and strength of the contractions could be determined by abdominal palpation. The more experienced practitioner should be able to detect the head. If it is very tight, the more experienced practitioner can divide the cord between two clamps.

THE SHOULDERS

The anterior shoulder will deliver spontaneously, perhaps with the aid of gentle posterior flexion of the head. The posterior shoulder then follows, again aided by anterior flexion of the head. The rest of the baby will now follow.

THE BABY

The baby should be delivered on to the mother's abdomen, where she may hold it, or, on to the bed. It is wise not to hold the baby for too long: babies are quite slippery. The baby is dried and wrapped in a blanket. Despite copious secretions, suction of the baby's airways is rarely necessary when the baby appears to be in good condition.

It is important to record the time of birth. The umbilical cord may now be cut between two clamps or pieces of string. This is usually done a couple of minutes after the birth of the baby. It is preferable to leave a reasonable length of umbilical cord, about 5 cm, attached to the baby.

The baby's condition – the Apgar score

The Apgar score correlates with the condition of the newborn. It is recorded at 1 and 5 minutes. A baby with a score of 7 or above is in good condition. The Apgar score is based on the five parameters given in Table 42.1.

When the Apgar score is below 6, three basic resuscitative measures should be taken (according to what equipment is available):

- Dry the baby in a warm towel
- Oxygen
- Bag and mask ventilation.

The subject of neonatal resuscitation is covered in more detail in Chapter 43.

The third stage

The third stage of labour is from the delivery of the head to delivery of the placenta. The placenta will usually deliver itself within 5–20 min and controlled cord traction is best avoided. Sometimes, expulsion is aided by rubbing up a uterine contraction or putting the baby to the breast.

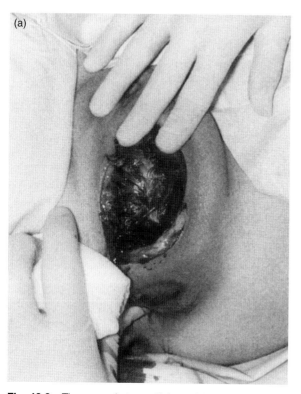
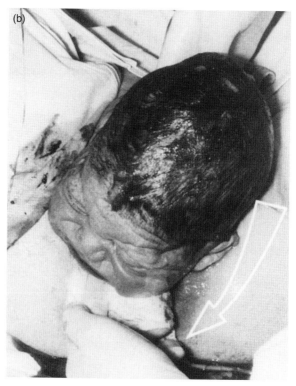

Fig. 42.2 • The second stage of labour. (a) Normal delivery in the lithotomy position. (b) The head is born; restitution of the head has undone the twist on the neck.

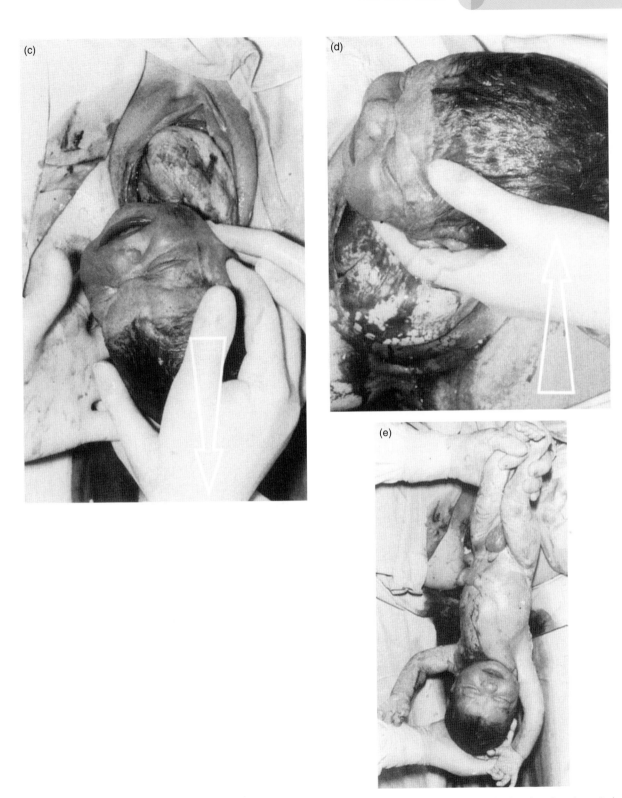

Fig. 42.2 • (c) The anterior shoulder is being released from under the symphysis pubis by directing the head and neck posteriorly. (d) The posterior shoulder is delivered by lateral flexion of the trunk in an anterior direction. (e) The baby is delivered. (With permission from Beischer et al 1997.)

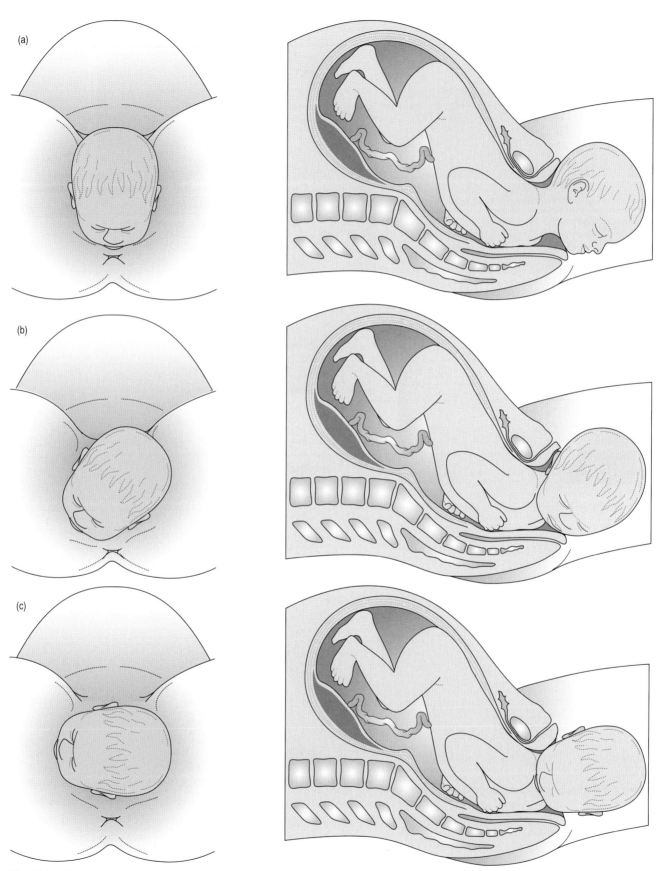

Fig. 42.3 • Delivery of the head.

Table 42.1 Apgar scores

Sign	Points		
	0	**1**	**2**
Colour	Pale	Blue	Pink
Pulse	0	<100	>100
Respiration	None	Irregular	Good
Tone	Limp	Some flexion	Active flexion
Reflex	No	Limited	Cry/active
Irritability	Response	Response	Movements

POSTPARTUM HAEMORRHAGE

Retained placenta and postpartum haemorrhage are the main reasons for calling an obstetric flying squad. If the blood loss is greater than 500 ml then the following action should be taken:

- Rub up a uterine contraction
- Put the baby to the breast
- Give Syntometrine (1 ampoule) or ergometrine (0.5 mg) intravenously if available
- Set up an intravenous infusion (give 1 litre of crystalloid or colloid)
- Notify the nearest obstetric unit and transfer patient.

Abnormal deliveries

Some problems allow enough time for transfer to an obstetric unit (e.g. delay with an occipitoposterior position or brow presentation). Shoulder dystocia is associated with a slow first stage with a big baby. Because there may well have been delay in such a case and the patient will have usually been transferred to hospital, shoulder dystocia is rarely encountered in the prehospital setting. In a case of transverse lie of the fetus, the mother and baby should be transferred to hospital because operative delivery will be required.

The four main abnormalities that may happen suddenly and require immediate attention are:

- Pre-term delivery
- Prolapsed cord
- Twin delivery
- Breech delivery.

PRETERM DELIVERY

Management of the first and second stages is as above. These babies have a large surface area relative to their body weight and are prone to rapid heat loss and its ensuing complications. The most important first-aid action is to wrap the baby up to prevent this heat loss. A baby that is much smaller than expected should alert the attendant to the possibility of twins.

PROLAPSED CORD

The sudden appearance of the cord at the vulva (or its palpation in the vagina below the presenting part) should be managed as follows:

- Position the mother (to take pressure of the cord) left lateral and head down
- Cover the exposed cord with a large warm swab and minimize handling
- Transfer to hospital immediately.

TWIN DELIVERY

Delivery can be rapid but relatively straightforward and is essentially conducted as the delivery of two babies. The babies are usually smaller and often preterm. If the second twin does not appear within 15 min, there is often time to transfer the mother to hospital for the birth of the second baby. In this era of ultrasound scanning, undiagnosed twins are a rarity. The main risk is the high incidence of postpartum haemorrhage.

BREECH DELIVERY

Breech presentation is more common below 37 weeks' gestation and the babies may be small. It may not be diagnosed until the buttocks or feet appear at the vulva. Breech deliveries in multiparous patients can be quite rapid and in these cases entrapment of the aftercoming head is quite unusual. Sudden decompression of the head is best avoided. In a primigravida, the second stage often lasts several hours, giving time to transfer the patient to an obstetric unit.

The basic rule for the attendant is 'hands off the breech'. No attempt should be made to pull the baby out.

Babies born before arrival

Babies born before arrival at hospital have an increased perinatal mortality compared with hospital-born infants. Most of these babies have arrived quite suddenly and are often preterm. In the case of a planned hospital birth or concealed pregnancy, no preparations will have been made by the community midwife for home delivery. Concealed pregnancy is usually accompanied by considerable delay before informing the emergency team. Spillane et al (1996) reviewed 106 babies born before arrival in 1988–91. They represented 0.4% of the births and preterm birth was the major factor contributing to increased mortality. There were two distinct groups of patients. The first consisted of 14 women who had neither booked nor attended for antenatal care. Ten of these were first-time mothers, 13 were unmarried and seven were under 27 years of age. The second group was made up of 92 women booked for antenatal care: only four of these 92 were first-time mothers. Many of the multiparous women had a history of preterm spontaneous rupture of the membranes but delayed coming into hospital.

Bhoopalam & Watkinson (1991) reviewed 31 140 consecutive births and found 0.44% (137) BBAs. The perinatal mortality rate in the BBA group was nearly six times as high as for hospital births. Hypothermia was the commonest morbidity problem. The survey, in the Birmingham area, noted that women delivered before arrival tended to be either multigravid inner-city Asians living a long way from the hospital or unmarried, unbooked younger white Europeans. They concluded that the high perinatal mortality was related to immaturity and low birthweight rather than to birth before arrival itself.

Confidential Enquiry into Maternal and Child Health

Confidential Enquiry into Maternal and Child Health (CEMACH) is a self-governing body that runs confidential enquiries into maternal, perinatal and child health. It has taken over the role previously filled by the Confidential Enquiries into Stillbirths and Deaths in Infancy conducted by the Department of Health.

Perinatal mortality has been falling since the 1950s, with stillbirths accounting for 70% of perinatal deaths in 2004. Multiple births have an incidence of stillbirth three times, and a perinatal mortality rate seven times, that of singleton births. The preinatal mortality rate in the UK in 2003 was 8.6 per 1000 births (CEMACH 2005).

It is recommended that all community professionals should be trained in the management of the more common emergencies that may arise, including an unexpected breech delivery, shoulder dystocia and neonatal resuscitation. Multidisciplinary training sessions, improvement in risk recognition, good communications and instruction in the management of rare serious complications are recommended.

Concealed pregnancy

Concealed pregnancy is often disastrous both for mother and baby. Babies have been born in toilets or abandoned

at various locations and are at serious risk from hypothermia. The mother, often young and frightened, requires medical and social help. Brezinka et al (1994) reported a high incidence of preterm birth and perinatal death among 27 women who professed that they did not know they were pregnant until labour began.

Conclusion

Choice and woman-centred care are leading to an increase in home births. The debate about the safety of home birth will go on. Unexpected birth before arrival in hospital will continue to occur. Childbirth will always produce surprises, including the sudden onset of emergencies threatening the lives of the mother and baby. Professionals must respond to the challenge of managing these emergencies. The traditional physician-manned obstetric flying squad is being superseded by front line emergency paramedic unit teams providing skilled aid to the attending midwives and GPs.

The key to successful provision of emergency domiciliary obstetric services lies in the provision of a team capable of advanced obstetric and paediatric life support followed by rapid transport to a receiving specialist unit.

References

Beischer NA, Mackay EV, Colditz P 1997 Obstetrics and the newborn, 3rd edn. Baillière Tindall, London

Bhoopalam PS, Watkinson M 1991 Babies born before arrival at hospital. British Journal of Obstetrics and Gynaecology 98: 57–64

Brezinka C, Huter O, Biebl W et al 1994 Denial of pregnancy: obstetrical aspects. Journal of Psychosomatic Obstetrics and Gynaecology 15: 1–8

Confidential Enquiry into Maternal and Child Health 2005 Stillbirth, neonatal and post-neonatal mortality 2000–2003, England Wales and Northern Ireland. Royal College of Obstetricians and Gynaecology Press, London

Department of Health 1993 Confidential inquiry into stillbirths and deaths in infancy. Annual report. HMSO, London

Departments of Health 1996 Report on confidential inquiries into maternal deaths in the United Kingdom, 1991–1993 (Department of Health, Welsh Office, Scottish Home and Health Department, Department of Health and Social Services Northern Ireland). HMSO, London

Spillane H, Khalil G, Turner M 1996 Babies born before arrival at the Coombe Women's Hospital, Dublin. Irish Medical Journal 89: 58–59

Further reading

Andina MM, Fikree FF 1995 The Faisalbad Obstetric Flying Squad. Mother Child International. World Health Statistics Quarterly 48: 50–54

Bullough CHW 1992 Action in international medicine and maternal health care in developing countries. British Journal of Obstetrics and Gynaecology 99: 358–359

Douglas KA, Redman CWG 1992 Eclampsia in the United Kingdom. The 'BEST' way forward. British Journal of Obstetrics and Gynaecology 99: 355–359

James DK 1977 Obstetric flying squad service – a defence. British Medical Journal 1: 217–219

Liang DYS 1963 The emergency obstetric service–Bellshill Maternity Hospital, 1933–1961. Journal of Obstetrics and Gynaecology of the British Commonwealth 70: 83

McCloskey KAL, Orr RA 1995 Pediatric transport medicine. Mosby–Year Book, St Louis, MO

Saunders E 1989 Neonaticides following secret pregnancies: seven case reports. Public Health Reports 104: 368–372

Suzuki T, Ikeda N, Umetsu K, Kashimura S 1986 Fatal case due to atonic haemorrhage with giant placenta following concealed delivery. Medicine, Science and the Law 26: 295–298

Neonatal resuscitation and transport

43

Introduction 448

Physiology of the neonate 448

Normal physiological values 449

Resuscitation 449

Meconium aspiration 451

Transport 452

References 452

Introduction

Because the vast majority of births in this country occur within hospitals, the need for neonatal resuscitation is rarely encountered within prehospital medicine. However, every year a number of infants are born prior to their mother reaching hospital for a planned delivery. In addition, there is an increasing trend towards planned home deliveries, at which a midwife and usually a GP will be present. In these settings a practitioner in prehospital medicine may be asked to assist in the resuscitation of the newborn infant.

Physiology of the neonate

The fetus in utero is totally dependent on maternal circulation via the placenta for oxygenation. Therefore the entire respiratory and circulatory systems of the fetus are designed to allow for this. At the time of birth, however, newborn babies must establish adequate physiological changes within the respiratory and circulatory systems so that they can oxygenate themselves independent of the maternal/placental unit (Caroline 1991).

The majority of newborn babies can establish spontaneous respiration at birth because of physical stimuli at that time and also because clamping of the umbilical cord leads to hypoxaemia, which is a stimulus for the newborn baby to breath on its own. During these first few minutes of spontaneous ventilation, numerous changes take place in the newborn lung. The alveoli, which have been filled with fluid in fetal life, now expand with air, which also helps displace the fluid. Thus, within a short space of time the alveoli are filled with air during inspiration.

In addition, a compound called *surfactant* is produced within the alveolar epithelium. Its function is to reduce alveolar surface tension and prevent the alveoli collapsing completely during expiration (this would increase the work of each breath that the infant takes). Levels of surfactant may be low or non-existent in premature babies and this is one of the major causes of respiratory problems in the preterm infant.

In addition to changes within the alveoli of the lung, there are also changes in the pulmonary circulation. During fetal life the pulmonary circulation is bypassed, because it is not required, by the ductus arteriosus. However, with clamping of the cord and the child initiating its own breaths, it is important that the pulmonary circulation is established. This is achieved by blood flowing through the pulmonary trunk and the arterioles in the lungs beginning to open simultaneously with alveolar opening; as a result oxygen is transferred from the alveoli into the pulmonary

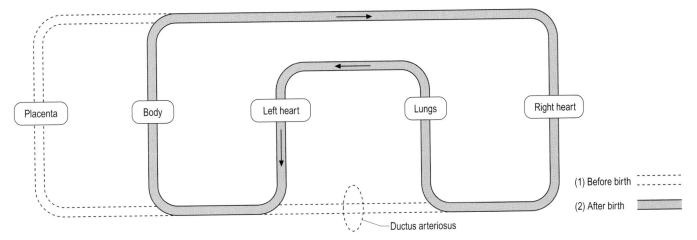

Fig. 43.1 • The neonatal circulation before and after delivery.

vasculature. As this begins to occur the ductus arteriosus constricts and begins to close so that a normal circulatory pattern can be established (Fig. 43.1).

In order for the newborn child to take its first breath it must have a functioning central nervous system with a functioning respiratory centre within the brain to drive ventilation. Newborns who have suffered intrauterine asphyxia or have been exposed to central nervous system depressant drugs (such as opiates) during the delivery may have such a depressed conscious level they cannot initiate or continue ventilations and may develop periods of apnoea.

Normal physiological values

Most infants at birth are vigorous and crying, quickly establish respiration, have a steady heart beat and are able to clear their central and peripheral cyanosis rapidly. Normal values for heart rate are 120–140 beats min^{-1} palpated at the apex beat, the brachial artery or the umbilical artery palpable in the umbilical stump. The normal values for respiration are a respiratory rate of approximately 40, with an upper limit of normal of 60 breaths min^{-1}. In addition to the rate, the breaths should be regular and there should be no periods of apnoea. The normal systolic blood pressure is 60 mmHg (Table 43.1).

In an effort to combine these physiological parameters, a scoring system termed the Apgar scoring system has been established as an aid to scoring and describing the child's wellbeing in the minutes after birth (Roberton 1992). The parameters of the Apgar scoring system are shown in Table 43.2 and it is normally applied at 1 min and 5 min after birth, although it is perfectly permissible to use it thereafter, particularly if resuscitation has been undertaken.

Table 43.1 Normal physiological values in the neonate

Heart rate	120–140 beats min^{-1}
Respiratory rate	40–60 breaths min^{-1}
Blood pressure (systolic)	60 mmHg

Table 43.2 Apgar scores

Sign	0	1	2
Heart rate (min^{-1})	Absent	Slow (< 100)	> 100
Respirations	Absent	Slow, irregular	Good, crying
Muscle tone	Limp	Some flexion	Active motion
Reflex irritability (catheter in nares)	No response	Grimace	Cough or sneeze
Colour	Blue or pale	Pink body with blue extremities	Completely pink

Resuscitation

The vast majority of newborn babies require no resuscitation. However, a small number of babies remain limp after birth, have difficulty establishing their first breath or a normal cycle of respirations and therefore become at risk of failing to maintain their heart rate. The common causes for an infant requiring resuscitation at birth include:

- prematurity
- congenital malformations
- intrauterine asphyxia drugs given to the mother during birth (Roberton 1992).

In most cases the newborn infant will respond to basic resuscitation measures such as drying with a dry cloth and towel. This stimulates the baby and also helps to prevent the rapid heat loss that newborn babies can suffer, which is a cause of acidosis. In addition, other forms of tactile stimulation, including slapping the sole of the foot, flicking the heel or rubbing the back of the infant may be effective (American Heart Association 1994).

Do not allow the baby to become cold!

Occasionally, as a result of secretions in the lung and upper airway, cyanosis fails to resolve. These secretions, as mentioned previously, are due to the fluid that was in the alveoli and airways prior to the first breath. The use of gentle suction to help clear these secretions also acts as a type of tactile stimulus. It should be stated that the use of *vigorous* suctioning has a harmful effect on the baby and can initiate a slow heart rate as a result of increased vagal tone; apnoeic spells may also occur. Ideally only soft suction catheters should be used.

While any of these procedures are being employed, the use of supplemental oxygen should be considered and can usually be applied by a face mask (Boychuk 1991). Oxygen 100% may safely be given to all babies, including preterm ones, for short periods.

These measures need to be undertaken rapidly after birth and are appropriate for mild to moderate distress (e.g. the infant who is slow to establish a normal respiratory pattern but can maintain a normal pulse rate). Clearly, these measures will be ineffective if the infant is born in severe distress when there is no respiratory effort, cyanosis and bradycardia. In this situation, more advanced methods of resuscitation are required.

Advanced resuscitation continues along the paradigm of ABC (Airway, Breathing, Circulation). Therefore, it is important that, at a very early stage in neonatal advanced resuscitation, the neonate is intubated. Normally a size 3.0–3.5 endotracheal tube is sufficient for a term neonate. Smaller sizes down to a 2.5 endotracheal tube may be required in the preterm infant. It is important to confirm that the chest is inflating bilaterally and symmetrically and ventilation can then be continued at a rate of approximately 40 min^{-1}.

Use a 3.0–3.5 endotracheal tube in a term neonate.

Once ventilations have been established, a quick assessment of the pulse rate is required. If it is below 60 beats min^{-1} or initially between 60 and 80 min^{-1} but does not increase with the first minute of ventilation, then external cardiac massage should be instituted. Adequate chest compressions can be achieved either by using two fingers on the sternum, placed one fingerbreadth below the nipple line, or by circling the torso with both hands so that both thumbs are placed on the sternum, again at a site one finger breadth below the nipple line (Fig. 43.2).

The compression rate should be approximately 100 min^{-1}. In order to achieve this and the requisite 30 ventilations min^{-1}, it is necessary to carry out three compressions to one ventilation cycle. Thus, the aim is to compress the chest three times and ventilate once in every 2 s period.

Neonatal resuscitation: three compressions to one ventilation.

If these measures fail to initiate adequate respiration, and in particular fail to increase the heart rate or establish spontaneous circulation, then the use of drugs will be required for advanced life support. The drugs most commonly used are as follows.

ADRENALINE (EPINEPHRINE)

The first dose of adrenaline (epinephrine) is 10 μg kg^{-1} (which is 0.1 ml kg^{-1} of 1:10 000 strength adrenaline). This should be given by the intravenous or interosseous route but, if these cannot be established, a higher dose (100 μg kg^{-1} (0.1 ml kg^{-1} of 1:1000 adrenaline) can be given via the endotracheal route.

If the baby requires further doses of adrenaline, doses of 10–30 μg/kg should be used IV or IO. Higher dose adrenaline (100 μg/kg) is no longer recommended.

INTRAVENOUS FLUIDS

The asphyxiated infant may require additional intravascular volume in order to assist resuscitation. An infusion rate of 20 ml kg^{-1} is appropriate.

GLUCOSE

The small-for-dates or preterm infant is susceptible to profound hypoglycaemia, which causes central nervous system (CNS) depression and seizures and may be the cause of inadequate respiration.

Therefore a bedside BM Stix should be taken early in resuscitation and, if the child is hypoglycaemic, intravenous dextrose given. The infant will usually require 3–5 ml kg^{-1}

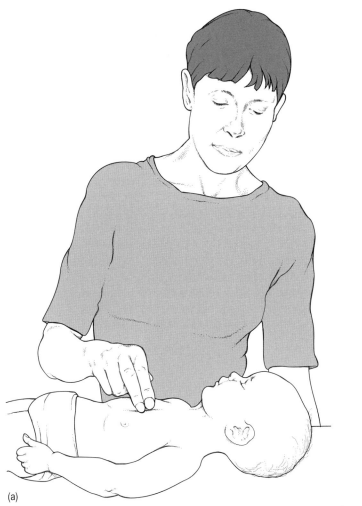
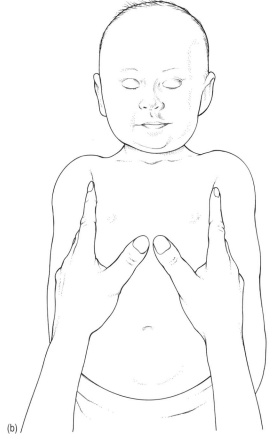

Fig. 43.2 • Two methods of external cardiac compression in the neonate.

of a 10% solution. The use of 50% dextrose is difficult, because of the size of neonatal veins, and appropriate dilution is indicated.

BICARBONATE

Although cautious administration of sodium bicarbonate is used in hospital practice for the treatment of neonatal acidosis, its use in prehospital care is not recommended.

NALOXONE

As previously stated the use of opiates during delivery or indeed by mothers who have a drug dependence problem may result in an infant being born with inadequate respiration secondary to CNS depression. This is treated with naloxone, a dose of $0.1\,ml\,kg^{-1}$ as an intramuscular injection is usually effective.

VASCULAR ACCESS

In attempting to establish vascular access, the practitioner should consider peripheral intravenous lines, including scalp veins. In the newborn the use of the umbilical vein as an access point can be considered, although this approach is likely to be difficult in the prehospital environment. Alternatively, intraosseus access should be obtained. If intraosseous access is not available, no delay while prolonged and inappropriate attempts at access are carried out should be incurred in transferring the infant to hospital.

Meconium aspiration

This condition is unique to newborn babies. It occurs when there has been fetal distress during the labour and the amniotic fluid surrounding the baby has become contaminated by meconium, which is the first form of stool that the baby passes per rectum. Meconium is highly toxic to the infant lung and therefore efforts to prevent the newborn infant aspirating any meconium are important.

It is usually possible to suction meconium from the baby's nose and mouth as soon as the baby's head is born (Suri & McFarlane 1997). In addition, once the infant has been born it may be possible to suction meconium away from the upper airways and trachea by using direct laryngoscopy. This will usually require an endotracheal tube with suctioning on the tube as it is withdrawn. Clinical judgement is then required to decide whether it is in the infant's best interest to have further meconium suction from the trachea or whether positive pressure ventilation is required to assist the child's resuscitation.

Transport

As these measures are being undertaken in an out-of-hospital setting, it is important that once resuscitation has been established prompt transfer to an appropriate hospital is organized. The prehospital practitioner will need to summon a paramedic ambulance to bring the neonate to the most appropriate facility. This will usually be the local emergency department, particularly if there is an associated paediatric/maternity service on site. In some cities it may be more appropriate to bring the child and mother to the local maternity hospital. In either instance it is important that the prehospital practitioner is aware of what facilities are available and communicates with the receiving hospital and receiving doctor, so that the receiving facility can be prepared.

Transport of the ill neonate occurs in two settings. The first is the baby born outside hospital needing transfer to hospital – as already described in this chapter. In this instance the child is brought to hospital by ordinary ambulance. The key roles of the prehospital practitioner are the simple measures of keeping the baby warm throughout transport and ensuring adequate oxygenation, that the endotracheal tube and intravascular access, if sited, are secure and that there are enough assistants to continue cardiopulmonary resuscitation if that is on-going.

However, the most common setting for neonatal transfer is where an infant is being transferred from a hospital to a neonatal referral centre, either for intensive care facilities or for neonatal surgery (Miller & Macrae 1994). The prehospital practitioner may become involved in this situation.

The practitioner will ensure that the referring and receiving hospitals have been in communication with each other, that the referral has been properly sanctioned and that the exact destination (intensive care ward, theatre or emergency department) at the referral centre is known.

In this setting the use of a portable incubator may be required. The usual requirements of a portable incubator are:

- mains or battery power
- maintenance of a temperature of at least 36°C
- ease of observation
- easy access
- space for a suitably sized oxygen cylinder to allow for 100% oxygen for up to 6 h (Chiswick 1992).

Paramedic staff are the normal prehospital practitioners involved in these situations and it is essential that they are aware of and familiar with such transport incubators. A doctor or nurse either as part of the referring team or as part of the retrieval team will also be present.

References

American Heart Association 1994 Textbook of neonatal resuscitation. American Heart Association, Dallas, TX

Biarent D, Bingham R, Richmond S, Maconochie I, Wyllie J, Simpson S, Rodriguez Nunez A, Zideman D. European Resuscitation Council Guidelines for Resuscitation 2005. Section 6. Paediatric life support. Resuscitation (2005) 67S1, S97–S133

Boychuk R 1991 The critically ill neonate in the emergency department. Emergency Medicine Clinics of North America 9: 507–522

Caroline N 1991 Neonatal care and transport in emergency care in the streets. Little, Brown, New York, p 801–813

Chiswick M 1992 Regional organisation of perinatal care. In: Roberton N (ed) Textbook of neonatology. Churchill Livingstone, Edinburgh, p 1133–1146

Miller O, Macrae D 1994 Newborn emergency transport. British Journal of Intensive Care 4: 226–229

Roberton N 1992 Resuscitation of the newborn. In: Roberton N (ed) Textbook of neonatology. Churchill Livingstone, Edinburgh, p 173–198

Resuscitation Council (UK). Resuscitation Guideline 2005: newborn life support. Resuscitation Council; London, 2005

Suri S, McFarlane P 1997 Survey of delivery rooms management of the infant born through meconium stained liquor. Paediatrics Today 5: 76–80

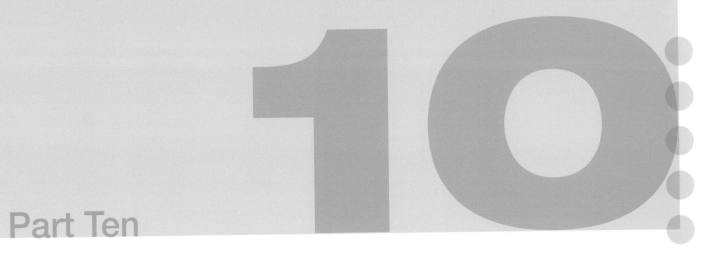

Part Ten

44 Psychiatric emergencies 455

45 Human reactions to trauma: their features and management 465

46 Dealing with the violent or uncooperative patient 476

Psychiatric emergencies 44

Introduction 455

What is a psychiatric emergency? 456

Essentials of assessment 456

Psychosis: recognition and treatment 457

Parasuicide: recognition and treatment 458

Depression and mania 459

Anxiety disorders 460

Physical causes of psychiatric emergencies 460

Personality disorder 461

The Mental Health Act 1983 461

Common law and informed consent 462

Managing the aggressive and uncooperative psychiatric patient 463

Conclusions 464

Further reading 464

Introduction

Psychiatric emergencies present immediate risks to the patient's health, wellbeing and safety, as well as to the safety of others. Despite these apparent risks and their immediacy, admission to hospital is not always indicated. The vast majority of psychiatric emergencies are not immediately life threatening and there is usually time in which to plan a coordinated and careful response. Unfortunately, perhaps because of ignorance, there is a tendency to over-react and look on hospital admission as the only option. This may result in unnecessary use of expensive resources but, more importantly, may have a profound and long-lasting detrimental effect on the patient.

Stigma associated with mental illness remains rife, as does that associated with psychiatric hospitals. Many psychiatric services are promoting the use of alternative community facilities for the management of people with mental disorders, and it is likely that many people who in the past would have been admitted to hospital can now be managed at home or in an alternative community facility that does not carry with it the same prejudice as is linked to more traditional psychiatric settings. This applies no less to patients presenting as an emergency, who are often subject to the fear and apparent helplessness of carers or authorities, who in turn may have become blinded by their desire to react quickly and remove the person from the crisis situation without first considering other options that may be available. Nevertheless, serious mental illness and significant risk must be taken seriously, and hospitals are the first choice for those patients who require intensive support, treatment and supervision. Admission to hospital should not be avoided because of ideological considerations.

Most psychiatric emergencies involve patients who are distressed and helpless, and who may appear dangerous or at risk of harm (Table 44.1). Most psychiatric patients are not dangerous and it is important to counter the myth that uncritically associates dangerousness with psychiatric

Table 44.1 Some mental health emergencies

Immediate risk to a patient's health and well-being

- Nihilistic delusions or depressive stupor (stops eating and drinking)
- Manic excitement (stops eating, becomes exhausted and dehydrated)
- Self-neglect
- Vulnerability to assault or exploitation
- Sexual exploitation

Immediate risk to a patient's safety

- Suicidal intentions
- Deliberate self-harm
- Chaotic behaviour

Immediate risk to others

- To family (as a result of depressive or paranoid delusions)
- To children, who may be neglected as a result of parent's erratic behaviour (in schizophrenia or mania)
- To newborn baby (in postnatal depression or puerperal psychosis)
- To general public (as a result of paranoid or other delusions)

disorder. It is particularly important to be aware that, as a result of their behaviour (deeming them to be at risk to themselves or others), mentally ill patients may be admitted to hospital involuntarily on a section of the Mental Health Act. This results in their loss of liberty and may have a profound effect on how they are treated in the immediate and long term.

Dealing with psychiatric patients requires skills of counselling, empathy and negotiation, and ability to liaise with different professional groups (the police, social workers, nurses, doctors). The general public too have a role, as their concerns may have precipitated the response from health or social services. It is especially important to support and inform relatives, who are often somewhat bemused and upset at the situation. They may harbour strong feelings of anger, guilt and sadness, and require reassurance and understanding.

What is a psychiatric emergency?

A psychiatric emergency can be defined as a situation involving someone exhibiting psychological distress that exceeds the coping strategies of that individual, or their carers, or society and/or that involves a possible risk to themselves or others and requires immediate attention to avert a serious outcome.

The causes of psychiatric emergencies are manifold and varied. Some will be described below. However, it is important to note that many apparent emergencies can be resolved without necessarily resorting to the powers of the Mental

Health Act or the facilities of the local hospital. They often arise out of particular social difficulties (e.g. running out of money or electricity, homelessness, lack of food), breakdown in relationships or altercation with the police. Some may occur as a result of a physical disorder or be related to medication or use of illicit drugs. Some may result in a psychiatric patient being scapegoated or otherwise becoming a victim of public overconcern, fear, ignorance and overreaction. All require an assessment that may be prolonged and involve psychiatrists, social workers and relatives. At the end of this assessment the result may be a loss of someone's liberty if they are admitted to hospital against their will.

Essentials of assessment

The essentials of any assessment of a psychiatric emergency are to obtain all relevant information, engage the patient, undertake a mental state and physical examination, support any relatives or carers and, above all, to remain patient and unflustered. Ensuring the safety of everyone involved is paramount and if there is any doubt as to the level of risk towards those undertaking the assessment no attempt should be made to continue it without further assistance.

GATHER INFORMATION FROM PATIENT AND INFORMANT

All psychiatric assessments (and emergencies are no exception) should begin with gathering as much information as possible about the patient (Table 44.2). The nature of the presenting symptoms (whether gradual or sudden onset), past medical and psychiatric history (including substance misuse), present medication (both prescribed and non-prescribed) and level of support at home are essential elements of an accurate assessment and should be obtained both from the patient and from an informant.

This initial assessment may not be straightforward. For example, a patient may not allow access to his/her residence. In this case it may be possible to conduct a reasonable appraisal of the situation through the letter box, thereby persuading the patient to open the door or gathering enough information to make a decision regarding admission under the Mental Health Act. Neighbours can be extremely useful informants who, as well as providing background information about the patient, have often noticed recent changes in behaviour. Close relatives are often available to give detailed information.

MENTAL STATE EXAMINATION

Mental state examination is the term given to observation of the patient's behaviour, mood and speech in order to gather

Table 44.2 Taking a psychiatric history

- Presenting symptoms
- Past medical history
- Past psychiatric history (including substance misuse)
- Medication
- Available support

Table 44.3 Organic causes of psychiatric emergencies

- Hypoglycaemia
- Infection
- Cardiac failure
- Delirium tremors
- Subdural haematoma
- Substance abuse

evidence of mental disorder. It is important that a mental state examination is objective and not subjective or based on supposition. A comprehensive mental state examination should be carried out in all cases. The usual procedure is to subdivide the examination into a number of categories:

- appearance and behaviour
- speech form (i.e. coherence) and content
- beliefs and thoughts expressed
- overall mood state and whether it is congruent with the thought content
- any observable abnormal perceptions or experiences (e.g. hallucinations)
- assessment of level of consciousness, orientation in time, place and person, concentration and short-term memory
- presence of insight (the acknowledgement by the patient that they are having psychological problems that need to be resolved)
- suicidal ideation should always be evaluated.

PHYSICAL EXAMINATION

This should be carried out in every case as far as is possible, even if there appears to be no apparent physical disorder. Common organic causes of psychiatric emergencies (e.g. hypoglycaemia, infection, cardiac failure, delirium tremens, subdural haematoma) should be rigorously and systematically searched for (Table 44.3). Breath odour may reveal solvent or alcohol misuse, and recent skin puncture marks suggests drug misuse.

Psychosis: recognition and treatment

Psychosis refers to disturbances in thinking and behaviour usually involving delusions, hallucinations and thought disorder. Where these symptoms are sufficiently recognizable and characteristic, they may be attributable to a diagnosis such as schizophrenia, mania or psychotic depression. However, psychiatric diagnosis is complicated and bedevilled by problems of definition and applicability, and it is usually simpler just to describe symptoms expressed and signs observed.

ASSESSMENT OF PSYCHOSIS

Delusions

A delusion is a firmly held but false belief that is out of context with the person's social and cultural background, not amenable to any logical argument that is presented to refute it and based on spurious and inappropriate evidence. There is often an element of persecution accompanying the belief but patients may express delusions that they have special powers or are invested with great authority or fame. Examples include delusions that they are being persecuted or hounded by others (often the police or other authority figures), that others are watching or listening to them through bugging devices, that presenters on the television are referring directly to them or that items in newspapers or the media have special significance to them, beliefs about bodily malfunctions (e.g. bowels seizing up or interference with particular organs) or excessive guilt or self-blame for particular life circumstances. Often it is impossible even to attempt to confront the reality of the belief and there is a danger in so doing of losing rapport with the patient, resulting in argument.

Hallucinations

Hallucinations refer to the experience of perceptions (e.g. hearing voices or noises, seeing vivid images, or tasting particular flavours) in the absence of a stimulus causing the perception. They can occur in any sensory modality. They are not imagined experiences and to the patient appear real. Often, a delusional explanation of the hallucination may be put forward. For example, voices may be explained in terms of transmitters through the electric cable or bugging devices in the pipes. Hallucinations are often frightening and distressing, and patients may be observed to be responding to apparent hallucinations, especially if they appear to be distractible, preoccupied, or talking or muttering inappropriately. Rarely, patients may act on their hallucinations in an impulsive manner.

Psychotic behaviour

Often this is the reason why an emergency has arisen. Patients suffering acute psychological distress may act in unusual, bizarre or even frightening ways. They may shout and swear, gesticulate in a threatening way and indulge in antisocial behaviour. Their speech may be incoherent and their thoughts disjointed. They may be preoccupied with delusions and responding to hallucinations. They may attempt to harm themselves or appear to be endangering others. On the other hand, they may become withdrawn and uncommunicative.

Dangerousness

It is important early in the assessment of a psychotic patient to be aware of any propensity to dangerousness. It is a common fallacy that all psychotic patients are dangerous. While this is not true in the overwhelming number, there are a minority who have a propensity to be violent, usually as a direct consequence of their illness. Part of the initial assessment should include an appraisal of the presence of any aggressive or violent behaviour. Pointers that indicate whether a patient is likely to be violent are a past history of violence, whether violence has already occurred, the patient's appearance and behaviour, whether the patient is intoxicated by alcohol or drugs, and the content of any delusions. Clearly, it is inadvisable to enter a situation that may result in physical danger and in the community, if there is a likelihood that this will occur, the police should be involved.

As a general rule it is inadvisable to assess an acutely psychotic patient alone because of the risk of unpredictable behaviour that may lead to injury. The assessment should be carried out in an area from which it is easy to escape, and the assessor should be placed between the patient and the exit. Although sitting down is sufficient in many cases to defuse the situation, if necessary the interview should be conducted standing up. It should be noted that much aggression in these situations is born out of fear, and it is helpful to be as reassuring, empathic and non-confrontational as possible in order to try and establish a rapport.

MANAGEMENT OF PSYCHOSIS

The key to managing an acutely psychotic patient is to be able to control behaviour. This can often be achieved by use of good interpersonal skills of empathy and reassurance, a non-threatening posture and an air of calmness and confidence. For any patient, but particularly one who is paranoid (who believes fervently that individuals or groups are against them), distressed and reacting to threatening hallucinations, the use of inappropriate force, verbal aggression and impatience is distressing and may be seen as confrontational. This may invite retaliation, further compromising any established therapeutic relationship and resulting in a greater use of force. Worse still, the display

of aggression by the patient is very likely to be attributed to 'illness', and this will influence others' assessment and lead to the patient being labelled as aggressive and, perhaps even, as a troublemaker.

If sedative medication is required this will usually take the form of antipsychotic drugs (also called neuroleptics or major tranquillizers), of which there are several different groups.

Antipsychotic drugs

These drugs have an initial sedative action that precedes any antipsychotic effect. The safest group to inject are the butyrophenones – haloperidol 2–10 mg or droperidol 5–10 mg. It may be necessary to repeat the dose if the initial dose has been ineffective. *Haloperidol* can be given in doses up to 30 mg for emergency control. *Chlorpromazine* has been associated with fatal cardiovascular collapse when given by intramuscular injection and should not be given by this route. However, it is the most sedative neuroleptic and effective when given orally in doses of 25–100 mg. *Thioridazine*, in doses of 25–100 mg, is effective for severe psychomotor agitation. It is important to be aware that neuroleptics can precipitate severe extrapyramidal side effects in the form of acute dystonia, tremor, muscular rigidity or motor restlessness. This can be treated symptomatically or prophylactically with *procyclidine* 5–10 mg intramuscularly. One rare but potentially fatal consequence of using antipsychotic medication is *neuroleptic malignant syndrome* (Table 44.4). This is characterized by a rapid onset, over 1–3 days, of acute autonomic instability (with marked swings in blood pressure, tachycardia, excessive sweating, salivation and urinary incontinence), hyperpyrexia and muscular rigidity. The mortality is 10–15%. Treatment is symptomatic. The patient should be cooled and fluid balance maintained. Often there is an intercurrent infection, which should be treated.

Parasuicide: recognition and treatment

Evaluating suicide risk is one of the hardest, yet most pertinent, parts of any psychiatric assessment. In an emergency situation (e.g. following a suicide attempt) the first consideration must be to safeguard the physical welfare of the patient and this will usually entail transporting him/her to the local emergency department. It is important to be alert to the suspicion of a suicide attempt, especially if the patient has a past history of psychiatric contact, is drowsy or unconscious and/or is drunk. Do not be deceived by any apparent evidence that only a small quantity of tablets has been ingested or the patient's protestations that the overdose was not life-threatening. A significant proportion of

Table 44.4 Neuroleptic malignant syndrome

- Labile blood pressure
- Tachycardia
- Excessive sweating
- Excessive salivation
- Urinary incontinence
- Hyperpyrexia
- Muscle rigidity

Table 44.5 Risk factors for successful suicide

- Present or past psychiatric illness, especially depression
- Schizophrenia or eating disorder
- Personality disorder
- Family history of suicide
- Single status
- Unemployment
- Social isolation
- Problem drinking
- Previous attempts at self-harm
- Recent 'loss' events
- Older age

Table 44.6 Signs and symptoms of depression

- Sadness
- Low self-worth
- Lethargy
- Lack of motivation
- Disturbed sleep and appetite
- Lack of libido
- Anxiety symptoms
- Guilt and self-blame
- Self-neglect
- Poor appetite

those who attempt suicide will make further fatal attempts and often patients are not aware of the lack of toxicity of the medication that they have taken and believe that the quantity ingested was sufficient to cause death. In particular, do not be sidetracked by the responses of others, who may minimize the importance of a person's actual or threatened attempt at self-harm and give explanations or interpretations of behaviour (most commonly in terms of manipulativeness, acting out or attention seeking). More violent methods of attempted self-harm (hanging, shooting or deep lacerations) should always be assessed by a psychiatrist.

Self-harm is not a mental illness.

It is important to be aware that self-harm is not in itself a mental illness and that the majority of people who harm themselves have no psychiatric illness. Moreover, there is no good evidence that psychiatric treatment will prevent the repetition of self-harm behaviour in the absence of psychiatric illness. Nevertheless, the most important intervention in the management of the suicidal patient is the treatment of any psychiatric illness.

If a person has not made an attempt at self-harm but is expressing suicidal ideation then a thorough assessment, as outlined above, should be carried out. Risk factors of eventual suicide such as present or past psychiatric illness (especially depression, schizophrenia and eating disorder), personality disorder, family history of suicide, single status, unemployment, social isolation, problem drinking, previous attempts at self-harm, recent 'loss' events and older age should be noted (Tables 44.5 and 44.6). If the person agrees to admission to hospital, and this is appropriate, then it should be expedited. If the person does not agree but is detainable under the Mental Health Act then the appropriate procedure should be followed, with the patient being closely supervised until admission takes place. Before leaving the situation the patient should be supervised until another professional can take over. If the person is deemed not to be detainable under the Mental Health Act but still expresses suicidal ideation, there is an ethical dilemma. Strictly speaking, the patient cannot be prevented from leaving. However, if the person appears actively to be attempting to end his life, or to be about to do so, then he can be restrained from so doing (under common law) pending a further psychiatric assessment.

Depression and mania

Suicide is most commonly associated with depression, although people with serious and long-standing mental disorders such as schizophrenia, manic depression, alcohol dependence and chronic anxiety are at increased risk of suicide. Clinical depression refers to a persistent and debilitating disorder of mood characterized by sadness, an inability to get pleasure out of any activity, low self-worth, lethargy and lack of motivation. Other common symptoms include disturbed sleep and appetite, lack of libido, anxiety symptoms and thoughts of guilt and self-blame. Patients may neglect themselves and become physically at risk through not eating or drinking. Often depressed mood is associated with poor social circumstances and deprivation.

Occasionally, patients with a history of depression may become elated and overactive with increased speed of thought and excessive, expansive speech. They may appear to be overcheerful or irritable, or their mood may swing between the two emotional states. They may express grandiose delusions of excessive self-importance or unwarranted ability, and there is often a history of increased spending (sometimes extravagantly) and sexual excesses or disinhibition. They may see themselves as famous or as having particular powers and may experience hallucinations that reinforce their behaviour. This is a presentation of mania and it is often difficult to manage outside hospital. Such individuals may become so preoccupied with their beliefs and behaviour that they neglect their appearance or dress in florid but totally unsuitable clothing, stop eating and drinking and pay little attention to their living conditions. If their mood state progresses unchecked they may develop a manic stupor in which they appear mute and motionless but in full consciousness. Stuporose state can also occur in depression.

Anxiety disorders

These include disorders such as anxiety states, phobias and obsessive compulsive disorder. They rarely present as a psychiatric emergency but anxiety commonly accompanies other psychiatric disorders and may exacerbate a patient's distress. Anxiety can be defined as the combination of psychological symptoms of fearfulness, irritability, difficulty in concentration, sensitivity to noise and a feeling of restlessness with physical symptoms of sympathetic nervous system overactivity such as sweating, increased heart rate, churning stomach and dry mouth (Table 44.7).

Acute anxiety is extremely distressing and may occur in normal people, especially victims of or witnesses to traumatic events. It is manifested in a psychological and physiological response, the most important form of which is hyperventilation. Hyperventilation is the result of excessive breathing and results in hypocapnia. Hypocapnia causes tinnitus, tetany, tingling, weakness and chest pains. The experience of the physical symptoms may exacerbate the feeling of anxiety, causing more hyperventilation. The best way to counteract acute anxiety is to induce relaxation and control hyperventilation. An explanation of the patient's symptoms and reassurance that the patient will not come to any harm as a result of them is the first step and may need to be repeated frequently and authoritatively. Hyperventilation is effectively managed by getting the person to rebreathe into a large paper bag for several minutes or until the breathing begins to regulate. Ensure that patients are sitting or lying in a supported posture and impress upon them the need to regulate their breathing by breathing slower and taking shallower breaths (not

Table 44.7 Signs and symptoms of anxiety
● Fearfulness
● Irritability
● Poor concentration
● Sensitivity to noise
● Restlessness
● Sympathetic nervous system overactivity

deeper ones), ideally until they can breathe through their nose. Demonstrating how they can breathe using their diaphragm by placing one hand on their chest and one on their abdomen is useful. The hand on the abdomen should move more than the one on their chest.

These measures may obviate the need for pharmacological treatment. If treatment is required, benzodiazepines are the drugs of choice for acute short-term anxiety. The intravenous or rectal route is the most effective for administration. Diazepam should not be given by intramuscular injection because of its variable absorption rate but can be given intravenously in the form of Diazemuls. Doses vary considerably between patients with a range of 2–20 mg. Lorazepam ($25-30 \mu g \, kg^{-1}$) is a short-acting benzodiazepine and is effective for panic attacks (episodes of acute anxiety associated with overpowering thoughts of dying or imminent physical ill health, and the desire to escape).

Physical causes of psychiatric emergencies

There are numerous physical causes of psychiatric emergencies that manifest as an acute toxic confusional state. The cardinal features of this state, also called delirium, are clouding and fluctuation of consciousness (patients have periods of drowsiness, poor concentration and lack of lucidity), increased arousal (often manifested in acute anxiety and fearfulness), disturbances in perception (in the form of illusions or hallucinations) and disorientation in time, place and person. As a result of these experiences, a person may become extremely distressed and liable to misinterpret the actions of others. Often, the elderly present as an emergency in this way, and it is important to be aware that many drugs to which the elderly are sensitive can precipitate delirium. An elderly person suffering from dementia may develop a toxic confusional state as a complication. Differentiation of dementia and delirium is not difficult – the latter has an acute onset with an abrupt change in behaviour, whereas dementia is altogether a more gradual deterioration in functioning and behaviour and does not fulfil the criteria for delirium (Table 44.8).

Table 44.8 Signs and symptoms of delirium

- Fluctuation of consciousness
- Poor concentration
- Lack of lucidity
- Increased arousal
- Disturbances in perception
- Disorientation

ALCOHOL AND ILLICIT DRUGS

The assessment and appropriate management of intoxicated individuals poses particular problems for all health service staff. It may not be easy to decide whether an intoxicated individual requires hospital assessment or, if causing a disturbance, whether police custody is more appropriate. On the one hand, intoxication is not uncommon, is sanctioned by society and in most cases leads to no harm. On the other hand, intoxicated individuals may be at considerable risk to themselves, especially if they have a history of alcohol dependence, and therefore require some assessment in a hospital setting. If it is felt that intoxicated and incapacitated individuals are likely to suffer from physical effects of the intoxicating substance (e.g. delirium tremens, withdrawal fits or septicaemia) such that they need to be monitored, then such people should be taken to hospital, if necessary against their will. Clearly, as soon as they are no longer at physical risk they must be allowed to leave, unless they are liable for detention under the Mental Health Act. Admission to a psychiatric hospital, on the other hand, may be indicated for assessment of a suspected underlying mental disorder. In this case it may be possible to apply the Mental Health Act. Certain hallucinogens (e.g. lysergic acid diethylamide (LSD) or magic mushrooms) can trigger off a psychotic reaction in a previously undiagnosed or vulnerable person, or they may worsen pre-existing states of psychosis.

Delirium tremens, which occurs some hours or days after the cessation or reduction of drinking, is characterized by tremulousness, disorientation, vivid hallucinations or illusions and autonomic overactivity, is associated with a mortality of 10% and should always be managed in a general hospital. Acute withdrawal can be managed with long-acting benzodiazepines such as chlordiazepoxide. However, it should be noted that many problem drinkers will supplement benzodiazepines with alcohol, and only a small quantity should be prescribed at any one time. Clomethiazole should not be used for outpatient or community detoxification, or treatment of withdrawal.

Personality disorder

One of the most difficult categories of patient to assess is those with a diagnosis of personality disorder. The validity and meaning of this term is a matter of some debate and it is often used as a pejorative and demeaning label (along with other discredited terms such as manipulative, hysterical, attention seeking and inadequate). These patients often harm themselves or express suicidal ideation and have often had multiple admissions to hospital. They may be hostile and impatient, and lack the ability to form a rapport. They appear to induce feelings of irritability and antagonism in staff and it is easy to lose an objective approach to their problems. This may result in an inadequate assessment and a failure to recognize serious psychiatric illness. There may be a tendency to minimize these patients' risk of eventually committing suicide because of the number of previous attempts, which are often not life-threatening. However, a proportion of these patients do succeed in ending their lives and it is important therefore to be aware that personality-disordered patients do develop other psychiatric disorders (e.g. depression), which may predispose them to making a more serious attempt to end their life. Therefore it is vital that patients with personality disorders are assessed thoroughly if they are expressing suicidal ideation. Professionals who may be involved include social workers, community psychiatric nurses and the patient's GP, as well as family and friends or voluntary agencies. It is often more worthwhile to the patient if these other professionals are involved sooner rather than later, as they are likely to be extremely familiar with the patient's history and may obviate the need for the patient to go to hospital for assessment.

The Mental Health Act 1983

If, after assessment, it is felt that a patient needs to be in a psychiatric hospital, and admission is refused, then compulsory admission can be arranged under the provisions of the Mental Health Act 1983. The sections that are most likely to be used in an emergency are sections 2, 3, 4 and 135. The section papers must be filled in before the patient is taken to hospital but it should be noted that the section only comes into force when all the forms have been accepted by, or on behalf of, the hospital managers after the patient arrives in hospital.

It is important to note that the Mental Health Act does not apply to people who are intoxicated by alcohol or drugs. However, if it is felt that there is an actual or possible underlying mental disorder in someone who is intoxicated, or that intoxication has precipitated a mental disorder and that person is at risk to him/herself or others, then admission under the Act may be appropriate.

SECTION 2: ADMISSION FOR ASSESSMENT

This section is for assessment in hospital, or for assessment followed by treatment, and it is usually applied when a patient has no past history of mental disorder or is not known to the local psychiatric service. The grounds for detention are that the patient must suffer from a mental disorder that warrants the patient's detention in hospital and that admission is necessary in the interests of the patient's own health or safety or for the protection of others. A specific diagnosis is not a prerequisite for detention – indeed the rationale for detention is to make a diagnosis. The section is valid for 28 days. The procedure requires an application by an approved social worker or nearest relative and medical recommendations by two doctors, one of whom must be approved under the Act (usually a consultant psychiatrist). The approved social worker must have seen the patient within the last 14 days and should, so far as is practicable, consult the nearest relative. The approved social worker can be contacted at the local Social Services Department.

SECTION 3: ADMISSION FOR TREATMENT

This section allows the compulsory admission of a patient and treatment for up to 6 months. It is usually applied when there is a known diagnosis. In order for this longer-term order to apply, the patient must suffer from a mental disorder, specified as mental illness, severe mental impairment, psychopathic disorder or mental impairment, that is of a nature or degree which makes it appropriate for the patient to receive medical treatment in a hospital. In the case of psychopathic disorder or mental impairment, treatment should alleviate or prevent a deterioration of the patient's condition. In addition, in all cases, it must be necessary for the health or safety of patients or for the protection of others that they should receive such treatment and that it cannot be provided unless they are detained under this section. The application is made by the patient's nearest relative or an approved social worker. The latter must, if practicable, consult the nearest relative before making an application and cannot proceed if the nearest relative objects. The medical recommendations are as for section 2. In addition, the recommendations must state the particular grounds for the doctor's opinion, specifying whether any other methods of dealing with the patient are available and, if so, why they are not appropriate. The doctor must specify one of the four types of mental disorder (see above).

SECTION 4: ADMISSION IN AN EMERGENCY

If there is difficulty in obtaining a second medical application from an approved doctor to detain the patient under Section 2 and the situation is an emergency, then an emergency order for assessment (Section 4) can be completed by the approved social worker and a doctor, who need not be approved under Section 12 of the Act. Application is made by the approved social worker, who must have seen the patient within the previous 24 h, or the nearest relative. The patient must be admitted within 24 h of the medical examination or application. The duration of the order is 72 h and it is expected that it will be converted to a Section 2 as soon as possible after the patient has arrived in hospital.

SECTION 135

If a social worker believes that someone is suffering from a mental disorder and is unable to care for himself, or is being ill-treated or neglected, he may apply to a magistrate for a warrant for that person's removal to a place of safety.

SECTION 136

It is possible that some emergency situations (e.g. road traffic accidents) will necessitate the removal of apparently mentally ill people to a place of safety without being able to get applications from social workers or psychiatrists. Under Section 136, police constables have the power to remove to a place of safety a person whom they find in a public place who appears to be suffering from a mental disorder and to be in need of care and control in the person's own interests or for the protection of others. These persons should be taken to the nearest convenient place of safety (usually a hospital or police station) where they can be detained for a period not exceeding 72 h for the purpose of examination by a doctor and interview by an approved social worker.

SECTION 5(2)

This section allows an inpatient to be prevented from leaving hospital on the recommendation of one doctor, providing the patient is under the care of a psychiatrist. If the doctor in charge of treatment is not a psychiatrist, he should act in person and should obtain a psychiatric opinion as soon as possible. *Section 5(2) cannot be applied in outpatient clinics or emergency departments under any circumstances.* Treatment cannot be given involuntarily to patients detained under Section 5(2).

Common law and informed consent

Any interaction between a health service worker and a patient is assumed to occur with the patient's informed consent. If a patient does not give consent for a particular examination or intervention, however minor, and is capable of consent, then the worker can be charged with assault. If a patient is unable to give consent because of mental illness then a person can act against the patient's wishes but only in certain circumstances; the treatment or investigation must be seen to be life-saving or necessary to prevent immediate serious harm to the patient or others and should be given in good faith. Clearly, if at all possible, treatment should be given under the provisions of the Mental Health Act 1983. However, in certain circumstances this will not be possible and emergency treatment (usually an injection) can be administered against the patient's will under common law. It is good practice always to make a contemporaneous note as to the reasons for any treatment given without the patient's consent, as well as recording the names of witnesses.

Managing the aggressive and uncooperative psychiatric patient

Safety is of paramount importance when dealing with violent and aggressive patients and those with acute psychiatric symptoms whose behaviour may be unpredictable and exaggerated. Prevention of violence has two components – preparation and prediction – and requires a knowledge of the risk factors for violent behaviour (Table 44.9).

When dealing with an aggressive psychiatric patient, whatever the cause, try to obtain unobstructed access to the patient and ask onlookers to leave quietly, ensuring that adequate staff remain for protection. Do not rush and do not give non-verbal indications that you are short of time, such as looking at your watch or a clock or fidgeting. Keep a sideways posture to the patient, as this is less threatening and presents a smaller target. Keep hands visible so that it is obvious that you are not concealing a weapon. Engage the patient in conversation, allow the patient to explain or vent the problems and initially do not interrupt too soon with solutions. Talk calmly and remind the patient that you are there to help. Acknowledge with them that they may feel out of control, frightened and overwhelmed, and that if necessary you will help them regain control. Be honest, clear, direct, non-threatening and non-confrontative. Do not give promises that you cannot keep but give some assurances, especially if these result in a change in behaviour. Do not criticize. Try to keep the momentum going and have an idea what your objective is, such as to get the person to sit down, drop a weapon, accede to a demand or prevent self-harm. Have an idea of what circumstances warrant retreat or use of restraint, and plan the next step beyond that. Always try to understand the context of aggressive behaviour, identify the causes and deal with them as far as possible.

RAPID TRANQUILLIZATION

Rapid tranquillization is the short-term use of tranquillizing drugs to control potentially destructive behaviour. It should

Table 44.9 Some important risk factors for violent behaviour

Psychological

- Anxiety or fears for personal safety
- Anger or arguments
- Feelings of being overwhelmed or unable to cope
- Learned behaviour
- History of physical or sexual abuse

Organic

- Intoxication with alcohol or illicit drugs
- Side effects of medication
- Inadequate control of symptoms
- Delirium

Psychotic

- Delusional beliefs of persecution
- 'Command' hallucinations to harm others
- Depressive or nihilistic delusions and intense suicidal ideation

Social

- Group pressure
- Social tolerance of violent behaviour
- Previous exposure to violence

The most consistent risk factor is a personal history of violent behaviour

only be used under medical supervision and when other, non-pharmacological, methods have failed. Before administering drugs, ensure that the patient is securely restrained as injecting a struggling patient risks inadvertent intra-arterial injection (causing necrosis), damage to the sciatic nerve for injections to the buttock or other injury to the patient or health worker. After intramuscular or intravenous administration of drugs, patients should be restrained until they show signs of sedation. When sedated, patients should be placed in the recovery position and their heart rate, respiration and blood pressure should be monitored.

Any patient who requires rapid tranquillization as a result of behaviour consequent to psychiatric symptoms should be reviewed by a psychiatrist as soon as possible. The psychiatrist will then be in a position to advise on the future management in the short and long term. Rapid tranquillization should not normally be used in the community.

- *Always consider* non-drug measures ('talking down').
- *Give either* droperidol 10 mg intramuscularly + lorazepam 2 mg intramuscularly. Wait 30 min for a response;

  or

  haloperidol 10 mg intravenously + diazepam 10 mg intravenously. Wait 10 min for a response.

Table 44.10 Precautions with rapid tranquillization

- Intravenous administration only under medical supervision
- Administer intravenous drugs slowly
- Ensure that resuscitation equipment is available
- If antipsychotic drugs are used, have an antimuscarinic drug (e.g. procyclidine) available in case of acute dystonia
- If benzodiazepines are used, have flumazenil available in case of respiratory depression (give 200 μg intravenously over 15 s if respiratory rate falls below 10 breaths min^{-1})
- Use a lower dose in:
  - older patients
  - patients not previously exposed to drug
  - patients intoxicated with drugs or alcohol
  - patients with delirium
- Avoid intramuscular clopromazine (risk of hypotension and crystallization in tissues)
- Avoid long-acting antipsychotic drugs (including zuclopenthixol acetate)
- Avoid antipsychotics in patients with heart disease (use benzodiazepines alone)

- *Repeat* the same drugs as above. Wait 30 min for a response. If necessary, repeat doses to maximum of 40 mg haloperidol + 40 mg diazepam in 24 h.

- *Make clear notes.* Detail why injection was necessary, the risk that would have resulted if the patient was not sedated and what other measures had been tried.

After a violent incident any physical injuries should be treated and the details of the incident should be recorded and reported to the relevant authorities. The police should always be informed if a criminal offence has been committed or weapons have been used. All staff involved should assemble 1 or 2 days later to discuss the incident, support each other and identify any changes that should be made resulting from the incident. Acknowledgement should be made that those involved in an aggressive incident may be profoundly affected and may suffer psychological distress. Some may be unable to resume work for hours or days, and anxiety symptoms may remain for some time.

Conclusions

Assessment and appropriate management of a psychiatric emergency requires time, patience and common sense. It is a dynamic process in which negotiation and arbitration may have to take place not only between patient, relative or carer and professionals but also among the professionals involved. Time should be taken to gather information and decisions should be reached as a result of objective appraisal of that information as opposed to arbitrary, hasty and ill-informed opinion. A basic knowledge of psychiatric disorders and the psychopathology that accompanies them, and an understanding of the risk of psychiatric patients losing their right of autonomy and advocacy as a result of misplaced stigma and prejudice, will increase the likelihood of a thorough assessment.

At the end of the assessment it should be possible to decide whether the patient is presenting with an organic, functional or predominately social problem. The decision then needs to be made as to whether the patient requires further assessment in hospital or a local community facility, or whether it would be more appropriate for other agencies (e.g. social services) to review the situation. It may be more appropriate for the patient to make contact with voluntary agencies or self-help groups. These have been established for many of the problems that can present as psychiatric emergencies and include substance misuse groups such as Alcoholics or Narcotics Anonymous and Aquarius, helplines for drug addicts, rape victims or battered wives, church organizations and marriage guidance (Relate).

If patients do appear to require further assessment and agree to go to hospital, then they should be taken there. If patients refuse and appear to be at risk to themselves or others, either the police can take them to a place of safety (if they are is in a public place) or a Mental Health Act assessment will need to be arranged by the local social services team.

Further reading

Atakan Z, Davies T 1997 ABC of mental health: mental health emergencies. British Medical Journal 314: 1740–1742

Royal College of Psychiatrists 1996 Assessment and clinical management of risk of harm to other people. Council report CR 53. Royal College of Psychiatrists, London

Thompson C 1994 Consensus statement. The use of high-dose antipsychotic medication. British Journal of Psychiatry 164: 448–458

Westcott R 1994 Emergencies, crises and violence. In: Pullen I, Wilkinson G, Wright A, Pereira Gray D (eds) Psychiatry and general practice today. Royal College of Psychiatrists. Royal College of General Practitioners, London, p 170–179

Human reactions to trauma: their features and management

45

Introduction   465

Pathological reactions to trauma and severe
stress   466

Normal reactions to trauma   468

Interventions in the acute phase following trauma   470

Grief reactions and their management   471

Breaking bad news   473

The effect of trauma care on staff   473

Summary and conclusions   474

References   475

Further reading   475

Introduction

The medical and surgical care of trauma patients has advanced impressively over the last 30–40 years; the psychiatric and psychosocial care has lagged behind. The overall management of the trauma patient would be improved by the closer integration of these dimensions.

To this end, this chapter will describe:

- the historical background to our understanding of trauma
- pathological reactions to trauma and their prognostic indicators
- normal reactions to trauma
- interventions in the acute phase following trauma
- grief reactions and their management
- breaking bad news
- the effect of trauma care on staff.

This chapter also contains a list of voluntary organizations that deal with survivors of different kinds of trauma.

HISTORICAL BACKGROUND

The earliest military chronicles (e.g. those of the Graeco-Roman Wars) are rich in their description of the psychological effects of one kind of trauma, namely, military combat.

During the Napoleonic Wars physicians and surgeons were challenged by the depletion of the fighting forces through 'nostalgia' (also called *Heimweh* and *maladie du pays*), a condition characterized by anergia, melancholy and a preoccupation with home. A similar phenomenon was also reported during the American Civil War, but a new diagnosis was coined, 'soldier's heart', and in the First World War the fashionable diagnosis was 'shell shock'.

Over this period the list of possible aetiological culprits hypertrophied but scant attention was paid to the possible role of psychological ones associated with combat. The proposed contenders included fever, 'a derangement of stomach and bowels', alterations to atmospheric pressure caused by artillery fire, carbon dioxide poisoning, hyperthyroidism and even cigarette smoke. Not surprisingly, in view of this prevalent ignorance, treatments were ill founded and, at times, barbaric and even life-threatening. These included ether injections, electric shocks and cigarette burns to the tongue. No doubt the horrors of the battlefield must have offered some respite from the 'care' of the physicians!

The Second World War effected a shift in emphasis by identifying combat per se as the key factor, as was revealed by the emergence of the terms 'combat exhaustion' and 'battle fatigue'. The emphasis was still on physical factors and 'fatigue' and 'exhaustion' almost trivialize the nature of the reactions and seem to imply that they can be relieved merely by rest.

The civilian world offered fewer insights into the effects of traumatic events. Although, in his famous diary, Samuel Pepys does describe the impact on him of the Great Fire of London, and his subsequent nightmares, insomnia and irritability (symptoms he could perhaps have escaped had he not gone out in a rowing boat to obtain a better view of the fires). Stierlin, a Swiss researcher, investigated the effects of mining disasters in the early 20th century and the English surgeon Erichsen described 'railway spine', from which victims of railway crashes in the late nineteenth century appeared to suffer (Charles Dickens being the most celebrated victim of this condition). Its associated symptoms of anergia, insomnia and loss of appetite were, however, generally thought to have a physical cause.

ORDER OUT OF CHAOS

The proliferation of diagnoses confirmed the ignorance as to the cause of posttraumatic reactions and sustained a durable prejudice against those reporting such symptoms.

Reluctance to acknowledge the genuineness of psychological reactions has taken a long time to erode and some sceptics claim that those who report such symptoms are either 'weak' or motivated by ulterior motives, such as a desire for compensation. (In fact there is very little evidence to suggest that trauma patients frankly exploit the opportunities for compensation. On the contrary, there is some evidence that the legal processes themselves may exacerbate the patients' situation.)

A major initiative, which imposed some order on the prevailing chaos regarding the classification and aetiology of post-traumatic reactions, was inspired by the Vietnam War. Concerned about the prevalence of psychopathology and problems of psychosocial adjustment reported among Vietnam veterans, the US government charged the American Psychiatric Association with investigating this phenomenon. As a result of their enquiries, the Association introduced the new diagnosis of post-traumatic stress disorder (PTSD) into the third edition of the *Diagnostic and Statistical Manual* (DSM-III, American Psychiatric Association 1980). Since then it has undergone revisions (DSM-III R, American Psychiatric Association 1987, DSM-IV, American Psychiatric Association 1994) and it was introduced into the 10th Revision of the International Classification of Mental and Behavioural Disorders (ICD-10, World Health Organization 1992).

The term has its critics. It could be legitimately argued that the introduction of this diagnosis owes more to socio-political pressures (particularly from some who opposed the war) than to clinical science. Also, there are those who criticize the diagnostic criteria, while others regard it as a psychiatric concept that has 'medicalized' normal reactions and one that may be culture-bound and therefore has no relevance outside contemporary Western cultures. Their criticisms are not without foundation (nor are they exclusive to PTSD). However, it can be argued in particular that the diagnosis has reduced the extent to which victims are blamed for their own emotional state and has encouraged research into post-traumatic reactions across many domains, including the biological one. Thus, some very interesting findings have been made in terms of cortical changes (Bremner 2005) and biochemical changes (Sutherland et al 2003). Another problem is that the DSM and the ICD use different definitions of what constitutes a sufficiently disturbing event to justify the diagnosis of PTSD. As can be seen from Box 45.1, the DSM refers to the 'objective' features of the event as well as to the individual's 'subjective' reactions to it. The ICD-10 is the taxonomy used most commonly in the UK; reference will therefore be made to post-traumatic conditions classified therein.

Pathological reactions to trauma and severe stress

ICD-10 recognizes:

- acute stress reaction
- post-traumatic disorder
- adjustment disorders
- dissociative disorders
- enduring personality change after catastrophic experience.

Box 45.1

The 'stressor' criteria according to DSM-IV and ICD-10

DSM 4

The person experienced, witnessed, or was confronted with an event that involved actual or threatened death or serious injury, or a threat to the physical integrity of self or others.
The person's response involved intense fear, helplessness or horror.

ICD-10

A stressful event or situation (either short- or long-lasting) of an exceptionally threatening or catastrophic nature, which is likely to cause pervasive distress in almost anyone.
The person's response involved intense fear, helplessness or horror.

ICD-10 CLASSIFICATION

Acute stress reaction (F43.0)

This is a transient disorder, the onset of which is usually within minutes of the exposure to the trauma and usually subsides within a few days of the event. Typically, it involves an initial state of shock and numbness or disorientation, followed by a fluctuating picture that includes depression, anxiety, anger and social withdrawal. Autonomic overreactivity is also common.

Post-traumatic stress disorder (F43.1)

This may be an acute, chronic or delayed condition. The characteristic symptoms are:

- intrusive re-experiences of the original trauma, e.g. flashbacks and nightmares, against a background of numbness, and emotional blunting, detachment from other people, unresponsiveness and anhedonia
- 'commonly', there is avoidance of reminders of the event
- 'usually', there is hyperarousal and hypervigilance, an exaggerated startle response and insomnia.

These symptoms must have endured for at least a few weeks, and the diagnosis is not usually made unless the symptoms occur within about 6 months of the trauma.

Adjustment disorders (F43.2)

These states of distress and emotional disturbance, following a significant life event (including the possibility of serious physical illness), interfere with the patient's functioning. The onset is normally within 1 month of the event, and they remit within about 6 months (with the exception of 'prolonged depressive reaction' – see below).

Different subcategories, reflecting the primary emotional disturbance, are as follows:

- brief depressive reaction
- prolonged depressive reaction
- mixed anxiety and depressive reaction
- with predominant disturbance of other emotions
- with predominant disturbance of conduct
- with prominent disturbance of emotions and conduct.

Dissociative disorders (F44)

The common denominator among these disorders is 'a partial or complete loss of the normal integration between memories of the past, awareness of identity and immediate sensations, and control of bodily movements' (ICD-10, p151).

The conditions include dissociative amnesia, dissociative fugue and dissociative disorders of movement and sensation (formerly labelled 'hysterical conversion symptoms').

These occur in response to an overwhelming stress (which may be a single event or an enduring one). The onset is acute, beyond conscious control and tends to remit after a few months.

Patients with these symptoms often display a 'striking denial of problems or difficulties that may be obvious to others' (ICD-10, p 152).

Enduring personality change after a catastrophic experience

Certain events or experiences are so severe and/or prolonged (e.g. being taken hostage, major catastrophes and being incarcerated in a concentration camp) that they can induce permanent personality change. These changes are:

- a hostile and pervasive suspiciousness
- social withdrawal
- feelings of emptiness or hopelessness
- chronic 'edginess'.

PREVALENCE OF POST-TRAUMATIC SYNDROMES

Epidemiological data have been reviewed elsewhere (Klein & Alexander, in press). There has been no specific UK survey of such syndromes. 12-month prevalence rates for PTSD have been found to range from 1.3% in Australia to 3.6% in the USA. PTSD after road traffic accidents has been reported at 12% and female rape yielded a higher figure (50%).

Depression, substance misuse and anxiety very commonly accompany PTSD, although it should be noted that those conditions may also be triggered as primary disorders following trauma in patients who do not develop PTSD.

Psychological adjustment following man-made trauma, e.g. terrorist acts, is generally more complicated and lengthy than that following natural disasters (North et al 1999).

TRAUMA AND CHILDREN

The diagnosis of PTSD in children may be difficult (partly because of language problems and the lack of suitable measures).

- Children may display their emotional distress by 'acting out' rather than through symptoms. (This may be misinterpreted as 'deviant' or 'bad' behaviour.)
- The onset of problems may be delayed. Thus, careful and extended attention to children is required following trauma.
- Children are particularly vulnerable if they witness violence (including sexual violence) to parents.
- They may also be adversely affected by media presentations of major trauma.

CHRONICITY OF POST-TRAUMATIC CONDITIONS

According to ICD-10, PTSD is generally a short-lived condition but the figures above confirm that, for some individuals, the symptoms may become chronic.

Symptoms may worsen after discharge from hospital because of:

- repeated re-exposure to reminders of the trauma
- maladaptive methods of coping (e.g. alcohol abuse)
- realization of the longer-term consequences of physical injuries
- specific prognostic indicators (see below).

Untreated or chronic cases may be associated with a decline in social, family and employment circumstances and with the development of secondary problems of adjustment and psychopathology.

PROGNOSTIC FACTORS

According to a meta-analysis by Brewin et al (2000) certain factors increase the likelihood of trauma survivors developing PTSD. These are:

- female gender
- younger age
- lower socioeconomic status
- lack of education
- lower intelligence
- minority status
- psychiatric history (personal and familial)
- childhood abuse
- previous trauma
- adverse childhood upbringing
- severity of trauma (see below)
- lack of social support
- life stressors (in addition to the trauma).

Clinical experience suggests that other factors may play a role in determining adjustment. These are:

- the meaning of the trauma (the death or injury of a child are particularly disturbing)
- the meaning to the victim of a physical injury (according to the ISS the injury might not be defined as 'severe' but the impact of the injury on the individual's self-esteem, self-image or level of functioning may be great)
- prolonged exposure (see 'Enduring personality change after a catastrophic experience', above)
- multiple deaths and/or mutilations
- previous adverse life events to which the individual has not fully adjusted

- man-made trauma (e.g. terrorist events or other acts of personal malevolence)
- chronic pain (there may be a vicious cycle between pain and intrusive phenomena such as flashbacks).

In general terms, pretraumatic factors seem to play less of a role in determining outcome than the peri- and post-traumatic ones.

At present, there is no universally accepted screening measure for post-traumatic conditions but two invite further research: the Trauma Screening Questionnaire (for PTSD only) by Brewin et al (2002) and the Aberdeen Trauma Screening Index (for general post-traumatic psychopathology) by Klein et al (2002).

Normal reactions to trauma

With the exception of rare psychotic reactions to trauma, normal and pathological reactions are generally distinguished by:

- the intensity of the reactions
- the duration of the reactions
- the extent to which they render the survivor dysfunctional.

Unless there is good evidence to the contrary, it generally helps to reassure patients in the acute phase that their reactions are normal (Table 45.1)

NUMBNESS AND DENIAL

This is a natural protection against being overwhelmed (but it may prevent patients from taking in what staff tell them). (See the section on 'Breaking bad news', below.)

Table 45.1 Common normal reactions to trauma

- Numbness
- Fear
- Depression
- Elation
- Anger
- Helplessness
- Guilt
- Irritability
- Cognitive changes
- Impaired sleep
- Flashbacks
- Autonomic hyperarousal (and hypervigilance)
- Avoidant behaviour

FEAR

Fear is essential to the initiation of the 'flight–fight' response. Patients should be reassured that there is no need to feel ashamed of being afraid.

NB. Panic is not a common reaction to traumatic events.

DEPRESSION

Depression is commonly seen in relation to loss and trauma and generally entails some kind of loss. (See the section on 'Bereavement', below.)

ELATION

This is similar to the 'combat rush' described by fighting troops, probably due to a combination of psychological factors (e.g. at having survived) and neuroendocrinological ones that may implicate the production of the natural opiates (these may lead temporarily to a raised pain threshold).

ANGER

Anger may be redirected at those staff who carry out painful procedures or who have to break bad news. (See the section on 'Breaking bad news', below.)

HELPLESSNESS

A sense of powerlessness and helplessness is almost pathognomic of the traumatized victim.

GUILT

'Survivor' guilt occurs, for example, after multiple fatalities when survivors believe (usually wrongly) that they were responsible for the deaths of others. Parents may experience this in relation to the death of a child.

IRRITABILITY

Irritability can be a pernicious problem at home and at work that strains otherwise good relationships. It is probably due to a combination of anger, frustration (at the trauma) and autonomic hyperreactivity.

COGNITIVE CHANGES

Victims commonly misperceive the order in which, and the speed at which, events occur during trauma (most commonly they see everything as having been slowed down).

In addition, they frequently display 'tunnel vision', such that even important events and circumstances occurring peripherally may not be registered. The focus of their attention is usually the source of threat. They may also experience impaired memory and concentration.

IMPAIRED SLEEP

This is associated with autonomic hyperarousal and hypervigilance. Sleep is commonly punctuated by nightmares, which may deter patients from trying to sleep. The sleep architecture is altered resulting in an increased proportion of light sleep (stages 1 and 2); decreased deep sleep ('delta' sleep) and increased REM sleep.

FLASHBACKS

These are involuntary re-experiencings of the original trauma and its associated emotions. They may involve any or all sensory modalities. They may be triggered by reminders of the trauma.

AUTONOMIC HYPERAROUSAL (AND VIGILANCE)

These may have biological survival value but they can be distressing to patients, causing them to overreact to sensory input. Hyperarousal is characteristically revealed by an exaggerated acoustic startle response; hypervigilance defines itself by a heightened sense of vulnerability. (Alcohol is commonly used as a form of self-medication for this symptom.)

AVOIDANT BEHAVIOUR

Patients seek to avoid reminders of the trauma by, for example, not talking about it, not reading about it, avoiding situations or people associated with the trauma. (Because this can become a major problem in the longer term, collusion by staff with patients' total avoidance is not usually helpful.)

The last three reactions (flashbacks, hyperarousal and avoidance) are the distinguishing core features of PTSD according to both DSM-IV and ICD-10, but only if they have endured for about a month.

Note. While one never 'gets over' a serious trauma, most individuals do come do terms with and adjust to what has happened. Even more reassuring is the fact that many individuals, families and even communities come through all the stronger. Resilience is therefore the most likely general outcome rather than psychopathology after traumatic experiences. This principle should encourage optimism but not complacency; we still need to identify how best to facilitate the adjustment of individuals, families and communities after particularly disturbing events.

Interventions in the acute phase following trauma

The contribution of mental health specialists must not overshadow what others (including families and friends) can do in the earliest phase following trauma (Table 45.2). However, the following principles of *Psychological First Aid* (Raphael 1986) are particularly appropriate to managing victims of major trauma in the field.

PSYCHOLOGICAL FIRST AID

Comfort and isolation

Basic needs for comfort and safety are pre-eminent after trauma. The determination to survive will subordinate higher order needs. Physical contact is often more consoling than words.

Protect from further harm

Particularly because of the influence of shock, trauma victims may expose themselves inadvertently to further risk.

Counteract helplessness

It is best, especially when there are multiple casualties, to involve those who are physically and emotionally competent in purposeful duties (comforting others, rendering physical aid, etc.).

Re-establish order

Trauma implies a temporary sense of loss of order and control. Try to establish time scales, e.g. for eating, meetings and transportation, and it is helpful to minimize unforeseen change, e.g. in relation to theatre lists following hospital admission (Alexander 1993).

Table 45.2 Psychological first aid

- Comfort and isolation
- Protection from further harm
- Counteract helplessness
- Re-establish order
- Expression of feelings
- Provision of (accurate) information
- Reunion with significant others
- Identification of support

Expression of feelings

Beyond gentle probing, deeper feelings should be left alone until the patients feel more secure and until their physical state is stabilized. Listening is usually more helpful than asking questions and running the risk of saying 'the wrong thing'.

It is not best to take sides on issues of culpability with regard, for example, to a road traffic accident because, during the recovery phase, patients themselves frequently change their own opinions as to responsibility and culpability.

It is also important to note that in certain cultures, e.g. those of the Indian subcontinent, people may not easily express their feelings orally but tend to somatize.

Provision of (accurate) information

Information helps to re-establish a sense of order and control but bear in mind that shock, numbness and impaired concentration and/or memory will delimit what survivors can take in. (See the section on 'Breaking bad news', below.)

Survivors generally appreciate being told what has happened and what will happen to them and their loved ones.

Reunion with significant others

Whenever possible, it is generally helpful to allow survivors to meet with not only their loved ones but also fellow survivors. Victims of shared trauma appear to forge powerful bonds; these bonds may be particularly helpful in the wake of a trauma (Alexander 1993).

Identification of support

Establish who and where are the sources of support of victims. Information should also be made available about voluntary and professional sources of help in the community (Table 45.3).

PSYCHOLOGICAL TRIAGE

Survivors of traumatic events are not equally at risk of developing post-traumatic psychopathology. The list of prognostic indicators given earlier in the subsection on 'Prognostic Factors' will help to identify high-risk patients.

Psychotic reactions are uncommon after trauma and their occurrence requires expert psychiatric help, particularly in the case of head injury or seriously burned patients. Suicidal ideation should always be taken seriously; one can have no faith in the adage: 'If they speak about it, they won't do it'. Suicide risk is heightened by profound low mood, guilt and a sense of hopelessness. It should be borne in mind that the most overtly distressed patients may not be those in most need of comfort and support: be aware of the silent sufferer.

'Watchful waiting'

The guidelines produced by the National Institute for Clinical Excellence (2005) recommend that for most trauma survivors there should be a period of about a month of 'watchful waiting' before instituting any formal treatment. All that is required is support, comfort and 'psychoeducation' (the last-named includes information about normal reactions and their course, and how survivors can help themselves). It is important not to pathologize normal reactions or to interfere with normal methods of adjustment.

It should also be remembered that drugs will never combat all the primary or secondary symptoms following trauma, although they may stabilize patients so that they benefit from other forms of help and treatments.

Formal treatment methods

Psychotherapies

Particularly for PTSD, the National Institute for Clinical Excellence (2005) recommends as the treatment of choice two psychological therapies: trauma-focused cognitive behavioural therapy (TF-CBT) and eye movement desensitization and reprocessing (EMDR; Shapiro 2001). Both need to be administered by appropriately trained mental health personnel.

Table 45.3 Voluntary organizations

Organization	Address
Compassionate Friends (for parents following the death of a child)	53 North Street, Bristol B53 1EN, UK
CRUSE Bereavement care	Head Office, 126 Sheen Road, Richmond, Surrey TW9 1UR, UK
Roadpeace (for victims of road traffic accidents through bereavement or injury)	PO Box 2579, London NW10 3PW, UK
Samaritans	PO Box 9090, Stirling FK8 2SA
Trauma After Care Trust (TACT)	Headquarters, Buttfields, The Farthings, Withington, Gloucester GL54 4DF, UK
Victim Support England and Wales	National Office, Cranmer House, 39 Brixton Road, London SW9 6DZ, UK
Victim Support Scotland	National Office, 15/23 Hardwell Close, Edinburgh EH8 9RX, UK

Medication

These are only two psychotropics recommended in the guidelines for use by non specialists; these are paroxetine and mirtazapine. For specialists the recommended agents are amitriptyline and phenelzine.

The recommendations do not imply that other treatments may not be helpful for some individuals, it is just that their use would not be evidence-based (see also O'Brien 1998).

- *Benzodiazepines*: These may be helpful (short-term) measures to reduce marked anxiety, intrusive phenomena and impaired sleep. Caution, however, must be exercised because of:
  - the risk of tolerance and dependence
  - their disinhibiting effect on those with aggressive or 'acting out' tendencies
  - their tendency to lower mood
  - 'rebound' phenomena on discontinuation.
- *Beta-blockers*: Propranolol may reduce the autonomic hyperactivity but has little effect on anxious thoughts. Interesting research is investigating the prophylactic value of such medication.
- *Tricyclic antidepressants*: Amitriptyline is the most widely tested but there is some support for imipramine.
- *Monoamine oxidase inhibitors*: Treatment trials have yielded inconsistent results (apart from phenelzine) and the side-effects and dietary restrictions restrict their usefulness. The newer, reversible monoamine oxidase inhibitors may offer more hope.
- *Serotonin re-uptake inhibitor antidepressants*: Several open and controlled trials support the use of paroxetine and mirtazapine for the treatment of PTSD, although higher doses over longer periods may be required than for depressive disorders.
- *Anticonvulsants*: Carbamazepine has some support for its effect on insomnia and intrusive phenomena, and valproate may ease hyperarousal and avoidant/numbing symptoms.
- *Neuroleptics*: Unless there are psychotic symptoms, or marked aggressive and/or self-destructive behaviour, these have no specific role to play.

Repetitive transcranial magnetic stimulation

This new technique involves the use of an electromagnetic coil on the scalp and the administration of high intensity currents. At present, the evidence regarding its efficacy is inconclusive.

Grief reactions and their management

The death of a loved one is one of the worst traumas we can experience, particularly if the death is sudden, unexpected and untimely. In medicine, however, there are many 'little deaths' such as mastectomy, amputation, loss of function and loss of physical appearance (e.g. through severe burns). These events commonly provoke grief reactions.

NORMAL GRIEF REACTIONS

Few aspects of our wellbeing are not affected by a bereavement. Many of the experiences come in 'pangs' or 'waves', which are usually at their peak in the first few weeks after the loss but may be triggered by, for example, reminders of the deceased. Typical reactions to loss are set out in Table 45.4.

While most adjustment takes place within about 6 months, it takes about 2 years to adjust satisfactorily. Grief reactions may be triggered by the anniversary of the death or by other significant dates, including birthdays, wedding anniversaries and Christmas.

PATHOLOGICAL GRIEF REACTIONS

It must be remembered that grief is not an illness (most people adjust without medical help) and that there is no clear dividing line between normal and pathological grief. The concept of 'pathological grief' is probably a 20th century Western concept (Jacobs 1999). The distinction is usually made in terms of:

- the intensity of the reactions
- the duration of the reactions
- the effect of the reactions on the individual's level of functioning
- the delayed onset (this can be due to personality factors, exaggerated denial, a missing body or lack of opportunity to grieve).

POOR PROGNOSTIC INDICATORS

The determinants of a poor adjustment relate to the features of: (1) the death, (2) the bereaved; (3) the relationship between the deceased and the bereaved and (4) the circumstances of the bereaved (Parkes 1985) (Table 45.5).

CHILDREN AND BEREAVEMENT

Childhood bereavement (Black 1996) is often associated with psychiatric and adjustment problems in later life, especially if the loss involved the mother or is multiple (as in war and major calamity). The adjustment of children is compromised if those around them are failing to cope with the loss. Parents may often be too protective of bereaved children, who may have a better developed sense of death than they are given credit for. Occasionally, children falsely attribute a death to their own behaviour (e.g. 'not being good' or not saying their prayers). Expert help may be needed in such cases. Children may find it easier to express their grief non-verbally (e.g. through play or drawing).

THE MANAGEMENT OF GRIEF

Often the distress of the bereaved paralyses the onlookers or causes them to avoid the bereaved. Neither reaction is necessary or helpful. Even without the availability of an expert, we can:

- *Listen to the bereaved* – this is a better contribution than filling silence with irrelevant or, worse, insensitive comments. Avoid (at all costs) clichés. The following examples are likely to be hurtful or unhelpful or both:
  — 'You're lucky, you still have another son'
  — 'You can't live your life for the dead'
  — 'I know just how you feel'.
- *Provide time (and a suitable setting)* – busy ward rounds or surgeries are not the right time or place.
- *Tolerate their 'lack of gratitude', irritability etc.* – as was described earlier, the traumatized and the bereaved are frequently angry and irritable. These feelings may be

---

Table 45.4 Normal grief reactions

Emotional	Cognitive
● Depression	● Impaired concentration
● Anxiety	● Impaired memory
● Guilt	● Loss of faith
● Shock and numbness	● Bewilderment
● Denial	● Disorientation
● Anger	● Loss of meaning of life
● Apathy	
● Yearning	**Physical**
	● Insomnia
Social	● Anergia
● Withdrawal	● Loss of libido
● Conflicts (e.g. about new relationships, trying to enjoy life)	● Loss of appetite (or comfort eating)
	● Loss of weight (or weight gain)
	● Headaches
	● Chest pains
Behavioural	● Dyspnoea (and sighing)
● Searching/pining	
● Agitation	**Perceptual**
● Avoidance	● Misperceptions (or 'pseudo-hallucinations')
● Crying	● A sense of a 'presence' (of the deceased)
● Loss of interests	

directed at professional caregivers, although they are not usually the real 'targets' of such reactions.

- *Reassure them about the normality of their reactions* – it does not help if they feel they are 'losing their minds' or are 'being silly'. These are common fears amongst the bereaved.

MEDICATION

Because the peak for the normal acute reactions is a couple of weeks after the loss, antidepressants are not likely to be helpful in most cases because most compounds require 2–3 weeks before the antidepressant effect is experienced.

If, however, there are signs of deep and persistent low mood (with diurnal variation), early morning wakening and loss of weight, appetite and energy, antidepressant therapy may be required. Expert psychiatric opinion should be sought. It should also be requested when there is suicidal ideation.

It is generally believed that medication should not be used to suppress the natural and healing expression of emotions, but ensuring a good night's sleep through the short-term prescription of a night sedation can be restorative for the bereaved.

Table 45.5 Poor prognostic indicators in bereavement

Features of the death

- Sudden, unexpected or untimely
- A child or spouse
- Painful, horrifying, mutilating
- Mismanaged, e.g. in hospital (even if not founded in reality)
- Absence of a body (this increases the risk of denial of the death)

Features of the bereaved

- Insecure, anxious, poor self-esteem
- Previous psychiatric history
- Excessively angry or guilty (for the death)
- Sense of responsibility for the tragedy
- Physically disabled or ill
- Previous unresolved losses
- Unable to share and to express emotions
- Concurrent problems of living

Features of the relationship

- Highly dependent
- Characterized by extremes of mixed feelings (e.g. 'love-hate')

Features of the circumstances

- Unsupportive or unavailable family
- Lack of social, religious or other supports
- Low socio-economic status (probably because of association with other life stresses)

Breaking bad news

One of the most difficult challenges facing caregivers is how to convey unpalatable news to patients and their relatives (Klein & Alexander 2003). How this news is broken may have a major effect on those who receive it. The following guidelines may help when carrying out this difficult but important duty.

- *Initiate the conversation* – silences may create unnecessary anxiety and uncertainty.
- *Find out what the patient (or relative) wants to know*
  - there is no point in labouring what has been already established
  - the individual should have the chance to establish priorities.
- *Tailor the information and how you give it* – take into account such factors as age, gender, educational and social background, and the emotional state of the individual.
- *Pace the conversation*
  - our own anxiety usually causes us to speak too quickly
  - distressed individuals will not think as quickly and clearly as usual.
- *Find out what has been taken in*
  - reduced concentration and recall limit how much patients and relatives can absorb
  - distortions or misunderstanding may occur; these need to be corrected.
- *Try to have a member of staff remain with the individual after the bad news has been given* – avoid being interrupted while giving bad news. 'Pagers' have no respect for sensitive occasions!

The effect of trauma care on staff

Staff who care for trauma victims are usually inspired by a strong sense of altruism and aspire to high standards of professional practice. While these factors, in conjunction with the influence of training, experience and self-selection, may shield staff from the potentially deleterious effects of exposure to harrowing experiences, there is clear evidence that such factors do not confer an immunity against these effects (Duckworth 1986, Alexander & Atcheson 1998, Alexander & Klein 2001). This second study also dispelled the myth that senior and more experienced staff are unaffected by the emotional impact of their work. Figley (1995) has also introduced the concept of 'compassion fatigue' in recognition of the fact that caring for the seriously injured takes its emotional toll.

Trauma care staff should be willing to acknowledge the emotional impact of their work on them. The factors that are likely to increase that impact are:

- injuries to or death of children
- multiple exposure to mutilation and death
- prolonged and/or serial exposure (without respite) to mutilation or death
- lack of support (at work and at home)
- personal life stresses.

PROTECTION OF TRAUMA CARE STAFF

Such personnel have devised their own methods to shield themselves against distress. These include:

- talking openly amongst themselves
- mutual support
- good teamwork
- a clear definition of duties and responsibilities
- a sense of purposeful commitment
- 'black' or 'gallows' humour*.

* Interestingly, black humour does not appear to be used in relation to trauma involving children.

CRITICAL INCIDENT STRESS DEBRIEFING

While peer and family support is probably the most potent psychoprophylaxis against adverse reactions to the stressfulness of work, extensive use is made of critical incident stress debriefing, particularly by the military and emergency personnel (Mitchell & Everly 1995, Dyregrov 1997). 'Critical incidents' are those events that trigger emotional reactions powerful enough to overwhelm staff and to compromise their ability to fulfil their duties. There are different models of debriefing, but common denominators include opportunities to:

- normalize emotional reactions after critical incidents
- enable emotional expression
- identify what went well
- identify problems and solutions
- help staff to disengage from their duties
- conduct triage (using the prognostic indicators described earlier).

While those who undergo debriefing generally report high levels of satisfaction, the few systematic attempts to evaluate debriefing as a prophylaxis do not endorse the enthusiasm underlying its use (Rose et al 2004). Some have challenged the quality and relevance of the studies in the Cochrane Review, but one principle that has gained widespread acceptance is that mandatory one-off debriefings are contraindicated.

If debriefing is used the following points should be noted:

- It should be conducted by a professional who is familiar with reactions to critical incidents and with group dynamics.
- It is not a treatment for 'sick' people; it is for normal individuals who have undergone an abnormal event.
- The proceedings must be confidential.
- Participants should not be forced to speak.

WARNING SIGNS

Most staff, even after particularly disturbing critical incidents, will come through these using their own well tried methods of coping. However, the following are guidelines for identifying those who may require personal help. Should such help be necessary these members of staff should not be regarded as 'wimps' and they should not be subject to gratuitous and hurtful remarks, such as 'If you can't stand the heat, get out of the kitchen'. For reasons described above, we are all potential 'victims'; none of us carries a special immunity. If you can care, you can hurt. Guidelines for identifying staff who may be in need of personal help are:

- excessive use of alcohol (and other substances)
- unusual poor timekeeping and work performance
- unusual carelessness and proneness to accidents
- excessive irritability and moodiness.

Summary and conclusions

- Human reactions to trauma are complex, and much has yet to be done to understand their origin and the best way to manage them.
- Psychological distress and psychiatric symptoms are not the hallmark of the weak-willed, the naive, the manipulative or those bent on financial gain; they are genuine phenomena to which all of us are potentially susceptible. Total trauma care must address the emotional and psychological needs of victims (and their families).
- While no single trauma is a necessary and sufficient condition for the development of any post-traumatic syndrome, there are guidelines as to who is at most risk of adverse reactions after trauma.
- Grief reactions are not confined to the loss of a loved one, as trauma commonly engenders many kinds of loss, each of which may provoke grief in those affected.
- Family support (and peer support particularly in the case of trauma care staff) should be encouraged and should not be supplanted by 'experts' in the counselling and debriefing.

- Psychological first aid should be used to shield victims from further harm, re-establish order in their world and stabilize their emotional reactions.
- 'Breaking bad news' can be stressful for the professional, but providing such information sensitively is essential to total trauma care and may do much to facilitate the successful adjustment of victims and their families.
- Psychopharmacological agents also require a more rational basis but there are guidelines as to suitable compounds for the management of post-traumatic reactions.
- Surgical, medical, nursing and emergency personnel should not underestimate how much they can do in terms of the palliation of the impact of traumatic events without specialist psychiatric help. However, they must also consider their own welfare.

References

Alexander DA 1993 Burn victims after major disaster: reactions to patients and their caregivers. Burns 19: 105–109

Alexander DA, Atcheson SF 1998 Psychiatric aspects of trauma care: a survey of nurses and doctors. Psychiatric Bulletin 22: 132–136

Alexander DA, Klein S 2001 Ambulance personnel: the impact of accident and emergency work on mental health and well-being. British Journal of Psychiatry 178: 76–81

American Psychiatric Association 1980 Diagnostic and statistical manual of mental disorders, revised 3rd edn. American Psychiatric Association, Arlington, VA

American Psychiatric Association 1987 Diagnostic and statistical manual of mental disorders, revised 3rd edn. American Psychiatric Association, Arlington, VA

American Psychiatric Association 1994 Diagnostic and statistical manual of mental disorders, 4th edn. American Psychiatric Association, Arlington, VA

Black D 1996 Childhood bereavement (Editorial). British Medical Journal 312: 1496

Bremner JD 2005 Does stress damage the brain? Understanding trauma-related disorders from a mind-body perspective. WW Norton, New York

Brewin CR, Andrews B, Valentine JD 2000 Meta-analysis of risk factors for post-traumatic stress disorder in trauma-exposed adults. Journal of Consulting and Clinical Psychology 68: 748–766

Brewin CR, Rose S, Andrews B et al 2002 Brief screening instrument for post-traumatic stress disorder. British Journal of Psychiatry 181: 158–162

Duckworth D 1986 Psychological problems arising from disaster work. Stress Medicine 2: 315–323

Dyregrov A 1997 The process in psychological debriefings. Journal of Traumatic Stress 10: 589–605

Figley CR 1995 Compassion fatigue. Coping with secondary traumatic stress disorder in those who treat the traumatized. Brunner/Mazel, New York

Jacobs S 1999 Traumatic grief. Diagnosis, treatment and prevention. Brunner/Mazel, Philadelphia, PA

Klein, S, Alexander, DA 2003 Good grief: a medical challenge. Trauma 5(4): 261–271

Mitchell JT, Everly GS 1995 Critical incident stress debriefing: CISD. An operations manual for the prevention of traumatic stress among emergency service and disaster workers. Chevron Publishing, Ellicott City, MD

North CS, Nixon SJ, Shariat S et al 1999 Psychiatric disorders among survivors of the Oklahoma City bombing. Journal of the American Medical Association 282: 755–762

National Institute for Clinical Excellence 2005 Post-traumatic stress disorder. The management of PTSD in adults and children in primary and secondary care. National Clinical Practice Guideline 26. Gaskell/British Psychological Society, London

O'Brien LS 1998 Traumatic events and mental health. Cambridge University Press, Cambridge

Parkes CM 1985 Bereavement. British Journal of Psychiatry 146: 11–17

Raphael B 1986 When disaster strikes: how individuals and communities cope with catastrophe. Basic Books, New York

Rose S, Bisson J, Wessely S 2004 Psychological debriefing for preventing post traumatic stress disorder (PTSD) (Cochrane review). Cochrane Library, Issue 3. John Wiley, Chichester

Shapiro R 2001 Eye movement desensitization and reprocessing: basic principles, protocols, and procedures, 2nd edn. Guilford Press, New York

Sutherland AG, Alexander DA, Hutchison JD 2003 Disturbance of pro-inflammatory cytokines in post-traumatic psychopathology. Cytokine 24: 219–225

World Health Organization 1992 International classification of mental and behavioural disorders, 10th edn. World Health Organization, Geneva

Further reading

Alexander DA 1996 Trauma research: a new era [Invited editorial.] Journal of Psychosomatic Research 41: 1–5

Black D, Newman M, Harris-Hendriks J, Mezey G (eds) 1997 Psychological trauma: a developmental approach. Gaskell, London

Cramer D 1996 Post-traumatic stress counseling: benefit or indulgence? British Journal of Hospital Medicine 56: 567–568

Hind CRK 1997 Communication skills in medicine. BMJ Publishing, London

Jones E, Wessely S 2005 Shell shock to PTSD. Military Psychiatry from 1900 to the Gulf War. Psychological Press, Hove, Sussex

Mitchell M 1997 The aftermath of road accidents. Routledge, London

Royal College of Physicians and Psychiatrists 1995 The psychological care of medical patients. Council Report CR35. Royal College of Physicians and Psychiatrists, London

Wilson JP, Raphael B (eds) 1993 International hand-book of traumatic stress syndromes. Plenum Press, New York

Dealing with the violent or uncooperative patient

46

Introduction 476

What is anger? 476

What is violence? 476

Verbal and non-verbal communication 476

Principles of assessment 477

What to do after a violent incident 479

Staff training and education 480

Summary 480

References 480

Introduction

The majority of our interactions with people will be friendly, courteous and polite. However, there will be times when people will be angry, violent and uncooperative. It is essential to know how to deal with these patients so as to prevent harm to ourselves, others and the patient. Each individual will have their own background, culture, standards and beliefs. These characteristics will affect the manner in which they deal with a situation.

What is anger?

Anger is an emotion or a feeling. It is normally a response to something that is said or that has happened. It can be:

- visualized – gritted teeth, clenched fists, loud speech
- felt – tachypnoea, tachycardia, tense muscles.

Anger sometimes leads to aggression.

What is violence?

The Health and Safety Executive defines violence at work as:

any incident in which an employee is threatened or assaulted by a member of the public in circumstances arising out of the course of his or her employment.

Violence can be verbal or physical. Both, but especially verbal aggression, are often under-recognized and poorly recorded.

It must be accepted that repeated exposure to violent episodes can have a cumulative effect on health-care workers that may ultimately affect both their professional and personal lives. The effects of violence on the carer are listed in Table 46.1.

Verbal and non-verbal communication

This is a skill that is developed over time. Once developed, it can be a powerful tool.

When making an assessment of a violent or uncooperative person, verbal communication must be appropriate

Table 46.1 Symptoms of stress due to exposure to aggression

- Agitation
- Disturbed sleep pattern
- Loss of appetite
- Loss of concentration
- Feelings of paranoia

Table 46.2 Non-verbal communication

- Facial expression
- Limb movement
- Head movement
- Body posture
- Interpersonal distances

to the situation. The pitch of speech should be slightly higher than normal but the volume should be normal. The speed should ideally be slower than normal conversation. By adopting these guidelines, verbal communication will be more effective.

Non-verbal communication is often referred to as 'body language'. This is made up of the external signs that we exhibit when communicating. It is vital to be aware of these when dealing with a person in crisis. Examples are given in Table 46.2.

POSITIVE METHODS OF VERBAL AND NON-VERBAL COMMUNICATION WHEN DEALING WITH THE POTENTIALLY VIOLENT PATIENT

The following suggestions may be useful in dealing with violent patterns.

- Listen to what the person is saying. Anger and then aggression can be the product of somebody not listening. Listening is an excellent defuser.
- Communicate clearly. This is obvious, but it is not always easy to do. Do not use jargon that only confuses the situation further, e.g. 'This is the ASW' (approved social worker).
- Display understanding. This is done by reflecting or mirroring what is being said. This technique is used to check that one has understood what has been said, e.g. 'You were not able to get an appointment this week'.
- Acknowledge the crisis. This shows the person that you are willing to help them, e.g. 'I can see that you are in pain; I can help you'.
- Body space. People have different optimal body space. The 'invasion of personal space' is likely to be perceived as threatening by the patient.
- Maintain eye contact for a few seconds at a time. Staring at the person can be perceived as threatening. When

breaking eye contact, look at the person's body, never look away. Eye contact can then be re-established.
- Never stand straight in front of the person. Stand at an angle. This is less confrontational (Mehrabian 1972).
- Hands are very powerful tools in communication. Raising the hands with fingers open and palms pointing towards the ground may have a calming effect. Never point a finger, this is very threatening and can cause a situation to escalate. Hands should be held in front of the body with the fingers interlinked.

Principles of assessment

IN THE HOME

Home visits are among the occasions when there is a higher risk of assault (Brown et al 1986). Given this, some questions must be asked. Is the visit really necessary? Could the person come to the practice?

As much information as possible should be obtained relating to the person's medical and psychosocial circumstances. Who are you going to visit? It may be another member of the family who has made the appointment; e.g. a wife concerned about her husband's ill health: does the husband know of the intended visit? Similarly, parents might be concerned about their teenage son or daughter whom they suspect to be taking illicit drugs. Once this information is available an objective decision can be made about the home visit. If it is a first home visit, absence of information regarding the personal or domestic circumstances of the family calls for a certain degree of caution before confirming the appointment.

It is important to make appropriate introductions. Bona fide identification should always be offered.

On entering a person's house it is easy to forget that it is their home and you are a visitor. However, there are some precautions you can make for home visits (Table 46.3).

It the planned time for a visit is exceeded, it should be arranged that someone will call to ensure that no problem has arisen. A code can be agreed over the phone:

- If you say 'I can't make that visit' – you need help.
- If you say 'I can make that visit' – you are all right.

If there is no answer on the telephone then the practice/home should call the police to your last known whereabouts.

If after assessment it is clear that a home visit is necessary but doubts remain over safety, consideration should be given to taking a colleague along or seeking police attendance.

AT THE SCENE OF AN ACCIDENT/INCIDENT

Prior to arriving it is necessary to ensure that communication equipment works. A test call should be performed.

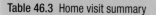

Table 46.3 Home visit summary

- Plan your visits
- Let someone know your whereabouts at all times of day or night
- Plan your communications
- Agree a fixed time for a visit, e.g. 30 min
- If you go over this time then the surgery/home calls you
- Agree a code for use over the telephone
- If there is no answer on the telephone the police should be called to the address (it could be the person has taken your telephone!)
- Take somebody with you

Table 46.4 Accident/incident scene summary

- Is it safe to approach?
- Where is the patient: standing, sitting or lying?
- Is the person calm, upset or angry?
- Are their potential objects they could hurt themselves or you with?

On arrival at the scene of an accident or incident safety clothing should immediately be put on, including a safety helmet, gloves and a high-visibility jacket with 'DOCTOR' displayed.

It is important to remember that some equipment may be used as weapons. Examples include mobile phones/pagers, torches, equipment bags, scissors and stethoscopes.

On arrival at the accident scene, appropriate vehicular exit points should be identified. It is essential that the emergency services are aware of any medical personnel present and that doctors know the rules of those emergency services. Any services that are required but not present should be called.

For the person(s) involved it may have seemed quite a time from point of injury or distress to the arrival of the emergency services. The arrival of health-care personnel may be greeted with a variety of emotions including anger, fear, frustration, joy and relief.

To deal with these feelings it is important to remain alert and flexible. If a crowd has gathered jobs should be delegated, e.g. sending for help, traffic control and reassuring victims. This will disperse the crowd, preventing frustration and verbal abuse. If a passenger involved in a car accident is uninjured but angry, distraction by giving the passenger a job may defuse the incident.

'John, I can see you're angry. I need your help in supporting your wife's arm. Can you hold her arm while I get her a painkiller?'

When the statutory services arrive command and control can be handed over. Treatment of the injured then becomes the priority.

IN THE PRACTICE

The design of the practice premises has a major contribution to make in preventing anger and aggression (Hobbs 1990).

Parking should be accessible, with a separate entrance for staff into the practice. External lighting should be in place to provide safety and also to support closed-circuit television (CCTV).

Access to the practice should be controlled, so all persons entering can be accounted for. This can be accomplished by limiting the entrances and exits. The security of each of these entrances/exits should be assessed. Internal doors should have limited access, e.g. a key pad or swipe card (bearing in mind fire regulations). External doors should be monitored by CCTV or be observable from the reception desk.

On entering the premises, clear, concise information boards should direct patients to the reception area. The reception area should ideally be easily identifiable and easily accessible. Open-plan layouts with a deep counter provide some protection but not to the same degree as is provided by a screen. Such a screen, if used, should be of modern design (as seen in banks) for ease of communication. Alternatively, raising the height of the counter improves security but can be perceived as intimidating and not easily accessible by the general public. The design should take into account the needs of the disabled. Panic buttons and alarms must be available for reception staff.

Internally, environment issues including good lighting, air conditioning and soft music should be considered. Decor should reflect tranquillity (Hobbs 1991). An effective method of communicating with patients should be considered (e.g. personal address system.)

Notices should be displayed advising patients and visitors that any form of threat or violence will not be tolerated and that the police will be summoned if this occurs. CCTV is used successfully in many situations and is effective in improving safety. Careful consideration should be given to the positioning of the cameras. A recording facility must be available for reviewing potential and actual incidents. A sign stating 'CCTV in use at all times' can act as a deterrent. CCTV can also be a source of annoyance to some people. There are ethical issues concerning observation of people without their knowledge. A local assessment must be made of the benefits and problems of overt or covert CCTV surveillance (NHS Executive 1997).

If appointments are running late, verbal violence is often directed to the reception staff. Guidelines should be in place to deal with this. For example, if appointments are running 10 min or more late, an announcement should be made to the people waiting. Anyone who is concerned about their condition or circumstances should be asked to come to the reception desk and discuss the matter. Hobbs (1991) stated that the most common quoted cause of verbal abuse was an anxious patient. Proactive communication with people waiting is the gold standard and will go a long way in decreasing verbal violence.

The waiting area

A seating area should be provided with up-to-date magazines catering for a wide range of interests and age groups. Health promotion material and information relating to the services offered by the surgery might also be beneficial.

Children require special consideration (Audit Commission 1996): low seats, colourful walls with durable, easy to maintain toys, accessible toilets and changing facilities should be provided.

Adolescents have different needs from adults and children (Rush & Knight 1997). Surveying adolescent attendees might give insight into what they would like to see in the practice. This survey could also identify service needs, such as alcohol services.

As adults accompany children, if the latter group are well catered for this will ensure a stress-free time for the parent/guardian and so cut down on the potential for anger and/or violence in the practice.

The consulting room

The room should be designed to ensure privacy and safety for the doctor and patient (Fig. 46.1).

The consulting room should be conducive to a relaxed atmosphere. Thought should be given to decor and lighting (Woodson 1981). Careful consideration should be given to a colour scheme – some colours such as green, bluish-green and yellowish-green have a calming effect, while some, e.g. bright yellow and red, have an irritating effect. Other colours, e.g. brown, black and grey, may be depressing.

When considering the colour scheme, give thought to the materials. Paint is cheaper than paper and easier to maintain if damaged.

Pictures may be added to walls. These should be securely fixed to prevent them being used as weapons. The glass should be shatterproof. Pictures may also help exert a calming effect on the room. Scenic pictures should be used instead of abstract ones.

Lighting is an important consideration, with natural light used to a maximum. Blinds slightly tilted can promote greater privacy and allow natural light to enter the room. If using artificial light, it should be of good quality. To avoid glare, use matt finishes on the furniture and floor.

By giving some thought to the decor you can transform your room into a tranquil environment.

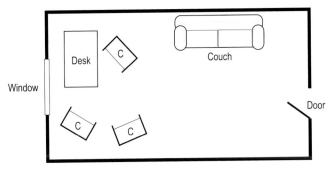

Fig. 46.1 • A layout for a consulting room.

As you can see from Fig. 46.1, the layout of furniture is important. The entrance should be accessible to doctor and patient. In the heat of a moment a person may just want to leave. If a clear path is available this reduces the risk of violence and damage. The door should provide privacy but should not be able to be used against the clinician in a hostage situation. Do not have keys in the locks, as a person may lock the door and then take the key. One option is to have a manual digital lock. This allows access to your room without the use of a key. The combination can be changed regularly to minimize unauthorized access. If the lock has a snib inside, this allows the door to be locked or put on the latch. Making an exit is simplistic as a key is not required.

The desk in Fig. 46.1 is against the window in the top right-hand corner of the room. With seats positioned to the side, both parties have access to the door. The seats should be of equal height to allow equality in the conversation rather than talking down to the patient; this prevents frustration. The desk should not have picture frames or solid statues. These can be used as weapons.

Introduction of panic buttons should be considered. These can be silent or audible. Silent alarms at the reception desk allow a staged response to be initiated. Loud alarms are useful, as they cause an ear-piercing noise and also summon help. They can act as a distraction, allowing a safe exit to be made. Thought should be given as to where in the room they are placed or whether staff carry an alarm on their person.

What to do after a violent incident

It is important not to deny that the incident took place: 'I'm all right, forget the incident.' Do not blame yourself: 'It was my fault, I shouldn't have been there.'

A physical examination should be arranged as soon as possible by an independent practitioner (bruises and marks soon fade), and an incident form should be completed in detail. Clinical photographs may be taken.

Following such an incident some will prefer to carry on working, others to return home. People deal differently with situations. Arrange a lift home rather than driving.

Incident reporting is vital. The form should be simple. Once completed the form should be sent to the line manager and senior partner. Incident forms should be reviewed by senior managers. What could have prevented the incident taking place? Was anyone injured? Are they all right? A check should be made to ensure that someone has made contact if the person is off work sick. Consideration should be given to involving the occupational health team.

It may be desirable to talk the incident over with a friend or work colleague. People who were present may understand what it felt like to be subjected to the violence. Sometimes there are difficulties at home. If the situation is not improving at home or the practice then there is a need to seek expert advice.

Staff training and education

All staff should be trained appropriately in the management of the violent and/or uncooperative patient (NHS Executive 1997). Communication skills and defusing techniques should be included in the content.

Training should be mandatory. Once trained, staff will feel better equipped to deal with a violent or uncooperative patient. This training may defuse the situation and so prevent an escalation of anger to aggression. This ensures that staff are not injured and patients feel safe. Staff morale will also be raised, as a commitment to training in

dealing with the violent and/or uncooperative patient is often neglected.

Summary

- Prevention of violence is vital.
- Training is a necessity not a luxury.
- Support is vital in the short and long term.

References

Audit Commission 1996 By accident or design: improving accident and emergency services in England and Wales. HMSO, London

Brown R, Bute S, Ford P 1986 Social workers at risk. Macmillan, Basingstoke

Hobbs FDR 1991 Violence in general practice: a survey of general practitioners' views. British Medical Journal 302: 329–332

Mehrabian A 1972 Non-verbal communication. Aldine-Atherton, Chicago, IL

NHS Executive 1997 Effective management of security in A & E. HMSO, London

Rush H, Knight S 1997 Adolescents in accident and emergency. Southampton University NHS Trust, Southampton

Woodson WE 1981 Human factors design handbook: Information and guidelines for the design of systems, facilities, equipment and products for human use. McGraw-Hill, New York

Part Eleven

11

47 Major incidents 483

48 Triage 493

49 Chemical incidents 503

50 Radiation incidents 514

51 Mass gathering medicine 529

52 Medicine at sporting events 534

53 Disaster medicine 540

Major incidents

47

Definition	483
Classification	483
History	484
Major incident planning	484
Prevention	484
Preparation	485
Response	487
Recovery	491
Reference	492
Further reading	492

Definition

A major incident in *health service* terms has been defined in many ways. Perhaps the best definition is:

Any incident where the number, severity or type of live casualties, or by its location, requires extraordinary resources.

It is not, therefore, simply the number of casualties that is important. A single hospital may cope with 50 patients with minor injuries, but 50 polytrauma cases would paralyse a network of general hospitals. Equally, a smaller number of casualties with specialist injuries (burns, spinal injuries, head injuries), or injured children, would rapidly swamp limited regional resources. The location is important as an incident in a remote area (mountain, desert, sea) with difficult access will often require extraordinary resources even for relatively few casualties.

A criticism of this definition has been that it does not directly take into account 'psychological' casualties. These people may not have been physically injured, but require extraordinary support from the voluntary aid societies (Red Cross, St John's and St Andrew's ambulances) at the scene, or from social services in the community. In the latter case this may be required for many weeks or months.

A major incident for the health services may not be a major incident for the other emergency services, and the converse is also true. For example, an industrial fire may occupy multiple fire appliances without any casualties whereas a passenger aircraft crash where all passengers are killed will be a major incident for the police casualty retrieval and identification teams, but not for the health services. Furthermore, a hospital may initiate its major incident plan without being notified of a major incident by the ambulance service – this has happened in the UK when, for example, in December 1995 an unanticipated episode of freezing rain over a densely populated area resulted in multiple walking wounded with predominantly orthopaedic injuries.

Classification

Major incidents may be classified as *natural* or *man-made* (Table 47.1).

Each incident may also be *simple* or *compound*. A compound major incident occurs when:

● the lines of communication are disrupted (mobile telephone or radio does not work at the scene, or land-lines are broken)

Table 47.1 Types of natural and man-made incident

Natural incident	Man-made incident
Earthquake	Transport (road, rail, air, sea)
Volcano	Terrorist (bomb, shooting)
Tidal wave	Industrial (chemical, nuclear)
Tornado	Mass gathering (sport, concert)
Bush fire	War

- the lines of transportation to hospital or between hospitals are disrupted (road or rail links impassable; weather prohibits flying)
- the hospital is part of the incident.

A compound incident is more likely to occur when the incident is natural – although war is a prime example of a man-made compound incident.

Finally, major incidents may be subclassified as *compensated* or *uncompensated*. An uncompensated incident is one where whatever extraordinary resources are made available, the incident still cannot be managed adequately. The term *disaster* may, therefore, be used synonymously with an uncompensated major incident, although published definitions of a 'disaster' do vary considerably.

A major incident may be:

- **natural or man-made**
- **simple or compound**
- **compensated or uncompensated**

Most major incidents in the developed world are man-made, simple and compensated.

History

War has provided much experience in the management of mass casualties. One of the earliest military medical support systems was to the Macedonian army in 350–320 BC. Personnel were deployed specifically to evacuate the Byzantine injured in their campaigns from 600–1071 AD and were paid per capita as an incentive. Baron Dominique Jean Larrey, Napoleon's surgeon marshal, is attributed with first applying the principles of triage on the battlefield in the 1790s, which are now an essential element of the health service management at the scene (Ch. 48). Percy, Napoleon's physician-in-chief, would deploy surgeons to the forward edge of the battle area. He also introduced *wurstwagens*, which transported eight medical orderlies to forward areas to provide first aid.

The American Civil War of 1861–65 resulted in the first documented protocols for the treatment of mass casualties. This same conflict highlighted the importance of early surgical treatment of battlefield casualties. Regimental surgeons would apply dressings, attempt to arrest haemorrhage and perform some surgical procedures prior to expedient transfer to a nearby field hospital. A similar system was followed in the First World War, where the introduction of the Thomas splint brought about a dramatic reduction in the mortality rate from femoral fractures. These principles of early life-saving treatment were taken several steps further in the Vietnam conflict with the forward deployment of surgical teams.

In peacetime, it is a sad fact that many of the fundamental errors in major incident management are repeated. This is understandable when it is remembered that major incidents will rarely affect the same community twice, and emergency personnel (other than those directly involved in major incident planning) often adopt the attitude that 'It will never happen to us'. This results in poor preparation.

Major incident planning

There are four milestones in the history of each major incident:

- *Prevention*: could this incident have been prevented?
- *Preparation*: were the emergency services prepared to respond?
- *Response*: how did the emergency services manage the incident?
- *Recovery*: what ongoing resources are required to allow the community to return to normality?

Each of these will be discussed in this chapter. The emergency services will focus much of their attention on the *preparation* and *response* elements. It is worth considering first, therefore, how forethought may prevent the incident from occurring or how it might mitigate the effects.

Prevention

The prevention of major incidents is often beyond the influence of health professionals. Man-made incidents may be prevented by legislation for safety standards, an example of which was the implementation of the Taylor Report (Lord Justice Taylor 1990) following the Hillsborough football stadium crowd crush in 1989. The report required football stadia to be all-seater and outlined the minimum medical support criteria for a football match (one 'first aider' per 1000 crowd, one 'crowd doctor', one defibrillator and one ambulance per 10000 crowd).

Natural incidents may be anticipated but are not preventable: their effects, however, can be mitigated by early warning (allowing public evacuation or action to limit property damage) and the introduction of various illness prevention strategies following the event (immunization, sanitation, refuse disposal, vermin control, public warning notices, education campaigns).

Preparation

Adequate preparation is the cornerstone of an effective major incident response. Preparation has three prongs and involves:

- planning
- acquisition of equipment
- training of personnel.

PLANNING

As it is rarely possible to predict the nature and precise location of a major incident, major incident plans must be flexible and adaptable to all instances – the 'all-hazard' approach. Guidance exists for the health services on how to prepare plans. It is important that planning committees are multidisciplinary (involving representatives from other emergency services, and the local authority) as contacts established at such meetings (and knowledge gained from an understanding of other services' roles) will be vital to the smooth running of the incident on the day. There are three key levels of planning:

- national
- regional
- local.

Examples of these levels are given in Table 47.2 for England (and Australia for comparison).

Department of Health supplements exist to guide planning for chemical and nuclear hazards.

EQUIPMENT

Equipment that must be acquired in the preparatory phase is divided into *personal* and *medical*. It is essential that health workers at the scene have adequate personal protective equipment (PPE). An ambulance officer in shirt sleeves, a doctor in a white coat or theatre 'greens' or a nurse in uniform should not be the television images of the scene response. Regrettably, this may still be seen despite national recommendations for standards of PPE. The areas of the body that must be protected are:

- head
- face

Table 47.2 Planning guidance in England and Australia

England	Australia
National	
- Health Circular number 25 (1990) - *Handbook of Guidance*, 1996 Revision (vols 1 and 2) - *Dealing with Disaster*, 2nd edn (Home Office guidance)	- *Disaster Medicine* (Commonwealth guidance produced by Emergency Management Australia)
Regional	
- Health Emergency Planning Area guidance - County Ambulance Operational Plan - State Ambulance Operational Plan	- State Disaster Plan (omniagency directives) - State Health Plan
Local	
- Hospital Major Incident plans - Ambulance plans for local high-risk events or installations	- Hospital Major Incident plans - Ambulance plans for local high-risk events or installations

- eyes
- ears
- torso
- hands
- legs
- feet.

The head is protected with a rigid plastic or Kevlar-composite helmet, with a three-point chin strap to discourage the user from discarding a loose helmet. A torch can be attached to leave both hands free in the dark. Ambulance helmets are white with green lettering; medical and nursing helmets are green with white lettering. The face can be protected with a visor but this does not provide adequate eye protection: additional goggles or safety glasses should be worn, as sparks or fragments may still fly under the visor. The ears should be protected by foam plugs, or ear defenders, which can be mounted on the helmet. A high-visibility jacket is required in temperate climates but a tabard (vest) may be more practical in warm climates; both should be labelled with the user's appointment ('Paramedic', 'Doctor' or 'Nurse'). The generally accepted health service colour is green, and almost all health service personnel are identified by a yellow jacket with a green yoke (some services use a red yoke, which is the traditional fire service colour). High-visibility trousers are also required, or a one-piece high-visibility jumpsuit may replace both the jacket and trousers. The hands should be protected from injury when moving about the scene (heavy-duty gloves), and from the patient's blood (latex gloves). Strong footwear should be worn. Identification should be carried, together with a small amount of money (in case the paramedic, doctor or nurse is used as an escort to a distant location and has no return transport).

Ambulance services rarely provide personnel with adequate personal protective equipment to operate in a fire, chemical or nuclear environment. Only personnel who have been trained to use breathing apparatus should be expected to use it. The fire service will therefore assume the responsibility for treatment and rescue of casualties in a hazardous environment.

Officers in administrative (command) roles would find the following supplementary items of personal equipment useful:

- notepaper and pen, or dictaphone to record decisions
- hand-held radio with headset and spare battery
- aide-mémoire
- pocket binoculars
- whistle.

Medical equipment may be considered in four tiers:

- triage labels
- life-saving first aid
- advanced life support
- specialist medical.

The first requirement is for triage labels, a small number of which should be carried on every emergency ambulance and in bulk on the emergency equipment vehicle. The type of triage label used is less important than the need for all who are using it to understand it, and particularly to understand its limitations. However, the label should be highly visible, dynamic and simple to use. The plethora of available labels (approximately 120 systems in the UK) underlines the problems of designing the ideal label. Triage labels are discussed in detail in Chapter 48.

Life-saving first-aid equipment will include portable suction apparatus, simple airway adjuncts (oropharyngeal, nasopharyngeal), semirigid cervical collars and dressings to arrest haemorrhage. Advanced life support equipment (some of which may only be carried by a mobile medical team from a hospital) is listed in Table 47.3.

Specialist medical equipment will usually only be carried by the hospital mobile medical team, for use by a doctor. This is listed in Table 47.4.

Equipment carried by a mobile medical team (MMT) should be compatible with that carried by the ambulance

Table 47.3 Advanced life support equipment

- Oxygen, and high concentration masks
- Bag–valve–mask apparatus
- Needle cricothyrotomy*
- Endotracheal tubes, or other airway adjunct (laryngeal mask, Combi-tube)
- Portable ventilator*
- Chest drains*
- Intravenous cannulae and fluids
- Intraosseous needles*
- Box splints
- Long spinal boards with integral headbox
- Traction splints*
- Extrication device
- Entonox
- Intravenous analgesia (nalbuphine, morphine,* ketamine*) and anaesthesia*

May only be carried by a mobile medical team

Table 47.4 Specialist medical equipment

- Surgical cricothyrotomy set
- Intravenous cut-down set
- Rapid infusion devices
- Amputation equipment

service. If different cervical collars or intravenous cannulae are used this will cause difficulties when equipment is pooled and shared. It is important that the MMT equipment does not simply duplicate that carried by the ambulance service but reflects the additional skills of the doctor and the doctor's complimentary role to the ambulance service at the scene.

Equipment should be carried in secure, highly visible containers that provide ready access to the contents. Rucksacks are commonly used for these reasons.

TRAINING

It is unwise to presume that staff have read and understood the major incident plan (ambulance operational plan or hospital plan), no matter how well constructed the plan is. If action cards have been produced noting an individual's key responsibilities and priorities, staff will often be unfamiliar even with these. It is therefore essential to ensure that staff receive regular education and exercise.

Education may take the form of a lecture, seminar or formal course. There are several structured major incident courses in the UK. One particular course, 'Major Incident Medical Management and Support' (MIMMS), is designed to be multidisciplinary and trains paramedics, doctors and nurses on the same course. The course runs for 3 days and teaches a systematic approach to the scene management of a major incident.

Education should precede exercise. Without a knowledge of basic principles an exercise can be at best frustrating but at worst it will reinforce poor practice. It is important that the objectives of the exercise are clear and the temptation to make the scenario too complicated is avoided. When planning an exercise, ask yourself, 'What aspects of the response is the exercise testing?'. The opportunities for exercising a major incident response are great, and methods include:

- paper exercise (triage, casualty flow, command and control)
- communications exercise (test availability, practice radio voice procedure)
- practical exercise without casualties (test command and decision-making)
- practical exercise with casualties
  - restricted to the health services
  - multiagency.

Response

In order for the emergency service response to a major incident to be immediately effective, a simple, systematic, all-hazard approach is required. The system for the health services is taught on the MIMMS course and is:

- command
- safety
- communication
- assessment
- triage
- treatment
- transport.

COMMAND

There is a subtle difference between *command*, *control* and *coordination*. *Command* operates vertically within each emergency service at the scene. Each service has a 'commander' or *incident officer* who is responsible for the deployment of all personnel within that service. *Control* operates horizontally across the services. The police are in overall control at the scene. An analogy is the service chiefs (commanders) of each armed service (Navy, Army and Air Force), who are responsible to the monarch or president (controller). The police are often uncomfortable with being labelled 'in

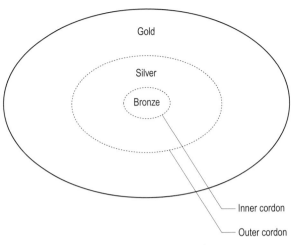

Fig. 47.1 • Cordons and tiers of command.

control', as they prefer to see themselves as facilitators or *coordinators* of the other emergency services. But remember that it is the police who have complete authority to restrict access to the scene and to preserve the forensic evidence – they have ultimate control.

Control is achieved by establishing an *outer cordon* and an *inner cordon*. The outer cordon is a physical barrier at the entrance of the scene: a police officer or vehicle in the road, blue and white police minetape, cones or temporary metal fencing. If required, the surrounding air space can also be restricted. All doctors arriving at the scene of an incident must 'log in' at the control point and then report to the medical incident officer.

The inner cordon surrounds the immediate area of the incident and may be a physical barrier if a hazard, such as fire or chemical, exists. In this case the fire service may control this cordon and may restrict the access to the hazardous area. A tagging system can be used to be certain of who is in the area, should the incident suddenly escalate.

The cordons are, convenient boundaries to the *tiers of command* at a major incident (Fig. 47.1). These are:

- operational (or *bronze*)
- tactical (or *silver*)
- strategic (or *gold*).

The area inside the inner cordon is the operational (*bronze*) area, the area inside the outer cordon is the tactical (*silver*) area and the area outside the outer cordon is the strategic (*gold*) area. The incident officers are *silver commanders*; their deputies, the forward incident officers, are *bronze commanders*. There may be any number of operational areas within a single tactical area. In a natural disaster, with damage over a wide area, there may be a number of tactical areas. There is only one strategic control, where senior officers of the emergency services, together with local authority representatives, gather to determine the resources that will be released in support of the major incident.

The first vehicle of each emergency service will act as the control unit for that service. The attendant will act as the ambulance incident officer and provide a conduit for information to ambulance central control. The duties of the first ambulance crew at the scene do not include triage, treatment or transport of the injured. Each service will despatch a dedicated control and communications vehicle, which will park close to each other within the tactical area. All other emergency vehicles should extinguish their beacons to allow the control units to be seen (the ambulance control unit may be identified by a steady green light or a green and white chequered dome).

A single doctor will be identified as the medical commander (or medical incident officer (MIO)) and will be responsible for the medical response within the outer cordon (at silver level). The medical commander may appoint a forward medical commander to work at bronze level. The role of medical commander is taken by the first doctor to reach the scene but is usually handed over to one of a small number of doctors in each area who have been tasked for this role and have received appropriate training.

The role of the medical commander is to coordinate the medical aspects of the emergency services response in conjunction with the ambulance commander (or ambulance incident officer (AIO)), police commander (or police incident officer (PIO)) and fire commander (or fire incident officer (FIO)) at silver command. The medical commander commands all other medical and nursing staff on the scene (a nursing incident officer may be appointed to assist) and reports to the strategic (gold) command.

The medical commander therefore works in very close cooperation with the ambulance commander in coordinating all the aspects of the medical response. The medical commander acts as a source of medical advice to the ambulance commander regarding treatment and patient evacuation, although s/he may delegate these tasks. Statements to the media on medical aspects of the incident are usually made by the ambulance commander or medical commander.

SAFETY

Personal safety is paramount at the scene of a major incident. A member of the rescue services who is injured can no longer contribute and will require additional medical resources. Each individual must take responsibility for his/her own safety. The incident officers must also ensure safety of their own personnel. The responsibility for monitoring the safety of health service personnel is often given to the ambulance safety officer. This officer may refuse entry to the site to doctors and nurses who have inadequate personal protective equipment.

The outer cordon has the important function of preventing unauthorized personnel from entering the scene

---

Table 47.5 Hazards at a rail incident

- Fire and smoke
- Chemical, if the incident involves a cargo train
- Electricity:
  - live rail
  - overhead power lines
- Other trains (diesel trains even when power neutralized)
- Unstable wreckage
- Glass and sharp metal
- Elements:
  - sun, rain, snow
- Patients' blood
- Downdraught from helicopters

---

and potentially becoming part of the incident. Casualties in immediate danger require a 'snatch rescue' from the hazardous environment. This is the responsibility of the fire service and rescue will be achieved without any prior first aid, and specifically without spinal immobilization.

These priorities can be summarized as the '1, 2, 3 of safety' – yourself, the scene and the casualties. An assessment of the safety risks at the scene of a rail incident is given in Table 47.5.

STRUCTURE OF A MAJOR INCIDENT

There are certain standard components of the structured emergency services response to a major incident. These are shown diagramatically in Fig. 47.2.

The casualty clearing station is the location for the majority of medical interventions carried out on-scene (a few procedures may be carried out on trapped patients before they are extricated). It also provides a facility for the *triage sort* (see Ch. 48). The ambulance service will appoint an ambulance parking officer and ambulance loading officer to establish casualty flow from the scene. Forensic examination takes place at the temporary mortuary, which is usually remote from the scene.

A body holding area will be identified for the short-term placement of bodies while initial legal formalities are completed.

Other clearly defined areas include those for press briefings, shelter for involved but uninjured victims of the incident, and staff rest points.

Communication

Poor communication is the commonest failing at the scene of a major incident. There is a failure of incident officers to brief and update their own personnel, a failure to communicate adequately with agencies outside the scene and a failure to liaise with each other.

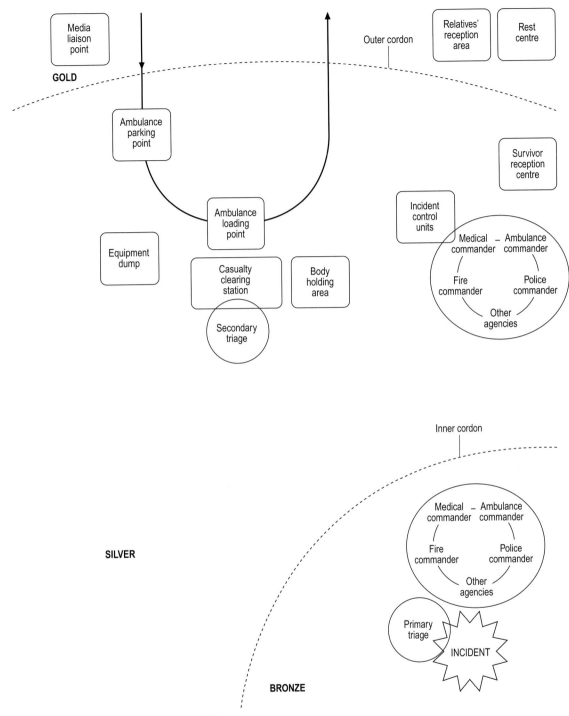

Fig. 47.2 • The structure of a major incident.

Communication failure can be categorized in the following manner:

- *A lack of information* – if the need for further equipment or personnel is not communicated, no-one will know there is a problem.

- *A lack of confirmation* – if the message is not verified (in writing) it may be misinterpreted – 'I need Entonox' ('*I need an empty box*'), 'I need morphine' ('*I need Maureen*').

- *A lack of coordination* – if health service messages are not all passed through the ambulance control vehicle at the

489

scene, messages will not be logged and requests may not be followed through (or may be duplicated).

There are a number of important methods of communication at the scene of a major incident. These are listed in Table 47.6.

Regular face-to-face discussions between the incident officers is encouraged. These may be hourly to begin with. The radio is a commonly used communication tool but its effective use requires the operator to be familiar with the radio working parts, the principle of a radio net (who the operator can talk to on that frequency) and a reasonable mastery of radio voice procedure (including a knowledge of key words, message construction and the use of the phonetic alphabet). The first time a doctor or nurse uses a radio should not be at the scene of a major incident.

A runner may, in some instances, be faster than using the radio. If the radio channel is particularly busy or a long message needs to be sent, a written message delivered by runner is a useful alternative. But who should be the runner? Emergency service staff will have important primary roles to fulfil. Voluntary aid society staff (St John's, Red Cross) can be usefully employed in this task.

An established public address or information system should not be ignored as an opportunity to pass group messages. In addition, either individual or group messages can be sent to emergency service personnel using the radio pagers that most officers carry.

Telephones are a mixed blessing. A field telephone system may be established within a few hours by contacting the operating agency (e.g. BT). This will provide communication between key fixed points at the scene (e.g. between the joint emergency services control point, the casualty clearing station and the survivor reception centre) and reduces the amount of information that needs to be passed by radio. The telecommunication service agencies may also assist by providing a supply of mobile phones, by enabling pay-phones

to be direct-dial lines and by laying cable for supplementary land-lines in protracted incidents. The principal problem with mobile phones is a loss of coordination of messages. If messages are not logged they cannot be followed through. All health service messages should be passed via the ambulance emergency control vehicle at the scene. This may mean it is necessary to duplicate a message passed by mobile phone. A secondary problem with mobiles is the saturation of available cells, often by the media. In this instance the police incident officer may authorize the institution of the 'ACCOLC' system (ACCess OverLoad Control), whereby modified phones may operate on a restricted number of cells.

Hand signals are commonly used by the military to communicate over distances where personnel can see each other but cannot hear each other. If the system is to be effective, it must be practised in advance. A whistle is used by the fire service to indicate the need to evacuate the rescue area because of an escalating hazard. Any other use of a whistle may be misinterpreted.

Communication with the media is essential. Local media representatives will respond very quickly and will be followed by representatives of national and international radio, television and newspaper agencies. Control is important but must be balanced against a genuine requirement to report the event. The police will appoint a media liaison officer who is responsible for ensuring that regular bulletins are issued, and ideally timed to allow preparation for broadcast at peak times. There is no absolute need for the ambulance or medical commander to provide a statement, but one will always be welcomed. Initially, a simple presentation of the facts will satisfy. This will give way to the desire to find out the circumstances surrounding the incident, and ultimately who is to blame. A prepared written statement may avoid the potential embarrassment of an inappropriate response.

Assessment

The scene must be assessed for:

- new and continuing hazards
- the number and severity of casualties
- the requirement for ambulance personnel
- the requirement for hospital mobile medical teams
- the requirement for specialist medical support (a mobile medical team with a surgical capability)
- the requirement for equipment resupply, and relief personnel.

There will be an assessment by the forward ambulance and medical incident officers within each operational area, and by the ambulance and medical incident officers within the tactical area. The assessment is likely to be refined as more information is gathered. It is important that ambulance and medical officers in these key appointments work as a team, thus avoiding making any decisions in conflict.

Table 47.6 Methods of communication

- Face to face
- Radio
- Runner
- Public address system (e.g. at a sports stadium)
- Radio pager
- Telephone:
  - mobile
  - field telephone
  - land-line
  - INMARSAT
- Hand signals
- Whistle

Triage

The sorting of casualties into priorities for treatment and evacuation is required when the number of victims exceeds the number of skilled rescuers available. The aim is to ensure that the most severely injured patients receive their potentially life-saving treatment early. Those with minor injuries, or those individuals whose injuries are so severe that they have a low probability of survival even if they are the only casualty (the expectant category), may not be treated at the scene or must wait for treatment.

There are certain features that are fundamental to effective triage:

- The aim of triage is to do the 'most for the most'.
- Triage is rapid.
- Triage is dynamic.
- Triage is reproducible (and therefore safe).

The initial *primary triage* is performed where the victim is found. Once the casualty has been evacuated to the casualty clearing station (CCS) a more detailed assessment (*secondary triage*) is made to determine the priority for treatment within the CCS. This will be repeated at every stage of the evacuation process to identify any change in the patient's condition. The triage priorities and labelling systems are discussed in detail in Chapter 48. Triage methodology and, specifically, the *triage sieve* and the *triage sort* are also discussed in detail in Chapter 48.

Treatment

The principles of treatment at the scene of a major incident are simple. They are:

- **Control of exsanguinating external haemorrhage**
- *Airway*, **with control of the cervical spine where appropriate**
- *Breathing*, **with oxygen where available**
- *Circulation*, **with control of external blood loss always.**

Major external bleeding must be controlled.

Simple airway adjuncts will be utilized. Intubation will rarely be appropriate. A patient who is not breathing when the airway is opened is dead (see Ch. 48) and in the presence of mass casualties should not be intubated. If a patient is electively anaesthetized and intubated at least one nurse or doctor will be needed to continuously monitor the patient and provide assisted ventilation.

The degree of treatment is a balance of doing the best for the most patients and ensuring that patients are safe to transport to hospital as quickly as possible.

Transport

In a developed country most patients will be transported to hospital by road ambulance. These vehicles may accommodate one or two stretchers and will provide a high specification of resuscitation equipment. They should be reserved for the immediate and urgent priority cases. Alternative transport should be considered for the delayed priority cases. Outpatient minibus ambulances, coaches or trains are all suitable. If casualties are to be transported any distance then medical support should accompany the casualties, lest an immediate or urgent case unmasks itself.

The responsibility for selecting the transport and determining the destination rests, in England and Wales, with the ambulance incident officer. There is sense in developing a system whereby decisions on casualty destination are made at a strategic level, so removing the difficult and time-consuming liaison between the scene and a number of hospitals. If direct communication by hospitals with the scene is discouraged, this will release the incident officers to direct their efforts to optimize the casualty care and flow at the scene. A hospital does not need to know the clinical details of individual casualties but simply the number of casualties of each priority it will receive and their estimated time of arrival.

Recovery

The recovery phase may be divided into the following components:

- operational debriefing
- emotional debriefing
- community reconstruction
- emergency planning.

OPERATIONAL AND EMOTIONAL DEBRIEFING

Operational debriefing refers to the analysis of the mechanics of the rescue response. Emotional debriefing provides a forum for individuals to express their fears or doubts about their performance and to rationalize what happened and how it was managed. Although the aims are distinct, it is likely that in early debriefing sessions there will be considerable overlap.

Debriefing can start during the rescue process. Some authorities (e.g. New South Wales, Australia) provide disaster counsellors who respond to the scene, support the rescuers emotionally and can identify to the medical incident officer those who are struggling to cope psychologically at the scene. Less formally, volunteer welfare organizations provide the 'tea and sympathy' environment at the scene for rescuers to begin to talk about their experiences.

Immediately following the incident stand-down commanders at all levels outside hospital and in hospital will debrief their staff. This may only be for a couple of minutes, to thank everyone for their work, as people will be tired and anxious to seek the support of their families. Importantly, a time should be set for a more formal debriefing ('critical incident stress debriefing') within the next 48 h. Notice should be taken of those who fail to attend or those who are significantly disturbed. Counselling can be offered, and a small minority may require psychiatric help. The majority of emergency service personnel will cope with the incident because of their supportive group dynamics or an understanding spouse. Those who have difficulty should not regard seeking help as a failure. The need for the commander to be debriefed must not be overlooked.

Some weeks following the incident there will be a joint emergency services debriefing. A similar pattern of recommendations can be expected. Many of the problems will relate to poor communication. These will be highlighted again at any public inquiry or subsequent prosecution.

COMMUNITY RECONSTRUCTION

Many incidents will damage or destroy property. This may be widespread following natural incidents. Displaced persons will require shelter, food and clothing. In a simple, compensated incident it is likely that the local authority resources will find rigid temporary shelter and will be able to provide hotel-style accommodation for those with longer-term needs. Following a natural incident many thousands may be displaced. Accommodation may then be under canvas. Public health crises should be anticipated and an appropriate infrastructure established for adequate sanitation and primary care.

The mental reconstruction of a community may take much longer than the physical reconstruction. Community centres may be required to provide support for years. Additional support at the time of an anniversary of the incident is predictable.

EMERGENCY PLANNING

Here the loop closes. Lessons learned from practical experience must be used to improve the planning for any subsequent major incident. Publication of recommendations will enlighten those distant from the incident and remind them – 'It could happen to you!'.

Reference

Home Office 1992 Dealing with disaster. HMSO, London

Further reading

Advanced Life Support Group 2002 Major incident medical management and support: the practical approach, 2nd edn. BMJ Publishing, London

Triage

48

Introduction	493
Triage at a major incident	494
Triage method	495
The expectant category	496
Triage labels	498
Prioritized despatch	499
Trauma scoring for triage	499
The Trauma Score and the Revised Trauma Score	501
Conclusion	501
References	501

Introduction

The word *triage* is derived from the French verb *trier*, which means to 'sort' or 'choose'. It was a French surgeon, Baron Dominique Jean Larrey, who first prioritized medical care when faced with an overwhelming number of casualties, developing a system that we would recognize today as triage. Larrey was surgeon marshal of Napoleon's Imperial Guard and as well as being a highly gifted surgeon he was a formidable medical administrator. Rather than leaving casualties on the battlefield until the end of the day's fighting (in the hope that they might be rescued by their comrades under the cover of darkness), Larrey established a system of fast-moving, horse-drawn ambulances, which would evacuate casualties during lulls in fighting. These were known as *ambulances volantes* (Fig. 48.1). Casualties were prioritized according to injury severity, with the aim of treating only those with a high probability of survival and especially favouring those with the potential to return to action.

In a contemporary developed medical system, 'triage' is now practised on a daily basis to prioritize patients for treatment within the emergency department or even to prioritize injuries within an individual patient. Traditionally, however, the term triage has been applied to situations where the number of casualties exceeds, or threatens to exceed, the capacity of the local medical support. It is in

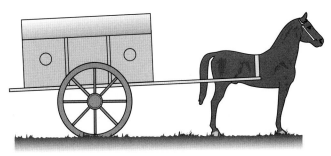

Fig. 48.1 • Larrey's flying ambulance.

this context that this chapter discusses various triage tools and systems.

The systems of triage for mass casualties were developed throughout the 20th century as a result of natural and man-made disasters and two world wars. The methodology used has inevitably been driven and advanced by military doctors – in particular in the First World War, the Spanish Civil War, Korea and Vietnam. Ryan (1984), reporting on the experience of the British Army in the Falklands War in 1982, reinforced the need for dynamic triage at all levels of medical care from the time of injury to surgical care at the field hospital so that changes in the casualty's condition are appreciated early. This is especially important in the military setting because of the potential delay in evacuation from the battlefield. Importantly, Ryan noted the effectiveness of dental officers used as triage or resuscitation officers.

To understand the need for prehospital triage, one has to first appreciate the trauma system in which the patient is managed. A *trauma centre* has traditionally meant a hospital that deals solely with trauma. Other smaller hospitals will be bypassed when the prehospital triage criteria suggest severe trauma. This trauma system is operational in North America. In communities where trauma (in particular, penetrating trauma) is less common, e.g. in the UK and Australia, the trauma system may consist of a regional major trauma receiving hospital that accepts both medical and surgical emergencies but has an augmented trauma response. A number of smaller hospitals will again be bypassed.

All injured patients cannot be assessed and treated in a trauma centre, or a major trauma receiving hospital, and a decision must be made in the prehospital setting as to which patients would benefit from transportation to such a unit if this facility is available. Attempts have been made to develop prehospital triage criteria to separate severely injured patients from those who are likely only to require care in a non-specialist hospital. The validation of such criteria in the UK, at the present time, may be of largely academic value other than to select patients for transfer to hospitals with certain specialities 'on site' (e.g. burns or neurosurgery).

A valuable aspect of triage is deciding the level of prehospital response to an individual casualty, or to an incident, based on information received in the telephone call from the public. This is known as *prioritized despatch*. This has been given a higher profile outside the UK, particularly in the USA – but this is now changing with the introduction of prioritized despatch in some counties in the UK.

One of the potential advantages of *prioritized despatch* is that an ambulance response, a medical response or a combined response may be assigned depending on the needs of the patient. In France it is felt that doctors should have a greater role in prehospital care. The result has been the development of the Service d'Aide Medicale Urgence (SAMU), which ensures that a doctor is available to attend prehospital emergencies at any time. A doctor also stays in the control room monitoring all emergency calls to make best use of medical resources, although this doctor will rotate to clinical duties to ensure that practical skills are maintained. In the UK the presence of a doctor at an incident depends on the voluntary commitment of members of the British Association for Immediate Care (BASICS), unless a medical team is specifically requested from a hospital.

Triage at a major incident

The Advanced Life Support Group (2002) have developed a system of managing major incidents, in conjunction with the other emergency services, which now forms the basis of the 'Major Incident Medical Management and Support' (MIMMS) course in the UK and Australia. This is currently thought of as the 'gold standard' of major incident management in these countries. The MIMMS triage methodology is discussed in this chapter.

Triage is required at *any* incident where the casualties outnumber the skilled rescuers available. There are important principles that should be adhered to:

- The aim of triage is 'to do the most for the most'.
- Triage is to be performed by one of the most experienced members of ambulance or medical staff.
- Triage is rapid.
- Triage is dynamic.
- Triage is reproducible (safe).

The initial (*primary*) triage is performed where the casualties are found. It is a task delegated by the ambulance incident officer or the medical incident officer to a senior member of the ambulance or medical staff. This 'primary triage officer' will initially be a paramedic or a senior ambulance officer, but the task may be handed over to a doctor or nurse depending on the resources that become available.

Primary triage should represent a 'snapshot' of the victim's condition at the time of assessment. As this assessment is performed in seconds it is inevitable that it will not pick up every life-threatening injury, and it is essential that triage is thought of as a continuous, dynamic process. Repeated assessment is the only way to guarantee that changes in physiological status will be identified. The second, and more detailed, assessment will often be deferred until the casualty reaches the casualty clearing station (CCS) (see Ch. 47) and should be performed by another senior member of the ambulance or medical staff.

P	T	Description	Colour
1	1	Immediate	Red
2	2	Urgent	Yellow
3	3	Delayed	Green
	4	Expectant	Blue
Dead	Dead	Dead	White

Fig. 48.2 • Triage categories.

Triage method

It is the aim of any triage system to accurately label each casualty. This ensures that the casualty is treated and evacuated at a time appropriate to his/her needs and the needs of the collective patient body. It would also be desirable to have a common system of labelling with international acceptance and validation, but this has not yet been achieved.

In the UK the accepted methods of labelling are (Fig. 48.2):

- colour coding
- descriptive
- the 'P' (priority) system
- the 'T' (treatment) system.

Life-threatening airway, breathing and circulation problems will be given the highest priority (red, immediate, P1 or T1) – e.g. airway obstruction, tension pneumothorax or critical hypovolaemia. Patients requiring treatment (surgical *or* medical) within 4–6h are classified as second priority (yellow, urgent, P2 or T2) – e.g. a compound fracture. Those patients with 'minor' injuries who can wait for more than 6h are classified as third priority (green, delayed, P3 or T3) – e.g. small burns, superficial lacerations, minor fractures. The *expectant* category (sometimes referred to as the 'fourth priority') is discussed later in this chapter.

The rapid 'first look' assessment is the *triage sieve* and can be performed in seconds (Fig. 48.3). Casualties are prioritized according to their ability to walk and maintain their own airway, respiratory rate and capillary refill. Victims who have no respiratory effort despite a simple airway manoeuvre are labelled dead. If capillary refill cannot be used to assess circulation, e.g. in the dark or very cold weather, then a pulse rate of 120 beats min^{-1} is used as the marker of potentially life-threatening haemodynamic compromise. Capillary refill is timed after compression of a fingernail bed for 5s and should not exceed 2s. If the triage officer times their own capillary refill before assessing

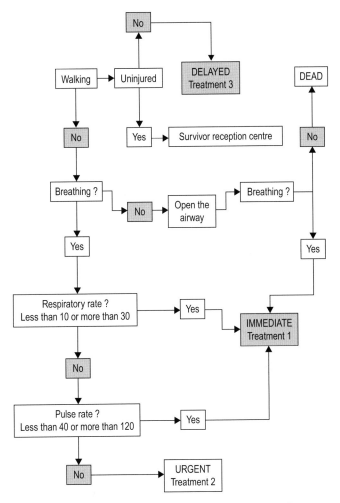

Fig. 48.3 • The triage sieve. (Reproduced with permission from Greaves et al 2006.)

the victim then a limited adjustment can be made for local temperature.

The *triage sieve* may be repeated if the casualty cannot be moved from the point of injury within a few minutes, and an appropriate change in triage priority must be made if there is a significant deterioration in his/her physiological status. Once the casualty is removed from the point of injury s/he is taken to the CCS. It is here that advanced treatment procedures are ideally performed (rather than in the difficult environment of the wreckage, unless absolutely essential). The *triage sort* is a more detailed triage assessment that is made on arrival at the CCS (secondary triage) and repeated before evacuation to hospital.

The Advanced Life Support Group has suggested that an appropriate triage tool for the triage sort is the Triage Revised Trauma Score (Champion et al 1989) (Table 48.1).

The Triage Revised Trauma Score (T-RTS) was developed for use by paramedics in the USA to assist in identifying those patients who should receive care in a trauma

Table 48.1 Triage Revised Trauma Scoring system

Physiological variable	Measured value	Score
Respiratory rate (mmHg)	10–29	4
	>29	3
	6–9	2
	1–5	1
	0	0
Systolic blood pressure (beats min^{-1})	>90	4
	76–89	3
	50–75	2
	1–49	1
	0	0
Glasgow coma scale	13–15	4
	9–12	3
	6–8	2
	4–5	1
	3	0

Table 48.2 Triage Revised Trauma Score (T-RTS) and priority

Priority	T-RTS
T1	1–10
T2	11
T3	12
Dead	0

centre rather than a general hospital. The score has three physiological components:

- Glasgow coma scale
- Respiratory rate
- Systolic blood pressure.

Coded values are given for each component from 0 to 4, and then added to vgive a maximum score of 12. The Advanced Life Support Group has recommended a T-RTS of 1–10 to indicate the 'immediate' priority, 11 to indicate the 'urgent' priority (there is a statistically significant increased mortality if there is a drop of 1 point in *any* parameter), 12 to indicate physiologically normal or 'delayed' priority and a score of 0 to identify the dead (Table 48.2).

Champion et al (1989) found that a T-RTS of 10 had a specificity of 0.92 for detecting patients with an Injury Severity Score (see Ch. 66) of 16 or more but a relatively low sensitivity of 0.49. Overtriage occurs when a patient

is given a higher priority than their injuries require. An example of overtriage is the small child, who will normally have a low blood pressure and a high respiratory rate. Undertriage (T-RTS of 12), on the other hand, will, for example, occur in the early stages of a 30% burn.

It is therefore advocated that a limited anatomical assessment is combined with the T-RTS, allowing the triage officer to use his/her discretion and make allowances for potential rather than immediate problems. This examination should take the form of an abbreviated secondary survey, as complete exposure of the casualty at this time is both time-consuming and might aggravate hypothermia.

A North American alternative to the triage sieve is the Simple Triage and Rapid Treatment system (START, Fig. 48.4) developed at Hoag Memorial Presbyterian Hospital, California by Super et al (1994). This system also rapidly identifies those who can walk, before going on to assess breathing. If there is no respiratory effort after a simple airway manoeuvre the victim is labelled as dead. Anybody who requires opening of their airway to initiate breathing is labelled as immediate (red), even if their respiratory rate is normal (unlike the triage sieve). Those who do not require any airway support have their respiratory rate counted. A respiratory rate of more than 30 breaths min^{-1} is an indication for immediate care. Victims with a normal respiratory rate have their circulation assessed by examination for the radial pulse. If this is absent then external haemorrhage is controlled and their status is immediate. If the radial pulse is present, a simple neurological assessment is made based on the ability to follow commands. If victims are able to follow commands they are labelled as 'urgent' (yellow), otherwise their status remains immediate.

The expectant category

Inevitably when a very large number of people have been injured there will be a small subgroup who stand a low chance of survival even when considerable resources are diverted towards them. This is seldom a problem where local medical facilities and infrastructure remain intact but in war and other *compound* disasters this apparent waste of time, equipment and expertise on victims with a low probability of survival cannot be justified. This severely injured category of patients is referred to as expectant.

There is no consensus on how to identify expectant patients by triage labelling. A well-accepted method is to use a green label, with the label endorsed 'expectant'. Blue is also used. With a cruciform label it is possible to fold the corners of the green label back and allow red 'ears' to show. In the 'T' system expectant patients are coded T4, and in the 'P' system they are coded 'P1 hold'. Expectant patients

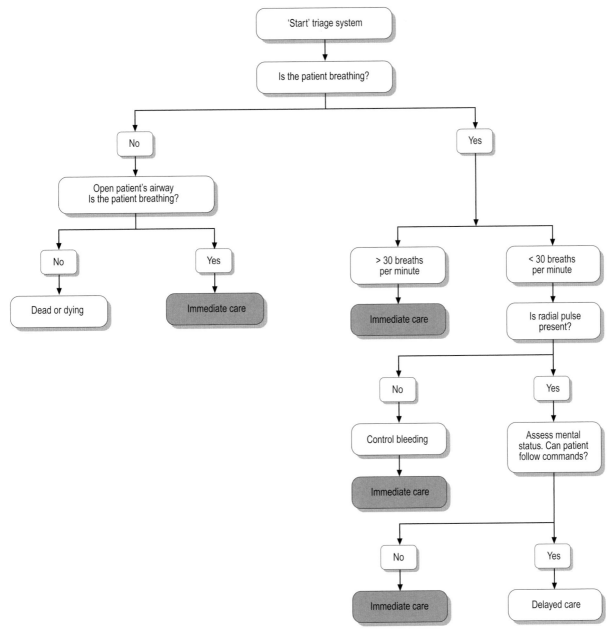

Fig. 48.4 • The simple triage and rapid treatment system.

are kept to one side, where they are monitored and their symptoms are controlled. If there is a change in physiological status or more resources become available, their triage status may change.

> **The labelling system for expectant patients is not important. What is important is that everyone is aware of the local system.**

The decision to invoke the expectant category should be taken at the highest level (ambulance and medical incident officers). Failure to invoke this priority at the appropriate time is likely to result in more loss of life.

Schultz et al (1991) as part of their earthquake disaster response model recommended that victims with a greater than 50% probability of survival should receive treatment when the severity of the disaster warranted the use of the expectant category. The probability of survival could be estimated using the T-RTS (63% survival rate if T-RTS is 6).

Triage labels

Once a decision has been made concerning an individual's triage category it must be made clear to other rescuers so that treatment and evacuation may proceed in an appropriate order. The most effective means to do this is some sort of highly visible label attached to the victim. It is also desirable that this label has space for recording a limited, but vital, quantity of clinical information.

There are approximately 120 different triage labels in use around the world. Within the UK alone there is considerable variation between ambulance services. This is at best unnecessary and at worst dangerous, as the multitude of systems will inevitably lead to confusion when health-care workers move from one region to another. Which label is adopted is less important than the need for familiarity with their meaning and format by all personnel who are likely to

use them. This includes staff at the receiving hospitals, not just prehospital workers.

There are two major forms of triage labelling card in use: single and cruciform. Single cards (multiple cards with one colour each) are generally colour-coded, with the descriptive category also written in bold letters. There is space for clinical information. The major problem arises when the victim's triage category changes, as this requires the card to be changed. The information written on the card may have to be transferred to the new card (some systems have an extra card for patient information only) or both cards left in place, possibly leading to confusion as to the true current priority.

The Mettag label (Fig. 48.5) gets around this problem by having coloured strips at the bottom of the card that are ripped off in sequence. Two disadvantages remain:

- The strips are difficult to see from a distance (the whole card is only postcard size) and in the dark.

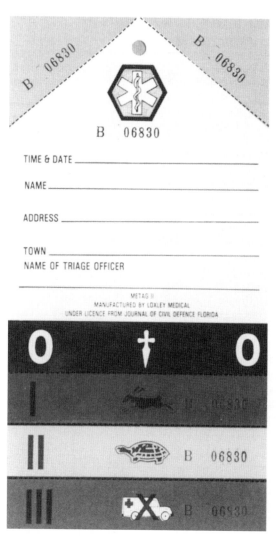

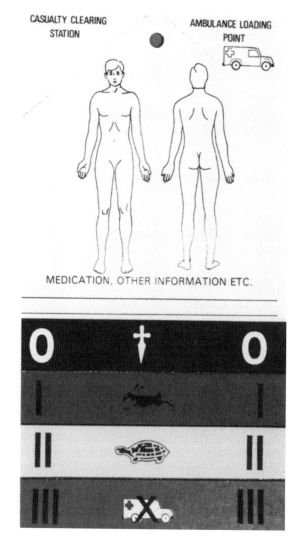

Fig. 48.5 • The Mettag triage sieve.

- The card only makes allowances for victims deteriorating, as the strips cannot be reattached once removed.

The label that fulfils the most requirements at the present time is the cruciform or Cambridge card (Sherriff & Wallin 1989) (Fig. 48.6). When folded correctly, the shape of the cruciform card allows only one coloured surface to be visible. When a victim's triage category changes the card is simply re-folded to show the new priority. There is considerable space for clinical information and it is intended that the card acts as a record from the time of initial triage to arrival in hospital. A potential disadvantage is that the victims might change their own priority by folding the card themselves. The expectant category is denoted by the green card over the red card, with the corners of the green card turned back.

BASICS, the International Committee of the Red Cross (Coupland et al 1992), the Armed Forces and SAMU are some of the prominent organizations who have developed their own triage labelling system. Although each labelling system has its own particular advantages, they all represent a failure to create a unified and internationally accepted approach.

Prioritized despatch

It is fundamental to any emergency system that a seriously ill patient is transported to hospital by the most rapid and appropriate means. Some patients may require life-saving treatment before they reach hospital, whereas others may simply require reassurance and monitoring. Emergency medical despatch (EMD) systems are designed with the aim of minimizing the prehospital time of the most seriously ill while making the best use of the enhanced prehospital skills and equipment that are available.

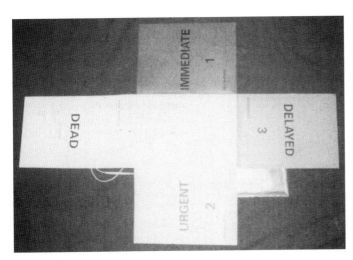

Fig. 48.6 • The Cambridge cruciform triage card.

There are two main priority despatch systems: Advanced Medical Priority Despatch (AMPDS) and Criteria Based Despatch (CBD). The Medical Care Research Unit (MCRU) have already studied the safety and reliability of AMPDS and CBD (Medical Care Research Unit 1996).

Both AMPDS and CBD employ a rigid sequence of questions. Questions are directed to determine the patient's respiratory status and conscious level, and ultimately produce a despatch priority of high, medium or low:

- High – emergency response (Advanced or Basic Life Support vehicle) with lights and sirens
- Medium – immediate response without lights and sirens
- Low – respond as soon as possible but not necessarily immediately.

The CBD system has been operating in King County in the USA since 1990 and has been shown by Culley (1994) to reduce the number of inappropriate Advanced Life Support vehicle despatches. Whether this benefit will be reproduced in the UK, where the number of paramedic crews is increasing all the time, is uncertain but there is the potential to save life and reduce morbidity by the focusing of resources and their more rapid deployment. It has been estimated by the Medical Care Research Unit that, with some modification to the two systems, a rate of serious (life-threatening) underprioritization of 1 in 2200 will be achieved.

Trauma scoring for triage

Each ambulance crew must decide the most appropriate destination for its patient. In the UK specialist trauma facilities are very scarce and in most cases a severely injured casualty will simply be transferred to the nearest emergency department. This hospital may or may not have enhanced facilities, such as a well-practised trauma team, or the presence of certain regional specialities on the same site (neurosurgery, burns and plastic surgery, spinal injuries). The decision to bypass a local hospital is therefore only going to be made in a very few areas of the country (e.g. the Helicopter Emergency Medical Service in London and the Medical Care Research Unit pilot Trauma Centre in Stoke-on-Trent). It has been demonstrated that severely injured patients have a significantly improved outcome if they are treated in a multidiciplinary trauma centre rather than the nearest general hospital. West et al (1983) observed a reduction in mortality from 74% to 20% in Orange County, California, when local hospitals were bypassed and severely injured casualties were taken directly to a trauma centre.

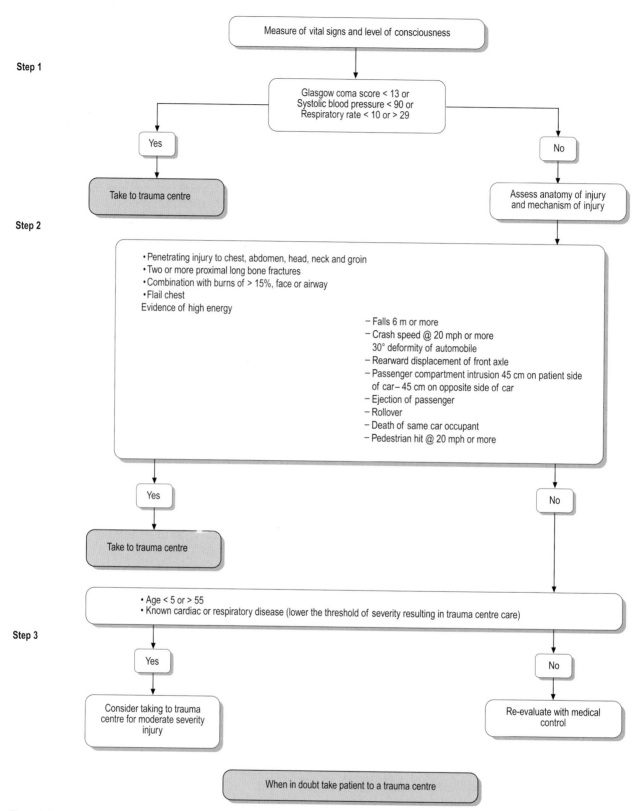

Fig. 48.7 • The triage decision scheme.

The methodology by which patients are triaged directly to a trauma centre has been developed principally in the USA (see below). Following the recommendations of the report by the Royal College of Surgeons of England (1988) on major trauma, and the follow-up report, *Trauma: Who Cares?* by NCEPOD (2008), the UK may move towards regionalization of trauma care. These principles of prehospital triage may then be more relevant to our practice in the UK.

The Trauma Score and the Revised Trauma Score

The Trauma Score (TS) is a dynamic assessment of injury severity based on the patient's physiological response to that injury. It is comprised of coded values for respiratory rate, respiratory effort, systolic blood pressure, capillary refill and the Glasgow coma scale, which are added to give a maximum of 16 (see Ch.66). A Trauma Score of 13 or less is associated with a mortality of at least 10%, and has been used by some paramedic services in the USA as the cut-off for triage directly to a trauma centre.

The Trauma Score has been shown to correlate well with mortality (Sacco et al 1984) and also to have low inter-rater variability (Moreau et al 1985). However, its field use has been hampered by difficulties in assessing capillary refill and respiratory effort, particularly at night. This prompted Champion et al (1989) to simplify the Trauma Score by deleting both these parameters in creating the Revised Trauma Score (RTS) and the Triage Revised Trauma Score (T-RTS).

The T-RTS (Table 48.1) combines three coded variables whose maximum total score is 12. A fall of only one point is associated with an increased mortality and will identify 97% of all fatally injured patients. This has been used as an indication for transfer to a trauma centre. A number of high-risk patients will, however, not be identified by the T-RTS because of a lack of physiological disturbance at the time of assessment, despite underlying severe injury. This will occur when the ambulance attends a severely injured patient rapidly, before the patient has physiologically decompensated.

For this reason the American College of Surgeons Committee on Trauma (1990) published a Triage Decision Scheme (Fig. 48.7) that combined physiological assessment in the form of the T-RTS with a stepwise analysis of anatomical derangement 'mechanism of injury' and, finally, individual patient factors (such as age and comorbidity) that might warrant direct transfer to a trauma centre.

Mechanism of injury alone as a criterion for transfer or *trauma team* activation results in significant levels of overtriage. Studies such as Cooper et al (1995) in Charleston, South Carolina found that mechanism of injury alone had a positive predictive value of 6.9% for identifying patients with an Injury Severity Score of 16 or more. Shatney & Sensaki (1994) came to a similar conclusion.

Conclusion

Triage takes place at all levels of medical care and can save lives. An improvement in mortality is the result of casualties with life-threatening problems being treated and/or evacuated before those with lesser injuries. When the number of casualties overwhelms the medical facilities, the use of the expectant category will prevent time and resources being wasted on patients with little chance of survival.

References

Advanced Life Support Group 2002 Major incident medical management and support: the practical approach, 2nd edn. BMJ Publishing, London

American College of Surgeons 2004 Advanced trauma life support for doctors: student course manual, 7th edn. American College of Surgeons, Chicago, IL

American College of Surgeons Committee on Trauma 1990 Resources for optimal care of the injured patient. American College of Surgeons, Chicago, IL, p 17

American College of Surgeons Committee on Trauma 1993 Resources for optimal care of the injured patient. American College of Surgeons, Chicago, IL, p 20

Champion HR, Sacco J, Copes WS et al 1989 A revision of the Trauma Score. Journal of Trauma 29: 623–629

Cooper ME, Dabney R, Yarbrough MD et al 1995 Application of field triage guidelines by pre-hospital personnel: is mechanism of injury a valid guideline for patient triage? American Surgeon 61: 363–367

Coupland RM, Parker PJ, Gray RC 1992 Triage of war wounded: the experience of the International Committee of the Red Cross. Injury 23: 507–510

Culley L 1994 Increasing the efficiency of emergency medical services by using criteria based despatch. Annals of Emergency Medicine 24: 867–872

Greaves I, Hodgetts T, Woollard M 2006 Emergency care: a textbook for Paramedics, 2nd edn. Saunders

Medical Care Research Unit 1996 The safety and reliability of priority despatch systems. Final report to the Department of Health. University of Sheffield, Sheffield

Moreau M, Gainer PS, Champion HR 1985 Application of the Trauma Score in the pre-hospital setting. Annals of Emergency Medicine 14: 1049–1054

Ryan JM 1984 The Falklands War triage. Annals of the Royal College of Surgeons of England 66: 195–196

Royal College of Surgeons of England 1988 Commission on the Provision of Surgical Services. Report of the Working Party on the Management of Patients with Major Injuries. Royal College of Surgeons of England, London

Sacco WJ, Champion HR, Stega M 1984 Trauma care evaluation. University Park Press, Baltimore, MD

Schultz LH, Dilorenzo RA, Koenig KL 1991 Disaster medical direction: a medical earthquake response curriculum. Annals of Emergency Medicine 20: 470–471

Shatney CH, Sensaki K 1994 Trauma team activation for 'mechanism of injury' blunt trauma victims: time for a change? Journal of Trauma 37: 275–282

Sherriff H, Wallin C 1989 The Cambridge Casualty Card – a triage card for multiple casualties. Journal of the British Association for Immediate Care 12: 30–33

Super G, Groth S, Hook R 1994 START: simple triage and rapid treatment plan. Hoag Memorial Presbyterian Hospital, Newport Beach, CA

West JG, Gales RH, Cazaniga AB 1983 Impact of regionalisation. The Orange County Experience. Archives of Surgery 18: 740

Chemical incidents

49

Introduction 503

Planning and preparation for chemical incidents 504

Operational management of chemical incidents 505

Management of casualties from chemical incidents 508

Conclusions 512

References 512

Table 49.1 Types of chemical incidents reported to the Health Protection Agency in 2008 (HPA 2009)

- Leaks (18%)
- Spills (14%)
- Fires (33%)
- Explosions (2%)
- Release (10%)
- Deposit (7%)
- Land (1%)
- Other (14%)
- Unknown (1%)

Introduction

Every day in Britain, serious chemical incidents occur which threaten the health of the population (HPA 2010). Such potential health threats might involve chemical fires, chemical contamination of the environment, or the deliberate release of chemicals and poisons. Old tyres catch fire releasing clouds of toxic smoke, acid leaks out of a tanker creating noxious gas or an explosion rips through an industrial plant. The UK Office of Security and Counter Terrorism (2010) considers that chemicals, combined with explosives, may be used as small-scale (assassination or poisonings) or large-scale (mass casualty) weapons. Some chemical weapons have used toxic industrial compounds; others have deployed agents specifically developed for warfare. For example, chlorine gas, an industrial chemical, was used during the First World War to kill or debilitate troops. During and after the Second World War, more sophisticated chemicals (such as the nerve agents sarin, tabun and VX) were developed for use in weapons.

Since chemical incidents are so varied in nature, they are difficult to define. As a result, several definitions are used:

- The Health Protection Agency (HPA), UK, defines them as all incidents representing 'an acute event in which there is, or could be, exposure of the public to chemical substances which causes, or has the potential to cause, ill health'. All incidents with an off-site impact, as well as on-site incidents where members of the public are affected, are included in this definition and, for the purposes of the definition, hospital staff and emergency services personnel should be regarded as members of the public (HPA 2008) (Table 49.1 summarizes the types of chemical incidents identified by HPA and Table 49.2 summarizes the chemicals involved in chemical incidents reported to the HPA in 2008 (HPA 2009)).

- The International Programme on Chemical Safety (a joint activity of World Health Organization, the International Labour Organization and the United Nations Environment Programme) provides the following three definitions:
  - Chemical incident: an uncontrolled release of a chemical from its containment that either threatens

Table 49.2 Chemicals involved in chemical incidents reported to the Health Protection Agency in 2008 (HPA 2009)

- Acids (5%)
- Ammonia (2%)
- Asbestos (3%)
- Carbon monoxide (5%)
- CS (<1%)
- Cyanides (1%)
- Halogens (3%)
- Metals (6%)
- Natural gas (1%)
- Other inorganic (14%)
- Other organic (12%)
- Particulate (<1%)
- Pesticides (<1%)
- Petroleum oils (5%)
- Products of combustion (36%)
- Unknown/other (8%)

to or does expose people to a chemical hazard (WHO/IPCS 1999). Such an incident could occur accidentally, e.g. a chemical spill, or deliberately as in the release of the nerve agent sarin on the underground railway system in Tokyo in 1995 (Okumura et al 2005). In both cases, the release of the chemical or chemicals is usually obvious either from smell and other physical properties or from its effects on exposed persons.

- Chemical emergency: a chemical incident that has passed the control capability of one emergency service.
- Acute public health chemical incident: a public health chemical incident where the exposure dose is rising or is likely to rise rapidly and where rapid public health measures may limit the exposure.

The IPCS definition of a chemical emergency above has important implications for practical health care in that a chemical incident that has passed the control capability of one emergency service.

This reflects the need for multiple agency response to a serious chemical incident.

This chapter provides a pragmatic approach to chemical incidents which can be adapted flexibly to individual circumstances.

Planning and preparation for chemical incidents

Planning should be meticulous. It provides an opportunity to understand and integrate the roles and responsibilities of other medical professionals, agencies and organizations that are part of the response (OSCT 2010) provide summary information on the roles of Government Departments,

Devolved Administrations and Agencies. Local needs and logistics can heavily influence the organization of major incident strategies and plans (HM Government 2005). The development and use of emergency plans should be assessed by regular meetings of the core group. Many of these activities can be facilitated by the local emergency planning officer of the health authority, local authority or industry. Plans can be divided into the following areas:

- Prevention
- Preparedness
- Response
- Recovery.

PREVENTION

This section of the plans allows for improved incident documentation to identify and provide strategies to reduce incidents. It should also include hazard prevention, surveillance and identification of incidents, and the development of strategies to reduce hazards, along with education.

PREPAREDNESS

Plans for chemical incidents should include active preparation in a number of areas, e.g. patient decontamination. Health and safety issues of responders and personal protective clothing provision should be planned for, and documented by availability and location. Other areas that should be considered include general sampling requirements that may occur during incidents for both biological and environmental samples. Training in the use of these plans and specific aspects, such as when to wear and how useful is personal protective clothing, is essential. Various levels of training have been described and the study of reference texts is highly recommended (Borak et al 1990, Briggs & Brinsfield 2003, Heptonstall & Gent 2006).

RESPONSE

Within the plans should be included documentation needed during the response, including incident logs, checklists and material related to specific sampling, public safety and clean-up measures.

RECOVERY

This deals with reviewing the incident and auditing the response, legal proceedings and feedback on processes (lessons identified). It can be invaluable in determining any risk to the responders and in improving plans for the future.

MAJOR CHEMICAL INCIDENT EXERCISES

All exercises provide an opportunity for learning about the roles and responsibilities of other agencies. In particular, they offer a chance to meet, in advance, others who may be part of the response in a 'real' incident, and facilitate an understanding of the detailed working practices of individual services. All exercises take a considerable amount of preparation and none really reflects a 'real' incident. However, if there is a duty to respond to a chemical incident, it is important to make the time to attend and to share in an exercise and its debrief. There are various paper, table-top or simulated 'actual' exercises. These can involve the whole spectrum of personnel from single department to full multiservice exercises (Advanced Life Support Group 2002). Exercises can concentrate on one area (e.g. triage, communications or decontamination procedures) or on a complete incident.

Table-top exercises are usually run in accelerated time so that actions that in real life last several days are discussed in just a few hours. These often provide a means of assessing communication difficulties and may allow for a better understanding of how and by whom a press release may be prepared most effectively. Exercises involving the use of 'made-up' casualties and real equipment such as ambulances and decontamination facilities are usually played over a longer time frame. However, these types of exercises often promote systems for a 'seamless' response while spreading best practice and helping to identify organizational weaknesses.

Operational management of chemical incidents

SAFETY

Safety is of paramount priority in any major incident. Personal safety must take precedence over patient safety. If rescuer safety is maintained and injury or contamination does not occur, the provision of medical aid to others can then be assured. This order of priorities is just as important for chemical incidents as for other types of major incident and may even be more important because any potential hazard may not be visible or obvious. Consequently, before approaching an incident, it is vital to make sure that it is safe to do so. Previous experience, unfortunately, has shown that secondary contamination of responders and emergency services personnel is all too common (Thanabalasingham et al 1991, Baker 2005). This leads to an unnecessary magnification of the size of the incident and a needless waste of scarce resources, time and personnel, as well as additional health consequences.

In the UK, the Civil Contingencies Act, and accompanying non-legislative measures, delivers a single framework for civil protection capable of meeting the challenges of the twenty-first century (Cabinet Office 2010). In the UK, any terrorist incident is regarded as a crime scene and the Police Incident Commander remains in operational command (Home Office 2003). Indeed in the first instance site security at the scene is as a result often the primary responsibility of the police working together with other emergency services, while the fire service is responsible for containing any hazard and making the scene safe. Therefore, only when permission has been given by the relevant authority, is it safe to approach the scene of an incident. At this time appropriate personal protective equipment (PPE) should be worn, if required, in order to minimize any risk of hazard exposure. It cannot be emphasized too much that it is only by ensuring the safety of rescuers that the maximum benefit to any potential or actual casualties can be achieved.

If you are told to stay away, then do so!

ESTABLISHING A CHEMICAL INCIDENT: RECONNAISSANCE AND REPORTING

Chemical incidents are often complex in nature and may lead to a disproportionate amount of disruption compared with other emergencies. In addition, many different emergency and rescue services may become involved, along with other agencies and authorities such as the wider National Health Service (NHS), HPA, the Health and Safety Executive (HSE), the Environment Agency (EA), meteorology, utilities and local councils, ministerial departments, private companies and voluntary agencies (OSCT 2010). In fact, this interagency partnership is characteristic of the response to chemical incidents. As a result of these factors, collaboration and efficient communication with all the involved units is crucial as it allows uniform and correct knowledge to be disseminated to all concerned. In the UK, this is now co-ordinated via the Civil Contingencies Act and the Category 1 and 2 responders (MacDonald & Pettis 2006). Likewise, flexibility, teamwork and planning enhance the effective management of the incident. All these factors help to simplify the complexities of the incident by identifying the responsibilities and lines of authority of those involved and clarifying any potential problems. A breakdown in communications can quickly lead to a reduction in the efficiency of the emergency response.

An important responsibility of those arriving by chance at the scene of a chemical incident is to ensure that the appropriate help has been summoned. If it has not, this should be done immediately. It is also essential to pass on information about the exact location and type of incident, hazards, casualties present and access. Several aids for reporting exist as mnemonics with the most commonly used summarized in the graphics box (Heptonstall & Gent 2006).

Mnemonics for rapid incident assessment

'METHANE'
My call sign/major incident alert
Exact location
Type of incident
Hazards at the scene
Access
Number of casualties and severity
Emergency services present or required

'CHALETS'
Casualties, number and severity
Hazards, present and potential
Access and egress
Location – exact
Emergency services – present or required
Type of incident
Safety

If called to a scene, if possible emergency responders should approach from upwind and at a safe distance. On arrival, all staff should identify themselves to the individual in charge or proceed to the initial control point or the incident command centre if it is already set up. The presence of each worker and any special skills, equipment or knowledge that they have can then be logged. It may also be necessary to consider wearing PPE at this time, if it is required. No personnel should use self-contained breathing apparatus (SCBA) unless specifically trained beforehand in its use.

At this time, individuals will be given a precise role, e.g. medical commander, hazard advisor or triage officer. It is important to keep to this allocated role so that duplication and confusion are minimized. If involved in the positioning of any medical facilities, it is important to take into account current wind direction and strength, and any possible changes to these, as well as considering any other geographical factors. If possible, these facilities should be upwind and uphill from the incident scene and at a safe distance (Borak et al 1990, Advanced Life Support Group 2002).

Once the overall scene has been assessed by the individual in command, implementation of any local pre-agreed on- or off-site plans or major incident policies can be instituted. Communicating these plans to all agencies involved is the key arrangement at this stage of an incident (HM Government 2005). One of the main difficulties of a chemical incident is in obtaining rapid information on the identity of the chemical or mix of chemicals involved and their health hazard. Disseminating this information is vital and allows medical management to proceed on an adequately informed basis (Thanabalasingham et al 1991, HM Government 2005).

Unfortunately, a comprehensive health risk assessment is not available for the majority of chemicals and details regarding human toxicity data may be sparse. Toxicological information can be obtained from the National Poisons Information Service (NPIS), which is a Department of Health approved, and HPA commissioned – national service that provides expert advice on all aspects of acute and chronic poisoning (NPIS 2010) and where appropriate from the HPA itself (HPA 2010). Early contact with them and their resources and experience is highly recommended. NPIS can provide clinical advice and the location and availability of certain specific antidotes, and HPA-specific chemical incident management information. Even if the chemical incident has involved an acute exposure, it is important to consider any potential for delayed or long-term effects because these can occur occasionally in the absence of acute toxicity.

There are a number of published documents that provide guidance on the general management of chemically contaminated casualties. These documents can be helpful when organizing and taking part in preparatory planning for a potential incident (Department of Health 2005). This advance planning is a major determinant of the successful management of an actual incident. Regular review, updating and amending of the local major incident plans by involved parties is always worthwhile (HM Government 2005), and it also facilitates collaboration, teamwork and understanding of the plans.

EVACUATION OR SHELTER?

In practical terms, the police, in conjunction with the fire brigade, usually decide what action is needed and whether to evacuate or shelter. Local information (e.g. whether there are any nearby industrial or major chemical sites) and the geography and topography surrounding the incident are all invaluable and help to decide on the appropriate strategy. There are many arguments for and against an evacuation or shelter strategy. Pragmatically, there has to be a sensible balance between the risks (potential amount of chemical, its toxicity and the expected duration of exposure), costs, advantages and disadvantages (timing, communication, transportation and population factors) of either approach. This complex balance may well be decided by the individual circumstances, practicalities and difficulties of the incident. Often decisions are based on experience and value judgements although Kinra et al (2005) provides an evidence base for sheltering.

As a general rule, however, unless there is an explosive or radioactive risk or substantial environmental contamination, evacuation is a *measure of last resort*. In most incidents, the best advice is usually for the population at risk from chemical accidents to shelter at home, close and seal their windows and doors, and stay inside until they are advised that it is safe to go outside. Listening to the local radio station will help keep individuals informed and updated. This has been summarized as a message of 'go in, stay in, tune in' and has been promoted by several local authorities, in collaboration with local industries and emergency services (Directgov 2010). If evacuation is recommended, then accommodation and subsistence for the displaced persons will be needed.

RISK ASSESSMENT

The potential hazard of a chemical is a function of its toxicity and exposure (Baker et al 2008). The latter is a function of both the chemical's bioavailable concentration and time. Circumstances and environmental factors can affect any or all of these factors, making a risk assessment a complex process (Baker et al 2008). Importantly, an incident risk assessment starts as soon as the first information about the incident becomes available. It is not a one-off exercise but a continuing process and is updated as the situation unfolds and as more information about the incident and hazards become available. Some pre-planning and assessment of obvious potential local sites may allow a preliminary risk assessment to be made from 'off-the-shelf' information; however, the more likely situation is that the assessment evolves as details become apparent.

Once an incident has occurred and been recognized, a preliminary evaluation of risks and assessment of hazards must take place in conjunction with the HPA. The circumstances surrounding an incident are crucial to making an informed evaluation. The key details are the nature and amount of the chemical or toxin involved, its toxicity (known human acute and chronic effects), storage, degradation and persistence factors (dilution, dispersion, diffusion) (Table 49.3).

Likewise, details concerning mixtures of chemicals are important because they can lead to unexpected effects, making an assessment more complex (Baker et al 2008). The variety of incident mechanisms also form part of the assessment, e.g. was the incident a fire; explosion; transport accident; spill or leak; malicious act; air, water or land pollution; waste, food or medicine contamination? Another vital factor is the timescale of the incident and whether it is acute or chronic.

Other details needed include any reactions observed between the released material and the environment, as well as the number of exposed or symptomatic casualties, any relevant clinical details and the route or routes of exposure (contact and cutaneous absorption, inhalation or ingestion).

Data about potentially hazardous chemical processes at the site are highly valuable (e.g. information about manufacturing, storage, transport or waste disposal). Other useful facts are the exposure conditions and site details, including location, meteorological conditions (atmospheric and temperature conditions, rivers and tides), topography (housing, schools, hospitals, nursing homes), agriculture and food chain factors, industry and transport, population factors (susceptible groups) and any sentinel cases or clusters.

Finally, information on any available analyses, specific antidotes and treatments can be important. Using information on all of these factors, as it becomes available, it is possible to formulate an assessment and extrapolate the probability of short- and long-term toxicity for the hazard exposure.

INCIDENT DOCUMENTATION

Good on-site documentation of an incident is essential, although the rewards for this are often only seen at meetings, enquiries or appraisals some time after the event. Accurate, clear and informative, but concise, notes are required. The time, date and source of any information should always be clearly recorded. It is important to bear in mind that any incident may become the subject of a public enquiry, coroner's inquest or even criminal investigation. Consequently, legible writing, understandable diagrams and signed notes are essential, as well as keeping duplicate copies on file. If notes are amended later, it is important that any changes should be timed and dated.

Writing notes during the incident is important, otherwise information overload and fatigue take their toll on memory. It is best to complete necessary documentation as soon after the end of the incident as possible, otherwise details are likely to be forgotten or even remembered erroneously. Notes will be particularly useful at any debriefing or feedback sessions that are undertaken and are also an excellent subject for audit.

DEBRIEFING AND FEEDBACK

All incidents are unexpected and often require the use of already overstretched resources. Medical professionals may be concerned about the effectiveness of the response. A 'hot debrief' after the incident can often identify problems not identified by advanced emergency planning and allow an opportunity for early remediation. Most importantly,

Table 49.3 Details of toxic chemicals
● Nature
● Amount
● Toxicity
● Storage
● Degradation
● Persistence

concerns may exist about the hazard and any risk to workers that might have arisen during the response. It is essential where such risks are identified that medical help is sought. This help may include a proper medical assessment and even triage along with other casualties, which may lead to referral to hospital, GP or occupational health department depending on the severity of any illness.

A 'hot debrief' also allows individuals concerned in the response to express any anxieties or fears over their ability to respond. For instance, it may highlight problems in identification of the hazard. Further investigation may be required by other collaborating agencies or organizations. Planned interagency debriefing helps to identify communication issues and clarify roles and responsibilities. It also allows an appropriate team to continue any longer-term investigation into an incident. It is vital that all those who have played a part in the response to an incident make the time to participate in the appropriate debriefing process in order to ensure an ability to contribute more effectively next time, and that plans can be improved. Good documentation facilitates debriefing and feedback.

Management of casualties from chemical incidents

GENERAL CONSIDERATIONS

If possible, the number of emergency personnel involved in the management of contaminated casualties should be kept to the minimum in order to contain any potential risks of secondary contamination. It is also important to be alert to the dangers of the spread of contamination throughout all stages of extrication, resuscitation and treatment of casualties. Circumstances, weather conditions and information on contamination can all change, so it is vital to stay in communication with the incident control unit. Similarly, it is also important to be aware that there is always potential for exposure to cocktails of chemicals to lead to the development of unpredictable or unexpected toxic effects. Vigilance is crucial.

One of the main aims of management of contaminated casualties is for them to be managed as close to the scene as feasible without compromising patient care or putting responders at undue risk. This minimizes the potential spread of contamination while also allowing early resuscitation. Combined with decontamination, this approach optimizes the chances for recovery of casualties. It is also important to remember that casualties of a chemical incident may also have sustained trauma either as a primary or secondary feature. This trauma is treated in a conventional manner. Casualties may have pre-existing medical illnesses or have conditions that may be precipitated or exacerbated by the chemical contamination. The management of

patients at a chemical incident can be a complex process and may involve many areas of medical expertise.

In the UK, the management of chemical casualties within a contaminated zone is now the responsibility of the ambulance service Hazardous Area Response Teams (HART) (Ambulance HART 2010). These comprise specially trained paramedical personnel who are equipped to work in contaminated zones and provide essential advanced life support and antidotes to casualties before and during decontamination when there is a risk of respiratory distress and failure.

Recent plans by the Department of Health for NHS organizations to assist in developing and deploying Medical Emergency Response Incident Teams (MERITs) are being prepared. It builds on the guidance given in the underpinning section of the NHS Emergency Planning Guidance: immediate medical care at the scene. The purpose of a MERIT response is to provide advanced medical care on scene at a range of emergency incidents, up to and including major and mass casualty incidents (Department of Health 2010).

PROTECTION OF EMERGENCY RESPONDERS

During an incident, PPE should be available in adequate amounts, accessible and appropriate for the hazards present. Consequently, prior planning with regard to PPE and the ensuing logistics is an essential priority in any major incident plan, policy or strategy. Prior to using any PPE, training is essential (Borak et al 1990).

PPE for emergency medical responders consists of low-flammability clothing and masks that protect, as far as reasonably possible, the individual from exposure by inhalation, absorption or physical contact with the chemical hazard present. It can also be used for protection against physical and biological hazards. It is vital to choose the appropriate level of PPE for each individual incident, and this will depend on the level and type of chemical hazard, taking into account the particular risks from dermal or inhalational contamination. Although no combination of PPE protects against all hazards, it is important to be as safely protected as possible. There must be a compromise between levels of protection and visibility, dexterity, manoeuvrability and flexibility to carry out tasks. Consequently, expert advice on the appropriate PPE to wear should always be sought, although there are still a number of controversies over the specific details. In addition to these controversies, different countries have varied needs for PPE, and as a consequence there are no universally applicable standards.

Respiratory protection can be provided by appropriate masks and filters and by two main types of respirator mask – atmosphere-supplying (positive pressure) air respirators and air-purifying respirators. The latter type acts by filtering air through various types of chemical filter canisters. The canisters chosen for each respirator depend upon the nature of the toxins present. Atmosphere-supplying respirators are either SCBA, using time-limited and often heavy cylinders, or supplied air respirators (SARs), using an air hose from an external source. Use of this type of PPE should always be under the careful guidance of the fire service and SCBA should never be used by emergency responders unless they have received special training.

PPE is divided into groups that provide four broad levels of protection (Borak et al 1990):

- Level A (maximal) is used when there is a highly toxic chemical environment and provides maximal vapour and splash protection. SCBA is used with a body suit that is fully encapsulated and is made of impermeable and chemical-resistant materials.
- Level B also provides maximal respiratory protection but only provides splash protection using chemical-resistant clothing and overalls. This level of PPE is used when less skin and eye protection is required.
- Level C is appropriate when the identity of the chemical is known and its exposure risk is low. This level of PPE provides similar skin protection as level B but the air-purifying respirators give less respiratory protection.
- Level D is used when there is no danger of chemical exposure and usually consists of work clothes without a respirator.

There are three levels of PPE (high, medium and low) that may be appropriate to the emergency services' practice. High protection is required when chemicals are of high or unknown toxicity and when there is a vapour or aerosol hazard. A respirator with eye protection and a light-weight, chemical-resistant oversuit, gloves and boots are recommended. Medium protection is needed when there is a skin contact hazard, and eye protection, gloves, boots and an oversuit are used. Low protection for minimal hazards consists of normal work clothes and gloves. Ordinary hospital gowns, latex gloves, theatre masks and clothing fall into this latter group.

As an incident evolves, increasing information may become available about the chemical hazards present and may allow the level of PPE used to be adapted. If little or no information is available and there are presenting toxidromes in casualties from the site of release, then staff should assume that any chemicals present are highly toxic and wear the appropriate PPE.

Regular changing of PPE during an incident is helpful in minimizing exposure; a 'no touch' surgical technique is also useful while dealing with casualties so that potential contamination is minimized.

TRIAGE

Triage of casualties is an essential preliminary part of treatment. Casualties are sorted into order of priority, taking into account their level of contamination. This facilitates the work of responders so that resources can be directed towards patients most in need and also to patients who are most likely to respond to help. Consequently, in the setting of a mass casualty incident, triage may direct treatment priorities away from the most severely ill patients and aims to do the greatest good for the greatest number. Triage should be carried out in a safe environment by suitably trained personnel. There are three broad triage categories for chemically contaminated casualties (Heptonstall & Gent 2006).

- P1 – resuscitation required *before and during decontamination* in a stretcher facility.
- P2 – treatment may be delayed until *after decontamination* in a stretcher facility.
- P3 – minor injuries, may walk unaided to an *ambulant decontamination* facility.

Triage of chemical casualties is a continuous process, and casualties need to be re-evaluated at each stage of their management so that any toxic effects that develop can be recognized early and treated appropriately. Casualties are usually assessed at the scene and then again on arrival at hospital (secondary triage) using the same triage methodology. Individual patients may need to be triaged a number of times over the time span of an incident and may change triage group more than once.

DECONTAMINATION OF CASUALTIES

As a first step in the decontamination process for casualties, it is important to identify contaminated 'dirty' areas and uncontaminated 'clean' areas. Ideally, these should be separate and there should be monitoring of flow of individuals between the two areas in order to reduce cross-contamination. Decontamination prior to transfer of casualties to hospital is the best method but is not always possible (Clarke et al 2008). This can be due to adverse weather conditions, lack of equipment, training or facilities. Despite this, decontamination may be undertaken by the fire service, often using copious quantities of cold water from hoses or temporary shower units. The decontamination procedure has been summarized as 'rinse–wipe–rinse', which is repeated as many times as is required to achieve decontamination. Large amounts of water are particularly important and relevant if the water reacts with the contaminant exothermically. Wet decontamination can either be 'non-contained', where the contaminating substance is diluted and washed down the drainage system into the water system and water courses, or 'contained' where residual water containing the contaminants is collected for later supervised disposal (Home Office 2004). Hypothermia is a predictable risk from the decontamination process and should be actively sought and treated. After decontamination, casualties should be wrapped up and kept as warm as possible. Particular care should be taken with decontamination of the eyes. Copious irrigation is required while making sure that contamination is not washed from one eye into the other. It is critically important to initiate this irrigation process as soon after the exposure as possible because this reduces the potential for damage and its extent.

Another area requiring particular care is wound management. Any foreign material in wounds should be removed carefully and treated as an ongoing source of contamination.

A dry decontamination procedure, using special vacuum cleaners or fuller's earth, can be used when the chemicals involved react with water. Clothing for disposal should be put in sealed, labelled and double clear bags in order to prevent further exposure or secondary contamination, and also for medico-legal or forensic purposes. Any other decontaminated waste should be disposed of in a similar way.

RESUSCITATION

Resuscitation is provided along established guidelines using standard methods. It follows the accepted 'ABCDE' priorities of airway, breathing and circulation. As noted above, resuscitation may have to proceed concomitantly with decontamination. Thus, resuscitation personnel should be aware of the potential for contamination via skin or mucosal contact and use appropriate PPE. This is particularly important if basic life support measures are being considered. Mouth-to-mouth resuscitation is contraindicated. Manual ventilation bags can be fitted with absorbent canisters if resuscitation is needed in a toxic environment (Baker 1999). The HARTs are equipped with specially adapted portable gas-powered ventilators which can operate safely in a contaminated zone. For safety, if electrical defibrillation is required, the patient's chest should be dried to prevent arcing of the electricity between the defibrillator paddles and also to prevent burns to the casualty. Emergency responders also need to be as dry as possible in order to prevent electrocution or injury to themselves during resuscitation. Expert advice on management may be needed if the chemical is explosive or combustible. Safety is of vital importance in order to prevent any additional casualties.

SPECIFIC TREATMENT

The preliminary part of treatment for any contaminated victim is to remove the patient from any ongoing exposure to the chemicals or toxins if this has not already been done. This simple manoeuvre significantly reduces the hazard to the casualty. Any contaminated clothing or possessions should be removed. This one action may reduce contamination by as much as 70–80%.

Treatment then consists of general supportive care along with any available specific measures for individual toxins. Attention to the airway, breathing, ventilation and support of the circulation are mandatory. Treatment of other concomitant medical conditions and injuries and attention to possible hypothermia are essential. These are usually managed along conventional lines. Overall, general supportive treatment is usually all that is needed for the majority of patients, but a low threshold should be kept for seeking expert advice or mobilizing trained mobile medical support. Specific antidotes can be despatched to the scene if required. Information regarding their use can be obtained from the Health Protection Agency with support from the NPIS (2010). Previous preparatory planning and the major incident plan should provide information concerning local sources and stores of antidotes.

In general, the majority of chemically contaminated casualties are treated symptomatically with supportive care only. There are a few specific antidotes and treatments for a small number of toxins. Information regarding these and their use can be obtained from the Health Protection Agency with support from the NPIS (2010). Previous preparatory planning and the major incident plan should provide information concerning local sources and stores of antidotes.

Collection of appropriate biological samples at an early stage is invaluable in order to confirm exposure and determine the degree of absorption of toxic chemicals.

TRANSFER TO HOSPITAL CARE

There is a delicate balance between early transfer of casualties to hospital and the treatment of casualties at the scene. The latter may lead to delays in patients being transferred to hospital, while the former may delay instituting early decontamination and treatment. These issues are open to judgement and often depend on individual circumstances, e.g. the number and severity of contaminated casualties, location of the incident, weather conditions, distance to the appropriate medical facilities and resources available. As mentioned above, the HART paramedic teams are trained to provide essential advanced life support at the point of injury before decontamination and hospital transfer.

Vehicles taking casualties to hospital should take a route that does not pass through any contaminated areas or plumes. Vehicles used to transport contaminated casualties should be separated from other vehicles and used only for the incident. All equipment and devices used during the incident should be kept together in order to facilitate comprehensive decontamination at the end of the incident. Past experience has shown that there can be secondary contamination from use of contaminated equipment, clothing or vehicles.

Advance warning for any receiving hospitals is essential so that emergency procedures can be implemented. It is important to note that casualties may have self-evacuated and may arrive at hospital or the emergency department without warning. Consequently, prompt action is always necessary. Information is needed as to whether casualties have been decontaminated at the scene or whether decontamination will be needed at the hospital. A separate area for ambulances used in the incident should be allocated so that they can be decontaminated after the incident.

HOSPITAL CARE

If separate facilities for the management of contaminated casualties are not available, then the clinical areas should be divided up into clean and dirty areas in order to prevent cross-contamination (Clarke et al 2008). These should be clearly labelled clean and dirty areas.

Decontamination of casualties should be undertaken before being taken to the hospital. If this has not happened at the scene, it should happen outside the department or in an allocated and separate well-ventilated area of the emergency department, ideally close to the entrance of the department. Tepid water and soap or mild detergent may be needed at this stage, with special attention being paid to the eyes, skin and hair. The official recommendations require the decontamination section to have outside stretcher access with self-contained ventilation and drainage. This facility should be tiled and the coverings should be acid-resistant. Unfortunately, as in America, very few emergency departments have these facilities and so makeshift arrangements are usually necessary. Staff must not move from dirty to clean areas without themselves being decontaminated. PPE should be used when moving from clean to dirty areas, if the type of contamination requires it. If the contaminating substance is not known, staff should assume patients are contaminated with toxic agents until proved otherwise. Patients' clothing and property must be bagged and kept in a secure dirty area.

During and after the preliminary resuscitation and decontamination, a detailed and precise history must be taken. New information may be elicited at this stage, including the patient's individual susceptibility to toxins and personal medical history. Specific information should be asked about drug and allergy history so that drug–poison interactions or allergic reactions can be predicted and managed (Clarke et al 2008).

The doctor looking after each casualty should perform a general examination (primary and secondary survey) and look for specific features of chemical toxicity that may suggest ongoing exposure or a predisposition to the effects of exposure. This examination may also reveal the amount of exposure and the underlying level of reserve against toxicity.

Staff should be aware that what appears to be a relatively minor exposure, e.g. phenol, chromic acid or phosphorus contamination of the skin, can lead to severe systemic and organ toxicity. Similarly, phosphorus burns need to be kept moist until particles are removed as phosphorus ignites on exposure to air.

General investigations, depending upon the circumstances, may include physiological observations and monitoring, biochemical (glucose, electrolytes, renal and liver function tests), haematological (blood count and differential, clotting tests), arterial blood gases and carboxyhaemoglobin levels, chest X-ray, electrocardiogram, peak flow and spirometry. Toxicological samples of blood, urine, vomit or other relevant biological or environmental materials may be needed but results will not be available immediately.

Special tests depend upon the chemicals involved or potentially involved (Clarke et al 2008). This may include tests for specific toxins, biological sampling or testing of sentinel cases. Sometimes, however, specific information about the contaminating chemicals may not be initially available, in which case suitable samples, after discussion with the Health Protection Agency or NPIS, should be taken for screening and for future tests.

Most patients will not require admission as exposure will usually have been small, especially if effective decontamination has been carried out. However, it is important to be aware of the potential for delayed effects from chemical exposure, e.g. delayed pulmonary oedema from inhaled toxins, which may necessitate 24-hour admission for observation (Clarke et al 2008). It is important not to discharge individuals back to a previously contaminated area without prior checking that it is safe to do so.

FOLLOW-UP

The site clean-up operation at the end of the incident may well be time-consuming, using many personnel, facilities and resources. Staff involved in this operation may need follow-up at their own occupational health department or other specialist services. Particular follow-up may be needed for any exposed individuals or emergency services personnel. High-risk groups who may require follow-up include the young and elderly, pregnant women and those with pre-existing illness. Patients may need referral and follow-up at a review clinic, out-patient department, burns unit or toxicology centre. It should be noted that long-term follow-up of exposed individuals is important A high level of suspicion should be maintained for acute psychological illness immediately following an incident and other more long-term psychological sequelae, including post-traumatic stress disorder, in all the above groups and also in any distressed relatives.

Timely and proactive research into the long-term effects of chemical incidents is essential and can be very informative (Anto 1997, Landi et al 1997). A multidisciplinary approach is advocated and a variety of different methodologies can be used to extract the information needed. Epidemiological surveillance may be invaluable.

Conclusions

Every day in Britain, chemical incidents occur which threaten the health of the population. Practical prehospital care offers considerable value in minimizing harm to those exposed within the context of a multidisciplinary emergency response. This chapter provides a pragmatic approach to chemical incidents which can be adapted flexibly to individual circumstances.

The chapter is divided into three main sections. First, planning and preparation for chemical incidents are discussed briefly including the value of participation in chemical incident exercises. Secondly, operational management of chemical incidents is reviewed. This includes consideration of responder safety, recognition of a chemical incident, issues relating to evacuation or shelter, risk assessment, incident documentation, debriefing and feedback. Finally, the specific aspects of chemical incident management are examined including protection of emergency responders, triage, decontamination, resuscitation, specific treatment, transfer to hospital care, hospital care and follow-up.

References

Advanced Life Support Group 2002 Major incident medical management and support: the practical approach, 2nd edn. BMJ Publishing, London

Ambulance HART 2010 Hazardous Area Response Teams. Available at http://www.ambulancehart.org/ (accessed 15 April 2010)

Anto JA 1997 Health effects due to inhalation of oilseed rape emissions. Lancet 350: 458–459

Baker DJ 1999 Management of respiratory failure in toxic disasters. Resuscitation 42: 117–124

Baker DJ 2005 The problem of secondary contamination following chemical agent release. Critical Care 9: 323–324

Baker DJ, Fielder R, Karalliedde L, Murray, VSG Parkinson N (eds) 2008 Essentials of toxicology for health protection: a handbook for field professionals. Cambridge University Press, Cambridge

Borak J, Callan M, Abbott W 1990 Hazardous materials exposure: emergency response and patient care. Prentice Hall Inc., New Jersey

Briggs SM, Brinsfield KH 2003 Advanced disaster medical response manual for providers. Harvard Medical International Inc.

Cabinet Office 2010 Civil Contingencies Act web site. Available at http://www.cabinetoffice.gov.uk/ukresilience/preparedness/ccact.aspx (accessed 11 April 2010)

Clarke SFJ, Chilcott RP, Wilson JC et al 2008 Decontamination of multiple casualties who are chemically contaminated: a challenge for acute hospitals. Prehospital and Disaster Medicine 23(2): 175–181

Cullinan P, Acquilla S, Ramana Dhara V on behalf of the International Commission on Bhopal 1997 Respiratory morbidity 10 years after the Union Carbide gas leak at Bhopal: a cross sectional survey. British Medical Journal 314: 338–343

Department of Health 2005 The NHS Emergency Planning Guidance 2005. Available at www.dh.gov.uk (accessed 13 April 2010)

Department of Health 2010 NHS Emergency Planning Guidance: planning for the development and deployment of Medical Emergency Response Incident Teams in the provision of advance medical care at scene of an incident. Available at http://www.dh.gov.uk/en/Publicationsandstatistics/Publications/PublicationsPolicyAndGuidance/DH_114464 (accessed 13 April 2010)

Directgov 2010 Public services all in one place. General advice about what to do in an emergency. Available at http://www.direct.gov.uk/en/Governmentcitizensandrights/Dealingwithemergencies/Preparingforemergencies/DG_175910 (accessed 11 April 2010)

Fisher J, Morgan-Jones D, Murray VSG, Davies G 1999 Chemical incident management for accident and emergency clinicians. Stationery Office, London

Health Protection Agency 2010 Chemical and poisons. Available at http://www.hpa.org.uk/ProductsServices/ChemicalsPoisons/ (accessed 11 April 2010)

Health Protection Agency. Chemical incidents surveillance review. January 2006–December 2007, 2008. Available at http://www.hpa.org.uk/web/HPAwebFile/HPAweb_C/1211184033548 (accessed 11 April 2010)

Health Protection Agency Chemical Hazards and Poisons Division 2008 Chemical incidents surveillance review. 1 January–31 December 2008. Available at http://www.hpa.org.uk/web/HPAwebFile/HPAweb_C/1259152298305 (accessed 11 April 2010)

Heptonstall J, Gent N 2006 CBRN incident: clinical management and health protection. Health Protection Agency, London. Available at http://www.hpa.org.uk/web/HPAwebFile/HPAweb_C/1194947377166 (accessed 11 April 2010)

Home Office 2003 The release of chemical, biological, radiological or nuclear (CBRN) substances or material guidance for local authorities, p. 15). Available at http://www.cabinetoffice.gov.uk/media/132655/cbrn_guidance.pdf (accessed 11 April 2010)

Home Office 2004 The decontamination of people exposed to chemical, biological radiological or nuclear (CBRN) substances or material: strategic national guidance, 2nd edn. Available at www.cabinetoffice.gov.uk/media/132883/peoplecbrn.pdf (accessed 15 April 2010)

International Programme on Chemical Safety (WHO/ILO/UNEP) 2010 Key definitions. Available at http://www.who.int/ipcs/emergencies/definitions/en/index.html (accessed 11 April 2010)

Kinra S, Lewendon G, Nelder R et al 2005 Evacuation decisions in a chemical air pollution incident: cross-sectional survey. British Medical Journal 330: 1471–1474

Landi MT, Needham LL, Lucier G et al 1997 Concentrations of dioxin 20 years after Seveso. Lancet 349: 1811

MacDonald G, Pettis T 2006 Civil Contingencies Act. Health Protection Agency: Chemical hazards and poisons report 6: 20–21. Available at http://www.hpa.org.uk/web/HPAwebFile/HPAweb_C/1194947321801 (accessed 11 April 2010)

National Poisons Information Service 2010 Available at http://www.npis.org/ (accessed 11 April 2010)

Office for Security and Counter-Terrorism (OSCT) 2010 Home Office: The UK's strategy for countering the use of CBRN by terrorists. Available at http://security.homeoffice.gov.uk/news-publications/publication-search/cbrn-guidance/strat-countering-use-of-CBRN.html (accessed 13 April 2010)

Okumura S, Okumura T, Ishimatsu S et al 2005 Clinical review: Tokyo – protecting the health care worker during a chemical mass casualty event: an important issue of continuing relevance. Critical Care 9: 397–400

Okumura T, Nomura T, Suzuki S et al 2007 The dark morning: the experiences and lessons learned from the Tokyo subway sarin attack. In: Marrs TC, Maynard RL, Sidell FR (eds) Chemical warfare agents: toxicology and treatment, 2nd edn. John Wiley and Sons, Chichester, UK, pp 277–286

Thanabalasingham T, Beckett MW, Murray VSG 1991 Hospital response to a chemical incident: report on casualties of an ethyldichlorosilane spill. British Medical Journal 302: 101–102

WHO/IPCS 1999 Public Health and Chemical Incidents: Guidance for National and Regional Policy Makers in the Public/Environmental Health Roles. Available at http://www.who.int/ipcs/publications/en/Public_Health_Management.pdf (accessed 11 April 2010)

Radiation incidents

50

Introduction	514
Basic physics	515
Biological effects	518
Radiation protection	520
Types of radiation accident	521
Plans, special arrangements and advice	522
Packages and source identification	523
Safety – scene, self and the casualty	524
Medical management of radiation casualties	525
Information to hospitals/triage	527
Public protection in radiation accidents (Emergency Reference Levels)	528
References	528

Introduction

Almost the first principle that any first aider or immediate carer learns is safety; their own and that of their casualty. Compliance with this principle requires the recognition of potential hazards and the assessment of risk in the particular situation in which we find ourselves.

Despite the fact that the vast majority of man-made radiation exposure occurs as a result of medical practice, the average knowledge of radiation hazards by health professionals is not high. We are not, therefore, well equipped to make such risk assessments. While the treatment of radiation injury has changed significantly and improved in recent years, there remain no vital specific skills that the immediate carer must master to treat these casualties. Although this section does include some consideration of the treatment of radiation injury and contamination, it concentrates on the provision of information on radiation hazards, as well as identifying sources of expert advice available to the immediate carer responding to a radiological incident.

It is a popular myth that the terms 'radiation incident' and 'nuclear incident' are synonymous. Sources of ionizing radiation are ubiquitous in our society, being used in many industrial and research activities, medical and dental practice, as well as in everyday items such as light sources, smoke detectors and valves. It is highly probable, therefore, that in a lifetime of immediate care all of us may have to respond to an accident where ionizing radiation is present. This view determines that all immediate carers need some basic knowledge on radiation and their hazards.

The aim of this chapter is to provide immediate carers with basic information on:

- ionizing radiations and their biological effects
- basic radiation protection considerations
- sources of expert advice available in radiation accidents
- concepts involved in the initial treatment, decontamination and public protection following radiation accidents.

Basic physics

IONIZATION

Most people are familiar with the Bohr concept of an atom as a relatively small central nucleus composed of protons and neutrons, orbited by electrons in a series of concentric shells. Most of the mass of the atom is in the nucleus, as the electrons are relatively light compared with protons and neutrons. The negatively charged electrons are held within the atom by the equal but positive charge of the protons.

Radiation can be defined in terms of the transfer of energy from one source to another. What then separates 'ionizing radiation' from other types, such as heat and light? If an electron is given enough energy to break its bond to the atom, this is referred to as ionization. The results of ionization are free electrons and positively charged ions, both of which can go on to take part in other reactions, causing biological effects. Radiation with enough energy to split away an electron and cause ionization is, by definition, ionizing; forms with insufficient energy are non-ionizing.

Short of full ionization, radiation may give energy to an electron that, while insufficient to break it away from the atom, is enough to push it out to a shell further out from the nucleus. This process is known as excitation and the resultant atom is left in an energized or excited state (Fig. 50.1).

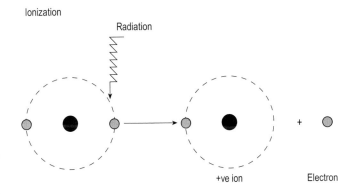

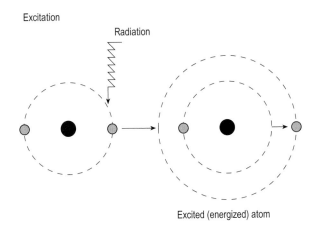

Fig. 50.1 • Ionization/excitation.

RADIATION AND RADIOACTIVITY

Where then does this ionizing radiation come from? As all health professionals know, we can make it in machines; X-ray generators are based on excitation. A metal target is bombarded with radiation, exciting the metal atoms. As the electrons fall back from their excited state to their original position, they give off the extra energy in the form of electromagnetic radiation – X-rays. Man-made machines can also produce and accelerate particles such as neutrons and protons as ionizing radiation.

In addition to these generated radiation, ionizing radiation is also given off by radioactive material. Radioactive atoms have unstable nuclei. Radioactive forms of almost all elements exist or can be produced. The basic concepts are best illustrated by looking at hydrogen. It is the number of protons in the nucleus that determines the element. If an atom has a single proton it is hydrogen (Fig. 50.2), if there are two it is helium, and so on. Most hydrogen atoms consist of that single proton with its circulating electron. If a neutron is also present in the nucleus, the atom is still hydrogen (by virtue of its single proton). Its physical properties are very slightly different, based on the increased mass of its nucleus, but chemically it is indistinguishable from the common form. This form is heavy hydrogen or

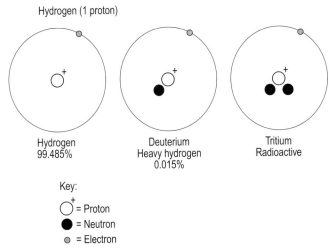

Fig. 50.2 • Hydrogen (one proton).

deuterium. If a second neutron is introduced into the nucleus the atom is still, of course, chemically hydrogen but is now unstable, the radioactive form of hydrogen, tritium.

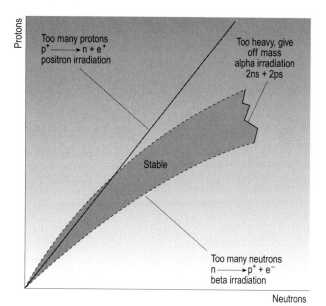

Fig. 50.3 • Relationship between nuclear protons and neutrons with stability.

Table 50.1 Uranium decay chain

Radionuclide	Uranium-238 (99.3% of natural uranium)	→ Thorium-234	→ Protactinium-234
Radiation	1α energy 4.197 MeV 2γ 49.6 MeV	1β 0.198 MeV 2γ × 3 − 63.3, 92.4 and 92.8 MeV	1β 2.29 MeV γ × 2 − 100 and 766.4 MeV
Half-life	4.47 × 10⁹ years	24.1 d	1.17 min

Fig. 50.3 shows a basic graph of neutrons against protons in the nucleus. In simple terms, atoms with broadly equal numbers of each particle are stable up to a maximum size, beyond which all atoms are radioactive. Unstable atoms are radioactive, giving off ionizing radiation in order to become stable. Three situations can be identified.

- For nuclei that are beyond the maximum mass for stability, the most usual type of radioactive emission is to give off a large amount of mass, two protons and two neutrons, in a single particle, termed alpha-radiation.

- In the zone where the nuclei have too many neutrons, the nucleus transforms a neutron into a proton, giving off additional mass and the negative charge as an electron, termed beta-radiation.

- In the zone where the nuclei have too many protons, a proton transforms to a neutron, giving off a positively charged electron termed a positron, or beta⁺-radiation.

In addition to these particle radiation, the new nucleus may be left with some additional energy. These exited nuclei give off the energy as electromagnetic radiation, termed gamma rays.

A radioactive atom is, therefore, one that is unstable and gives off mass or energy by emitting particles and/or electromagnetic rays. This process is called radioactive decay. Radioactive materials are termed radionuclides. The type of radiation given off and its energy are specific for each radionuclide. All radionuclides decay at a characteristic exponential rate, producing a constant time for the amount of radionuclide to be halved. 'Half-lives' for different nuclides vary from a few seconds to many thousands of years. Radionuclides some distance from the stable zone in Figure 50.3 will not reach it by a single transformation. Here the new element formed will also be radioactive, giving off its own characteristic radiation of specific energy, a half-life. The process of a number of radioactive transformations to eventual stability is termed a decay chain. The first three steps of the uranium-238 (^{238}U) chain are shown in Table 50.1.

RADIATION AND CONTAMINATION

Radiation is the hazard we are concerned with, but we can see that we can be irradiated from a number of sources, including radioactive materials. These materials can be in any physical form, including liquids and powders. Material can therefore be deposited on to the surface of our bodies or even taken internally. This is termed internal and external contamination.

Where irradiation is taking place from *a distant source*, protection can be achieved by basic considerations of:

- time
- distance
- shielding,

i.e. limiting the time spent in the radiation field, increasing your distance from the source or placing shielding between you and the source. Once *contamination* has taken place, radiation will continue until either decontamination is accomplished or the radioactive material decays away. For internal contamination, decay depends not only on the physical half-life of the radionuclide taken in but also a biological half-life for elimination from the body. Like other toxic materials, the effect and dose from internal contamination depends on the chemical form of the radioactive material that has been taken in.

Contamination therefore is a specific consideration where radioactive materials are present. Individuals are not contaminated with radiation such as alpha or beta particles but with radionuclides that emit these, such as plutonium or tritium.

RADIATION CHARACTERISTICS

Having established the sources of ionizing radiation, it is important for the carer to appreciate some of their physical characteristics, as these are crucial to understanding the resultant health effects.

Alpha particles, we have said, consist of two protons and two neutrons; they are therefore heavy and charged. They cause dense ionization and accordingly their range is very short. They are easily stopped by a thin layer of paper. Alpha-radiation therefore is no hazard from distant sources. If external contamination occurs with an alpha-emitter, such as plutonium, the radiation can hardly penetrate the superficial dead layer of skin, hence it presents no hazard. If internal contamination takes place, the cells immediately around the contamination will receive dense irradiation; hence, health effects will be based on the specific organs that have been contaminated.

Beta-particles and positrons are also charged particles. They too cause dense irradiation, but their range is somewhat longer. They can be stopped by relatively thin sheets of metal such as aluminium. Like alpha-irradiation, therefore, beta-irradiation is not a hazard from distant sources. If external contamination occurs, the beta-irradiation does have the range to reach the first layer of live skin cells. The so-called beta-burns seen in some of the emergency workers at the Chernobyl accident resulted from the deposition of beta-emitting radioactive material on their skin. In the event of internal contamination, again, it is the cells immediately around the material that are irradiated, and health effects are determined by the pattern of contamination.

X-rays and gamma-rays are penetrating electromagnetic rays. They are relatively sparsely ionizing, and their range is long and exponential within the medium. In other words, for rays of a given energy 50% attenuation can be achieved by a specific distance of shielding material. So-called 'half value layers' can thus be used for shielding calculations. By virtue of their range they pose a 'whole body' hazard whether the source be distant or from external or internal contamination.

The different characteristics, ranges and energies of radiation have resulted in many monitoring instruments being developed to detect them (Fig. 50.4). *Care must be taken to use monitoring equipment that will detect and respond to the type of radiation or contamination involved in any accident.*

RADIATION UNITS

The sheer number of units involved in radiation can be intimidating and cause concern, particularly where some individuals and the media continue to use old pre-SI titles or, worse still, jump between the two systems. A detailed description of radiation units is outside the scope of this

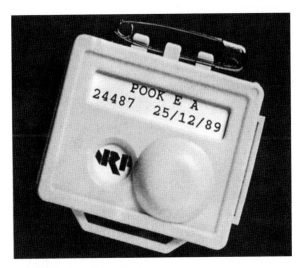

Fig. 50.4 • A radiation dosimeter.

section; however, the immediate carer should have some basic knowledge of the units important in determining hazard to themselves and their patients.

Activity

The amount of radioactive material present in a sample changes with time, depending on its half-life. Conventional measures such as weight are therefore not useful. Radioactivity is thus measured in terms of the number of atoms undergoing decay at that particular time. The SI unit of activity is the becquerel (Bq), which equals one disintegration per second. In the accident situation, where irradiation has occurred from a distant source, the size of that source is given as its *activity*. Where contamination has taken place, either internal or external, the amount of material is again measured as *activity*. In order to gain information regarding the hazard, the actual radioactive material involved needs to be identified. A very large sealed source of a pure alpha-emitter will, as we have said, provide no distant hazard at all to the carer, whereas a source of similar *activity* of a high-energy gamma-ray could very quickly pose a threat to the life of both carer and patient.

Dose

Radiation has its effect by passing energy to its target. The energy deposited to a unit mass of target is therefore a useful quantity of measure. In the SI unit here would be $1\,J\,kg^{-1}$ of target, and in radiation protection this is called the gray (Gy). The gray is a measure of absorbed dose. In the health profession we are, of course, interested in a particular target: humanity. Unfortunately, the biological effects of radiation are more complicated than simple energy deposition calculations at the macroscopic level, and different types of radiation vary in their biological effectiveness. This is dealt with in the system of radiation units by multiplying the absorbed dose by a radiation weighting factor for the radiation involved. The new term is called the equivalent dose:

$$\text{Absorbed dose} \times \text{Radiation weighting factor} = \text{Equivalent dose.}$$

The unit of equivalent dose is the sievert (Sv).

In summary, therefore, we can measure the amount of radioactive material present as its *activity* and its biological effect to man in terms of *equivalent dose*. The derivation of sieverts (to a person) from becquerels (of a given radioactive material) can be relatively simple in cases of direct irradiation from sealed sources, or much more complex in cases of contamination, where chemical and physiological considerations also need to be modelled.

HUMAN RADIATION LEVELS

It is a popular misconception that before the discoveries of Curie, Becquerel and Roentgen we lived in a radiation-free world and that radiation is a 20th century phenomenon. Nothing could be further from the truth. We have lived with radiation since the beginning of time and we will continue to do so for as long as we can envisage. Natural sources of ionizing radiation remain by far the dominant cause of radiation exposure to the UK population.

Over 80% of the radiation dose to the UK population comes from natural sources. The majority of natural radionuclides are included in two decay chains based on uranium and one on thorium. In addition, there are some other natural radionuclides, the most important being potassium-40, which forms about 0.01% of all potassium in the world. This, of course, is a significant source of internal contamination within ourselves. Some naturally occurring radionuclides are constantly being formed by the impact of cosmic radiation, the most important example being carbon-14. The majority of the natural dose comes from radon and its daughter decay products. Other radiation sources from naturally occurring radionuclides come from gamma-rays from soil, rocks and building materials. In addition to potassium-40 and carbon-14, natural radionuclides are present in most food and drink, producing internal contamination. The other principal source of natural irradiation is from cosmic rays produced in the upper atmosphere from interactions of high-energy particles from space. Cosmic radiation increases with latitude and altitude.

Almost all the rest of UK radiation exposure comes from medical irradiation, which appears to increase every year. Occupational exposure is very small, and even here three-quarters of UK exposure comes from natural sources such as cosmic irradiation of air crew and radon and gamma exposure in mines. It is important for the carer to understand, therefore, that the concept of zero levels of radiation and/or contamination is impossible, even in accidents where ionizing radiation is not involved.

Biological effects

GENERAL

Having looked at some basic physics and the sources of ionizing radiation, attention can now be turned to the most important aspect, their biological and health effects. From natural background radiation our bodies have to deal with millions of radionuclide disintegrations within us and gamma-rays passing through us. All the cells in our body probably suffer ionization damage every year. Natural radionuclides have been decaying since the beginning of the Earth and thus were at higher levels in the past. It is not surprising, therefore, that cells have evolved efficient mechanisms for radiation repair. The majority of radiation damage is repaired by these systems without generating health effects.

Where damage is not effectively repaired, textbooks of radiation protection describe two types of radiation effect:

- *deterministic* (previously called non-stochastic), where the severity of the effect varies with dose
- *stochastic* (random), where it is the probability of the effect occurring rather than its severity which is dose dependent.

At the level of this text it is simpler to consider these effects in terms of cell killing (deterministic) or cell damage (stochastic). There are also whole-body reactions to these effects on cells.

CELL DEATH EFFECTS (DETERMINISTIC)

Cells vary in their sensitivity to killing by ionizing radiation. In broad terms undifferentiated, rapidly dividing cells are most sensitive (Fig. 50.5). There are, however, some exceptions, such as mature lymphocytes, which are readily killed despite their long life and differentiation. Most organs and tissues are unaffected by the loss of substantial numbers of cells. Only if the loss is sufficient will there be visible injury or loss of function.

Cell death effects from radiation can be equated with an S-shaped curve. There is some individual variation in sensitivity but, most importantly, there is a clear threshold for these effects. If radiation doses do not reach these thresholds, the effect cannot occur.

Typical effects that fit this cell death (deterministic) model include sterility, cataract, skin burns and teratogenic effects *in utero*. Additional body reactions to the cell killing may be an important part of the clinical picture, e.g. the

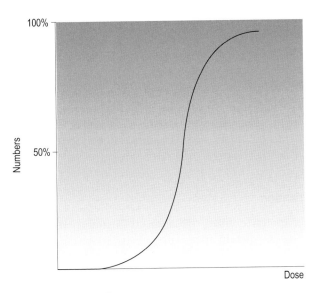

Fig. 50.5 • Cell death.

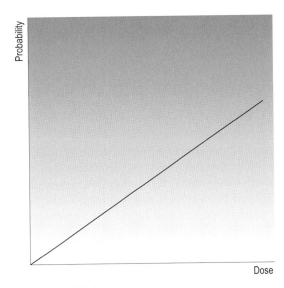

Fig. 50.6 • Cell damage.

acute pneumonitis or chronic fibrosis that high-dose irradiation of lung tissue can produce. Death is also, of course, a cell death effect. At doses above about 500 mSv the general body response to irradiation produced the classical prodrome 'radiation sickness' of vomiting and diarrhoea. The threshold for death is in the region of 2 Sv. Here it is the killing of bone marrow progenitor cells that is the key insult. The circulating granulocytes, platelets and red blood cells are not replaced, and death occurs 30–60 days after the irradiation from infection and bleeding as the shortages of functional cells and platelets become apparent. At higher doses (over 8–10 Gy), death occurs sooner from infection and electrolyte imbalance. The critical cells here are in the gut epithelium. The stem cells at the bases of the pits are killed and hence the microvilli are not replaced. At even higher levels, many body cells are killed and death occurs rapidly from raised intracranial pressure, the so-called central nervous system (CNS) syndrome.

Important cell killing (deterministic) effects are completely avoided if radiation doses are kept below 500 mSv.

CELL DAMAGE (STOCHASTIC) EFFECTS

Depending on the type of cell damaged, ionizing radiation exposure is associated with an increased probability of an individual developing cancer, or the development of hereditary defects in subsequent generations (Fig. 50.6). Radiation protection is based on the assumption that there is a straight-line relationship between this increasing probability and radiation dose. This line goes through the origin without a threshold, so that all radiation exposure is considered to add additional risk.

While there is some variation between tissues in their radiation sensitivity to cancer induction, most types of

cancer can be caused by ionizing radiation. Exceptions include chronic lymphatic leukaemia and malignant melanoma. Radiation's prime role is believed to be as a cancer inducer, and this corresponds with the observed latent periods between exposure and clinical diagnosis. These periods are a minimum of 2 years for leukaemia and 5–10 years for solid tumours. Of course, cancer is a common disease without radiation exposure: current research suggests that, while for leukaemias the risk of radiation is additive to the 'natural incidence', for solid tumours a multiplicative model fits better. Young children and babies in utero are considered to be more sensitive to the carcinogenic activity of radiation.

RISK ESTIMATION

Ionizing radiation is perhaps the most studied human toxic agent. In vivo and in vitro radiobiological work is also bolstered by epidemiological research into exposed populations. All these data are reviewed at intervals by the following international expert groups, with the aim of establishing radiation risk estimation:

- International Commission on Radiological Protection (ICRP) (established in 1928 – its recommendations are binding on the UK through the EURATOM Treaty)
- Biological Effects of Ionizing Radiation (BEIR) (US Advisory Group)
- United Nations Scientific Committee on the Effects of Atomic Radiation (UNSCEAR).

In addition, in the UK the National Radiological Protection Board (NRPB) also gives advice to the government on radiation risk.

Table 50.2 ICRP radiation risk estimates			
	Fatal cancer	**Severe hereditary effect**	
Adult worker	4	0.8	$10^{-2}\,Sv^{-1}$
Population	5	1.3	$10^{-1}\,Sv^{-1}$

The survivors of the atomic bombs in Japan remain the most important human data input into radiation risk estimation, although other important studies have taken place on groups exposed to significant medical irradiation. With regard to cell death effects, the bombs are estimated to have killed 200 000 people from a mixture of blast, radiation and conventional injury. In addition, skin burns and teratogenic effects (particularly microcephaly) were seen. For cell damage effects, the approximate 100 000 surviving population have experienced about 400 additional cancer deaths. No significant increase in hereditary conditions has been seen, although this effect is considered to have been masked by population movement considerations.

Current world-wide radiation risk estimates from the ICRP are given in Table 50.2.

The difference between the population and occupational figures is accounted for by the presence of children in the general population. UK figures provided by the NRPB are a little higher based on the UK's 'national cancer' rates.

HORMESIS AND ADAPTIVE RESPONSE

In recent years, ideas of radiation hormesis, i.e. that very low levels of radiation exposure could be beneficial, have received some attention. Like many other stressors, such as hypoxia and heat, there is evidence of an adaptive response to radiation cell killing from a preinsult lower level radiation dose, but it is difficult to see the relevance of this finding to cancer causation. The thresholdless straight-line dose response remains the consensus view for cell damage radiation effects and the basis for radiation protection considerations.

Radiation protection

PRINCIPLES

Radiation protection is a specialized occupational hygiene task. Its systems must address the nature of the hazard, which as we have seen has both threshold and thresholdless effects. This system is embodied in the three principles of protection recommended by the ICRP:

- Justification
- Optimization
- Limitation.

Justification

If there is no safe dose of radiation, its use must be justified and practices should not be adopted that produce no benefit to society. Justification decisions are for society to consider. However, it is clear that benefits can arise from the use of radiation – examples include appropriate use in medicine for diagnosis and treatment, as well as the use of sources in equipment such as smoke detectors that save many lives each year.

Optimization

Even if practice using radiation is justified, protection requirements dictate that work needs to be assessed to ensure best use of the resources in reducing radiation risks. The phrase 'as low as reasonably achievable' (ALARA) or the comparable 'as low as reasonably practicable' (ALARP) are the bywords of radiation protection. Of course, continued dose reduction meets with diminishing returns, and the ALARA/ALARP definition includes the need to take into account social and economic factors in the process. It would clearly be inappropriate to place individuals at greater risk by efforts to reduce radiation exposure. Similarly, the spending of huge sums of money to stop individuals incurring a trivial radiation dose, e.g. in relation to air travel, would also be inappropriate.

Limitation

The adoption of strict dose limits achieves two separate purposes. First, they ensure that deterministic (cell death) effects do not occur. Second, they give an upper limit of risk from radiation to the groups exposed. The definition of 'unacceptable' is a judgement for society. It is important not to consider these limits as an abrupt change in biological risk or a demarcation between safe and dangerous. Current limits are set in terms of unacceptable risk based on a working lifetime exposure at such levels. While breaches of an annual limit are significant regulatory events, it is important to assess the resultant increase in risk when counselling the individual concerned.

Dose limits in the UK were laid down in the Ionizing Radiation Regulations (IRR) 1985. Recommendations were published in 1990 (ICRP 60; International Commission on Radiological Protection 1990), and a new EU Directive has been adopted as the basis of new UK legislation (EU Directive 1996). IRR and ICRP limits are listed in Table 50.3.

For internal contamination, control is based on a system of annual limits of intake (ALI). This is the assessed level of nuclide that, if taken every year for 50 years, would not cause a breach in a primary dose limit. For nuclides with short half-lives, this effectively means doses up to the limit

Table 50.3 Annual dose limits (mSv)

	IRR 85	ICRP 60
Whole body		
Occupational (18+ years of age)	50	20 per year averaged over 5 years
		50 maximum in any year
General population	5	1
Organs and tissues		
Occupational (18+ years of age)	500	Skin – 500
		Hands/feet – 500
Population	50	Skin – 50
Lens of eye		
Occupational (18+ years of age)	150	150
Population	15	15
Woman of reproductive capacity		
Worker	13 in any 3 months	As other workers
Fetus	10 mSv	As member of public

in each year. For nuclides with long half-lives, the future dose commitment needs to be included. For example, internal plutonium, to give a dose of 1 mSv in the year it is taken in, will continue to irradiate at 1 mSv year^{-1} for the next 50 years. ALIs are set to ensure that in *no* year of occupation is the primary limit breached.

Types of radiation accident

GENERAL

Having established the nature of ionizing radiation and its health hazard, we can now move on to consider the accident situation. We can define such accidents as 'unforeseen occurrences', either actual or suspected, involving irradiation and/or contamination of individuals or the environment. In what situations can these accidents occur? It is convenient to consider them under three headings:

- Radiation devices
- Radionuclide release
- Criticality excursions.

Radiation devices

Probably the most common type of radiation accident involves radiation devices such as X-ray machines, particle accelerators or sealed radioactive sources. Irradiation is used extensively in clinical practice, and also in industry for sterilization and non-destructive testing. Units are normally located at fixed irradiation sites, although industry makes extensive use of site radiography, particularly in the non-destructive test area.

So long as any radioactive material or source remains 'sealed', radiation device accidents represent a pure radiation hazard, with no consideration necessary for contamination. Individuals may be subject to high doses of radiation and, unless the machine can be switched off or the source reshielded, high radiation dose rates will continue to exist in the vicinity.

Very-high-activity sealed sources can, in fact, be physically very small, allowing them to be put into pockets or bags, with resultant high-dose radiation to legs or arms.

Radioactive material release

Man-made radioactive material is also commonly used in medicine, laboratories and industry. In most cases it remains contained, although if that containment is breached the material is released into the atmosphere, with the potential to cause direct irradiation of individuals in the vicinity, as well as external contamination and, possibly, internal contamination.

Releases of radioactive material can occur at the site where work is taking place, although as material is also moved around the country it may be involved in transport accidents, also with the potential of release. It is important to emphasize that transport of radioactive materials is governed by strict regulations, and correctly packaged material is safe. Even if a package has been involved in an accident, no measures will be required unless the package itself has been damaged.

The release of radioactive material category includes two potential types of accident that receive significant public and media interest. The first is the so-called nuclear weapon accident, which, despite its name, is not the detonation and explosion of a nuclear weapon. Rather, it is the release of the radioactive contents of the weapon (plutonium and uranium) potentiated by fire or the detonation of conventional explosive within the weapon. The second is the possible release of radioactive material from the transport of spent nuclear fuel. Spent fuel contains radioactive material produced by the nuclear fission of uranium, which occurs within the reactor. Fuel transport takes place in specially constructed fuel flasks. The potential accident is therefore once again not a nuclear explosion but the release of radioactivity to the environment.

> ### Box 50.1
> - Direct radiation from material in the air
> - Inhalation of material in the air
> - Direct radiation from material deposited on the ground or surfaces
> - Ingestion of contaminated food/water
> - Inhalation of material resuspended from the ground

Accidents involving the release of radioactive material have the capacity to result in a radiation dose to man by the routes shown in Box 50.1.

The accident scenario and the material released determine the predominant hazard. For example, direct radiation hazards are of no importance if a pure alpha-emitter is released, while they could be the dominant hazard from high-energy gamma material.

CRITICALITY

Criticality is the term given to the instigation of a chain reaction causing the splitting of a large nucleus, such as a uranium atom, into two, with the release of energy and radiation. This process is called nuclear fission, and the radiation given off in the form of particles called neutrons can go on to split further uranium atoms, with more release of energy and radiation. The two nuclei produced by the splitting of the uranium are called fission products, and they are invariably radioactive in their own right.

As with the other types of accident, criticality accidents can be of hugely different scales, ranging from simple laboratory/lecture room demonstrations through research assemblies to considerations of nuclear reactors themselves. Criticality accidents are usually self-limiting, as the maintenance of the chain reaction is very dependent on the geometry of the system. Individuals involved in criticality accidents may have been subject to direct irradiation and contamination. In certain circumstances individuals very close to criticality events may be subject to neutron activation (i.e. some of their tissues may be made radioactive by the neutron irradiation).

Following an accident, additional problems may occur because of the release of the radioactive material produced, resulting in the hazards and considerations described in the previous section.

Plans, special arrangements and advice

THE IONIZING RADIATION REGULATIONS 1985

The number of incidents involving ionizing radiation in the UK dropped significantly following the introduction of the Ionizing Radiation Regulations 1985. Important aspects of these regulations included statutory requirements for radiation protection advice and supervision, and for detailed local rules to be promulgated and put into operation. The legislation also requires proper accounting for radioactive substances. Another important aspect of the legislation is in relation to contingency planning for accidents. These are required for all reasonably foreseeable accidents and involve, where appropriate, consultation with emergency services. Plans must also include arrangements for people likely to be affected, as well as naming people authorized to implement the plan and the individual with responsibility for safety.

In radiation accidents the carer should, therefore, arrive in a situation where a plan has been or is in the process of being instigated, and a source of advice on the specific radiological considerations should either be present or contactable.

TRANSPORT PLANS

The availability of detailed contingency plans and the availability of expert advice greatly facilitates the immediate carer role at any fixed site radiation accident. The situation is more difficult at remote operations, such as non-destructive testing, etc., although again the plan must exist and specify how to contact those responsible for safety and advice. For transport arrangements, once again there are specific considerations for contingency planning. These range from situations where detailed plans are produced and expert advice is available as part of the transport escort, such as the case within the Ministry of Defence Nuclear Accident Organization, to circumstances such as the Nuclear Industry Road Transport Emergency Plan (NIREP), where expert radiation protection advice can be provided at very short notice.

NATIONAL ARRANGEMENTS FOR INCIDENTS INVOLVING RADIOACTIVITY

In addition to the statutory obligations on users and operators, the National Arrangements for Incidents Involving Radioactivity (NAIR) was established as a mechanism to provide the civil police with advice and resources for the protection of the general public. The arrangements are managed through the National Radiological Protection Board.

The police may invoke NAIR in any circumstances where they feel a need for radiological assistance. Other bodies, including the other emergency services and those carrying out immediate care, can request the police to summon NAIR assistance if they believe it applicable. The arrangements cover the whole of Great Britain based on the areas of the police forces. Assistance is provided at two levels or stages.

Stage 1

Stage 1 assistance is provided by a radiation protection expert, who will arrive supported by relatively simple monitoring equipment. The most important element of this task is to form a view as to whether there is a radiation hazard and advise the police on appropriate immediate action. Stage 1 assistance can only carry out very small-scale recovery operations and is not equipped to cope with spreading of radioactive contamination, except of a very minor nature. Where the incident is beyond Stage 1 capability, advice is given to the police on the steps necessary to prevent undue exposure while Stage 2 assistance is awaited.

Stage 2

Stage 2 assistance is normally a team of up to four people, including suitable monitoring equipment, special clothing and decontamination facilities. It is provided by all the major nuclear establishments in the UK, and the team includes an operational health physicist linked to a base and able to call further resources as considered necessary.

Hospitals

In addition to the stage 1 and stage 2 NAIR responses, the system also identifies hospitals prepared to accept contaminated casualties or to advise and assist with decontamination of personnel. A separate list is also provided of hospitals prepared to provide advice on the treatment and admission of casualties exposed to large doses of radiation. As with the stage 1 and stage 2 responses, the hospitals are listed on a regional or area basis.

Packages and source identification

As in the contingency plan area, the packaging and labelling for radiation hazards are governed by strict regulations. The general trefoil sign (Fig. 50.7) is specific for ionizing radiation. It is seen illuminated in situations where X-rays are on, or sources exposed, and a direct radiation hazard exists. In certain circumstances there may be the clear identification of a radiation dose rate beneath the sign quantifying the hazard.

In relation to packaging and transport, various standards of package are designated according to their differing capabilities of surviving accidents and the greater quantity of

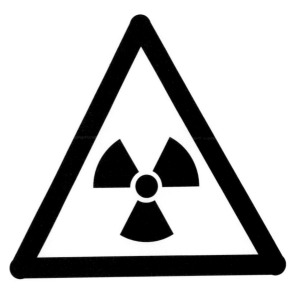

Fig. 50.7 • Trefoil nuclear hazard label.

hazard of the contents. Increasing in their robustness, four types of package are categorized:

- exempted
- industrial
- type A
- type B.

EXEMPTED PACKAGES

Exempted packages provide no special protection for the radioactive contents and are used for very small quantities of radioactive material that present negligible hazard even if the package were destroyed. Packages of this type carry no external labelling. They do, however, cause some NAIR scheme calls, where packages are broken and the contents are then identified as being radioactive.

INDUSTRIAL PACKAGES

Industrial packages are normally used for large items of low radioactive content. They are designed only to prevent the loss of material under normal conditions of transport. Specific labelling states low specific activity, or surface contaminated object.

TYPE A

Type A packages are designed to provide containment and shielding for radioactive materials. Their testing includes drop, compression and penetration tests. In addition, there are regulations limiting the quantities of material that can be carried in such a package. The packages carry a label bearing the trefoil sign, as well as a category (I, II or III in red). The numbers show increasing radiation levels at the surface of the package and/or 1 m from it.

TYPE B

Type B packages are intended to withstand severe accident conditions and are extensively tested on this basis. The large flasks used by the nuclear industry are Type B packages, although there are many much smaller Type B containers used for the transport of radioactive sources.

In addition to the labelling of the packages themselves, transport regulations require some placarding of vehicles. Vehicles may carry exempted packages without any such considerations, but placards bearing the trefoil sign are required on each side and rear, and a fire-resistant notice in the driving compartment, where Type A and Type B packages are being carried.

Safety – scene, self and the casualty

SCENE SAFETY

Possible radiation accident scenarios display the whole range of safety considerations considered in the other sections of this book. Precipitating causes for accidents include fires, pressure releases, explosions and impacts, all capable of having significant impact on the safety of the scene and of the rescuers and casualties. It is only by carrying out a proper scene hazard evaluation that the carer may conclude that ionizing radiation is involved in the accident at all.

Looking specifically at radiation and contamination issues, these range from situations where there is no residual hazard to those where direct irradiation continues or radioactive material is still being released. Looking first at hazards posed by a device or sealed source, these can be eliminated if the device is switched off or the source reshielded. Under no circumstances should radioactive sources be handled or moved in the accident situation without the advice of health physics experts, either present at the scene through existing contingency plans or arriving as part of a NAIR scheme response. If irradiation is continuing, accident management should be coordinated from a safe distance where radiation levels are low. Hazards from devices may be very direction-specific, although most radiation sources will emit ionizing radiation in all directions. Distance and shielding are the important protection principles in establishing the extent of a safe cordon. Again, advice should be sought from the radiological expertise available.

The radioactive material released in contamination incidents can be in the form of dusts, liquid gases or vapours.

Scene and safety considerations are therefore dependent on the scale of the release and its physical form. The extent of any contamination needs to be assessed and the accident control and coordination should take place from a location outside the demarcated cordon area. An important aspect is to try and ensure that the contamination is not spread unnecessarily by those involved in the accident response. On this basis a single point of entry in and out of the contaminated area should be established, with monitoring and decontamination facilities available. In large-scale contamination incidents, where the release of radioactivity is continuing, it will be dispersed in the downwind direction and therefore the entry point to the cordon and the control facilities should be upwind.

SELF

While radiological sources are commonplace in our society, accidents producing life-threatening radiation exposure are very rare indeed. Real or perceived hazards to the carer are a vital aspect of the successful management of any radiation accident. The carer needs to be provided with information regarding the hazard and confirmation of their own continued safety. In a pure external radiation hazard accident, radiation dose is the hazard to the carer. In addition to the considerations of distance and shielding already mentioned in defining a safe cordon, the other radiation protection principle, that of time, forms an essential part of radiation protection for individuals who may be deployed into the cordon for rescue or immediate treatment.

The basic principles of radiation protection in the non-accident situation are discussed above. Once an accident has occurred it is those principles that need to be applied. Two areas need specific consideration in relation to the role of the immediate carer:

- Life-saving immediate care and rescue
- Other immediate care following life-saving action.

For individuals involved in life-saving aid, it appears inappropriate to specify maximum levels of radiation dose. Current UK advice from the National Radiological Protection Board is only that substantial efforts should be made to keep doses to such individuals below levels where serious deterministic (cell death) effects may occur. In practice, emergency services in the UK have developed their own guidelines for these events, and carers may feel it appropriate to work under these systems. An important part of working in such conditions is good-quality hazard advice; the rapid movement of an individual from a high radiation field out of a beam to a well-shielded area can make significant reductions both to that individual's dose and to the dose of individuals carrying out the treatment function. Clear instructions as to the time constraints applicable to working in any particular area are also an important element of overall dose control.

In the non-life-saving area, the carer may still be exposed to a radiation dose above normal background levels. The National Radiological Protection Board advises that workers taking action to protect the public in the event of an accident should be allowed to receive doses up to dose limits for those occupationally exposed, and only in exceptional circumstances to receive doses that are above such limits.

In situations where radioactive contamination is also involved, the basic dose restrictions described above remain. In the event that the released material poses a direct radiation hazard, then distance shielding and time considerations remain valid. In addition, however, the carer may need specific protection from becoming contaminated.

Protection from external contamination is best achieved with protective clothing. This term is particularly badly understood by the public and hence by carers, who occasionally believe that it offers some magic protection from ionizing radiation. The function of the clothing is to provide a barrier between the contamination and the wearer's skin. On leaving the contaminated area, the clothing can be discarded, leaving the individual uncontaminated. Any clothing can therefore fulfil this function. The best forms of protective clothing are easy to dispose of and relatively loose fitting to allow easy movement. Hoods are particularly useful in restricting contamination to hair. Entries into the suit at ankles and wrists should be taped, and overshoes or washable boots worn. Hand contamination would be particularly common for carers, and therefore disposal gloves (two pairs if possible) should be worn, again taped in place over the taped wrists of the clothing.

Internal contamination is also a hazard that needs to be considered and for which protection should be provided. Clearly there should be no eating, drinking or smoking within areas considered to be contaminated. On this basis, ingestion should be completely avoided. Appropriate use of protective clothing should avoid considerations of contamination through intact or even broken skin. With regard to inhalation, the appropriate respiratory protection will again be determined by the type and scale of the accident. Advice should be sought from the health physics expertise provided by the plan or through the NAIR scheme. Possibilities range from the need for no protection whatsoever through simple masks to more complicated dust masks and respirators, up to the need for specialist breathing apparatus.

Finally, in relation to contamination, in the specific situation of a reactor accident where new fission products being discharged to the environment form the major hazard, specific treatment can be provided to carers to mitigate the most important health consequence. In this situation the predominant hazard would come from the release of radioactive iodines. Like stable iodines, these would be concentrated in the thyroid glands of those individuals inhaling them, hence causing a significant radiation dose to that gland with an associated increase in the probability of developing thyroid cancer. Increases in thyroid cancer among children have been noted in relation to the release of radioactive iodine from the Chernobyl accident. If a large dose of stable iodine is administered by mouth before, or shortly after the inhalation of radioactive iodine occurs, the stable iodine saturates the thyroid gland, enhancing the excretion of the radioactive form. Licensed preparations of stable iodine in the form of potassium iodate are available in the UK and form part of emergency response considerations and public protection action within contingency plans where iodine release would pose a hazard. The tablets are safe to take for all members of the public, with the exception of those known to suffer from iodine allergy, or the rare diagnoses of dermatitis herpetiformis and hypocomplimentaemic vasculitis.

THE CASUALTY

Safety for the casualty in relation to radiation injury needs only the briefest mention, corresponding to those considerations already mentioned for the carer. In direct contrast to conventional accidents, immediate danger to life is not likely to be a presenting feature of radiation accidents. In the very rare cases that it is, medical treatment could not affect the prognosis. It is vitally important therefore in all radiation accidents that consideration and treatment of coexisting conventional life-threatening injuries must take precedence over any radiation- or contamination-specific management for the casualty. Only when immediate care management of conventional injury has ensured the individual's survival should attention pass to the radiation aspects of treatment.

Medical management of radiation casualties

CLASSIFICATION OF RADIATION CASUALTIES

It is convenient to consider radiation accident casualties in the categories shown in Box 50.2.

In practice this classification is an oversimplification, as any or all of these conditions may occur singly or in any combination.

Whole body irradiation

The treatment of whole body irradiation has made significant advances in recent years, with a high probability that the bone marrow effects can be successfully managed

Box 50.2

- **Whole body irradiation**
- **Local external irradiation**
- **External contamination**
- **Internal contamination**

using cell growth factors. Detailed treatment protocols are beyond the scope of this chapter, but prehospital treatment is relatively simple. An important element of management is the assessment of dose. This can be accomplished by reading dosimeters the casualty was wearing, or by calculation by radiation protection experts based on the casualty's movements in radiation and contaminated areas. Clinically, the onset of the prodrome of nausea and vomiting within 2 h of irradiation provides the best indication that life-threatening irradiation has taken place. Patients should be transferred to specialized units with reverse barrier facilities. Such units are listed in the NAIR scheme.

Early on-site treatment consists of basic care, with suppression of unpleasant prodromal symptoms by sedatives and antiemetics. 5-HT$_3$ antagonist preparations such as ondansetron are dramatically effective in radiation-induced vomiting, although control can be achieved with older antiemetics. Haematological investigations form an important guide to the management of radiation casualties, and early samples form useful baseline results:

- Full blood count: changes in peripheral blood may occur very rapidly depending on dose.
- Cytogenetic dosimetry: peripheral lymphocytes can be cultured and studied for chromosomal damage to give an indication of radiation doses received.
- Peripheral blood CD34$^+$ cells: in the future measurement of circulatory CD34$^+$ cells may be used to assess the potential for marrow regeneration using growth factors.
- Blood grouping and HLA typing: later treatment may include platelet transfusion, immature haemopoietic stem cells or, rarely, bone marrow transplantation.

Local irradiation

Very high doses of irradiation of localized parts of the body can take place without the prodromal symptoms of whole body irradiation. The casualty may therefore have no signs or symptoms and could be unaware that the exposure has occurred. Liaison between the doctor and radiation protection staff is important to reconstruct a dose estimate. Biological dosimetry such as lymphocyte culture is much less specific in cases of partial body irradiation. Outside the focused beams of radiotherapy or radiography, it is highly likely that the skin would be the most vulnerable tissue to local irradiation. A transient erythema may appear within 2–3 h, to be followed after a variable dose-dependent period by fixed erythema. This may proceed

to vesiculation, as an ordinary burn, but at a much slower pace (sometimes) after the exposure. High doses will cause epilation after 2–3 weeks, and this is permanent at even higher doses. Pain, infection, failure to heal, fibrosis and malignant change are longer-term complications of high-dose skin irradiation.

Health professionals need to remember the extended time frame of radiation 'skin burns' if they are not to be missed and their causation is to be properly identified. Detailed history taking and appropriate review dates are required.

External contamination

The purpose of external decontamination is to remove the radioactive material from the individual and hence prevent further irradiation. The presence of contamination determines the need to consider protection of carers as well as the casualty. It is highly desirable to remove as much external contamination as possible prior to the despatch of casualties to hospital. Such action greatly facilitates their treatment and management at hospital, as well as concentrating the released radioactivity at the accident site. In order to carry out on-site decontamination, radiation protection advice should be available and staff carrying out the role should be equipped with protective clothing. In practice, simple theatre wear with a dust mask and double gloves is more than adequate. The area where decontamination is to take place should be designated as a contamination area, with appropriate communications and entry and exit controls (including ventilation and drainage). No eating, drinking or smoking is to be allowed in the area.

Before decontamination is considered, adequate monitoring of the skin should be carried out. With careful undressing (scissors, inward folding, etc.) almost 90% of contamination can be removed. Some rules of decontamination are as follows:

- Total body survey and demarcation of contaminated areas.
- Breaks in skin should be identified and covered.
- Decontamination procedures are carried out starting at the periphery and working towards the centre.
- Monitoring should be carried out and recorded after each attempt at decontamination.

Soap and water is the initial decontamination choice, with the use of soft brushing, so long as redness is avoided. In the event that full decontamination is not achieved, specialist advice should be sought.

Internal contamination

In most cases treatment decisions are based on efforts to reduce the future risk of cancer. Optimization is therefore the important principle and it would clearly be

Box 50.3

- **Reduced absorption – strontium is absorbed from the intestine in competition with calcium. Intestinal uptake of radioactive strontium can be reduced using aluminium-containing antacids or alginates**
- **Reduced internal deposition – radioactive iodines, like stable iodine, are concentrated in the thyroid gland. Stable iodine is administered to saturate the gland and hence reduce the uptake of the radioactive forms**
- **Enhance elimination – tritium, as tritiated water, is completely absorbed. Forcing of fluids (3–4 l day^{-1} by mouth) will reduce the clearance half-life significantly**
- **Enhance excretion – a number of heavy metal radionuclides such as plutonium can be bound by chelating agents, which are readily excreted by the kidney**

Table 50.4 Radiation categories

- RP – the individual is potentially irradiated but no action has been taken to confirm this status
- R1 – the individual is believed to have received a dose in excess of 2 Sv and hence has potentially life-threatening radiation exposure. Needs specialist hospital attention
- R2 – is assessed as receiving a radiation dose between the threshold for significant deterministic (cell death) effects and 2 Sv. The individual will suffer the radiation prodrome and require admission to hospital
- R3 – the individual is estimated to have received a dose in excess of statutory dose limits but deterministic (cell death) effects are not anticipated
- R0 – the individual is believed to have received radiation exposure less than statutory limits

Table 50.5 Contamination categories

- CP – potentially contaminated but no assessment has taken place
- C1 – significant external and internal contamination is believed to have taken place
- C2 – significant external contamination has occurred, although there is confidence that no internal contamination took place (the individual was wearing satisfactory respiratory protection at the time of the accident)
- C0 – the individual was not contaminated

inappropriate to put the casualty at greater risk by therapeutic agents and procedures than would be saved by the removal of the radioactive material. Clinicians must therefore not only be aware of the costs and side-effects of treatment but also have a very accurate assessment of the radiation detriment associated with the intake their patients have experienced. This assessment needs the input of radiation protection expertise and may require specialist monitoring equipment, as well as biological sampling of excreta, etc. It is important that excreta produced during the immediate care period is retained, if possible, for later monitoring.

As with any toxic material, radioactive contamination can enter the body by ingestion, inhalation or through damaged or intact skin. The amount taken in and the amount retained are dependent on the chemical and physical nature of the material. The aim of treatment for internal contamination is to remove it from the body, hence preventing further irradiation. The general principles of treatment are as follows:

- Reduce absorption or internal deposition.
- Enhance elimination or excretion.

Detailed treatment protocols are outside the scope of this unit but the general principles are highlighted in Box 50.3.

Information to hospitals/triage

Ambulance services and disaster plans already have triage categories for casualty sorting and the provision of information to receiving establishments based on conventional injury. As yet, there is no standard UK system for categorizing radiation and contamination information in this way. There is, however, a real need for the carer on site to provide information back to the receiving hospital about the nature of the radiological conditions so that the hospital may prepare adequately for the casualties it will receive. Within Scottish Nuclear accident plans this is achieved by two further triage categories based on radiation and contamination status subservient to the overall conventional system (Kalman et al 1998).

The radiation categories are given in Table 50.4.

Contamination categories are given in Table 50.5.

In addition to these categories, further suffixes have been introduced as follows:

- D – complete external decontamination was accomplished at the accident site.
- DR – external decontamination took place, although residual contamination remains.
- W – denotes the presence of a contaminated wound.

Using such systems, a full picture can be provided to the receiving unit in good time. For example, an individual with severe conventional injuries requiring immediate transfer to hospital could be transferred as Triage Category 1, RPCP, where there is no time to assess their radiation or contamination status. At the other end of the spectrum, an individual with an injury that would necessitate transfer

Box 50.4

- Shelter – staying indoors with doors and windows closed and ventilation turned off
- Evacuation – rapid removal of people from the affected area
- Administration of stable iodine – if radioactive iodine has been released

Box 50.5

- Relocation – slow planned movement from the affected area
- Food/water controls
- Decontamination

Table 50.6 Emergency Reference Levels (ERLs) for early countermeasures

Measure	Organ/body	Averted dose (mSv)	
		Lower level	Upper level
Shelter	Whole body	3	30
	Single organ	30	300
Evacuation	Whole body	30	300
	Single organ	300	3000
Stable iodine	Thyroid gland	30	300

to hospital, although there is time for more treatment and evaluation at the accident site could be transferred as Triage Category 2, R0C1D, where there is confidence that the individual has not received a significant radiation dose and is believed to have been internally and externally contaminated, although external decontamination has been completed.

Public protection in radiation accidents (Emergency Reference Levels)

The release of radioactive material to the environment during an accident has the capacity to irradiate the public. The criteria for taking measures to protect the public in such situations are based on consideration of the potential health effects of such exposure. Health professionals should therefore have some knowledge of the basis of such decision-making so that they can provide comment on public protection advice given by the police.

A radiation accident causing a release of radioactive material to the environment determines the need to consider measures to protect the public. Three urgent early measures may be appropriate: these are given in Box 50.4.

Unlike conventional fires and other emergencies, such measures are not to protect the public from the chance of immediate death but are in relation to an increased probability of developing cancer in years to come. In addition to the early urgent measures, other recovery measures may be appropriate (Box 50.5).

While the normal system of radiation protection and dose limits can form the basis for implementation criteria of the longer-term measures, triggers for early urgent measures need further consideration.

The general principle of optimization means that radiological work is planned and practised in detail to ensure that doses are ALARP. In the accident situation, however, dose will continue unless action is taken, unless *intervention* takes place. As in medical practice, the decision to intervene is a balance between the risks of implementing the measure (treatment) and the risks of not doing so. The nature of this balance determines that intervention criteria should not be set as dose limits that individuals can receive but in terms of dose avoided or averted by the countermeasure, if put into effect. Within the UK, quantitative criteria are recommended by the NRPB and are termed Emergency Reference Levels (ERLs) (National Radiological Protection Board 1990). They are set for each countermeasure, because the harm associated with each measure is different. ERLs are a range bounded by an upper and a lower level of averted dose. At the lower level the NRPB judges that the countermeasure is unlikely to be justified. At the upper level the NRPB judges that every effort should be made to introduce the measure (Table 50.6).

References

EU Directive 1996 Safety standards for the protection of health of workers and the general public against the dangers arising from ionizing radiation. European Union, Brussels

International Commission on Radiological Protection 1990 Document 60 (ICRP 60). International Commission on Radiological Protection, Stockholm

Kalman C, McVey A, Mann J et al 1998 Triage of nuclear/radiation casualties. Pre-hospital Immediate Care 2: 160–165

National Radiological Protection Board 1990 NRPB Board statement on Emergency Reference Levels. Documents of the NRPB 1. National Radiological Protection Board, London

Mass gathering medicine

51

Introduction   529

Legislation concerning medical cover at mass
gatherings   530

Medical skills for mass gathering medicine   531

Equipment, clothing and documentation for
mass gathering medicine   532

Conclusion   532

References   533

Introduction

Mass gathering medicine is seen as a relatively new variation of prehospital care in the UK but has been developing throughout the last three decades. It was formalized in the USA and defined as *'medicine for people attending a mass gathering'*, a 'mass gathering' being defined as a crowd in excess of 1000 people.

Within the UK, mass gathering medicine has grown in response to a litany of tragedies at sporting and concert venues. Although most of the increased medical support at mass gatherings now is the result of Lord Justice Taylor's report into the Hillsborough Stadium tragedy in 1989 (Taylor 1989), that was the ninth official report covering crowd safety and control at football grounds, and the third crowd accident at Hillsborough. This is not to say that the Sheffield Wednesday ground was in a worse state than most; indeed, it was considered one of the best grounds at the time by the authorities, who had chosen it as a neutral venue with appropriate crowd capacity to host the semi-final of the FA Cup between Liverpool and Nottingham Forest.

In 1914, 75 fans needed hospital treatment after a wall collapsed and again in 1981, in another Cup semi-final, there was a crowd surge and 38 fans were injured. At least 35 serious incidents and 4000 injuries had occurred at 29 different British sports grounds before the surge by late arrivals at the match on 15 April 1989 caused 95 deaths before the eyes of those controlling the event.

Perhaps the universal horror generated, both at home and abroad, in the vast audience not only in the ground but on world-wide television screens was the final catalyst in ensuring that the recommendations in the report were taken seriously, although there are still those who subscribe to the view that 'it will never happen here'.

Sadly, history repeats itself at other crowd-related incidents. How often have we heard of crowds crushed trying to escape from cinemas or clubs when the safety doors have been locked and barred – as far back as 1845 a theatre fire in Canton, China, saw the deaths of 1670 people. In Sunderland in 1883, 183 people died in a fire, and in the 20th century 71 children died in a Paisley cinema fire in 1929. In 1942, 488 died in the Coconut Grove Night Club in Boston. The horror continued: Nuneaton Co-op dance (1961 – 16 dead), Beverley Hills Supper Club, Kentucky (1977 – 164 dead), Stardust Club Disco, Dublin (1981 – 48 dead), Statuto Cinema, Turin (1983 – 48 dead), the litany continues.

Almost all the matters Lord Taylor was asked to review and all his recommendations had been considered in detail over the previous 60 years, as had the recommendations by Lord Justice Popplewell (1985) following the Bradford stadium fire in 1985.

Both these enquiries had been preceded by the publication of *The Guide to Safety at Sports Grounds* (commonly known as the Green Guide), which was first produced in 1973 following the Wheatley Report (Wheatley 1972) into crowd safety at sports grounds after 66 people died at Ibrox Park, Glasgow in 1972. Ibrox was also the site of the first football disaster in 1902, when 25 people died and 500 were injured as the result of 'crowd pressure'. The Green Guide was completely revised in 1997 by the Department of Culture, Media and Sport. It has no legal force, but is a voluntary guide with recommendations on perceived best practice for ground management, local authorities and technical specialists (including the medical profession) for the improvement of crowd safety. The guide was shortly followed by the Safety at Sports Ground Act 1975, requiring the licensing of certain grounds as well as safety inspections. Many grounds had been built long ago and had little investment, and remedial action was expensive. Most important of all, there was a lack of a safety philosophy or culture, with little willingness to invest in safety measures. Following the Bradford fire, the Fire Safety and Safety of Places of Sport Act 1987 came into force, and then the Football Spectators Act 1989 commenced its course through parliament before Hillsborough. After much heated debate, the recommendation for a national membership scheme, starting with football clubs, was thrown out as being unlikely to further the course of safety.

One recommendation in the Taylor Report that was implemented was the establishment of a Football Licensing Authority to oversee the implementation of the advice within the report. This body consists of a board with a wide range of expertise – sport, law, accountancy, management, medicine and engineering – and a cadre of inspectors who ensure the safety of grounds within their regional area. This body, although established for football, provides advice to other sports both at home and abroad, and has ensured a reduction in accidents at many grounds. Members regularly travel to Europe to provide help in preparation for European and World Cup events and provide their expertise to enquiries or wherever it is deemed appropriate.

Sadly, history continues to repeat itself in areas where a safety culture is not the norm. In Guatemala in October 1996, 85 football fans died and a further 200 or more were injured in an incident reminiscent of Hillsborough when a late surge of fans, perhaps augmented by those who had bought forged tickets, pushed into the National Sports Stadium to see a World Cup qualifying match.

Such incidents illustrate the importance of the following aspects of safety management:

- strict control of ticket production, with forgeries being easy to recognize
- need for turnstiles that monitor crowd capacity
- computer control of the total distribution of spectators
- effective communication networks between stewards inside and outside the ground
- attractive prematch entertainment, which encourages fans to arrive early.

In addition to this, there is the obvious need to move towards all-seater venues or at least safer terracing with effective crush barriers, appropriate gradients to allow good sight lines from all angles (to avoid 'huddles' of spectators at the best viewing angle) and either total weather protection or none (to prevent people crowding into the partially protected areas with weather changes).

Legislation concerning medical cover at mass gatherings

Lord Justice Taylor's report was far more wide-reaching than just dealing with the stadium tragedy itself. He was asked to prepare an interim report into the disaster and make recommendations on short-term safety measures before the start of the football season but was also instructed to conduct a wider and deeper investigation into crowd control and future safety for his final report. Visits were made to compact sports grounds (such as rugby, football and cricket grounds, and tennis clubs) as well as those less contained (such as golf courses and racing tracks), both at home and abroad. Consultation was wide, but unfortunately only the opinions of the voluntary and statutory ambulance services were sought on medical matters. Subsequently, Mr Myles Gibson was asked to chair a group of doctors and ambulance service representatives to review the medical arrangements for football league grounds following the report (Football League 1990). The views of this committee have since been extended to other venues.

Towards the end of his report, Taylor considered first aid, medical facilities and ambulances. He called for one first-aider per 1000 spectators, one or more first-aid rooms at each ground (the number of such rooms and the equipment within them being a condition of the annual safety certificate issued by the local authority) and introduced the concept of a 'crowd' doctor to be present at the ground if a crowd above 2000 is expected.

The Gibson Report expanded upon Taylor's requirement for the doctor to be competent in advanced first aid and suggested that such a doctor should be competent at immediate care and that the ultimate goal should be to appoint a crowd doctor who holds the Diploma in Immediate Medical Care (issued by the Royal College of Surgeons of Edinburgh) or equivalent.

From the 1998–99 season any doctor employed as a crowd doctor within the Premier League must have successfully undertaken the two 1-day Football Association courses in Immediate Medical Care (see below) or equivalent, and any doctor thereafter appointed must hold the Diploma in Immediate Medical Care.

If a crowd of less than 3000 is anticipated at any event the club doctor can take on the role of crowd doctor, provided he is suitably trained and makes the crowd his first responsibility.

It was originally agreed that, when the crowd was expected to exceed 5000, an ambulance with two paramedics would be required; the number of ambulances to be in attendance for larger gatherings being decided by the local ambulance service and being a condition of the safety certificate. It was also decided that a major incident vehicle should attend when crowds were expected to exceed 25 000 (Table 51.1).

The responsibility for the ambulances rested with the NHS ambulance service, but they were allowed to devolve responsibility to private or voluntary sector vehicles provided that the statutory service was satisfied that such additional vehicles were equipped to the required standard and their crews suitably trained.

The 1997 revision of the Green Guide (Department of Culture, Media and Sport 1997) was amended to allow for these suggestions but the words 'a paramedic crew' were substituted for 'two paramedics with each vehicle' to comply with current ambulance service practice – some using one and others two paramedics on different shifts. Both the Taylor Report and the Green Guide recommend an increasing number of first aiders and ambulances as the crowd size increases, but only one crowd doctor is stipulated. This underlines the management role of the doctor, who will coordinate the medical cover, distribute the problems amongst the staff present and see only the more serious patients himself. Once a major incident is anticipated he has the facility to call for further medical resources as outlined in the district plans. Some clubs appoint more

than one club doctor, although it is unusual for more than one to be at the ground at the same time.

Medical skills for mass gathering medicine

Most of the preceding discussion has focused on major incident preparation and planning but the day-to-day work of the crowd doctor is not the management of victims of multiple casualty incidents or the usual trauma expected by an immediate-care practitioner but the management of minor acute (or occasionally acute on chronic) episodes.

Reviewing the medical records over 10 years of one GP's attendance at the Open Golf Tournament, 22% of patients had an exacerbation of an existing problem. Commonly, they had forgotten medication and needed prescriptions for replacement therapy, but it was not uncommon to see hypoglycaemia in patients who had dutifully taken their usual insulin and had then been held up in the traffic for longer than expected. Again, in the excitement of going off to a major championship, patients with epilepsy occasionally forgot their tablets and then had a fit, needing care during this and the postictal phase.

Many mass gatherings take place in the open and problems relating to extremes of temperature are not uncommon, from sunburn and sunstroke at one extreme to frank hypothermia in a patient sleeping off an excess of alcohol at the other. Again, at such venues there are catering outlets, and minor scalds and burns are common. At the 1995 World Cup football matches in the USA, special areas with fine water mist jets were established to deal with the problems of excessive heat. The public were encouraged to enter these areas to cool down and to leave their skin or clothes covered in water to continue the cooling process by evaporation. Such areas were extremely popular and probably reduced the volume of heat-related illness. In Saudi Arabia, heat-related problems are responsible for thousands of incidents at the annual pilgrimage to Mecca, although this pilgrimage entered the history books after the deaths of over 2000 people from crushing in the tunnel approaching the central square in 1990.

Comparing statistics gathered from many events, the patterns are very similar. As well as the groups of incidents described above, there are the expected minor injuries, with 3–5% of patients suffering ankle sprains or fractures. Figures from the United States Air Show (De Lorenzo et al 1993) revealed that 9% of patients had fractures and lacerations (not subdivided), 5% had eye injuries (similar to the Open Golf Tournament, as there are high winds, debris and dust at both) and 7% required transport to hospital, compared with 4% at the Open and at Indianapolis Speedway.

Published records from the 1982 US Festival (a 3-day outdoor rock concert) were similar (Ounanian et al 1986).

Table 51.1 Current recommendations for medical cover at sporting events

- One first-aider per 1000 spectators
- One or more first-aid rooms with appropriate equipment
- A crowd doctor if the attendance is above 2000
- One ambulance with a paramedic crew if the crowd is above 5000
- A major incident vehicle where the crowd is expected to exceed 25 000

At the two American events and the Open (as well as other events taking place over a longer period, such as the Wimbledon Tennis Championship and outdoor festivals) about 1–2% of the attending population will make contact with the medical services, although many will only be requesting simple analgesia for headaches.

Perhaps the biggest nightmare for any organizer is an outbreak of gastroenteritis. Despite public health advice, education and legislation, small outbreaks of food poisoning are common, although fortunately large outbreaks remain rare. In 1988 over 3000 women contracted shigellosis at a music festival in Michigan. The outbreak was traced to a tofu salad and was thought to be transferred by the food handlers. A lack of washing facilities for the staff preparing food was identified, although hand-washing has been observed to limit secondary transmission (Lee et al 1991).

The value of public health measures is demonstrated in a 1991 paper in the *West African Medical Journal* (Bito et al 1992) when an outbreak of *Vibrio metschnikovii* (not *Vibrio cholerae* as anticipated) broke out at a village festival in Nigeria. A local stream was found to contain the organisms and also traces of faecal contamination. A multifaceted programme was initiated with chlorination of water sources, chemoprophylaxis, intensive health education to key groups in the community and immunization of contacts.

Equipment, clothing and documentation for mass gathering medicine

In addition to the standard equipment for classical immediate care, the crowd doctor will need to adapt his/her equipment to the length and type of event, the environment (whether indoor or outdoor, spring, summer, autumn or winter), the type of crowd (mobile or static, predominantly young or an older population) and the facilities provided by the organizers. These can range from sophisticated hospital-type establishments (such as at Wembley Stadium) to a small shack, tent or just a designated space. However, more and more events conform to the Green Guide and temporary sites often provide excellent mobile cabins with all the necessary facilities. A typical GP's visiting bag, with arrangements for resupply of drugs and dressings with a local pharmacy or hospital, is the usual practice. Plenty of simple analgesia, together with drugs and equipment to deal with the conditions likely to be met, will be needed. If opiates are to be carried, the legal requirements for their storage must be met.

Prescribing is a problem. Some establishments allow local GPs to undertake the role of crowd doctor, and patients are treated under the emergency regulations of the NHS, but most use private prescriptions for all drugs and dressings other than those used for immediate treatment. Often, at

events lasting a few days, a local pharmacist will be on site or offer a good delivery service.

The clothing required will depend on the venue. Modifications of standard immediate-care clothes are most appropriate. At the North West 200 and Isle of Man TT races, where doctors and paramedics use motorcycles as well as helicopters, both clothing and communication equipment need to be modified. At pop festivals and indoor events, personnel may well need only identity badges and tabards or arm bands. Ease of immediate identification by other emergency colleagues is most important, both in person and over the radio. Personal communication equipment, therefore, should be integrated both with the statutory services and the venue's own internal system.

Documentation will need to be planned well in advance of the event. Apart from confidential medical records, data may be required by non-medical club personnel, as well as the press and local authority. Standard letters will be needed both by the family doctor and the hospital if a referral is being made. An ongoing register of attenders at each medical facility helps in future planning and, if based on a numerical code, can be released to event organizers without loss of confidentiality.

As with all events, it is preferable not to become involved with the press but to refer them to the appropriate press officer, who will involve you when required. The importance of good record-keeping cannot be over emphasized. The doctor should keep a copy of all records, as patients often take action against clubs for lack of safety standards some considerable time after the event, as well as against staff for the usual medico-legal reasons.

Interpersonal skills are paramount to reduce the need for medical intervention to a minimum. The doctor will need to liaise with the event staff (who tend to put health and safety matters low on their list of priorities), with catering and exhibition staff and with club stewards who, if trained to the new programme for stewards (Football League 1996), will have some basic patient handling skills from their first-aid module. The doctor will also have to deal with public health physicians, health emergency planning officers and their entourages, and the usual security and statutory services. Being aware of the skills of the ambulance and voluntary service personnel will make your task easier, and involving them in patient care, using their skills to the full and teaching them on other areas will foster good team relationships.

Conclusion

This chapter has reviewed the history of mass gathering medicine, the special needs of the medical teams undertaking the role of crowd doctor and opportunities for suitable training. Mass gathering medicine is an interesting and rewarding side of immediate care provided that one does not attend the event with the prime aim of being a spectator. In discussing medical care at football matches, Lord Justice Taylor might be said to have summed up our current hopes for the future of mass gatherings:

It is not enough to aim only at the minimum measures for safety. That has been, at best, the approach in the past and too often not even that standard has been achieved. What is required is the vision and imagination to achieve a new ethos on football.

References

Bito AO, Kale OO, Oduntan SO 1992 Epidemiological survey of an outbreak of gastroenteritis in a rural community in Oyo State. West African Journal of Medicine 11: 34–38

De Lorenzo RA, Boyle MF, Garrison R 1993 A proposed model for a residency experience in mass gathering medicine: the United States Air Show. Annals of Emergency Medicine 22: 1711–1714

Department of Culture, Media and Sport 1997 Guide to safety at sports grounds (the Green Guide). HMSO, London

Football League 1990 Report of the Medical Working Party to Review Lord Justice Taylor's Recommendations. Chairman Mr Myles Gibson. Football League, Lytham St Anne's

Football League 1996 The Stewards Training Pack. Staffordshire University, Stoke on Trent

Lee LA, McGee HB, Johnson DR et al 1991 An outbreak of shigellosis at an outdoor music festival. American Journal of Epidemiology 133: 608–615

Ounanian LO, Salinas C, Shear CL, Rodney WM 1986 Medical care at the 1982 US Festival. Annals of Emergency Medicine 15: 520–527

Popplewell OB 1985 Committee of Enquiry into Crowd Safety and Control at Sports Grounds: (i) Interim report 1985: MD9585; (ii) Final report, Cmnd 9710. HMSO, London

Taylor P 1989 The Hillsborough Stadium Disaster – 15 April 1989. An inquiry by The Rt Hon Lord Justice Taylor (i) Interim report, August 1989. Cmnd 769; (ii) Final report, January 1990 Cmnd 962. HMSO, London

Wheatley J 1972 Report of the Enquiry into Crowd Safety at Sports Grounds (Cmnd 4952). Home Office, Scottish Home and Health Department. HMSO, London

Medicine at sporting events

52

Introduction   534

Cause of injury   535

Nature of sports injuries   536

Injury profiles   536

The management of sports injuries   538

Drugs and the sportsperson   538

References   539

Introduction

In the affluent and leisure-activity-oriented society in which we now live, there is considerable scope for participating in an ever-growing range of sports and outdoor activities. Many of these are recognized as being dangerous. Contact team sports contribute the highest rate of injury, with association football, followed by rugby football, being the worst offenders. This is due to the fact that they are among the most popular sports. Combat sports and horse riding carry a high risk of injury and, while they are not common, the injuries sustained are often more severe.

No major studies have ever been carried out to investigate the true extent of the problem of sports injuries in the UK. A study in Scotland (Campbell 1995) showed that there were nearly 6 per 100 new attendances at emergency departments for sports- and leisure-related injuries. The financial cost of this is huge: when extrapolated to take account of the population of the whole of Britain it accounts for up to £303 million (Campbell 1996).

Many of the deaths that occur in the sports arena are wholly unrelated to the sport itself. We are all familiar with the golfer having an infarct on the 17th green or the spectator dying in the crowd at a large event. In addition, there is a small number of deaths each year in fit young people who have congenital heart diseases such as hypertrophic obstructive cardiomyopathy. Some deaths do arise directly from participation in sports (Office of Population Censuses and Surveys 1991) (Table 52.1) despite the government's intention to reduce injury in its well-publicized Accident Prevention Charter (Secretary of State for Health 1991).

Table 52.1 Fatal accidents in sports (per annum)

Sport	Number of fatalities
Air sports	13
Horse riding	12
Mountaineering	11
Motor sports	10
Ball games	6
Watersports	6
Winter sports	5
Athletics	4
Cycling	1
Shooting	1

Source: Office of Population and Census Studies 1991

Sportsmen now expect their injuries to be treated expertly, and it is therefore incumbent upon the provider of prehospital care to be fully conversant with the assessment and treatment of those injuries. No longer can the 'good Samaritan' doctors turn up at a sporting event with the intention of having a nice day out. They must be suitably equipped and trained to deal with all the potential problems that may befall the participants and the crowd. If they are not prepared, they are likely to be sued.

Cause of injury

The cause of injury can be classified as extrinsic or intrinsic.

EXTRINSIC FACTORS

Extrinsic factors in sports injury include:

- Nature and type of the sport
- Venue
- Equipment
- Weather
- Conduct and control of the event.

Nature of the sport

The nature of the sport affects injury rate. For example, contact and combat sports predispose to direct injury while other sports, such as scuba diving or parachuting, carry risks that involve the elements and the environment.

Venue

The venue for sports predisposes to injury. An icy pitch can lead to severe injury for rugby players, while footballers who play on artificial surfaces suffer a high rate of superficial skin injury if they fall on the abrasive surface. The safety standards at a venue may have a bearing on the injury rate for participants and spectators. A well designed motor racing track will have numerous safety devices to try and prevent injury to drivers and spectators in the event of a crash, while the safety standards on the track at a rally do little to protect either the drivers or the spectators to any great extent. Mass gathering medicine (Ch. 51) is a burgeoning field and many new initiatives are being developed to try to prevent tragedies such as the Hillsborough football stadium disaster.

Equipment

The equipment used in sports can be a major factor in causing injury; hockey sticks and racquets, for example, can lead to severe injury to head and face; eyes are at risk in games such as squash and badminton; lack of adequate protection for hockey goalkeepers predisposes them to serious injury. Equipment failures such as a broken rope in mountaineering or a failed demand valve for divers could lead to a fatal accident. Safety checks on all equipment are therefore essential.

Weather

The weather is no respecter of human life. Many walkers and mountaineers are caught out by sudden changes in the weather. The sea can change cruelly in minutes to endanger sailors, and long-distance runners can suffer heat exhaustion in warm weather if adequate allowances for fluid intake are not made.

Control and conduct

The control of the referee in contact sports is a vital element in injury prevention. A poor referee will allow excessive contact and even violence, which may lead to unnecessary injury. A rugby union referee was recently found guilty in court of causing injury to players, fined and banned when his poor control of the scrummage resulted in serious injury. Poor crowd control can lead to injury to spectators and players at a football match where hooligans are allowed to throw objects into the crowd or on to the pitch.

INTRINSIC FACTORS

Intrinsic factors include:

- Sex
- Age
- Previous injury or illness
- Physical fitness.

Sex

No clear difference in injury rate per 100 participants is observed between the sexes; however, boys over the age of 14 years are three times more likely to be injured in sport than girls of the same age because of the increased participation of boys in contact sports at this age.

Age

The age of an athlete influences the type of injury that develops; e.g. younger athletes can develop stress fragmentation of apophyses and avulsion of bone around the hip and pelvis as a result of excessive strain, whereas older athletes tend to develop tendon injuries. In addition, younger, less experienced sportsmen tend to take greater risks, with an increased injury rate in the younger age groups.

Previous injury

Previous injury predisposes to further injury. Sportsmen or women 'carrying' an injury are prone to exacerbating the problem or developing further injuries as their techniques and movement will be affected.

Physical fitness

Physical fitness is important in the prevention of injury. Unfit sportsmen/women are more likely to pull muscles when they do not warm up properly. Many develop knee injuries because quadriceps muscle tone and power, and thus knee stability, is poor. Professional sportsmen/women are prone to injury through overuse.

Nature of sports injuries

The vast majority of sports injuries are soft tissue injuries. Lower limb injuries are most common, followed by upper limb, head and face, then chest and abdomen. The majority are minor and self-limiting; however, serious injuries such as ligament and tendon tears, fractures, head and spinal injuries and damage to internal viscera do occur and all prehospital physicians should be alert to the possibilities. Reading the scene and obtaining a clear history of the injury is of paramount importance. The decision whether to refer and transport to hospital or not is fraught with danger for the unwary. Many injuries do not require referral to hospital but can be treated simply with *r*est, *i*ce, *c*ompression and *e*levation (RICE).

Injury profiles

Certain sports predispose to a particular injury profile. A number of these are outlined below.

ASSOCIATION FOOTBALL

The majority of football injuries are to soft tissues. Partial and complete tears of muscles and tendon are common, especially in the unfit occasional player. Severe ligamentous knee and ankle injuries occur less commonly. Meniscal damage can occur when a knee is twisted. Head and neck injuries occur in clashes of heads and bad falls. Facial injuries are not common but when they do occur may compromise the airway.

RUGBY FOOTBALL AND AMERICAN FOOTBALL

The pattern of injury in these two games is similar. Minor soft tissue injuries predominate but injuries to bone and ligament are not uncommon. Players are liable to suffer fractures of the upper limb, with damage to hands, wrists and clavicle being most common. Lower limb problems include meniscal and knee ligament damage, ankle ligament damage and ankle fractures. Fractures to long bones occur also. Head injuries are common. Bruising, lacerations and fractures to facial bones can often be clues to more serious head injury, and are often associated with concussion and loss of consciousness. Neck sprains and severe damage to the cervical spine occur in collapsed scrums and head-on tackles, when hyperflexion of the neck combined with axial loading together create significant damage. Chest and visceral damage can occur in the crush at the bottom of pile-ups and rucks. The medical attendant must maintain a very high level of suspicion in the treatment of any rugby player.

CRICKET AND HOCKEY

Players in these games are prone to minor sprains and strains. Additional risk is present from the hard ball, which travels towards players at speeds approaching 100 mph. The bat and stick can also make direct contact and cause severe injury to whatever part is hit. Fractures to the facial bones are common and, although major advances in safety equipment have reduced the incidence of severe injury, it can still happen to unprotected players.

HORSE RIDING

Horse riding is the sport that has one of the highest fatality rates in the UK (Office of Population Censuses and Surveys 1991). Falls from horses causing severe head and spinal injury may lead to as many as 50% of these deaths. All riders who suffer a fall should be examined carefully.

Spinal injury must be anticipated and adequate methods of immobilization must be available and used. Many competitive riders will try to remount and continue after a heavy fall – if there is *any* doubt that they may be concussed, have been knocked out or have suffered a neck injury they should be prevented from continuing. Facial injuries from kicks can lead to major airway problems. Heavy kicks to the chest and body can cause severe visceral damage, as illustrated by the famous jockey Willie Carson in 1996. Crushing injuries are commonplace when horses fall and then roll over the rider, and should be treated with the utmost suspicion. Chest and abdominal injuries should be anticipated and sought.

ATHLETICS AND FIELD SPORTS

The majority of athletes suffer soft tissue injury and sprains. Overuse predisposes athletes to chronic muscle and ligament problems that can be exacerbated in competition. High-jumpers and pole-vaulters are liable to severe neck and spinal injury if the landing area is badly prepared or if they fall awkwardly. Spectators are at risk from flying missiles such as javelins, shots and hammers. Heat exhaustion is a constant worry in hot climates. Never forget that the apparently injured sportsperson may be suffering from a coincidental medical problem.

BOXING AND COMBAT SPORTS

There is considerable anxiety amongst the public about the dangers of boxing and combat sports. While participation in such sports undeniably leads to injury, the death rate is very low compared to motor sports, rugby and mountaineering (Hamlyn 1995). The most serious, immediately life-threatening problem is that of an unconscious fighter with an obstructed airway. Competent ringside care should prevent all deaths from this. Acute subdural haematomas can occur. These will, if not rapidly treated, lead to significant disability or death. Rapid resuscitation with management of the airway and cervical spine is paramount in the pre-hospital phase. Definitive care is in the hands of the hospital specialist. It is important to beware of the lucid interval, which may lull the unwary into a false sense of security. Chronic problems can occur when fighters become 'punch drunk' as a result of repeated and progressive neuronal loss from multiple small intracerebral injuries. Neck injuries can occur from blows that impart rotational forces in boxing. In addition, head, neck and spine injuries must be anticipated in sports such as judo, where players are thrown and may land awkwardly. Visceral damage can also occur when a player follows through a throw and lands forcefully on their opponent. Eye, facial and soft tissue, and bone injuries are common in 'punching' sports such as boxing and karate. A vital role of the ringside doctor is in the recognition of a fighter who has taken enough punishment; s/he should not be afraid to stop a bout.

MOTOR SPORTS

Motor sports as a whole are amongst the most dangerous (Office of Population Censuses and Surveys 1991). In recent years numerous improvements to trackside safety and vehicle design have led to significant reductions in deaths; however, they still occur. High-speed accidents predispose to severe multiple injury. Deceleration injury is a major factor in motor racing as, although carbon fibre monocoque design of cars has led to a reduction in direct injuries, there is little that can be done to markedly diminish deceleration forces when a car comes into contact with a brick wall. Not all racing tracks are safe, moreover. The Isle of Man TT races and the Great Northern 2000, both examples of motorcycling races held on normal roads, take a steady toll. Rally drivers are at risk from trees and cliffs, and the spectators of this sport appear to have a strange desire to stand in the way of cars hurtling towards them at great speed. Head and neck injuries are common in open racing cars.

Doctors should approach the scene and read the wreckage of a motor sports incident in the same way as any other road traffic accident. Personal safety is the paramount concern, as the race is very likely to continue. Thereafter, treatment must follow the basic tenets of control of exsanguinating external haemorrhage, airway maintenance, cervical spine control, breathing and circulatory control with arrest of external bleeding. Rapid evacuation to definitive hospital care is essential, as internal vascular and visceral damage will need urgent surgery.

WATERSPORTS

In the UK hypothermia poses the greatest risk to water sportsmen. Many sailors are ill prepared for sudden changes in the weather. Drowning is an ever-present risk. Head and limb injuries from falls on wet decks are not uncommon, and a flailing boom poses significant risk of serious head injury. Jetskiers risk head and neck injuries in falls at high speed. Water skiers can suffer severe rectal and vaginal lacerations when they fall and receive a forceful injection of water. Propeller injuries, although rare, can be very severe. Head and neck injuries are common in those who risk diving into shallow water.

Diving emergencies are covered in detail in Chapter 37.

RACQUET SPORTS

Soft tissue sprains and strains are common, the upper limb being most often injured in these sports. Facial and eye injuries are of great concern. A squash ball can do untold damage to an unprotected orbit. The familiar picture of unfit players collapsing on the court as they play squash to get fit is an all too common a sight.

MOUNTAINEERING AND HILL WALKING

The weather poses the greatest threat to these sportsmen. Minor sprains and strains take on massive significance if they occur miles from home in hostile terrain with the weather closing in. Hypothermia and frostbite are an ever-present risk. Falls do cause serious injury and death;

however, the commonest cause of death in the hills is myocardial infarction.

The management of sports injuries

The management of a sports injury is no different from that of any other in a non-sporting environment. The overall tenets of assessment of airway, cervical spine, breathing, circulation and disability are just as important on the sports field as in the road accident. A knowledge of the sport and possible injury patterns is very important for medical attendants. An accurate history is essential, and witnesses must be closely questioned. The mechanism of injury will often lead to a diagnosis. A thorough examination and repeated reviews are vital to detect hidden or latent injuries. It is important to remember that most sportsmen/women will try to belittle their injury in an attempt to continue with the game. If serious injury is suspected the medical attendant must insist that the player is removed from the game, despite protest.

Most players will have soft tissue injuries that may require no more than advice and treatment in accordance with the RICE principles. The application of cold compresses may help considerably in the early management of a soft tissue injury. If there is any doubt about the nature of the injury, especially if joints are involved, then removal to hospital for further examination and X-ray is appropriate.

Dislodged teeth can be stored in milk as they can readily be re-implanted if stored safely in this way.

All suspected head and neck injuries should be dealt with in the normal manner. In-line immobilization, cervical collars and long spinal boards should be utilized. All injuries, whether they be head and neck injuries or fractures or haemorrhage, should be treated in accordance with the guidelines in the specific chapters in this book. The basic essentials of basic life support, advanced life support and advanced trauma life support must *never* be ignored.

Drugs and the sportsperson

Most competitive sports are governed by very strict rules about the use of drugs. Considerable publicity is given to those drugs that are banned and advice is available from sports governing bodies. It is essential that medical attendants are aware of the rules so that they do not inadvertently provide players with banned substances.

It is perfectly in order to give narcotics in the case of major injury. Steroids can be used topically and in intra-articular or local injections. They cannot be used intramuscularly. Local anaesthetics are permitted by local or intra-articular injection. If such drugs are used the medical attendant must provide details of reason, dose and route of administration to the event medical officer before the competition begins (Budgett 1996).

Table 52.2 Banned and restricted substances

Prohibited substances

- Stimulants – cocaine, amfetamine, ephedrine, pseudoephedrine, adrenaline (epinephrine)
- Narcotics – pethidine, diamorphine, dextropropoxyphene, codeine, dihydrocodeine
- Anabolic agents – steroids, beta-2-agonists
- Diuretics
- Hormones and analogues (growth hormone, erythropoietin, adrenocorticotrophic hormone (ACTH))
- Hormone antagonists and modulators

Prohibited methods

- Blood doping (enhancement of oxygen transfer)
- Altering urine samples by chemical and physical manipulation
- Gene doping

Drugs subject to some restriction

- Alcohol
- Marijuana and other cannabinoids
- Beta-blockers

Source: World Anti-doping Agency prohibited list 2008

The International Olympic Committee publish a list of banned and restricted substances and this is summarized in Table 52.2 (International Olympic Committee 1995).

References

Budgett R 1996 How to play fair. Medicom, (UK), London

Campbell H 1995 Leisure accidents in Scotland. Health Bulletin, London

Campbell H 1996 Preventing sports and leisure injuries. BMJ Publishing, London

Department of Trade and Industry 1993 Home and leisure accident research: 1993. HMSO, London

Hamlyn P 1995 A fight to the death. Medicom, (UK), London

International Olympic Committee 1995 IOC medical code. International Olympic Committee, London

Office of Population Censuses and Surveys 1991 HMSO, London

Secretary of State for Health 1991 Health of the nation. HMSO, London

Disaster medicine

53

Introduction 540

Natural disasters 540

Man-made disasters 540

Armed conflict 540

Complex emergencies 541

The impact of a disaster 541

International medical aid 548

Prepare, practise and have a plan 549

Communications 550

The future 551

Further reading 551

Table 53.1 Natural disasters

- Drought/famine
- Earthquake
- Flood
- High wind (cyclone, hurricane, storm, typhoon)
- Landslide
- Volcano
- Avalanche
- Cold wave
- Epidemic
- Food shortage
- Heat wave
- Tsunami

Introduction

When the response to a crisis fails to match the needs of the victims, disaster ensues. The difference between the size of the disaster and the scale of the response determines the *impact* of the disaster.

Disasters can be classified in many ways. Traditionally, large-scale events have been divided into natural and man-made. War and armed conflict should also be considered disasters, and increasingly it has been recognized that all the above can combine to form a complex emergency.

Natural disasters

A summary of the causes of natural disasters is given in Table 53.1. Some idea of the enormous impact in terms of mortality and morbidity can be gained from Table 53.2.

Man-made disasters

Causes of man-made disasters are summarized in Table 53.3 and their impact is indicated in Table 53.4.

Armed conflict

Armed conflict still remains a major cause of death both among combatants and involved civilians. The Gulf War in

Table 53.2 The human impact of natural disasters from 1970 to 1994

	Earthquake	Drought/famine	Flood	High wind	Landslide	Volcano	Total
Killed	21 593	73 606	12 361	28 194	1560	1014	138 328
Injured	30 952	N/A	17 910	7668	247	280	57 057
Affected	1 768 695	58 622 156	52 543 433	11 107 110	137 613	94 030	124 273 037
Homeless	232 406	22 720	3 502 014	1 111 092	107 434	14 764	4 990 430
Total	2 053 646	58 718 482	56 075 718	12 254 064	246 854	110 088	129 458 852

N/A: not applicable
Source: data from the Centre for Research on the Epidemiology of Disasters (CRED), Department of Public Health, Catholic University of Louvain, Belgium

Table 53.3 Man-made disasters

- Accidents (transport accidents, structural collapse)
- Technological accidents (chemical, nuclear and mine explosions, chemical atmospheric, and oil pollution)
- Fire

Table 53.4 The human impact of man-made disasters from 1970 to 1994

	Accident	Technological accident	Fires	Total
Killed	3667	617	3333	7617
Injured	1701	5583	751	8035
Affected	17 290	53 558	44 125	114 973
Homeless	868	8517	8939	18 325
Total	23 526	68 275	57 148	148 950

1991 and the war in Yemen in 1994 claimed many lives, and the death toll in Afghanistan has continued to ravage Asia. The wars in Ethiopia, Somalia, Angola, Liberia, Sudan and Algeria have served to ensure that Africa has kept pace with Europe at least in the numbers killed on the battlefield. Up to 1 million people are believed to have died in Iraq since the Allied Invasion of 2003 and more than 8000 in Afghanistan in 2007 alone.

Complex emergencies

This describes the situation where political institutions within a country have failed to respond to natural or man-made disasters or emergencies. This failure may be deliberate or unintentional, but the political constraints of the area place considerable obstacles in the path of the normal delivery of humanitarian aid and an intermediary is required.

The most common type of complex emergency accompanies civil conflict where the lives of non-combatants, often trapped between opposing forces, are threatened but humanitarian aid is severely hampered by the conflict itself and the actions of the combatants. Large numbers of people may be displaced from their homes and add to the problems of those communities they attempt to join.

Not all complex emergencies start with conflict. Any mass movement of people, following a natural disaster for example, can precipitate a political crisis, which in turn may precipitate a conflict. At the root of understanding a complex emergency is the recognition that an emergency has arisen that requires humanitarian assistance where the political authorities have neither the will nor the means to help.

The victims of complex emergencies may be:

- trapped in combat areas where assistance is not available
- forced to cross international borders and become refugees
- forced to move to safety within the confines of their country and become internally displaced.

The impact of a disaster

THE NUMBER OF CASUALTIES

The first and obvious measure of the size of a disaster is how many victims have been involved. The greater the number, the higher the potential impact. However, it must be appreciated that apparently small numbers will overwhelm poor or underprepared facilities, and larger numbers will be safely absorbed into a well-resourced and well-prepared response. The overwhelming of facilities by numbers is, however, always at the root of a disaster. It can be mitigated by *triage*, where patients are sorted into categories of individual need measured against the needs of

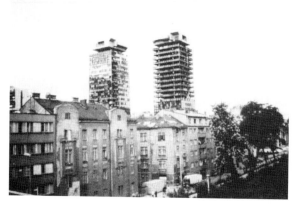

Fig. 53.1 • Fighting in a built-up area – former republic of Yugoslavia.

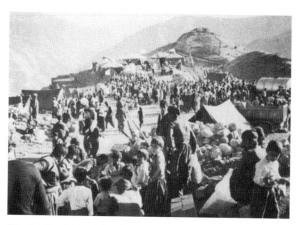

Fig. 53.2 • A Kurdish refugee camp.

others and the resources available. This process is an every-day occurrence in day-to-day emergency medical practice, where patients' needs are classed as 'immediate', 'urgent' or 'delayed'. The skill acquired in weeding out the minor, non-life-threatening conditions at a very early stage is often the most crucial factor in reducing the immediate impact of a disaster. However, in large-scale disasters a fourth category – 'expectant' – may be required. This is more familiar to military doctors, where the contingencies of the battlefield might dictate that those in need of immediate treatment but with a very poor prognosis will be put to one side while those with less serious but eminently salvageable conditions are treated first. This process is amongst the most difficult in medicine, and those who do it must be experienced and senior enough to combat the doubts and recriminations of others, and at times themselves, that may surface in the aftermath of these terrible events.

THE NATURE OF THE CASUALTIES

Next to the number of casualties, the nature of the casualties will determine the impact of the disaster.

Disease

Non-traumatic medical conditions are the most common medical problems encountered in disaster medicine. They mostly affect the very young and the very old and complicate the effects of injury. They may be the source of the disaster but more usually complicate a non-medical catastrophe such as the sudden mass migration of people.

Diarrhoea, dehydration and respiratory tract infections are the commonest killers. Outbreaks of specific diseases such as cholera can complicate the mass migration of people. Where there are a large number of unburied bodies, such as after an earthquake, there is often a fear of epidemic. In practice, any epidemic is more likely to accompany the movement of people into unsatisfactory, unsanitary, temporary accommodation.

Malnutrition

Lack of food can often complicate the early stages of disaster. Otherwise healthy adults can tolerate an acute loss of several kilograms without ill effect. The very young, the old and the already sick can often tolerate little in the way of acute weight loss and quickly become vulnerable to disease. Wasting in young children is, not surprisingly, a poor prognostic sign. However, when already stressful situations are compounded by a fall in calorie intake to below $1500\,\text{kcal}\,\text{d}^{-1}$ there is an associated increase in mortality. Maintaining calorie intake at above $2000\,\text{kcal}\,\text{d}^{-1}$ is associated with a much lower mortality. Tolerating more prolonged undernutrition depends, in addition, on the starting weight of individuals in the population. This was a critical factor in surviving the siege of Sarajevo, where the population as a whole was overweight initially.

Data from the subcommittee on nutrition of the United Nations (UN) administrative committee on coordination indicate that more than 0.75 million people lack sufficient food energy for productive lives and 184 million children under the age of 5 years are underweight for their age. Since the 1970s the world has produced 3% more food every year – enough food to provide 10–20% more than its population needs with everyone still receiving an adequate calorie intake of $2350\,\text{kcal}\,\text{d}^{-1}$. There has been a fall in the overall number of malnourished people in the world during this period but improvements in nutrition in some areas (e.g. Asia) have been offset by worsening conditions in others (e.g. Latin America and sub-Saharan Africa).

Famine

Large-scale severe undernutrition has plagued humankind since biblical times. The short-term solution is food but the longer-term answers lie in politics and world economics. Emergency food aid through the World Food Programme is amongst the most important of all the aid programmes. Attempts have been made to identify trigger levels for urgent action. These include a rise in crude mortality to 1 in $10\,000\,\text{day}^{-1}$; wasting greater than 15% and energy supply less than $1500\,\text{kcal}\,\text{d}^{-1}$.

Injury

In developed countries major motorway pile-ups have the potential for creating huge disasters each winter but often the nature of the casualties is such that relatively few high-demand patients are sandwiched between the dead and those with minor injuries. But should even four multiply-injured patients arrive together at a well-staffed and well-equipped modern western emergency department their presence will threaten available resources, if only temporarily. These patients will be on the brink of disaster until the response grows to match their needs. A realization of the huge demands that the treatment of severe injury can place upon a system leads to an appreciation of how quickly an apparently small number of injured casualties can overwhelm and create disaster. This situation should not be seen as something that happens elsewhere and particularly to poorer countries. The overwhelming of facilities for the care of the severely injured remains a feature of health care throughout many areas of the world, including the UK.

Because the demands of severe injury are so great and the window of opportunity for life-saving treatment is sometimes small, the chance to avert or limit the initial impact of such disasters is often very limited. If life-saving surgery is required it can usually only be offered by those close to the incident. This appreciation will ensure that outside assistance to disasters involving injured patients focuses mostly on secondary management.

However, the secondary demands of severely injured patients can be enormous and adequate treatment in the early stages after injury may avert or reduce a lifetime of disability. The impact of a large number of injured patients on a health service will be felt for a long time, and material and manpower assistance can be required long after the media spotlight has moved on.

Land mines

The aftermath of military conflict can leave huge areas blighted for generations by unmapped land mines. The World Health Organization has estimated that the conflict in the former Yugoslavia alone had caused at least 5000

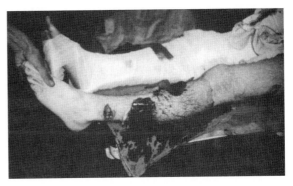

Fig. 53.3 • Fragment injuries to the lower limbs.

mine-related amputations by 1995. Worse still, this figure excludes deaths and fragmentation injuries and completely excludes data from Serb-controlled areas. It is estimated that 110 million land mines are scattered across 64 countries. The International Committee of the Red Cross (ICRC) estimate that they kill or maim 2000 people every month.

Untreated illness

The longer a crisis persists the more the population can be deprived of basic medical care. Intercurrent but untreated illness will complicate the effects of the disaster and recovery.

The dead

Corpses are not usually a health risk to the living but may become infested and a source of infection (e.g. typhus and plague). Extreme care must be taken in the presence of viral haemorrhagic fevers.

There is a recurring myth that the unburied dead pose a serious risk to health and are the potential source of epidemic after a disaster. The fear is usually fuelled and, perhaps, even created by the media. Yet pestilence after disaster is usually a function of *Vibrio cholerae*, *Salmonella typhi* and *Yersinia pestis* and not the bacteria of putrefaction. In other words, it is water-borne, food-contamination-related and vector-related.

The fact that there are no live casualties, or that there are unlikely to be any, does not exclude a need for medical support. The identification of human remains is a difficult task, and extremely stressful and confusing for those unused to dealing with injured body tissue. A piece of coloured cloth covered in brick dust can appear remarkably similar to lung or other internal body tissue in these circumstances. Dealing with a large number of dead can paradoxically require a great deal of medical support. Furthermore, the rescue workers labour on in the faint hope of finding someone in the carnage who might possibly have survived. They are greatly reassured by the presence of medical support just in case they find such a person. In addition, they harbour a fear of finding someone clinging on to life only to lose them for lack of immediate medical support.

THE NATURE OF THE EVENT

Certain catastrophes have predictable consequences for which preparations and plans can be made.

Earthquake

Movements of the Earth's crust cause tremors (ground shaking), liquefaction (upward movement of moisture turning soil to quicksand) and vertical and horizontal ground disruption from surface faulting and tectonic uplifts. Falling buildings and masonry trap, injure and kill.

The onset of the catastrophe is sudden but may be prolonged thereafter by aftershocks, which can occur for several hours or even days afterwards. When earthquakes occur at night and most people are in their homes the death toll will be higher. The combination of entrapment and injury sets a limit on the severity of injury that can be survived in these circumstances. By and large, most of those with severe injuries to the head and chest will perish before rescue or transport to an adequate facility. Some abdominal and most limb injuries will survive. The bulk of injured survivors have peripheral limb injuries. As a rule of thumb, there are three times as many injured as dead, but this is obviously only a guide.

Widespread muscle injury, particularly when accompanied by prolonged compression, will lead to 'crush injury'. The characteristic feature of this is breakdown of muscle tissues (rhabdomyolysis), skin necrosis and sometimes, but by no means always, underlying bony injury.

The release of muscle breakdown products into the circulation can produce 'crush syndrome' leading to renal failure, hyperkalaemia and death. Large amounts of myoglobin in the kidneys lead to renal failure, which in turn leads to further accumulation of myoglobin. Potassium is released into the circulation from damaged muscle but is not excreted by the failing kidneys, compounding the already rising potassium levels consequent upon the renal failure itself.

'Crush injury' is not synonymous with 'crush syndrome' but the former is a precursor of the latter. The likelihood of one following the other is proportional to the degree and duration of crush. The sooner the casualty is released, the less the chance of crush syndrome. The risk of developing crush syndrome is obviously increased if the patient is already in renal failure. Hypovolaemia from blood loss and/or dehydration will provoke prerenal failure and compound

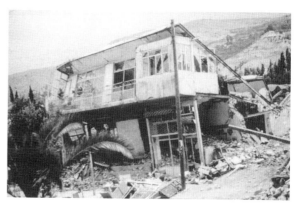

Fig. 53.4 • Structural damage following an earthquake.

the effects of the renal damage that accompanies the release of myoglobin into the circulation. Prolonged entrapment is usually associated with water deprivation and injury. The potential for crush syndrome lies within everyone released during rescue from an earthquake.

The treatment of established crush syndrome involves intravenous volume replacement, alkalinization of the urine and possibly renal dialysis. Vigorous volume replacement should begin before release and continue during and after extrication. This is perhaps the most important role for the prehospital doctor in the rescue of those trapped after an earthquake. Increasing the circulating volume before release and titrating volume infused against blood pressure during and after release will maintain blood pressure, reduce the concentration of potassium by increasing the circulatory volume and reduce the risk to the kidneys by diluting the myoglobin load. Prehospital alkalinization of the urine is impractical without laboratory control. Dialysis is often rationed at the best of times and, once crush injury has deteriorated into a full-blown crush syndrome with established renal failure, the prognosis is grave. In fact, the latter may constitute a triage group that is viewed as 'expectant' in these circumstances.

The vulnerability of an area to the effects of earthquake is related to the siting of human settlements, industrial plants, dams and infrastructure. Chemical and nuclear plants pose specific and potentially catastrophic problems when sited in earthquake-prone areas. The resistance of buildings is a critical factor in determining loss of life. The earthquake in Armenia in 1988 claimed at least 25 000 lives, due in no small part to the propensity for poorly built modern apartment blocks to crumble when vibrated. In contrast, an earthquake of less but not too dissimilar force shook the west coast of the USA in 1989 but killed only 300 people and injured 400. Many of those who died in the Loma Prieta earthquake were killed when roadways collapsed, apparently because their structure had not complied with building standards for that earthquake-prone area. The vast majority of buildings did meet building regulations and mitigated the effects of the quake. What begins as a natural disaster is too often compounded by a much greater man-made disaster, involving poor building construction and inadequate building regulation.

The destruction of roads, bridges and railways compound medical problems. The injured cannot be evacuated and the helpers cannot get in. Damage to pylons leads to power failure and loss of communication.

Water supplies may be disrupted and water contaminated, but to date no significant outbreaks of water-borne diseases have been documented following an earthquake. The fear of epidemic is always high and is inevitably fuelled by uninformed media speculation but the evidence to date is that threats to public health after earthquake come from the mass movement of people, particularly into temporary camps, rather than from the earthquake itself.

When considering aid to stricken areas the following must always be borne in mind:

- The majority of rescues will have taken place in the first 2–3 h and will have been accomplished by local people. Those who survive and constitute the largest initial group of casualties are the less seriously injured and those who were not trapped.

- Survival from entrapment is rare beyond 2 days.

- The national response will be mobilized in the first 48 h. In the following days and weeks further medical aid will be made available, perhaps from neighbouring states or the international community, but largely to treat a self-selecting group of survivors, most of whom have relatively minor injuries.

- There will be survivors, with severe limb injuries in particular, who will benefit greatly from reconstructive surgery.

The local medical services will be consumed by the disaster and may require international help to maintain routine health facilities for conditions unrelated to the earthquake as well as with the aftermath of the disaster.

The impact of the disaster on health services will last months or even years, and a much overlooked aid need lies in the rehabilitation of those disabled by the disaster.

Medical aid to earthquakes is not without physical risk and danger to the rescuers. Buildings damaged by earthquakes are inherently unstable and one must be aware of the risks involved in entering such places. One should only enter with the express permission of those in charge of the rescue services. Aftershocks continue for some time, and buildings already weakened by the initial earthquake can tumble quickly and without warning. Damage to industrial plants can pose particular and potentially extremely serious problems. In Armenia, for example, there was considerable concern over possible damage to chemical plants in

the area and concern even about the status of local nuclear reactors.

Unfortunately, many areas prone to earthquake are also prone to civil unrest. The civil disruption caused by the earthquake can lead to a rapid breakdown of law and order, particularly in areas that were already teetering on the brink of civil disturbance. This is an added burden and danger for the rescue workers. Fortunately, such problems are not common but must always be borne in mind.

Of more importance is to understand that the greatest risk to foreign rescue workers is that posed by road accidents. When surrounded by an increased level of risk it is surprising how often human beings abandon the normal safety procedures they would follow at home. A certain degree of recklessness seems to accompany increased risk-taking and this can be reflected in driving habits. Furthermore, the combination of tired rescue workers driving unfamiliar four-wheel drive vehicles over rough and now damaged terrain combines to form a potentially lethal cocktail.

Tsunami

Earthquakes are, in fact, very common but mostly occur out at sea. However, seismic activity under the sea bed can produce huge walls of water that wreak havoc when they hit land. These seismic sea waves are sometimes called tidal waves but are usually referred to as tsunami. Such a wave may travel in deep ocean at speeds up to $800\,\mathrm{km\,h^{-1}}$. The speed slows in shallower water and the energy is transferred into creating a steep front of water as high as 30 m. A train of waves may come one after the other, perhaps up to 10 over a period of 20–30 min. Low-lying coastal areas are obviously the most vulnerable. When the wave subsides the drag of water returning to the sea can erode building foundations and cause buildings and sea walls to collapse. When the wave has gone completely there is still serious danger from residual flooding and in particular floating heavy debris, often moving at speed. Over 100 000 people are thought to have perished as a result of the Asian tsunami in December 2004, the biggest humanitarian disaster of our time.

Rescue workers will face the consequences of damage to buildings and utilities. Many will have drowned, and dealing with the dead and the bereaved may play a large part in aftercare. Once again, the mass migration of people both before and after the event will pose the biggest medical problem.

Landslide

Landslides can follow heavy storms, earthquakes and volcanic eruptions. They can incorporate rock falls and mud flows. Rivers of mud will also flow after tsunami, flood and sometimes earthquake. They are powerful and destructive, and sweep buildings and people before them. The weight of the mud that encases a body immersed in it makes extrication extremely difficult. Victims should be considered to be at risk of crush syndrome and, in particular, of a sudden fall in blood pressure when the pressure of surrounding mud is suddenly released. Fluid loading before, during and after rescue may be required.

Floods

In addition to the obvious threats of drowning and injury, floods damage agriculture, housing and transport, which may conspire to precipitate acute food shortages. A large number of drownings occur when people are trapped in their cars.

There are three main types of flood:

- river floods
- flash floods
- coastal floods.

Dam breaks can lead to flooding and this can obviously complicate earthquakes.

Storm surges

These occur when the sea level rises, usually as a consequence of a tropical storm. As with a tsunami, the force of the flow back to the sea can be as damaging as the original surge.

Volcano

An erupting volcano emits ash and gas into the atmosphere and pours molten rock (magma) on to the Earth's surface. The greatest threats to life come from ash falls, pyroclastic flows (horizontal blasts of gas containing ash and larger fragments in suspension), mud flow and tsunami. Volcanic earthquakes can also occur. There is a greater risk from injury than burns. Falling rocks and frantic escape lead to falls and injury. Burns may occur but those left very close to the lava may not effect an escape. Hot ash in the air can produce inhalation burns but only the most superficial to the very upper airways are likely to be survived in this scenario.

Ash at normal temperature will produce acute respiratory problems, and coughs and running eyes are common. Asthmatics are particularly vulnerable. The sheer volume of ash at the time of eruption can produce asphyxia in those close to the eruption and is the most frequent cause of immediate death. Even without a volume effect, the irritant ash will provoke excessive mucus production, which,

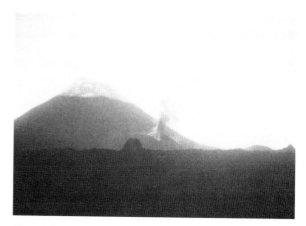

Fig. 53.5 • A recent volcanic eruption.

when mixed with the ash, forms obstructive mucus plugs. In those who survive a significant exposure, acute respiratory distress syndrome (ARDS) may ensue. The silica content of the ash may lead to long-term problems. Early evacuation away from the contaminated area is required.

Volcanic gases include carbon monoxide, hydrofluoric acid and sulphur dioxide, all of which are toxic in themselves and compound the effects of the ash.

Volcanic ash eventually provides a very fertile soil and areas vulnerable to repeated volcanic activity are paradoxically often well populated. When activity occurs the panic can be immense, and the overriding and lasting medical problems are related to the mass migration of people, homelessness, refugees and inadequate temporary accommodation becoming inadequate permanent homes.

Pyroclastic flows are the most dangerous consequence of a volcanic eruption. The speed of movement can be several hundred kilometres per hour and the temperature of the moving material can be up to 1000°C. These flows can last several minutes and be repeated for prolonged periods.

Mud flows may also occur. They usually occur after heavy rain has emulsified ash and loose volcanic material. The mud, with a consistency of wet concrete, can flow rapidly downhill, reaching speeds of over 100 km h^{-1}.

Lava flows will destroy everything in their path but their predictability and slow speed of movement (in sharp contrast to pyroclastic flows) significantly reduce the risk to human life. However, the heat of the lava flow will ignite vulnerable structures, and death and injury occur from secondary fires.

Direct exposure to a large amount of volcanic gas is very hazardous but only those very close to the volcano are at risk.

Tropical storms

When these occur in the Indian Ocean, convention dictates they are called *cyclones*. This same convention dictates

Table 53.5 The Saffir/Simpson hurricane scale

Grade	Speed (mph)
I	74–95
II	96–110
III	111–130
IV	131–155
V	>155

Table 53.6 Other conditions associated with refugee status (see text)

- Cholera
- Diphtheria
- Infestation
- Intestinal parasites
- Meningitis
- Polio
- Skin infection
- Tetanus
- Tuberculosis
- Typhoid
- Whooping cough

that when they occur in the north Atlantic, Caribbean and south Pacific they are termed *hurricanes* and when in the north and west Pacific they are called *typhoons*. Whatever they are called, they involve humid air twisting upwards from warm seawater (27°C) into cooler air above and moving erratically at speeds of up to 50 km h^{-1}. That is the speed of progress over land; the air itself may be swirling at speeds of over 300 km h^{-1}. In the northern hemisphere the wind moves anticlockwise (like the water from a bath) and the storm generally drifts in a north-westerly direction. In the south the rotation is clockwise and the drift generally south-westerly. A classification of hurricanes is given in Table 53.5.

The wind itself is not necessarily harmful but flying debris is. Secondary flooding may provoke later disease if the water supply is contaminated by sewage. In keeping with other disasters, it is often the effects on communication and transport that pose the greatest risk to health, although initial mortality is often the result of drowning.

Refugees and internally displaced persons

The 1951 Convention and the 1967 Protocol define a refugee as

[Any person who] … owing to a well founded fear of being persecuted for reasons of race, religion, nationality, membership of a particular group or political opinion, is outside the country of his nationality and is unable or, owing to such fear, is unwilling to avail himself of the protection of that country, or who, not having a nationality and being outside the country of his former habitual residence as a result of such events, is unable or, owing to such a fear, is unwilling to return to it.

The UN High Commission for Refugees (UNHCR) recognizes refugees as forcibly displaced people who have crossed an international border. Those who flee but stay within their country are internally displaced people. It is true that increasing numbers of people flee their countries for environmental and economic reasons. Equally, millions are displaced because of urban development and the expansion of transportation systems. It might seem semantics to label each group separately but the Red Cross emphasizes that misuse of the term refugee will erode the protection rights of those truly in need. On the other hand, it remains essential to regard as special those who flee across borders because of fear of violence or human rights abuses, even those connected with development programmes or environmental catastrophes.

The numbers of refugees and internally displaced people have increased dramatically. There were 22 million in 1985 and over 36 million in 1995 (14.5 million refugees and asylum seekers and 21.5 internally displaced persons). The principal causes of this increase are internal conflicts resulting from ethnic and religious tensions and the greater number of collapsed states. In 1990 there were an estimated 22 million internally displaced persons, and in 1994 there were about 26 million.

The five major killers associated with the sudden mass movement of people are:

- malnutrition
- measles
- acute respiratory infection
- diarrhoea
- malaria.

These five conditions account for up to 90% of all deaths in these populations. Other conditions to be particularly aware of in these circumstances are listed in Table 53.6.

Refugee camps

These inevitably generate their own special medical problems:

- Food shortage
- Poor shelter

- Lack of fuel for cooking, washing and cleaning
- Lack of water
- Camp violence – aid workers are vulnerable but those most at risk are the camp members themselves, especially the young, the sick and the old (groups already vulnerable)
- Disease – large numbers of people living cheek by jowl in unsanitary situations quickly become vulnerable to infectious disease. Establishing clean water and sanitation are the first priorities
- Lack of usual/adequate health-care provision
- Break up of family units, and unaccompanied children and elderly.

The most important measure of the rising pressures on a displaced persons camp is the mortality rate. If the camp is coping then mortality rates should be within 1.5 times that of the host population. If initial efforts to curb mortality are working, very high mortality rates should fall below 1 per 10 000 d^{-1} by the first month or so of operation. A serious crisis is represented by a mortality rate of 2 per 10 000 d^{-1}.

International medical aid

If the presence of an aid worker at a disaster is to relieve rather than add to the number of homeless in need of food and shelter it is imperative only to attend in response to a specific request for help from an authoritative body. This will ensure that particular skills will plug any local gaps and that local resources will not be diverted to looking after the needs of aid workers rather than those of the victims. Time spent at home negotiating a clear route through to the target area is time saved waiting at airports, embassies and road sides while visas, accommodation and local transport are arranged. All aid workers should be self-sufficient, understanding that this might involve food, water and shelter. Aid workers should always carry a supply of their own medication.

It is imperative that doctors understand that the most important needs for victims of a disaster might be food, water, shelter, clothing and blankets, and that such needs have a much greater priority usually than strictly medical needs. Doctors must understand where purely medical problems fit into the overall scale of priorities.

Furthermore, doctors can come under immense pressure from the media to respond to disasters overseas. The cries of 'something must be done' can be loud and persuasive. However, local facilities may be more than adequate. Often what is most needed is financial support to enable the local authorities to mobilize local resources. The unheralded influx of outside aid can divert attention and resources at a time of greatest need and must be avoided. There

are recognized channels through the UN and government departments in tandem with the large aid organizations through which doctors and medical teams can direct their efforts. There will be times when outside help is asked for and clearly required. If the benefits of such outside help are to outweigh the costs, then there must be coordination and the local authorities must retain control. There is no place for competitive humanitarianism, only cooperation.

It is always best to use local supplies and distribution channels. All medical personnel are hostile to using drugs and equipment with which they are unfamiliar. Unfortunately, local and national supplies can become exhausted quite quickly after large-scale disasters. The World Health Organization has developed special kits that are prepackaged and ready for use. Each kit is composed of a basic unit and a supplementary unit. Each of 10 basic units is intended for primary health-care workers to assist a population of 1000 for 3 months. They weigh 45 kg and are 0.2 m^3 in size. They contain only oral medications. The supplementary kit is also designed for a population of 10 000 for 3 months. It weighs 410 kg and is 2 m^3 in size. It is for the sole use of professional health-care workers. It does not duplicate any of the contents of the basic unit and cannot be used alone. The entire kit will fit on the back of a standard pick-up truck.

It is always a somewhat precarious exercise to plan for the next disaster solely on the experiences gained from the last. However, the medical responses to international disasters can be seen to fall into certain groups.

ASSESSMENT

This is the most important function, usually of those who respond in the immediate aftermath of a large-scale disaster. While the local authorities are dealing with the immediate casualties and consequences of a disaster, outside medical help can make assessments of the degree of sophistication of pre-existing facilities, the impact of the disaster upon those facilities and the degree of sophistication of the local response. When making assessments it is usually helpful to identify an area of the medical services with which one is already familiar and work outwards from there. Reports should be made to the on-site operations and coordination centre (OSOCC) of the UN disaster assessment and coordination team, and briefing sessions from other non-governmental organizations and government agencies should be attended. Information should be shared freely and the time of local officials should not be monopolized, as this will divert their attention away from the disaster. When attending meetings it is useful to have at least two people there. One can do the talking while the other listens, observes and takes notes. In this way nothing is missed or misinterpreted.

The local government agencies will carry out the most important assessment of medical needs. Donor agencies and aid agencies will wish to carry out their own assessments as well. This can lead to a frustrating period for the stricken country when international aid *appears* to be piling in but all that looks to be happening is one assessment after the other. On the other hand, if aid is to be most effective and not wasted it must be appropriate and well targeted. Unnecessary duplication of effort can be avoided by sharing information. In particular, the coordinating role of the host government and UN agencies must be recognized. The Department of Humanitarian Affairs of the UN has established a disaster assessment and coordination team (UNDAC) that will respond immediately the UN is asked for help. One of its first priorities will be to establish an OSOCC, to which you must report.

Immediate health assessment needs must include a judgement as to whether the remaining facilities in the affected area are sufficient to meet immediate or predicted demands. The status of material facilities must be established both in the affected area and in areas to where victims are being evacuated.

In addition to the number and nature of casualties and the availability of and need for medical materials, it is important to check whether the infrastructure has been affected. Does the hospital have power and water, for example?

When receiving information from local agencies it must be established how the information was collected and what mechanisms for health surveillance were in place prior to the accident. Estimates of the medical effects of disasters can vary wildly, particularly in the early stages, and the degree of certainty surrounding statistics and information must always be checked and confirmed.

Assessments should not be duplicated – this is wasteful of time, effort and money, and infuriating for the local authorities.

THE PROVISION OF SURGICAL TEAMS

These are rarely required in the immediate aftermath of disasters, even after earthquakes. Survival after prolonged entrapment is unusual, and casualties are usually those with minor injuries and those who have not been trapped. However, large numbers of patients with peripheral limb injuries will quickly overwhelm the local or even national facilities, and help with the planned surgical treatment of these patients is often needed and very welcome. There may be no rush to do this immediately after the incident, allowing time for careful negotiation with hospital authorities. A commonly overlooked form of aid is the support that can be given to medical authorities in stricken areas by outside doctors taking over the normal day-to-day duties in the non-affected areas while local doctors attend to the specific needs of the disaster.

THE PROVISION OF MEDICAL TEAMS

Very occasionally medical, non-surgical teams may be required. This is usually for secondary and tertiary care (e.g. help in treating large numbers of patients who need dialysis after crush syndrome). Again, there is often no rush to do this within the immediate aftermath of an incident, and time can be spent very usefully making contacts with the medical authorities in that country.

PRIMARY CARE

This is probably the type of medical response that is most often required. The mass migration of people and their location in refugee camps precipitates enormous needs for primary care, particularly for children and the elderly. Even relatively well-resourced areas can experience a dramatic increase in the need for primary care when facilities have been destroyed or disrupted in earthquake-stricken or other disaster-struck areas. A combination of emergency and general practice can provide very powerful support to a wide range of large-scale emergencies. Such support may be needed for several weeks or months, and sometimes even longer.

SPECIALIST SUPPORT

Requests may be made for public health advisers or reconstructive surgeons when local authorities and/or the UN or other large agencies have identified a specific need. These specialists may serve a dual function of assessment and immediate help followed by the organization of a more prolonged structured programme of support.

Prepare, practise and have a plan

The following suggestions might be useful for those intending overseas aid work.

- Enquire about usual and expected weather conditions in the areas where you will be travelling. Actively seek and contact those who have been before or have just returned.

- Ensure your own health is in order. If you become unwell while on mission you will compound the problems of those already afflicted by the disaster and jeopardize the efforts of your colleagues. Failing to reveal a serious medical or psychiatric problem to your colleagues to ensure selection for a team is an act of unforgivable selfishness.

- Pay attention to simple things. Dental hygiene can be difficult to maintain in adverse conditions and can fall as a consequence of stress. Toothache can be very disabling at the best of times but catastrophic when in isolated adverse conditions. Keep your teeth healthy! Take at least one pair of spare spectacles.

- Pay rigid attention to malaria prophylaxis. Mosquito repellent is forgotten at your peril. Mosquito nets can help.

- Maintain your vaccinations and be honest when they have lapsed. In particular, maintain your tetanus, polio and hepatitis B status.

- When on mission be aware that working under adverse conditions is tiring. Poor decisions are made by the tired. Take adequate rest and work in rotation. Not everyone can take the first shift. Establish an order and routine as quickly as possible – this increases effectiveness and reduces stress.

- Look after one another. Appoint someone as a clear leader and do what they say. Set up a series of meetings so that everybody gets a chance to air their views and concerns, and try and reach a consensus. Ultimately, the leader may have to make an executive decision which the team should be prepared to accept. If you are not prepared to work under a fairly rigid command structure, then you should not put yourself forward for working in a team in these circumstances.

- Pair people off in a 'buddy' system: make sure one person is always responsible for another. In this way people are unlikely to get lost so easily or be misplaced! Make it clear to members of the team before leaving that it will be other people, particularly your buddy, who will determine whether or not you are becoming stressed and need a rest. In fact, often the first sign of stress is to fail to recognize that you are becoming stressed and respond angrily to any suggestion that you might need to take a rest. People must sign up to clear 'rules of engagement' that, in addition to including acceptance of a command structure, will also include an agreement to take time off and rest when a colleague, leader or buddy expresses concerns.

- Eat a balanced but standard diet. Boil all drinking water. Some degree of gastrointestinal upset is almost inevitable but diarrhoea and vomiting might render your efforts worthless. Make sure all your food has been thoroughly cooked and is hot when served. Avoid uncooked foods. Peel fruit and shell nuts.

- If diarrhoea develops increase your intake of (boiled) water and take oral rehydration salts.

- Maintain a strict personal hygiene. Avoid alcohol. It may be culturally unwise in any case, but the stress of the situation can easily lead to over indulgence. Unwind later at home by all means, but abstinence is the best policy on mission. For emotional and medical stability abstinence from other pleasures is also advised!

- Make sure your passport is always up to date and you have it with you. You will need visas and international certificates of vaccination for some countries. Even though you are on a humanitarian mission, the law still applies and you will need all your papers. Do not forget a driving licence, pens, paper, toilet paper and other sanitary requirements.

- The journey to and from the area may be prolonged and tortuous. Take credit cards. You will need at least one change of clothing. A collar and tie will make any official meetings marginally less stressful. Always be prepared for being stranded. Have emergency food rations and a sleeping bag. Matches, a torch and spare batteries are essential. The commonest symptom of stress in the field is headache. Take paracetamol. You may wish to take your own cup and plate, and personal tool with blades and other instruments.

- In rushing to respond to the needs of others do not forget a personal first-aid kit. Blisters, and minor cuts and bruises, can be very disabling when you are already stressed. You may wish to consider taking a sterile syringe, needles and cannula for personal use should you become ill or injured.

- Do not forget water purification tablets and sunscreen.

- Finally, do label yourself with a 'dog tag' that includes name, nationality and blood group. The unthinkable can happen.

The mission is not over until a formal debriefing session has been completed. Everyone must attend. Again, attendance at the debriefing session is something that everyone must sign up to before leaving. It is extremely important that all members of the team learn from every other member of the team exactly what they did, so that each member of the team has a final picture of the sum total of their activity. When faced with these stressful events people can erroneously assume that they have 'missed out' on the overall activities of the team or fail to appreciate the overall impact of their mission. Furthermore, a great deal of stress is unloaded when people talk together and recount all the events of the exercise. It is not always necessary to have formal 'counselling' but anyone who does appear to be suffering adversely as a result of the mission is likely to be spotted at the debriefing session and suitable psychological support can be offered. It is important also that the intense experience is not allowed to evaporate too quickly and that a further meeting or reunion is organized some weeks after return home. The most practical timetable is to allow people to meet immediately with their loved ones on the night they return home but to honour a commitment to a debriefing session the following day, and to meet 2 or 3 weeks later for a reunion.

Communications

One of the earliest casualties of many a disaster is communications and in some areas there may have been little in the way of communications to begin with. It is important to be familiar with hand-held portable radios and to use them as one would in the prehospital arena at home. The same messages and codes should be used, and approval sought from all the appropriate authorities.

Satellite technology is used increasingly in remote or isolated areas, and one should have at least a basic knowledge of its workings.

- Inmarsat A – is a portable system for voice data. To process data it needs an additional PC or fax.
- Inmarsat C – is a portable system that can process data only and is therefore cheaper than Inmarsat A.
- Inmarsat M – is highly portable and can process voice and data. It is contained in a briefcase but needs an additional PC or fax to process data.

The future

Information is power. The Centre for Research on the Epidemiology of Disasters (CRED) at the Department of Public Health, Catholic University of Louvain, Belgium has developed a system of databases for global disaster management. There is now a disaster events database EM-DAT, developed by CRED with sponsorship from the International Federation of Red Cross and Red Crescent Societies. It has more than 10 500 records of disasters from 1900 onwards. The criteria for entry is 10 deaths and/or 100 affected and/or an appeal for assistance. The following definitions apply:

- The date the appropriate authority declares an official emergency: there has to be some recognized start point even though it is understood that some disasters such as famine may have been running silently for a long time before the event is recognized officially.
- Those killed in disasters include all confirmed dead, and all missing and presumed dead. Those simply missing will not be included initially but may be added later.
- Injured describes physical injury, trauma or illness requiring medical treatment as a result of the disaster. There is as yet no consensus on whether treatment from first aiders and volunteers should be included.
- Homelessness refers to those who need immediate assistance with shelter. It may be necessary to use average family sizes for the region to calculate the total individuals affected.
- The total number of persons affected inevitably relies on some sort of estimate.

Information is received regularly from:

- UN Department of Humanitarian Affairs (UNDHA) situation reports (SitReps)
- International Federation of Red Cross and Red Crescent Societies SitReps
- Lloyds of London Insurance Underwriters; the Lloyds Casualty Week gives information on weather events, earthquakes, volcanic eruptions and other events/accidents world-wide
- The Internet.

Ultimately, the way forward is to improve the availability and quality of training. Disaster medicine is increasingly recognized now as a subspecialty of emergency medicine, and this is to be encouraged and developed further. This will allow the recognition of a core curriculum and international qualifications that will ensure that in the future those who put themselves forward to respond to international medical emergencies will be suitably trained and experienced. The Diploma in the Medical Care of Catastrophes of the Society of Apothecaries of London, UK and the European Academy of Disaster Medicine (EURADIM) are some of several steps now being taken by the international community in this direction.

Further reading

Baskett P, Weller R 1988 Medicine for disasters. Butterworth, London

Cahill K (ed) 1993 A framework for survival: health, human rights and humanitarian assistance in conflicts and disasters. Council on Foreign Relations, New York

International Federation of Red Cross and Red Crescent Societies 1996 World disasters report 1996. Oxford University Press, Oxford

James WPT, Schofield C 1990 Human energy requirements. Oxford University Press/FAO, Oxford

Sanderson D, Davis I, Twigg J, Cowden B 1995 Disaster mitigation, preparedness and response – an audit of UK assets. Oxford Centre for Disaster Studies, Oxford

UNICEF 1995 The state of the world's children. UNICEF, New York

Part Twelve

54   Immobilization and extrication 555

55   Transport in prehospital care 568

56   Aeromedical evacuation 572

57   Aviation medicine 581

58   Structure and function of the ambulance service 594

59   The fire service: structure and roles 603

60   Police force: structure and roles 614

61   The role of other agencies at a major incident 625

Immobilization and extrication

54

Introduction 555

Basic principles of immobilization 556

Basic principles of extrication 556

Methods of immobilization 557

Cervical immobilization 557

Limb immobilization 559

Traction splints 561

Pneumatic antishock garment 563

Extrication devices 563

Log rolling 565

Rapid extrication 565

Vacuum splints and mattresses 566

References 566

Introduction

When confronted with a prehospital emergency situation involving casualties, it is essential to follow the conventional pathway of safety, then primary survey and necessary resuscitation before performing a secondary survey, if appropriate. Rescuers must continually remember that definitive patient care takes place in hospital. Immobilization and extrication in order to move the casualty to hospital, although not at the forefront of activities during the initial casualty contact, must be an early priority in the rescue effort and appropriately planned in order to achieve the most effective and expeditious result for the patient.

The nature of the entrapment (if any), local circumstances, distance to hospital and suspected injuries may all influence not only methods of immobilization and extrication but modes of transport also. Alternatively, the method of transport may influence patient packaging. By that, it is meant that it is of little benefit to prepare a casualty in such a way that the use of certain immobilization equipment may prevent the casualty being transported in the way that had been planned. Equally, intending to use a certain method of transport may dictate which pieces of equipment may be used in the rescue. Early and careful planning are essential to marry together the various options as far as immobilization and extrication are concerned in order to ensure safe and speedy onward passage for the casualty while maintaining casualty comfort, preventing further injury or damage and allowing full monitoring to take place.

The basic prehospital approach of primary survey, resuscitation and stabilization is even more important when dealing with trapped casualties. The <C>ABC principles apply and continuing reassessment will be required during the rescue. With a trapped casualty, problems created by a missed critical injury cannot be retrieved by early evacuation to hospital (Karbi et al 1988).

Basic principles of immobilization

The principles of immobilization are relatively simple and reflect the concepts of first aid – maintain casualty safety and comfort and do no harm. It is important here to reiterate the principle that during patient 'packaging' the casualty should be repeatedly reassessed and any necessary interventions performed. This is particularly important when dealing with unstable injures for example, or moving injured limbs before applying a splint, or moving the casualty from the accident scene to an ambulance or helicopter.

Reduction and immobilization will be required in prehospital settings:

- to prevent further injury to other structures close to the fracture site, such as nerves or blood vessels
- to provide pain relief
- to reduce blood loss
- to reduce the risk of fat emboli
- to facilitate extrication and rescue.

PREVENTION OF FURTHER INJURY

Appropriate immobilization of a fracture will reduce the risk of damage to adjacent structures including nerves, blood vessels, muscles and skin due to movement of bone ends. Occasionally, reduction of a fracture will be necessary in order to reduce pressure on one or more of these structures from displaced bone (e.g. potential skin necrosis secondary to complex displaced ankle fractures).

PAIN RELIEF

Immobilization of a fracture reduces painful movement of bone ends as well as irritation of the sensitive periosteum. It may also reduce painful spasm in adjacent muscle groups. In the case of some fractures, immobilization may relieve local painful pressure on a nerve.

REDUCTION OF BLOOD LOSS

Traction splintage of long bone fractures of the lower limbs reduces the internal volume of the affected part of the leg and thus reduces the volume available for haematoma formation. In addition, it acts to close large venous channels by restoring muscle tension, thus reducing bleeding further.

REDUCTION OF FAT EMBOLI

Immobilization of fractures reduces the incidence and magnitude of fat emboli, which occur when marrow fat enters the venous circulation. An additional theory suggests that fat emboli occur as a consequence of biochemical changes in circulating chylomicrons.

FACILITATION OF EXTRICATION AND RESCUE

This is discussed in detail below. When applying immobilization techniques it must be remembered that, if possible, the fracture site should be supported on either side of the fracture rather than directly over the fracture site, and that the joints above and below the injury should be immobilized.

All open fractures must be surgically explored and cleaned. If the fracture was reduced at the scene then it is mandatory to ensure that the receiving doctor is completely aware that the fracture was open. (If possible, take a photograph before manipulating the leg or applying a dressing.)

The principles of equipment design suggest that the equipment should be:

- simple
- easy to use
- lightweight
- easily cleaned following use
- damage-proof.

In addition, the equipment used in the prehospital and hospital settings should be interchangeable and should be familiar to both groups of personnel. New equipment or modifications to existing equipment should only be introduced after appropriate training. Equipment needed for immobilization and extrication purposes should be designed in such a way that it will not prevent any immediately necessary treatment or procedure from being performed.

Basic principles of extrication

Entrapment is relatively common in high-speed road traffic accidents but can also be encountered in industrial, recreational, aircraft, rail, farming or domestic incidents. In dealing with the trapped casualty the prehospital worker's role is vital. The time-specific responses previously mentioned cannot always be applied when casualties are trapped but the concept of the 'golden hour' is still important and therefore the medical priorities must be determined at a very early stage.

It is important that early consultation takes place between all the emergency services working at the scene to establish the priorities. It must be appreciated that this involvement may include the hospital staff, first to alert them of the possible problem so that they may be prepared and second to seek their help if extra equipment or skills are required. If a casualty is not trapped but has a time-critical injury or the environment is hazardous, a snatch rescue may be needed with minimal preceding medical intervention.

DEFINITIONS

Entrapment itself may be:

- actual
- relative.

Actual entrapment

Actual entrapment occurs when victims are physically enclosed or held in a vehicle or area by the structure impinging on their body (examples include a deformed vehicle following a road traffic accident, a roof fall following a mining or caving accident, building collapse following an explosion or bomb blast where masonry may be lying on the casualty).

Relative entrapment

Relative entrapment occurs when the victim's condition renders him/her unable to be extricated. The physical environment may play an important role in the entrapment. No actual physical entrapment is present. Examples include the fitting patient at the top of winding stairs, the victim of a traffic accident with pain due to a fractured femur.

PREPARATION AND APPROACH

Preparation includes training, and a knowledge of the rescue teams and other services. It is important to know the equipment they carry and their potential. Personal equipment must be regularly checked and in working order, and drugs in date.

Each group of professionals must recognize their own limitations and know how they can assist the other emergency services. In the case of the fire service, this may mean giving early access to medical workers to stabilize the casualty. It may then be possible for the medical workers to stand back, perhaps monitoring the casualty remotely through pulse oximetry and non-invasive blood pressure monitoring, while other aspects of the rescue take place.

Working with a trapped casualty is one of the most challenging and rewarding areas for prehospital personnel: it is noisy, dangerous and difficult, and is not without risk to the rescue worker. Strong team bonds can be formed in such rescue situations.

PAIN RELIEF

Although applying traction to an injured lower limb may in itself give significant pain relief to a casualty, it should be clearly borne in mind that moving injured limbs or extricating casualties may produce pain. Unless the patient's life is in danger and a snatch rescue is necessary, extrication should be performed in a controlled manner. Appropriate pain relief should always be given before attempting a potentially painful extrication. Methods include Entonox, titrated intravenous analgesia, ketamine and local blocks.

Methods of immobilization

The ability to adapt and improvise is the hallmark of the prehospital care provider. Any device that immobilizes a fracture or suspected fracture is a splint. These may at times include rolled newspaper, canes or broom handles, the casualty's body or commercially produced splints. These methods are discussed below.

Cervical immobilization

MANUAL IMMOBILIZATION

Approach from behind

This situation commonly occurs in road traffic accidents, with the rescuer approaching the casualty from the rear seat. The rescuer places his hands on either side of the neck with the thumbs pointing upwards; the other fingers will point forward and will naturally encase the neck and cervical spine, reaching to the lower jaw, which can be controlled, giving airway support.

Approach from in front

This might be necessary, for example, when immobilization is only possible through the shattered front windscreen of a car. The rescuer places his hands round the casualty's neck so that the little fingers pass behind the neck of the casualty. The other fingers will lie over the sides of the face and neck (taking care not to block the ears) and the thumbs can then hook behind the angle of the jaw, pushing it forward if necessary.

Approach from the side

The cervical spine can be immobilized from the side but it is essential that the casualty does not attempt to turn his head towards the rescuer. The rescuer places one hand behind the casualty's neck in such a way that the palm of the hand lies over the cervical spine at the base of the skull. The fingers are then fanned out to support the occiput. The other hand is placed under the lower jaw.

When handing over cervical spine immobilization between rescuers there are two ways in which this move can be safely achieved. Either the second rescuer places his/her own hands exactly over the first rescuer's hands and then the first rescuer removes his/her hands, or alternatively, the second rescuer may place his/her fingers between those of the first rescuer and when in control allow the first rescuer to remove his/her own hands.

CERVICAL COLLARS

Any casualty with an injury above the clavicle, or who is unconscious or who has sustained a mechanism of injury likely to result in cervical spine damage must be assumed to have sustained a cervical spine injury. This statement highlights the problem of the cervical spine injury and has, it might be argued, led to a degree of overemphasis on the possibility of cervical spine injury in recent years. It must be accepted that full cervical spine immobilization can delay patient extrication and transfer to definitive care. A sensible decision must therefore be taken regarding the possibility of cervical spine injury. In general, if the patient is fully conscious and if there is no neck pain or tenderness, no complaint of paraesthesia and neck movements are not restricted, cervical immobilization is not necessary.

In the prehospital setting it is necessary to place considerable reliance on the mechanism of injury in deciding whether to apply a collar. It is better to assume a cervical spine injury than to put the casualty's wellbeing at risk. The head is held and moved to the neutral in-line position unless this results in increased pain, results in any tingling in the arms of the patient or is met with physical resistance suggestive of a facet joint dislocation. If the neck cannot be moved into a neutral position, a collar cannot be applied and the neck must be immobilized as effectively as possible, usually by manual in-line stabilization in the best achievable position. Once manual stabilization is in place, a cervical collar can be applied. Cervical collars do not completely immobilize the cervical spine but they do reduce the potential for neck movement. Manual stabilization is still required after a collar has been fitted (Liew & Hill 1994).

The collar should be correctly sized. Inappropriate collar size will either be ineffective or potentially dangerous (Blaylock 1991), particularly in the unconscious (Dodd et al 1995). There is strong evidence that cervical collars increase intracranial pressure (Craig & Nielson 1991, Raphael & Chotai 1994). However, this observation is not relevant in prehospital care providing transport times are relatively short. Following any manoeuvre involving the head and cervical spine or the application of a collar, the casualty should be reassessed in order to ensure that there have been no changes in his/her neurological status.

Two types of collar are in general use (although many types have been evaluated (Podolsky et al 1983), the NecLoc® collar and Stifneck®, both being widely used by doctors and the ambulance services. Both these collars are available in a range of sizes. More recently, a number of collars, such as the Sure-loc®, that are adjustable over a range of neck sizes have been introduced.

The Stifneck® is a single-piece collar and comes in a range of sizes. The method of sizing a collar is important. The key dimension on a casualty is the distance between an imaginary line drawn across the top of the shoulder where the collar will sit and a parallel line running backwards from the tip of the chin. It can be difficult at times to determine these points but in doing so the head should be in a neutral position. The measurement is usually made using the fingers of the rescuer. The collar is then sized using the distance between the sizing post and the lower edge of the rigid plastic encircling band, which should accommodate the same number of fingers (Fig. 54.1).

The selected collar is formed by inserting the fastener into the hole and is then gently flexed or rolled to aid application and pliability. Depending on the position of the casualty, the front piece is applied under the chin, or if the casualty is supine the rear piece is slid behind the casualty's neck before the front piece is brought up under the

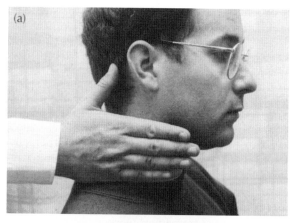

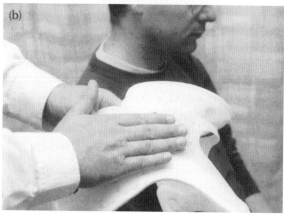

Fig. 54.1 • Sizing a Stifneck® collar. (Reproduced with permission of Medekit.com.)

chin. Finally, the Velcro strap is firmly fastened. The rescuer holding the neck in the neutral position may have to adjust his/her hand position but should not let go, so maintaining neutral alignment throughout the procedure.

The NecLoc® collar (Fig. 54.2) comes in a number of sizes. Each collar has two parts, a front and rear portion. The correctly sized collar should rest on the casualty's shoulders and the casualty's chin should sit comfortably in the chin support. There is a sizing strip on each collar and the upper border of the sizing strip should extend to but not above the line of the bottom of the chin. The front half is applied first. With the correctly sized front half in place, the Velcro strap is passed round the back of the neck and loosely attached to the other side of the front half. The rear piece (similar colour code) is placed behind the casualty's head and, after it has been centred, the two sides are folded round the neck and attached to the front half with Velcro straps.

The best method of cervical spine immobilization is a combination of a cervical collar together with a long board or similar device and this will be discussed later.

Recent work looking at the optimal position for cervical immobilization suggests that in healthy adults a slight

degree of flexion, equivalent to 2 cm of occiput elevation, produces a favourable increase in spinal canal/spinal cord ratio at the level C5 and C6, a region of frequent unstable spine injures (De Lorenzo et al 1996).

Recently, a number of collars have been marketed that obviate the need to carry a series of sizes in order to fit the full range of adults. In general, these collars have an adjustable chin piece, allowing them to be fitted to an individual patient.

VACUUM SPLINTS

Vacuum splints have been developed to fit around the neck. When a vacuum is applied they form a very rigid support to the neck. Rosen et al (1992) suggested that they provide the most effective restriction of the cervical spine.

Limb immobilization

SIMPLE METHODS

Slings for the upper arm can be improvised using the casualty's clothing (the arm may be tucked into a jacket). The lower half of a jacket or jersey can be folded over an injured arm and either buttoned or pinned in such a way as to support the arm. Ties and scarves can also be used as improvised slings.

Alternatively, a tabloid newspaper rolled around a forearm provides an effective temporary splint. Simple methods for immobilization of the lower limbs include tying shoe laces together, improvised padding with clothing and using a tie or scarf to secure the injured to the non-injured limb.

MANUAL METHODS

The casualty may support an injured arm or hold the chest wall over a fractured rib. A rescuer may at times support a damaged limb before a more formal splint or means of support is applied. The most widely used method of manual immobilization or stabilization is that for the cervical spine (see above).

TRIANGULAR BANDAGE

To provide simple prehospital care for upper limb injuries, the triangular bandage, the mainstay for many years of the first-aid societies, offers the easiest method available. The triangular bandage as described by Esmarck is made from calico. It can be used as a conventional broad arm sling, a high arm sling or a collar and cuff sling. When tying the ends of a triangular bandage that is being used as a sling, it is best to use a reef knot, as this will tend to lie flat and, most importantly, will not slip.

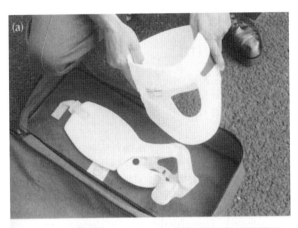
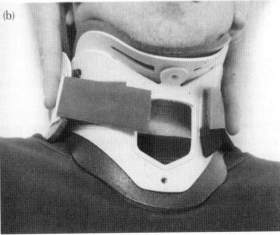

Fig. 54.2 • Stifneck® and NecLoc® collars. (Reproduced with permission of Medekit.com and Jerome Medical.)

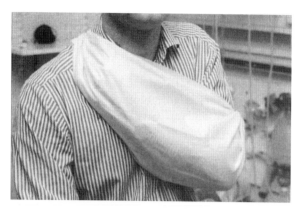

Fig. 54.3 • The high arm sling.

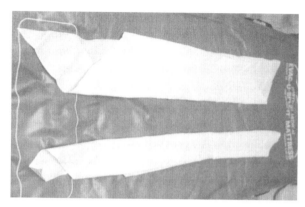

Fig. 54.4 • Forming broad and narrow bandages from a triangular bandage.

A *broad arm sling* rests the limb with the elbow at a right angle. The sling supports the whole arm, including the wrist. When the sling is being applied, the casualty supports the injured arm and the triangular bandage is passed between the injured limb and the body, with the right angle towards the elbow. The sling is then passed over the arm and the two ends are tied around the neck. The point of the triangular bandage is then secured to the bandage in front of the elbow using a safety pin or tape.

A *high arm sling* supports the limb with the hand raised towards the opposite shoulder. Again, it is important that the hand does not dangle out of the sling so causing pressure at the wrist. To apply a high sling, the casualty places the fingers of the injured arm over the opposite clavicle while supporting the injured arm at the elbow with the opposite hand. The triangular bandage is then placed over the injured arm with the 90° corner to the elbow and the long axis parallel to the patient's forearm. The free edge is tucked under the forearm for support and the lower corner is then brought under the arm and passed behind the casualty's shoulder and tied to the free end of the sling behind the neck. The 90° corner is secured to the front of the sling (Fig. 54.3).

A broad or narrow bandage formed from a broad arm sling by simple folding (Fig. 54.4) can be used to bind the legs together in association with other forms of support, or to hold a wound dressing in place including injuries to a hand or scalp. Alternatively, they can be used to augment the immobilization of a humerus fracture in conjunction with a broad arm sling.

FRAC STRAPS®

These commercially available straps that fasten with Velcro can be used to fasten one leg to another or immobilize an arm to the side of the chest.

NEIGHBOUR STRAPPING

Injured fingers may be bound to the fingers on either side or a lower limb may be bound to the other limb in order to provide support. In the latter case, this may allow a casualty to be moved to a less precarious situation, at which point a more appropriate form of immobilization may be applied.

INFLATABLE SPLINTS

These splints are clear plastic, double-walled tubes that come in two sizes, one for an arm and a longer one for legs. When produced it was thought that they would be used to treat fractures of the lower limb below the knee and upper limb below the elbow (Inflatable splints 1966), but it has become evident that they have little to contribute to fracture management. However, they still retain a use in the treatment of soft tissue injury.

The injured limb is slid into the inflatable splint and the splint is inflated. This should only be done by the rescuer blowing up the splint like a balloon (Shakespeare et al 1984). Under no circumstances should any pump or compressor be used to inflate the splint, as this can lead to tissue ischaemia (Christensen et al 1986). Because they are clear plastic, any wound can be observed, as can the circulation of the limb. Because they are stored folded, these splints often crack or perish and tend to leak. The pressure should therefore be regularly checked following application. Inflatable splints are also vulnerable to damage from sharp objects.

THE BOX SPLINT (LOXLEY SPLINT)

This is a simple device that consists of three long, padded pieces of board joined to form an open oblong together with a foot support at one end (Fig. 54.5). Where possible,

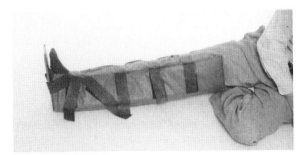

Fig. 54.5 • A box splint.

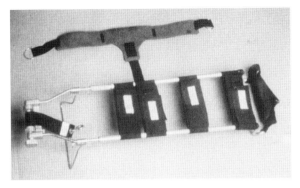

Fig. 54.6 • Hare traction splint.

the casualty's footwear should be removed (although pain and time may prevent this) and any wounds dressed before the splint is applied. The injured leg is placed in the splint. The foot support holds the foot at right angles and the outer sides of the splint are folded round the leg. Velcro straps are fixed across the leg, holding the outer sides of the splint tight. The foot support is then fixed again using Velcro straps. Care must be taken to attach the Velcro straps to the attached Velcro pads.

This splint comes in two sizes, suitable for adults and children. After the splint has been applied, care of the limb includes checking the distal pulses. A watchful eye must also be kept on the splint to ensure that blood from any wound does not gather unnoticed within the splint.

Some box splints have a side pocket into which a long wooden board can be inserted forming a long leg splint suitable for immobilizing a fractured femur. The limb is secured to the long wooden board using triangular bandages or Frac Straps®.

SAM® SPLINT

The SAM® splint is built from a thin core of aluminum alloy, sandwiched between two layers of closed-cell foam. Freshly unrolled from storage, the splint is extremely pliable. Bent into any of three simple curves, it becomes extremely strong and supportive for any fractured or injured limb. It is extremely mouldable and soft enough to cut with ordinary household scissors. Additional benefits of the SAM® splint are:

- Waterproof
- Lightweight and compact
- Radiolucent
- Can be rolled or folded for easy storage in emergency kits/backpacks
- Fastens in place with tape or wrap
- Not affected by extreme temperatures or altitudes – even works underwater!
- Reusable

- Closed-pore, impermeable foam surface allows easy cleaning and disinfection. Material is compatible with all standard cleaning solutions
- Will not puncture.

Traction splints

THE HARE TRACTION SPLINT

The Hare and Trac III traction splints are very similar and can be considered together; both splints can be used with traction to maintain a reduced fracture of the lower limb or without traction for support (Fig. 54.6).

Indications

With traction:

- Closed and open fractures of the femoral shaft
- Closed and open fractures of the shafts of the tibia and fibula.

Without traction:

- Fractures around the knee.

Contraindications to traction

These are:

- Dislocation of the hip
- Fracture dislocation of the knee
- Ankle injuries.

Simple undisplaced fracture of the lower third of the tibia and fibula may be better immobilized with a box splint.

Function of the traction splint

The primary function of the traction splint is to immobilize the fracture in a reduced position. This will greatly reduce the patient's pain but, more importantly, will also prevent further neurovascular damage, reduce the severity of shock by reducing blood loss and reduce the likelihood of significant fat embolism.

Application

Correct application of the splint requires two people. This splint can only be applied after extrication from a vehicle.

1. Appropriate analgesia should be given before the splint is applied.
2. With open fractures, external haemorrhage should be controlled. Routine exposure of the fracture site is not necessary.
3. Footwear should be removed (otherwise it may be pulled off by the splint after the application of traction) and the neurovascular status of the injured limb assessed.
4. The appropriate ankle hitch is selected and the splint is adjusted for length against the normal leg. The straps are opened and placed at the correct intervals down the splint. Some of the traction strap is unwound.
5. The hitch is placed under the ankle and the straps are then tightly folded across the front of the ankle and the rings are brought together below the foot.
6. Manual traction is started with one hand. The leg is supported while the splint is put in position. Circumstances will dictate to an extent how this is done, but the best method is to roll the patient away from the splint and then slide the splint under the patient. The top padded ring must fit under the ischial tuberosity. The patient is then rolled back on to the splint. Manual traction must be maintained throughout this procedure.
7. The top strap is then done up, avoiding the external genitalia.
8. The traction hook is then put through the D rings and traction is taken up, ensuring that manual traction is not released before the traction is tightened. Traction is applied until the limb is comfortable. The neurovascular examination is repeated.
9. The leg is elevated by raising the foot stand and the Velcro straps are positioned and tightened.

The neurovascular status of the limb should be regularly reassessed following application of the splint, and the straps checked and loosened if swelling occurs. The tension of the traction should be reassessed, as reduced spasm in the muscles can result in tension being lost.

The two splints have slightly different release mechanisms. In both cases, manual traction is first applied, after removal of the Velcro straps. The Hare splint has a pull ring that releases the traction suddenly, whereas the Trac III has a knob that has to be unwound to release the traction and is less likely to be accidentally released, as well as allowing a more controlled release of traction.

Complications

The only significant complication that can occur is damage to the neurovascular supply to the leg. This can be prevented by careful and repeated examination of the distal limb function. These splints can result in pressure sores in patients with sensory loss.

Absence or changes in distal function must be reported to the hospital emergency department. If it is found that the distal pulses diminish or are absent after traction has been applied, the tightness of the straps should be checked in case circumferential occlusion has occurred and, if this is not the case, under manual control, traction is reduced until the pulse returns. The use of an oximeter can detect alterations in the blood flow if the probe is placed on one of the toes of the fractured leg, but the reading should be compared with a reading from an uninjured limb.

Because these splints extend beyond the casualty's foot there may be problems with certain forms of transport if the space around the casualty is limited.

SAGER® TRACTION SPLINT

The Sager® traction splint, weighing less than 1.3 kg, can be used to treat single or bilateral fractures of the lower limb, especially of the femur (Fig. 54.7). The Sager® can be applied with the patient in any position so long as the leg can be straightened. A further advantage is that the splint does not extend beyond the end of the casualty's leg following application. For all these reasons, the Sager® traction splint is perhaps the splint of choice in many prehospital settings.

Method of application

1–3. Follow steps 1–3 for the Hare splint, above.

4. The cushioned end of the splint is placed between the patient's legs against the perineum and symphysis pubis,

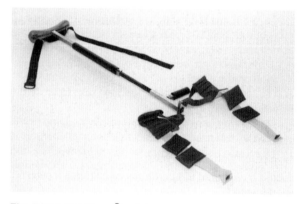

Fig. 54.7 • The Sager® splint.

avoiding the external genitalia. The S strap is fastened around the top of the thigh of the injured leg.

5. The splint is extended so that the ankle hitch lies at the normal heel position.

6. The ankle harness is applied behind the heel and wrapped around the malleoli, adjusting the cushions on the strap to fit the size of the leg.

7. The traction is applied until the patient is comfortable (recommended at 10% of body weight) and the leg cravats are applied.

8. The bridle around the thigh is tightened if necessary and the cravats are secured. The neurovascular status is reassessed.

The same method is used if the splint is being applied to bilateral fractured femurs.

To release the traction, manual traction is applied and the cravats are removed. Along the shaft of the splint there is a small, sprung piece of metal, which is lifted to release the tension in the splint.

DONWAY SPLINT

This splint is used to treat fractures of the lower limb and employs a pneumatic method to provide the traction force. It is a relatively lightweight splint that comes in two halves (upper and lower) and is packed into a neat carrying case. It can only be applied to one leg and, as it protrudes beyond the patient's foot, may not be compatible with some ambulance designs (Fig. 54.8).

Application

1–3. Follow steps 1–3 for the Hare splint, above.

4. The ischial ring component is slipped under the thigh and the strap and buckle are loosely fitted around the front.

5. The lower end of the splint is checked (by depressing the air release valve) to ensure that there is no pressure

in the system and the locking screws are unlocked. The footplate is raised and the splint is passed under the leg so that the casualty's foot rests on the foot support. The splint is attached to the ischial ring. The side arms from the lower end are extended trombone-fashion.

6. The casualty's foot is then strapped to the footplate using the side straps and the figure of eight straps provided. As a result, when traction is applied the pull should be through the whole foot along the axis of the leg.

7. The pump is then used to apply pneumatic pressure. The operating range of the splint is 10–40 lb. Enough pressure is applied to make the casualty comfortable (again, approximately 10% body weight). Manual traction should be applied and maintained until the pneumatic traction has taken over.

8. The supports are now positioned under the limb at mid-thigh and mid-calf. Finally, the knee support is secured.

9. The stand can now be lowered, the limb rechecked and the tension adjusted. The locking nuts (collets) are now turned into the locked position and the pressure is released from the system by depressing the air-release valve.

If at any time it is necessary to adjust the tension then the system should be repressurized and manual traction applied while the adjustment is made. A paediatric version of this splint is available.

Pneumatic antishock garment

The pneumatic antishock garment (PASG), originally known as the MAST (military antishock trousers), is an inflatable garment that surrounds the legs and abdomen. Following a Cochrane review of the evidence supporting its use, it was found that it is associated with a worse outcome (Dickinson & Roberts 2004) and is therefore no longer recommended for routine use. Indeed, in a survey of all 31 ambulance services in the UK (Roberts et al 2003), none routinely carry this piece of equipment.

Extrication devices

There are a number of different types of extrication device available. In current use are the Kendrick extrication device (KED), the Russell extrication device (RED; Fig. 54.9) and the ED2000. These have replaced the short wooden board, which was always difficult to use and became increasingly so as car seats became shaped (Howell et al 1989).

These devices are used to provide support and stabilization to the upper spine. Manual in-line cervical stabilization should be performed, followed by the application of a cervical collar; an extrication device will then allow the patient to be moved more easily.

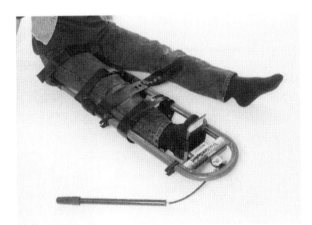

Fig. 54.8 • The Donway splint.

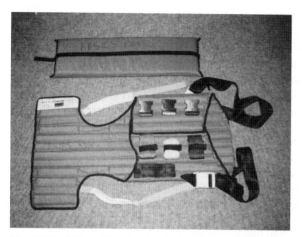

Fig. 54.9 • A Russell extrication device (RED)

These devices all have a similar method of application but each has its own particular characteristics. The devices are, to an extent, flexible and can be positioned between the casualty and the seat, being passed behind the casualty, ensuring that the various straps do not become snagged or tangled in any wreckage. The device is then positioned correctly in relationship to the casualty's head and shoulders.

The wings of the device are drawn around the sides of the casualty's chest and are then tightened using the straps (the matching straps are colour-coded). The wings must be applied carefully so as not to cause any respiratory embarrassment. The leg straps are passed under the casualty's legs and then correctly fitted to the splint and tightened.

The shoulder straps are placed across the body and fixed to the opposite side of the device. Care must be taken that these straps do not interfere with the cervical collar. Finally, the head straps are applied, after making sure that any space behind the neck or head is filled with an appropriately sized pad supplied with the device. These will hold the head and cervical spine firmly, allowing manual immobilization to be withdrawn. All straps are rechecked for tightness and adjusted accordingly before the casualty is lifted out of the vehicle. As the casualty is placed on a trolley or vacuum mattress, the leg straps will have to be loosened to allow the legs to lie flat.

SCOOP STRETCHER

The scoop stretcher provides a means of lifting a patient on to a trolley or trolley cot. It is not designed for the transfer of patients over long distances. The scoop stretcher can be split into two halves longitudinally. The length of the stretcher can be adjusted according to the height of the patient by pulling the lower portion of the splint further out of the upper portion.

The scoop should be laid beside the casualty and extended to the required length. The two halves in turn are slid underneath the casualty, taking care not to pinch the casualty

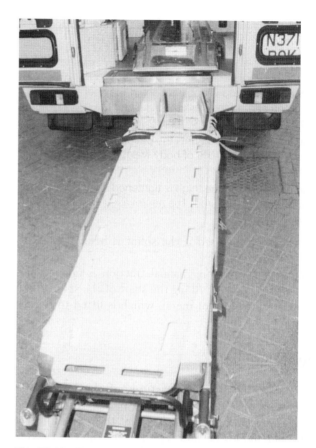

Fig. 54.10 • The long spinal board.

between them. The casualty may have to be rolled slightly to allow the half stretcher underneath. The pelvis may have to be lifted to allow the two halves to lock together.

Once the patient is on the stretcher and the two halves are locked together, the head cushion is secured and the casualty can then be lifted on to the trolley cot.

Once the casualty is on a trolley, the scoop stretcher should be removed to prevent pressure sores developing, unless travel time is short and a further lift may be needed at the hospital from the trolley cot on to the accident service trolley.

The other use of a scoop stretcher is to allow a casualty to be turned over. A scoop stretcher is placed underneath the casualty and a second scoop is placed on top, forming a sandwich with the casualty in between the two scoops. The two stretchers are tied together and the casualty can be lifted and rolled over before the scoops are untied and removed.

LONG SPINAL BOARDS

Long spinal boards are used to assist in the movement (extrication) of patients from an accident scene. They provide a secure stable base on to which a patient may be strapped, so providing spinal stabilization (Fig. 54.10).

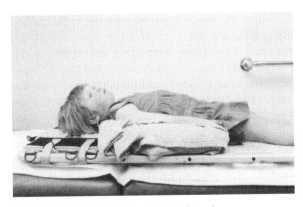

Fig. 54.11 • A child on a long spinal board.

A long spinal board requires a minimum of four operators if a patient needs to be carried any distance.

Despite concern that patients may develop pressure sores from prolonged use of spinal boards (Cordell et al 1995, Walton et al 1995), they still provide the best form of protection in the prehospital field (Chan et al 1994). However, it is possible that vacuum mattresses may provide an alternative method of spinal protection with improved casualty comfort (Chan et al 1996, Johnson et al 1996).

A spinal board may be used to secure and move a casualty who is on the ground, to assist in the extrication of a casualty or, if time is a critical factor, to extricate a casualty rapidly from a vehicle.

The use of a long spinal board requires teamwork. If the patient is being extricated using a long spinal board, the board can be placed behind the patient and the patient lowered on to it, or it can be passed through the door of a vehicle to the side of the patient so that the patient is carefully rotated and lowered on to the board.

If the board is not being used for extrication, the casualty may be rolled on to it or lifted on to it using a scoop stretcher.

Manual in-line cervical stabilization will be required until the casualty is secured to the board.

Once the patient is on the board, the head should be supported in a head immobilizer using the head straps provided. The straps on the board are applied according to the manufacturer's instructions.

If a child is placed on a long board, because of the relatively larger size of the child's head, a pad may be required underneath the shoulders to prevent any forward flexion of the neck (Huerta et al 1987, Herzenberg et al 1989, Curran et al 1995; Fig. 54.11). Before a patient is placed on a long spinal board, all articles that might cause the development of pressure sores should be removed.

If transport times are likely to be long, consideration should be given to transferring the patient from a long spinal board to vacuum mattress or trolley cot after extrication. Use of a scoop stretcher will facilitate this.

Log rolling

Log rolling is a method of turning a casualty without compromising the spine. To perform a log roll, a minimum of four people are needed.

The casualty should, if possible, have his arms by his sides with the palms placed against the legs, but if this is not possible then the arms should be placed across the abdomen. It is essential to keep the whole spine in alignment, and to achieve this the cervical spine is stabilized by the team leader and the casualty is moved keeping the neck, shoulders and pelvis in the same plane (McGuire et al 1987).

A second person holds the casualty's further shoulder and arm and a third person the patient's pelvis, while the fourth person takes the legs, placing one hand under the opposite thigh and the other on the opposite shin. When all are ready the person at the head calls the instructions and the whole body of the casualty is rolled over, ensuring that the spine does not twist. The amount of roll is kept to a minimum, allowing enough movement to inspect the back or insert a long board underneath the casualty. The patient is then rolled back on the command of the team leader. The patient can be rolled back on to the spinal board or the board can be applied to the back of the patient. Whichever method is used, the board must be held firmly by a further rescuer.

Rapid extrication

Access to a casualty trapped in a vehicle is obtained either by springing the front door of the car, by removing the roof of the vehicle or through the rear window, or, if the car is a hatchback, through the rear hatch. If the roof of the car has been removed, the long board can be slid behind the casualty.

Approaching from the side, one person maintains in-line cervical stabilization from behind the casualty. A second person applies a cervical collar while the third brings the long board, which is placed firmly on to the seat under the casualty. If room is tight then the long board should not be put under the patient until later in the procedure.

The casualty's feet and legs are then freed. The first rescuer maintains manual in-line cervical stabilization. The third rescuer should be beside the casualty ready to lift the casualty's legs across the other seat. The second rescuer assumes the command of all movements and places one hand on the mid-thoracic spine and the other on the sternum of the casualty.

The second rescuer uses both hands to sense any twisting of the casualty's spine and directs the movement of the casualty. The legs are swung on to the seat so that the casualty's back faces the open door. Depending on the position moulded around the injured part. Suction is then applied to the bag, creating a vacuum, and the contents of the splint take up a rigid form, supporting and splinting the injured part or body.

Vacuum splints can be used to immobilize the limbs, the cervical spine and other spinal injuries (Hamilton & Pons 1996). The vacuum mattress is laid on to the trolley and the casualty is laid on the mattress, which is then secured around the casualty's body using Velcro straps or a continuous webbing strap. The mattress is actively moulded around the casualty. Care must be taken to support the head as the mattress is moulded around the casualty's neck and head. The rescuer's hands should be carefully moved to support the casualty's head through the upper portion of the mattress.

A vacuum is then created inside the mattress using the suction pump provided. The mattress will conform to the casualty and provide whole body support (Fig. 54.12). The valve mechanism is secured and the pump is removed.

The splint can be removed by opening the valve and allowing air into the mattress. A vacuum mattress is a good immobilization device but is not a lifting device.

References

Blaylock B 1991 Solving the problem of pressure ulcers resulting from cervical collars. Ostomy Wound Management 42: 26–33

Chan D, Goldberg R, Tascone A et al 1994 The effect of spinal immobilisation on health volunteers. Annals of Emergency Medicine 23: 48–51

Chan D, Golberg RM, Mason J, Chan L 1996 Backboard versus mattress splint immobilisation: a comparison of symptoms generated. Journal of Emergency Medicine 14: 293–298

Christensen KS, Trautner S, Stockel M, Nielsen JF 1986 Inflatable splints, do they cause tissue ischaemia? Injury 17: 167–170

Cordell WH, Hollingsworth JC, Olinger ML 1995 Pain and tissue interface pressures during spine board immobilisation. Annals of Emergency Medicine 26: 31–36

Craig GR, Nielson MS 1991 Rigid cervical collars and intracranial pressure. Intensive Care Medicine 17: 504–505

Curran C, Dietrich AM, Bowman MJ 1995 Paediatric cervical spine immobilisation achieving neutral position. Journal of Trauma 39: 729–732

De Lorenzo RA, Olson JE, Boska M et al 1996 Optimal positioning for cervical immobilisation. Annals of Emergency Medicine 28: 301–308

Dickinson K, Roberts I 2004 Medical anti-shock trousers (pneumatic anti-shock garments) for circulatory support in patients with trauma (Cochrane Review). The Cochrane Library, Issue 3, 2006. John Wiley, Chichester

Dodd FM, Simon E, McKeown D, Patrick MR 1995 The effects of a cervical collar on the tidal volume of anaesthetized adult patients. Anaesthesia 49: 437–439

Hamilton RS, Pons PT 1996 The efficacy and comfort of full body vacuum splints for cervical spine immobilisation. Journal of Emergency Medicine 14: 553–559

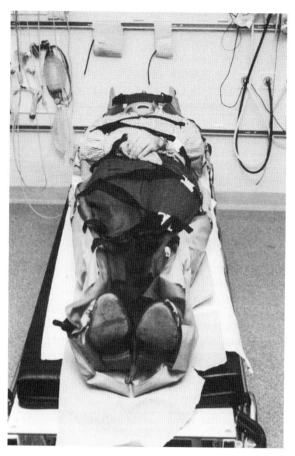

Fig. 54.12 • A vacuum mattress.

of the first rescuer, another rescuer may have to control the casualty's neck while the first rescuer negotiates the door post.

Once the casualty is sitting across the front seat the long board, if not already in place, is pushed well under the casualty's buttocks and the casualty is lowered on to the board. The casualty is then slid in small movements up the board. To achieve this, rescuer 1 maintains in-line cervical stabilization. Rescuer 2 places his hands in the casualty's armpits and rescuer 3 steadies the patient's hips, pelvis and legs. Once the casualty is on the long board he can then be moved from the immediate area. He can then be properly stabilized on the long board.

Vacuum splints and mattresses

Vacuum splints provide rigid support to the body and can be very comfortable. They are bags of polystyrene beads enclosed in tough plastic. The injured limb or the whole patient can be placed on to the splint, which is actively

Herzenberg JE, Hensinger RN, Denrick DK, Phillips WA 1989 Emergency transport and positioning of young children who have an injury of the cervical spine. Journal of Bone and Joint Surgery 71: 15–22

Howell JM, Burrow R, Dumontier C, Hillyard A 1989 A practical radiographic comparison of short board technique and Kendrick extrication devices. Annals of Emergency Medicine 18: 943–946

Huerta C, Griffith R, Joyce SM 1987 Cervical spine stabilisation in paediatric patients: evaluation of current techniques. Annals of Emergency Medicine 16: 1121–1126

Inflatable splints 1966 Inflatable splints. Drug and Therapeutics Bulletin 4: 87–88

Johnson DR, Hauswald M, Stockhoff C 1996 Comparison of a vacuum splint device to a rigid backboard for spinal immobilisation. American Journal of Emergency Medicine 14: 369–372

Karbi OA, Caspari DA, Tator CH 1988 Extrication, immobilisation and radiologic investigation of patients with cervical spine injuries. Canadian Medical Association Journal 139: 617–621

Liew SC, Hill DA 1994 Complication of hard cervical collars in multi-trauma patients. Australian and New Zealand Journal of Surgery 64: 139–140

McGuire RA, Neville S, Green BA 1987 Spinal instability and log rolling manoeuvre. Journal of Trauma 27: 525–531

Podolsky S, Baraff LJ, Simon RR et al 1983 Efficacy of cervical spine immobilisation methods. Journal of Trauma 23: 461–465

Raphael JH, Chotai R 1994 Effects of the cervical collar on cerebro-spinal fluid pressure. Anaesthesia 49: 437–439

Roberts K, Allison KP, Porter KM 2003 A review of emergency equipment carried and procedures performed by UK front line paramedics. Resuscitation 58: 153–158

Rosen PB, McSwain NE Jr, Arata M et al 1992 Comparison of two new immobilisation collars. Annals of Emergency Medicine 21: 1189–1195

Shakespeare DT, Henderson NJ, Sherman KP 1984 Transmission of pressure into the human limb from pneumatic splints. Injury 16: 38–40

Walton R, DeSalvo JF, Ernst AA, Shahane A 1995 Padded vs unpadded spine board for spine immobilisation. Academic Emergency Medicine 2: 725–728

Transport in prehospital care

55

Introduction 568

Medical transport 568

Patient transfer vehicles 569

Summary 570

Further reading 571

Introduction

Transport in prehospital care is usually taken to refer to transport of a patient, but transport of staff to the site of the accident is of equal concern. It is essential that every doctor involved in prehospital care is aware of the law relating to travelling to an incident. Similarly, doctors need to understand the requirements for safe patient transfer in order to ensure the best possible outcomes for their patients.

Medical transport

Traditionally, prehospital care doctors have used their private motor vehicles to get them to the site of incidents. Originally, there was no identification of the doctor and no standard marking for cars. The first help through traffic was a flashing light that showed green to the front and red to the rear, devised by Dr Roger Snook of Bath. In 1976 the Road Traffic Act was amended to allow all registered medical practitioners proceeding to an emergency to use a rotating green beacon visible through 360°, supplemented with either grill-mounted or dashboard-mounted green strobes.

The question of an audible warning has been controversial, although some police forces have been prepared to allow immediate care doctors to use two-tone horns as a special dispensation. There is, however, no provision in the Road Traffic Act to support this. There has always been discussion as to whether it would be safer and more appropriate for doctors to use blue flashing lights. Under the current law this would be a contravention of the Road Traffic Act. However, in some areas, notably central London where there are problems of traffic and security, there is a special arrangement allowing doctors acting as agents of the ambulance service to use blue flashing lights when responding to calls. There is no universal permission for this and the London case cannot be used as a precedent.

The BASICS Equipment Committee has produced standards for the identification of immediate-care doctors' cars. These vary according to the number of calls attended and the other uses for the vehicle, and it is suggested that all doctors using their own private cars should use this system. Hospital flying squads have either had dedicated vehicles for their own use or rely on the ambulance service (or in some cases the police) for transport. The advantage of this is that it does allow a fully trained professional driver to be in charge of the vehicle. Since the inception of BASICS there have been concerns about the driving skills of immediate-care doctors, and many doctors have obtained qualifications through the Institute of Advanced Motorists or ad hoc advanced driving courses arranged by their local police or ambulance service. More recently BASICS itself has introduced a training course in conjunction with the Royal Society for the Prevention of Accidents.

In other parts of the world it is routine for doctors to attend the site of the accident. In Germany the *Notartz* is simultaneously mobilized with the ambulance service and will attend the incident with the aim of providing immediate care. A *Notartz* is only present during the transfer of the patient in about 30% of cases. In France the Service d'Aide Medicale Urgence (SAMU) has used motorcycles to transport the immediate care doctor to the site of accidents. An alternative approach in France, Germany and Switzerland is to deliver skilled medical aid to the site of the incident by helicopter and for only a relatively small percentage of cases to be transported by helicopter – the vast majority being treated by the helicopter doctors but transported by the ground ambulance.

Patient transfer vehicles

The ground ambulance was introduced in the early part of the last century, predominantly for the transfer of patients with infectious diseases. Following this, local authorities took on responsibility for the transport of patients to hospital. The attendants were local authority manual workers and were trained by the voluntary aid societies. As a result of the fragmentation, first of the local authorities and later of the ambulance services, there has never been a standard UK ambulance chassis design.

The development of ambulances has tended to run parallel with that of light vans, the traditional model being a light van chassis with a coach-built body. At one time, demountable bodies were popular, on the grounds that the chassis of the vehicles lasted less time than the coach-built body, but this has been superseded by a move towards conversions of commercial light vans. However, this raises a fundamental problem, in that the chassis was never designed for the problems of transporting sick patients. This was recognized early by Gissane and his co-worker Bothwell at the Birmingham Accident Hospital, who produced a prototype design for an ambulance, the most important advance in the design being the ability to lower the floor of the vehicle to the ground in order to facilitate access to the vehicle and patient handling. This design is now incorporated into many new front-line ambulances and patient transport service vehicles.

While there have been some improvements in ambulance design over the years, these have been mainly in the addition of extra equipment and redesign of cabin layout, which has greatly reduced the physical demands of patient loading and reduced the incidence of back injuries among ambulance service personnel.

The original specification for ambulance body design in the UK required that every ambulance should be capable of carrying two stretcher patients or six seated patients at all times. An inevitable consequence of this was that the stretchers were placed against the sides of the vehicle, reducing the access of attendants to the patients. More recently, this demand has been relaxed and the majority of emergency ambulances have a single centrally placed trolley.

Although this arrangement is ergonomically more sound, it still takes little account of the forces experienced by the patient, in particular the forces of acceleration and deceleration. Most road vehicles (and, indeed, aircraft) brake with a much higher G-force than they accelerate. If the patient is loaded head to the front then the maximum acceleration forces are directed toward the brain, increasing intercranial pressure. The human body is much more able to withstand acceleration directed towards the feet and therefore it would seem preferable for patients to be loaded into ambulances feet first, and for the attendant to sit by the rear doors. Unfortunately, this has the disadvantage that the necessity to have the loading doors at the rear means that it would not be possible for the attendant at the head end to have appropriate access to any necessary equipment. In addition, such an arrangement would make communication between the attendant and the driver much more difficult.

Vertical acceleration, when the vehicle goes over a pothole, is even more of a problem than deceleration. For this reason, in the ideal situation, the patient is accommodated within the area of the wheel base of the vehicle rather than over the rear suspension. Most ambulance vehicles have a suspension designed to function best at around 30 mph and there is therefore no justification for very slow transfers of patients with actual or suspected cervical spine injuries.

In a UK ambulance the are usually two ambulance personnel. As one has to drive, this only leaves one person to care for the patient. In complex situations an extra person may be needed in transport. Thus, in many cases immediate-care doctors should become part of the transport team accompanying the patient to hospital. This should improve the quality of care en route and also provides a much more effective handover for the patient in hospital. Current thinking on care of both trauma and cardiac patients would suggest that management should be confined to airway and breathing on scene but that cannulation should take place in the back of the ambulance en route to hospital.

It has taken many years to provide adequate lighting within ambulances but this is now occurring, with spotlights being common for interior lighting and also to illuminate the scene immediately surrounding the vehicle. Inadequate thought has been given to the restraint of patients, attendants and equipment within ambulances. The doctor who is not restrained within the vehicle must be careful to brace him/herself when performing procedures on the patient. Equally, any medical equipment needs to be carefully secured to prevent movement during transport. A particular problem in this respect are infusion fluids, which are often hung from hooks on the ceiling and develop a pendulum effect, making accurate control of flow rates difficult.

Motion and vibration effects on equipment and passengers must be considered. Many electrocardiogram monitors have cables that are very susceptible to picking up electromagnetic radiation and vibration. This interference can pose a particular risk if advisory defibrillators are to be used, and indeed there is evidence to suggest that if these are used then the vehicle must be stationary before defibrillation. In the same way as there is no standardization of ambulance bodies and chassis, there is similarly no standardization regarding equipment and it is therefore important that immediate-care practitioners check that their equipment, high-pressure oxygen connections and electrical connections are compatible with those of the transport vehicle.

The road ambulance does not always reflect the ideal method of transporting patients. In mountainous terrain the standard road ambulance may not have access or, frankly, may be dangerous. The mountain rescue service often uses four-wheel drive vehicles. In Lancashire, for example, there is an arrangement between the ambulance service and the mountain rescue service to make four-wheel drive vehicles available should the paramedics require them. In island areas, particularly in the Channel Islands, the use of ambulance launches operated by St John Ambulance personnel has been common, and the question of air transport is becoming more and more topical. This usually occurs in relation to helicopters, with many ambulance services either operating helicopters, as in Kent and Northumbria, or working with a multiservice helicopter, as in Lancashire, East Sussex and Wiltshire. The Helicopter Emergency Medical Service (HEMS) in London offers an alternative model for helicopter-based prehospital care.

Helicopters offer a convenient, although expensive, method of transporting patients. There may, however, be problems with landing sites, and most hospitals in the UK do not have dedicated helipads. When loading patients into helicopters it is necessary to be very aware of their dangers. These are discussed fully in Chapter 56. In particular, the helicopter must only be approached from a safe direction under the direct supervision of the pilot; the rear tail rotor is particularly dangerous and care must be taken with the downwash from the rotor causing flying debris. In mountainous areas or on soft ground it may not be possible to shut down the engine to load the patient, thus increasing the risk further. The lack of hospital helipads in many areas means that it is impossible to transfer the patient to the emergency department from the helipad, and there has to be liaison between the helicopter and a road ambulance, further delaying the transport of the patient. In mountainous areas and on the sea the question of winching patients has to be considered. Patients are usually lifted in a strop or on a Stokes litter. In a Sea King helicopter, the hover is usually some 75 m above the ground. The winchman has a trailing wire that acts as a static discharge for the aircraft, and under no circumstances should anyone on the ground touch this. The patient must be totally packaged prior to winching and particular attention must be paid to preserving the patient's body temperature, both in the winching phase and during transport, as helicopters tend to be draughty and cold.

In the UK fixed-wing aircraft are used on a relatively small scale, except in areas such as Scotland where they are used for both primary evacuation and secondary transfer. The advantage of fixed-wing aircraft over helicopters is their higher speed, smoothness and lower cost. Their main disadvantage is the necessity for an appropriate predetermined landing area, and the fact that secondary transfers by road ambulance will almost certainly be necessary at both ends of the journey.

Summary

The keys to successful patient transport as far as the immediate care practitioner is concerned, might be summarized as:

- an awareness of the limitations of the vehicle being used
- an awareness of the effects of the mode of transport on the patient
- an awareness of the effects of the mode of transport on the medical equipment being used during transfer
- an awareness of the effects of the mode of transport in limiting possible medical interventions
- an awareness of the importance of correct patient packaging, handling and loading.

If the immediate care doctor remains aware of all these factors and sees the provision of the best possible quality of patient care during transfer as a component of his/her responsibility, the outcome for the patient can only be improved.

Further reading

Fairhurst R, Ryan JH 1998 Principles of first aid for the injured. Trauma care. Butterworth Heinemann, London, ch 24

Tinker J, Browne DRG, Sibbald W 1966 Critical care standards audit and ethics. Edward Arnold, London, ch. 3

Aeromedical evacuation

56

Introduction 572

Fixed-wing operations 573

Rotary-wing operations 573

Indications for aeromedical evacuation 573

The clinical rationale for helicopters expanded 574

Funding and planning 575

Tasking 575

Medical crew configuration 575

Planning of missions 576

Clinical care en route 576

Equipment 576

Data collection 576

Regulation 576

Safety 577

At the scene 577

Landing sites 577

Choice of aircraft 577

Aircraft used in the UK 578

Hours of operation 579

Helicopter operations in the UK 579

The proof 579

References 580

Introduction

Often considered a North American or military institution, aeromedical evacuation or 'medevac' is an integral feature of health-care services in Europe, Asia, Russia, South America and Australasia (Passini 1997). The variety of activity is enormous, from commercial fixed-wing flights to access specialist medical care (e.g. a patient living on an island attending a mainland transplant clinic) to those with multiple injuries being airlifted by helicopter from the scene of a road traffic accident. In all cases the fundamental theme is to bring the patient closer to an appropriate level of medical care while minimizing the risks or problems en route. It is the unique ability of aircraft to reduce this gap between the medical problem and the appropriate treatment that allows aircraft to transform health-care delivery.

The aim of this chapter is to provide the reader with a rationale for aeromedical evacuation and give an insight into some of the operational issues that ensue. The focus is on helicopter retrieval, which forms the majority of aeromedical activity in the UK.

Table 56.1 Air ambulances in Scotland

- The Scottish ambulance service is one of the few British medevac operators funded from central government funds
- An air desk based in Aberdeen receives requests from doctors all over Scotland
- Aircraft from local coastguard and Ministry of Defence search and rescue aircraft are also used
- 2000 missions per year, of which 650 are for emergencies

Fixed-wing operations

For obvious reasons, fixed-wing aircraft (aeroplanes) are more common in areas such as North America and Australia, where distances are large, but even in the UK aeroplanes are used to move patients off coastal islands, such as the Isle of Man or Shetland, to mainland facilities. In some cases patients may simply use seats on commercial flights, in others a dedicated medical fit such as some of the aircraft used by the Scottish ambulance service (Table 56.1) may be required.

The need for a landing strip usually restricts the role of aeroplanes to secondary transfer work, although in some areas such as Australia fixed-wing aircraft have been used in primary transfers. Where operators have the facility of both helicopters and fixed-wing aircraft the distance threshold for using fixed-wing aircraft rather than rotary is in the region of 150 miles.

Repatriation of injured or sick visitors from abroad is another important role of fixed-wing aircraft. There are many repatriation organizations throughout the world, some with their own aircraft, others acting as medical agencies leasing aircraft when required. Funding for this work usually comes from holiday and health insurance cover. A full spectrum of medical care is provided, for the patient recovering from a myocardial infarction who returns on a commercial flight with a nurse escort or for the multiply injured, anaesthetized and ventilated patient transferred from a remote area in a developing country. Several companies in the UK provide such services but finding high-quality staff who are free to leave the country at 12 hours' notice and be gone for 5 or 6 days can be difficult. Consequently, the quality of escorts can, and does, vary enormously.

Rotary-wing operations

Unlike their fixed-wing counterparts, helicopters are well suited to both the primary and secondary roles. It is beyond the scope of this chapter to describe at length the enormous variation in helicopter operations throughout the world but it is important to have a feel for the different ways helicopters are employed.

In France a centrally funded helicopter system provides over 50 airbases nation-wide. Emergency calls are screened by a doctor, who decides the appropriate resource to send. If an aircraft is despatched it will carry a doctor to the scene of the incident. Scene time is not considered as important as getting the right patient to the right hospital facility. A similar situation is found in Germany (Earlam 1997).

In comparison, it is not unusual for a US aircraft to concentrate on secondary transfer work between hospital facilities. In 1996 a survey of 204 US hospital-based helicopter units showed 63% of activity to be interhospital transfer and 34% scene (primary) work (Mayfield and Lindstrom 1996). The flight crew would normally consist of a paramedic–paramedic or paramedic–nurse team. When used on primary (scene) work it was usually in response to a land-based crew requesting air support.

There are many reasons for such a wide variation but differences in workload and workforce infrastructure are fundamental. In the USA high volumes of penetrating injury requiring surgical care, particularly for vascular haemostasis, have focused medical input on the operating room. Where blunt trauma predominates (e.g. the UK and Europe) historically, an emphasis on reduced scene time has been considered less important.

Indications for aeromedical evacuation

The concept that aircraft should evacuate only specific sorts of 'critically ill' patient has dogged the acceptance of aircraft into health-care pathways for many years. All too often hospital clinicians or health-care purchasers have been 'outraged' because simple, non-life-threatening cases have been airlifted. It is important to understand that the term 'aeromedical evacuation' does not define a specific type or severity of disease where an aircraft should or should not be used. The decision to use an aircraft depends on many factors, including important system and patient factors.

THE PATIENT PERSPECTIVE

The primary reasons for using an aircraft for transporting a patient are clinical. Those responsible for care should have a firm understanding of the disease process, the rate at which deterioration may occur, the risks that may ensue en route and the time that will be required to reach the receiving unit.

For example, a patient with appendicitis may deteriorate over hours. Geographical isolation from appropriate medical care will compromise outcome. An aircraft can usefully reduce a journey of several hours by land or sea to minutes, minimizing the time to assessment and treatment. In this case moving a patient from an island off the coast of Scotland to a mainland surgical facility is a natural and humane choice. Other conditions deteriorate more rapidly. Outcome from a serious road traffic accident is quickly compromised by a flail chest, a tension pneumothorax or other ventilatory abnormalities. If death does not occur immediately it may ensue in days or weeks later from an initial oxygen debt accrued at the scene. Minimizing the time to time-critical interventions such as controlled ventilation and anaesthesia, thoracocentesis or removal of extradural haematoma is vital, and rapid transportation is essential in the delivery of these endpoints.

Where doctors are not part of the helicopter team, clinical indications for using an aircraft must be clearly defined by the responsible clinicians and despatch protocols defined. Sadly, in many areas in the UK, medical input into the use of aircraft is tenuous and limited to an advisory role.

THE SYSTEM PERSPECTIVE

Clinical urgency is not the only indication for using an aircraft: operational or logistical reasons are also important. This system perspective is often misunderstood by hospital clinicians and all too often causes unnecessary 'bad press' and fuels ill-informed debate. To understand the system perspective and why it might be necessary or indeed preferable to use a helicopter for minor injuries, a fundamental understanding of the provision of emergency medical services (ambulance services) is necessary.

In the UK, ambulance operators in rural areas are obliged to provide a response to all calls within 19 min. A fully staffed land-based ambulance costs in the region of £250 000 per vehicle per year; a *daylight* helicopter service may cost as little as £350 000 per year. The area covered in 19 min by a helicopter flying at 130 knots as the crow flies is far greater than that of an ambulance. To cover the same area the ambulance service would need many ambulances to meet the same response times.

Similarly, an aircraft can be moved to cover sickness or staffing shortages, and can offer the system an unrivalled degree of flexibility when trying to meet its statutory responsibilities. An aircraft can be used in the secondary transfer role. Using front-line ambulance vehicles and staff to do long-distance transfers may take a vehicle and crew out of their primary '999' role for up to a day. Occasionally, an overnight stop is required. An aircraft could carry out the same transfer and possibly several more in the same period. This allows the system to maximize its resources

for primary emergency responses and avoids the other economic costs of secondary transfers by ambulance, such as multiple police escorts and accommodation and wage costs.

The clinical rationale for helicopters expanded

Major trauma is the disease process that most UK aeromedical operators consider to be the primary target, and even in the urban environment there are compelling reasons for using helicopters.

The concept of the 'golden hour' is widely accepted; however, it is important to realize that much of this period is not a 'hospital event'. Even in the urban environment the time for a doctor to reach a multiply-injured patient has been documented in several studies as some 45 min (Nicholl et al 1995, London Ambulance Service 1997). Where patients are trapped by wreckage this figure may be considerably longer. In this environment a helicopter has been shown to be able to deliver a senior doctor to the patient 10 min after injury and provide critical life-saving intervention up to 30 min before the land-based model of care (Nicholl et al 1995).

Prehospital ambulance staff may only expect to see a multiply-injured patient every 1–2 years and the average district general hospital perhaps only once every 2 weeks (Airey & Franks 1995). Performing well as a trauma team member on such a rare occasion is an unreasonable expectation. Recognition of this 'skill utility' issue came from the Royal College of Surgeons of England (1988) and the American College of Surgeons Committee on Trauma (1998) and along with it recommendations relating to the number of patients individual doctors or institutions should see. A helicopter allows the trauma system to concentrate medical skills in both the prehospital provider (the person who carries out the care in the streets) and those in the receiving hospitals.

Several workers have demonstrated that time to neurosurgery is important. Data from several authors indicate that surgery within 3–4 h of injury produces better outcomes (Seelig et al 1981, Stone et al 1986, Wilberger et al 1991). In the UK, time to intracranial haematoma removal has not been well documented. In London, flying patients directly to a neurosurgical centre has resulted in a mean time of 177 min to haematoma removal (Wright et al 1996). Given that most patients with severe head injuries are secondary transfers to specialist centres, the window of opportunity is being lost. If striking changes like this can be established in the urban environment then the requirement for a similar system in the rural situation is obvious.

Those who use helicopters do so on the basis that they are logical enhancements to the process of patient care. Too often, diseases are forced to conform to systems of care. Logically, the system should be designed to accommodate the best possible management of the disease. For the disease of multiple trauma, helicopters have allowed the system to work around the disease and not the other way round.

Funding and planning

Funding for aeromedical activity may come from a variety of sources: central or local government, insurance agencies, hospitals or health-care purchasers. In most European countries operations have developed with central planning and funding. Mature systems are based on local geography and health-care facilities.

In Germany, the first airbase was developed in 1970 in response to rising accident statistics and was initiated by ADAC (the German Automobile Association). In 1974 the introduction of emergency medical service (EMS) legislation meant funding for the system came predominantly from the public purse and that every emergency call for help evoked a doctor-based response within 12 min. Now 50 airbases are located all over Germany. Each unit has a radius of 50–70 km with average flying times of 8 min (Earlam 1997).

In France a similar infrastructure exists (Service d'Aide Medicale Urgence (SAMU)), where 48 centrally funded bases are spread over the country. Like Germany, this structure is required by legislation.

In stark contrast, most aeromedical activity in the UK operates from charitable funds with little or no central planning. As a result, the integration of helicopter emergency medical service (HEMS) systems into clinical pathways has been neglected. Even today helicopters remain the source of much ill-informed debate. The National Association of Air Ambulance Services, a body that aims to represent UK helicopter air ambulance operators, provides a unified voice to bring forward the debate to encourage coordinated progress between various parties.

Tasking

Tasking is of little consequence for helicopter operations providing a secondary transfer service. However, if a helicopter is used as a front-line primary response to an emergency call from the general public, as in France and Germany, then tasking is of enormous importance.

Many despatch systems such as Medical Priority Despatch and Criteria Based Despatch, or modifications thereof, classify large proportions (30–70%) of cases into the top priority 'urgent category' (Stratton 1992, Curka et al 1993). The small numbers of patients who benefit from special resources tasking are not identified with high specificity. Under these

systems 'abort rates' for helicopters are extremely high. Specific tasking protocols have therefore been developed to address this issue.

In France and Germany doctors scrutinize all calls directly. In London a flight paramedic vets all emergency calls according to a clear despatch policy. There are few data available on the European systems but work from London suggests that one-quarter of all missions will be to a patient with an injury severity score (ISS) of more than 15. On 60% of missions, the doctor felt it necessary to stay with the patient. With these tailored despatch systems abort rates can be as low as 18–20% (Earlam 1997).

Where aircraft are used as part of a tiered response to ground crew requests, several scoring systems (Rhodes et al 1986, Wuerz et al 1996) have been developed to help ground crew identify the multiply-injured patient. Using clinical findings and mechanism of injury, the despatch of the aircraft can work to defined levels of specificity and sensitivity of injury severity score.

The trauma triage system of the American College of Surgeons is a system that uses both clinical findings and mechanism of injury. Wuerz et al (1996) found that this system identified 58 out of 67 patients with major injury (ISS > 15) and triaged them to a level 1 trauma centre, but 125 patients were overtriaged (a specificity of 7.6% and sensitivity of 97.4%).

Medical crew configuration

In the USA paramedics and nurses predominate. The majority of operations (95%) use two attending crew; 60% being nurse–paramedic and 26% nurse–nurse. Only 6% use physicians. In Europe and Australia, medical care is routinely provided by a doctor.

Evidence for the best crew configuration within the medical literature is weak and often conflicting. Baxt & Moody (1987) have suggested that physicians provide a higher level of care, while other studies (Hamman 1991) have suggested the converse. There are no satisfactory and objective studies that conclusively answer this question.

Aircraft can be used for a wide variety of cases, from minor patients with difficult access to the multiply injured. The level of medical care will be different for each case. While a fractured ankle may not require a doctor in the first hour, the mortality from multiple injury (> 10%) most certainly does. The aim of an emergency medical system must be to get the patient to a doctor in the first place. Multiply injured patients deserve and often get consultant-delivered care following arrival in hospital; quite why the most 'important' hour of the disease process is devoid of invasive medical care is difficult to understand. It is vital that the system fits the disease and not the disease the system. A helicopter gives the system the flexibility to deliver the appropriate resources in a cost-effective manner.

In most UK operations the choice of crew is the decision of the ambulance service operating the aircraft. For the most part, this means a paramedic, although many carry doctors occasionally and some routinely (e.g. London HEMS, Great North Air Ambulance). No service routinely carries nurses.

Planning of missions

Planning for helicopter missions is essential. When undertaking hospital transfers it is essential to be sure that both accepting and referring units have spoken. Preformatted checklists go some way to avoiding the uncomfortable position of turning up at hospital where there is no longer a bed or perhaps there never was one. Helicopter services must talk to both the referring and receiving clinicians and confirm the clinical status of the patient. The time of departure and estimated time of arrival at the accepting unit should be clearly communicated.

Clinical care en route

The noise and cramped space of most helicopters makes the routine work of patient care considerably more difficult. Access to the patient is difficult in all but the largest helicopters. Listening to the chest with a stethoscope is impossible. Observing for movement of the chest may be difficult. Patients should be appropriately monitored to compensate for the problematic environment.

Intubation is almost impossible in small helicopters. Even in middle-size helicopters, such as a Dauphin, it is extremely difficult in most cabin configurations. It is therefore essential to think ahead and to consider what could go wrong and what could be done about it. Anticipation of potential problems is fundamental to all transfer and prehospital work.

The intubated and ventilated trauma patient with fractured ribs is at significant risk of a tension pneumothorax. Pleural decompression via a needle may prevent an impending cardiac arrest but will do little to re-expand a lung. A low threshold for tube thoracostomy or thoracostomy alone is therefore prudent.

Establishing an intravenous drip in the back of an ambulance is difficult at the best of times. In flight there is no possibility of pulling in to the roadside for a few minutes to have a more 'steadied' attempt. It is always necessary, therefore, to have a reserve access line ready to run if the patient requires ongoing intravenous therapy.

Equipment

When most operations start there is a tendency to overstock on the range and type of equipment carried. Visiting other units helps to minimize this problem. All electrical equipment must be certified for use in a particular type of aircraft. It is not unusual for medical equipment to interfere with vital aircraft systems such as navigation equipment. Manufacturers should be able to tell you whether the country's regulatory authority has certified an individual piece of equipment.

Like all prehospital work, it is important to plan for equipment failure and in particular electrical failure. Battery-operated suction may be routine but hand-operated suction must be available. Similarly, duplication of crucial pieces of equipment, such as laryngoscopes, is mandatory.

The volume of supplies, such as oxygen and drugs, should be calculated and should include appropriate reserves in case the flight is diverted or a vital vial is smashed.

Data collection

In the age of evidence-based medicine it is vital that those using expensive resources are able to account for their expenditure. If the aircraft function is to deliver advanced medical aid to the scene of an accident then the information collected should reflect this. If its aim is to reduce the time to neurosurgery then it should reflect this. If an aircraft is being used for secondary transfer work then its effects on releasing ground units should be demonstrable.

Regulation

Each country has a body that regulates its aircraft industry. Much of this regulation is found in legislative acts. In the UK the Civil Aviation Authority (CAA) governs aviation. Strict definitions apply to mission types, crew types and how and when an aircraft can be used. Each medevac operation must have an Air Operator's Certificate (AOC). This defines nearly every aspect of the operation from an aviation point of view, from hours of operation to types of landing and who can fly in the aircraft. In recent times there has been a move to unify regulations throughout Europe with the creation of the Joint Aviation Authority (JAA). According to JAA there are two types of crew and two types of mission.

- *HEMS crew member* – a person who is assigned to a HEMS flight for the purpose of attending to any person in need of medical assistance carried in the helicopter and assisting the pilot during the mission. This person is subject to specific training. In such a role the crew member will help with navigation and the aircraft radios. To minimize cost, this could be a paramedic or doctor.

- *Medical passenger* – a medical person carried in a helicopter during a HEMS flight, including but not limited to doctors, nurses and paramedics. The role of this individual should focus on patient care. No specific training is required other than the usual preflight briefing.

- *Helicopter air ambulance flight* – a flight usually planned in advance the purpose of which is to facilitate medical assistance where immediate and rapid transportation is not essential. A planned transfer of a patient between designated landing sites.

- *HEMS flight* – a flight by helicopter the purpose of which is to facilitate emergency medical assistance where immediate and rapid transportation is essential by carrying medical personnel, supplies or ill or injured persons.

Safety

The safety record for medevac operations varies from country to country and partly reflects the number and frequency of flights and the variety of conditions in which they are flown. The worst period for rotary wing operators was in the late 1970s and early 1980s when there was a proliferation of operations in the USA. Accident rates were as high as 13.4 per 100 000 flight hours, with approximately 50% of these being fatal. In 1988 a report produced by the National Transportation Safety Board (NTSB) identified many of the issues that were thought to contribute to the situation (National Transportation Safety Board 1988). Commercial pressure was thought to drive many operators to fly when conditions were marginal. Few pilots were instrument-rated and many could not cope if they suddenly found themselves in poor visibility. By the early to mid-1990s the incidence of crashes had fallen to 3.1 per 100 000 flying hours (Reeder 1995).

Safety issues do not simply relate to the flight crew. All emergency service personnel should be briefed on ground safety issues. In all but one commercial aircraft there is a risk of walking into the tail rotor. The noise of a helicopter is deafening at the best of times. At the rear of the aircraft the exhausts of the jet engines are directed backwards toward the tail rotor making the invisible rotor inaudible. Similarly, one should never walk under the disc when the rotors are starting up or stopping. When the disc is at full speed, the blades are sent out straight and flat by centripetal force. As they slow down they sag. When it is windy a sudden gust can blow the blades below head height. On sloping ground the uphill part of the rotor disc will be closer to the ground and may be below head height. One should always exit and approach from the downhill side. On the whole it is best not to enter the area under the disc unless absolutely necessary. Trained aircrew should be allowed to move equipment and patients in and out of the aircraft where possible. One should never approach unless the captain gives a clear indication to do so.

Never approach a helicopter without a clear signal from the captain.

At the scene

Landing at the scene of an accident is always the captain's decision, irrespective of the ground crew's training and perception at the time. However, if acting as a member of land-based response and an aircraft has been despatched to the scene, being able to identify a likely landing site is extremely helpful. An ideal landing site has a minimum clear area of twice the diameter of the rotating blades ($2D$, where D is the rotating blade diameter). This depends on the type of aircraft involved but for smaller helicopters (Bolkow 105 or Squirrel) it would be about 25 m in diameter – approximately the size of a tennis court. The land should be firm and flat, and ideally cleared of loose debris. People should be positioned away from the area and instructed to shield their eyes as the aircraft descends its last few metres to avoid foreign objects blowing into their eyes.

Landing sites

The CAA lays down strict definitions relating to landing sites. Few hospitals have dedicated helicopter landing facilities and even fewer have purpose-built helipads. Wherever possible, landing sites at hospital facilities should be within a 'trolley push' of the emergency department. Loading and unloading patients into and out of vehicles destabilizes the already unstable patient and produces unnecessary delays.

Choice of aircraft

Throughout the world just about every type of helicopter has been used for medevac purposes. Given the huge variation in aircraft type it is obvious that operations work in very different environments and meet very different endpoints. When considering an aircraft for a medevac operation many factors need to be considered before an ideal can be selected.

Large aircraft such as the Sea King, used in search and rescue operations, require larger landing sites than aircraft such as the Bolkow 105 or Aerospatiale Squirrel, and could not be used as a primary resource in the urban environment. However, if large distances and winching capability are envisaged then this sort of aircraft is an obvious choice. Similarly, the number of patients and crew may affect aircraft size. Small helicopters such as the Squirrel limit the number of pilots and crew that can be carried (see below).

Aircraft performance is similarly important. In the event of an engine failure a helicopter must be able either to land or fly away safely. Not all helicopters have the same engine performance. An aircraft with relatively weak engines must remain light to perform well in the event of an engine failure. If it is to remain light then there will be obvious restrictions on the number of crew or amount of equipment. A further complication is the environment. Wind speed, atmospheric pressure and temperature all affect performance. The safe weight that can be carried therefore varies from day to day. On very hot days when performance is reduced the aircraft must be lighter to compensate. To remain light and in a position to land safely the captain must get rid of either people, equipment or fuel. The weight of medical kit, number of staff and the area the aircraft is required to cover (amount of fuel required) will all affect the sort of aircraft used.

Aircraft used in the UK

AEROSPATIALE DAUPHIN

Advantages

The Aerospatiale Dauphin (Fig. 56.1) has a large medical cell to enable the carriage of two patients and two medical crew, or one patient, two medical crew and a trainee. There is a choice of single or twin pilot versions. Access to the patient is complete from head to toe from one side of the patient. In most fits, access to intubate the patient is limited. The tail rotor is enclosed and the disc height of the main rotors is well above head height. Large, spacious doors allow rapid loading and unloading of patients.

Disadvantage

The higher running cost of a larger aircraft.

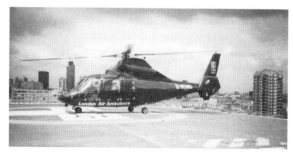

Fig. 56.1 • Aerospatiale Dauphin.

AEROSPATIALE SQUIRREL

Advantages

The Aerospatiale Squirrel (Fig. 56.2) is one of the most popular multirole commercial aircraft, with relatively low running costs. The disc height is high when configured with the 'tall' skids.

Disadvantages

The overall small size limits the crew to one pilot and two medical crew. There is usually one patient litter, although a double patient fit is available. Access to the patient is limited to one side of the upper body. Intubation en route is impossible. Assisted ventilation can only be done from the side. Equipment space is limited, as is the space for the two medical crew. In the dual patient configuration, access to the lower litter is virtually non-existent. The tail rotor is exposed.

BOLKOW 105

Advantages

The running costs of the Bolkow 105 (Fig. 56.3) are relatively low and the disc height high.

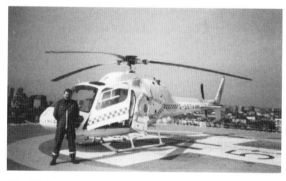

Fig. 56.2 • Aerospatiale Squirrel.

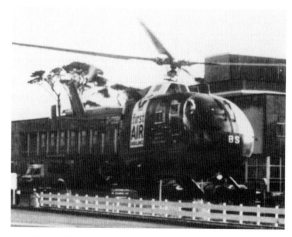

Fig. 56.3 • Bolkow 105.

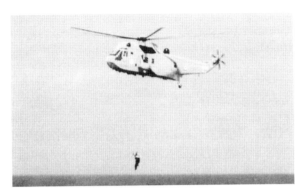

Fig. 56.4 • Sea King helicopter.

Disadvantages

This is a small, twin-engine aircraft with poor engine performance limiting helipad capability. The small interior cell limits the number of pilots to one and medical crew to two. It is usual for the second crew member to act as a navigator. There is limited access to the lower half of the patient in flight.

OTHER HELICOPTERS

Patients are occasionally evacuated from remote and offshore sites in Sea King (Fig. 56.4) helicopters of the Royal Navy and Royal Air Force. These helicopters are not primarily designed for 'medical' evacuation and do not form part of a regular medical service. Aircrew are trained in extended first aid, often to technician or paramedic level, and equipment scales are improving so that the majority of basic manoeuvres can be performed.

Advantages

Long ranges, rescue facilities and space.

Disadvantages

Landing difficulties due to size, noise and poor interior layout for medical purposes.

Hours of operation

The majority of operations provide daylight services only. In the USA only 35% of operators offer a night flight facility (Mayfield 1996). Landing at night is difficult. Wires and other obstacles are less easily seen – even with aids such as night-vision goggles or searchlights. Where night flight services are offered it is usual for this to be pure interhospital work flying between well-lit and presurveyed landing spots. Some operations, such as the Maryland state police, do provide 24h primary work at the scene, but unreconnoitred sites are considered too dangerous for most non-military operations. In the UK the majority of operations provide daylight coverage only.

Flying at night will put other constraints on an operation. For most regulatory authorities, such as the CAA, in the UK weather minimums are different, cloud level must be higher and forward visibility must be greater than in daylight. In some countries two pilots may be required at night. To remain serviceable, an operation might need to consider instrument rating its aircraft and pilots – itself an additional cost to the operation.

Providing a 24h service with one aircraft is not possible. Aircraft require regular maintenance and servicing schedules. A 24h service would require two aircraft and an increase in pilots and operations staff.

Helicopter operations in the UK

With the exception of the Scottish ambulance service, the Northumbria ambulance service and HEMS in London, most operators lease aircraft from third parties via charitable donations. This lack of central government funding has resulted in little geographical planning of operations. Nevertheless, it is estimated that 60% of the UK's population is covered by an air ambulance of some description during daylight hours.

Most operations run 10h a day, 365 days per year daylight services with an emphasis on rural operations. On the whole, a paramedic acts as the medical provider. In London and Lincolnshire a doctor is regularly used as part of the medical team. Where an ambulance service does not have its own dedicated aircraft it is common practice for them to use local police aircraft if the occasion requires it. Although far from ideal, patients can be evacuated to hospital more quickly.

Most aircraft are used in primary and secondary roles, although the relative proportions of this work vary from unit to unit. In Cornwall 20% of the work is secondary transfer (Nicholl et al 1994), whereas HEMS London transfers account for less than 5% of activity (Earlam 1997). A mixture of medical and surgical problems are encountered, although there is a tendency for the units to have a trauma bias. The unit in London is specifically targeted to treat major trauma patients in their primary phase.

The proof

There is no reliable research in the medical literature to demonstrate the contribution of a helicopter per se. Work by Sheffield University suggested that a physician-based helicopter system costing £1 million a year might save 13 lives per year.

It is essential to put the role of the helicopter in perspective. Helicopters form only a small link in a chain of medical care from the prearrival instructions of an emergency call-taker to a GP and practice nurse trying to integrate a patient back into society. Improvements anywhere in the system of care can be negated by deficits elsewhere. It is unrealistic to expect one small variable, such as a helicopter, to turn the system of care around and make up for the variation in surgeons, anaesthetists, physiotherapists and nurses who will all care for the patient along their way. Integrated systems of care save lives. A helicopter is simply one means of 'gluing' the system together and meeting the clinical needs of the patient.

References

Airey C, Franks A 1995 Major trauma workload within an English Health Region. Injury 26: 25–31

American College of Surgeons Committee on Trauma 1998 Resources for optimal care of the injured patient: 1999. American College of Surgeons, Chicago, IL

Baxt WG, Moody P 1987 The impact of a physician as part of the aeromedical pre-hospital team in patients with blunt trauma. Journal of the American Medical Association 257: 3246–3250

Blumen I 1996 Air medical physician handbook. Air Medical Physician Association

Curka P, Pepe P, Ginger V, Sherrad R, Ivy M, Zacharia B 1993 Emergency medical services priority despatch. Annals of Emergency Medicine 22: 1688–1695

Earlam R (ed) 1997 Trauma care. Saldatore, Bishop's Stortford, Herts

Hamman BL, Cue JI, Miller FB et al 1991 Helicopter transport of trauma victims: does a physician make a difference? Journal of Trauma 31: 490–494

London Ambulance Service 1997 Audit of prehospital care: time spent on scene for serious trauma patients. Clinical Audit Unit, London Ambulance Service NHS Trust, London

Mayfield T 1996 Annual transport statistics and transport fees. Airmedicine 2: 14–19

Mayfield T, Lindstrom A 1996 Medical crew survey. Airmedicine 2: 21–25

National Transportation Safety Board 1988 Safety study – commercial emergency medical services helicopter operations. NTSB/SS. National Transportation Safety Board, Washington, DC

Nicholl J, Beeby NR, Brazier JE 1994 A comparison of the costs and performance of an emergency helicopter and land ambulances in rural area. Injury 25: 145–153

Nicholl J, Brazier J, Snooks H 1995 Effects of London helicopter emergency medical service on survival after trauma. British Medical Journal 311: 217–222

Passini L 1997 Directory of air medical programmes. Airmedicine 3: 18–35

Reeder L 1995 EMS helicopter crash rates. Airmedicine 1: 36

Rhodes M, Perline R, Aronson J et al 1986 Field triage for on-scene helicopter transport. Journal of Trauma 26: 963–969

Royal College of Surgeons of England 1988 The management of patients with major injuries. Royal College of Surgeons of England, London

Seelig J, Becker P, Miller D et al 1981 Traumatic acute subdural haematoma, major mortality reduction in comatose patients treated within four hours. New England Journal of Medicine 304: 1511–1518

Stone J, Lowe R, Jonasson O et al 1986 Acute subdural haematoma: direct admission to a trauma center yields improved results. Journal of Trauma 26: 445–450

Stratton S 1992 Triage by emergency medical despatchers. Prehospital and Disaster Medicine 7: 263–269

Wilberger JE, Harris M, Diamond D 1991 Acute subdural haematoma: morbidity, mortality and operative timing. Journal of Neurosurgery 74: 212–218

Wright KD, Knowles CH, Coats TJ, Sutcliffe JC 1996 Efficient timely evacuation of intracranial haematoma – the effect of transport direct to a specialist centre. Injury 27: 719–721

Wuerz R, Taylor J, Stanley Smith J 1996 Accuracy of trauma triage in patients transported by helicopter. Air Medical Journal 15: 168–170

Aviation medicine

57

Introduction   581

The atmosphere   581

The physiological effects of altitude   582

The biodynamics of flight   586

Clinical considerations during aeromedical
transport   587

Conclusions   592

References   592

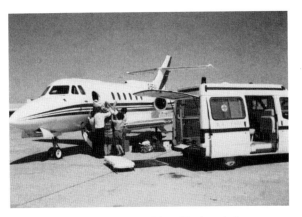

Fig. 57.1 • British Aerospace BAe 125 air ambulance.

Introduction

Research in aviation medicine developed originally from the needs of military flying during the First World War and continued to make many major advances during the golden age of experimental high-altitude and high-speed flight in the interwar years. The needs of the 1939–45 conflict ensured that research continued and the major physical, physiological and psychological stresses of flight are now reasonably well understood.

This chapter summarizes those aspects of altitude physiology and flight medicine that are most relevant to those who transport the sick and injured by air, whether at low level (by helicopter) or at higher altitudes (usually in the pressurized cabin of a passenger-type fixed-wing aircraft). Clearly, there is a great difference between the operations of an urban HEMS helicopter used for primary responses (where the aircraft serves as the means of patient transport from the scene of an incident to a receiving facility) and an air ambulance company that specializes only in long-distance repatriation. Aircraft involved in secondary and tertiary missions usually transport patients from outlying emergency facilities where some degree of stabilization has already been performed; the patient is then delivered into the care of a higher level facility (Fig. 57.1). This chapter will also be of interest to medical and paramedical personnel who may encounter illness or injury among those who fly, either professionally or as passengers.

The atmosphere

The atmosphere is a flexible, gaseous envelope that surrounds the Earth. It extends to an upper limit of around 800 km and is retained by the gravitational attraction of the planet. Conventionally, there are three layers, which are of variable depth depending where on the Earth's surface the measurement is taken. The most important, from an aviation point of view, is the *troposphere*. Reaching about 6000 m at the poles and 20 000 m at the equator, it is here that the phenomena collectively known as *weather* (activity such as clouds, precipitation and turbulence) occur. The major components of air are oxygen (21%) and nitrogen (78%). These proportions are constant throughout the troposphere because of the mixing actions of the vertical air currents. Air consists of matter: it has the properties of mass and density and can be compressed. If the atmosphere is considered as a column (Fig. 57.2), it can be seen that the pressure at any point in the atmosphere is proportional to the weight of all the molecules above it and therefore decreases as altitude increases (Fig. 57.3). Ambient pressure is halved at 5500 m (18 000 ft) (380 mmHg) and halved again at 10 200 m (33 400 ft) (190 mmHg).

The physiological effects of altitude

Boyle's law states that, at constant temperature, the volume of a given mass of gas is inversely proportional to

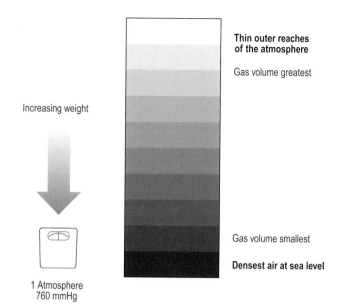

Fig. 57.2 • The atmosphere as a column. (© Aeromedical *transportation: a clinical guide*, Martin & Rodenberg, 1996, Ashgate Publishing, reproduced with permission.)

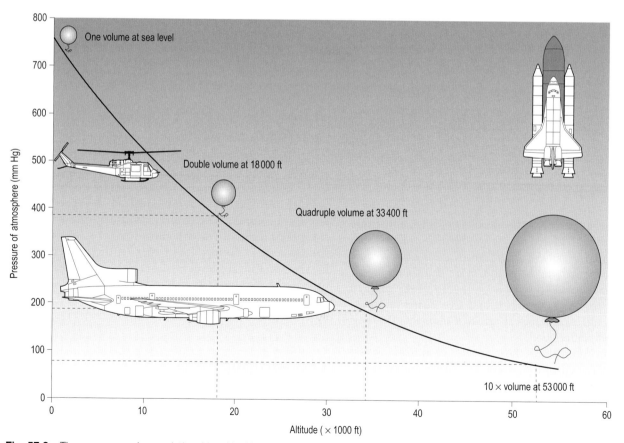

Fig. 57.3 • The pressure–volume relationship with altitude. (© Aeromedical *transportation: a clinical guide*, Martin & Rodenberg, 1996, Ashgate Publishing, reproduced with permission.)

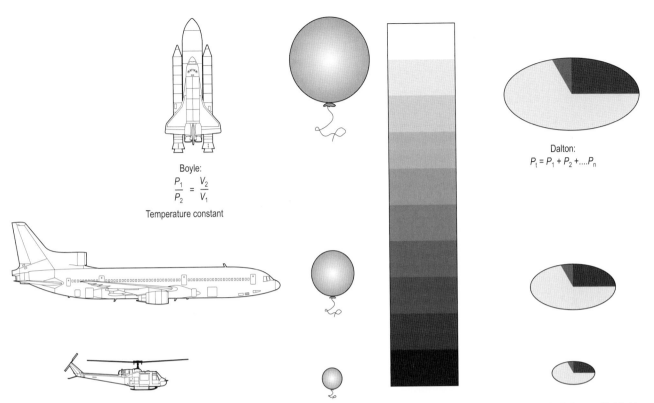

Fig. 57.4 • Boyle's law and Dalton's law. (© Aeromedical *transportation: a clinical guide*, Martin & Rodenberg, 1996, Ashgate Publishing, reproduced with permission.)

the pressure exerted upon it. It follows that, as density and pressure decrease with increasing altitude, the volume of gas will increase. Dalton's law describes *partial pressure*. It states that the pressure exerted by a mixture of gases is the sum of pressures that each would separately exert if it alone occupied the space filled by the mixture (Fig. 57.4).

As altitude increases, fewer oxygen molecules are available for metabolic use, precipitating anaerobic metabolism with the subsequent production of lactic acid.

Alveolar gas is air fully saturated with water at body temperature. The vapour pressure of water remains a constant 47 mmHg at all altitudes. The carbon dioxide (CO_2) fraction of alveolar gas is soluble and diffuses readily, so that the partial pressure of carbon dioxide in blood leaving the pulmonary capillaries (P_aCO_2) is almost in equilibrium with that of alveolar gas. At ground level pulmonary ventilation is automatically regulated to keep pace with CO_2 production and the alveolar partial pressure (P_aCO_2) is kept constant at around 40 mmHg. At altitude, however, P_aCO_2 is reduced because of the hypoxic drive to increase pulmonary ventilation, effectively washing carbon dioxide out of the lungs. The partial pressures of the components of the alveolar gas mixture at sea level and at 8000 ft (2450 m) are shown in Fig. 57.5.

The relationship between oxygen saturation (quantity of oxygen combined with haemoglobin (Hb)) and oxygen tension (partial pressure of oxygen in the blood) is

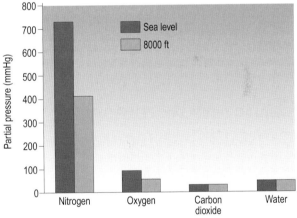

Fig. 57.5 • Proportions of alveolar gas at sea level and 8000 ft. Total atmospheric pressure at sea level and 8000 ft is 760 and 565 mmHg, respectively. At 8000 ft, the partial pressure of oxygen in dry air would therefore be 21% of 565, i.e. 119 mmHg. However, alveolar gas is fully saturated and the vapour pressure of water remains a constant 47 mmHg at body temperature at all altitudes. The partial pressure of carbon dioxide is slightly reduced (37 mmHg) because of the hypoxic drive to increase pulmonary ventilation. The partial pressure of oxygen in alveolar gas is therefore lower than in dry air at the same altitude.

described by the sigmoid-shaped oxygen dissociation curve (Fig. 57.6) The shape is of great importance: the flat upper portion ensures that moderate variations of alveolar oxygen tension around the norm (103 mmHg at sea level)

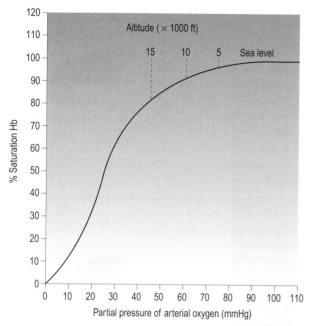

Fig. 57.6 • The oxygen–haemoglobin dissociation curve at 37°C and pH 7.4.

have little effect on the amount of oxygen combined with Hb in arterial blood (i.e. its saturation). This allows normal, healthy individuals to exist comfortably up to 3000 m (10 000 ft) without overt signs and symptoms of hypoxia. The steep portion at lower oxygen tensions ensures optimal dissociation of oxygen from Hb into the tissues. A large drop in saturation (as a large quantity of oxygen is given up to the tissues) results in only a small fall in tension. This is important in maintaining oxygen tension at tissue level.

HYPOBARIC (HYPOXIC) HYPOXIA

Hypobaric hypoxia is caused by an inadequate partial pressure of oxygen in inspired air (and inadequate gas exchange at the alveolar–capillary membrane) sufficient to cause impairment of physiological function. Except when emergency rapid decompression occurs, hypoxia is usually insidious in onset and there is considerable variation in its effects between individuals. The appearance of signs and symptoms, and their severity, depends on the altitude to which the individual is exposed, the rate of ascent and the time spent at that altitude. In addition, extremes of ambient temperature and the physical activity of the individual may make demands on available oxygen, as will a number of other personal factors. Over and above pathological conditions (even minor infections), these include fitness, previous acclimatization, metabolic rate, diet, nutrition, emotional state, fatigue, some medications and alcohol. Transport in a pressurized cabin will reduce the likelihood of hypoxic complications, but medical escorts must be aware of predisposing conditions which can exacerbate

hypoxia at altitude. These pre-existing conditions include any which interfere with gaseous exchange, or oxygen carriage, delivery or demand.

Signs of cerebral hypoxia begin when the alveolar partial pressure of oxygen ($P_A\text{CO}_2$) falls to 50–60 mmHg (Ernsting et al 1988). Cerebral blood flow is affected by the partial pressures of both oxygen and carbon dioxide. Hyperventilation (a normal response to hypoxia) will induce hypocapnia sufficient enough to cause cerebral vasoconstriction and decreased perfusion. When arterial P_{CO_2} falls to 45 mmHg, a hypoxia-driven vasoconstriction also occurs. Below 45 mmHg the reverse happens and increased cerebral blood flow results from the vasodilatory effects of extreme hypoxia attempting to offset the vasoconstriction caused by the hyperventilatory response (hypocapnia).

The symptoms of hypoxia in normal individuals have been described according to the level of altitude (Blumen 1995) and are shown in Table 57.1 but aeromedical personnel and patients will not be exposed to altitudes above 10 000 ft except in the event of an emergency rapid decompression of an aircraft cabin when flying above that altitude.

GASEOUS EXPANSION

There are several gas-containing organs in the body. They may be filled with saturated air (in the middle ear cavities and paranasal sinuses), alveolar gas (saturated air enriched with carbon dioxide in the lungs) or a mixture of air and gases generated by digestive processes (in the gut). These cavities communicate with the atmosphere with varying degrees of efficiency, and the gas contained within them obeys Boyle's law. If increased volume cannot be vented, stretching of the walls of the cavities may cause considerable discomfort. Two common examples are barotitis (otic barotrauma) and barosinusitis (sinus barotrauma).

Gas expansion in the middle ear with increasing altitude escapes through the eustachian tube every 150–300 m (500–1000 ft) (felt as a 'popping'). On descent gas volume contracts, creating a negative pressure within the middle ear that pulls the tympanic membrane inward. The eustachian tube will not normally allow the passive movement of air into the middle ear but it can be actively opened by elevating the pressure in the nasopharynx by moving the jaw, swallowing or the Frenzel manoeuvre ('pinch the nose and blow'). Any inflammation of the mucosa can cause obstruction and equalization may be impossible, resulting in barotitis with severe pain, vertigo, nausea, perforation and bleeding. Similarly, air can usually pass in and out of the sinus cavities freely but, if the mucosa is swollen, trapped air will expand as altitude increases. As a consequence, the Frenzel manoeuvre is not effective and symptoms of barosinusitis (predominantly pain in the cheek or forehead) soon develop.

Table 57.1 The symptoms of hypoxia in normal individuals

Altitude (ft)	Stage	% saturation of arterial blood (S_aO_2)	Symptoms
Up to 10 000	Indifferent	90–98	No awareness of symptoms and no noticeable impairment
10 000–15 000	Compensatory	80–90	Increase in respiratory rate, heart rate and systolic blood pressure to offset the decrease in oxygen carriage. Normal individuals may remain asymptomatic or begin to experience nausea, dizziness, lethargy, headache, fatigue and apprehension. Poor judgement, decreased efficiency, impaired coordination and increased irritability may become obvious after a 10–15 min exposure at 12 000–15 000 ft
15 000–20 000	Disturbance	70–80	Physiological mechanisms can no longer compensate for the oxygen deficiency. Air hunger, headache, amnesia, decreased level of consciousness and nausea are more pronounced. The senses are diminished, with impairment of visual acuity due to blurring or tunnelling of vision, and loss of colour clarity. There may be weakness, numbness, tingling, and decreased sensation of touch and pain. Reaction time, working memory and speech may be greatly impaired. Behaviour may appear aggressive, belligerent, euphoric, overconfident or morose, and impaired muscular coordination makes delicate or fine movements impossible. Despite a noticeable increase in respiratory rate, central cyanosis may be obvious and muscular spasm and tetany may result from hypocapnia
Above 20 000	Critical	60–70	Higher mental functions and neuromuscular control decline rapidly. In addition to the features of the disturbance stage, objective findings now escalate to include myoclonic jerking of the upper limbs, grand-mal-type seizures and, often with little or no warning, unconsciousness. Unless the hypoxia is relieved immediately, irreversible cerebral damage will increase and death will follow

As the stomach and intestines normally contain up to 1 litre of gas, expansion on ascent can cause abdominal pressure with pain, shortness of breath or hyperventilation (from diaphragmatic splinting), and nausea. Prevention is the key. The most notorious gas producers are beans and pulses, green vegetables and other high roughage foods. Loose non-restrictive clothing may also be of benefit, and sufferers should not be modest about venting expanding gas to relieve discomfort.

Table 57.2 lists items of equipment that are susceptible to the effects of altitude. Gaseous expansion may lead to damage or failure of equipment, or to loss of accuracy of measuring or monitoring devices. Most incidents are predictable, such as when air is instilled into the cuffs of endotracheal and tracheostomy tubes. Some anaesthetists argue that the best solution is to fill the inflatable cuff with sterile water, which, as liquids are non-compressible, does not change volume with altitude (Martin & Rodenberg 1996).

Air splints may also expand and contract with altitude. The danger here is either of producing a compartment syndrome or of providing inadequate immobilization and support. The pneumatic antishock garment (PASG) may also cause compartment syndrome at altitude. On descent, relative deflation may cause inadequate pressure support, both to the circulation and to pelvic and lower extremity fractures.

Table 57.2 Equipment susceptible to gaseous expansion

- Glass intravenous fluid bottles
- Intravenous administration sets
- Pressure bags
- Chest drainage bags
- Nasogastric tubes and other closed drains
- Endotracheal tube cuffs
- Tracheostomy tube cuffs
- Catheter balloons
- Sphygmomanometer cuffs
- Pneumatic antishock garment
- Air splints

© Aeromedical transportation: a clinical guide, Martin & Rodenberg, 1996, Ashgate Publishing, reproduced with permission.

Expansion of gas in unvented glass bottles of fluid causes a build-up of pressure that may eventually shatter the container. Whenever possible, fluids contained in plastic bags should be used in preference to those in glass bottles, but they still require venting if significant pressure changes are encountered. Intravenous fluids and medications that require exact titration should be regulated by electronic pumps to avoid the artificial increases in flow

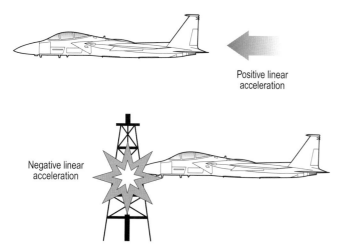

Fig. 57.7 • Linear acceleration. (© Aeromedical *transportation: a clinical guide*, Martin & Rodenberg, 1996, Ashgate Publishing.)

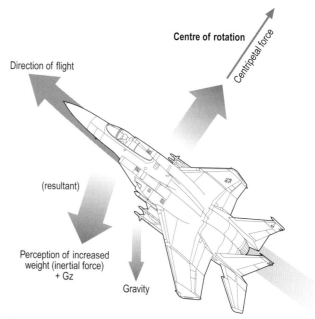

Fig. 57.8 • Radial acceleration. (© Aeromedical *transportation: a clinical guide*, Martin & Rodenberg, 1996, Ashgate Publishing.)

rate that follow gaseous expansion and overpressure within the bag.

The biodynamics of flight

THE EFFECTS OF ACCELERATION

Life within the gravitational envelope of the planet exposes us all to an acceleration of $9.81 \, \mathrm{m \, s^{-2}}$ ($32 \, \mathrm{ft \, s^{-2}}$) directed towards the centre of the Earth. This gravitational pull gives rise to the force we know as weight. All life forms have evolved to operate in this '$1g$' environment. However, modern means of transport can expose us to much greater accelerations, which may have either physiological or pathological effects, depending on their duration, direction and magnitude. *Short-duration accelerations* (less than 1 s) very often result in injury or death. Examples include forces experienced during crashes or ditching and, for the military pilot, the operation of ejection seats.

Long-duration accelerations result in physiological changes as body organs and fluids obey Newton's third law of motion and respond with an equal and opposite reaction to the applied acceleration. However, under normal circumstances, medical crew and patients will experience only mild accelerations compared with the aircrew of modern agile military aircraft. Two types of acceleration may be experienced: linear acceleration and radial acceleration.

Linear acceleration results from an increase or decrease in the rate of movement along a straight line (Fig. 57.7). This will be encountered on take-off and is also felt as jets are reversed during the landing run of large passenger aircraft. No physiological consequences occur in normally seated individuals.

Buffeting is a sequence of irregular linear accelerations operating in the long axis of the seated occupant. It is often experienced when flying at high speed in turbulent conditions, especially through or under storm clouds, but it can be just as bad at low level, in hot climates and when flying over mountains. These rapidly alternating vertical accelerations may reach a magnitude of up to $3g$ and are extremely fatiguing.

Radial acceleration results from a change in direction of motion of the aircraft (Fig. 57.8). The unbalanced force acts towards the centre of a circular path but is perceived as an increase in weight by occupants of the aircraft. At low levels of acceleration the hydrostatic effects of positive g are minimal and unlikely to be a serious cause for concern (Glaister 1988). However, repeated fluctuating manoeuvres are fatiguing and may increase the risk of motion sickness, and flight medical personnel should be aware of the effects of increased g on equipment such as free-hanging traction weights.

VIBRATION

The main sources of vibration in fixed-wing aircraft are the engines and turbulence. Helicopters are a special case with vibration frequencies also associated with main and tail rotors, and the gearbox. Different parts of the human body have *natural frequencies* and therefore oscillate at distinct frequencies within the spectrum. The most significant frequency range lies between 0.1 and 40 Hz (Stott 1988). For instance, the head resonates at about 6 Hz and the forearm at around 40 Hz. The result is discomfort and fatigue as muscular effort is required to stabilize the body.

Low frequencies can also cause blurred vision, shortness of breath, motion sickness and chest or abdominal pain.

NOISE

The vibration of air (sound) is one of the most irritating factors encountered in the cockpit. Noise is generated by aircraft engines, propellers, the friction of air as it passes over the aircraft fuselage, and radios. It is worse in helicopters and in some military transport aircraft. There is great individual variation in tolerance of the effects of noise and what is considered to be unpleasant, but the longer the exposure and the more intense the noise, the greater the annoyance, as well as being a cause of potential damage. Prolonged and intense exposure may also result in ear discomfort, deterioration in performance of tasks, headaches and fatigue (Rood 1988). Such a background level of noise also prevents the use of a stethoscope. It is therefore important for medical crew to use other means to monitor the patient. Hearing protection may be needed by both the medical crew and patient. Simple earplugs or ear defenders will usually suffice, but headsets and helmets offer better noise attenuation and will improve communications.

MOTION SICKNESS

Individuals vary in their response to motion stimuli and, although some may be very tolerant of the provocation caused by aircraft movement, if the stimulus is intense enough all will eventually succumb. The underlying mechanisms are not understood, but sickness tends to occur when visual and vestibular evidence of motion are in conflict, or when signals from the semicircular canals and otoliths do not conform to expected patterns (Benson 1988). Some aircraft manoeuvres are more provocative than others, and unintentional, unexpected motion (such as turbulence) may provoke both nausea and an anxiety overlay. In addition, an overly warm or stuffy environment, or the sight or smell of food (or of others vomiting), can be enough to turn even the strongest stomach. The symptoms are probably familiar to every reader. Before vomiting, sufferers may describe an increased 'stomach awareness', nausea or retching. They may be apathetic, malaised or fatigued. A feeling of overwhelming warmth, headache, pallor and sweating are common. Those who succumb may receive some comfort if their anxieties can be allayed and if they are able to concentrate on an activity (although not reading, which tends to worsen the symptoms). Antiemetics may be ineffective once nausea has started but relief may be achieved by reducing further sensory conflict, either by fixing the gaze outside of the aircraft if the horizon is clearly visible or by lying flat with the head still and eyes closed. Any patient susceptible to motion sickness, or in whom vomiting would cause considerable medical problems, should be given an antiemetic prior to departure.

Clinical considerations during aeromedical transport

The initial approach to any ill or injured patient who requires transportation by air should follow the familiar ABCDE assessment. This is not only key to initial patient assessment but provides a template for the care of patients should in-flight problems or complications arise. By consistently examining all patients using this system, life-threatening problems can be anticipated and dealt with at the earliest opportunity.

AIRWAY CONSIDERATIONS

Any patient who is obtunded and unable to maintain the patency of the upper airway is at serious risk of obstruction, especially during movement and transport. Such patients should have a patent airway (cuffed endotracheal or tracheostomy tube) prior to flight. Once checked to ensure correct placement, it should be secured against accidental dislodgement. To replace a malpositioned tube is difficult enough in the protected environment of a hospital; it is even more so in the confines of an aircraft cabin moving in three axes at once. With respect to the tube, even with high-volume, low-pressure cuffs, air expanding under the influence of lowered ambient pressure is likely to increase pressure on the tracheal wall and may result in necrosis if pressures are of sufficient intensity (more than 20 mmHg or 3.0 kPa) and duration. If the medical escort recognizes this potential problem and releases some of the air in the cuff on ascent, but subsequently forgets to reinflate it on descent, an air leak will occur, oxygenation may be impaired and the airway will no longer be protected. Similarly, a pressure-limiting pilot balloon will prevent overinflation at altitude, but it cannot prevent an air leak on descent.

Care of the cervical spine is an integral part of airway management. All primary transfer trauma patients should be fully immobilized with a hard cervical collar and head restraint applied. Immobilization will simplify lifting and loading, but restrained patients are at risk of aspiration after emesis, and of pressure sores at points of prolonged contact.

RESPIRATORY CONSIDERATIONS

Patients with problems of oxygenation at ground level are likely to exhibit increased difficulty at altitude. These patients must be identified before departure so that adequate oxygen supplements and/or mechanical ventilation can be provided. Whatever the disease process, if oxygen is required at ground level the requirement for oxygen at altitude can be calculated using the percentage of inspired oxygen (F_iO_2) required by the patient to maintain an alveolar partial pressure of oxygen ($P_{A}O_2$) of 100 mmHg, as measured at the originating hospital. Even if a patient does not appear to require oxygen at ground level, there may be enough respiratory impairment to reduce $P_{A}O_2$ to such an extent that the patient is, from a respiratory point of view, already equivalent to being at altitude. With a knowledge of expected $P_{A}O_2$ at various altitudes, it is simple to estimate the effects of a 'further' 1800 m on oxygen tension (Rodenberg 1992, Berg et al 1993, Vohra & Klocke 1993). Whichever method is used to screen pulmonary patients for flight, $P_{A}O_2$ at sea level should be at least 70 mmHg. This will yield a $P_{A}O_2$ at cruise altitude of 50–55 mmHg and will preserve oxygen–haemoglobin saturation at or above 90%.

Pneumothorax, from whatever cause, will be exacerbated by the effects of altitude if not properly drained. Although surgical emphysema may worsen alarmingly, it is the potential for impairment of gaseous exchange and life-threatening tension pneumothorax that is of most concern. If a thoracostomy drain has been recently removed, a suitable delay should elapse before flight is considered, and then only with radiographic evidence of a fully expanded lung. If in doubt, it is better to keep the drain in place during the transfer, as an open, draining air leak is preferable to a closed, expanding lesion. Chest tubes should be fitted with a functioning Heimlich valve or a valved drainage bag. Fluid draining from the chest may demonstrate faster flow at altitude if the pleural cavity contains free air.

CARDIOVASCULAR CONSIDERATIONS

The American College of Chest Physicians (1960) developed a list of altitude limitations for cardiorespiratory disease (Table 57.3). The cardiac patient is at risk from the reduction of $P_{a}O_2$ that occurs within the aircraft cabin but may also be affected by fear of flight, the stress of travel, time zone changes, gastric distension and confinement in the aircraft cabin. It has been suggested that those who have suffered a myocardial infarction should not be transported by air until after at least 1 week of complication-free recovery (Kaplan et al 1987, Alexander 1995), although there is no clear medical evidence to support this recommendation. Like all such rules, much depends on the facilities at the patient's location, the capabilities of the transferring aircraft and the skills of the in-flight team. It may be necessary to transfer patients earlier, especially if they are in a remote place or at a location that cannot offer specialty cardiac care (Fig. 57.9).

A preflight assessment of postinfarct patients is necessary to detect dysrhythmias, cardiac failure, pain and anaemia.

Table 57.3 Altitude restrictions for patients with cardiopulmonary disease flying without supplemental oxygen

Altitude limitation (ft)	Patient condition
10 000	Mildly symptomatic cardiopulmonary disease
8000	Moderately symptomatic cardiopulmonary disease Significant ventilatory restriction
6000	Angina pectoris Sickle cell anaemia Cyanosis of any aetiology Respiratory acidosis of any aetiology Cor pulmonale
4000	Severe cardiac disease with cyanosis or decompensation Patients with two of the following: • cyanosis • cor pulmonale • respiratory acidosis
2000	Congestive heart failure Within 8 weeks of myocardial infarction if there is concurrent: • cyanosis • cor pulmonale • respiratory acidosis

Source: after American College of Chest Physicians 1960

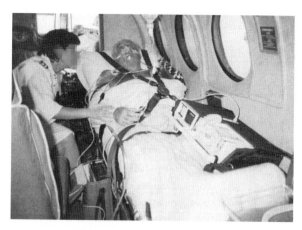

Fig. 57.9 • In-flight cardiac care can be achieved even within the confines of the small cabin of an air ambulance.

Review of the latest electrocardiogram, chest X-ray, biochemistry and haematology results allows anticipation of potential problems and treatment of any dangerous instability before departure. As with cardiac care on the ground, the aims of management should be to prevent hypoxia (with subsequent myocardial ischaemia) and metabolic acidosis, to promote cardiac contractility, prevent cardiac failure and treat pain and anxiety (Bellinger et al 1988).

Any deleterious changes in cardiac rhythm at altitude may be due to hypoxia, and supplemental oxygen should be immediately administered or increased. Although much has been written about the use of defibrillators in aircraft (Dedrick et al 1989, Martin 1993), there is no evidence that aircraft or occupant safety is at risk. However, because of the possibility of stray electric fields affecting aircraft avionics, it is mandatory to warn the flight crew before defibrillation or synchronized cardioversion is performed. The overall treatment of dysrhythmias is no different from that which would occur at ground level.

Pacemaker oversensing can occur in the presence of extraneous electromagnetic fields and stray currents, which are common in aircraft and around airport security devices (Sumchai et al 1988, Gordon et al 1990). The possibility of lead movement and dislodgement always exists. While little can be done for internal pacemaker problems in the transport setting, failure of external pacemakers should dictate that leads be checked before an attempt to regain capture is made by increasing the pacing output and before the use of inotropic agents.

The efficient carriage of oxygen by blood depends on the quantity and quality of haemoglobin (Hb) in the circulation. Because pulse oximetry can be misleading, a knowledge of the most recent Hb level is mandatory for proper interpretation. Although increases in cardiac output and ventilation can compensate for some reduction in haemoglobin, these mechanisms may themselves be subject to the adverse effects of hypoxia. For instance, myocardial ischaemia will be exacerbated by anaemia, and poor cardiac reserve will minimize the compensatory capability of increasing cardiac output. Compensatory effects are more efficient with chronic anaemia but a small degree of acute blood loss may also be beneficial. The most efficient haematocrit is 35% (this level represents the maximum oxygen-carrying capacity of blood). Ideally, all patients for aeromedical transport should have a stable haematocrit of at least 35% and a minimum haemoglobin level of $7.5\,g\,dl^{-1}$. Patients with an acute haemoglobin level lower than $7.5\,g\,dl^{-1}$ will require continuous oxygen support throughout the flight and possibly preflight transfusion.

Sickle cell anaemia is a specific problem. Sickling crises may be provoked by hypoxia and circulatory stasis exacerbated by enforced immobility during flight. Patients particularly at risk are those with haemoglobin C (Hb C) disease and sickle cell beta-thalassaemia. If air travel cannot be avoided, cabin pressure should be as high as possible, supplemental oxygen should be administered throughout the journey and patients should be encouraged to increase their intake of non-alcoholic fluids (Green et al 1971, Michel et al 1992).

Finally, postoperative cardiac patients are often much fitter than they might have been before operation. As long as the patient is stable, asymptomatic and free of trapped pleural or mediastinal air, there is no specific contraindication to flight.

NEUROLOGICAL AND NEUROSURGICAL CONSIDERATIONS

The major consideration for any patient suffering neurological illness or injury is to prevent secondary damage by cerebral hypoxia and the effects of cerebral compression. A preflight Glasgow coma score (GCS) should be documented in the notes, along with the date and time of the examination, and used as a baseline for further GCS monitoring in transit.

Patients with closed head injury or tumour may be carried safely by air, as long as cerebral metabolism and oxygenation are ensured and close observation is maintained for sudden elevations in intracranial pressure. However, as air in the cranium will expand at altitude, any patient who has had a craniotomy should not fly before the seventh postoperative day unless the aircraft is pressurized to the altitude of the site where the operation was performed. Similar care should be taken for those who have recently undergone an air encephalogram or ventriculogram, suffered a penetrating head injury or have had cerebrospinal fluid (CSF) leakage from the ears or nose suggesting a basal skull fracture. If a CSF leak is present at ground level, it will drain slightly faster at altitude.

Facial injuries may also complicate head trauma and may compromise airway patency. Any patient who has had external fixation of the jaws must have either a quick-release device fitted to the apparatus or have wire or band cutters easily accessible, preferably affixed to his/her person for the duration of both ground and air phases of the transfer. Prior to the start of the journey, patients with facial and mandibular immobilization may benefit from a suitable antiemetic and the placement of a nasogastric tube through which the stomach can be aspirated or drained. The deranged anatomy and inflammation of a severely injured face may disrupt the sinuses and their drainage, causing subcutaneous emphysema and sinus pain, which will worsen with altitude.

Many aspects of the aviation environment can predispose patients to seizure activity (e.g. hypoxia, psychological stress and excitement). Known epileptic patients may require premedication prior to departure. Previously prescribed anticonvulsants may be given 1 h before departure, regardless of the time of the last dose. Patients known to be at risk should travel as stretcher patients, and convulsions occurring during flight should be treated in the same way as they would be on the ground.

The clinical features of an acute cerebrovascular accident (CVA) are likely to be exacerbated by hypoxia, and continuous supplemental oxygen will be required for all patients during transport. For those with proven CVA, transfer is recommended after 14 days, as long as deterioration or complications have not occurred (Dan Air Services Limited 1989). Hard and fast rules cannot be enforced as much of the transport decision relies on the facilities of the referring hospital, the condition of the patient and the capabilities of the in-flight team. Acute subarachnoid haemorrhage is more difficult to manage because rebleeding is common. Recommended times for patient transfer after the acute event are either during the first 48 h or after 2 weeks have elapsed.

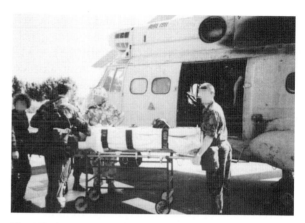

Fig. 57.10 • A Povey frame being used for the transportation of a spinally injured patient in a helicopter.

SPINAL INJURIES

In the early transfer of spinal patients to the primary receiving facility, those who are at risk of cervical injury should have the neck and back immobilized on a rigid spine board and supported in the neutral position. This is best done with a hard collar and sand bags, rolled towels or foam blocks placed on either side of the head. Tape should be placed over the forehead to secure the head to a spinal board or the stretcher upon which the patient is lying. A vacuum-mattress-type neck collar may also be used but all the air must be evacuated as residual air will expand with altitude, causing the collar to lose its rigidity.

If the flight is likely to exceed 4 h, arrangements for the safe turning of the patient must be made. This may be possible by using a rigid backboard, cervical collar and head restraint. The board–patient unit is periodically turned from side to side. Although transfer on a spinal board is preferable for prehospital patients being moved to an initial receiving facility, this mode of carriage is uncomfortable for those with residual sensation and may cause pressure sores in patients with sensory loss. A Stryker or Povey frame might seem ideal but these devices are bulky and heavy, and can only be accommodated in larger aircraft (Fig. 57.10). Most patients on short-haul transfers can be transported satisfactorily on a vacuum mattress conformed to the patient's body contours and lined with a sheepskin blanket.

The patient whose cervical spine has already been stabilized may well have traction tongs in situ. Cervical traction must be maintained by a closed system. Free-hanging weights are susceptible to movement in all three axes of flight and to the effects of increased gravitational forces. During acceleration or turning manoeuvres exerting a force of 2 g, a 1 kg mass will weigh 2 kg, a 3 kg mass will weigh 6 kg, and so on. The extra 'weight' may result in distraction injury.

Spinal cord injuries have the potential for major derangements of normal physiology. The nature of the dysfunction will depend on the level and severity of the damage. Paralysis of intercostal muscles and the diaphragm will impair ventilation and lead to hypoxia. A full pre-flight assessment is essential to ensure that those patients requiring supplemental oxygen or ventilation are identified and appropriately managed. Close monitoring of oxygen saturation is essential, and measurement of end-tidal carbon dioxide will help to identify hypoventilation in those at risk.

It is advisable to decompress stomach gas, which may otherwise splint the diaphragm and impede adequate ventilation, or may cause regurgitation and aspiration. A freely draining nasogastric tube may be placed before flight. In the presence of ileus, persistent abdominal distension may be due to the expansion of intestinal gas. This may be relieved by the passage of a flatus tube.

When the sympathetic chain is also damaged, vasomotor control becomes unbalanced. The combination of unopposed vagal stimulation and loss of vascular tone results in neurogenic shock. Such 'relative' hypovolaemia caused by vascular dilation and venous pooling will exacerbate the effect of any true fluid losses. Intravenous access is essential and should be in place before the journey is started. In addition, the lack of opposition to vagal influence on the heart produces a bradycardia that may progress to asystole when the vagus is further stimulated by the placement of an oropharyngeal or nasopharyngeal airway, nasogastric tube or urinary catheter. Atropine, a potent parasympatholytic agent, may be administered prior to all such manoeuvres, and the electrocardiogram should be monitored throughout the transfer.

Care should be taken to ensure that the temperature of the aircraft cabin is comfortable, as vasomotor lability and sensory deficits also prevent adequate thermoregulation. The patient may also require thermal protection (from both heat and cold) during the ground phases of the transport.

BURN INJURIES

Minor burns (less than 15% of body surface area) should not present physiological problems during flight, although patients with injury to cosmetic areas, or when appearance or odour may cause offence to other passengers, may be refused permission to fly on commercial aircraft. Patients with major burns often have severe derangements of normal anatomy and physiology. The simplest approach to these patients is the familiar ABCDE method.

Laryngeal oedema following a respiratory tract burn should be considered in all patients being transferred to a primary receiving centre and those being transferred to a burns unit within the first 12 h of injury (Baack et al 1991). It is essential to provide a definitive airway before complete laryngeal obstruction occurs and neck oedema distorts anatomic landmarks. Bronchodilators may be necessary for those with troublesome airway spasm and are best given as nebulized solutions. Continuous monitoring of oxygen saturation is essential for all patients, and intubated burn victims may benefit from continuous end-tidal carbon dioxide measurement to ensure correct tube placement and adequacy of ventilation. Patients should ideally be nursed in the head-up position, and chest physiotherapy, bronchial lavage and suction may be necessary to maintain airway patency in the dry atmosphere of the aircraft cabin.

Patients with less severe inhalation injury may not develop significant signs for several days but even the patient without a respiratory tract burn is at risk of pulmonary dysfunction as part of an overall systemic response to major injury. Severe necrotizing parenchymal damage is frequently seen with large burns and appears to be related to immunosuppression. It is vital that all patients have an evaluation of pulmonary function prior to departure (including arterial blood gases if possible) so that appropriate equipment and facilities can be provided in flight (Judkin 1988).

Although hypovolaemia is expected in the early hours after a significant burn injury, an additional fluid volume load should be considered to counter enhanced fluid losses at altitude.

With loss of the normal physical barrier against microbial infection (skin) and the presence of a medium for bacterial culture in revitalized tissues, resistance to infection is low. Although the burn is sterile soon after the injury, the gradual fall in immune responses means that infection will inevitably follow. Wounds must be redressed under sterile conditions prior to transfer as the inside of an aircraft is a less than ideal place for the prevention of contamination. Any seepage of dressings during the journey should be covered with sterile cotton wool and bandages.

Temperature regulation is also likely to be disturbed. Loss of skin and subcutaneous tissue results in a deficit in body insulation. Loss of body heat is made worse by the evaporation of fluids from the surface of the burn wound. Evaporation will be exacerbated by the dry atmosphere of the pressurized aircraft cabin. Covering the wound at all times to prevent excess fluid loss is the key. The use of warming or reflective ('space') blankets may prove useful in maintaining an adequate thermal environment.

MISCELLANEOUS CONDITIONS

Orthopaedic

Plaster of Paris casts may contain air pockets, which may expand at altitude, causing pressure to the underlying skin and disrupting the structural integrity of the cast. Compressive effects from the expansion of soft tissues at subatmospheric pressures may also occur. Bivalving the cast down to the layer of the skin cover may eliminate these risks, but exchanging full circular casts for backslab splints before transport is preferred.

Because of the confined cabin space and the effects of acceleration, all forms of traction should use closed systems, such as springs or cords under tension. Free-hanging weights must not be used. External fixators must be checked for security prior to departure, and care should be taken in the movement of patients (and people around the patient) to avoid jarring the metalwork.

Ophthalmic

Although a recent study has failed to demonstrate any appreciable effect of the expansion of gas within the eye during flight below 900 m (3000 ft) (Kokame & Ing 1994), traditional aeromedical wisdom holds that patients who have suffered penetrating eye injury, or who have been subject to surgery where an air bubble remains in the eye, should not fly until at least 1 week after surgery, or otherwise only when the aircraft cabin altitude can be maintained at sea level (Jackman & Thompson 1995). In theory, expansion of gas bubbles within the eye may precipitate acute glaucoma.

Abdominal

The main considerations in patients with abdominal injury are gaseous expansion and haemorrhage. Patients who have had a laparotomy or repair of the gastrointestinal tract should preferably not fly until the seventh postoperative day, as volume expansion may weaken or disrupt sutures. Similarly, expansion of intraluminal gas may cause secondary haemorrhage in healing wounds and peptic ulceration. A decision to transport the patient earlier should be made in conjunction with the referring surgeon and only then if there is no evidence of ileus or gross abdominal distension and no risk of wound dehiscence. Patients who require urgent transport despite these conditions may require placement of an orogastric, nasogastric or rectal tube prior to flight, and cabin altitude should be maintained as close to sea level as possible. Patients who have undergone laparoscopic examination will be fit to fly 48h after surgery, assuming an uneventful postoperative period.

Endocrine

During long flights, diabetic patients may require feeding, insulin administration and assessment of serum glucose levels at specific intervals (Gill & Redmond 1993). Similarly, patients on supplemental corticosteroids may require their medication to be administered at specific intervals in order to avoid precipitating an adrenal crisis. The prevention of many in-flight problems related to endocrine disorders lies in maintaining the patient on the local (overseas) time, irrespective of the number of time zones crossed in flight. Gradual adjustment of medication and routines to home local time is best achieved at the accepting hospital.

Infectious diseases

Infectious diseases have implications for the aeromedical team, flight crew, other passengers, aircraft and equipment on board. Even if the condition is not critical, the possibility of spreading infection and the often unpleasant sights and smells of some infectious diseases cause most airlines to be reluctant to accept these passengers, and the only means of transport may be by dedicated air ambulance. The nature of the illness dictates the level of precautions to be taken in the care of the patient. Clearly, patients with tuberculosis require appropriate respiratory precautions while those with acquired immune deficiency syndrome (AIDS) or hepatitis need thorough care in disposal of blood, body fluids and contaminated medical material. While the use of barriers such as gowns, gloves and goggles may seem intimidating and uncaring, safe practice dictates their use in the unknown or undiagnosed patient. In-flight personnel may also be required to take prophylactic medications to counter exposure to infectious disease.

Psychiatric

Any psychiatric patient considered to be a danger to him or herself or others should be sedated before flight and should ideally travel as a stretcher patient. Location within the cabin is also important. It is unwise to place the violent or suicidal patient next to an emergency exit or close to emergency equipment such as flares and axes. Appropriate manpower and restraints should be available in the event that patient control is lost (Jones 1980). Other patients who may react adversely to air travel should be identified by the flight team and considered for mild sedation prior to flight. Special concern should be given to those patients who have been involved in any form of recent transport accident, regardless of their apparent willingness to fly.

Conclusions

When deciding to transport any patient by air, an understanding of the physical, physiological and psychological constraints imposed by travel and the flight environment will allow anticipation of any problems that may occur en route. The atmosphere is a hostile place. As we have seen, air pressure declines with increasing altitude, less oxygen is then available for cellular metabolism, and gases trapped within body cavities will expand. Although passenger-carrying aircraft maintain a cabin altitude that rarely exceeds 1800m, there is a measurable decline in alveolar partial pressure of oxygen (from 103mmHg at sea level to about 75mmHg at 1800m) even in healthy passengers. At the same altitude, gas volumes will expand by about 30%. There may also be problems with motion sickness, vibration, noise, cold or humidity. In addition to clinical concerns, flight medical crew should plan for logistic factors such as the duration of out-of-hospital time, time zone changes and the actual time of arrival (and the weather) at the destination facility. The overall aim is to deliver the patient from point of origin to destination, safely and causing no further harm.

References

Alexander JK 1995 Coronary problems associated with altitude and air travel. Cardiology Clinics 13: 271–278

American College of Chest Physicians 1960 Committee on Physiologic Therapy, Section on Aviation Medicine. Air travel in cardiorespiratory disease. Diseases of the Chest 37: 579–588

Baack BR, Smoot EC, Kucan JO et al 1991 Helicopter transport of the patient with acute burns. Journal of Burn Care and Rehabilitation 12: 229–233

Bellinger RL, Califf RM, Mark DB et al 1988 Helicopter transport of patients during acute myocardial infarction. American Journal of Cardiology 61: 719–722

Benson AJ 1988 Motion sickness. In: Ernsting J, King PF (eds) Aviation medicine. Butterworth, London

Berg BW, Dillard TA, Derderian SS, Rajagopal KR 1993 Hemodynamic effects of altitude exposure and oxygen administration in chronic obstructive pulmonary disease. American Journal of Medicine 94: 407–412

Blumen IJ 1995 Altitude physiology and the stresses of flight. Air Medical Journal 14: 87–99

Dan Air Services Limited 1989 Guidelines for carriage of passengers with medical conditions. Dan Air Medical Section Handbook. Dan Air Services Limited, London

Dedrick DK, Darga A, Landis D, Burney RE 1989 Defibrillation safety in emergency helicopter transport. Annals of Emergency Medicine 18: 69–71

Ernsting J, Sharp GR, Harding RM 1988 Hypoxia and hyperventilation. In: Ernsting J, King PF (eds) Aviation medicine. Butterworth, London

Gill GV, Redmond S 1993 Insulin treatment, time-zones and air travel: a survey of current advice from British diabetic clinics. Diabetic Medicine 10: 764–767

Glaister DH 1988 The effects of long duration acceleration. In: Ernsting J, King PF (eds) Aviation medicine. Butterworth, London

Gordon RS, O'Dell KB, Low RB, Blumen IJ 1990 Activity-sensing permanent internal pacemaker dysfunction during helicopter aeromedical transport. Annals of Emergency Medicine 19: 1260–1263

Green RL, Huntsman RG, Serjeant GR 1971 The sickle cell and altitude. British Medical Journal 4: 593–595

Jackman SV, Thompson JT 1995 Effects of hyperbaric exposure on eyes with intraocular gas bubbles. Retina 15: 160–166

Jones DR 1980 Aeromedical transportation of psychiatric patients: historical review and present management. Aviation, Space and Environmental Medicine 51: 709–716

Judkin KC 1988 Aeromedical transfer of burned patients: a review with special reference to European civilian practice. Burns, Including Thermal Injury 14: 171–179

Kaplan L, Walsh D, Burney RM 1987 Emergency aeromedical transport of patients with acute myocardial infarction. Annals of Emergency Medicine 16: 55–57

Kokame GT, Ing MR 1994 Intraocular gas and low-altitude air flight. Retina 14: 356–358

Martin TE 1993 Transportation of patients by air. In: Harding RM, Mills FJ (eds) Aviation medicine. BMJ Publishing, London

Martin TE, Rodenberg HD 1996 Aeromedical transportation: a clinical guide. Ashgate, Aldershot

Michel JB, Hernandez JA, Buchanan GR 1992 A fatal case of acute splenic sequestration in a 53-year-old woman with sickle-hemoglobin C disease. American Journal of Medicine 92: 97–100

Rodenberg H 1992 Aeromedical transport and inflight medical emergencies. In: Rosen P, Barkin R, Baker FJ et al (eds) Emergency medicine: concepts and clinical practice. Mosby, St Louis, MO

Rood GM 1998 Noise and communication. In: Ernsting J, King PF (eds) Aviation medicine. Butterworth, London

Stott JRR 1988 Vibration. In: Ernsting J, King PF (eds) Aviation medicine. Butterworth, London

Sumchai A, Sternbach G, Eliastam M, Liem LB 1988 Pacing hazards in helicopter aeromedical transport. American Journal of Emergency Medicine 6: 236–240

Vohra KP, Klocke RA 1993 Detection and correction of hypoxemia associated with air travel. American Review of Respiratory Disease 148: 1215–1219

Structure and function of the ambulance service

58

Introduction   594

The ambulance service as an NHS trust   594

The functions of the ambulance service   595

Ambulance vehicles   595

Ambulance service control and communications   597

Ambulance service training   598

Contracting for ambulance services   599

Performance standards for ambulance services   599

Ambulance system design   600

The high-performance system   600

Conclusion   601

References   602

Introduction

It seems ironic that many of the originating strands of the current ambulance services have their origins in times of war. Organized care of those injured on the battlefield was almost certainly a feature of parts of the Roman army, but Napoleon's senior battlefield surgeons are traditionally credited with the first coordinated battlefield medical plan, involving ambulance transportation of the injured.

In the UK, current ambulance service National Health Service (NHS) trusts deliver emergency and routine pre-hospital patient care and transportation. These have evolved from the post-war Civil Defence provision of ambulance services, through local authority ownership, and the major move in 1974 to become an integral part of the NHS. There are now 11 ambulance services, compared with 46 in 1990.

The moves in the 1990s to NHS trust status dramatically altered the demands placed on ambulance service managers, as well as road staff. These moves coincided with a national commitment to a paramedic-led service, with the target of ensuring that a qualified paramedic was a member of the crew on each emergency ambulance by the beginning of 1996.

Paramedic training resulted in increasing involvement of the medical profession in the training and clinical practices of ambulance services. For the first time it necessitated ambulance staff undertaking more comprehensive in-hospital training under medical supervision. This has quietly resulted in better clinical skills, coupled with a more professional approach to providing patient care. Each ambulance training school accredited to train paramedics by the Institute of Health Care Development (IHCD) is required to have an independent Local Advisory Paramedic Steering Committee. Most ambulance services have full-time medical directors.

The ambulance service as an NHS trust

NHS ambulance trusts are managed by a chief executive and have to provide their own operational, finance and human resources services. They have a trust board with a chairman, appointed by the Secretary of State, and both

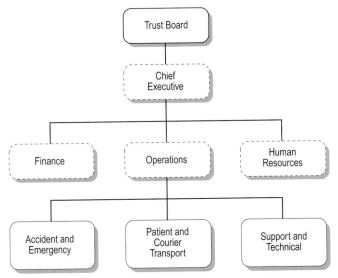

Fig. 58.1 • The structure of an NHS ambulance service trust.

executive and non-executive directors. A typical trust structure is shown in Fig. 58.1.

Traditional ambulance trusts are typically organized into emergency services (dealing with emergency and urgent cases) and patient transport services (dealing with non-emergency and outpatient cases). Fleet, estates and supplies services are usually managed collectively under the support services function. Other non-patient transport functions, such as courier transport and communications services, are provided by many ambulance trusts. Training, which usually includes internal and external functions, may be an operational or human resources function.

The functions of the ambulance service

EMERGENCY AMBULANCE SERVICE

The primary function of this service is to respond to emergency calls arising from the public, other health-care professionals and other emergency services. A service is also provided to transport urgent cases to hospital at the request of doctors and other authorized health-care professionals. Transfers to hospitals, and other treatment centres, of cases requiring more specialized care than is provided locally are also undertaken, along with specialized retrieval services such as paediatric intensive care, where a specialist team is transported to retrieve seriously ill or injured patients.

NON-URGENT PATIENT TRANSPORT SERVICE

The ambulance service, through its patient transport services division, also provides non-urgent outpatient transport for a variety of other NHS and social service agencies. Voluntary car services are also provided for more ambulant cases.

MAJOR INCIDENT RESPONSE

The ambulance service has the statutory requirement to provide the front-line NHS response to major incidents. This includes the provision of transport, patient triage and treatment facilities, medical support and communications at the site of the incident. It must have plans coordinated with other ambulance and emergency services, hospitals, BASICS schemes and other agencies, such as local authorities.

Ambulance vehicles

There are five basic vehicle types:

- Emergency ambulance
- Patient transport ambulance
- Paramedic/Emergency Care Practitioner (ECP) response vehicle
- Support vehicle
- Air ambulance.

THE EMERGENCY AMBULANCE

The emergency ambulance is becoming an increasingly sophisticated vehicle, often with ramps or a single self-loading stretcher cot. Adequate space, lighting and storage are essential, as are rear saloon radio communications, powered suction, in-built ventilation and a fluid warmer. The provision of adequate splinting and patient handling equipment (such as traction splints and long spinal boards, straps and head restraints) is essential, along with pulse oximetry and cardiac monitor–defibrillator units.

Complex electrical systems are required to provide external 'shore line' mains power to maintain charge to batteries and on-charge units, such as defibrillators and fluid warmers, when the vehicle is not in use. Emergency audible and visual warning systems and external lighting need to be increasingly sophisticated with denser traffic situations, and mains power must be available from voltage inverters to power intensive care unit equipment for inter-hospital transfers (Fig. 58.2).

Diesel power is an inevitable requirement for emergency ambulances, as vastly superior fuel consumption and associated engine longevity is irresistible in view of the continuing pressure to reduce recurring costs and provide cost-efficiencies for purchasers. Fortunately, current diesel turbo technology provides a largely acceptable compromise of economy and performance for emergency ambulances.

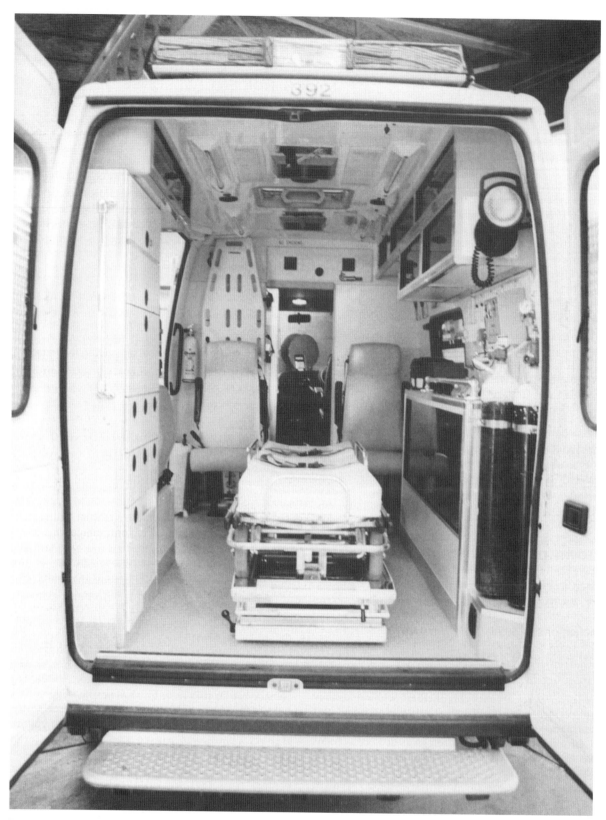

Fig. 58.2 • Modern emergency ambulance with central self-loading cot, in-built suction and ventilator, and sophisticated electrical support system.

PATIENT TRANSPORT AMBULANCES

These ambulances are also more sophisticated than previously, with stretcher-carrying ability and oxygen therapy provision for transporting high-dependency cases. The ability of these vehicles to carry automatic defibrillators for first response to cardiac cases must also be considered when designing this type of ambulance.

PARAMEDIC (ECP) RESPONSE VEHICLES

The paramedic response vehicles vary from the saloon car through the four-wheel drive vehicle to high-powered motorcycles. Their function is to provide a rapid single paramedic response to the scene, with adequate resuscitation equipment for first response. They have advantages of more rapid response in mainly urban areas, and the provision of an additional paramedic to assist with patient management in cardiac arrest and major injury cases. However, an ambulance is still required to transport the patient and there are stresses caused by being a single responder, such as finding difficult locations and dealing with critical cases alone with no support from colleagues. ECP response vehicles vary from the four-wheel response vehicle to a small van-type vehicle that allows a patient to walk in and lie down so that the ECP may treat the patient on scene (e.g. perform a diagnostic test or wound care). It would also be equipped with extra lighting, which would allow the ECP to examine wounds. The role of the ECP is to treat at the scene if appropriate and refer to other primary care professionals to prevent avoidable emergency department attendances or admissions to secondary care.

SUPPORT VEHICLES

These include specialized four-wheel drive ambulances, control vehicles and equipment carriers. Most of these suffer from 'occasional use syndrome', in that they are essential when needed but may be relied upon never to start or to be miles away from wherever they are required. As a means of tackling this, Staffordshire Ambulance Service NHS Trust has a combined unit that carries resupply of long spinal boards, D- and F-sized oxygen, intravenous fluids and drugs for day-to-day incident support. It is fitted with a radio system, for both large and major incident command and control, incident lighting, and has the ability to deploy a single Aireshelta tent. This vehicle is fitted with sophisticated systems to provide mains power and is shore-lined to provide mains charging of all batteries when not in use.

HELICOPTER SUPPORT

Helicopter support is provided from a number of agencies, including the armed forces, the coastguard, police and dedicated ambulance aircraft. Dedicated air ambulance resources are probably the best solution, as they are permanently rigged for air ambulance duties and staffed accordingly.

In some cases, the provision of helicopter services has developed more in response to charitable intent and public pressure than genuine operational need. However, there is no doubt that the provision of these expensive facilities is becoming increasingly focused under medical direction.

There is no doubt that in more rural areas, and in some urban areas, helicopter transportation of patients with specific needs to the most appropriate hospital is desirable and the most effective use of this resource to improve outcomes. Major trauma and severe burns cases are obvious candidates but require prearranged bypass protocols in order to be most effective. The use of an aircraft that provides room and equipment for in-flight care is essential, as is the appropriate skill level for the flight paramedics manning the aircraft.

Operating hours, radius of operation and ability to operate in less than ideal flying conditions are also considerations that should be considered in the planning stages, as should the primary role of the aircraft. Interhospital transfers are often beneficial in terms of quality of ride and shortened duration but highly dependent intensive-care patients cannot safely be transferred by paramedics, so staffing of the aircraft is an important issue. If the aircraft is frequently used for transfer work it is less available for primary response and cannot provide a reliable rapid response to serious incidents.

All these issues need to be addressed if a successful air ambulance operation is to function as a key part of ambulance provision. The likelihood of fewer fully functional district general hospitals, with more resources being transferred to a few larger tertiary centres, is high in the next decade, and this will necessitate an effective air ambulance provision.

Ambulance service control and communications

The ambulance control centre is becoming an area of increasing technological innovation, with significant developments in communication and information technology having a major effect on ambulance service command and control processes.

Call receipt is the entry into the system for the vast majority of demands for assistance. BT provides access from all its landlines to its computerized database of subscribers and their addresses via digital exchanges (Call Line Identification (CLI)), which enables the ambulance control centre to visually display the caller's number and address details virtually as the telephone rings. With modern computer-aided despatch (CAD) systems, once verified, these details can be passed, via an interface, directly into the appropriate fields in the call details screen.

Computer-aided despatch (CAD) systems are becoming very sophisticated and are now interfaced with various mapping products and automatic vehicle location systems (AVLS). This allows the precise location of the address on a display. The CAD can then locate the nearest ambulances to respond. Sophisticated CADs can store these locations for further planning of ambulance response locations. By allocating the precise despatch triage code to the call, along with retrospective plotting of defined major trauma and cardiac arrest cases, it is possible to use these historical data to plan ambulance provision to reach life-threatening cases in the critical 8 min.

The use of data transmission and digital paging can transmit call details to the responding crew, either to a data pager or to a data terminal in the ambulance. Transfer of these data into appropriate fields in electronic patient report forms is now possible, as is transmission of data from recording devices on the ambulance to the receiving hospital.

Current analogue radio systems will be replaced with a trunk digital radio system in the not too distant future. This will revolutionize the provision of efficient speech and data transmission and provide a much more sophisticated communications network.

Mobile telephones are in regular daily use within services, and are equipped with an access override control system (ACCOLC) to allow access to reserved channels in major incident situations where the systems tend to overload rapidly. A mobile emergency control facility is essential to provide adequate communications in cases of major or special incidents. This may be in the form of a dedicated or multirole vehicle.

Finally, the provision of one of the two available medical priority despatch systems is an essential requirement in the modern control centre. The ability to be able to place calls in a medical triage category will enable a decision to be made regarding a 'lights and sirens' or 'no lights and sirens' response by the crew. In addition, it provides prearrival first-aid instruction for callers and better patient information for the responding crew.

Ambulance service training

The current staffing requirement on an emergency ambulance is a crew of two, at least one of whom is a paramedic. Most services can meet this requirement and the national training standard is the IHCD awards of ambulance technician and paramedic (National Health Service Training Division 1991, 1995).

Technicians complete a 6-week ambulance aid course, followed by a 2-week advanced driving course and a 9-month continual assessment process to qualify and to become eligible for consideration of progression to paramedic training. Paramedic training comprises a 2-month preclinical and clinical course with a supervision period to follow. Refresher training comprises a 2-week course every 5 years, with additional refreshers for paramedics yearly and a 3-yearly hospital review.

Paramedic training is moving from in-house training under the umbrella of the IHCD to universities. It is anticipated that paramedics training will be at diploma or foundation degree level. Ambulance services, universities and the Health Professional Council (HPC) are working to develop pre- and postregistration training programmes.

ECPs are one of a number of new roles to emerge following the publication of the NHS Plan (Department of Health 2000) and more recently *Transforming Emergency Care* (2001; Department of Health 2007). ECPs were developed out of the Practitioner in Emergency Care concept, which was first suggested by the Joint Royal Colleges Ambulance Liaison Committee and the Ambulance Service Association. ECPs are required to have completed an accredited clinical education; this will have been evidenced by a paramedical or from a registered nurse background, followed by 3–5 years experience working in the field of emergency or acute clinical care.

Clinicians may then progress to the role of ECP by commencing a recognized university degree BSc programme, modular based over a period of 2 years, as recently established by a Department of Health consultation document implemented by Skills for Health, based on the *Competence and Curriculum Framework for the Emergency Care Practitioner* (2006). The main focus of the ECP role is to enhance the patient experience through their emergency and urgent care journey by providing emergency assessment, diagnosis, treatment and aftercare. ECPs provide a rapid response to an episode of urgent care, in a number of different environments (e.g. ambulance services, general practice, urgent care centres, out of hours service, rapid response vehicles, walk in centres and emergency departments), treat at the scene if appropriate and refer to other primary care professionals to prevent avoidable emergency department attendances or admissions to secondary care.

The critical care practitioner, involved in the transfer of critically ill patients, may well be the next development in ambulance personnel.

In trauma, for instance, Pre-hospital Trauma Life Support (PHTLS), promoted by the Royal College of Surgeons of England (1998) in partnership with the Advanced Trauma Life Support course (ATLS) for physicians (American College of Surgeons 2004) has become quite widely used. This course upgrades clinical assessment and management skills to dovetail with current hospital practice.

In paediatrics, Pre-hospital Paediatric Life Support (PHPLS) is another essential course for paramedics, and has been recently launched to complement the Advanced Paediatric Life Support course (APLS) for physicians (Advanced Life Support Group 2001). This is an area poorly covered in current paramedic training and one in which many paramedics feel a great vulnerability.

Advanced life support (ALS), with its emphasis on current ALS skills and in particular early defibrillation, is another area of essential skills development for paramedics (Resuscitation Council (UK) 2004).

The increasing demands of patient care will require paramedics with augmented abilities, especially in patient assessment and management of trauma, paediatric and cardiac cases. The courses discussed above will provide the basis of this.

University courses for certificate and diploma awards are currently offered at many universities for existing paramedics, and undergraduate courses leading to a degree in Paramedical Sciences are being offered in many UK universities. This higher education base for future paramedic education is undoubtedly the way ahead for the existing paramedic.

Contracting for ambulance services

Contracts are negotiated for emergency services directly with health authority purchasers and for non-emergency services directly with other acute, mental health and community trusts. These contracts are usually for 3–5-year terms but subject to annual review of performance, activity and quality targets.

Performance standards for ambulance services

Audit of the performance of the emergency ambulance service against contracts by purchasers has to date been crude and based on adherence to response time performance requirements established nationally and generally adopted by purchasers locally.

These standards (ORCON) originated in 1974 and were not in any way based on any clinical assessment of patients' needs. They required the emergency ambulance to reach the patient in 50% of cases within 8 min, and in 95% of cases within 14 min in urban areas and 19 min in rural areas.

To date, these have been the baseline performance standards for UK ambulance services, and any additional quality standards have been variable and at the discretion of individual purchaser. These standards tend to be related to paramedic manning levels and provision of suitable vehicles.

Measures and targets based on clinical performance have been conspicuous by their absence, which should be of great concern in the front-line emergency service of the NHS.

In 1996 a joint working party, with ambulance, clinical and other health-care representation, was convened with a remit to revise emergency ambulance performance standards. It published a series of proposals to substantially improve emergency ambulance performance (Steering Group on Ambulance Performance Standards 1996), which are at last related to the clinical needs of patients.

The proposed standards require priority attendance at life-threatening emergencies within 8 min. These cases include patients with chest pain, evidence of cardiorespiratory arrest, some types of penetrating trauma, and ill or injured children under the age of 2 years.

The 8 min standard relates to achieving improved outcomes from cases of prehospital sudden cardiac death. As the majority of cases involve ventricular fibrillation within the first few minutes following collapse, the provision of bystander cardiopulmonary resuscitation, followed by the arrival of a defibrillator and immediate defibrillation largely determine the outcome for the patient. Clearly, in other cases where life is at threat, an 8 min response is likely to improve survivability.

The Bradley report (Department of Health 2005) set ambulance performance targets in response to 999 emergency calls based on the clinical need of the patient. The calls are prioritized according to the seriousness of the patient's condition:

- *Category A*: Immediately life-threatening
- *Category B*: Serious
- *Category C*: Not life-threatening/serious

Category A patients, i.e. those with immediately life-threatening conditions, should receive a response within 8 min for 75% of all cases, irrespective of location. Presenting conditions that require a fully equipped ambulance vehicle to attend the incident must in 95% of cases have an ambulance vehicle arrive within 19 minutes of the request for transport being made.

Category B patients, i.e. those with serious but not life-threatening conditions, should in 95% of cases receive a response within 19 minutes.

Category C calls are considered non-life-threatening and non-serious. For these calls the response time standards are not set nationally but are locally determined. Some of these are dealt with over the telephone by a clinical advisor within the accident and emergency control.

Urgent transport requests are those received from a doctor, midwife or health-care professional to transfer a patient to hospital. From 1 April 2007 these calls have been prioritized and classified in the same way as emergency 999 calls. Because most urgent requests are now categorized as Category C calls the performance standards for this group cannot be reported upon until agreement has been reached with the service commissioners.

Ambulance service performance is also judged by how quickly patients receive thrombolysis (clot-busting) treatment. This should be received within 60 minutes of the 999 call.

Ambulance system design

Changes in the performance requirements for ambulance services will demand a substantial review of how these services are provided. If the emergency ambulance response is to achieve the 75% life-threatening emergency target, irrespective of location, substantial changes in operating methods are essential.

The high-performance system

An ambulance system can claim to be operating to high performance standards when it achieves:

- reliable and consistent response times
- high clinical quality
- high customer satisfaction
- high economic efficiency.

In effect, when that service provides the combination of rapid response times, excellent clinical care, high patient satisfaction for the most cost-effective price, it is providing the basic requirements of high performance.

THE SCIENCE OF LOCATING AMBULANCES

Recent changes include the introduction of some of the very successful methods employed in high performance ambulance systems in the USA. Comprehensive assessment of historical patterns of patient demand, both by hour of day and geographical location, allows matching of ambulance provision to patient demand. Map plotting of emergency and urgent call locations by hour of the day allows accurate siting of ambulance standby locations in order to allow calls to be reached most rapidly. An ambulance siting plan, based on the volume and location of emergency and urgent case demand, can be formulated and is called a system status plan. It will vary the chosen locations in accordance with demand on an hourly basis. This is only one of the changes necessary, which, in general, require a radical openness of management style and very good industrial relations, as substantial operational changes are necessary in current ambulance practice.

Many ambulance services place ambulances on standby in places selected by a computer that predicts where the next emergency might come from, on the basis of rolling 60-week statistics held by the computer program. It is well proven that an ambulance on standby will take less than 30 s to respond to a call compared to 1–2 min if the ambulance is based at a station. Moving from the relative comforts of an ambulance station base to free-standing standby locations is a significant change for crews and they must be closely involved in this process as local knowledge is essential when siting such locations.

DESPATCHING AMBULANCES AND PRIORITY-BASED DESPATCH

Changes in control procedures and the employment of quite sophisticated computer-aided despatch and automatic vehicle location systems are essential in evolving a high performance system. Much, however, can be done by simple procedural changes, such as mobilizing the ambulance immediately the approximate geographical location of the call is known. The vehicle is updated with call details en route.

The employment of a medical priority-based despatch system has been viewed as an essential component in achieving the 8 min standard in life-threatening cases. This is supported by a report from the Medical Care Research Unit (MCRU) at the Sheffield Centre for Health and Related Research, University of Sheffield (Nicholl et al 1996), which suggests that on assessment, both systems currently in limited use in the UK, the advanced medical priority despatch system (AMPDS), and criteria-based despatch, are equally effective at triaging emergency cases into life-threatening and non-life-threatening categories.

However, there are problems; the primary one being the decision at which point to mobilize the ambulance. To achieve an 8 min response, the ambulance must be mobilized as soon as the approximate location of the emergency call is known. This is possible within seconds of the call reaching the control centre but if the despatch is delayed until the exact nature of the call is defined by the medical priority despatch system questions then at least 2 min will be lost before the vehicle mobilizes. This may be critical survival time in cases of cardiac arrest, and the only safe solution is to aim for an 8 min response for all emergencies. While this may be viewed as ambitious, it is entirely possible with adoption of 'high performance' methods. The ability to retrospectively plot the times and locations of cardiac arrest cases may be used to refine the system status plan to being more sensitive to cardiac arrest cases.

Two hidden elements of medical priority-based despatch systems are perhaps the most valuable. First, the uniform reception by telephone of all emergency calls, with the use of prearrival instruction up to and including telephone cardio-pulmonary resuscitation (CPR) instruction to the caller, has been a revelation in providing enhanced CPR rates in cardiac arrest cases. It also leads to a huge response from the public in terms of gratitude for 'staying on the line' while the ambulance is en route, giving advice and reassurance. Second, the provision of a call summary to the crew prepares them better when they arrive at the scene and allows appropriate equipment to be taken immediately to the patient.

AMBULANCE VEHICLES AND SUPPORT SERVICES

Reliable, well-equipped ambulance vehicles that provide good performance and economy, coupled with a first-class patient treatment environment, are essential, as are well-organized support services such as supply and fleet. Vehicle defects causing failure during an emergency call are as lethal as a faulty defibrillator or poorly performing paramedics.

If one were to start all over again, it would be with a single central ambulance depot with a single control centre, centralization of training, supply and fleet services, and administration. This would allow a coordinated 'make ready' function for ambulances so that the oncoming crew would collect a cleaned, fuelled and fully stocked vehicle and leave the depot at the start of a shift ready to respond immediately or move to the nearest high priority standby point. Ambulance vehicles in some areas are being fitted with electronic patient record systems, which will mean that there is capability for ambulance staff to have the necessary information to provide appropriate patient care. The patient care record summary will eventually be available at the point of care. Work should be undertaken to establish the degree to which this can currently be achieved and the connectivity medium to allow the ambulance clinician at the scene to access the NHS care record service.

MEDICAL DIRECTION AND CLINICAL QUALITY

All the developments described above will be of limited value in effecting improved patient care and outcomes if the key area of clinical quality and audit are ignored. Simply getting the ambulance there more quickly will not alone save more lives unless the crew perform to the highest standards clinically, taking advantage of the time window gained by a better response.

As an example, the audit process in Staffordshire showed no significant improvement in cardiac arrest survival during the first year despite radical improvements in response times. Only after clinical review, including the assessment of crews' clinical performance, noted delays in applying immediate defibrillation and subsequent retraining of all emergency staff did a significant improvement in survival occur. Without the presence of medical direction and a clinical services department, this key deficit would have remained elusive and lives would have been unnecessarily lost.

CLINICAL AUDIT

Many services rely on currency of paramedic qualification and basic recertification of paramedic and technician staff as their hallmarks of clinical quality. The inadequacy of this is rapidly illustrated when the processes involved in clinical audit are introduced.

In attempting to introduce clinical audit, the first stumbling block is the lack of protocols that define the standard to audit against. The second is frequently the low compliance with data recording on patient report forms. Without a standard, audit is impossible. All ambulance services use clinical audit as a quality improvement process that seeks to improve patient care and outcomes through systematic review of care against explicit criteria and the implementation of change. Aspects of the structure, processes and outcomes of care are selected and systematically evaluated against explicit criteria. Where indicated, changes are implemented at an individual, team or service level and further monitoring is used to confirm improvement in health-care delivery.

Development of effective improvement strategies is a key component of clinical audit. Recommendations from audit projects are considered by the local clinical governance group, which has responsibility for monitoring clinical improvement strategies. Audit is undertaken to improve the care and services offered to patients, who may be involved with the audit process and outcomes. An environment to support the participation of staff with clinical audit is necessary within ambulance services.

PATIENT SATISFACTION

Finally, the assessment of patient satisfaction is essential. Scant attention has been paid to the quality of customer care provided by our ambulance crews, and in an increasingly demanding and litigation conscious environment the need to provide good-quality care to both the patient and their relatives is an obvious component of effective ambulance care.

Conclusion

The UK ambulance service has a proud history and has progressed in line with its evolution as an integral part of the NHS since 1974. The adoption of the rigours of trust status have established further pressures, both in financial and patient demand terms. In the next 2–3 years, to respond to the further challenges of more demanding performance standards, further fundamental changes will be necessary in operating methods and improved clinical performance.

The concept of high performance ambulance systems has been developed over some years in the USA. These methods have been similarly evolved in some services in the UK over the last 4 years. Some or all of these methods will need to be introduced across the UK if services are to progress in response to these new challenges.

By cooperation with primary care and community-based services, developments such as ECPs will provide a wider array of mobile health-care services, as out-of-hospital health care expands in the near future. In the meantime, an improvement in the care of the acutely ill and injured remains the main goal. This may well lead to the development of critical care practitioners.

References

Advanced Life Support Group 2001 Advanced paediatric life support, 3rd edn. BMJ Publishing, London

American College of Surgeons 2004 Advanced trauma life support for doctors: student course manual, 7th edn. American College of Surgeons, Chicago, IL

Department of Health 2000 The NHS Plan: a plan for investment, a plan for reform. Stationery Office, London

Department of Health 2005 Taking healthcare to the patient – transforming NHS ambulance Services. Stationery Office, London

Department of Health 2007 Reforming emergency care in England: a report by Professor Sir George Alberti. Stationery Office, London

National Health Service Training Division 1991 Ambulance service paramedic training. National Health Service Training Division, Bristol

National Health Service Training Division 1995 Ambulance service basic training. National Health Service Training Division, Bristol

Nicholl J, Gilhooley K, Parry G et al 1996 The safety and reliability of priority despatch systems. Medical Care Research Unit, Sheffield Centre for Health and Related Research. University of Sheffield, Sheffield

Operational Research Consultants 1974 Minimum standard performance measures and targets for emergency, urgent and non-emergency patients. Operational Research Consultants, Cranfield Institute of Technology, Cranfield, Bedfordshire

Resuscitation Council (UK) 2004 ALS manual, 4th edn. (revised). Resuscitation Council (UK), London

Royal College of Surgeons of England 1998 Pre-hospital trauma life support manual, 4th edn. Royal College of Surgeons of England, London

Steering Group on Ambulance Performance Standards 1996 Review of ambulance performance standards. Final report of the Steering Group. NHS Executive, London

The fire service: structure and roles

59

Introduction   603

Organization and structure   603

The fire service role at road traffic accident
entrapments   605

Medical training levels in the fire service   607

Equipment carried by the fire service   607

The fire service role at major incidents   609

The fire service role at incidents involving
hazardous materials   611

Summary   613

Further reading   613

Introduction

Most individuals operating in the field of prehospital medicine at some time will find themselves working alongside their colleagues from the emergency services. Although each service has its own area of expertise and contribution to make at these incidents, a seriously injured casualty's recovery will often depend on the successful teamwork employed. Nowhere is this demand for a 'team approach' more apparent than at road traffic accident entrapments. Rescue times can be significantly reduced by improved teamwork and by each service having a clear appreciation not only of their own role but also of that of their emergency service colleagues. This chapter intends to provide an insight into the structure and role of the fire service, with particular reference to its organization, attendance at road traffic accidents and involvement in prehospital care.

Organization and structure

The Fire Services Act 1947 returned the fire service to local authority control following nationalization during the Second World War. Subsequent local government reorganization has resulted in the UK fire service currently consisting of 57 brigades. While in England these are mainly county or metropolitan brigades, in Wales the three brigades that now exist are controlled by joint boards made up of representatives from the various unitary authorities. A similar situation exists in Scotland. The Northern Ireland fire brigade provides cover for the entire province and is funded directly from central government.

Under the Fire Services Acts 1947 and 1959, the Home Secretary has responsibility for the fire service in England and Wales. The Fire Department of the Home Office consists of the Fire Service Inspectorate, which carries out annual inspections of brigades, and two administrative divisions that provide support to the Home Secretary in respect of his responsibility for fire matters. Although central guidance is exercised by the Home Secretary in coordinating the development of the service and ensuring that the operational efficiency of brigades is maintained, fire authorities have complete discretion in the day-to-day administration of their brigades.

In Scotland, ultimate responsibility for the fire service falls to the Secretary of State for Scotland, while inspections are carried out by fire service inspectors who are members of the Scottish Office Home and Health Department. In Northern Ireland these responsibilities fall to the Permanent Secretary of the Department of the Environment for Northern Ireland and the Fire Service Inspectorate, respectively.

Under the command of the chief fire officer (firemaster in Scotland) each fire brigade has its own headquarters housing its principal officers and associated support staff. Each brigade also has its own control room for receiving emergency calls and mobilizing resources. These control rooms are able to access and transmit an enormous amount of information to fireground commanders via radio, fax or computer terminal. As well as recording the relevant details of all emergency calls received, fire control can provide information regarding:

- plans of individual premises and their risk assessments
- location of hydrants and open water supplies
- availability of additional resources.

They are also able to provide:

- contact with other emergency service control rooms
- contact with other support services

- guidance on hazardous materials via Chemdata and CIRUS (the Chemical Information Retrieval Update Scheme).

Although an increasing number of brigades are adopting functional management systems, most brigades are organized geographically into divisions under the command of a divisional officer. Each division in turn consists of a number of fire stations, normally under the command of a station officer, and each station is staffed by four watches. Each watch is usually commanded by a sub-officer, who is in turn assisted by one or more leading firefighters (Fig. 59.1).

Figure 59.2 illustrates the various uniform and helmet rank markings. It may be useful to note that at operational incidents firefighters can be easily identified by their helmets. Officers above the rank of sub-officer have white helmets, while sub-officers and below have yellow. The greater the number and width of the black bands around the helmet, the higher the individual's rank (Fig. 59.2).

White hats outrank yellow hats; the greater the number and width of black bands, the higher the rank.

Although the majority of firefighters in the UK are full-time professionals, *retained firefighters* who have other full-time jobs are also employed – either as back-up to their full-time colleagues in larger towns and cities, or in rural areas where the prevailing risk and number of fire calls is insufficient to justify employing full-time firefighters. These retained firefighters respond to fire calls via radio-pagers, with the first to arrive forming a crew and riding the fire pump (engine).

Although the fire service has no statutory obligation to attend incidents other than fires, and receives no direct funding for doing so, under Section 3.1.(e) of the Fire Services Act 1947 the fire authority is empowered to use the fire brigade and its equipment for purposes other than firefighting. This has led to the role of the fire service gradually evolving so that each fire brigade now provides a range of emergency services over and above the statutory provision of fire cover. Indeed, since 1968, nearly half have changed

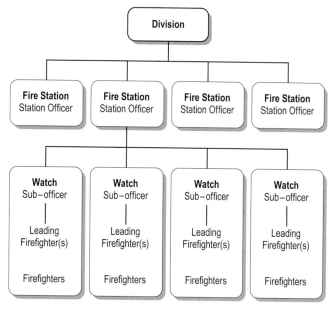

Fig. 59.1 • The fire station (schematic).

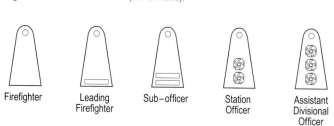

| Firefighter | Leading Firefighter | Sub–officer | Station Officer | Assistant Divisional Officer | Divisional Officer | Senior Divisional Officer | Assistant Chief Officer | Chief Officer |

Fig. 59.2 • Fire service rank marking.

their name to 'the fire and rescue service' in order to more accurately reflect the changing nature of their work.

This work includes:

- providing a rescue service for persons trapped in road, rail or aviation incidents
- rescue of persons trapped in lifts, and in agricultural and industrial accidents
- dealing with hazardous materials
- providing personnel and equipment to deal with a diverse range of other emergency incidents.

Since the Second World War these non-fire-related emergencies, so called 'special service calls', have risen to the extent that they now account for 16% of all emergency calls. Despite this changing role, the principal aims of the fire service remain largely unaltered. They are: to save life; to protect property from fire; to render humanitarian services; and to protect the environment.

- **To save life**
- **To protect property**
- **To render humanitarian services**
- **To protect the environment**

The fire service's role as the principal rescue service is confirmed by the official figures issued annually by the Home Office. Each year some 4000 rescues are carried out from fires, some 22 000 from lifts and over 7000 other rescues are carried out from a range of different incidents.

In addition to all of the above, in the year 1996/97 in England and Wales the fire service rescued well over 10 000 people trapped in vehicles following road traffic accidents. It is a strange anomaly that, in a decade that saw safety features such as airbags, seat belt pre-tensioners and side impact bars become commonplace, and in which serious injuries and deaths due to road accidents fell steadily, the number of rescues carried out by the fire service at road traffic accidents increased by 56%. No other type of incident brings the emergency services together more often, so it is important that those involved in prehospital care appreciate the fire service role at road traffic accidents, their medical training levels, the equipment they carry and their working practices.

The fire service role at road traffic accident entrapments

The Fire Service College is the UK's central training establishment for fire officers and has a central role in providing road traffic accident training via instructor courses and the 'core progression' system of training that all junior officers and officers experience. As part of its commitment to improving the road traffic accident training it provides for the fire service, the college has compiled an entrapment database believed to be the largest of its kind in the world. This database provides unique information about the nature of vehicle entrapments and has led to the development of a systematic approach to effecting rescues from road traffic accidents. This system is particularly appropriate for single casualty entrapments, which account for over 70% of incidents, and is designed to assist fire officers in achieving safe, time-effective, casualty-centred rescues. Based around the recognition that several distinct phases exist at a well-controlled rescue, these 'key' phases act as a checklist for fire officers to complete systematically and provide prehospital carers with a useful insight into the fire service's role at these incidents. Viewed in simple terms, the six phases of a road traffic accident rescue are:

- scene assessment and safety
- stabilization and initial access
- glass management
- space creation
- full access and immobilization
- extrication.

SCENE ASSESSMENT AND SAFETY

During the initial moments of any road traffic accident rescue, incident commanders must ensure that their assessment includes both a close-up check of individual vehicles and a wider appraisal of the entire incident scene. In effect, this could be described as an inner circle, outer circle survey. The inner circle survey confirms the number of casualties trapped and identifies immediate hazards such as fuel leaks, live electrics and so on. The outer circle survey establishes the full extent of the incident, existing traffic hazards and walking wounded. This method quickly identifies the safety precautions necessary to protect the scene and establishes priority working areas. The fire service will automatically lay out firefighting equipment to reduce the risk from fire.

STABILIZATION AND INITIAL ACCESS

The general guidance given to firefighters is that all persons involved in road traffic accidents must be treated as if they have spinal injuries. As a general rule, therefore, the fire service will stabilize vehicles before committing rescuers inside or before commencing rescue efforts. Perhaps the only exception to this would be where a snatch rescue were required, as in the event of fire or exposure to chemicals, or were there to be doubt as to the casualty's airway. Quite obviously, an obstructed airway is a life-threatening situation and any steps necessary to check, clear and maintain an airway must not be delayed. As a general guide when dealing with the more common types of entrapment, the vehicle stabilization phase will take a trained crew about 1 min to achieve using various blocks and chocks that are routinely carried on fire appliances. The effective stabilization of vehicles results in a safe, solid platform for rescuers to work on and prevents movement being transmitted to casualties trapped inside.

GLASS MANAGEMENT

The hazards posed by toughened or laminated glass are often overlooked during rescue operations. Badly managed, it remains a hazard to rescuers and casualties alike throughout the entire incident. The fire service's aim, therefore, is to reduce the hazard in one continuous phase at the earliest opportunity. Ideally, this phase should take only 2–3 min at the beginning of the rescue, and is achieved by winding down windows, cutting bonded laminated windscreens, completely removing glass panels or controlled breakage – whichever option is most appropriate.

In situations where immediate access to casualties is required and conventional access through doors is denied, rescuers will find tools such as automatic centre-punches and glass hammers invaluable. These inexpensive tools facilitate the rapid accessing of casualties via the controlled breakage of the toughened glass panels found in the side windows and rear screen.

SPACE CREATION

Fire officers are taught that the three problems common at all difficult entrapments are:

- the presence of casualties requiring urgent medical attention
- difficulty gaining access to casualties
- the absence of space in which to work.

They are taught that the solution to these problems centres on space creation, with one of the hallmarks of professional rescuers being the early and adequate creation of space around victims. The fire service's ability to systematically dismantle vehicles has improved dramatically in recent years through the use of powered hydraulic rescue equipment. A few years ago, only a limited amount of this equipment would be strategically sited in a brigade and it would therefore be some minutes before it would arrive at an incident. The availability of this equipment, however, has risen to the extent that it is now carried on most first attendance fire pumps.

When faced with a casualty severely trapped by the door, by the pedals and footwell, and by the steering wheel and dashboard, it is sometimes difficult to know where to begin. Firefighters are taught as a general guide to make the *biggest* space *first*, that is, to remove the roof rather than the door as this provides medical rescuers with better all-round access to casualties and generally results in quicker, more effective rescues.

FULL ACCESS

While in the 1970s few fire brigades were equipped with powered hydraulic rescue equipment, the exact opposite is the case today. Gaining full access to victims, therefore, requires little more than the systematic dismantling of the vehicle – something unimaginable a few years ago. Firefighters are taught that *full* access to *all* entrapment victims should be their realistic goal, and that *limited* access invariably results in poor patient handling and can compound the injuries a casualty may be suffering. Fire service personnel are taught to 'make the hole fit the casualty, not the casualty fit the hole!'

EXTRICATION

Owing to the forces to which road traffic accident victims are frequently subjected, fire service rescuers are taught to assume that casualties have sustained spinal injuries and to err on the side of caution. Indeed, more and more fire brigades carry cervical collars and spinal immobilization devices to protect casualties during the rescue process. Although the extrication phase of the rescue will invariably proceed under the direction of the senior ambulance paramedic or doctor present, the correct use of extrication devices and long spinal boards is labour-intensive. With this in mind, fire service personnel may well provide useful additional help.

MAKING THE SYSTEM WORK

This systematic approach to effecting rescues provides useful guidance for those faced with the challenge of a difficult road traffic accident entrapment. It should be appreciated, however, that mere recital of a system is of no value unless the system is made to work. Fire officers are taught that the common faults at poorly managed rescues are:

- The notable absence of a clearly identifiable officer in charge.
- The absence of liaison (typically between medical rescuers and physical rescuers).
- The notable absence of 'simultaneous activity'.
- General confusion, congestion and clutter around the entrapment vehicle.

The following guidance is given to fire officers in command at road traffic accidents to enable them to *avoid* these common faults. While providing further insight into the fire service's procedures for dealing with road traffic accident entrapments, much of the advice is relevant to the other services involved in the rescue.

- Liaise with paramedics – the casualty's condition should always determine the exact rescue method adopted.
- Preplan and delegate routine tasks in advance; brief individuals on the sequence of events – do not assume they know what you are thinking.
- Control events by remaining 'hands off' rather than becoming 'hands on'. Put yourself in the best position to see the full picture.
- Control both the quality of the work and the *tempo* that your personnel work at. It can be as necessary to slow a crew down during the extrication phase as it can be to inject urgency into rescue efforts.
- Do not be reluctant to encourage or discipline personnel as appropriate. These are important leadership functions.
- Continuously assess and evaluate proceedings, asking yourself the important questions: 'Is this the best option? What other options are there? What if plan A does not work?'
- Take advantage of any opportunity to do two or more jobs at the same time. *Simultaneous activity* or *multitasking* is the best way of reducing on-scene time and may make the difference between life and death for patients with time-critical injuries.
- Eliminate congestion and clutter by establishing equipment pools. These, ideally, should be situated within a few metres of the entrapment vehicle, close enough to be used but far enough away so as not to constitute a trip hazard.
- Remove anyone who is not contributing to the rescue from around the entrapment vehicle – they only serve to further congest the scene.

Medical training levels in the fire service

The question, 'What is an appropriate level of medical training for the UK fire service?' has long been the subject of discussion and debate, with differing standards of training apparent across the brigades.

In 1993 the Home Office issued guidance to fire brigades via Fire Service Circular 9/93, as to the minimum level of first-aid training they should provide to satisfy the Health and Safety (First Aid) Regulations 1981 Approved Code of Practice. It recommended to brigades *as a minimum* that 25% of all firefighters should be qualified to 'trained first-aider' standard and should requalify every 3 years and that all remaining firefighters should be trained to 'emergency first-aider' standard. It also emphasized that

Table 59.1 Fire service attendance times

Risk category	Attendance
A	Two pumps in 5 min plus one further pump in 8 min
B	One pump in 5 min plus one further pump in 8 min
C	One pump in 8–10 min
D	One pump in 20 min
Special	Unspecified
Remote	Unspecified

the long-term aim was for all firefighters to become trained first-aiders and remain qualified throughout their careers.

While a minority of brigades are unable to fulfil this recommendation at present, the majority of brigades train their firefighters to first-aider level, with an increasing number providing medical training to a higher standard. This higher standard includes training personnel to 'first responder' level and even, in some instances, training selected individuals to 'emergency medical technician' (EMT) level. A number of other brigades provide firefighters with short courses in trauma management. The provision of 'advanced first-aid training' is a response to the fire service's faster attendance times, which frequently result in firefighters having to deal with the victims of fires and road accidents prior to the arrival of the ambulance service. Table 59.1 indicates the fire service's attendance times for different areas of risk and provides a further insight into their role.

Table 59.1 identifies only the *minimum* fire service attendance within each risk area. It is commonplace, for example, for many brigades to send *two* pumps to any property fire occurring in C and D risk areas. Furthermore, as the fire service has no statutory obligation to attend incidents other than fires, there are no specified attendance times for special service calls such as road accident entrapments.

Equipment carried by the fire service

Just as medical training levels in fire brigades differ markedly, so does the medical equipment carried on fire appliances. However, all brigades carry first-aid kits and resuscitators, with 51 of the 57 brigades in the UK carrying oxygen resuscitators in preference to compressed air. The majority also carry suction, together with simple airway adjuncts such as oropharyngeal airways.

Recent guidance issued via a 'Dear Chief Officer...' letter (the standard route of communications between the Home Office/Scottish Office and the fire service) provides advice to fire brigades as to the equipment that should now be carried on pumping appliances (pumps) attending road traffic accidents. These recommendations were designed to ensure that the first pumps to arrive at an incident have sufficient equipment to render help to persons trapped or injured and to obviate the need to await the arrival of a specialist rescue/emergency tender, which invariably has a much longer distance to travel. As the overwhelming majority of pumps attend road traffic accidents, this letter provides a reliable indication of the trend that brigades are likely to follow when equipping vehicles. The list below provides a useful guide as to equipment, other than for firefighting, that is likely to be available on-scene. Although this equipment is carried primarily for use at road traffic accidents, it will, of course, be available at *any* incident the fire service attends. This additional equipment falls into the following categories:

- lifting, spreading and cutting equipment
- personal protective equipment
- medical equipment
- communications
- miscellaneous equipment.

LIFTING, SPREADING AND CUTTING EQUIPMENT

A set of portable powered lifting, spreading and cutting equipment, with a minimum capacity of 4 tons.

PERSONAL PROTECTIVE EQUIPMENT

A range of equipment which could include high-visibility jackets, chemical protection suits, protective gloves, eye protection, head protection and ear defenders. Similar equipment should also be provided to protect casualties when appropriate.

MEDICAL EQUIPMENT

This includes resuscitation equipment (in fact, all but six brigades already carry oxygen resuscitators; the remainder carry compressed-air resuscitators), cervical collars, spinal boards, stretchers, blankets and enhanced first-aid kits containing large dressings and other first-aid equipment.

COMMUNICATIONS EQUIPMENT

This includes hand-held portable radios and loudhailers.

MISCELLANEOUS

This includes lighting (both powered and portable), lighting tripods, blocks and chocks, road cones, accident warning signs, stationery to include labels for body tagging, road marking equipment, warning beacons and hand-cleaning solution.

In addition to the equipment carried on fire pumps, most fire brigades still provide a number of specialist rescue/emergency tenders carrying a comprehensive range of rescue equipment. However, the trend has been towards reducing the number of these vehicles as more rescue equipment is carried on fire pumps. As mentioned previously, there will invariably be a delay of some minutes before these vehicles arrive due to the large geographical area they cover. Although in theory brigades design and equip these vehicles to suit their own individual circumstances, in practice the type of equipment carried is very similar. Table 59.2

Table 59.2 Fire service equipment

Name of equipment	Common name	Description/use
Powered hydraulic rescue equipment	Cutters, spreaders, rams, combi-tools, 'jaws of life'	Heavy rescue equipment used to push, pull, lift, spread or clamp
Cengar saw	Cengar saw	Air-powered saw used to cut thin-gauge metal and timber
Pneumatic chisel	Zip gun, ripper gun, air chisel	Air-powered chisel designed to cut holes in metal panels
Pneumatic lifting units (high pressure)	High-pressure airbags or air cushions	Air lifting units of varying sizes with lifting capacities up to approx. 100 tons
Pneumatic lifting units (low pressure)	Low-pressure airbags	Air lifting units of about 3 ton capacity – useful where conventional jacking is inappropriate
Tirfor	Hand-operated winch	Multi-purpose hand-powered winch capable of hoisting approx. 3 tons
Hot cutting equipment	Thermic arc, thermic lance, oxyacetylene, oxypropane	Cutting equipment typically used on heavy-gauge metal where other equipment is too slow/ inappropriate

provides those working in the prehospital environment with a brief description of this equipment and the uses to which it may be put.

The fire service role at major incidents

This section is designed to provide an overview of the fire service role at major incidents and enable those from the other emergency services to integrate their own preplanning into an overall framework that complements joint operations. Although by their very nature major incidents are invariably different and will require different responses and some flexibility, many elements are common to all circumstances and will be outlined in the paragraphs below.

For the purposes of this section, the term 'major incident' is taken to mean any emergency that requires the implementation of special arrangements by one or more of the emergency services for the following:

- the initial treatment, rescue and transport of a large number of casualties
- the involvement either directly or indirectly of large numbers of people
- the handling of large numbers of enquiries likely to be generated both from the public and the news media (usually the responsibility of the police)
- the need for the large-scale combined resources of the emergency services
- the mobilization and organization of the emergency services and supporting organizations, for example, the local authority, to cater for the threat of death, serious injury or homelessness to a large number of people.

Not all of these requirements would necessarily apply to the fire service and, of course, major incidents can have many causes. Those most likely to involve the fire service in large-scale operations would normally result from fires, explosions, release of hazardous substances or transportation accidents whether by air, sea, road or rail. It must also be recognized that the fire service attends large fires and other incidents where resources often equal those required at a major incident, but which do not fall within the above definition.

The fire service role at a major incident is at the centre of the scene of disaster where effective command and control of operations must be exercised. Beyond this, the overall responsibility for coordinating the strategic roles of the emergency services lies with the police for land-based incidents and the coastguard for coastal areas and cliffs. It is recognized, however, that because of the nature of certain major incidents or natural disasters this coordination role may be handed over to another more appropriate service or agency. At all times, however, fire service personnel remain under the command of their senior officer. In discharging the coordinating role, account is taken of the features of a particular incident, together with the expertise of each of the emergency services and their statutory duties. As well as their statutory responsibility for fighting fires, the fire service is recognized as the principal rescue service and will have responsibility for the rescue function.

PRINCIPAL RESPONSIBILITIES

The role of the fire service at major incidents is derived from its long experience of firefighting and rescue operations of all types. Fire service major incident plans are designed to cover the following:

- the rescue of trapped people
- preventing further escalation of the incident by tackling fires, dealing with released chemicals and other hazardous situations
- information gathering and hazard assessment to give advice to the police and enable them to advise the public regarding evacuation
- liaison with the police regarding the provision of an inner cordon around the immediate incident to enable the fire service to exercise control
- the safety of all personnel involved in rescue work
- consideration of the effect the incident may have on the environment and the action to be taken to minimize this
- liaison with the medical incident officer and other medical services, and liaison with the ambulance service with regard to providing assistance at ambulance loading points and the priority evacuation of injured persons
- assisting police with the recovery of the dead
- participating in investigations as appropriate, and preparing reports and evidence for enquiries
- if necessary, to standby during the non-emergency recovery phase to ensure continued safety at and surrounding the site.

This division of responsibility allows the fire service to make a significant impact in preventing escalation of the incident and gives casualties and others at risk the greatest chance of survival.

THE FIRE SERVICE RESPONSE

Fire brigade plans include a predetermined response to a major incident message. This response will vary depending on the resources of individual brigades but should include sufficient pumps, emergency tenders and other vehicles to make a significant impact in terms of personnel and equipment.

This initial response should also include a mobile control unit and appropriate staff, together with officers of suitable ranks to enable the necessary levels of command to be set up and liaison officers to be provided. Owing to the considerable increase in telephone calls to the fire service control, arrangements are normally made to increase the availability of personnel and equipment to meet this demand.

Although initial fire appliances are directed to the immediate scene of the incident as soon as practical, full use should be made of rendezvous points and marshalling areas. The aim of these measures is to control the responding appliances, reduce congestion around the incident and establish a pool of resources that can be ordered on to the incident without delay when required.

INITIAL ACTIONS BY THE FIRST FIRE OFFICER ON-SCENE

Although there may be considerable pressure to commence rescue and other operations, the first officer to arrive on-scene must not become involved in rescue efforts. Instead, this officer's primary function is to determine the size, scope and nature of the emergency, and convey this information to control. It is therefore important that the scale of the incident be thoroughly assessed and the correct level of response initiated. On receipt of the standard phrase 'major incident', fire control will mobilize the appropriate pre-determined attendance and inform both police and ambulance controls.

COMMAND STRUCTURES

In order to ensure a common approach to the management of a major incident, many fire brigades have now adopted the police force's 'gold, silver, bronze' concept of command as follows.

- **Gold (strategic): overall incident officer determines the strategy**
- **Silver (tactical): incident commander determines tactics within the parameters set by gold**
- **Bronze (operational): sector (or functional) commanders implement the tactics set by silver**

Gold control is normally sited remote from the incident, while silver control is normally sited close to the incident (Ch. 47). It may be difficult for the fire service command structure to accurately reflect these levels of control, particularly in smaller brigades, as the principal officer is likely to be at the scene of the incident. It may be the case, therefore, that at any discussions held by the 'gold' senior

coordinating team at a remote location, the fire service is represented by a senior liaison officer, with the fire and rescue commander attending meetings of the on-site coordinating group.

THE FIRE SERVICE ROLE

The senior fire service officer present at the scene at any given time will become the fire and rescue commander of the incident. This officer will take control of firefighting and rescue operations in the immediate area of the disaster. As resources increase, responsibilities will normally be apportioned to officers who may take control of fire and rescue operations in particular areas of the incident (sector officers), or carry out specific duties (functional officers). The fire and rescue commander should appoint a coordinator to run the incident control post once it is established.

In the initial stages of a major incident, the emergency services are likely to be confronted with a scene of confusion and uncoordinated activity. It is essential to establish control of the immediate area of the incident and anyone who is assisting with rescue work. If there is a fire, chemical or explosive hazard, or if a situation exists where the incident may escalate, an inner cordon will normally be established to enable the fire service to exercise control of firefighting and rescue operations.

The fire service is responsible for safety at the scene of a major incident.

The fire service has responsibility for the safety of all persons within this cordon. This entails:

- as soon as practical, clearing all non-essential personnel from within the inner cordon
- briefing personnel entering as to fire service safety procedures
- briefing personnel entering as to the evacuation signal and nominal roll procedures
- booking in all non-fire-service personnel entering the inner cordon
- ensuring these people are aware of, and conform to, fire service safety procedures
- ensuring the correct equipment is used within the cordon in the event of a flammable atmosphere with the risk of explosion
- where appropriate, ensuring that only intrinsically safe or explosion-protected equipment is used
- ensuring that those entering the risk area are dressed in appropriate personal protective equipment.

Initially all efforts will be directed at preventing an escalation of the disaster by controlling fire or the release of dangerous materials and rescuing trapped casualties. During this phase the fire and rescue commander will take direct control of firefighting operations within the inner cordon. Second only to the prevention of further catastrophe (e.g. gas or other explosion), priority will then be given to the treatment and recovery of casualties from the site. A system of marking should be established to prevent unnecessary second searching of the site.

Early liaison with the NHS ambulance service and medical officers will provide advice on medical aspects of recovery, the evacuation of casualties and the protection of personnel carrying out this work. Fatalities will normally be left in position unless in danger of being lost or impairing the rescue of live casualties. Fire service personnel may become involved in the labelling of fatalities using a standard 'fatality identification system'.

CONTROL POINTS

Dependent on the size and nature of the incident, several levels of control may be established by the fire service and other emergency services. These may consist of:

- forward control point
- incident control post (silver)
- fire service control room
- major incident control room (gold).

A *forward control point* is normally the first control point established and will be sited close to the scene of the incident. It will usually consist of the first fire appliance to arrive.

An *incident control post* will be established as more resources arrive. Normally this will be a mobile control unit positioned away from the immediate centre of operations and will usually be adjacent to the police and ambulance controls. Its functions include:

- the booking in and management of all fire service personnel
- liaison with the fire and rescue commander, sector and functional officers
- liaison with other emergency services and support services
- making a plan of the rescue area showing the deployment of resources
- logging all messages and occurrences
- providing situation reports as required
- ensuring adequate relief of personnel and equipment.

The *fire service control room* is responsible for the mobilizing of the necessary resources, and alerting the other emergency and support services.

A *major incident control* (gold control) may be established by the police depending on the size of the incident. This control will be under the command of the police. In general, however, command of fire service operations will remain at the incident.

The fire service role at incidents involving hazardous materials

This section is designed to provide an overview of the fire service role at incidents involving hazardous materials. It should enable those attending such incidents to integrate their own preplanning into an overall framework that complements joint operations.

It is recognized that a disorganized response to a hazardous materials incident can easily place both the personnel responding and members of the public in unacceptable positions of risk. This could result in major injury, unnecessary contamination or even death. The principal aims of the fire service, therefore, are to gain rapid control of these incidents and to achieve a segregation of the public and responding personnel from the problem – whatever it may be.

Apart from those large incidents that arise as a result of a catastrophic failure of plant or equipment, many incidents start off as small ones and develop as a result of inadequate management and lack of anticipation during the early stages of the event. This escalation can often be so rapid as to confront fire officers with a planning task of potentially bewildering proportions. In order to assist them in this task, the fire service have developed a standard system of incident management that can be used at any hazardous materials incident. This system of management is based around six major tasks:

- Assuming command of the incident and establishing a supporting organization
- Ensuring that the incident scene is approached in a safe manner
- Establishing a security perimeter around the incident scene
- Establishing restricted areas (or hazard control zones) by the use of cordons
- Assessing the incident with regard to the need for immediate action (rescues and other initial actions to protect life and the environment)
- Establishing a system to control oncoming resources via staging areas, rendezvous points and equipment pools.

ASSUMING COMMAND OF THE INCIDENT AND ESTABLISHING A SUPPORTING ORGANIZATION

This entails the fire officer in charge assuming command and establishing a command structure that ensures that everyone at the incident knows who is in overall command and which individuals they answer to. Central to this command structure is the appointment of sector commanders and functional officers. A command post will be established, together with communications between fireground control, brigade control, fireground personnel and other agencies. A means of requesting and managing additional resources will then be set up.

ENSURING THAT THE INCIDENT SCENE IS APPROACHED IN A SAFE MANNER

The initial approach route and setting-up area chosen by the initial attendance is critical to the success or otherwise of operations at the incident. Points that should always be borne in mind are:

- If possible always approach from uphill and upwind. If this is not possible, consider rerouting or skirting the area at a distance. Avoid approaching through any area where there is the possibility of coming into contact with a vapour cloud – visible or invisible!

- Clues as to the extent of any release may be provided by wet areas, visible condensation or fumes, spilt materials, etc. Assess the situation using biological indicators – are there any dead animals or birds in the vicinity? If so, there is probably a toxicity problem. If it is impossible to approach the area without compromising crew safety then the fire service will establish a restricted area and deploy personnel in protective clothing and breathing apparatus.

ESTABLISHING A SECURITY PERIMETER AROUND THE INCIDENT SCENE

After the approach has been made, the next action immediately necessary will be to establish and identify the boundary of the area directly affected by the hazard. This will consist of an *outer cordon* sufficiently large as to exclude all unauthorized personnel and to allow emergency service personnel to function without hindrance.

ESTABLISHING RESTRICTED AREAS (OR HAZARD CONTROL ZONES) BY THE USE OF CORDONS

Within this outer cordon will be the *inner cordon* or 'hot zone' proper, within which the hazard is present. The exact configuration of the 'hot zone' will depend on factors such as the type of material involved, weather conditions, wind directions, slope of the ground, etc. It is essential to ensure that the area outside the cordon is safe.

The fire service may also establish additional outer cordons surrounding the hazard area, in effect creating a 'warm zone'. Access to this area is restricted to emergency response personnel supporting operations in the hot zone to allow them to proceed without outside interference. Crews working inside the hot zone will be dressed in appropriate protective clothing. Decontamination facilities, if appropriate, will normally be sited at the boundary between the hot zone and the warm zone.

The establishment of cordons and delegation of cordons officers are designed to isolate hazardous materials incidents from the public and to provide the fire service with complete control over events.

ASSESSING THE INCIDENT WITH REGARD TO THE NEED FOR IMMEDIATE ACTION

Immediate action will normally include:

- Life saving and preservation, to include the rescue/removal of those endangered by the incident and the treatment of the injured
- The safety and welfare of responding personnel throughout the duration of the incident
- Incident stabilization by the implementation of activities designed to minimize the potential of additional danger or harm to either humans or the environment.

One of the earliest actions of the incident commander will be an initial scene assessment, or 'size up' as it is known. This process consists of rapid but deliberate consideration of all factors at the scene which will have either a direct or potential impact on the development of the incident, and consequently the actions needed to mitigate it. These factors include the geographical size of the incident, the complexity of the event, the availability of resources and the anticipated duration of the incident. Consideration must also be given as to whether the incident is *static* or *dynamic*. An example of a *static* incident might be a spill of hazardous material which is no longer spreading; while a *dynamic* incident may develop rapidly as, for example, at a large fire involving liquified petroleum gas (LPG) storage bullets, where there is the potential for catastrophic escalation.

ESTABLISHING A SYSTEM TO CONTROL ONCOMING RESOURCES VIA STAGING AREAS, RENDEZVOUS POINTS AND EQUIPMENT POOLS

At many incidents, the arrival of large numbers of personnel and appliances together with large amounts of specialist equipment can prove extremely difficult to control. In these circumstances, typically, the fire service would establish rendezvous points and staging areas close to the incident where personnel and equipment can be held ready for deployment. Equipment pools are normally strategically sited to service the scenes of operations. The use of these pools serves to increase efficiency by reducing foreground clutter and maximizes valuable resources.

The fire service has a variety of methods of dealing with incidents involving hazardous substances. These methods include sealing tanks and plugging leaks, the isolation of valves, containing spillages, dilution or absorption. All these methods would be first assessed as to their effect on the environment; indeed close liaison has resulted in a recent memorandum of understanding between the fire service and the Environment Agency.

Summary

This chapter has provided an introduction to the structure and role of the fire service – an organization providing a range of emergency services over and above its statutory obligation to fight fires. While its role will continue to evolve in line with the demands placed upon it, the fire service is likely to remain a national service, locally delivered.

Knowledge of the structure and role of the UK fire service, together with an appreciation of its operational procedures, will greatly increase the effectiveness of all those involved in the delivery of prehospital medicine.

Further reading

Fire Service Circular 9/93 (Home Office document)

Fire Services Act 1947

Health and Safety (First Aid) Regulations 1981 Report of HM Chief Inspector of Fire Services for England and Wales. HMSO, London

Police force: structure and roles

60

Introduction   614

Introduction to the police service   614

Management of the police service   615

Rank structure   616

Specialized duties   617

Complaints and discipline   617

Civilianization   617

Other police forces   618

Image   618

Statutory obligations   618

The process of law   618

Road traffic law   619

The role of the scene of crime officers and
how medical staff can help   620

Major incidents   622

Phases of a major incident   623

References   624

Introduction

This chapter is intended to provide an insight into various aspects of the police service, specifically for those people who have little or no knowledge of the subject. Areas that will be discussed include the structure of the service in the UK, specific duties performed by police officers, the specialist areas of forensic science, the examination of scenes of crime and the handling of major incidents.

Introduction to the police service

There are 43 police forces in England and Wales, which operate on a tripartite basis under the direction of the Home Office, local police authorities and chief constables. Individual forces vary in size quite considerably; the largest is the Metropolitan police force in London, with 31 000 officers.

The statement of common purpose and values of the police service defines its purpose as follows (Association of Chief Police Officers 1990):

> To uphold the law fairly and firmly, to prevent crime; to pursue and bring to justice those who break the law; to keep the Queen's Peace; to protect, help and reassure the community; and to be seen to do this with integrity, common sense and sound judgement.
>
> Officers need to be professional, calm and restrained in the face of violence, and apply only that force which is necessary to accomplish their lawful duty.
>
> They must be compassionate, courteous and patient, acting without fear or favour or prejudice to the rights of others. The police service must strive to reduce fears of the

public and, so far as they can, to reflect their priorities in the action they take and respond to well founded criticism with a willingness to change.

Each police force is responsible for the maintenance of law and order within its geographical area and also attempts to address issues of specific local concern. This involves police officers operating in a variety of roles within the community.

A fundamental principle of British policing embodied in Section 96 of the Police Act 1996 is that police forces are required to consult with the public they serve, thus strengthening the role of the police within the community.

A partnership approach involving the police working closely with other community agencies is being used increasingly: for example, many forces have schools liaison programmes where officers attend local schools in order to discuss issues affecting pupils, and many are formalizing 'community safety partnership strategies' with unitary authorities.

Management of the police service

One of the most far reaching reforms affecting the management of the police service is the Police and Magistrates' Courts Act 1994. This Act changed the composition and functions of police authorities and placed emphasis on the production of local policing plans and the setting, by the Home Office, of national objectives and corresponding performance indicators.

The Act sets out the roles and responsibilities of the tripartite power structure comprising the Home Office, the police authority and the Chief Constable, as indicated below.

HOME OFFICE

General duty

The Home Office is responsible for promoting the general efficiency and effectiveness of the police service, as well as for the specific areas listed below.

Finance

The Home Office is responsible for determining the aggregate grant and capping level for individual force budgets and issues guidance to police forces encouraging internal budget delegation.

Personnel

The Home Office arbitrates in disputes over management of civilians and approves the appointment of chief and assistant chief constables, and can require them to retire in the interests of efficiency.

Objectives and targets

National objectives are set by the Home Office, which can direct the police authority to establish levels of performance for them.

Local policing plans

A copy of the annual plan of each police force is sent to the Home Office, but it does not resolve disputes over the content.

Deployment of resources

The Home Office can issue directions on performance targets in relation to national objectives that may impact upon the use of resources.

POLICE AUTHORITY

Composition

The majority of police authorities have 17 members comprising nine councillors, three magistrates and five independent members. The chairperson is elected by the authority members.

General duty

The duty of the police authority is to secure the maintenance of an efficient and effective police force for its area.

Finance

Ultimate responsibility for all expenditure rests with the police authority. Its financial regulations determine the degree of delegation of this to the chief constable, it agrees a budget and issues precepts upon the constituent unitary authorities.

Personnel

The police authority employs all civilians and places them under control of the chief constable, except where agreed otherwise. It also appoints chief and assistant chief constables, and can call upon them to retire in the interests of efficiency.

Objectives and targets

Local objectives and performance targets are set by the police authority after consultation with the chief constable and the community.

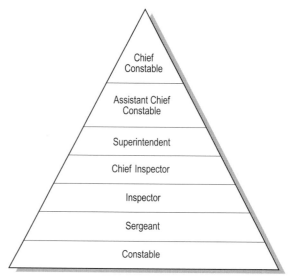

Local policing plans

The police authority must issue a local policing plan, and if this differs from the draft submitted by the Chief Constable must consult him or her regarding any changes. In the final analysis, however, responsibility rests with the police authority. As soon as possible at the end of each financial year the authority must publish a report relating to the policing of its area, including an assessment of the extent to which the local policing plan for the year has been carried out. A copy must be sent to the Secretary of State.

Deployment of resources

The local policing plan may specify the proposed allocation of resources and, in addition, the police authority controls funding for additional resources.

CHIEF CONSTABLE

General duty

The chief constable is responsible for the direction and control of the force.

Finance

A draft budget is prepared by the chief constable, who is responsible for day-to-day financial management of the force within regulations drawn up by the police authority.

Personnel

Police officers and civilians are under the control of the chief constable, except those civilians whom the police authority wishes to manage directly.

Objectives

The chief constable must have regard to national and local objectives in discharging his or her functions.

Local policing plans

The chief constable must draft a local policing plan on behalf of the police authority setting out policing priorities and arrangements for the forthcoming year. The police authority has the final say on the content of the plan.

Deployment of resources

Responsibility for operational control over how resources are deployed rests with the chief constable.

Fig. 60.1 • Police rank structure.

Rank structure

The police service is a disciplined organization and the rank structure is as shown in Fig. 60.1.

Each provincial police force is headed by a chief constable and, dependent on its size, may have more than one assistant chief constable. Of these one is designated as the deputy to the chief constable, the others having areas of responsibility such as operations, training and support services. Chief officers in the City of London and Metropolitan police forces are known as commissioners and commanders; the ranks of superintendent and below are, however, the same.

Police forces, for the purposes of command, are usually divided into geographical areas known as divisions. Each division and most specialist departments are under the command of a superintendent and a chief inspector.

Inspectors are responsible for a shift of officers and the day-to-day management of a police station, a sector or specialist department. Constables form the bulk of the service and are generally supervised by a sergeant (Fig. 60.2).

Opportunities for promotion are open to all officers who have passed the appropriate examination and are assessed as having the necessary skills for the next rank. Examinations only apply for promotion to the rank of sergeant and inspector: promotion to the ranks of chief inspector, superintendent and above is by selection. Officers must have completed a 2-year probationary period as constable before they can qualify for promotion; however, there is a system for accelerated promotion. All officers, including chief constables, are still required to progress through each rank in the structure.

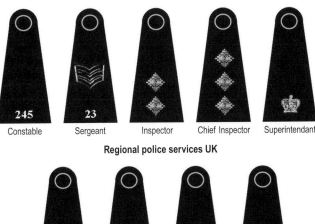

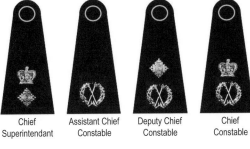

Regional police services UK

Chief Superintendant · Assistant Chief Constable · Deputy Chief Constable · Chief Constable

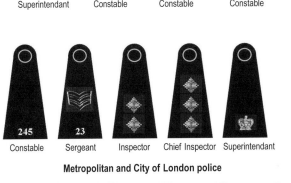

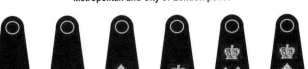

Metropolitan and City of London police

Constable · Sergeant · Inspector · Chief Inspector · Superintendant

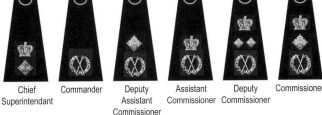

Chief Superintendent · Commander · Deputy Assistant Commissioner · Assistant Commissioner · Deputy Commissioner · Commissioner

Fig. 60.2 • Police service rank markings: (a) Regional police services UK; (b) Metropolitan and city of London police.

Recruits to the service undergo a rigorous programme involving classwork, self-defence and fitness training. They deal with simulated incidents and spend time at the division to which they are to be posted on completion of training.

Specialized duties

There is no direct entry into specialist areas of the police service and officers must have completed their probationary period before being considered for specialist duties.

CRIMINAL INVESTIGATION DEPARTMENT

Detective officers work in plain clothes and investigate all serious crime such as burglary, rape and murder. Such enquiries are generally protracted and involve working long hours. Under the umbrella of the CID, other specialist units such as the Drug Squad and Scenes of Crime Department also operate.

TRAFFIC DEPARTMENT

This duty involves mobile patrol of our roads and motorways. Specialist units within this department deal with accident investigation and vehicle-related crime.

OPERATIONS

Most forces have an 'Operations' or similarly named department, which has a mixture of uniformed support staff. These can include *response groups* such as:

- firearms teams
- dog handlers
- mounted police
- underwater search teams
- air support.

Complaints and discipline

DISCIPLINE CODE

Police officers are subject to a strict code of discipline, and any breach of that code may result in the officer concerned appearing before the chief officer and being punished. Such punishment can range from caution to dismissal.

The offences against the discipline code include discreditable conduct, neglect of duty, disobeying orders and racially discriminatory behaviour (Discipline code, Police (Discipline) (Senior Officers) Regulations 1985).

Civilianization

There has always been a civilian staff in the police service carrying out administrative and other duties. In recent years, however, the trend has been for civilians to replace police officers in all non-operational roles, ranging from senior management posts to operators in the control rooms, as well as other traditional administrative tasks.

Other police forces

Apart from the 43 police forces under the umbrella of the Home Office, there are a number of others that have a specialist responsibility. These include the British Transport Police, which has responsibility for our railways and train stations, and the Ministry of Defence Police, which has responsibility for key areas of the defence estate, Crown property and other places.

SPECIAL CONSTABULARY

Mention should also be made of the Special Constabulary, volunteer police officers who turn out for duty alongside their regular colleagues and greatly assist in the policing function. They have their own rank structure and wear the same uniforms as regular officers.

Image

While retaining some elements of tradition in both style and image, today's police officers are uniformed and equipped appropriately to meet current demands. The original 'appointments' of wooden truncheon, whistle and note-book have been replaced by long batons and, in some forces, CS gas incapacitation sprays. Accountability of the police service to the communities it serves has greater recognition and forces are constantly researching methods of providing enhanced information, e.g. through the publication of annual policing plans and performance indicators. The use of scientific aids and advanced information technology is widespread in an effort to reduce and detect crime, to police more effectively and to meet public expectations.

Having considered briefly the structure of the police service and its individual forces, the following part of this chapter concentrates on the statutory obligations placed on the police.

Statutory obligations

Lord Chief Justice Parker (Parker 1966) stated that:

> It is clear that it is part of the obligation and duty of a police constable to take all steps which appear necessary for keeping the peace, for preventing crime and for protecting property from criminal injury.
>
> There is no exhaustive definition of the powers and obligations of the police, but they are at least those and they would further include the duty to detect crime and bring an offender to justice.

In essence, this summary of a police officer's obligations is a popular and historical view of what many would consider to be the core functions of a constable.

There are, however, many more duties including the enforcement of road traffic legislation, enforcement of licensing laws, the police role at major incidents and other major events, and the police role as officers of the coroner.

Police authority is, in the main, bestowed by a bank of legislation that defines the role, responsibilities and powers of the police in dealing with specific offences.

There are three main streams to the origins and history of British law, as detailed below.

COMMON LAW

Common law is that part of the law which has grown out of the customs of the people through judicial decisions from the 12th century onwards, and has been modified and defined over the years. The obligations imposed on the police service by common law include the prevention of any breach of the peace, and the recording and investigation of crime.

EQUITY

Equity is law as applied in all civil cases.

STATUTE LAW

The main source of English law today, statute law is that legislation passed as an Act of Parliament, subject to evolution, revision or amendment. For example, the provisions of the Police and Criminal Evidence Act 1984 have had a radical influence on a police constable's dealings with suspects and prisoners, effectively eroding some common law powers (particularly in relation to the rules allowing an officer to enter a premises without judicial warrant and to stop and search members of the public).

Statute law also clearly defines the rights and entitlements of people in police custody and governs the conditions of their treatment and detention.

As legislation is passed to combat changes in social behaviour, so demands on the police service increase.

While the police are concerned with each of the provisions of criminal (as opposed to civil) law, they cannot enforce all the law all of the time; police officers must increasingly rely on the expertise of other outside agencies (such as Customs and Excise or Social Services, among others) as appropriate in the execution of their duties.

The process of law

ARREST

The power to arrest a person originated through common law and later became defined by statute to include the authority to act with and without judicial warrant. An arrest is the taking of a person's liberty and should only be exercised when there is no viable or reasonable alternative.

An arrest may be effected for an offence concerning the prevention or breach of a common law or for the contravention of a statutory 'arrestable offence' or through the enactment of a judicial warrant.

The term 'arrestable offence' is given to those offences where either the sentence on conviction is fixed by law (e.g. murder, manslaughter) or where legislation has categorized those offences as *arrestable*.

The Police and Criminal Evidence Act 1984 simplified, clarified and rationalized the previously existing power of arrest, bringing some common law offences not previously covered that by their very nature are considered serious (e.g. kidnapping) within the definition.

The provisions of this Act also determine the code of practice that must be applied in all cases when such an arrest has been made.

It states that any person arrested must be taken to a police station as soon as possible, where a designated custody officer, at least of the rank of sergeant, will enquire into the circumstances of the case and determine whether detaining the prisoner further is justified or whether justice is best served by releasing him/her with or without charge.

DETENTION IN POLICE CUSTODY

The code of practice governing the conditions under which a 'suspect' may be held in police custody was recently revised following the recommendations of the Royal Commission on Criminal Justice, which implemented changes in the law brought about by the Criminal Justice and Public Order Act 1994.

This code of practice regulates the practices in relation to the treatment and questioning of persons by police officers, clarifies identification procedures and clarifies the procedures in relation to taped interviews by the police.

Every person in police detention must be clearly informed in writing of his or her entitlements:

- the right to have someone notified of the arrest
- the right to free legal advice
- the right to examine the codes of practice.

Only in exceptional circumstances with a superintendent's authority may these entitlements be delayed (e.g. under the Prevention of Terrorism Act).

Once a custody officer considers that there is sufficient evidence to charge a prisoner, this must be expedited without further delay and the detainee either held in custody or bailed to the appropriate magistrates' court.

DECISION PROCESS

In 1986 the government established the Crown Prosecution Service, an independent body acting as decision-maker in criminal cases (Decision Process – Section 3(2) and Section 23 Prosecution of Offenders Act 1985). While the police actually commence criminal proceedings, the Crown Prosecution Service has an obligation to assess the weight of evidence before deciding whether or not there is a case for the defendant to answer in court.

After this decision has been made the matter may be scheduled for listing before either a crown or a magistrates' court.

Road traffic law

Traffic law constantly falls under the spotlight for reform. It is complex legislation which seeks to govern all aspects of vehicular law, and its primary purpose is to reduce the number of fatalities, casualties and accidents that occur daily throughout the country.

The police service is often criticized for what the public perceive to be an overzealous concentration on road traffic offences. However, with over 5000 fatalities a year on our roads, many of which are as a direct result of unforced driver error or vehicle defect, it would be irresponsible of the police not to execute the law vigorously. It is often the likelihood of detection and the conviction of offenders that prevents a far greater number of serious accidents.

Any person who is involved in the field of medical care will have been involved in the treatment of road accident casualties, and will be aware of the extent of the problem.

ROAD ACCIDENTS

In common with the other emergency services, the paramount responsibility of the police is the preservation of life. Invariably at road accidents this responsibility is best exercised by enabling medical staff and the other services who will utilize their experience and training.

The police, while under an obligation to investigate the probable cause, will concentrate their initial efforts in securing and managing the accident site, gathering information and preserving the scene if necessary for forensic or accident investigation.

They will not interfere with any ongoing medical care or treatment but will seek to establish the restoration of normality and to co-ordinate the efforts of all the emergency services.

The police are also able to provide essential communication links to hospitals, additional medical staff or other outside services and, when necessary, to provide either fast or slow escorts of casualties to hospitals.

DRINK DRIVING

It is unfortunately the case that a great number of road accidents are caused by drivers who have consumed alcohol. The Road Traffic Act 1988 defined the powers available to police officers to arrest any person suspected of driving, attempting to drive or being in charge of a vehicle while under the influence of drink or drugs.

Uniformed officers may require any person they suspect of such an offence to provide a specimen of breath for a breath test. If that screening test proves positive, or if the alleged offender refuses or fails to provide it, he may be arrested.

At road accidents any person whom an officer suspects of being the driver of a motor vehicle involved in the collision may be required to provide such a specimen of breath. Any person arrested for a drink driving offence will be asked to provide two further samples of breath at a police station. These samples are instantly analysed and the lower of the two readings is used in evidence. Alternatively, a suspect may be asked to provide a sample of blood or urine for laboratory analysis.

Occasionally a person who has been taken to hospital as a patient may be asked to provide either a specimen of breath or a blood or urine sample for analysis.

However, this can only be requested by a police officer if the medical practitioner in immediate charge of the case consents to the process. He may object if it is considered prejudicial to the proper care and treatment of the patient.

The role of the scene of crime officers and how medical staff can help

The police service has always been acutely aware that the scene of a crime (or other incident), interpreted correctly, has the potential to provide the investigator with a retrospective view of what happened and when. Indeed, painstaking scene exploration and evaluation, using a wide range of scientific disciplines, has often resulted in dramatic reconstructions of events and even of victims.

In a well-publicized case in Cardiff the exhumed skeletal remains of a young female were, using medical facial reconstruction techniques, eventually identified as being those of Karen Price, who, it was later established, had been unlawfully killed and buried many years prior to discovery of the grave. Owing to the passage of time the perpetrator may have believed that his actions would go unpunished. However, sufficient material of evidential value was recovered and ultimately a man was sentenced to life imprisonment for this offence.

While this case was fairly exceptional, the end result was by no means unique, with many convictions being achieved each year wholly or partly as a consequence of the scene being induced to give up its secrets.

In recognition of this potential, UK police forces have for many years employed specialist *scenes of crime officers* to carry out this work. They may, depending on the individual force, be specialized police officers, civilian employees recruited and trained for the specific role or else a mixture of both within the same unit. Irrespective of their designation, they will have in common an eye for detail, the ability to work in a methodical manner (often in the most unpleasant of circumstances), an investigative mind and total objectivity. The National Training Centre for Scientific Support was established in Durham in order to ensure that individuals selected for such tasks are able to achieve the level of expertise necessary to obtain optimum results from crime scenes and other similar non-crime occurrences (e.g. suicides, some accidental deaths, fires of unknown origin, etc.), and to develop this in line with advances in science.

Scenes of crime officers undertake a wide range of duties, with perhaps slight changes of emphasis from one police force to another. Their core function is to visit known or suspected crime scenes and to identify, record (including photography) and, where appropriate, recover evidential matter to determine what has happened.

It is, of course, possible often either to incriminate or exclude individuals by means of fingerprints or the presence of certain forensic material discovered at the scene.

Fingerprints (and this includes the palm ridged surface area) have long been relied upon by law enforcement agencies throughout the world to provide positive evidence of identity, and a Fingerprint Bureau was established as long ago as 1901 at New Scotland Yard. The first successful prosecution rapidly followed when a Harry Jackson was charged with burglary of a house in Denmark Hill, South London, on 27 June 1902 (Harry Jackson was tried in the Central Criminal Court, London, 13 September 1902). A plea of 'Not Guilty' was entered but, unfortunately for Mr Jackson, an imprint of a fingerprint had been found in wet paint on a window sill by a Sergeant Collins. This was subsequently proved to match Jackson's left thumb. He was found guilty and sentenced to 7 years penal servitude, an excellent early illustration of what can be achieved when efficient action at the crime scene is reinforced by effective work in the Fingerprint Bureau.

Since then millions of fingerprint comparisons have been made. Fingerprints have also on occasions been employed to establish the innocence of suspects and clearly, in a democratic society, this function is equally, if not more, important.

The basic techniques employed in confirming identity are largely unchanged and rely on the opinion of the fingerprint expert following painstaking evaluation of both the crime scene mark and the recorded impression of the suspect's fingerprints. Comparisons are routinely subject to rigorous checking procedures but once the identification has been agreed, by the experts, 'the Court may accept the evidence of fingerprints though it be the sole ground of identification' (R v. Castleton (1909) – Court of Criminal Appeal). This case was followed in 1915 by R v. Bacon (Court of Criminal Appeal), which reiterated the strength of fingerprint evidence, stating 'identification of fingerprints by a person expert in such matters is allowed and may be the only source of identification'.

While the value of fingerprint evidence to the investigator has not changed in the intervening years since those judgements, the techniques available for developing and recovering fingermarks (or palm marks) have been subjected to ongoing development and refinement, with the result that surfaces that were unproductive in the past can now yield positive results. Similar progress has been achieved in the Fingerprint Bureau, where the capacity to search outstanding crime scene marks in far greater quantity, across national databases, has been provided by the implementation of computerized search systems. The more sophisticated of these operate through a system of matching algorithms that has the potential to search fingermarks of a poorer quality than was previously viable using manual systems alone. Indeed, it is not always necessary to recover complete fingermarks as adequate ridge detail for positive identification is often present in quite small fragments.

Unfortunately, fingermarks left at scenes can be fragile and in some circumstances are easily destroyed or damaged by the activities of people who may be legitimately at the crime scene. The need for caution at such scenes cannot be overemphasized.

Crime scenes also have the potential to yield valuable trace evidence that may prove contact between persons and objects (e.g. burglary offences) or else contact between individuals (e.g. sexual offences or offences of violence). A long established principle known as Locard's law states that 'when A and B come into contact, something from A is transferred to B and vice versa' (Locard 1928). Scenes of crime officers remain alert to the possibility of recovering material that may have been removed from a scene by the culprit(s) on clothing, footwear or perhaps on any instrument or weapon used in the commission of the offence. For example, a screwdriver or jemmy used to force entry may retain particles of paint and will almost certainly have left an indentation at the scene, which a forensic scientist may be able to match to the suspected instrument.

Similarly, it may be possible to physically fit small fragments of paint (or glass) to the area that was attacked, again proving the connection between any recovered item and the scene. The possible ways in which persons or instruments can be connected to the scene, or vice versa, are legion, and items of particular importance include footwear impressions (which may be in blood), fibres from clothing and body fluids, including blood and semen.

The advent of DNA profiling has revolutionized the importance and value to the investigator of body fluids, which may have been left at crime scenes by the culprit or perhaps the blood of the victim has contaminated the clothing of an assailant. Following the achievements of Professor Alex Jeffreys at Leicester University in the mid-1980s, DNA profiling has been extensively adopted and developed for forensic use (Jeffreys et al 1985). Not only is it now possible to identify known individuals through the use of this technique with a far greater degree of certainty than was previously possible, but the establishment of the national DNA database facilitates the search of profiles achieved from recovered material and comparison against samples from potential suspects. However, the continued storage of DNA data from innocent persons is currently (in 2008) being challenged in the European Court of Human Rights.

The sensitivity of the systems continues to improve enabling ever smaller deposits of blood, semen and other fluids to be successfully profiled, with the end result that offenders are being identified who were not previously thought to be connected with the offence.

While the evidential value of the scene examination relies on both the skill of the scenes of crime officer (SOCO) and the expertise of the scientist and fingerprint expert, ultimately the results that can be achieved are highly dependent on the integrity of the scene being maintained. All scenes of crime officers and police officers are trained in taking effective measures to preserve scenes and prevent contamination. They will ensure that people with a legitimate requirement to enter a scene (e.g. a Home Office pathologist, medical practitioner or forensic scientist) do so in a manner and by a route commensurate with minimizing any risk to evidential material that may be present.

Difficulties can arise, however, where people legitimately enter a crime scene (often before it is known or suspected that a crime has taken place) prior to the presence of the police. Such categories may well include doctors (possibly a police surgeon but more probably a GP), ambulance staff (including paramedics) and neighbours, friends and relatives. While in most cases little can be realistically done to prevent damage to, or loss of, evidence by the actions of the latter group, some care exercised by medical staff attending in uncertain situations could significantly reduce the likelihood of such loss. The preservation of life will clearly be the paramount objective of doctors and medical teams but elementary precautions such as reducing any handling or moving of items (particularly anything bloodstained) to an absolute minimum and restricting the numbers of persons who enter the scene where such measures are compatible with their core function, will considerably improve the prospect of the scenes of crime officer recovering good evidence.

Instances where medical assistance is summoned to a dwelling where the occupant is found to be dead can sometimes very quickly escalate from a routine sudden death to a murder enquiry, and in such circumstances it will be of particular importance to know whether doors or windows were open or perhaps locked from the inside, whether televisions or other electrical appliances were switched on, whether the house lights were on or off, whether the gas cooker was on, and so on. Such seemingly mundane information can be crucial in formulating police lines of enquiry and in the ensuing trial of offenders where crime has taken place.

Occasions may arise where, perhaps to render appropriate medical response or for other compelling reasons such as safety, it is absolutely necessary to switch off lights or appliances, handle or move articles, or perhaps even to force entry. In such cases it is imperative that, should a police investigation ensue, immediate steps are taken to ensure that the police, and ideally the scenes of crime officers concerned with examining that particular scene, are informed of what has taken place. It is vital that details of all personnel who attend are provided as it may be necessary to eliminate their fingerprints from any recovered from the scene. While the wearing of gloves (surgical type) may be essential for reasons of hygiene, it should be borne in mind that fingermarks will be lost if articles bearing them are carelessly handled, irrespective of whether or not gloves are worn. Similarly, forensic trace evidence and body fluids, particularly where the quantities are minute, are easily lost or contaminated.

All persons entering crime scenes should be aware of the fragile nature of much of the evidential material that may be present and how easy it is for unnecessary activity to cause irreparable damage to the chances of accurate reconstruction by the scenes of crime officer. A little care will go a long way towards ensuring a satisfactory outcome.

Major incidents

A major incident (Association of Chief Police Officers 1991, Home Office 1994) can be described as one:

- that involves a large number of members of the public, as casualties or as a result of their lives being otherwise disrupted
- where the three emergency services together with the local authority commit many resources and implement special arrangements to cope with the incident
- that produces a large number of enquiries from both public and media surrounding the event.

This definition can be seen to encompass all incidents, e.g. an aircraft accident, a train crash, widespread flooding or freak storm, all of which have been the cause of major incidents during the last 20 years in the UK.

The purpose of this section is to outline the roles and responsibilities of the police service in relation to a major incident, and to discuss the initial response and subsequent action.

The main areas of police responsibility in relation to a major incident can be summarized as follows:

- The primary duty of every police officer is the protection of life, and this is the paramount consideration at every major incident. It is not the responsibility of the police to engage in rescue operations: they are not trained for that purpose nor do they possess the necessary equipment. The role of the police is to ensure that the rescue services can operate effectively by coordinating the response to the incident of those agencies and to ensure that, at the scene of the incident or elsewhere, effective communication is maintained.

- Protection of the scene is undertaken by the setting of cordons at predetermined distances from the incident:

    — An *inner cordon* affords immediate security to the incident scene and allows emergency service personnel the opportunity to carry out the tasks of rescue and firefighting without hindrance by unauthorized personnel. The cordon also provides protection at the scene of any evidence, at those major incidents that are initially treated as a crime. If this is not done, that evidence may be lost.

    — An *outer cordon* enables the police to provide a controlled zone between the two cordons. This area is used to marshal resources in close proximity to the incident, allowing the emergency services the facility to respond appropriately. All access points to this zone will be controlled by the police, who ensure that only authorized personnel are allowed entry. Within this controlled zone each of the emergency services will set up their command and control vehicles. Ideally, these vehicles will be situated as close to one another as possible to enable the incident commanders to communicate and facilitate cooperation between the relevant services.

    The outer cordon absorbs pressure away from the inner cordon, allowing those involved in the rescue operation to get on with what they have to do. It also provides a secure environment for the command vehicles and the forward control point. Consideration must also be given to diverting traffic over a wider area to prevent a build-up of vehicles in the vicinity due to a possible influx of onlookers. It is essential that the emergency services' vehicles can both enter and leave the scene without hindrance.

    The area within the inner cordon is referred to as the *bronze* area, that within the outer cordon the *silver* area.

- There is invariably an investigation following a major incident. That responsibility rests primarily with the police. However, in certain circumstances, other investigative bodies have a statutory responsibility to investigate. In the case of an incident at an oil refinery, the Health and Safety Executive would be the appropriate agency; in the event of an air incident the Air Accident Investigation

Branch of the Department of Transport would conduct their enquiry. In all cases, a senior police officer, usually a detective, will work in close liaison with the overall police incident commander, ensuring that all possible evidence that remains at the scene of the incident is discovered and preserved.

It is incumbent on the police, together with the other investigating agencies, to provide the best evidence at any subsequent legal proceedings, whether they be public enquiries, criminal trials or coroner's court hearings. An investigation can continue for many months, if not years, after the actual incident has occurred, with the painstaking enquiries resulting in files of evidence being presented at the relevant hearing. It is therefore vitally important that initially all possible evidence, including dead bodies, remains in situ until photographed for the purpose of the investigation, unless this actually hinders the saving of lives or puts the evidence at risk of destruction by fire or other hazard.

- In all incidents, from road traffic accidents to major incidents involving a large number of casualties, the police are responsible for collating the details of those casualties and disseminating this information to the relatives. The focal point of this activity is the casualty enquiry bureau, which is set up at a predetermined location, usually the headquarters of the police force in which the incident occurs.

- The police are also responsible for the identification of the deceased on behalf of HM Coroner. Once the scene of the incident has been declared safe, specialist *body and property recovery teams* will sweep the area to recover all the dead bodies, parts of bodies, property and evidential exhibits. Arrangements are made for the removal of the bodies to a recognized mortuary or, in the case of an incident involving many casualties, to a premises identified as a temporary mortuary. The premises are likely to have been selected by the police and local authority at the planning stage and will ideally have among other things a large impervious floor space, good ventilation, lighting and drainage, and hot and cold running water. These temporary mortuaries will be staffed by police personnel and it is here that the post-mortem examinations and identification of the deceased will take place in suitably screened areas.

- The police will be heavily committed to a multitude of tasks at a major incident. One such task is to prevent crime at the scene. It is a distressing fact that there may be those who will take advantage of the circumstances by preying on the bodies and belongings of the casualties. The scene of flooding, for example, which often involves the evacuation of families, leaving homes empty, may create an easy target for criminals. It is in the setting of the inner and outer cordons that the police seek to establish a secure zone in an effort to prevent such criminal activity taking place. Unauthorized personnel will be identified at the control points and turned away from the scene, but it should be borne in mind that to maintain a secure zone is almost impossible. By its very nature the outer cordon will encircle a very large area and cover substantial areas of open terrain, which are often difficult to police effectively.

- The final area of police responsibility in relation to a major incident is to assist the local authority personnel and others in the restoration of normality.

- Senior coordinating group – where there is a major disaster it is now well-accepted practice that the response to it will be multiagency, with each agency having command of its own resources. The police have the coordinating role and this is achieved by setting up a multiagency senior coordinating group comprising senior representatives of the various agencies who have the power to make executive decisions. The objective of the group will be to determine the strategic approach of the overall response and to ensure it is accurately communicated to the tactical and operational commanders of their respective organizations.

  A senior coordinating group would typically comprise: chief constable, chief fire officer, chief ambulance officer, unitary authority chief executive, health authority chief executive, coroner, pathologist, senior police investigating officer and press officer. This coordinating group is often referred to as 'gold control'.

  The details of all discussions should be recorded and the minutes distributed to each organization.

The police procedures and working methods are identical in relation to every incident regardless of the gravity. It is only the scale of response which differs in the event of a major incident.

Phases of a major incident

FIRST OFFICER AT THE SCENE

The actions of the first police officer at the scene of a major incident are of utmost importance and affect the subsequent course of the investigation. Despite the temptation to become personally involved in any rescue work, the duty of this first officer is to assess what has happened and inform the police control room as to what has taken place. The gathering of this initial information is a priority and to assist the officer in this function a simple mnemonic – SAD CHALET – has been developed.

- **S** *Safety* – Maintain a safe location, do not become involved in the rescue effort.
- **A** *Assess and inform* – Pass the facts to the control room to facilitate the rescue effort.
- **D** *Declare* – Declare the incident a major incident.
- **C** *Casualties* – Give an approximate number of injured and dead.
- **H** *Hazards* – Notify hazards that exist at the scene, e.g. spillage of flammable material or fire.

A *Access* – Identify the easiest routes to the scene for incoming emergency vehicles.

L *Location* – Give the exact location of the incident; identify landmarks or road junctions.

E *Emergency services* – State which other services are at the scene and what is further required.

T *Type* – Relate a picture of the scene, what is involved, e.g. numerous vehicles, a train, aircraft, etc.

This first officer must also, if in a police vehicle, set up the police forward control point by illuminating the emergency blue lights on the vehicle. It is from here that the police operation during the incident will be directed, and the first officer on the scene will assume command of arriving police resources until a more senior officer arrives to take control.

CASUALTY ENQUIRY BUREAU

In the event of a major incident there are likely to be significant numbers of casualties, both dead and injured. The method used by police forces to cope with collating and disseminating information regarding those involved is to activate the *casualty enquiry bureau*. The bureau comprises both police and support personnel not normally engaged in operational policing working under the command of a departmental head or senior manager. Bureau work is extremely stressful and there is a need for the personnel to be trained in dealing with distressed members of the public. Supervisory personnel need to be aware of the signs of stress and to ensure that all staff are given adequate rest periods away from the bureau.

Once activated, dedicated telephone numbers are released by the bureau via the media. All incoming calls regarding the incident from distressed relatives, from local police stations, hospitals and ambulance stations, as well as other organizations, are then handled by the bureau. Information concerning casualties is gathered by police documentation teams attending at the scene of the incident, at receiving hospitals, and at survivor reception and rest centres. Descriptive forms are completed for each casualty and are transmitted to the casualty enquiry bureau. By collating all the information a comprehensive picture is built up, linking casualties and their location with passenger lists or manifests and with relatives. By becoming the central contact point, the bureau relieves the pressure placed upon police and hospital telephone switchboards.

Once the bureau has *verified* that a person is involved in the incident, then, depending on the circumstances, members of the immediate family can be informed. If the casualty proves to be fatal then the relatives are informed of the situation by trained personnel; if there is no serious injury involved some other appropriate means is used.

Should the casualty bureau become overwhelmed and fail to cope with the incoming calls, adjacent forces can be requested to activate their casualty bureaux to assist with the collation process. Regional training in this activity regularly takes place and procedures are identical from force to force, making the process a seamless operation.

THE MEDIA

The final area of major incident handling to be considered is the media. There is no doubt that a large-scale incident will attract local, national and international media coverage. Media reaction is likely to be immediate and massive. A resolute but managed response is required and to that end selected and specially trained police officers and support personnel from the public relations department will become involved and identify a *press centre* or *media centre*. Officers at the scene of the incident will inform members of the media that information can only be gained from this centre, and visits to the scene by the media can be controlled and managed so as to be safe and not disruptive or intrusive. The police will be responsible for providing the facilities required for regular press conferences.

Press liaison officers will also be despatched to the locations where casualties are sent and where relatives gather. Experience has shown the lengths to which some members of the media will go for a story, and efforts have to be made to ensure that appropriate privacy and dignity is maintained and that the scene of the incident is preserved for evidential purposes.

References

Association of Chief Police Officers 1991 ACPO emergency procedures manual. HMSO, London

Home Office 1994 Dealing with disaster, 2nd edn. HMSO, London

Jeffreys AJ, Wilson V, Thein SL 1985 Individual-specific fingerprints of human DNA. Nature 316: 76–79

Locard E 1928 Police Journal 1: 77 [1932 Traité de criminalistique. Desvigne, Paris]

Parker HL 1966 Rice v. Connolly [1966] 2 Law Reports, Queen's Bench Division 414; 3 Weekly Law Reports [1966] 17; [1966] 130 Justice of the Peace Law Reports 322; [1966] 110 Solicitors' Journal 371; [1966] 2 All England Law Reports 649

Police (Discipline) (Senior Officers) Regulations 1985 Statutory Instrument 1985/519. HMSO, London

R v. Bacon [1915] 11 Criminal Appeal Reports 90

R v. Castelton [1909] 3 Criminal Appeal Reports 74

The role of other agencies at a major incident

61

Introduction 625

The local authority 625

The armed forces 626

The voluntary services 628

Reference 630

Further reading 630

Introduction

While the police, fire and ambulance services are at the front line in dealing with the initial stages of major incidents, many other agencies play an essential role in mitigating the effects of disaster and ensuring a rapid return to normality. Local authorities should be alerted at an early stage and can make available a wide range of resources, including heavy plant, buildings for use as reception centres and other necessary functions, transport and social services staff. The role of voluntary services in major incidents can also be invaluable but is often underestimated. The Salvation Army and the Women's Royal Voluntary Service (WRVS) can provide essential on-scene refreshments and support for rescue workers and for survivors and relatives waiting at reception centres. The St John Ambulance Brigade and British Red Cross may be used in front-line rescue work, in giving assistance at reception centres and in supporting the ambulance service to maintain the day-to-day workload that will continue despite the disaster. The armed forces can offer

a vast range of expertise, manpower and equipment, and this is available to the civil community free of charge when human life is under threat. It is essential for those involved in disaster management to gain an understanding of these 'non-emergency' services if they are to make the best use of available resources in the event of a major incident.

The local authority

Local authorities often bear the brunt of the workload in dealing with major incidents, although this is rarely appreciated by many of those at the scene. In days gone by, the necessity for civil defence was the raison d'être for emergency planning by local authorities but with the end of the Cold War this type of planning has virtually disappeared. The focus of emergency planning has now shifted from dealing with war scenarios to assisting the community in the event of 'peacetime' emergencies.

Local authorities' responsibilities in this field stem from the Civil Contingencies Act 2004, which places an obligation on them to assess the risk of incidents, plan for them and run regular exercises in preparation for them.

Local authority emergency plans will usually include provision to bypass the council's generally slow and cumbersome decision-making process. In the immediate aftermath of a major incident the 'council' will have three principal aims: to provide support for the emergency services; to support and care for the local and wider community; and to coordinate the response by organizations other than the emergency services. As the incident progresses into the recovery phase the local authority will take the lead in rehabilitating the community and restoring the environment.

There will normally be a crisis management team, which will consist of key officers and will have authority to take immediate action despite financial implications. Local authorities have powers to raise as much credit as necessary to cover costs of dealing with emergencies, and in cases where the government declares a *Bellwin emergency* a large proportion of such costs will be recoverable from central government.

The local authority emergency plan is usually prepared by its *emergency planning officer* (EPO), who will ideally have forged good working relationships with the local emergency services and will have taken part in training exercises designed to test coordination and communications. The EPO provides a 24 h 365-days-a-year single point of contact in the event of emergency and will usually be the first point of contact for emergency services declaring a major incident. The EPO's aim will be to effect a rapid response from the local authority, bringing their substantial resources into use as soon as possible. As part of his or her contingency plan, the EPO will have put in place a system of communications, information gathering and analysis to provide an effective back-up to the crisis management team. A team member will usually be sent to police silver control to act as a liaison officer. During the incident the EPO will be on hand to assist and advise the team's officers and to monitor events as they develop.

Local authorities are large organizations and have access to a wide range of skills and resources that can be useful to the emergency services. The local authority can provide manual labour and heavy plant machinery such as diggers and lorries, as well as extensive technical advice and equipment and assistance with issues concerning environmental health. At the Clapham train crash in 1988 the local authority moved quickly to help the emergency services gain rapid access to the scene. It cut down railings and trees, and cut steps down a steep embankment to the trackside.

Another important role of the local authority is to provide access to buildings needed as survivor reception centres, relatives and friends centres, evacuation centres, temporary mortuaries and other functions required by the emergency services. It can also provide staffing for these centres, both from its own social services department and from voluntary organizations. Library staff have excellent information skills and can be invaluable in setting up information centres for the public during a prolonged period of disruption. After the Lockerbie bombing the local authority provided extensive support to the emergency services, releasing buildings for use as control rooms, reception centres and other important functions and providing emergency mortuary facilities. The authority had a long-term role in helping the Lockerbie community to return to normality, providing alternative accommodation where necessary and ensuring that long-term counselling was available to all local residents when required.

In many major incidents the majority of those affected are unscathed or suffer only minor injuries. In transport accidents large numbers of people may be stranded a long way from home and anxious to get in touch with relatives, and the local authority will take steps to meet these needs. It is a duty of the local authority to minimize the effects of a major incident on the local population immediately affected, and to coordinate arrangements to help, feed and, if necessary, accommodate those who are homeless or displaced. This can present a formidable task, as in the case of the Towyn flood, when more than 5000 people were unable to return to their homes for days, weeks and, in some cases, many months.

The local authority role continues long after the last emergency vehicles have left the scene and is concerned mainly with returning the area and its community back to normality. Many people may need counselling for post-traumatic stress, and the care of the public will fall upon the local authority and its social services department.

Of all the agencies involved in a major incident, the police and the local authority are likely to be engaged for the longest period in the aftermath. The 'council' will take a key role in clear-up operations, restoration and rebuilding. If buildings are involved the district surveyor, a local authority employee, will need to examine the structure and ensure it is safe before allowing the owners access. The exact nature of the council's work will obviously depend on the nature of the disaster but it will need to take a long-term view. If, for example, buildings or factories have been completely destroyed, the local authority will need to consider planning proposals for future development of the affected sites.

The general public often responds to news of a disaster by sending donations to help those affected and the local authority often takes the lead in setting up a disaster fund. Management of such appeals can be fraught with difficulties and can involve long-term commitment of staff and resources.

Local authorities must work on the principles of 'integrated emergency management', ensuring that their own emergency plans take into account the plans of the police, fire, ambulance and health authorities. They must aim to become an integral part of the emergency team and it is important for each council to establish mutual aid arrangements with neighbouring authorities so that additional resources can be made available when necessary.

The armed forces

The armed forces can play a key role in the management of major incidents, particularly those that are protracted and that demand high manpower and specialist skills, such as bridge building or setting up a communications network

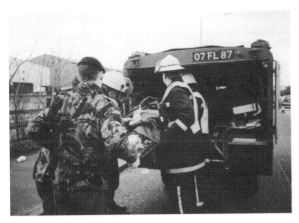

Fig. 61.1 • Armed forces assistance to the civil authorities.

(Fig. 61.1). The army has a long tradition of providing aid at disaster scenes. In 1864, for example, the military barracks at Woolwich organized a detachment of 1500 sappers and artillery troops to rebuild a section of the Thames embankment destroyed when a magazine packed with 115300 lb of gunpowder exploded. The detachment won a battle against time to repair the defences and save Plumstead from inundation at the next high tide. At the *Princess Alice* disaster in 1878, when a Thames pleasure steamer sank after collision with a collier, the same barracks sent its army services and army hospital corps to retrieve and assemble the 640-plus dead. More recent major incidents involving a significant input from the armed services include the Lockerbie jumbo jet crash, the Towyn and Chichester floods and the fierce snowstorms that isolated many parts of Scotland in 1996.

THE MAC 'A' SCHEME

The armed forces are unique in their ability to provide high levels of manpower, equipment and specialist skills. These resources are available to the civil community through the MAC 'A' scheme, which is divided into three distinct sections.

- *MAC P (Military Assistance to Civil Powers)* provides for support to civil authorities in countering insurgency, civil disturbances and terrorism, and ensuring national security.
- *MAC M (Military Assistance to Civil Ministries)* provides the government support in maintaining essential supplies and services, such as the prison, fire and ambulance service.
- *MAC C (Military Assistance to the Civil Community)* is the category that covers provision of military assistance at major incidents. Help is available under three main headings: at emergencies and disasters where life is in danger; at routine functions where there is no immediate threat to life, such as in providing communications equipment at large shows or delivering food to isolated communities; and providing specialists for attachment to civilian projects.

The army usually assumes the key role in MAC C work, taking a lead in tri-service operations and managing the coordination and allocation of resources. Military assistance is usually summoned by a direct call from a local authority in need of help but sometimes the initial call is from an individual. Requests for help can be made to any armed service establishment but the response will be fastest if it is directed to an army regional headquarters. These headquarters have communication systems, allowing them to effectively coordinate a response from all three services in their area and to call for resources from outside the area when necessary. The military can also be tasked to a particular role by the Ministry of Defence. An army liaison officer will be delegated to work closely with the local authority to explain the expertise and facilities available and to help ensure the best use of military resources. Military personnel and equipment always remain under the direct control of the military.

The armed services encompass a wide range of expertise and are able to draw on these resources in the event of a major incident. They can, for example, supply the full range of medical personnel, from doctors and dentists, nursing officers and general nurses to public health technicians and soldiers trained in basic pharmacy. They have mobile units able to establish field hospitals, field surgical teams, first-aid posts and medical reception centres. They have engineers, electricians, mechanics, logistics and communications specialists; and, perhaps above all, they have instant access to a large, highly disciplined and coordinated workforce.

The services can supply an extensive range of equipment, including ambulances equipped with advanced life support facilities, domestic ambulances, coaches fitted with stretchers, cargo vehicles, passenger transport vehicles, four-wheel drive vehicles for use in difficult terrain and helicopters for use in casualty evacuation, reconnaissance or rapid transport. They can provide special matting to provide temporary roadways and heavy-duty surface areas, generators to provide electricity, and tents for shelter and storage. They have the equipment and skill to install communication systems, build bridges, make safe dangerous structures and produce and store drinking water.

In cases of genuine emergency when there is a real threat to human life military assistance is free but in all other instances local authorities can expect to be charged. These charges can be on a 'no loss cost' or full-cost basis, and depend entirely on prevailing circumstances. Where there is still a conceivable danger to life and limb, military aid is charged as 'no loss cost', with the local authority footing the bill for expenses such as petrol. When there is no danger to life – even though there has been no return to normal – the charges are made at full cost, and will include the salaries of all personnel and costs of hiring and maintaining equipment. The difference between the scale of prices can be substantial.

A fixed level of response from the armed services can never be guaranteed, as the main priority of all forces is the defence of the realm, and commitments in this role obviously vary according to circumstances. In normal circumstances it is possible to mobilize a military response within 2–3 h of the initial request for assistance.

The voluntary services

Major incidents can overstretch the resources of the statutory emergency services and the efforts of voluntary organizations can provide invaluable assistance. The voluntary sector in the UK is highly organized, and many groups can offer the reliable, sustainable and consistent level of support that is essential for their resources to be included in emergency plans. The work of the voluntary services is usually coordinated by the local authority, but in some cases they may be alerted and controlled by the relevant statutory emergency service.

Dealing with Disaster (1997) categorizes voluntary assistance into four main groupings:

- established organizations such as the British Red Cross, St John Ambulance and the Salvation Army
- groups offering specialists skills such as the British Association for Immediate Care, and search and rescue organizations such as cave and mountain rescue teams
- organizations offering emotional support, such as the Samaritans
- skilled individuals, not necessarily members of voluntary organizations, whose help is offered or requested on the day.

ST JOHN AMBULANCE

St John Ambulance was founded in 1877 with the aim of providing a wide range of first-aid care to the public. Many of the initial branches were based in factories, shipyards and other businesses, offering free medical aid to injured workmen. One of the brigade's first major public appearances was at Queen Victoria's Golden Jubilee celebrations in 1887.

St John Ambulance now boasts more than 80 000 volunteer members, including 30 000 adults, and the organization provides first-aid cover at more than 80% of public events, from Royal weddings and marathons to village fêtes. This role has put them at the scene of several major incidents, including the Hillsborough tragedy, where 96 football spectators were crushed to death, the Poll Tax riots in central London and the stand collapse at a Pink Floyd rock concert.

St John volunteers include fully qualified medical practitioners, registered nurses and qualified first-aiders. They are organized locally at divisional level, then areas, counties and districts. They are a disciplined organization, with military-style rank markings. Brigade resources include fleets of ambulances and mobile first-aid units equipped with sophisticated emergency medical kit such as defibrillators.

St John has an Air Wing that transports donor organs throughout Europe and also operates an aeromedical service dedicated to bringing home British travellers who need urgent medical treatment in the UK. The brigade also provides a community care service for the elderly, sick and handicapped living in their own homes.

Another important function of St John Ambulance is to provide first-aid training for members of the public. It is the largest training agency in Britain and regularly works in schools, factories, offices and community halls, giving life-saving skills to well over 250 000 people every year.

BRITISH RED CROSS

The International Red Cross was founded after Swiss businessman Henry Dunant wrote a book describing battle scenes and calling for the formation of permanent aid societies to care for those wounded in war. Dunant had witnessed the terrible carnage at the Battle of Solferino in 1859 and the vivid scenes he portrayed spurred sympathizers to found the Red Cross Movement in Switzerland during 1863. A year later the Geneva Convention for War Wounded established the badge of the Red Cross as a sign of care for the injured and protection from attack.

Today, the British Red Cross has more than 100 000 volunteers dedicated to providing caring and emergency services to people in their local communities. As well as serving their own communities, Red Cross volunteers support the work of the international organization, providing money, materials and people as and when needed. This world-wide organization allows a rapid response to catastrophe in any part of the world.

There are nearly 100 British Red Cross branches, with approximately 1100 Red Cross centres and more than 5000 Red Cross groups. Each branch is managed by a committee of trustees responsible for ensuring that work is carried out in accordance with policies laid down by the national council. The national council is made up of Red Cross members and outside experts and meets regularly to determine policies.

The Red Cross aims to provide skilled and impartial care to people in need in their own homes and in the community, at home and abroad, in peace and in war. Policies adhere to the fundamental principles of the Red Cross Movement: humanity, impartiality, neutrality, independence, voluntary service, unity and universality.

The service provides 24 h cover at weekends and Bank Holidays and between the hours of 6 pm and 8 am on weekdays. Red Cross volunteers trained in crisis care form a rota that ensures attendance at a domestic fire within 90 min of a call. Each scheme has a mobile unit equipped with shower facilities, replacement clothing, blankets, baby milk and other refreshments, and the volunteers can offer on-the-spot practical help, advice and comfort. The volunteers can also, if necessary, take the family to temporary accommodation.

The fire victim support service is intended to supplement existing emergency support provided by local authorities and insurance companies.

AMBULANCE SERVICES' RESERVE

Red Cross and St John Ambulance Brigade units represent a trained pool of resources that can be called on for assistance whenever the statutory ambulance services are overstretched. This could be at major incidents or at times of particular stress such as New Year. Many ambulance services regularly deploy Red Cross and St John volunteers, usually in back-up roles or in helping to maintain normal services during the management of a major incident.

The principal function of reservists is to support the statutory ambulance service during a major incident or unusual circumstances, such as widespread celebrations. The exact role of the reservists is determined within individual ambulance service areas but it is envisaged they could drive ambulances, operate communications and assist in patient care. They could also provide support at the scene of the incidents, assist in receiving hospitals and at the ambulance control, and provide support to maintain normal services during the incident.

ST ANDREW'S AMBULANCE SERVICE

The St Andrew's Ambulance Association was established at the end of the 19th century with the aim of providing an ambulance service to cover the increasing numbers of accidents in the industrial areas of Scotland and to train the public in first aid.

After the Second World War the introduction of an NHS ambulance service allowed St Andrew's to concentrate on first-aid provision and today it has more than 3000 trained volunteers providing cover at public events including football matches and street demonstrations.

WOMEN'S ROYAL VOLUNTARY SERVICE

Members of the Women's Royal Voluntary Service – the WRVS – have given invaluable help to survivors and emergency workers at innumerable major incidents in the UK. The service, like many voluntary organizations, has its roots in the years before the Second World War when there was a perceived need to prepare for hostilities. In 1938 the WRVS was formed to assist local authorities with the recruitment of women for the 'air raid precautions service'. The role of its members was soon extended to include running nurseries, distributing clothing and organizing canteens and rest centres.

WRVS volunteers played a vital role in helping to maintain community morale during the blitz. In the East End of London, where the community was a sitting duck for endless volleys of German bombers intent on obliterating the docks, the WRVS did sterling work, running nightly tea and buns runs in the overcrowded shelters and helping the thousands of families who lost their homes and possessions in bombing raids.

The work of the WRVS has continued into peacetime and today the organization has more than 150 000 members organized into seven regional divisions. The group has a wide range of functions, including running old folks' luncheon clubs and hospital refreshment kiosks, and delivering meals-on-wheels. The emergency role of the WRVS is still important and a significant percentage of its members are trained and experienced in emergency services work. Teams can be provided to help in any disaster, whether that event affects a single person, a small community or the whole nation.

The type of help the WRVS can offer includes emergency feeding, setting up and running rest and reception centres, helping with essential documentation of survivors, providing refreshments for emergency service personnel and those affected by the incident, and providing clothing and bedding where needed. WRVS volunteers are also useful in manning information points and in giving general support and comfort to emergency service personnel and to victims, their families and friends.

THE SAMARITANS

The Samaritans have responded to all major disasters in the UK since the early 1970s. The organization specializes in giving emotional support at times of personal crisis and its trained volunteers are available 24 h per day, every day of the year and without time limit.

The Samaritans are organized into 13 regions that cover the whole of the UK and the Republic of Ireland, and its close coordination enables it to provide a disciplined and immediate response in any geographical area. If necessary, the organization can supply and work from a mobile Samaritan Centre, caravans or tents. Volunteers can also work in the open.

Samaritan volunteers are trained in counselling skills. They will help anyone affected by disaster, from the immediate victims to those who have no direct involvement but are nevertheless distressed. The support provided by the Samaritans is available in every part of the country

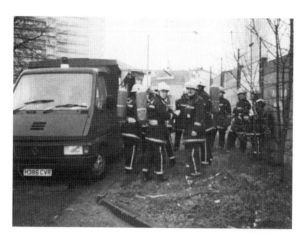

Fig. 61.2 • Providing refreshments at a major incident.

and can continue for months or years, depending on the needs of the client.

THE SALVATION ARMY

The Salvation Army also has a long tradition of service to the community and the emergency services during major incidents. In the Greater London area, and in some other areas of the country, mobile units are always prepared and equipped to be mobilized to provide refreshments, both food and drink, to the emergency services at the scene of any incident. Salvation Army officers also have a role in giving gentle encouragement and counselling support to those emergency rescue workers who are tired or stressed by the nature of their task.

The Salvation Army is also able to call on a large number of personnel who can assist with feeding, clothing and counselling at rest centres and evacuation centres.

The obvious overlap between services provided by the different voluntary organizations is beneficial in providing a seamless service that is adaptable to local needs.

Reference

Dealing with disaster 1997 Dealing with disaster, 3rd edn. HMSO, London

Further reading

Department of Health 1996 Emergency planning in the NHS: health service arrangements for dealing with major incidents. A handbook of guidance. HMSO, London

Ministry of Defence 1989 Military aid to the civil community: a pamphlet for the guidance of civil authorities and organisations. HMSO, London

Response of the faith communities to major emergencies: guidelines. General Synod of the Church of England Board of Social Responsibility, London

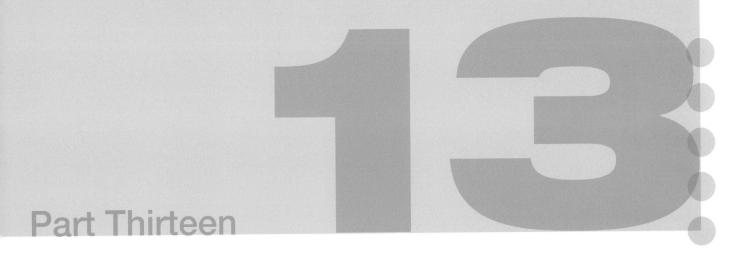

62 Legal aspects of immediate care 633

63 Record keeping in prehospital care 653

64 Communications and despatch 656

65 Trauma scoring 661

Part Thirteen

Legal aspects of immediate care

62

Introduction   633

The immediate care doctor and standards
of care   634

The Bolam test   634

Elective treatment, urgent treatment and
immediate care   635

Autonomy, beneficence and the patient's
best interest   636

Who obtains consent?   638

Treatment without consent   638

Medical negligence   647

Dealing with death/disposal of corpses   650

Conclusion   652

References   652

Introduction

The practice of immediate care is increasingly open to public scrutiny, with heightened interest and more public awareness, fuelled by the media, making health-care professionals working in the area of immediate care a target for interest and complaint by patients and observers alike.

Where in the past complaints and allegations of negligence were almost exclusively reserved for specialties such as obstetrics, neonatal care, and orthopaedic and trauma care, nowadays immediate care has become a focus for litigation.

Inevitably therefore, doctors undertaking immediate care work have to be more vigilant and to an extent more defensive if they are to remain clear of the law. In these days of increasing complaints, a combination of good practice and defensive medical technique, combined with a basic understanding and knowledge of the legal aspects of medical practice as they apply to the specialty is essential. Otherwise the doctor may be unable to achieve his or her objective of treating those patients in need of care while at the same time successfully defending allegations of poor or negligent treatment. This is particularly important where the outcome of the treatment may not have been successful, as unfortunately is sometimes inevitable in this kind of work. As death and disability are frequent consequences of the serious injuries that doctors in immediate care work are often called upon to deal with, it is inevitable that this specialty will bring with it distress, discontent and therefore complaint by those who suffer the injuries and those relatives and friends who suffer with them.

A basic general knowledge of such issues as consent, confidentiality and the criteria for medical negligence can only assist in improving the quality of care given and may help to reduce the likelihood of complaint or legal action against the medical practitioner.

A host of legal and ethical issues surround the provision of care by a doctor for his or her patient and some of these will be discussed in the context of immediate care. A central issue is the standard of care administered at the scene of an accident and the issues of consent to treatment, duty of confidentiality and clinical negligence are all relevant in respect of this.

The immediate care doctor and standards of care

The immediate care doctor is first a doctor and secondly a specialist in the field of immediate care provision at the scene of an accident or emergency situation. The care of the traumatized patient may require urgent life-saving treatment or less urgent but essential treatment at the scene while transport to hospital is being arranged.

In undertaking this work, the doctor commits him/herself to providing treatment for patients requiring immediate care to a standard that befits his/her specialist training and experience. In law, the standard of care given, in this country, currently is judged by the Bolam test. The standard of care identified in the case of *Bolam* v. *Friern Hospital Management Committee* (1957) was in the context of the tort of negligence and established the level of care necessary to defend an allegation of negligence. If care falls below the standard identified in the Bolam case, and damage is shown to have resulted from such care, then it would be difficult to argue against an action in the tort of negligence. The test as to whether care falls below a reasonable standard is referred to as the Bolam test.

The Bolam test

In the Bolam case, Mr J.H. Bolam, the plaintiff, claimed damages against the Friern Hospital Management Committee in respect of injuries he received while undergoing electroconvulsive therapy, on the basis that he had given consent to the procedure without having been warned of the risk of fracture during the convulsion that followed the electric shock if muscle relaxation was not given. There were divergent medical opinions as to whether muscle relaxants should or should not have been used, as well as over the question as to whether the patient should have been warned of the risks of the procedure. During the electroconvulsive treatment the patient suffered serious fractures of his pelvis, which were described as being an extremely rare complication, the risk of them occurring being put at 1 in 10 000. As part of his direction to the jury, the judge directed them to consider that:

in the case of a medical man, negligence means failure to act in accordance with the standards of reasonably competent medical men at the time.

He went on to express the following opinion:

to put it this way: a doctor is not guilty of negligence if he has acted in accordance with a practice accepted as proper by a responsible body of medical men skilled in that particular art... putting it the other way round, a doctor is not negligent if he is acting in accordance with such a practice, merely because there is a body of opinion that takes a contrary view.

In the case, the jury, perhaps not surprisingly, found the defendants not guilty of negligence on the basis that there was a body of expert medical opinion at the time that considered that it was reasonable to do what had been done. Until recent times in the UK, the Bolam test has been accepted as the test by which the law judges what is reasonable. It would apply to the standard of care given to the patient by the immediate care specialist and in the context of consent, might also be applied to the question of what is reasonable when obtaining such consent from the patient undergoing any form of immediate care. The question of the patient's competence to assess the situation and give consent, in the context of immediate care, will be discussed later.

More recently the case of *Bolitho* v. *Hackney Health Authority* (1997) has raised questions as to the validity of the Bolam test. This more recent case has modified our understanding of the Bolam test to the extent that the opinions expressed by the skilled medical practitioners have to be logically justifiable and defensible if they are to be valid and accepted. The case of Bolitho does not, however, apply to disclosure of information and is therefore not relevant to the question of consent. At the time of the Bolam test the issue was negligence in relation to the performance of a procedure. The issue of consent to the procedure was not specifically addressed, although mention was made of the disclosure of the risks involved. In considering the application of *Bolam* in the assessment of what is a reasonable standard of care, it must be accepted that part of that care is the disclosure of appropriate information to the patient as part of the process whereby consent to proceed with treatment is obtained. The problems of being unable to obtain consent in the context of immediate care will be discussed below. By using the Bolam test in setting what is or is not a reasonable standard of care, one is of course using the doctor's opinion, and those of colleagues the doctor chooses, to establish what is reasonable. Since it is the opinion of the doctor and the selected colleagues (the so-called responsible body of medical opinion) that determines the outcome, it might be claimed that it is somewhat biased in favour of the doctor. Hence the more recent case of Bolitho, in which mere acceptance by a responsible medical body of opinion was insufficient. In that case a defence of the views given by the expert was necessary, and was not merely accepted on the basis of the expert's standing as a professional person. It should also be remembered that the judge in the Bolam case indicated that

a doctor is not negligent ... merely because there is a body of opinion which takes a contrary view.

This simply adds further potential bias in favour of the doctor, but the recent Bolitho case does somewhat balance that out, in issues other than consent. In the case of *Sidaway* v. *Bethlem Royal Hospital Governors* (1985), the patient's right to receive information was questioned but, by a majority decision in the House of Lords, *Bolam* prevailed. In the UK, therefore, *Bolam* remains the test by which a reasonable standard of care is judged, leaving it in the hands of the medical profession to decide if care has fallen below a reasonable standard but now accepting that the medical profession have to justify their decision to accept a particular treatment as reasonable, in a court of law. In other countries, the use of a patient-oriented approach to the problem is adopted, as has been seen in cases such as *Canterbury* v. *Spence* (1972) in the USA, and *Rodger* v. *Whittaker* (1992) in Australia. These cases may well have relevance in the context of immediate care problems in the future, although currently *Bolam* and its modification by *Bolitho* remain untoppled.

Elective treatment, urgent treatment and immediate care

ELECTIVE TREATMENT

Elective treatment is treatment that is planned following the onset of a patient's symptoms or signs. In these circumstances, patients set in motion the process whereby they seek to have treatment in order to obtain relief from the symptoms of which they are complaining. Treatment may be considered to be elective when it is undertaken to alleviate symptoms, where such symptoms are a distress to the patient but where the continuation of the symptoms will not result in an irrecoverable problem relating to life or limb. In many instances where elective treatment is involved, symptoms are in a static state, or worsening slowly and there is no temporal deadline within which treatment must be undertaken. This kind of problem does not come under the remit of an immediate care specialist and it is therefore not specifically relevant to discuss this any further in the context of this chapter. It is, however, important to note that in elective work there is no temporal urgency or deadline, such that investigations and treatment may be undertaken or delayed as appropriate to individual patients' needs. This allows for the full scope of patient choice and permits as full an understanding as possible of the problems involved and of the objectives of the treatment to be undertaken.

URGENT TREATMENT

In a situation where a patient is in need of urgent treatment, such as in a condition requiring surgery to be undertaken quickly and where any unnecessary or inordinate delay might be detrimental, there is limited time and opportunity to discuss the treatment with the patient, including alternatives and any possible clinical consequence associated with undertaking or failing to undertake it. This will limit the time available to allow the patient to make a reasonable decision as to whether he or she would wish to proceed on the basis of the information presented. The urgency does, however, place a time constraint upon the patient in that a decision is required to be made without undue delay. There is usually, in these circumstances, time for the patient to discuss the problems with the physician, the patient's relatives, and indeed the patient's GP. Although more urgent than elective treatment, this situation is to a great extent also not relevant to the immediate care physician.

EMERGENCY TREATMENT/IMMEDIATE CARE

In this category of treatment, there is, by the very nature of the problem, little or no time in which to allow discussion between the patient and relatives or friends, GP or other interested parties. By its very nature, treatment is required to be undertaken immediately in order to avoid irrecoverable damage (Jardon et al 1973) such as limb loss, or indeed death. There may be some very limited time and opportunity for a rapid description of the problems, the proposed treatment and its objectives and risks, and the likely outcome. There is often, however, no such opportunity, and the patient is advised to have treatment, or indeed is given treatment without a good understanding of the procedure that is being undertaken. In most instances patients will accept the advice given, putting their faith in the doctor to do whatever is necessary in what the doctor believes to be the best interests of the patient. It is often the case that, in the role as an immediate care doctor, decisions of this kind are made. Invasive treatments, including the insertion of airways, intravenous infusions and chest drains are undertaken with minimal discussion or delay. In such circumstances patients and their relatives or friends do rely on the doctor to have, and to exercise, good clinical judgement and to act at all times in a way that is in the patient's best interests. They will normally assume that the doctor in these circumstances will have appropriate training and expertise to carry out the procedures being embarked on, without putting the patient at unnecessary risk from the procedures themselves.

In considering the question of emergency or immediate treatment, it should be understood that there is a significant common ground between these two kinds of treatment and, while it is reasonable for them to be considered as individual forms of treatment, in the context of immediate care, it is perhaps best to consider them under one heading, i.e. that of 'immediate care/emergency treatment', in so far as non-treatment will result in a deterioration of the problem that will not be in the patient's best interests and may result in a partly recoverable or indeed irrecoverable situation. As with all treatment, be it elective, urgent, emergency or immediate, the doctor will always be guided by:

- what the law permits
- what is in the patient's best interests
- clinical judgement
- the principle of never doing harm or mischief to the patient (the Hippocratic Oath).

It should also be remembered that there are no specific rules or laws for doctors, and they are obliged at all times to act within the law. Furthermore, there is no doubt that the Bolam test is a powerful influence on the doctor's working practice in determining the standard of care required in terms of the treatment he or she gives. An important component of this will be the method whereby consent is obtained from the patient for treatment to be given and the confidentiality with which the information received is held. The Bolam test is also important in assessing the question of negligence should a complaint or allegation be made at a later stage. Clearly, getting formal consent in the emergency situation may be irrelevant.

Autonomy, beneficence and the patient's best interest

AUTONOMY

There is a general perception that doctors practise in a world of beneficence where 'harmful offensive touchings are not to be found'. While this may or may not be a reasonable premise on which to base an argument that doctors should have a free hand in treating their patients, it cannot be used to suggest that patients should succumb to treatment by the doctor and give up their autonomy, to which they have a right, in circumstances where they have the competence to retain it. This applies equally in the case of immediate care as it does in any other branch of medicine. The patient's right of autonomy renders it wrong to override a person's preference. According to Beauchamp & Childress (1989), the word 'autonomy' derives from the Greek *autos*, meaning 'self', and *nomos*, meaning 'rule'. Beauchamp & Childress have stated that 'the autonomous person acts in accordance with a freely self-chosen and informed plan'.

In the context of giving consent to treatment, one refers to an autonomy of choice in deciding what action (i.e. what

treatment) will be carried out. To act autonomously, Beauchamp & Childress have agreed with the three-condition analysis, namely that the act must be:

- intentional
- understood, and
- without controlling influences determining the action.

In the context of immediate care, where treatment is required to be undertaken without necessarily having the option to discuss this with the patient and his/her relatives, autonomy may clearly be jeopardized. In this situation, the ability to give patients information such that they may act with free self-choice may be denied and autonomy will be replaced by the doctor's decisions made at the scene. The patient will inevitably expect that the doctor's actions will be governed by what is in the patient's best interests at that time. Autonomy is therefore often an unachievable goal in an immediate care situation and the paternalistic approach to treatment where the doctor knows best is frequently adopted. Often, however, the patient may have sufficient understanding or awareness, and indeed there may be sufficient time, for patients to exercise their autonomy in making a decision as to whether or not they would undergo life-saving treatment at the scene of an accident. In these circumstances patients may refuse treatment in a way that the doctor believes is to their detriment and, in these circumstances, to be discussed later in the chapter, the doctor may well be faced with the need to accept a patient's refusal to have treatment, if it is believed that the decision is made by a patient who is competent at the time of the decision.

BENEFICENCE

When one considers the question of beneficence, there is a general belief that doctors act to promote the welfare of patients and not merely to avoid harming them. In considering beneficence there are two principles that need to be outlined. The first is the provision of benefit, which includes the promotion of welfare as well as the prevention and removal of harm. The second is achieving the correct balance between benefit and harm. Consent to treatment on the basis of such benefit being a beneficent act must encompass both of these principles. The general belief that doctors act at all times to promote the welfare of their patients implies concurrence with both of these principles. In seeking consent, or treating patients without obtaining their consent when circumstances make that necessary, the patient and their relatives will assume that these principles underlie the doctor's advice and treatment. In considering this, patients do not distinguish between the moral basis and the legal basis of beneficence. From the moral standpoint there may be a moral obligation on the doctor to act in a beneficent way, where there in fact may be no legal obligation upon him or her to do so. There would, for example, be a moral obligation for a doctor to stop and help at the scene of an accident when asked to assist. In most instances of such an occurrence in the UK, there is no legal obligation on the doctor to do so. Interestingly, there is a legal obligation on the doctor to stop and assist such a case in the UK, if the doctor has reason to believe, or knows, that the victim is his or her patient. In France, however, there is a legal obligation on all doctors to stop and assist at the scene of an accident and proven failure to do so may result in legal and punitive action against the doctor. Such a legal obligation to act in these circumstances is called legally based beneficence.

Generally, where possible, the final decision as to what treatment should be undertaken should always be in the hands of patients and they, in giving consent, exercise their right to self-determination. In certain circumstances, particularly in immediate care, self-determination is not possible. In such circumstances the doctor takes on the responsibility of providing care that is in the patient's best interest. It should be remembered that obtaining consent has both a legal role in converting a battery or an assault into a legal act and a moral role in assuring the patient's autonomy. Where patient autonomy is not possible, the doctor's actions must be in the patient's best interests, and where there is no consent, the doctor does, ultimately, undertake to perform a battery or assault on the patient that would only not be considered a crime if the doctor is acting in what he or she considers to be the patient's best interests at all times. Clearly the doctor may have to justify and defend his or her actions at a later stage, perhaps at an inquest or in a court of law.

THE PATIENT'S BEST INTERESTS

Where it is not possible to obtain consent, as is frequently the case in immediate care situations, the term 'patient's best interests' is a phrase used to justify treatment undertaken. It is therefore a term frequently used in support of medical paternalism and in my view frequently means very little. What patients consider to be in their best interests (if they were given the chance to say) may not correspond with what the doctor believes to be so. In a situation where a patient has the right and facility for self-determination, the patient also has the right to decide what is in his or her best interests, although this can only be in so far as there is adequate information available to the patient, in association with adequate understanding by the patient of what is involved. In circumstances where the patient lacks the capacity to understand, or lacks awareness, autonomy becomes meaningless, paternalism takes over and the patient's best interests become the essence upon which treatment will be undertaken. Patient autonomy,

the patient's best interest, information disclosure and consent are all therefore complexly intertwined and have to be considered when treating patients.

When considering the immediate care situation, where time is of the essence, the patient is frequently incapable of understanding or making decisions and disclosure of information may not be possible. Consent may not be obtained and the only premise on which treatment is based is what is in the patient's best interests. Put more accurately, treatment will be determined by what the doctor believes is in the patient's best interests, given the circumstances of the case, based on clinical judgement, the doctor's integrity, his ethical code and moral practices. In considering the question of consent in the immediate care situation, it is frequently the case that treatment will proceed regardless of a lack of information disclosure to the patient. In these circumstances the purely legal role of consent in converting an assault or battery to a reasonable legal act becomes meaningless and is superseded by the doctor's decision to undertake treatment on the basis of what is in the patient's best interests.

It is important to recognize, though, that, when an immediate care situation arises where a patient has the facility to give appropriate meaningful consent, then such informed consent, either by implication or by verbal agreement, should be obtained. Conversely, where a patient refuses treatment and where such a refusal is made by a competent patient based on a reasonable understanding of what he or she is refusing and the consequences thereof, a doctor would find it difficult to justify proceeding with treatment on any grounds. One of the legal exceptions to this rule is therapeutic privilege.

THERAPEUTIC PRIVILEGE

When considering the legal exceptions to the rule of consent, care in the emergency situation, care of the incompetent and care in the presence of a waiver, along with therapeutic privilege, allow a doctor to proceed with treatment without the valid consent of the patient. In considering therapeutic privilege, Beauchamp & Childress (1989) describe it as 'the most controversial exception according to which a physician may intentionally and validly withhold information based on a sound medical judgement that to divulge the information would be potentially harmful to the patient'.

On the face of it, therapeutic privilege conflicts with the patient's autonomy (which may well have to be respected in the immediate care situation) but if it is accepted that it may only be used where it is considered that disclosure of the information in itself will do harm to the patient, thus making treatment unsafe, the benefits bestowed by nondisclosure outweigh the removal of autonomy. Therapeutic privilege in these circumstances becomes a beneficent principle. The idea of therapeutic privilege cannot be invoked if one argues that giving information will merely make patients react in such a way as to thereafter make them incompetent to decide. In such circumstances, where patient autonomy is not compromised and the timing of events allows, appropriate disclosure of information has to be given in order to obtain appropriate valid consent, as already mentioned.

Who obtains consent?

In the elective treatment of patients, the question of who obtains consent for treatment is still controversial. In the immediate care situation it is less so. The doctor is faced with the decision to undertake treatment on an emergency basis, with significant temporal restrictions, and is frequently faced with life and death decisions concerning his or her patients. In immediate care work, where the particular events allow for consent to be obtained by virtue of the fact that the patient retains competence to understand, and sufficient time is available, then verbal or implied consent should be obtained. This will inevitably involve the person about to undertake the procedure on scene. Written consent, or signed consent in circumstances of immediate care, does not arise. The already established American, and more recently British concept of 'physician-specific consent' and the idea of designer consent forms for individual problems, is not specifically relevant in this work.

Treatment without consent

In the medical and surgical treatment of patients, the majority of procedures are undertaken with the patient's consent, after appropriate explanations and discussions are held and formal consent has been obtained. In such circumstances, while written consent may be forthcoming in some situations, there is no legal requirement for consent to be written and most cases involve patients giving their implied or verbal consent for the procedures to be undertaken. There is, however, an increasing tendency amongst doctors to obtain written consent in order to protect themselves from later complaints, even where treatment is being performed on the competent patient without the use of sedation or anaesthesia.

In the case of immediate care, a significant percentage of procedures undertaken at the roadside or at the scene of an accident are carried out without patients' consent. There are a number of reasons why treatment without consent may have to be undertaken and the concept of treatment without consent needs to be addressed. There are perhaps three specific reasons why treatment without

consent would be undertaken in adult patients and these would generally come under the following headings:

- the unconscious patient
- the incompetent adult patient
- the patient who refuses to consent to treatment.

It is clear that the immediate care doctor is duty bound to provide care that promotes welfare and prevents harm, and balances the benefits against risk. In circumstances where the patient is unable to give his or her own consent, the doctor may seek to obtain consent for treatment from others, or may decide to proceed without any consent whatsoever. The common instances where consent from an adult patient may not be specifically forthcoming include:

- where an unexpected finding comes to light in a patient made unconscious by anaesthesia or sedation
- where a patient is already in an unconscious state as a result of an accident or brain disorder
- where the adult patient is incompetent, by reason of a mental disorder, or is incapable of understanding the nature of the treatment at the time.

It has to be said that the law is unclear as to whether a doctor is justified in treating a patient in the third group. The law does, however, accept such a justification on the basis of necessity. Lord Brandon in the case of *F* v *West Berkshire Health Authority* (1989), said about doctors' common law duties to their legally incapable patients that:

In many cases it will not only be lawful for doctors on the ground of necessity to operate on, or give other medical treatment to adult patients disabled from giving their consent: it will also be their common law duty to do so.

There is no specific 'definitive legal characterization', as described in *Mental Health Services, Law and Practice* (Gostin 1986), of such justification but 'merely a number of disparate judicial responses to specific factual circumstances'. In essence, this is what is still seen in case law in response to individual circumstances. It is, perhaps, because of these disparate judicial responses that one feels it necessary to look at and discuss specific circumstances in a moral as well as legal context.

Clearly in all circumstances the doctor undertaking immediate care work should consider what is in the best interests of the patient. It is also implicit that, in the absence of consent, medical paternalism will take over in the place of patient autonomy, assuming the patient has not previously indicated his or her unwillingness to have treatment in the event of the occurrence of the specific circumstances in question. Fennell (1990) has asked 'how can we be sure that decisions taken are genuinely in patients' best interests', pointing out that 'on its own, the best interest formula is so broad that it will give little guidance in the resolution of the ethical differences that may occur within care teams concerned with the treatment of incapable patients'.

Indeed it gives little guidance to the immediate care doctor when faced with making a decision as to whether to proceed with life-saving treatment in such patients. Fennell (1990) in his discussion of *F v West Berkshire Health Authority*, points out that it was held that:

> *doctors may lawfully give treatment to an incompetent patient without involving the court if it is in the patient's best interest. In order to be in the patient's best interests, the treatment must be carried out in order to save life, or to ensure improvement of or to prevent deterioration in his or her physical or mental health. In making decisions about treatment, the doctor must, to avoid liability in trespass, follow the* Bolam *formula.*

It is, of course, not unusual in immediate care situations to be undertaking treatment with the specific aim of saving life where consent cannot be obtained, and Fennell's discussion on this case is very relevant to what a doctor may lawfully do in these circumstances. The scope of this ruling is, of course, so wide as to be open to unlimited interpretation, allowing almost total freedom to practise unlimited medical paternalism. One could argue that doctors in exercising their belief that they are acting in the patient's best interests, are in fact returning to the paternalistic view that the doctor knows best.

THE UNCONSCIOUS PATIENT

There are two circumstances in which an immediate care doctor may be faced with an unconscious patient and in which a decision will need to be made about treatment in the absence of any form of reasonable consent. The first is where unconsciousness has been induced by anaesthesia or sedation at the scene of the accident, for the purpose of saving life, often in the presence of a chest or head injury, and where at that point the patient is discovered to have a further problem requiring immediate treatment, e.g. amputation. The second situation is where the patient is already in an unconscious state, usually secondary to the injury for which the doctor has been called to the scene, possibly with other injuries also requiring surgical treatment, or immediate care treatment at the scene.

In both instances it has to be accepted that treatment done to save life is reasonable, as described in Flemming's *The Law of Torts*, in which he states that a surgeon would be justified in proceeding 'without prior authority... when it is necessary to save life or preserve the health of the patient'.

There could be no argument as to the question of saving life. A procedure used to preserve the health of the patient may be another question. Since a doctor's whole approach to his or her work is based on preserving the health of the patient, it is unreasonable to suggest that doing so forms a reasonable basis upon which to undertake any form of treatment without prior authority. To accept that health preservation of itself should form a basis for unauthorized treatment would be to undermine the whole concept of autonomy and abolish the need for consent in the first place. One needs clearly to distinguish between a life-saving procedure and a procedure designed to preserve health. While the former is permissible without prior authority, the latter may not be. In the immediate care situation, therefore, it would be acceptable to assume that a life-saving immediate care procedure done at the scene would be justifiable, whereas anything other than a truly life-saving procedure would not be considered reasonable without some form of consent or further consideration at least. In considering the first situation mentioned above, that of the unexpected finding, once the patient has been anaesthetized or sedated, I would suggest that any further reasonable treatment to deal with the unexpected findings should only be undertaken if it is necessary to save life. To undertake any procedures not considered life saving would reasonably be considered as a trespass. This view is supported by Brazier in her book *Protecting the Vulnerable*, in which she states that 'save in circumstances of dire emergency, a patient's best interests are for the patient to define'. In applying such arguments to immediate care, one could argue that procedures necessary to save life are justifiable, while any other procedure would not be so.

In considering the second situation, the unconscious patient presenting in that state at the scene and requiring emergency treatment, there is no question of patient autonomy in so far as treatment to save life is concerned. Any treatment that can reasonably be delayed until restoration of consciousness should, however, be delayed and treatment should be confined to that which is necessary to save life. The question of necessity was discussed in the case of *Maynard v West Midlands Regional Health Authority* (1983), a case in which the difficulties of judging when a procedure is necessary were highlighted. Lord Scarman used the standard of *Bolam* and the exercise of clinical judgement to support his decision in the case. How does one judge what is a necessary procedure? It may be difficult to do so even when the patient exercises autonomy and gives consent. It is much more difficult where autonomy or consent are absent. Skegg (1990) in considering the circumstances in which a doctor is legally justified in proceeding without consent, distinguishes between:

> *those procedures which are intended to benefit the health of the patient, and those which are not intended to have this effect. In the latter group, where the procedure is not intended to benefit the patient, treatment without authority cannot be considered to be in the patient's best interests.*

He categorizes the procedures intended to benefit the health of the patient into four groups, based on the patient's capacity or incapacity to give consent; the presence or absence of another person authorized to give the consent of the patient; the patient's known or unknown views regarding any objections that he or she may have to the procedure being proposed; and the refusal of the patient to give consent. While this is a useful classification of the types of patient who will present to a surgeon or physician for elective or even semi-elective treatment, it does not distinguish between life-saving procedures and those that are merely advisable in pursuing the maintenance of health. The subdivisions Skegg describes are therefore of limited value in clearly identifying criteria for use in cases where it is proposed to undertake life-saving procedures.

In trauma cases of the kind we are discussing, the matter may be further complicated by the fact that the treatment, although not life-saving at the time of presentation, may, by not being undertaken, pose a potentially serious or fatal risk to the patient at a later stage and perhaps before he or she has regained consciousness, and thus competence, to consent to such further treatment. It could be argued that treatment to deal with such problems is justified on the basis of a direct necessity but indirectly on the basis of its need to be done to save life.

Skegg refers to short-term incapacity during which there would be no justification in doing everything in the interests of the patient's health 'for so broad a justification would create too great an inroad into the individual interest in deciding what is done to his or her own body'. In trying to clarify which procedures it would be reasonable to undertake in the absence of consent, in a situation where incapacity is temporary, Skegg argues that the question to be asked should be whether it would be unreasonable to postpone the procedure until a later stage rather than whether it would be reasonable to proceed immediately, the latter being too broad in terms of the tort of battery. He suggests that such an approach would avoid the possibility of the patient's life being put at risk for lack of consent but would 'encourage the doctor to limit intervention to that which could not reasonably be postponed'.

In essence, therefore, we see the concept of life-saving treatment being reasonable but only in so far as it is necessary at the time to undertake it in order to save life. The concept of undertaking immediate care procedures at the scene, where such procedures are not immediately life saving, must be carefully examined. Where a procedure can reasonably be undertaken on arrival at the hospital and failure to undertake it would not in any way jeopardize the patient's survival, then to undertake such a procedure might well be considered unjustified, particularly where the risks of its performance on scene are greater than those associated with its performance in the emergency department of a hospital to which the patient is to be transferred.

As already mentioned, the question of benefit versus risk has to be considered and unreasonable risk in the context of benefits to be obtained may well make the performance of such procedures at the scene unreasonable and the doctor liable to a justifiable complaint.

THE CONSCIOUS INCOMPETENT ADULT

In considering the emergency treatment of an incompetent adult, one can draw on the words of Lord Justice Brandon in the case of *F v West Berkshire Health Authority* (1989) where he said:

a doctor can lawfully operate on ... adult patients who are incapable for one reason or another of consenting to his doing so, provided the operation ... is in the best interests of such patients.

He went further in saying that:

the operation or treatment will be in their best interests only if it is carried out in order either to save their lives or to ensure improvement or prevent deterioration in their physical or mental health.

An analysis of the case of *F v West Berkshire Health Authority* (1989) reveals that it has relevance to the treatment of the adult patient incapacitated by unconsciousness following an accident, for a temporary or indeed a more permanent period of time. In the case, the plaintiff F was a severely mentally disabled female who since the age of 14 had been a voluntary inpatient in a mental hospital where she had formed a sexual relationship with a male patient. The medical psychiatric evidence was that a pregnancy was highly undesirable and that all ordinary methods of contraception were unacceptable. Medical staff decided that sterilization was the best course of action. The patient's verbal capacity was that of a 2-year-old and general mental capacity was that of a 5-year-old. She was therefore disabled from giving consent to the operation. Her mother sought a declaration making sterilization lawful in the absence of the patient's consent and, while accepting that the court had no power to give consent on F's behalf, the judge, Justice Scott Baker granted the declaration sought. The official solicitor on behalf of F appealed to the Court of Appeal, which affirmed the judge's decision, indicating that the court had the power to authorize such an operation and that the operation would not be unlawful by reason of the absence of F's consent. The official solicitor went on to appeal to the House of Lords on the grounds that sterilization would never be lawful in an adult mental patient who was unable to give her own consent. The House of Lords unanimously dismissed the appeal.

The case of *F v West Berkshire Health Authority* is an important one in respect of treatment being proposed and undertaken on incompetent adults. It raised and discussed a number of important issues that, although dealt with in terms of sterilization of the mentally incompetent adult female, can reasonably be applied to the incompetent adult in whom other forms of treatment are being considered. It therefore has relevance to the treatment of the adult patient incapacitated by unconsciousness following an accident for a temporary or indeed a more permanent period of time. Lord Bridge of Harwich pointed to 'a paucity of clearly defined principles in the Common Law which may be applied to determine lawfulness of ... surgical treatment ... in patients who lack the capacity to give consent'. He considered it axiomatic that the treatment that is necessary to preserve life, health or well-being of a patient may be lawfully given without consent. He rejected the rigid criterion of necessity as it would deprive such a patient of treatment that might be 'beneficial for them to receive'. He recommended the use of the *Bolam* standard to assess the lawfulness of treatment:

when undertaken in the belief that such treatment is appropriate to the patient's existing condition, or susceptibility to a condition in the future.

In immediate care application, the concept of treatment on the scene in order to avoid a condition to which the patient may become susceptible in the future (i.e. during transport to hospital) is encompassed. Lord Gough of Cheveley also rejected the idea that the operation must be necessary and recommended the use of the 'best interest' concept, arguing that the doctor should offer treatment 'just as if he had received the patient's consent' otherwise 'much useful treatment and care could ... be denied to the unfortunate'. Lord Jauncey warned that the law 'must not convert incompetents into second-class citizens for the purpose of health care'. Lord Brandon recommended leaving the matter entirely in the doctor's hands to decide what is in the patient's interests, allowing the common law to provide a solution in that under common law:

a doctor can lawfully operate on adult patients who are incapable ... of giving consent provided that the operation ... is in the best interests of the patient. The operation ... will be in their best interests if and only if it is carried out to save their life or ensure improvement or prevent deterioration in their physical or mental health.

The judgement in *F* v *West Berkshire Health Authority* is an important one in respect of the immediate care of incompetent adult patients on the roadside. The lawfulness of a procedure on an incompetent adult patient, on the basis of these recommendations, is up to the doctor to decide. The criteria for such lawfulness are so wide as to be justifiable in almost any circumstances. The judgement does not distinguish between necessity and convenience and one might ask the question 'whose convenience?' Where does one draw the line between necessity and convenience? Only Lord Justice Neal drew attention to the need 'to avoid the tendency for surgery to be done as a matter of convenience', suggesting that 'each case needs to be looked at individually to see if it is in the best interest of the patient'.

In the context of immediate care, clearly the court cannot be invited to make a decision, as time does not allow, and one has to accept the judgement of the House of Lords in the case of *F* v *West Berkshire Health Authority*, applying it to the immediate care situation in the context of the incompetent adult patient at the scene. In this context, Lady Justice Butler-Sloss summarized it neatly by saying:

the substantive law is that a proposed operation is lawful if it is in the best interest of the patient, and unlawful if it is not.

In considering what standard a court would accept as reasonable, when deciding what is in the patient's best interest, Lord Donaldson (MR) accepted the Bolam test, but went further in pointing out that 'the medical profession and the court have to keep the special status of such patients in the forefront of their minds'. In contrast to the Bolam test, he suggested that:

in exercising greater caution, the existence of a significant minority view would constitute a serious contra-indication [to treatment].

This is a slightly more constrained view of the doctor's freedom in deciding what he can or cannot do.

Lord Gough made the interesting distinction between a temporarily incompetent patient (e.g. the patient with short-term unconsciousness following a head injury) and the more permanently incompetent adult. In the temporarily incompetent patient, the surgery should do 'no more than is necessarily required in the best interest of the patient, until he regains consciousness'. It is left to the doctor to decide how long that may take and therefore what treatment may be considered reasonable in the circumstances. The distinction, however, between temporary and permanent incompetence, while in theory an important one, has little relevance when considering regulation of a doctor's activities when faced with the unconscious patient in the situation where the question of immediate care arises.

In considering the incompetent adult patient at the scene of an accident, we are therefore faced with the inevitable conclusion that treatment considered appropriate for whatever reason will ultimately find some justification in law and the doctor who treats the incompetent adult will in most circumstances be immune from a charge of trespass, or indeed negligence.

REFUSAL OF CONSENT

Where a patient refuses to give consent to a necessary treatment, for example, a life-saving operation, Skegg tells us that:

in all but the most exceptional circumstances, a doctor may not carry out treatment ... and the fact that the patient's health will suffer, will not of itself justify a doctor in overriding the patient's refusal

Even the certainty of a patient's death will not justify a doctor's intervention. The duty of care that a doctor owes to his or her patient does not override the obligation to accept the patient's refusal of treatment if the patient is considered competent to refuse such consent. If there is evidence of the patient's incompetence in his or her refusal to give consent, then the principles already considered above would apply and it would be considered reasonable to give necessary treatment without consent. In the immediate care situation it is much more likely that a patient be considered incompetent by reason of injuries, pain or other circumstances than to be presented with a situation where a doctor believes that a competent patient is refusing treatment. It is, however, clearly necessary to establish whether the refusal of consent is the act of a competent or incompetent person and this may be extremely difficult in an immediate care situation, where time is of the essence and a lack of it spurs on treatment within a matter of seconds or minutes of arrival on the scene. The case of *Re C* (1993) is useful in discussing this question. The patient was mentally ill and had gangrene of his leg. It was considered that he might die if his leg was not amputated but despite this he refused amputation. The hospital refused to undertake not to amputate if the patient's life was at risk and the patient therefore applied for an injunction to prevent amputation without his consent. Mr Justice Thorpe held that the question to be considered when establishing the capacity of individuals to refuse treatment was whether their capacity was so reduced (in this case by chronic mental illness) that they did not sufficiently understand the nature, purpose and effects of the amputation. He suggested that there were three parts in the decision-making process:

● understanding and retaining the information relating to treatment
● believing it
● assessing the information and comparing the risks in order to make a choice.

Mr Justice Thorpe held that, although the patient suffered from schizophrenia, he was able to understand the nature, purpose and effects of the amputation. He pointed out

that the application of this test had failed to displace the patient's right to self-determination and accordingly he allowed the application by the patient not to have the operation. It should be remembered that, as Lord Donaldson pointed out, consent may be refused for rational, irrational or even non-existent reasons, none of which detract from the validity of the refusal. It is clear that a refusal of treatment, regardless of how illogical this refusal may appear to the doctor, must be accepted if a patient is considered competent to refuse.

It could be argued that any adult suffering from the effects of injury and being in a state of mental shock is incompetent in respect of giving consent. One suspects that such a contention of itself might be difficult to uphold. It certainly could be regarded as reasonable to consider a patient who has been given an analgesic or hypnotic drug as incompetent if he or she subsequently refuses what the doctor considers to be reasonable treatment in terms of what is in the patient's best interests. Similarly, a patient who is in pain may also be considered incompetent. One could argue therefore, that all injured patients who have pain are incompetent by reason of the effects of the pain, or the drugs given to try and relieve it. This may be extremely relevant in the case of immediate care situations. In giving the necessary drug to combat pain, frequently without formal consent, the doctor is performing the very act that will in theory make patients competent, by relieving their pain, but in practice makes him incompetent by reason of the effects of the drugs on them. The immediate care situation does, therefore, give the doctor an opportunity to destroy patient autonomy and allow paternalism to take over. Crisp (1990) refers to this as 'capacity violation' and describes it as the most serious form of autonomy violation, by eliminating any possibility of the patient exercising choice. Lord Donaldson, in the case of *Re C* (1993) (where refusal of a blood transfusion followed erroneous information to the patient by the doctor and where a court order subsequently allowed its administration by reason of patient incompetence) accepted the 'well established' right of a patient as paramount but went on to say that, if there is any doubt about the patient's exercise of this right, then it should be resolved in favour of the sanctity of life. Lord Donaldson also felt that factors such as 'unconsciousness, confusion or other effects of shock, severe fatigue, pain or drugs' will act to reduce or deprive the capacity of a patient to give a valid consent. One could argue that this opens the floodgates for doctors at the scene of an accident to act in whatever way they feel is appropriate, on the basis that the patient in such a situation is inevitably affected by such factors as those mentioned above.

In considering the refusal of treatment by a minor at the scene of an accident, similar arguments as those given will apply. The situation is, however, complicated by the question of whether a child is competent to make a decision about refusal of treatment on the basis of his or her understanding of the treatment, its consequences, or refusal of such treatment, and the understanding of what is potentially a fatal outcome. It is unusual in the immediate care situation at the scene of an accident to encounter children who refuse consent, or indeed their parents refusing consent on behalf of their children. Time constraints will not allow the involvement of the courts in these circumstances and the doctor is left with the inevitable difficulty in balancing the sanctity of life against accepting a refusal of treatment. In circumstances such as these, it would be entirely reasonable for the doctor to proceed with life-saving treatment on the basis that the circumstances do not allow children, or perhaps indeed their parents, a proper understanding of the problem. By reason of this, one could consider most children in these circumstances to be incompetent. As the likelihood of refusal of treatment by a child or the parents at the scene of an accident is extremely low, this particular aspect of consent will not be discussed further here. It is sufficient to quote the words of Lord Templeman in the case of *Gillick*, where he stated:

> where there is no time to obtain a court decision, the doctor can safely treat in an emergency to save life, notwithstanding the opposition of a parent, or the impossibility of alerting the parent before treatment is carried out. In such a case the doctor must have the courage of his conviction that the treatment is necessary and urgent and in the interests of the patient. The court will, if necessary, approve after the event, any treatment which the court would have authorized in advance, even if the treatment was unsuccessful.

This ruling is interesting as it puts the question of emergency treatment of the minor firmly in the hands of the doctor, even in the absence of a parent or in the presence of a parent who objects to the treatment. It also gives authority to the doctor to treat as he or she sees fit, knowing that the backing of the court is there should it be required later. Clearly the doctor's clinical judgement and integrity will prevent the use of uncontrolled or innovative forms of therapy in these circumstances.

It will be clear from this section that the absence of consent is not a great hindrance to the doctor when trying to treat the patient. The intention to do what is in the patient's best interest, and the use of the concept of necessity, will allow the immediate care doctor to feel safe in the knowledge that he or she will ultimately probably be supported by the courts in trying to do what is in the best interests of his/her patient.

Probably the most important issue regarding legal aspects of immediate care relates to the question of treatment at the scene. The specific problems relating to consent have been discussed in detail. The other issues such as confidentiality and negligence will be discussed on the basis of general principles regarding these problems, rather than in the context of individual case law analysis, which I believe is necessary in the context of the particularly important issue of consent.

CONFIDENTIALITY

In caring for a patient the doctor is bound by a duty of confidentiality at all times. This duty obliges him/her to keep confidential all information pertaining to the patient, regardless of how this information came to be in his or her possession. Such obligations are no different in the context of immediate care from those in any other aspect of medicine. The circumstances as a result of which the doctor obtains this information are unique in the practice of immediate care and do present certain difficulties. The circumstances in which immediate care is provided (i.e. the emergency situation), frequently under the public's gaze, also present the doctor with certain difficulties in respect to the requirements to comply with police procedure and indeed the law. Maintaining confidentiality may also be a problem when the circumstances of an incident are so public such that by its very nature a large number of interested and uninterested parties will have access to information that the doctor might normally consider to be confidential.

While it is therefore accepted that in the practice of immediate care, particularly where such care is undertaken under the public gaze, a lot of information will be open to the public and the doctor will have had no hand in such openness; it also has to be accepted that the doctor will take reasonable care in trying to ensure that medical matters remain as confidential as possible and that s/he does not partake in activities that deliberately breach the duty of confidentiality towards the patient. It should also be remembered that the duty of confidentiality extends after death and, in the event that the injured person dies, the doctor remains under a duty of care to maintain confidentiality about the medical details regarding such a person permanently.

There are a number of instances where confidentiality may unwittingly or deliberately be broken and these will now be considered:

- Information transmitted over the airwaves
- Record keeping at the scene
- Police statements
- Press statements
- Discussions and debriefings
- Photography – its use and abuse
- Special circumstances requiring the doctor to breach obligations in respect of confidentiality.

INFORMATION TRANSMITTED OVER THE AIRWAVES

In the successful provision of immediate care, communication between any or all of a variety of agencies is utterly essential. Communications between doctors, the police force, the ambulance service, hospitals and a control centre of any or all of the emergency services are an essential part of any incident of the kind where immediate care may be provided. With the routine availability of transceivers and scanners, it is predictable that much of the information communicated over airwaves will be monitored by amateur and professional groups for a variety of reasons. In accepting that this is so, it is apparent that the material transmitted over the airwaves cannot be considered to have been transmitted in a confidential way. A doctor transmitting such information should do so in such a way as to provide anonymous, but appropriate essential information. Victims' names and other identifiable information must never be communicated and the condition of the victim should be communicated in a manner recognizable to those entitled to have such information. The KILO code is a method whereby the condition of the patient may be transmitted in such a confidential way. In some circumstances identifiable information may have to be transmitted, as for example the address where an incident is occurring, and clearly the use of such codes will minimize the available information to those monitoring the airwaves in these circumstances.

RECORD KEEPING AT THE SCENE

Keeping records at the scene of the incident is both good practice and essential to a successful outcome. Making such records does give rise to a number of issues in respect of confidentiality.

The first of these is the disposal of such records. It is the doctor's duty to ensure that these records are kept confidential and are passed on only to those entitled to see them. In many circumstances this means handing over the records to the appropriate ambulance personnel or to the hospital personnel where the patient is subsequently delivered. Under no circumstances should any records be left at the scene or given to persons not authorized to have them. The doctor is responsible for the disposal of records made and for ensuring that they become part of the patient's confidential records, be that in hospital or in their own practice.

The second issue that arises in respect of the records kept at the scene relates to the question of multiple copies of these records. In many instances the doctor at the scene, the ambulance and even the police take copies of records made. It should however be remembered that the medical information recorded at the scene by a doctor is confidential and that copies must not be handed out willy-nilly to all who ask for one. The disposal of records kept by police and ambulance services is clearly for them and will not be considered further here.

It is not unusual nowadays to dictate a report at the scene and keep records of on-going progress by means of voice dictation. Clearly any information kept in such form also comes under the term 'medical records' and the same rules of confidentiality apply to it. Any such records need to be appropriately transcribed, filed and kept in a way that affords them appropriate confidentiality. The doctor has the duty to ensure that recording devices, such as cassette tapes, are appropriately stored or erased once transferred, and the loss of such information may leave the doctor open to allegations of incompetence and poor practice.

Computerization of records is a separate, and indeed a very complex subject. It is not unusual for details of incidents, patients, their injuries, their treatment and ultimate disposal or final outcome to be kept on computer by doctors who regularly work in immediate care. Doctors who undertake to do this must comply with the Data Protection Act and all other regulations regarding the electronic storage of information. In the increasingly complex world of electronic data, confidentiality becomes increasingly difficult to maintain, but the doctor remains duty bound in respect of issues of confidentiality.

POLICE STATEMENTS

It is inevitable in this kind of work that the doctor will be required to provide statements to the police in respect of incidents, victims, their injuries, etc. Doctors have to be very wary of providing medical information to police, as to do so may put them in breach of their duty of confidentiality towards their patient. While it may be acceptable to make a statement regarding non-medical facts of an incident, in general it is unacceptable to make a statement that provides medical details without the patient's consent.

Exceptions to this will be discussed later under 'Special considerations'.

Where a police officer is acting as a coroner's officer, the enquiries are subject to the coroner's officers' jurisdiction and the doctor has no option but to respond. Confidentiality in these circumstances takes second place to the coroner's enquiry in the event of a fatal incident.

PRESS STATEMENTS

In general a doctor is advised to avoid making any form of press statement at the scene of an incident, or indeed subsequently. While a press statement may be acceptable that indicates the need for more vigilance on the part of individuals or groups, in order to avoid further problems, any details that may result in specific information becoming available to those who are not entitled to receive it can cause significant problems. It is all too easy to divulge information of a confidential nature without even realizing it, during the frenetic activity that frequently accompanies incidents of the kind where immediate care is provided. A doctor who is not careful may be caught off-guard and unwittingly provide information that may be the source of complaint at a later stage. The combination of the doctor unwittingly providing information to the press and the press's inevitable wish to sell copy, with possible distortion of the facts in the process, often combined with dramatic pictures of the scene, can result in considerable difficulty when later trying to defend a complaint against the doctor involving questions of confidentiality at the scene. In general, the advice that doctors should adhere to is that press statements should not be given at the scene and should be considered very carefully if provided later. Comments made to the press over the telephone, as frequently occurs after a serious incident, are even more prone to distortion and danger.

In essence, therefore, the need for the public to wallow in the difficulties produced by an incident in which people are hurt does not justify a breach of confidentiality by doctors aiming either to assist the press or indeed to get them off their backs.

DISCUSSIONS AND DEBRIEFINGS

Following incidents, particularly where a number of casualties are involved, it is not infrequent for debriefings and discussions to take place in respect of how the incident was handled. This is particularly so in the case of major incidents, where lessons are frequently learned. While these discussions and debriefings generally involve raking over the rights and wrongs of how things were done, how things might be done better and how best to avoid some of the problems often encountered, it is all too easy for doctors involved in such discussions to divulge information of a confidential nature and to become in breach of their duty of confidentiality towards their patients. While discussions of this sort in appropriate circumstances and with appropriate authorities and agencies is acceptable, it is important that confidential information is not divulged to those to whom it is not authorized. It is the doctor's responsibility during such discussions and debriefings to ensure that what is said does not breach the duty of confidentiality and to ensure as far as possible that comments are made only to those entitled to hear them. It is, unfortunately, all to common for such discussions to be held in an area where non-authorized persons have access to the discussions being held, and clearly that is something that a doctor has to be acutely aware of at such times.

Incidents involving immediate care do form interesting discussion points between doctors and their colleagues at a later time, and these discussions may take place in what may ultimately turn out to be totally inappropriate circumstances. It is unfortunately all too common for immediate care doctors to discuss what are often exciting exploits with colleagues or friends only to inadvertently divulge information that may subsequently prove to be their downfall. The often dramatic events surrounding incidents where immediate care is provided, while providing good material for after-dinner discussions, should be as confidential as the mundane discussions the doctor has with patients in a surgery. A doctor who fails to adhere to normal procedures in this respect and inadvertently divulges confidential information may find himself in breach of duty of confidentiality, even though the circumstances surrounding the event may be public knowledge and may have appeared in the newspapers at the time of the incident.

PHOTOGRAPHY

Photographic recording of injuries, damage and accident scenes is now routine for both medical and forensic work. In the context of the medical problems, however, the photographs of an injury, or the appearance of a patient following injury, constitute part of the medical records of the patient and must be treated with the same respect. There is no doubt that Polaroid or digital photography of, for example, a serious wound, or a compound fracture, can significantly assist in the management of these injuries by avoiding the need to repeatedly expose the injury for purposes of viewing. It is, however, unfortunately, all too easy to take multiple pictures at the scene, or subsequently, and to lose control of what happens to these images. If doctors authorize or take photographs for the purposes of recording a problem, they are duty bound to ensure that those photographs form part of the patient's records and are held in equal confidence to any other records. It must be ensured that the images are forwarded with the patient and the patient's records to the appropriate hospital, or kept in the appropriate place with other records. It is not permitted for such images to be given to police, the press, or indeed any other agency, for any purpose. Should the police require to take pictures of the scene of accident, which is frequently the case, then clearly those pictures belong to the police and will be used in their forensic and police investigations. The medical images, however, belong to the patient's records and must remain with them.

Photographs are often taken for purposes of later examination and teaching. There is increasing concern over the use of photographs for purposes of teaching or publication without a patient's consent. Photographs taken for the purposes of medical recording do not require the patient's consent. If, however, they are to be used for any other purpose, then the doctor is required to have the patient's consent before using such images in any other way. In the absence of consent, photographs cannot be used for purposes of presentation, teaching, lecturing or publication. In the event that they are, and the patient makes a complaint, the doctor will be liable for a breach of duty of confidentiality, as he or she will have chosen to use confidential material in a way for which no consent had been given. It should be remembered that there is no automatic right for a doctor to use medical records (in this case in the form of images) for the purposes of display, teaching or publication. Such a right is only granted to the doctor by use of valid consent, and in the event that such consent is not forthcoming it will be a breach of confidentiality to use images in these ways.

In some cases, it might well be said that images are unidentifiable and that therefore no case could be brought against doctors who used them. If, however, there is any way of identifying an individual image as belonging to an individual patient, or indeed of identifying it as *likely* to belong to an individual patient, by reason of a date, a registration number, a specific characteristic or such like, then doctors can find themselves in trouble if such images are published or presented without consent.

Since many incidents involve very specific, identifiable vehicles, situations or indeed injuries, the use of photographs for any purpose other than as patient records can result in significant problems for the doctor, who may be faced with allegations of a breach of the duty of confidentiality, and indeed, publication or presentation without appropriate consent to divulge such information.

In considering photography, therefore, the doctor has to take very seriously the responsibilities in respect of breaching confidentiality by discussing, presenting or publishing images that may prove identifiable in some way, even indirectly. It should be clearly understood that, while photography has a valuable part to play in medical investigation and treatment, in police investigation, and in forensic work, its use has to be carefully controlled in the context of presentations, discussions and publications where such are done without appropriate consent.

SPECIAL CIRCUMSTANCES REQUIRING A DOCTOR TO BREACH OBLIGATIONS IN RESPECT OF CONFIDENTIALITY

There are certain circumstances in which doctors are obliged to forego their duty of confidentiality and divulge information to appropriate agencies. Some of these may involve doctors involved in immediate care.

Fatal accident

In the event of a fatal accident, doctors are obliged, on the request of the police, to divulge appropriate information as may be necessary to allow the police to undertake their investigations. Doctors are not obliged to voluntarily provide information to police or other agencies in these circumstances. They are not permitted, however, to withhold appropriate information when requested to provide it in the event of a fatal accident.

Child safety

It may be reasonable to forego one's duty of confidentiality where the doctor has a reasonable reason to believe that a child's safety is at risk. Safety of a child, particularly regarding possible child abuse, is of paramount importance and the General Medical Council recognizes that there are circumstances in which a doctor's duty of confidentiality may be overridden by his or her concern over a child's safety. In these circumstances, divulgence of information to appropriate agencies to protect the child from potential or actual harm may well be justified. Where, while undertaking duties in immediate care, a doctor becomes aware of a potential risk to a child – as, for instance, in a household incident – the doctor may well consider it a duty to breach confidentiality in order to protect the child's interest. While each case has to be judged on its merits, it is likely that a favourable view would be taken if the doctor can show reasonable reason for believing the child's safety to be at risk.

The common good

Where a doctor becomes aware, through dealings with a patient, that there is a significant threat to the common good and that such a threat might be avoided by divulgence of medical information, it may be justified for information to be divulged in breach of duty of confidentiality towards an individual patient. While this is highly unlikely to result from an immediate care situation, it is an instance where a doctor may consider the duty of confidentiality to be overridden by the need to protect the common good. Once again, each case will be judged on its merits and, should the matter come before a court, it will be necessary for the doctor to justify his/her actions.

Terrorism

Under the Prevention of Terrorism Act, a doctor is obliged to voluntarily divulge information to the police authorities regardless of whether this constitutes a breach of confidentiality towards the patient. Doctors may be found to be in breach of the law if they do not volunteer to give information to the Police Authorities in the event that they suspects an act of terrorism. It will not be considered sufficient to await a police enquiry. This is perhaps the only instance where a deliberate breach of confidentiality, without being asked to give information, is required by law.

Insurance reports

It is not infrequent for insurance companies to request reports from doctors following accidents or incidents in which injury or death occur. In the absence of the patient's consent, a doctor may not divulge information to an insurance company, as to do so would involve a breach of duty of confidentiality towards the patient. The difficulty arises where the patient is unable to give consent, by reasons of incompetence, or indeed by reason of the fact that s/he is dead. In these circumstances, a doctor may have no option but to refuse to give information to an insurance company, regardless of the hardship that this may cause to the relatives. Many insurance policies taken out over the last 15 years will have the subscriber's consent for the doctor to divulge information in the event of the subscriber's illness or death, and this is usually sufficient to allow the doctor to prepare a report as requested by the insurance company. It is, however, important that the doctor is satisfied that the consent form being presented is valid. Simple things like ensuring that the date precedes that of the death of the patient and that the signature perhaps looks like the writing of the patient, if such is available for comparison, may be necessary to establish the bona fide nature of the consent form prior to submission of the report. In the event that the doctor has suspicions as to the validity of the consent, then the duty of confidentiality that pertains after the death of the patient will in fact prevent him or her from preparing a report for the insurance company.

Medical negligence

In providing patient care a doctor has a duty to act in accordance with good practice and to provide care of an appropriate and an acceptable standard. A failure to do so resulting in harm to the patient may result in an allegation of medical negligence.

As patients become more questioning, aware and autonomous, so the number of allegations of medical negligence made against doctors increases. As a consequence there has been an inevitable rise in the cost of medical defence insurance and an increasing tendency on the part of many doctors to practice defensive medicine. In the context of immediate care, this can be expensive, time consuming and, in some instances, counterproductive. Where time is of the essence, a concentration on a defensive form of practice may use critical time, which in turn may make the difference between life and death for the patient. In this respect, the use of defensive medicine may in itself result in allegations of negligence, where it may be considered that the

defensive practice itself resulted in irrecoverable damage or even death.

WHY IS MEDICAL NEGLIGENCE ON THE INCREASE?

There are many reasons why allegations of medical negligence are on the increase, many of which are unrelated to the incidence of medical negligence itself. A successful negligence action can result in high monetary awards for the patient and high fees for the solicitors and barristers involved in the case. Insurance companies, faced with large pay-outs following major serious injuries, are only too happy to see the burden shift towards medical defence insurance as an alternative to themselves paying out for injuries received. Furthermore, insurance companies are having to look carefully at their own financial state and are looking for contributory negligence as a way of reducing pay-outs. It is common practice for insurance companies and solicitors, when seeking medical reports in respect of injuries, to request the authors of such reports to specifically address the question of what care was given and whether it was appropriate. Clearly any suggestion that the final outcome following injury was adversely affected by the treatment given could significantly reduce the insurance company's contribution to the final pay-out and it is therefore not surprising that an allegation of medical negligence in respect of immediate care treatment following an accident may prove to be a godsend for the insurance companies concerned.

Solicitors acting on behalf of their clients clearly also have a duty to their clients to ensure the most advantageous settlement. In considering a true accident, where there is no attributable fault and therefore, perhaps, no reasonable source of compensation, it is perhaps not surprising that a solicitor will seek to establish that part of the ultimate problem was related to inappropriate medical action. While it is not yet routine current practice, it is becoming increasingly common for hospitals to receive requests for copies of entire medical records to be submitted to solicitors acting on behalf of their clients. Many of these requests are specifically geared at having the records carefully examined in order to try and identify specific instances of inappropriate care that might be considered relevant to the final outcome following injury and treatment.

Perhaps somewhat more disturbing is the increasingly common practice of seeking to blame doctors when an insurance claim in respect of an accident proves either too difficult to run or unsuccessful. Suing for damage allegedly caused by medical negligence becomes the backup should a claim for compensation through the usual insurance channels fail.

Immediate care, although not in the forefront of medical negligence, does have some very specific problems that will ultimately make it an attractive target for medical negligence allegations. Doctors undertaking to provide immediate care treatment should be aware of some of the pitfalls associated with their art, which may ultimately be used against them in a court of law. Before considering these, the specific criteria necessary to successfully prove negligence will be identified, without which an allegation of medical negligence would fail.

CRITERIA FOR MEDICAL NEGLIGENCE

The criteria for medical negligence are not specific to immediate care but apply across all medical treatment. Specific applications in respect of immediate care will be considered later in the chapter.

Currently in the UK, the criteria necessary to prove an allegation of medical negligence are threefold. They are:

- a duty of care
- a breach of the duty of care
- damage as a consequence of the breach of the duty of care.

In the absence of one or more of these criteria, an allegation of medical negligence will fail to be established.

Duty of care

Clearly the doctor treating a patient owes to that patient a duty of care. The duty of care begins when the doctor accepts to treat the patient and ends either when the treatment is complete and there is nothing further to be done or when care is handed over to another person who then takes on that duty from that point onwards. The doctor does not owe a duty of care to the general public as a whole. In the context of immediate care, the doctor may have a contractual duty of care to any patients who are the victims of accidents in the area to whom the doctor is called, or indeed if he or she happens to come across them at the scene of an accident. Individual doctors' contract terms will determine which of these is so. In France, there is an automatic duty of care inherent in being a doctor if a doctor arrives at or passes the scene of an accident. Failure to stop and assist at the scene of an accident can result in punitive action against the doctor regardless of any contractual obligations he may or may not have. This is not so in England, although clearly there may be a moral obligation on doctors to stop and assist at the scene of an accident. Failure to adhere to a moral obligation, however, cannot result in punitive action in the UK. Some contracts do specify that doctors will provide immediate emergency assistance to patients whom they believe belong to their practice. Precise policing of such contractual obligations may, however, be very difficult.

Where a doctor voluntarily opts to provide immediate care, be that as part of a recognized scheme of doctors providing such care or merely on the basis of serendipitous attendance at the scene of an accident, a duty of care is taken on towards the patients the doctor is opting to treat by reason of the very fact that the doctor has, voluntarily or otherwise, opted to do so. The idea that the doctor providing a 'good Samaritan' service does not have a duty of care towards the patients that he or she has voluntarily taken on to treat is nowadays untenable. The duty of care in these circumstances is no weaker than the duty owed by any doctor treating patients, regardless of the fact that the victim of the accident being treated is not the doctor's patient or was, up to that time, unknown to the doctor. The argument that the duty of care was merely provided on the basis of being a 'good Samaritan', will not be a satisfactory defence in the event that an allegation is brought against the doctor that he or she failed in the duty of care.

When does a duty of care terminate?

Clearly on the death of a patient, the duty to that patient terminates. It should, however, be remembered that the duty of confidentiality to a patient persists after death, unless there has been a specific premortal waiver, to keep confidential all medical matters relating to that person.

Other than in death, the duty of care that a doctor owes to a patient persists until it is reasonably taken over by another medical person or until the treatment for the specific problem is completed satisfactorily. Clearly in terminating his or her duty of care, it is the doctor's responsibility to ensure that the care of the patient has been satisfactorily transferred and taken over. In considering a failure to do so, the court will look at what is reasonable for a doctor to do to ensure that such a transfer has been properly effected. In the event of a patient's death, there is no obligation on the doctor, in terms of a duty of care, to interview or discuss matters with surviving relatives, although there may be a moral obligation or a feeling of the need to do so. Doctors do, however, have to be careful in respect of their duties of confidentiality, which were discussed earlier in the chapter.

Breach of duty of care

Once a duty of care has been established, the standard of care administered by the doctor concerned must be of a certain standard if it is not to be criticized. That standard in the UK is currently based on the Bolam test (discussed in the previous section) Every aspect of the care given to the patient must satisfy the Bolam test and failure to do so constitutes one of the three criteria of medical negligence. If any aspect of the care given by a doctor falls below the accepted standard, as based on the Bolam test, then it is considered that there will have been a breach of the duty of care owed to the patient in those circumstances.

In the context of immediate care, a failure to assess the scene properly on arrival, a failure to identify and treat the appropriate casualties, an inadequate knowledge of the equipment being used and failure to use it appropriately may all constitute a breach of the duty of care owed to the patient by the doctor concerned. Clearly it is necessary for the doctor to be in full control of the situation and have a full and satisfactory working knowledge of all the equipment under the doctor's control. It is not acceptable for doctors to have equipment with which they are not familiar and to try and use this on a patient at the scene of an accident in the hope that it will improve the situation. It is not an uncommon practice to provide doctors who undertake immediate care work within a group scheme with all kinds of interesting, sophisticated and indeed technologically advanced equipment. Simply having this equipment and using it, without the necessary skill that makes its use appropriate, will not satisfy the duty of care that the doctor owes to a patient. Appropriate training in its use, maintenance of the equipment and the ability to use it safely and correctly are essential pre-requisites for the use of any such equipment on the scene and the doctor may be called on to justify the use of the equipment at a later inquiry, in the event either of the death of a patient or of a complaint by patients or their relatives following the incident.

In considering whether a particular course of treatment, or a doctor's action during treatment, is to an acceptable standard, the Bolam test will be used. As already mentioned, the Bolam test is very physician-oriented and essentially allows for a group of appropriately skilled and qualified medical practitioners to decide whether a doctor's actions were or were not acceptable. The more recent case of *Bolitho* (1997) highlights, however, the fact that having a body of skilled medical opinion that agrees with the doctor's actions will not be sufficient to defend an action in court. The experts defending the doctor's action will need to logically defend their view that, in their opinion, what the doctor did was right and a failure to logically defend their view will result in an insufficient defence should the case come to court. Other than in the issue of consent, therefore, the Bolitho test alters *Bolam* in greater favour of the patient and, if there is an allegation that a breach of duty of care has occurred, the doctor may find it more difficult to defend actions nowadays than prior to the Bolitho case.

In considering the question, therefore, of a breach of the duty of care owed to the patient, the source of the allegation may be any aspect of the care given by the doctor, in respect of actual treatment, in respect of use of equipment and maintenance of the equipment used, particularly as this is so crucial to the successful outcome of care, as well as what may appear to be irrelevant issues such as training, experience and other aspects relating to the high technology equipment being used. An allegation that a duty of care has been breached may also even extend to the question of whether the doctor has acted defensively at the scene of the accident in order to prevent further injury to the patient, perhaps both in terms of how the vehicle was positioned and the equipment used, or indeed in relation to instructions s/he gave to other paramedics on scene relating to extrication, transfer and transport. Doctors undertaking immediate care work frequently underestimate their obligations and the potential for breaching their duty of care towards their patient. In coming years this will be increasingly highlighted by those making complaints and by those alleging medical negligence, particularly where a breach of the duty of care is an essential prerequisite to proving any such negligence. Doctors will be increasingly faced with the need to defend everything they do if inquiries are made later in respect of the care they have given.

Damage

This criterion is often the most difficult to prove and clearly, when it comes to negligence, may be the stumbling block at which the patient finally falls. In order to establish medical negligence it is necessary to show that, on the balance of probability, the breach of the duty of care, as already discussed, resulted in damage. The fact that the outcome following injury or treatment is poor, or indeed even that the patient has died, is not of itself proof of negligence. It has to be established that the damage was causally related to the breach of the duty of care and if this causal relationship between any breach in the duty of care and final outcome is not established then medical negligence will not be proved.

In the context of immediate care, the injuries suffered, and indeed the not infrequent serious permanent disability or death that is an inevitable part of some of the injuries being treated, in most instances have nothing to do with the care given by the doctor on scene. They are inevitable consequences of the injury rather than of the treatment given. In many instances, however, the final outcome is the result of a combination of the injuries received and the treatment given and in these circumstances it may be very difficult to establish the extent to which poor treatment contributed to the final outcome. It is not infrequent for medical negligence claims to come to a grinding halt on the question of the cause of damage.

Clearly if the patient can show that, on the balance of probability, the treatment or lack of it was specifically responsible for the damage that occurred, then a negligence action may well succeed. An example may be where a patient states that he had active controlled movements and sensibility in all his limbs until moved by a doctor or paramedic, following which he lost the use of perhaps his lower limbs. Clearly if there is a spinal injury that has resulted in paraplegia and the patient can convince all concerned that, up to the time he was moved, he did not have a cord injury but that after he had been moved he did, then damage may be accepted to be the result of poor handling or transfer by the doctor or paramedic concerned. In these circumstances, negligence might well be proved. A further example would be where at autopsy an endotracheal tube was found to be present within the oesophagus instead of in the trachea. If it can be shown that, on the balance of probability, a correctly placed endotracheal tube would have resulted in the patient's survival, then clearly a claim for medical negligence may succeed. If, however, death was due to a significant head injury and the correct placement of the tube would have made no difference to the final outcome, then, while the treatment given may have fallen below an acceptable standard and may be considered to be incompetent, negligence may not necessarily be proved. The provision of immediate care is one of those circumstances where causal damage may in fact be very difficult to prove in many instances, there being many other factors that might result in a similar outcome.

The knowledge, however, that patients may, in many circumstances, fail to prove negligence should not lull doctors into a false sense of security when treating patients at the accident scene, where incompetent or poor-quality treatment is always unacceptable, even if it does not ultimately lead to a proven allegation of medical negligence.

In providing immediate care, it is therefore essential that the doctor is properly trained in the use of all equipment, maintains the equipment properly and uses it in the correct way and for the right reasons. Good record keeping of the assessments and treatments administered will all assist in defending any allegation of negligence that is later made but there is no substitute for good training and good practice in defending against complaints and allegations made by patients and their relatives after what is frequently a very trying experience for them.

Dealing with death/disposal of corpses

In the practice of immediate care, death is unfortunately an inevitable consequence in many instances. The doctor may be faced with having to deal with a victim who has died prior to arrival on the scene, or who may die during the course of treatment. Apart from the inevitable difficulties in respect of relatives, friends and others present, doctors have to have a basic working knowledge of the practical procedures involved in dealing with a patient who has died either prior to their arrival on scene or during their management of the incident.

All deaths in such circumstances are unnatural and will therefore automatically come under the jurisdiction of the coroner. It is the coroner's duty to investigate where, why, how and when the death has occurred, should this be from unnatural causes, and inevitably a death at the scene of an accident will be subject to the coroner's investigation and enquiry, leading to an inquest.

The power of the coroner also exceeds that of the police and many other agencies, and a doctor faced with instructions from the coroner has to obey them. At an inquest a doctor may be faced with the need to provide extensive information, including information of a medical nature, and confidentiality in the face of a coroner's inquest goes by the board.

It should also be remembered that the coroner who will be responsible for the enquiry is the coroner in whose area of jurisdiction the death has occurred. This is clearly important in the context of road accidents, where a driver or passenger killed in an accident may not necessarily be from the area in which his or her death has occurred. The local coroner covering the area in which the death has occurred will have jurisdiction over the death and control of any subsequent enquiries. Immediate transfer of the body back to the area of residence of the dead person may not be permitted if this area is outside the coroner's jurisdiction.

An unnatural death in circumstances where an incident involves a doctor in procedures of immediate care is usually notified to the coroner through the police service. It may be necessary, however, for the doctor to undertake to inform the local coroner of the problem and provide information appropriate to the coroner's requirements. Clearly, these vary from one set of circumstances to another.

PRONOUNCEMENT AND CERTIFICATION OF DEATH

In the event of an unnatural death at the scene of an accident or an incident, a death certificate may not be produced by the doctor attending the incident. Certification of death will only be completed and the appropriate death certificate be provided once the coroner's autopsy has been undertaken and the coroner's enquiry completed. The pronouncement of death at the scene, however, where this is appropriate, is a doctor's duty.

Where a patient has died prior to arrival of the doctor at the scene of the accident then clearly it is the doctor's duty to pronounce that patient dead. It is important that, once this is done, the doctor diverts his or her attention to those requiring immediate care, where such care is necessary and can provide some benefit. It is important to resist any temptation to be sucked into arguments or discussions at the scene regarding the death of the victim as this can serve no useful function, particularly if other victims require assistance. Pronouncing a victim dead and then taking no further part in the management of the corpse, can often be extremely difficult in the presence of distressed relatives and friends but, while it may seem heartless at the time, it is in the best interests of the others for the doctor to carry on his or her duties by providing immediate care to those who might still benefit. A simple letter of condolence to the relatives of the dead victim at a later stage will often be sufficient to allay any concerns they may have had that their relative or friend was not dealt with in a manner that they considered appropriate. I have used this technique on a number of occasions and have always been surprised by the gratitude that relatives and others have expressed to me following the receipt of such a letter.

Similar principles apply to patients who die during the management of their injuries on the scene by an immediate care professional. Clearly in these circumstances it is important that the management provided was appropriate, as clearly this would be open to scrutiny at the subsequent coroner's enquiry. The natural and often extreme distress that frequently follows sudden deaths in traumatic circumstances is often reflected in allegations of negligence and complaint against the immediate care doctor, who may have to defend his actions against such allegations at a later time.

In pronouncing death the doctor has a duty to ensure that no mistakes are made and that a patient is not pronounced dead where any signs of life remain. It is surprising how difficult it may be to be certain of death when poor lighting, noise, cold, wet and other problems pertain. It is not unknown in the event of major disasters for victims to be pronounced dead only to find later that they have in fact survived. This is embarrassing for all concerned, is poor practice in the extreme and may result in avoidable problems for the patient should essential treatment have been denied. It is important that resuscitative measures continue until the pronouncement of death can be made with 100% certainty. It may be that this has to wait until arrival at hospital or assessment by another person. There is no shame in continuing to treat and resuscitate a victim whose death has not been confirmed. It is however undoubtedly a disaster if a patient who is still alive is pronounced dead and necessary treatment is discontinued if continuing treatment might have proved life-saving.

It should also be remembered, when pronouncing death, that the doctor may be requested to justify his or her decision that a patient was dead and may be asked to describe precisely how he or she came to that conclusion. A cursory examination in poor conditions may result in criticism of the doctor by relatives, who may incorrectly believe that their loved one could have been saved and that a life was lost as a result of a hurried and perhaps inappropriate decision that the patient was already dead. While pronouncements of death may be easy in the emergency room, where appropriate lighting and all of the facilities are available, it

may in fact be extremely difficult at the scene of an incident, where adverse conditions and frenetic surrounding activity make everything including the establishment of death infinitely harder.

DISPOSAL OF THE BODY

The precise way in which a body is disposed of from the scene of a fatal accident or incident will depend on local protocols and procedures. In the event that death has occurred prior to arrival of the doctor on scene and removal of the body is not necessary in order to save or assist other victims, it is generally accepted that the scene will be disturbed as little as possible to allow for appropriate forensic examination and photography. Clearly, leaving the body where it is found will not be a priority if the safety of others requires its movement. On moving a body for the purposes of assisting others, however, the doctor should try and recall as accurately as possible the position in which the body was originally found, the movements he or she undertook in order to assist others, and indeed the reasons for doing so. The doctor may be called upon later to identify these facts at an enquiry. Such an enquiry may not take place for some weeks or even months. The doctor should, at the end of the incident, make an effort to recount and keep records of what was undertaken and why, so as to assist in subsequent police and forensic enquiries.

As to the precise disposal of the body once the incident is complete, this depends on local procedures and protocols. In some centres the police take on this role and provide the appropriate vehicle to remove the corpse to the local mortuary or Department of Pathology where the autopsy will be undertaken. In some circumstances this may be via the ambulance service using one of their vehicles. Clearly in the event that other victims are being treated, appropriate priority will be given to them in their removal to a hospital prior to disposal of the body. In the event of a major accident a local temporary mortuary may be set up to deal with those who have died and appropriate facilities to confirm death will be necessary in order to ensure that mistakes of the kind already mentioned are not made.

In the event that treatment has been undertaken prior to death, as for example with the insertion of drips, drains, tubes, etc. it is essential that, once death has occurred, these tubes and other devices are left in situ. They will form part of the autopsy examination and the subsequent enquiry. A doctor who removes such devices may be severely criticized at an enquiry and questions may be asked as to whether the doctor's reasons for doing so related in any way to their incompetent insertion in the first instance and whether such incompetence contributed to the victim's death. Clearly it is in the doctor's interest to perform such invasive treatments at the scene confidently and to allow the evidence that this has been done to go with the body for later examination.

Conclusion

While a doctor undertaking immediate care at the scene of an accident or incident is faced with numerous problems, both medical as well as legal, this chapter has concentrated on the issues of consent to treatment and related topics. The issue of consent is a central legal, moral and ethical issue in the provision of immediate care. Clearly, considering these issues for the first time at the scene of an accident is inappropriate and hence it is undoubtedly the duty of a doctor providing immediate care to define his or her thoughts and beliefs in advance of attendance, although each individual case will provide its own challenges, often with the need for an immediate decision to be made and justification of that decision at a later stage. The increasingly public profile of immediate care treatment makes it necessary for doctors to have established reasonable views prior to their attendance at the scene of an incident or accident, if they are to avoid later criticism.

References

Beauchamp TL, Childress JF 1989 Principles of biomedical ethics, 3rd edn. Oxford University Press, Oxford, p 67

Bolam v Friern Hospital Management Committee [1957] 1 BMLR 1; [1957] 2 All ER 118; [1957] 1 WLR 582

Bolitho v City and Hackney Health Authority (1997) British Medical Journal 315(7119)

Canterbury v Spence (1972) 464 F 2d 772, US App DC; cert denied 409 US 1064

Crisp R 1990 Medical negligence, assault, informed consent and autonomy. Journal of Law and Society 17: 77–89

F v West Berkshire Health Authority [1989] 4 BMLR 1, [1989] 2 All ER 545

Fennell P 1990 Inscribing paternalism in the law: consent to treatment and mental disorder. Journal of Law and Society 17: 29–51

Gostin LO 1986 Mental health services – law and practice. Shaw and Sons, London

Gillick v West Norfolk and Wisbech Area Health Authority and another [1985] 2 BMLR 11, [1985] 3 all ER 402, [1986] AC 112, [1985] 3 WLR 830 HL

Jardon OM, Hood LT, Lynch RD 1973 Complete avulsion of the axillary artery as a complication of shoulder dislocation. Journal of Bone Joint Surgery 55: 189–192

Maynard v West Midlands Regional Health Authority [1983] 1 BMLR 122, [1983] HL 5 May

Re C [1993] Independent Law Report 15 Oct (Family Div Thorpe J)

Rogers v Whittaker [1992] 67 ALJR 47 (High Court of Australia)

Sidaway v Bethlem Royal Hospital Governors [1985] 1 BMLR 132; [1985] 1 All ER 643; [1985] AC 871; [1985] 2 WLR 480 HL

Skegg PDG 1990 Law, ethics and medicine. Clarendon Press, Oxford

Record keeping in prehospital care

63

Introduction 653

Record keeping 653

Log books 655

Research and audit 655

Reference 655

Further reading 655

Introduction

Record keeping is arguably the weakest point of prehospital care, being seen by practitioners as a distraction from patient care that is both bureaucratic and boring. The purposes of keeping records include:

- The provision of a contemporaneous record of events and actions. This serves as a template for producing subsequent handover to other practitioners and also facilitates the writing of medico-legal reports at a later stage.
- The collection of a series of patient records in order to produce a portfolio of experience for incorporation into professional log books.
- The provision of raw data that can subsequently be used for research or ongoing audit.

Record keeping

The problems of record keeping in prehospital care should not be underestimated. The patients are usually seen in poor environmental conditions where writing notes may be difficult because of poor visibility and inclement weather. The amount of time available for recording information is likely to be restricted because of time constraints associated with optimal patient care. Originally, notes were in the form of letters of referral to hospitals. These were often lost from the hospital records and even when they were preserved failed to provide a comprehensive record of events.

A particular difficulty of prehospital care is that several organizations are usually involved, all of which are required to complete their own records. The temptation for prehospital care practitioners is perhaps, therefore, to complete the ambulance service record rather than their own, which often renders it impossible for them to recover this information later.

In order to improve record keeping, patient report forms were devised. These usually consist of two-part forms so that a duplicate record can be kept by the practitioner (the 'top copy' remains with the patient). BASICS now offers a standard patient report form (Fig. 63.1).

One of the advantages of these forms is that, in addition to providing space to record data they act as an aide-mémoire regarding the data that should be collected. It is likely that some of the information required for the optimal completion of these forms will be added once the patient has been handed over to the hospital team. Only essential data should be recorded initially, but the temptation to estimate values retrospectively should be avoided.

Currently available forms still do not contain all the information that can be elicited by the 'AMPLE' mnemonic. Where necessary, this should be separately recorded.

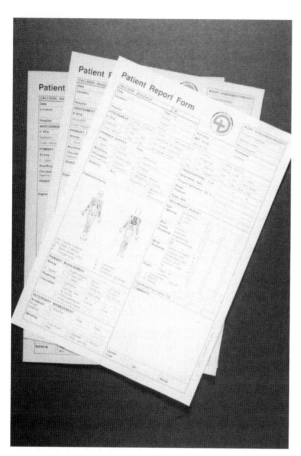

Fig. 63.1 • A BASICS report form.

- **A – Allergies**
- **M – Medications currently taken**
- **P – Past illness**
- **L – Last meal**
- **E – Events and Environment related to the injury.**

Polaroid photographs of the scene of an incident provide useful evidence of potential injuries. The photographs give the doctors in hospital a very clear impression of the mechanism of injury and can record the precise nature of wounds and on-site distortions of limbs. If possible, a second copy of the photographs should be taken for the practitioner's personal record.

Future developments include the increasing use of digital cameras, which allow images from the scene to be transmitted to hospital and the information to be digitally stored with the hospital record. Video recording of incident sites has been used to provide a record of the event that can also be valuable later as teaching material. This video work was originally performed by the fire service, the ambulance services being very concerned that videoing the incident could

be construed as a grave breach of confidentiality. However, with suitable procedural protection it is possible to maintain confidentiality and this valuable resource is being widely introduced. Retention of video records, however, requires the written permission of the patient (or next of kin in the event of the patient's death).

Some doctors have experimented with the use of hand-held tape recorders, which can be used either in the completion of a report form on arrival at hospital or in the preparation of a formal report at a later stage. Washable pads (sometimes attached above the knees of overalls) provide a further method of immediate data recording. The Smart Medimemo is similar.

With the development of the concept of triage in the management of multiple casualty scenarios, report forms have been incorporated into triage cards. A modified version of the BASICS report form is incorporated in the Cambridge cruciform triage card.

Recently trials have taken place in order to assess the use of portable computers in patient information recording. These systems allow a report form to be downloaded on to ambulance service computers or into a hospital accident and emergency computer system.

In a further study involving community nurses, their workload is allocated by computer and clinical interventions and care plans are recorded on portable personal computers. The information is then downloaded into health centre computers. This form of recording has great potential because it can accept digital information from patient monitors, such as the Propac, and also from digital cameras.

It is likely, however, in the current environment that paper-based records will remain standard at least in the near future.

A particular problem in prehospital care is the use and preservation of these records. As the requirement for data has increased the size of the record has increased; many are now of A3 size. The practicalities of completing the forms in a force 8 gale when it is already raining and dark cannot be overstated.

Ambulance service forms often contain more data than medical forms but there are equal problems with their completion and their emphasis is more often on paramedic interventions than on history and examination.

Some forms are for specific purposes and record data specific to the task. Such a form is used by the Scottish air ambulance.

Secondary transport from one hospital to another is often poorly documented or not documented at all. Transfer of information usually relies on a verbal handover. While this, in conjunction with the hospital medical records, may be adequate for short transfers, appropriate written documentation must be completed for longer journeys. Standard 'transfer forms' are available in some regions.

Log books

The keeping of the doctor's log book is now a part of normal professional life. BASICS first experimented with log books some years ago, and now considers the completion of a log book to be an essential component of the accreditation system. More recent developments include computer-based logs which will eventually allow the establishment of a national database.

Research and audit

There is undoubtedly a need in immediate care to establish both a system of audit and a comprehensive evidence base for clinical interventions. Without these, prehospital care will continue to be perceived by many as a second-rate, non-scientific, anecdotally-based specialty.

It is essential, therefore, when completing patient report forms that sufficient information is included to allow the subsequent calculation of simple and complex outcome measures ('trauma scores') that allow the effectiveness of interventions to be measured.

Following the *Trauma report* of the Royal College of Surgeons (1988) there has for the first time in the UK been an attempt to establish a National Trauma Registry. Hospitals have joined the Major Trauma Outcome Study coordinated from the Hope Hospital in Manchester and now known as the UK Trauma Audit Research Network.

These data now record the presence of a BASICS doctor in the prehospital phase.

In the future more consideration must be given to the problems of the prehospital environment when designing methods of capturing data. Far more thought must be given to what data are collected.

It must be remembered that data are needed for a wide range of purposes other than the treatment of the individual patient, they must therefore be correct, clear and concise as well as easy to access. With the increasing incidence of medical litigation, the completion of accurate signed reports is perhaps even more important than ever. Any action that was not recorded will be considered not to have been performed.

If it wasn't written down it wasn't done!

Reference

Royal College of Surgeons 1988 Report of the working party on the management of patients with major injuries. Royal College of Surgeons, London

Further reading

Greaves I, Porter KM 2007 Oxford handbook of prehospital care. Oxford University Press, Oxford

Communications and despatch

64

Introduction	656
Receiving the emergency call	656
Processing the emergency call – computer-aided despatch	657
Despatching the ambulance – contact with ambulance mobiles	658
Locating emergency ambulances – automatic vehicle locating systems	658
Assessing medical priority – medical priority despatch systems	659
Other areas of communication	660
Major incident communications	660
The future	660
References	660

Introduction

The need for rapid and effective communications within the ambulance service, in order to allow the provision of reliable and responsive emergency care, is obvious. The last few years have brought dramatic advances in communication technology and the next generation of Command and Control and digital communications systems is currently coming on line.

The simplest way to review ambulance service communications and despatch is to review the route that an emergency call takes as it passes through the system.

Receiving the emergency call

The first requirement is to have a secure control centre operating to established and proven operating procedures. The emergency control room must have a quiet and organized environment, with staffing levels appropriate to workload and demand (Fig. 64.1). The current targets

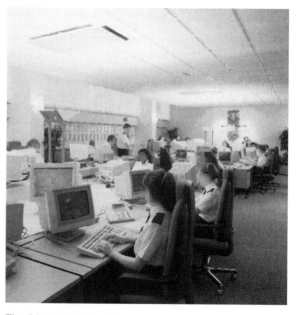

Fig. 64.1 • An ambulance service control room.

for 999 call answering (as set within *Taking Healthcare to the Patient*, Department of Health 2005) are for 95% to be answered within 5 s. Since the restructure of ambulance services in 2006 the chief executive group is now working on national standards for all aspects of communications, from key competencies to a performance management framework.

All incoming emergency and urgent telephone lines must be taped and there must be immediate access to playback tapes for review.

Currently, all emergency calls are directed to a BT emergency centre or service provider (e.g. Cable & Wireless) where they are then redirected to the appropriate emergency service control. This has the useful role of filtering out erroneous and clearly malicious calls but incurs some delay before the call reaches the emergency service concerned. Calls from mobile phones are redirected through the network's own emergency operators and other emergency service controls, such as fire and police, make contact on dedicated land-lines.

In the past the operator would pass the caller's telephone number verbally to the control room; now the call is put through with no handover as number and address are passed to services' computer systems. This information is known as caller line identification (CLI) and is available from all BT landlines and some other operators. All services are moving to an 'electronic handshake' between the telephone system and the command and control system (EISEC).

Once the address is confirmed by the ambulance service a vehicle is allocated, often automatically, and this decision is reviewed as further information is obtained during triage. After confirmation of the telephone number and the location of the incident all callers in the UK are asked 'What's the problem? Tell me exactly what has happened.' This is the first question in the Advanced Medical Priority Dispatch (AMPDS) triage system.

The NHS is developing its own triage system, called NHS Pathways, which will also cover other entry points to the NHS such as out-of-hours care. The system is currently under trial in the North East Ambulance Service (for 999) and Hampshire (for out-of-hours). It is anticipated that AMPDS will be the main system in the UK for some years.

Processing the emergency call – computer-aided despatch

The information from the telephone system (CLI) is passed to the CAD using EISEC, which generates an incident on the command and control system and populates the address and telephone number into the incident. As the call details are confirmed in the incident screen on the CAD, they appear on the despatcher's screen. The CAD has an integral mapping system with a database of address

locations for the county (a gazetteer) all provided with a map reference. As soon as the location is verified, the incident location illuminates on the mapping screen as an icon. Gazetteers can identify locations using post codes, map references, latitude and longtitude, street names or a combination of all of these.

Services use an automatic vehicle location system (AVLS), which, either by terrestrial or satellite triangulation systems, locates the ambulance vehicles. These locations are fed back into the CAD for display on the mapping screen.

Once the call is located, the CAD will offer up to the despatcher the nearest emergency ambulances, the 'as the crow flies' distance from the incident, an amended distance and time accounting for road conditions and the current operational status. Many services are moving to auto-allocation, with this decision being reviewed by the dispatcher as further information comes in.

The recommendation in *Taking Healthcare to the Patient* that response times are recorded from the time that the 999 call hits the switchboard of the service rather than once many details are confirmed has required some technological innovation. This change in performance measurement has cost services approximately 1 min in performance, which has led to demands for improvements in CADs and telephony to streamline reception and allocation of 999 calls.

Apart from its key role in processing calls, the CAD retains all call data in its database. These data form the basis of much of the performance information reported regularly to purchasing health authorities and the Department of Health. In addition, the management information contained within the CAD is vast, including data such as hospital turnaround times, crew workload and individual crews' activation performance.

Currently, ambulance services have performance standards, known as ORCON standards, that were established in 1974 (see Ch. 58). These govern, with the use of time standards, activation and response times on emergency cases with different urban and rural standards. There is a separate standard for urgent cases. These standards have been changed by *Taking Healthcare to the Patient* and are moving towards outcome-based as well as response-time targets.

Clinical information is currently limited on CAD systems but will improve with effective use of medical priority despatch. However, the best information these systems will be able to record in morbidity terms is that given by the caller at the outset of the emergency, and this may bear little resemblance to the final hospital diagnosis. However, support for the clinical audit function in areas such as retrospective audit of cardiac arrest cases is vital, and the response time records are easily extracted from the CAD system.

In services moving towards high performance methods of ambulance operation, analysis of calls by priority, hour of the day and location is an essential requirement in tailoring crews' shift rotas to patient demand. In addition, plotting the geographical location of all calls by hour of day is essential in formulating a system status plan, which hour by hour relocates ambulances into standby points in areas of high demand.

As virtually all the information required to generate a system status plan is held within the CAD, these data must be accessible. Once compiled, the CAD has to be able to assist despatchers in running a plan, which requires preordained ambulance movements to highest priority standby locations every hour.

The CAD is, therefore, a central tool in efficient and effective ambulance service despatching and management.

Despatching the ambulance – contact with ambulance mobiles

Currently all ambulance services operate a very high frequency (VHF) radio telephone system, utilizing the limited number of frequencies allocated to the NHS. These systems vary from simple voice-only systems to more elaborate systems offering data transmission and selective unit calling. A number of services operate short-range ultra high frequency (UHF) radio systems, either based on a VHF/UHF repeater set in the ambulance mobile (allowing use of a remote hand-portable radio) or for on-site use at major incidents based on a mobile control vehicle.

It is likely that all services will move over the next few years to the new Airwave digital system used by the police. This provides an integrated data and voice system to replace the current patchwork of data and voice systems. This system will allow voice calling between units as well as between units and communications centres, improving information flows throughout services. One major advantage of Airwave is the improved quality of data and voice transmission over the analogue systems used for voice radio. Most services currently use digital data transmission and this will also benefit from improved quality of transmission.

Using this link, the CAD can automatically transmit the call details to the vehicle's data unit (Fig. 64.2). This also sends the information to the satellite navigation system and allows this to guide the crew to the location determined by the CAD. AMPDS provides a case summary of the incident for the crew. The CAD system tracks the vehicle and automatically indicates to dispatchers their status, e.g. on scene.

The details of the 999 call can, therefore, be passed by radio, pager or data terminal to the tasked ambulance, or by land-line if the vehicle is on-base. The most rapid mobilization, however, is by data to a crew on standby in the vehicle. Once the vehicle is mobile, the crew confirm their status, either by verbal message or by status codes.

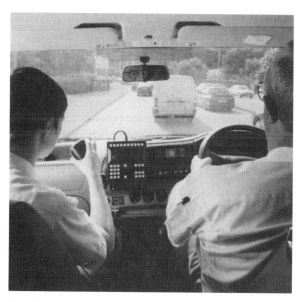

Fig. 64.2 • A vehicle-mounted data terminal.

Ambulance vehicles all have a fixed multichannel VHF radio. Some services use additional VHF hand-portable radios for crews and, although output is noticeably lower than the fixed mobile, they offer major advantages. More elaborate VHF/UHF repeater sets, with a UHF hand-portable, offer the advantage of using the more powerful vehicle VHF mobile to transmit back to control but are more complex and expensive. All resources also use mobile telephones; both radios and mobile phones will be replaced by the introduction of Airwave.

Data transmission from vehicles to hospital units (e.g. 12-lead electrocardiograms) are widely used and the future will see more electronic interaction between resources and other NHS areas using the electronic patient record.

Hospital emergency departments and other units that admit directly, such as medical admissions units, may have fixed VHF radios allowing direct contact with incoming crews. British Association of Immediate Care (BASICS) doctors and some hospital flying squads have ambulance service mobile and hand-portable VHF radios.

This commonality of radio provision permits easy communication between fixed and mobile locations and ambulance control.

Locating emergency ambulances – automatic vehicle locating systems

The AVLS systems provide a visual location of ambulances on mapping screens within the ambulance control centre. They are interfaced with the CAD to allow other data to be combined with the vehicle location (e.g. crew names and qualifications and vehicle status).

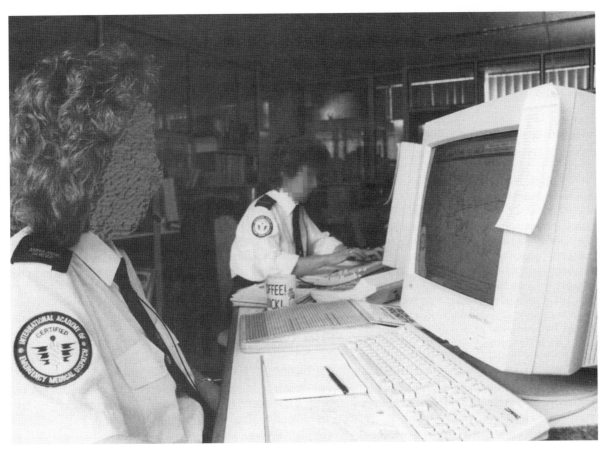

Fig. 64.3 • A call-taker gives advice to an emergency caller using the advanced medical priority dispatch system.

These systems are either terrestrial, using ground-based receivers that calculate, by an elaborate triangulation methodology, the vehicle location, direction and approximate speed, or satellite based, using global positioning system (GPS) technology.

The AVLS data are passed back, via an interface, into the CAD, and the mapping screen is updated with the vehicle position at regular intervals, varying from seconds to minutes depending on the system used.

The AVL system has a variety of other facilities, including the facility for the vehicle to obtain a map reference at its location and the ability to pass data via the AVL network back to control.

These systems have limitations, with periodic erroneous locations and poor performance in certain locations. Their value in locating the fleet automatically, however, far outweighs these occasional problems.

Assessing medical priority – medical priority despatch systems

There are two systems used in the UK that provide effective assessment of the medical priority of incoming telephone calls into life-threatening, serious and non-life-threatening categories. These are the advanced medical priority despatch system (AMPDS; Fig. 64.3) and NHS Pathways. Both are integrated into the call-taker's screen of the CAD. As previously indicated, only one service is currently using Pathways in a 999 setting.

AMPDS has a fully developed audit and quality assurance programme, with the requirement that the user attain certain quality standards before being awarded full certification.

These systems have structured question sets or protocols for a wide range of presenting conditions and can allocate a despatch priority to each call. If inadequate information or no information is available, the system defaults to a life-threatening recommendation. They have been independently evaluated by the Sheffield Centre of Health and Related Research (Nicholl et al 1996) and were found to be effective in safely triaging emergency calls.

Although attention has been focused on the use of these systems for prioritization, their contribution to patient care is fortunately not just limited to this currently popular function. The most important features of these systems are the provision of protocolized prearrival first-aid information to emergency callers and the provision of postdespatch clinical information to responding crews.

Prearrival instructions and 'staying on the line' with callers coping with critically ill or injured patients have a dramatic effect on how callers cope. For example, telephone cardiopulmonary resuscitation (CPR) instructions result in more patients getting essential CPR while the ambulance is en route. In addition, many alarmed and frightened callers are greatly reassured that an operator will stay on the line with them until the vehicle arrives. Furthermore, the crew are far better informed about the emergency to which they are responding. This has an effect on the stress levels of the crew, as well as letting them respond immediately on arrival with appropriate equipment.

The concept of prioritization has come to the fore in recent months, with the debate on inappropriate, and sometimes unnecessary, use of the emergency ambulance service.

Largely urban services have major problems with lack of, or inadequate, primary care community psychiatric and social services infrastructure, particularly outside working hours. The inappropriate use of ambulance resources is a major problem in these areas. In the rest of the UK the problem is relatively less acute.

One known benefit of prioritization is the ability to reduce the number of responses with blue lights and sirens to emergencies known reliably to be trivial, and hence to reduce unnecessary accidents involving ambulance vehicles en route to emergencies.

Calls are prioritized to Red (immediately life-threatening), Amber (not immediately life-threatening but serious) and Green (not immediately life-threatening or serious). Green calls are transferred to further triage using a variety of triage software (Psiam, TAS). Many of these calls can be provided with an alternative care pathway to 999 and/or allow for a further delay in response without light and sirens.

Other areas of communication

Ambulance control centres form a natural centre for NHS communications. Many control centres provide paging, messaging, radio and other communications services for its own officers, GPs, community nurses, midwives and other health service staff. Some control centres also perform bed bureau functions and, of course, all have to function on the front line, coping with the ever-expanding demands, as well as the curiosity of the media. The integration of out of hours, patient transport, NHS Direct and emergency ambulance control is turning the control room into a 'clinical hub' for the wider NHS operating 24/7.

Major incident communications

The ambulance service has a statutory obligation to provide communications on-site for the NHS response to a major incident. This is usually achieved by the provision of a mobile control unit. This unit must provide normal VHF communications, local incident control and radio and cellular telephone communications with other emergency controls and receiving hospitals. It must also provide facilities for support of the incident controllers for a period on-site.

Mobile control units are usually set up to utilize mains power facilities as well as connection to BT land-lines, where these facilities can be provided at the scene. They have facilities for fax transmission and receipt, and key cellular phones are equipped with access override (ACCOLC) to allow them to use reserved channels, accessible only to the emergency services, in the case of a major incident.

It is usual to use the emergency reserve channel (ERC) for all responding ambulance and medical vehicles en route to the incident, as this is the channel common to all UK services, specifically reserved for major incident use.

The future

The future lies in more seamless integration of modes of communication, and the developing digital technologies. Radio and telephone systems will be integrated to the extent that the user merely transfers from one to the other via touch-screen switching.

The development of trunked digital radio systems for combined emergency service use is well advanced, and this will allow the introduction of many new features with more effective and transparent use of radio channels. Direct entry from a vehicle hand-portable radio into the commercial telephone system and the ability to create discrete talk groups are two examples of the increased flexibility of digital systems.

Data transmission is becoming considerably easier. Transmitting patient data or video pictures from the scene of an incident to receiving hospitals will again be far more accessible to emergency services.

The implementation of these systems operationally is imminent. This will provide a revolution in effective communication.

References

Department of Health 2005 Taking healthcare to the patient. Stationery Office, London

Nicholl J, Gilhooley K, Parry G et al 1966 The safety and reliability of priority despatch systems. Medical Care Research Unit, Sheffield Centre for Health and Related Research. University of Sheffield, Sheffield

Steering Group on Ambulance Performance Standards 1996 Review of ambulance performance standards. Final report of the Steering Group. NHS Executive, London

Trauma scoring

65

Introduction 661

Physiological injury severity scores 662

Anatomical injury severity scores 665

Combined physiological and anatomical scores 666

The UK Trauma Audit Research Network 667

Conclusion 667

References 668

Introduction

WHY IS TRAUMA SCORING NECESSARY?

Simple systems have been used for some time, particularly in the USA, to aid prehospital triage. The aim of these systems is to identify severely injured patients and direct them to a hospital with enhanced trauma care facilities. The earliest of these to gain widespread acceptance by emergency workers was the trauma score (Champion et al 1981).

The care received by casualties once they come into contact with the emergency services should be of the highest standard. Retrospectively, trauma scoring systems (which indirectly assess injury severity) play a central role in the audit of this care, one aim being to identify the unexpected deaths and to promote further analysis of the trauma system.

Financial accountability is an inescapable part of modern medical practice, and it is no longer acceptable to divert large amounts of money into a highly expensive and labour-intensive field without evidence that the increased expenditure is resulting in improved patient outcome.

There is also a role for trauma scoring systems in major incident triage (Advanced Life Support Group 2002). This is discussed in Chapters 47 and 48.

HOW IS TRAUMA SCORED?

Trauma scoring systems are *physiological* or *anatomical*. Physiological systems are based on simple observations such as the patient's vital signs. They allow for ongoing or *dynamic* assessment.

Physiological data permit dynamic assessment.

An anatomical analysis of the injuries can only accurately be made once the patient has received definitive care or undergone a post-mortem examination. Anatomical characterization of injury severity is therefore *static*. Attempts have been made to combine static and dynamic indicators to provide a more accurate 'real-time' assessment of injury severity and these will be discussed.

WHAT MAKES A GOOD TRAUMA SCORE?

There are five criteria that have been suggested as the goals of any trauma scoring system (Gibson 1981):

- *Correlation with discrete outcome* – this includes death, survival and the requirement for surgery. The unpredictable course of long-term morbidity has so far prevented any scoring system from correlating well with subsequent disability.

- *Face validity* – a trauma score is only worth using if those applying it believe in it.
- *Criterion validity and mathematical consistency* – in simple terms, people with the same score should have the same severity of injury and, all else being equal, the same probability of survival. Someone with a 'worse' score must be more severely injured and have a lower probability of surviving.
- *Practicality* – the score should be precise even when applied under adverse circumstances, e.g. mass casualty situations. It must therefore be simple (with parameters which are easy to measure) and rapid if it is going to be an effective prehospital tool.
- *Reliability* – different observers should obtain the same score when rating the same patient. It should not be dependent on the level of skill or training of the observer but only on their familiarity with the scoring system.

Physiological severity scores can therefore be used as tools to aid the management of individual patients, but should require only the recording of simple observations and the minimum of data processing. Anatomical severity scores, on the other hand, are a much more detailed assessment of the victim's injuries which, in general, can only be determined retrospectively following hospital admission.

Physiological injury severity scores

THE GLASGOW COMA SCALE

The most durable of all the physiological scoring systems is the Glasgow coma scale (Table 65.1), which was first described by Teasdale & Jennett (1974). This score allows a patient's neurological function to be represented by a single number. The scale was initially developed for the assessment and monitoring of head-injured patients. However, the Glasgow coma scale has subsequently become the accepted means of classifying depression of conscious level from any cause.

The Glasgow coma scale has three components. Patients are assessed according to their best motor, verbal and eye-opening response to stimulation.

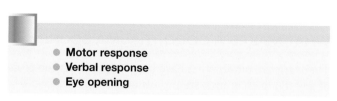

- Motor response
- Verbal response
- Eye opening

If there is a difference in motor response between the limbs the highest score is recorded. Some criticism has

Table 65.1 The Glasgow coma scale

a – Eye opening

Spontaneous	4
To voice	3
To pain	2
None	1

b – Verbal response

Oriented	5
Confused	4
Inappropriate words	3
Incomprehensible sounds	2
None	1

c – Motor response

Obeys commands	6
Localizes to painful stimulus	5
Withdraws	4
Flexion	3
Extension	2
None	1
Total (a + b + c) =	**15**

been lodged against the Glasgow coma scale because of interobserver variability, in particular when inexperienced personnel perform the assessment (Rowley & Fielding 1991). However, this should be placed in perspective as so wide is the acceptance of this score that it has been incorporated into other dynamic scoring systems, such as the Trauma Score, the Revised Trauma Score and the Triage Revised Trauma Score.

THE TRAUMA SCORE

The Trauma Score (Table 65.2) was developed as a dynamic indicator of injury severity by Champion et al (1981) and combines the Glasgow coma scale with coded values for respiratory rate, respiratory effort, systolic blood pressure and capillary refill. It is therefore the patient's *physiological response* to the injuries which is assessed. With increasing physiological disturbance the Trauma Score will fall, with a corresponding decrease in the probability of survival (Table 65.3). A Trauma Score of 13 is associated with a mortality of around 10% (Champion et al 1981). In recognition of this fact, a Trauma Score of 13 or less has been used by paramedics in some areas of the USA as an indication to bypass a local hospital in favour of a regional 'trauma centre'.

Table 65.2 The Trauma Score

	Rate	Coded value
A: Respiratory rate		
	10–24	4
	25–35	3
	≥36	2
	1–9	1
	0	0
B: Respiratory effort		
	Normal	1
	Retractive	0
	None	0
C: Systolic blood pressure		
	≥90	4
	70–89	3
	50–69	2
	0–49	1
	0	0
D: Capillary refill		
	≤2 s	2
	2 s	1
	None	0
E: Glasgow coma scale		
	14–15	5
	11–13	4
	8–10	3
	5–7	2
	3–5	1
Trauma Score =	A + B + C + D + E =	16

Table 65.3 Trauma Score and probability of survival

Trauma score	Probability of survival (%)
16	99
15	98
14	96
13	94
12	89
11	82
10	72
9	59
8	45
7	31
6	21
5	13
4	7.5
3	4.3
2	2.5
1	1.4

Although the Trauma Score has been found to correlate well with subsequent patient outcome (Sacco et al 1984) and have high interassessor reliability in the prehospital setting (Moreau et al 1985), the assessment of respiratory expansion and capillary refill has proved difficult, particularly when the light is poor. The Trauma Score was criticized for underscoring patients with an isolated severe head injury. This is because of the intervals that were chosen and the relative importance of the coded value of the Glasgow coma scale over other physiological parameters (see below).

In answer to these criticisms, the Trauma Score was revised in 1989.

THE REVISED TRAUMA SCORE

The revision of the Trauma Score was published by Champion et al (1989) (Table 65.4). The objectives of the revision were the following:

- the exclusion of capillary refill and respiratory expansion, making it a more effective prehospital tool
- the introduction of Glasgow coma scale ranges that correlate with and by convention define *mild*, *moderate* and *severe* head injury; the problem of underscoring head injuries should therefore be addressed
- the adoption of systolic blood pressure and respiratory rate values with similar survival probabilities to the new Glasgow coma scale intervals.

The Revised Trauma Score was validated using two large North American databases: the Washington Hospital Center database and the Major Trauma Outcome Study (MTOS). The combined dataset comprised more than 28 000 patients.

The Revised Trauma Score (RTS) has two configurations. When used as a tool to measure outcome, a requirement for precision necessitates the application of weighting coefficients to coded values of the Glasgow coma scale, systolic blood pressure and respiratory rate. These coded values

Table 65.4 The Revised Trauma Score

Glasgow coma scale (GCSc)	Systolic blood pressure (SBPc)	Respiratory rate (RRc)	Coded value for each
13–15	>89	10–29	4
9–12	76–89	>29	3
6–8	50–75	6–9	2
4–5	1–49	1–5	1
3	0	0	0

Revised Trauma Score = 0.9368GCSc + 0.7326SBPc + 0.2908RRc

Table 65.5 CRAMS (Circulation, Respiration, Abdomen, Motor and Speech) Score

Component	Score
A: Circulation	
Normal capillary refill and systolic blood pressure >100 mmHg	2
Delayed capillary refill and systolic blood pressure >85 <100 mmHg	1
No capillary refill	0
B: Respiration	
Normal	2
Abnormal	1
Absent	0
C: Abdomen	
Abdomen and thorax not tender	2
Abdomen and thorax tender	1
Abdomen rigid or flail chest, penetrating wound to the abdomen or thorax	0
D: Motor	
Normal	2
Responds only to pain	1
No response or decerebrate	0
E: Speech	
Normal	2
Confused	1
No intelligible words	0
Total CRAMS Score = A + B + C + D + E =	10
Score ≤ 8 Major Trauma	
Score ≥ 9 Minor Trauma	

range from 0 to 4 and when multiplied by their coefficients the sum of these calculated values has a range of 0–7.84, with a strong correlation with outcome. This sort of calculation is obviously inappropriate in the prehospital setting and the coded values are simply added together to give a maximum of 12. This is the Triage-Revised Trauma Score (T-RTS), and its role as a triage tool, in isolation and as part of the American College of Surgeons Committee on Trauma (1993) prehospital triage scheme, is discussed in Chapter 48.

The Triage Revised Coma Score (T-RTS) is the sum of the uncoded values of the Revised Coma Score (RCS).

CRAMS

Other physiological trauma scores have not gained the same international acceptance as the Trauma Score, Revised Trauma Score and Triage Revised Trauma Score. An example is the CRAMS (Circulation, Respiration, Abdomen, Motor and Speech) Score (Gormican 1982), which combines some features of the Trauma Score with a subjective assessment of abdominal and thoracic injury (difficult to evaluate accurately in the field). Each of the five components is scored from 0 to 2 to give a maximum of 10. Major trauma is regarded as a score of 8 or less, and in the USA this has been used as an indication for local hospital bypass to a trauma centre (Table 65.5).

CRAMS was originally studied prospectively using 500 patients transported by paramedics based at La Jolla, California, USA. The results were encouraging with a sensitivity of 92% for identifying major injury but as this represented only 11 out of 12 patients a much larger study would be indicated for validation. Ornato et al (1985) reported that CRAMS failed to identify as major trauma two out of three patients transferred directly to the operating theatre from the emergency department. This was based on a large, but retrospective, computer analysis of ambulance 'run sheets'. A possible explanation is that the paramedics recording the clinical information were not familiar with CRAMS and the prehospital assessment required. Any attempt to extract a subjective assessment from their records would therefore be flawed.

THE PAEDIATRIC TRAUMA SCORE

The Paediatric Trauma Score (PTS) is a combination of simple observations and a crude, subjective evaluation of tissue and bone disruption (Tepas et al 1987).

Table 65.6 Paediatric Trauma Score

Component	Score +2	Score +1	Score −1
Weight (kg)	>20	10–20	<10
Airway	Normal	Oral Nasopharyngeal	Intubated or surgical airway
Blood pressure (mmHg)	>90	50–90	<50
Level of consciousness	Alert	Obtunded or history of loss of consciousness	Coma
Open wound	None	Minor	Major or penetrating
Fractures	None	Minor	Open or multiple

Total = −6 to +12

A maximum score of +12 and a minimum score of −6 is obtained by the addition of the six coded values (Table 65.6). There is an inverse relationship with mortality. A score of +8 or less correlates with a mortality somewhere between 13% and 24% (Tepas et al 1987, Ramenofsky et al 1988).

Kaufmann et al (1990) evaluated the Paediatric Trauma Score compared with the Revised Trauma Score. They demonstrated an over-triage rate of 42.6% when using the Paediatric Trauma Score and 19.5% with the Revised Trauma Score – which might result in inappropriate triage to a hospital with enhanced trauma care facilities or unnecessary activation of the *trauma team*. However, in the same study the RTS was found to have an undertriage rate of 23.9% against 14.7% for the Paediatric Trauma Score, which was thought by the American College of Surgeons Committee on Trauma (ACSCOT) to be an unacceptable difference.

The Paediatric Trauma Score is therefore recommended as the paediatric prehospital triage tool by ACSCOT (American College of Surgeons Committee on Trauma 1997) using a score of +8 as the 'cut-off' for local hospital bypass to a trauma centre where such facilities exist.

Anatomical injury severity scores

THE ABBREVIATED INJURY SCALE

The definitive characterization of a patient's injuries is static. It is not something that can be done with any precision or reliability at the roadside as the data required can only be obtained after detailed investigation, operation or a post-mortem examination. Once the injuries have been evaluated they must be coded before being incorporated into a severity scoring system. The information generated is an essential component of the audit of a trauma system.

One of the earliest and most widely used anatomical scoring systems is the Abbreviated Injury Scale (AIS). It was originally developed for the specific assessment of injuries resulting from road traffic accidents by the American Medical Association's Committee on the Medical Aspects of Automotive Safety (1971).

Injuries are assigned to six anatomical regions:

- head and neck
- face
- chest
- abdomen and pelvic contents
- extremities and pelvic girdle
- external (i.e. skin).

The AIS scores injuries from 1 to 6 with increasing severity, a score of 6 denoting an injury that is almost invariably fatal. The latest revision of the AIS dictionary (AIS 90) has more than 1200 separate injury descriptions compared with 75 in the first edition. Attempting to apply Gibson's (1981) criteria for an effective Trauma Score, the AIS does not exhibit true mathematical consistency as it is not linear. In other words, a person who has an injury with an AIS code of 2 is not twice as badly injured as someone with an injury coded 1 (Petrucelli et al 1981).

Although AIS is able to characterize individual injuries it does not take into account the effect of multiple injuries on patient outcome. This led to the development of the Injury Severity Score by Baker et al (1974).

THE INJURY SEVERITY SCORE

The Injury Severity Score (ISS) uses the information contained in the Abbreviated Injury Scale but provides an assessment of outcome for patients with one or more injuries.

To obtain the ISS score for a particular patient the AIS is recorded for the most severe injury in the three most severely injured AIS body regions. These scores are squared and then added together. The maximum ISS for any one region, with any chance of survival, is therefore 25. The maximum overall ISS obtainable is 75. An AIS code of 6 in any region is automatically given an ISS of 75 and implies a fatal outcome. It is now accepted in the assessment of trauma outcome to regard an ISS of 16 or more as *major trauma*.

Although the ISS is the most widely accepted anatomical trauma score it is not without its critics. It does not take into account multiple injuries in the same body region (Champion 1989), and patients with the same ISS may not have the same probability of survival (Copes et al 1988). Zoltie & de Dombal (1993) noted an alarming degree of variation when 16 patients were scored by 15 observers. The probability of two observers agreeing on the ISS of an individual patient was found to be only 28%.

Combined physiological and anatomical scores

The Trauma Score, Revised Trauma Score and Injury Severity Score have all been shown to correlate well with patient outcome. A Trauma Score of 12, a Revised Trauma Score of 6 and an Injury Severity Score of 16 reliably predict a mortality of around 10%. Combining a physiological and an anatomical Injury Severity Score results in greater predictive power. This power is utilized in the audit of trauma systems by identifying unexpected outcomes.

By far the best known and validated methodology is TRISS (Trauma Injury Severity Score), which originally combined the Trauma Score, Injury Severity Score and the patient's age. The Revised Trauma Score has now replaced the Trauma Score because of its greater predictive accuracy (Boyd et al 1987).

A line can be drawn on a graph of ISS against RTS for a probability of survival of 50% (Ps_{50}). Survivors (L) who lie above and non-survivors (D) who lie below the Ps_{50} isobar are unexpected outcomes and should be investigated in a trauma audit.

The probability of survival (Ps) is calculated for each patient:

$$Ps = \frac{1}{1 + e^{-b}}$$

where e is the natural logarithm and

$$b = b_0 + b_1(RTS) + b_2(ISS) + b_3(A).$$

The coefficients used to calculate b (that is, b_0–b_3) were originally derived from a regression analysis of over 30 000 patients in the North American MTOS database and are different for blunt and penetrating trauma. A is 0 if the patient is less than 54 years old and 1 if s/he is 55 years or older.

Champion and his coworkers felt that if some of the ISS failings were addressed then a combined trauma score with even greater predictive value could be created. ASCOT (A Severity Characterization of Trauma – note the similarity in the acronym for the American College of Surgeons Committee on Trauma (ACSCOT); the two are often confused) was published in 1990 (Champion et al 1990).

ASCOT combines weighted values of the RTS codes for the Glasgow coma scale (G), respiratory rate (R) and systolic blood pressure (S), with a new *anatomic profile* (Table 65.7). The anatomic profile uses the Abbreviated Injury Scale codes for individual injuries but groups body

Table 65.7 The anatomic profile

Component	Injury	AIS (severity)	ISS body regions
A:	Head/brain	3–5	1
	Spinal cord	3–5	1, 3, 4
B:	Thoracic	3–5	3
	Front of neck	3–5	1
C:	Abdomen/pelvis	3–5	4
	Spine without cord change	3	1, 3, 4
	Pelvic fracture	4–5	5
	Femoral artery	4–5	5
	Crushing above knee	4–5	5
	Amputation above knee	4–5	5
	Popliteal artery	4	5
	Facial injury	1–4	2
D:	All other injuries	1–2	1–6

regions in a way that it is possible to make calculations based on more than one injury in a region.

The probability of survival (Ps) is calculated by the equation:

$$Ps = \frac{1}{1 + e^{-k}}$$

where

$$k = k_1 + k_2G + k_3R + k_4S + k_5A + k_6B + k_7C + k_8age \text{ (coded value)}.$$

The coefficients k_1–k_8 again depend on whether the mechanism of injury is blunt or penetrating trauma. A, B and C are the anatomic profile components illustrated in Table 65.7. If there is more than one injury in a region, A, B and C are calculated by taking the square root of the sum of the squares of the AIS codes for each injury in that region.

The coded values for age range from 0 to 4 and have the intervals shown in Table 65.8.

Comparing TRISS and ASCOT revealed only a modest improvement in the outcome analysis of blunt trauma using the newer score. ASCOT, however, performed substantially better than TRISS when the mechanism of injury was penetrating trauma (Champion et al 1990). More

Table 65.8 Coded values for age	
0	0–54 years
1	55–64 years
2	65–74 years
3	75–84 years
4	85 years or older

recently Champion et al (1996) published the results of a prospective study that again compared ASCOT and TRISS. Although the results were unspectacular, there would now appear to be evidence in favour of ASCOT.

The UK Trauma Audit Research Network

The UK Trauma Audit Research Network (UK TARN), formerly MTOS (Major Trauma outcome Study), is a study of injury severity and outcome that was started in the USA in 1982 by the American College of Surgeons Committee on Trauma. Within the USA it now includes more than 140 hospitals and has evolved into an enormous database. The methodology used to predict outcome has been TRISS.

As a result of the report of the Royal College of Surgeons of England (1988) on the management of major trauma, the UK TARN database was set up by the North Western Injury Research Unit (NWIRC) in Salford. The number of hospitals participating in the UK TARN has increased steadily such that more than half of all hospitals receiving major trauma are now enrolled. The admission criteria for a patient are the following:

- hospital admission for more than 3 days after injury, or
- death as a result of injury, or
- interhospital transfer for specialist care of injuries, or
- intensive care unit admission.

Patients who are more than 65 years old with an isolated fracture of a pubic ramus or femoral neck have now been excluded from the study.

The admitting hospital completes a datasheet, which provides enough information to calculate the Revised Trauma Score at the time of admission and the Injury Severity Score after definitive care or a post-mortem. Other factors, such as pre-existing morbidity, operations, complications and the seniority of the clinicians who were involved in the patient's care, are also recorded. An attempt is made to assess morbidity (in particular, locomotor and neurological) 3 months after injury.

The datasheets are analysed at the NWIRC by TRISS methodology using coefficients derived from the UK TARN

database. Reports are returned to the participating hospitals every 3 months. In addition to giving the probability of survival for every patient, information is supplied for local audit (e.g. audit of prehospital time, or excessive delay before a severely injured patient is seen by a senior doctor). The number of deaths more or less than the expected norm for a group of 100 patients treated in the UK (the 'standardized W statistic') allows a trauma system to compare its performance anonymously against its peers. The 'Z' statistic provides a measure of its statistical significance. The 'M' statistic compares the injury severity of the study population with the TARN group of patients to see whether the 'Z' statistic is applicable (it must be <0.88).

The first results of the UK TARN were published in 1992 (Yates et al 1992). The mortality of patients who had suffered severe blunt trauma was found to be significantly higher than a comparable North American dataset and inexplicable differences in mortality between hospitals were apparent. In many hospitals, severely injured patients were managed by very junior doctors. As a result of this study, the approach to the initial management of severely injured patients in many UK hospitals has changed.

Conclusion

Trauma scoring has a number of different applications depending on the scoring system in operation. Physiological scores have been shown to have a role in prehospital triage and in combination with an anatomical score more reliably predict outcome when used in trauma audit. It is easy to appreciate the relevance of physiological trauma scores to the prehospital worker when used as a triage tool. However, trauma audit must look at all aspects of a patient's care from the instant the patient comes into contact with the emergency services.

Physiological scores have been shown to have a role in prehospital triage.

Although the ability of injury severity systems to predict outcome is improving, it must be emphasized that decisions concerning an individual patient's management cannot be made based on the prognosis estimated by a trauma score.

The evaluation of injury severity is difficult enough. The evaluation of trauma scores is even more frustrating, often involving the retrospective analysis of data recorded incompletely and in adverse circumstances. The reliance on bewildering statistical methods makes critical analysis of study design by the interested 'amateur' almost impossible.

References

Advanced Life Support Group 2002 Major incident medical management and support: the practical approach, 2nd edn. BMJ Publishing, London

American College of Surgeons Committee on Trauma 1993 Resources for optimal care of the injured patient. American College of Surgeons, Chicago, IL, p 20

American College of Surgeons Committee on Trauma 1997 Advanced trauma life support student manual, 6th edn. American College of Surgeons, Chicago, IL

American Medical Association's Committee on the Medical Aspects of Automotive Safety 1971 Rating the severity of tissue damage: the abbreviated scale. Journal of the American Medical Association 215: 277

Baker SP, O'Neill B, Haddon W Jr, Long WB 1974 The Injury Severity Score: a method for describing patients with multiple injuries and evaluating their care. Journal of Trauma 14: 187–196

Boyd CR, Tolson MS, Copes WS 1987 Evaluating trauma care: the TRISS method. Journal of Trauma 27: 370–378

Champion HR 1989 Assessing the severity of trauma. In: Westeby S (ed) Trauma, pathogenesis and treatment. Heinemann, Oxford

Champion HR, Sacco WJ, Carnazzo AJ et al 1981 The Trauma Score. Critical Care Medicine 9: 672

Champion HR, Sacco WJ, Copes WS et al 1989 A revision of the Trauma Score. Journal of Trauma 29: 623–628

Champion HR, Copes WS, Sacco WJ et al 1990 A new characterisation of injury severity. Journal of Trauma 30: 539–546

Champion HR, Copes WS, Sacco WJ et al 1996 Improved predictions of severity characterisation of trauma (ASCOT) over Trauma and Injury Severity Score (TRISS): results of an independent evaluation. Journal of Trauma 40: 42–48

Copes WS, Champion HR, Sacco WJ, Frey CF 1988 The Injury Severity Score revisited. Journal of Trauma 28: 1

Gibson G 1981 Indices of severity for emergency medical evaluative studies: reliability, validity, and data requirements. International Journal of Health Services 11: 597–622

Gormican SP 1982 CRAMS scale: field triage of trauma victims. Annals of Emergency Medicine 11: 132–135

Kaufmann CR, Maier RV, Rivara P, Carrico CJ 1990 Evaluation of the Paediatric Trauma Score. Journal of the American Medical Association 263: 69–72

Moreau M, Gainer PS, Champion HR, Sacco WJ 1985 Application of the Trauma Score in the pre-hospital setting. Annals of Emergency Medicine 14: 1049–1054

Ornato J, Mlinek EJ, Craren EJ, Nelson N 1985 Ineffectiveness of the Trauma Score and the CRAMS Scale for accurately triaging patients to trauma centers. Annals of Emergency Medicine 14: 1061–1063

Petrucelli E, States JD, Hames LN 1981 The Abbreviated Injury Scale: evolution, usage, and future adaptability. Accidents, Analysis and Prevention 13: 29–35

Ramenofsky ML, Ramenofsky MB, Jurkovich GJ et al 1988 The predictive validity of the Paediatric Trauma Score. Journal of Trauma 28: 1038–1042

Rowley G, Fielding K 1991 Reliability and accuracy of the Glasgow coma scale with experienced and inexperienced users. Lancet 337: 535–538

Royal College of Surgeons of England 1988 Commission on the provision of surgical services. Report of the working party on the management of patients with major injuries. Royal College of Surgeons, London

Sacco WJ, Champion HR, Stega M 1984 Trauma care evaluation. University Park Press, Baltimore, MD

Teasdale G, Jennett B 1974 Assessment of coma and impaired consciousness: a practical scale. Lancet 2: 81–84

Tepas JJ, Mollitt DL, Bryant M 1987 The Paediatric Trauma Score as a predictor of injury severity in the injured child. Journal of Paediatric Surgery 22: 14–18

Yates DW, Woodford M, Hollis S 1992 Preliminary analysis of the care of injured patients in 33 British hospitals: first report of the United Kingdom major trauma outcome study. British Medical Journal 305: 737–740

Zoltie N, de Dombal FT 1993 The hit and miss of ISS and TRISS. British Medical Journal 307: 906–907

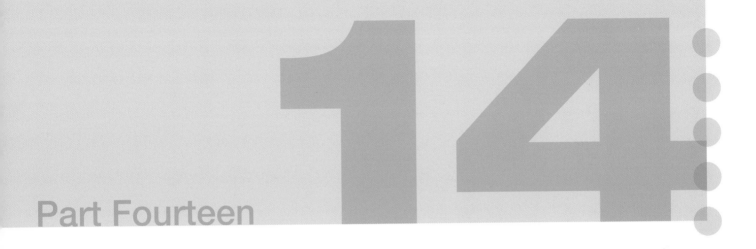

Part Fourteen

66 Training and education 671

67 Immediate care equipment 678

Training and education

66

Introduction   671

Adult learning   672

Adults as learners   672

Adult courses   672

Developing a course   673

Prehospital training and education   673

The Faculty of Immediate Care   676

The future   677

Introduction

When prehospital care was developing during the 1960s and 1970s, those involved in providing treatment to the sick and injured brought to this field of medicine their own experience from general or hospital practice or gained from a services background.

It was during the late 1970s and early 1980s that the need for particular training in this area of medicine was recognized. However, this training developed in a very haphazard way, mainly on a local basis, serving the needs of individual immediate care schemes.

The most significant advance came with the introduction of the Diploma in Immediate Medical Care by the Royal College of Surgeons of Edinburgh in September 1988 and the subsequent development of BASICS Education. A fuller explanation of the historical developments of the various educational and training activities will follow, but it is perhaps appropriate at this point to consider the meaning and implication of training and education.

It is very easy to use the terms 'training' or 'education' as though they are interchangeable but there is a considerable difference between them. Training is the acquisition of skills, whereas education also involves the promotion of understanding (knowledge) and awareness (attitudes).

Doctors involved in immediate care will have experienced the school system, a university or medical school and finally postgraduate education. From the prehospital point of view there are, however, two areas to be considered in this education process. First, when and how should the public be exposed to the concepts of prehospital (first-aid) care? Thus, one might advocate the teaching of first aid or acute life-saving skills in our schools so that everyone in the UK would be able to initiate the necessary care if they were first on scene following any accident or medical emergency: the first link in any prehospital chain of survival.

Second, it must be determined at what point in the medical education structure doctors should be exposed to training in methods of resuscitation. It is the responsibility of individual deans of medical schools who have to produce a medical course, while recognizing the many pressures placed upon them, to create an effective curriculum for their particular medical school. This might be considered the second link in the prehospital chain of survival. There is no doubt that there is great enthusiasm among students for education that they perceive to be directly relevant to daily clinical practice. This is, unfortunately, often not reflected by its prominence in the curriculum. A similar appetite for learning resuscitation skills has been shown by the many extracurricular school and community programmes that are run throughout the country.

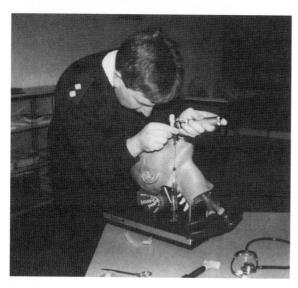

Fig. 66.1 • Practical skills teaching on a prehospital emergency care course.

In the University of Birmingham Medical School, a modified resuscitation course is offered to pre-final year medical students comprising a series of evening lectures and practical demonstrations followed by an assessment practical. On average 85% of the students in the year attend all the lectures on a voluntary basis and go on to take the course assessment. One would hope that, based on this experience, medical schools might introduce basic life support training (BLS) during the preclinical years and then advanced life support training (ALS) during the clinical period of training so that by the beginning of the pre-registration year newly qualified doctors would be able to build on this learning when exposed to the rough and tumble of the early years spent on the wards.

At present it must be recognized that for many doctors the first formal training in ALS occurs as a postgraduate, very often during a formal course. It is a recurring theme in the evaluation returns from the participants on many types of resuscitation course that the type of training provided on such courses could have been more usefully provided at an earlier point in the formal medical training and that the participants have found this type of course a most useful way to learn.

Some of the concepts of adult education need to be studied if an educational experience which will be both stimulating and practically useful is to be created.

Adult learning

The learning capacity of the brain, allowing for absence of disease or injury, continues into adulthood. Learning involves a change in an individual's knowledge, skills or attitudes that persists over time. There are three parts to this process.

- learning (acquisition)
- memory (storing)
- recall (retrieval).

Learning may be consciously undertaken through educational training or it may occur subconsciously from day-to-day experience.

However, memory and recall can be either reliable or unreliable. We may remember things that we see, hear, feel or otherwise sense but these memories may be coloured to a greater or lesser extent by our physical or emotional perceptions at that time. Similarly, our recall may be coloured or influenced by outside factors.

The other influence that plays an important part in the learning process is the basic interest of the participant in the subject under discussion. Learning is therefore more likely to occur when the information, material or attitudes taught are relevant to the participant, may be linked to what that participant already knows or may help that individual to expand their existing knowledge.

The skill of lecturing is to give participants the necessary time and help to recognize the interrelationship between the new concepts and knowledge presented during a course and what participants already know. However, there may be occasions when these two bodies of knowledge conflict. Participants' ability to learn may be blocked by their own anxieties about learning and concerns about their potential or imagined failure on the course. Fear of failure seems to be particularly associated with practical components of courses.

The participants should discover that learning is useful and rewarding and that they receive praise and just reward for their effort. This will in itself encourage and improve the participant's total learning.

Adults as learners

Adults bring established attitudes, patterns of thought and fixed ways of doing things to their new learning experience. Some of these pre-existing characteristics will help in the new situations and with the new ideas presented but they may also be a hindrance to the extension and alteration of the techniques, values and attitudes under discussion.

It must also be recognized that adults attending these particularly intensive courses may have many other commitments and as a consequence may not be able to devote additional time to their studies beyond the confines of the course, however interested or motivated they may be.

Adult courses

Adult participants on courses expect lecturers and demonstrators to know their subjects but they do not expect their teachers to be able to answer every single question that may be asked. Teachers should have a firm grasp and understanding of the subject of their lecture or demonstration and know where to find the answer to a question or to whom they should turn if the answer is not known. However, if the question does not have an obvious answer, the lecturer or demonstrator must be alert not to ignore or dismiss the question in case it may represent new thought on the subject under discussion.

Adults also expect their teachers to be enthusiastic about the subject and practically competent in skill teaching. In short, adults expect their teachers to be able to practise what they preach. During all forms of adult teaching, adults expect to be recognized and treated as adults and therefore they should not be harshly criticized, humiliated or patronized.

Adults come to a teaching session for many reasons. During any course adult participants may find that their motivation varies considerably. This variation may be brought about by problems related to the course, either because there is a lack of overall purpose to the course or unrealistic goals have been set, or because an unfriendly atmosphere has been created either in the course as a whole or in a particular demonstration or lecture.

In adult teaching it is evident that a lecturer's or demonstrator's personal style, commitment and enthusiasm are all major motivating factors in helping and encouraging adults to continue their learning. Adults will respond to teachers who show genuine interest in the candidates' or participants' achievements. Above all, adults will respond to a teacher who interacts with them on equal terms.

Lecturers and demonstrators must remember that in adult teaching any task or subject that is given to the participants must be seen to be relevant and meaningful to them as well as being presented in a useful and interesting way. Lecturers and demonstrators must also remember the vast and differing experience and knowledge that adult participants bring to the course, while recognizing that they often lack confidence in their own learning abilities.

Developing a course

Learning may be defined in many ways. Simplistically, it may be defined as a change of behaviour that is brought about by a planned experience. However, this only acknowledges the overt or planned curriculum (the actual content of the course) and in no way takes into account a fundamental additional factor particularly of residential courses, the hidden or unplanned curriculum (the interchange of ideas that occurs outside the formal course timetable). The changes that we are attempting to effect are in the areas of knowledge, skills or attitudes. The course must therefore create an atmosphere and give the participants an experience that will bring about the change in behaviour that is required by the course.

When considering course design the organizer should remember that a good course will be relevant to the needs of the participants. It will contain clear statements of purpose and have appropriate content that will be presented at the right level and pace for the participants in order to allow them the opportunity to try out new concepts and to gain feedback on their performance.

To achieve these goals it is essential that the course is well organized, provides appropriate refreshments and is conducted in a clean and comfortable environment. A good course or session, therefore, is one that helps the participants to engage in relevant learning in a variety of interesting ways and provides help from a responsive and supportive tutor.

In summary, learning depends on:

- motivation
- a capacity to learn.

The education experience must be meaningful, and learning depends on active involvement. The learning must be experience-centred. Feedback is essential to effective learning.

Prehospital training and education

Using the above background and brief educational synopsis let us look at the development of resuscitation training and particularly prehospital education. Many of the developments are so interrelated that it is difficult to separate each into a logical sequence.

Many local groups before the mid-1980s were teaching their own interested participants. These groups included some immediate care schemes, those involved in water, cave and mountain rescue, and the voluntary aid societies. There were a few central courses run from postgraduate centres, the best known of these being the courses held in Edinburgh.

BRITISH ASSOCIATION FOR IMMEDIATE CARE ANNUAL CONFERENCE

For many years from the mid-1970s the annual conference of the British Association for Immediate Care (BASICS) offered the only forum for training and the dissemination of new ideas and best practice. More recently, the conference has tended to look at the latest thoughts in the field of prehospital resuscitation and treatment, particularly as the BASICS Education courses have proliferated.

ADVANCED LIFE SUPPORT (ALS) COURSES

In the mid-1980s the first of the courses designed in the USA was introduced into the UK. This was the Advanced Cardiac Life Support (ACLS) course and it was designed to teach resuscitation techniques following a cardiac arrest, as well as postresuscitation care. David Skinner first introduced the ACLS course to the UK at St Bartholomew's Hospital.

The Resuscitation Council (UK) adopted, modified and updated the ACLS courses into the Advanced Life Support (ALS) course and is now responsible for the administration of courses, maintenance of standards and the running of the ALS movement. The course consists of lectures and practical sessions followed by a course assessment. The certificate gained on passing remains valid for 3 years when recertification is required.

THE DIPLOMA IN IMMEDIATE MEDICAL CARE (DIP. IMC RCS(EDIN))

There had been discussion between BASICS and the Royal College of Surgeons of Edinburgh for about 2 years before the first diploma examination was held at the college in September 1988. Since that date, the diploma examination has been held at least three times a year, with approximately 20 candidates attending each diet. Although the concept of the examination was a joint venture between BASICS and the Royal College, it is the college that conducts the examination and confers the diploma and those who pass are offered associate membership, which entitles them to receive the college journal. BASICS awards a medal to the most outstanding candidate each year.

The examination at first consisted of a number of slides of electrocardiogram (ECG) rhythm strips that had to be identified, then three written papers (multiple-choice, short-answer and triage question papers). These were followed by practical tests. There was a medical and a trauma practical test involving resuscitation skills demonstrated on mannequins, and patient assessment with physical examination involving casualty simulation. This type of practical assessment, which was first introduced in the immediate care diploma, has now been included in other diploma examinations.

Since its first introduction the time allowance for the various written papers has changed slightly and the slide show has changed from ECG rhythm analysis alone to include a whole range of prehospital slides, including accident scenes and equipment slides with a variety of questions being asked about each slide. The examination has been extended from just 1 day and is now held over 2 days, which has allowed an additional practical examination in the management of major incidents to be included.

The diploma examination looks at the prehospital management of traumatic and medical emergencies and has proved to be a hard hurdle to overcome. The pass rate since it started is only approximately 50%.

This examination is now well established and has been guided to this point of success by Mr Myles Gibson of the Royal College of Surgeons of Edinburgh. It provides a gold standard for those doctors working in the prehospital field.

The Diploma in Immediate Medical Care is also open to nurses and paramedics in addition to doctors. A Fellowship in Immediate Care has also been developed for practising prehospital care doctors. The Diploma in Immediate Care is the 'part 1' examination for the new fellowship.

ADVANCED TRAUMA LIFE SUPPORT (ATLS) COURSES

The problems of trauma management outside the large hospitals in the USA had been highlighted in 1976 by a Nebraskan surgeon following a light aircraft accident involving his family in which his wife was killed and he and his children were seriously injured. Following his recovery he has been reported as saying: 'When I can provide better care in the field with limited resources than my children and I received at the primary care facility – there is something wrong with the system and the system has to be changed.'

The ATLS concept of patient assessment and resuscitation developed from this incident and was adopted by the American College of Surgeons' Committee on Trauma. The ATLS course was introduced to Britain by David Skinner in 1988 and is managed by the Royal College of Surgeons of England. The introduction of this course had a profound effect on developing ideas in prehospital education, providing a significant directional push to the initial Cambridge Immediate Care course.

The concepts of assessment and resuscitation on the ATLS course are universally acknowledged but the ATLS course looks very much at the initial response following the arrival *in hospital* of a traumatized patient. The course therefore is aimed at the emergency department and hospital resuscitation during the first hours after the patient arrives in hospital. A further aspect of the ATLS concept that is worthy of mention, because it has become fundamental to other course design, is the progression from attending a course as a candidate and becoming a provider to becoming an instructor following selection.

This type of course is didactic and in order to obtain the best from such a course it is essential that all instructors talk 'with a single voice'. It is therefore essential that everyone experiences the course from the student's point of view before becoming an instructor.

The important additional component that ATLS insisted on between provider and instructor status is the introduction of an instructors' teaching course. All potential instructors must attend this course and therefore the standards of teaching methods and course content are maintained.

BASICS EDUCATION

Following the introduction of the Diploma in Immediate Medical Care in September 1988 there was a meeting of the Executive Committee of the Mid-Anglia General Practitioner Accident Service (MAGPAS) in November 1988 at which a decision was taken to organize a training course based on the syllabus of the Diploma in Immediate Medical Care examination.

The first course was held at Churchill College, Cambridge in April 1989. It was a 5-day residential course and covered all aspects of prehospital emergency medicine. During the following year two further courses were run and the venue was moved to Madingley Hall, Cambridge. Discussions had also taken place between the organizers of the course and BASICS, and from these discussions BASICS Education was established in 1990.

The Cambridge Immediate Care course is now run twice a year at Madingley Hall. Rather than being a didactic course, the aim of the week is to expose the participants to the fundamental skills and knowledge required in the field of immediate care and then to act as a catalyst for the many conceptual ideas that make this area of medicine so stimulating and exciting.

At first BASICS Education ran the 5-day Cambridge Immediate Care course and several ACLS courses but following an approach from the Royal College of Surgeons of Edinburgh a new type of course was developed. It had been recognized that people from several disciplines attended prehospital emergencies and that all were in need of training. A course was created that was multidisciplinary and that would be examined formally, with those who were successful in the examination being awarded a certificate by the Royal College of Surgeons of Edinburgh. This was the first time that a Royal College had awarded any form of academic recognition to those who did not possess a medical degree, as the course was designed to be open to doctors, nurses and paramedics.

This course is known as the Prehospital Emergency Care course (PHEC) and it is administered by BASICS. It has broken new ground because it not only looks at trauma but encompasses all areas of prehospital emergency care, as well as the problems encountered when dealing with multiple casualties.

The course is didactic and has its own course manual. At the end of two-and-a-half days of teaching there is an examination consisting of a projected material test, MCQ paper, multiple-choice paper and a brief triage paper. There is also a practical test on cardiac resuscitation and trauma assessment.

BASICS Education and the Royal College of Surgeons have formed other associations to create additional teaching courses, notably with the National Fire College at Moreton-in-the-Marsh, where a medical component for the fire service is now included in the Road Traffic Accident Instructors' course.

BASICS Education was at first organized and run by John Scott but gradually the need for administrative help became apparent and an office structure was set up. At the beginning of 1996 this administrative function was at last taken under the wing of BASICS headquarters and a management committee was established. This new committee are taking forward and developing the ideas and the educational programmes developed by BASICS Education. There is now an established position of director of education.

PREHOSPITAL TRAUMA LIFE SUPPORT (PHTLS) COURSES

The system of delivery of prehospital care is significantly different in the USA from that found in the UK. During the late 1980s a programme was being developed in the USA along the lines of the ATLS courses but for paramedics. This course was initially known as the 'ATLS course for non-physicians'. This developed into the Prehospital Trauma Life Support course, and now has a basic and advanced component.

The PHTLS course was introduced into Britain in the early 1990s in a number of centres and is now regulated in Britain by the Royal College of Surgeons of England. This course is concerned with the problems of trauma victims and teaches the skills required to deal with problems encountered in the prehospital situation, laying stress on the need to transport the critically injured patient to hospital as rapidly as possible. Although the method of delivering prehospital care is significantly different in the UK, this course is appropriate when looking at the rather narrow field of trauma, especially as trauma is the most important cause of death among young people in the UK.

MAJOR INCIDENT COURSES

Although major incidents happen rarely and any one person may only attend one such event in their lives, training is required. This rarity makes training and preparation even more essential.

The other problem in this area of training is that each ambulance service will have different views and operational methods for handling major incidents. There are general principles that can be applied to any incident, but failure to standardize the approach has bedevilled training.

The Postgraduate Centre at the Royal Hammersmith Hospital has run an annual 'major incidents' course but its vision has not been taken up elsewhere. BASICS Education has also run a number of major incident courses specifically to train doctors in the role of medical incident officer and has introduced the concept of precourse reading and postcourse exercises specifically to ensure that the participants on the courses make contact with the emergency service planners in their own area.

MAJOR INCIDENT MEDICAL MANAGEMENT AND SUPPORT COURSE

However, it was the Advanced Life Support Group (ALSG) in Manchester who created the foundation course in major incident training – Major Incident Medical Management and Support (MIMMS). This course is gaining wide acceptance across the whole of the UK.

The MIMMS course is a 3-day course that is structured so that the first 2 days give participants essential background information about the medical support at a major incident on which they are then examined. The final day gives the participants the chance to put their newly acquired knowledge into practice in a number of exercise settings. This course has now set a standard that can be taught anywhere and has a uniform and examinable outcome. Emergency planners can now build successful course participants into various emergency plans with confidence. A Special Incident Medical Management and Support (SIMMS) course has recently been developed for those who may be involved in incidents involving chemical and nuclear components.

DEGREE OR DIPLOMA COURSES IN MAJOR INCIDENT MANAGEMENT

There are a number of educational bodies that offer degree-type courses in this field. These courses are of more relevance to emergency planning officers than to those who may be at the front line in dealing with a major incident. Details of the best known of these courses may be obtained from the Society of Apothecaries, the University of Bradford and the University of Hertford.

ADVANCED PAEDIATRIC LIFE SUPPORT (APLS) AND PAEDIATRIC ADVANCED LIFE SUPPORT (PALS)

These courses cover the resuscitation of infants and children in a hospital setting. Although they both place considerable importance on preventing infants or children reaching the point of collapse, and are very much hospital-orientated, they offer the prehospital worker an insight into and practice in the methods of resuscitation appropriate to these patients.

TEACHING COURSES

Those involved in prehospital care have, until recently, had little experience of learning how to teach. At many levels of medical education, people are often asked to give talks, lectures or demonstrations and are simply expected to be able to perform to an appropriate standard.

With the introduction of didactic courses, this situation has had to change rapidly. Each course of this type has insisted that potential lecturers must have attended that particular course's instructors' training programme. Initially this was very sensible, and in particular the work of Professor Harris proved immensely valuable in the ATLS system. However, with the proliferation of this type of course, the problem of finding correctly accredited lecturers has arisen. There is often no cross-recognition of lecturers from one type of course to another. The effect of this is that a potential instructor in several of the types of course may spend much valuable time repeating 'how to teach' courses.

BASICS Education has always accepted that lecturers may participate on a course as long as they have attended the course and received formal teaching method instruction from any source. As well as the specific course teaching packages, BASICS Education offers occasional courses on adult education and teaching methods run by educationalists. These courses are open to anyone interested in educational methods.

Two distance learning packages leading to diplomas or master's degrees in medical education are offered by the universities of Dundee and Cardiff. These courses are designed so that they can be completed in 1 year but because they are modular the participants can take as long as their particular circumstances require.

The Faculty of Immediate Care

It had been a vision of a number of people for some years that there should be a central, respected body that could oversee best clinical practice and collate academic activities in this rapidly developing field. The opportunity to realize this vision came from the Royal College of Surgeons of Edinburgh, which in 1995 announced that it was setting up a Faculty of Prehospital Care. This Faculty is Chaired by Mr Myles Gibson and is open to anyone involved in immediate care. The aims of the faculty are:

- to set and maintain standards of practice in prehospital care
- to promote education in and teaching of prehospital care

- to initiate technical developments and research in prehospital care
- to integrate effectively the efforts of all participants in prehospital care to harmonize and facilitate the onward management of the sick and injured in whatever setting that may be.

The future

The Faculty of Immediate Care has an increasing influence on the direction of education and training in prehospital care. This should begin at a school level and involve the public, the voluntary aid societies and the emergency services, and should influence the formal medical education structure.

School programmes along the lines of the programme set up in Oxfordshire schools could be established. The programme, known as 'Injury Minimization Programme for Schools', (IMPS) is specifically designed to integrate injury prevention and simple resuscitation into the school curriculum wherever possible. The outcome of such an initiative may be to raise the level of awareness of resuscitation in our future adult population and might in the long run do more to reduce mortality and morbidity than any other aspect of prehospital training.

Reinforcement of these concepts will be needed not only in the secondary school system but also within the adult population. For those entering the emergency services, other than the ambulance service, there is a need to undergo basic training in resuscitation skills and for this training to be kept up to date both theoretically and practically.

The ambulance service will always need to receive detailed and careful resuscitation training but the input to this training should have a very strong medical lead and direction based on proper audit and outcome studies.

The nursing profession needs to continually encourage the updating of resuscitation skills in all branches of nursing but particularly among accident and emergency nurses, practice nurses, community nurses and those working in occupational health departments. Payment for courses for these particular groups should either be a condition of work for the employer or a system of bursaries and educational grants might be set up within the business community to benefit society as a whole.

In medical education it is necessary to ensure that, on entry to a medical school, undergraduates are rapidly taught or re-accredited in basic life support. On entry into clinical training they should be competent in BLS, patient assessment and the primary survey, while on starting the preregistration year they should be able to perform advanced life support in straightforward resuscitation scenarios.

The problem thereafter in training the young doctor further is one of cost. Having completed the preregistration year the doctor may be required to attend a number of resuscitation-type courses. To attend just three such courses will cost well in excess of £1500. A fresh approach will be needed. Many of the courses have considerable common ground and one possibility that is gaining some acceptance is the concept of having an intensive week that will cover the common core content of courses in trauma, cardiac and paediatric resuscitation. It has been suggested that the course should also include prehospital and major incident elements. Although this is a potentially exciting prospect for the future, no course designed using this template is currently available.

Finally, the establishment of the Fellowship in Immediate Medical Care of the Royal College of Surgeons of Edinburgh is perhaps the most exciting advance in prehospital care in recent years and offers enormous potential for future educational and other developments.

Initiatives in 2008 are targeted to the recognition of prehospital emergency medicine as a new subspecialty.

Immediate care equipment

67

Introduction   678

Safety equipment   678

Medical equipment   680

Communications equipment   683

Miscellaneous equipment   684

References   684

Introduction

A huge number of life-threatening problems are readily dealt with by using simple techniques once the initial problem has been identified; however, it must be accepted that to provide the *best* care it is necessary to have available the appropriate supportive equipment. Equally, it is important to consider the question of safety so that medical staff are safe and protected from the hazards at the scene. This chapter will therefore review both the safety and medical equipment that is essential for the provision of prehospital care.

Safety equipment

PERSONAL PROTECTION

It is essential that all those who attend incidents are protected from the hazards at the scene. There are many possible hazards but examples include lack of lighting, adverse weather, chemicals, falling masonry or rocks and rubble, vehicle wreckage, glass and spilt blood.

It is impossible to achieve total protection; however, with the provision of a few simple pieces of clothing it is possible to make the situation safer. The National Health Service Medical Executive (NHSME) has issued a document detailing its recommendations for hospital teams' protective clothing (Ambulance Policy Advisory Group 1994). The British Association for Immediate Care (BASICS) has produced specifications for protective clothing for its members (McNeil 1994). Both sets of guidelines are broadly similar. The British Standards Institute has revised its publication about high-visibility clothing (British Standards Institute 1994), upon which the NHSME and BASICS based their recommendations.

High-visibility jackets

The use of high-visibility clothing is vital for personal safety. Fluorescent jackets are now *de rigueur* and are readily available. It is recommended that medical personnel wear a yellow high-visibility jacket with green shoulder yolks. The jackets should have reflective strips attached – two round the chest, two round the arms, one round the bottom of the garment and a shoulder strip on each side. In addition, they should have a label on the front and rear denoting the status of the wearer. The jackets should meet British Standards BS EN 471 Class 2 as a minimum and should preferably meet Class 3. These standards take into account visibility, wearability and washability (Fig. 67.1).

High-visibility waistcoats

These are only appropriate for use in very hot weather as the protection they offer is limited. These should meet BS EN 471 Class 1 standards.

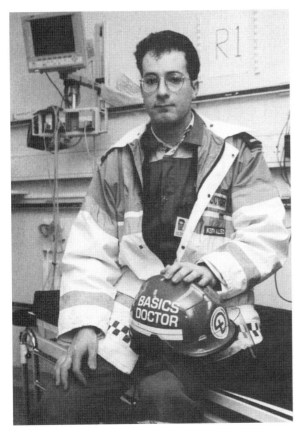

Fig. 67.1 • The BASICS recommended high-visibility jacket.

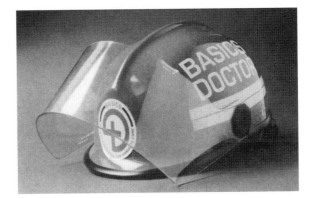

Fig. 67.2 • The BASICS approved helmet.

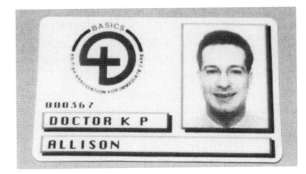

Fig. 67.3 • The BASICS identification card.

Overalls

The use of protective overalls is strongly recommended. Padded elbows and knees should be part of the specification. No overall currently available meets the standards required by BS EN 471 and they should thus be used in conjunction with jackets or waistcoats. The overalls should be hard-wearing and easily cleaned. They should have labels showing the status of the wearer. Two reflective strips should be placed on each arm and leg. Fireproof overalls are not mandatory except on motor-racing circuits.

Helmets

Head protection is essential. There is considerable risk of head injury from wreckage at road traffic accidents and in many other situations. Industrial bump hats are no longer regarded as adequate and it is recommended that rescuers use special application helmets such as the PACIFIC A3, RK70 Montgomery helmet. The most suitable is the Kevlar® aramid shell model A3k/2, which meets BS prEN 443 for European firefighters' helmets (Fig. 67.2).

Eye protection

Eye protection from direct injury and blood spray is essential. Many helmets provide inherent eye protection with visors; however, specifically designed safety eye wear is still recommended as visors do not provide complete protection. The use of glasses is not recommended. All eye protection should meet BS EN 166.

Hand protection

All rescuers should have access to leather debris gloves, latex rubber gloves and ideally blue nitrile gloves. 'Chain mail' gloves are available; these protect from slashing injuries but do not protect from stabbing injury from, f example, shards of glass.

Identification cards

All prehospital care practitioners should have appropriate official identification cards. The police may deny access to the scene if the prehospital physician is unable to prove his/her identity. Bogus doctors are often found at the scene of major incidents! BASICS produces identification cards for its members and all NHS trusts will provide appropriate cards for all their employees (Fig. 67.3).

VEHICLE PROTECTION

Most prehospital care practitioners will have to travel to the site of the incident unless they are attending an event as part of a predetermined on-site deployment. While some will be conveyed by the ambulance service there are many who will go in their own vehicle. The use of safety devices on such vehicles is essential if the driver is to get to the scene safely and quickly. To this end, many doctors use green beacons, audible warning devices, flashing headlights and reflective markings. There is considerable confusion about the legality of some of the methods used and the law is summarized below. It should be remembered that the use of warning devices does not confer any special privileges to the user with regard to exemptions from the Road Traffic Act.

BASICS has produced guidelines on the use of the devices detailed here (McNeil 1997).

Green beacons

The law relating to the use of green beacons is detailed in the *Road Vehicles Lighting Regulations* 1984, Statutory Instrument 812. It can be summarized as follows:

- Any vehicle being used by a registered medical practitioner for the purposes of an emergency may display one or more green lamps. Doctors who are not fully registered are excluded.
- Each green lamp or warning beacon is to be capable of emitting a flashing or rotating beam throughout 360° in the horizontal plane.
- Only those people entitled to use a green beacon may have one fitted to their vehicle.
- Each beacon must be visible a reasonable distance from the vehicle, must be mounted not less than 1200 mm from ground level and flash at a rate between 60 and 240 times a minute. Bulbs must not exceed 55 W.

The use of blue beacons is currently illegal in all areas of the UK. In Metropolitan London special dispensation has been given to some BASICS doctors to use blue lights when working for the London ambulance service.

Audible warning devices and flashing head lamps

There is no provision in law for doctors to use these devices, although many do so with the unofficial and usually unwritten consent of their local police force. The current best available types of audible device use the American-style wail and yelp siren. The traditional British two-tone horn is less often utilized nowadays. A new type of siren using short 'yelps' interspersed with 'white noise' is being trialled, and it is expected that this will become the device of the future as, in initial unpublished trials, they appear to be more directional and other drivers react to them more quickly.

High-visibility markings

The use of high-visibility vehicle markings is strongly recommended. They provide enhanced visibility to the vehicle and moreover help to portray a professional approach. The Road Traffic Act 1984 allows for the use of red reflective markings on the rear of a vehicle and any other colour, apart from red, on the front and sides.

Medical equipment

It is quite impossible to detail in one chapter all the medical equipment that is available for use in the prehospital field. Instead, an overview of the types of equipment that should be carried as a minimum is offered with further details of some of the more specialized equipment that may not be seen in hospital departments on a regular basis. Neither is this chapter intended as a training guide to the use of the equipment, rather it is an overview that highlights some advantages and disadvantages of the item in question.

Equipment must be compatible with that used by the local ambulance service.

When considering equipment it is essential that the equipment used by physicians should be compatible with that of the local ambulance service and emergency departments. In addition, purchasers should anticipate any additional training needs for all those who may come across the equipment. It is essential to test the equipment being purchased as manufacturers' claims are not always borne out in reality.

Equipment used solely for rescue and first aid can be bought free from value added tax by following the regulations in the Value Added Tax Act 1983, Schedule 5: Groups 14 and 16. An exemption certificate must be presented to the supplier.

AIRWAY SUPPORT

All prehospital physicians should carry a full range of airway adjuncts in a full range of sizes.

Airways

Simple oropharyngeal airways are the mainstay of oral airway maintenance. For patients with trismus, or who will not tolerate an oral airway, the use of a nasopharyngeal airway is recommended. Nasal airways are a much underused and undervalued tool.

Endotracheal tubes

Endotracheal (ET) tubes remain the gold standard for securing and protecting the airway. Physicians should carry a full range of ET tube sizes. Uncut tubes should also be carried in the event that nasal intubation may be required.

Miscellaneous adjuncts

Laryngeal mask airways (LMAs) have a well established role in modern anaesthesia. In recent years they have been used in resuscitation in hospital and their use is now being trialled in the prehospital field in both cardiac and trauma cases. It is hoped that the training requirements will be lower and the skill retention better for the occasional user compared to endotracheal intubation. The main problem with the use of LMAs is that the airway is still at risk from aspiration.

The Combitube®, a modern development of the now largely unused pharyngotracheal lumen airway, is a useful alternative for those patients in whom position precludes formal endotracheal intubation or in whom normal methods have failed to secure an airway. It consists of a double-lumen tube with cuffs that allows ventilation to occur whether it is placed in the trachea or the oesophagus. It can be inserted without the need for direct vision with a laryngoscope.

Cricothyrotomy kit

There are many available on the market, the most used is probably the Portex Mini Trach II, originally designed for bronchial toilet. All have the relevant equipment to carry out the procedure. It should be remembered that prolonged ventilation is only possible with an airway lumen of 6 mm or more. An alternative is the insertion through the cricothyroid membrane of a 6 mm endotracheal tube.

SUCTION

It is essential that suction is available to clear airways. All ambulances carry battery-powered suction devices. A number of hand-operated vacuum suction devices are available and there should be one in every prehospital physician's equipment bag. Those supplied by Vitalograph and Laerdal are probably the best currently available (Fig. 67.4).

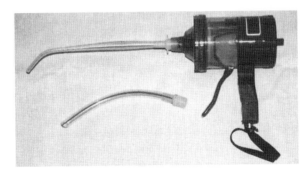

Fig. 67.4 • A hand-held aspirator.

Laryngoscopes

These are essential pieces of equipment. Many types are available and the choice should reflect the physician's own experience and preference. Metal laryngoscopes are more durable than plastic. Disposable units are available but are relatively expensive. A support pack of spare batteries, spare bulbs and various sizes of blade, including a straight paediatric blade, is essential.

VENTILATORY SUPPORT

Pocket mask/mouth-to-mouth resuscitators

The best and most used device is the Laerdal pocket mask with oxygen inlet which can, when used in conjunction with high-flow oxygen, deliver a concentration of 90% or more inspired oxygen. These are essential items of equipment for all prehospital practitioners.

Bag–valve–mask (BVM)

This is essential equipment for all who will provide ventilatory support. When purchasing a device it is important to ensure that the one purchased is the same as that in use by the local ambulance service. Silicone facemasks make better seals than those with inflated seals. The bag–valve–mask must always be used in conjunction with an oxygen reservoir. A paediatric bag–valve–mask is also mandatory.

Ventilators

Portable oxygen-driven ventilators are available from Pneupak. They are seldom used, with most practitioners opting for hand ventilation using a bag–valve–mask. They are, however, useful for those involved in long secondary transfers of ventilated patients.

Oxygen

All ambulances carry adequate supplies of oxygen. The prehospital physician therefore requires only a small size D cylinder which should give approximately 20 min of oxygen supply when used at $15 \, l \, min^{-1}$. All cylinders should be interchangeable with the local ambulance service. Maintenance of cylinders is important and evidence of regular testing of the cylinder's integrity is required before it can be recharged. Test dates are stamped on the neck of cylinders or put on a colour-coded ring applied around the pillar valve.

Oxygen masks

All oxygen therapy to seriously ill or injured patients should be at $15 \, l \, min^{-1}$ via a Hudson mask with attached oxygen reservoir bag.

Chest drains

A chest drain kit comprising scalpel, sutures, tubes, valves and collecting bag is available from Portex and Vygon. These kits are essential purchases for the regular immediate care practitioner (Fig. 67.5).

CIRCULATORY SUPPORT

Intravenous cannulas and giving sets

Supplies of cannulas, giving sets and tape are readily available. The choice of device is up to the individual. It is worth mentioning the Safelon intravenous cannula; this is a development of the much used Venflon that has a self-locating protective sheath and needle tip cover that automatically encloses the needle as it is withdrawn from the cannula. It represents a major step forward in sharps safety. The choice of giving set is dependent on local practice but ideally a blood-giving set, rather than a solution-giving set, should be used to avoid unnecessary changes of device if blood is required at a later date.

Intravenous fluids

The choice of intravenous fluids is dependent on local practice. Adequate amounts – at least 4 litres – should be carried.

Vein dilation devices

These devices use the Seldinger technique to dilate veins for rapid infusion. Size 8G devices are available and are relatively easy to use for those familiar with the Seldinger technique.

Intraosseous needles

These provide rapid access to the circulation of shocked children under the age of 6 years. Both drugs and fluids can be rapidly delivered using this approach. They are easy to use and are fast becoming the preferred device in paediatric resuscitation in emergency departments. The training requirement is minimal for physicians. A large-volume syringe and a three-way tap are required in addition to the needle if fluid resuscitation is needed.

Arm splints

These are required to immobilize limbs when intravenous lines are sited in the antecubital fossa. The Armlok splint is the easiest to use and is available in adult and child sizes.

Fluid insulators and fluid warmers

The rapid infusion of cold fluids leads to hypothermia and can precipitate cardiac dysrhythmias. Therefore it is necessary to ensure the fluids given are warm and are insulated from heat loss with a protective cover. A number of useful reusable devices that achieve this are available, including electric warm boxes and chemical heat packs. Insulating covers are also available for intravenous infusion tubing.

Drip stands

It is common to employ a firefighter in this role! Pieces of string, butcher's hooks, bent coathangers and the like have also been successfully used. Some devices are marketed but they are invariably expensive and are of no more use than the aforementioned home-made devices.

CERVICAL COLLARS AND EXTRICATION DEVICES

Cervical collars

Cervical spine immobilization is an essential component of the role of the immediate care physician. There are now a considerable number of cervical collars available; however, the two most commonly seen are the Stifneck and the Nekloc. Both are semirigid plastic collars. Newer systems such as the Sure-loc avoid the need to carry a selection of adult-sized collars. There is little to choose between them in terms of efficacy and speed of use. It is best to purchase those used by the local ambulance service. There is no place for a soft foam collar.

Extrication devices

These devices can be useful when moving casualties with suspected back or neck injuries as they provide reasonable back support and immobilization. There are again a large number

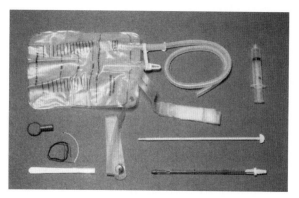

Fig. 67.5 • The Portex® chest drain kit. Reproduced with permission of Smiths Medical International Ltd.

of devices available. There is little to choose in efficacy. The most commonly seen are the Russell extrication device (RED), the Kendrick extrication device (KED) and the ED 2000. They are all similar and constitute a rigid plastic back brace with various forms of strapping that hold the patient in place. All have head restraints but it is essential to remember that they must all be used with a cervical collar. None of the available devices is able to fully support the lumbar lordosis.

Long spinal boards

The initial devices were made from polished plywood but now lighter and cheaper materials are used. All require sophisticated strapping devices to ensure that the whole casualty is immobilized. Some form of head immobilizer must be used to ensure adequate fixing of the cervical spine. While they can be used as a transport device there is a risk of pressure sores developing if a casualty is left attached for too long. They are extremely useful extrication devices but require teamwork and manpower to be used effectively.

Vacuum mattresses

These devices are extremely useful for packaging casualties with multiple injuries. They splint the whole body comfortably and effectively.

LIMB SPLINTAGE

There is a bewildering variety of splints available for the treatment of fractures. These include vacuum splints, inflatable splints, box splints, Frac straps and simple wooden or aluminium splints. The choice is very much an individual one.

Traction splints

There are three types available. The most versatile is the Sagar traction splint. This is a versatile spring-tension splint that provides dynamic, quantifiable traction to both lower limbs as required. It is easy to use, will splint both legs and fits into the profile of most ambulance trolley cots. The Donway splint is a more bulky device that uses pneumatic pressure to provide traction force against the pelvis. It can only splint one limb at a time and does not fit into the profile of some ambulance trolley beds. The Hare splint uses a ratchet winder to apply unquantified traction. It is bulky and can only splint one leg.

DEFIBRILLATORS

Defibrillators are now an essential part of a prehospital physician's equipment. Most are familiar with a number of

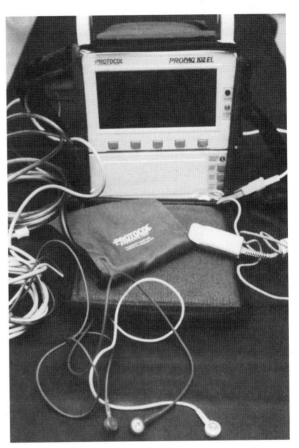

Fig. 67.6 • Robust portable monitoring. Reproduced with permission of Welch Allyn (UK) Ltd.

types. It is essential that all are fully familiar with the one they carry and those used by their local ambulance service. Maintenance can be a problem and it is essential that batteries are checked regularly. Spare batteries should be carried at all times. New devices are being developed all the time and some automatic devices are now no larger than this book.

ELECTRONIC MONITORING DEVICES

It must be remembered that these devices – be they pulse oximeter, capnograph or blood pressure monitor – are only tools. They are not substitutes for good clinical observation and examination. Devices such as those produced by Propaq (Fig. 67.6) are ideal.

Communications equipment

There is little point in carrying thousands of pounds worth of expensive equipment if the physician is unable to find out that his/her skills are required. Communications equipment is therefore a vital part of kit. All ambulance services are able to provide the necessary two-way radio and pager to ensure that contact is possible at all times. It is essential that the radio is fitted with the local ambulance service emergency channels and with the emergency reserve channel. Pagers should ideally be of the type that gives a written message. If the radio is part of the ambulance network there is no need for an additional licence. Mobile telephones, while useful devices, are unreliable and should not be relied upon as the main form of contact with ambulance control.

Miscellaneous equipment

There are a huge number of small miscellaneous items that should be included in a kit; these are listed alphabetically below.

- Aneroid sphygmomanometer
- Blankets – wool is best; space blankets do not protect against conductive, convective or evaporative heat loss
- Blood glucose reagent strips and meter
- Cases – a number of cases will be required to store all the equipment in. The choice is a very individual one
- Cling film – this makes excellent first-aid burns dressings
- Disposables – syringes, needles, blood sample bottles, cross-match request forms, casualty ID bracelets, wound dressings, sutures, Steri-Strips, copious amounts of Micropore tape, tapes to secure ET tubes, crepe bandages, OpSite, ECG electrodes, KY jelly, defibrillation gel pads, obstetric cord clamps
- Ear defenders – earphone-type or rubber plugs
- Eye protection – helmet guard, goggles. Spectacles are not adequate protection
- Fire extinguisher – consult your local fire brigade
- Gloves – rubber surgical, debris gloves, warm dry Gore-Tex gloves

- Incident report forms
- Indelible skin marker pen
- Life hammer – invaluable for breaking car windows
- Nebulizer – most ambulances have one, check compatibility
- Peak flow meter
- Plastic sheet or tarpaulin – keeps kit dry. May protect the patient from wind chill. Plastic bin liners work well as protection from the elements
- Safety knife
- Scissors – *two* pairs of Tufcut scissors
- Seat belt cutter
- Stethoscope – carry two
- Strong walking boots – wellingtons are cumbersome and uncomfortable when clambering over wreckage and do not give adequate support
- Surgical instruments – forceps, clamps, scalpels
- Torches – helmet torch (Petzl or LAGO), large waterproof torch, small penlight torch
- Triage cards – the Cambridge cruciform card is undoubtedly the best but is not used by many ambulance services.

References

Ambulance Policy Advisory Group 1994 Protective clothing and identification of ambulance, medical/nursing staff at major and serious incidents. NHS Medical Executive, London

British Standards Institute 1994 High visibility warning clothing. BSI, London

McNeil I 1994 Protective clothing for BASICS doctors. British Association for Immediate Care, Ipswich

McNeil I 1997 BASICS equipment directory. British Association for Immediate Care, Ipswich

Index

Note: Page numbers in *italics* refer to figures and page numbers in **bold** refer to tables.

A

Abbreviated Injury Scale (AIS), 665
ABC/ABCDE, basic life support, 18, **19**, 26,
    252, **252**
  chemical incidents, 510
  in children, 204–5
  see also Airway; Basic life support (BLS);
    Breathing; Circulation; Life support
Abdomen
  acute *see* Acute abdomen
  anatomy, 298–9
  aortic aneurysm *see* Abdominal aortic
    aneurysm
  auscultation, 142, 146, 301
  compression, basic life support, 21
  distension in abdominal injury, 238
  examination, 139, 142–3
  guarding, 143, 144
  injury *see* Abdominal injury
  mass, 139, 146
  pain *see* Abdominal pain
  palpation, 143, 146, 301, 424, 429
  rebound tenderness, 143, 144
Abdominal aortic aneurysm, 143–4
  acute abdomen, 140
  incidence, 143
  misdiagnosis, 143
  ruptured, 142, 143
  treatment, 148
Abdominal injury, 298–304
  air travel considerations, 591–2
  anatomy, 298–9, **299**
  associated penetrating chest injuries, 300
  blunt, 299
  bowel sounds, 142
  with chest and pelvic injury, 300
  in children, 238–9
  evisceration, 302
  examination and physical signs, 300–1

  genital injuries *see* Genital injuries
  genitourinary trauma *see* Genitourinary
    trauma
  impaled objects, 301–2
  life-threatening haemorrhage, **299**
  management, **304**
  mechanisms of injury, 299–300, *301*
  pelvic fractures *see* Pelvic fractures
  penetrating, 299–300, *301*
  prehospital fluid, 301
  treatment, 301–2
  unrecognized, 300
Abdominal pain
  abdominal aortic aneurysm, 143
  appendicitis, 144
  bowel obstruction, 146
  ectopic pregnancy, 145, 426
  gallbladder disease, 144
  gynaecological causes, 146
  history, 140–1
  medical causes, 146
  mesenteric infarction, 145
  pancreatitis, 144–5
  parietal, 140
  peptic ulcer disease, 145
  placental abruption, 429
  referred, 141
  renal calculus disease, 145
  time of onset, 141
  type of, 141
  of unknown aetiology, 139–40
  visceral, 140
Abdominal splinting, 152
Abdominal thrusts, 22–3, *24*
Abdominal wall, 298
Abortion, 426, *427*
  see also Miscarriage
Abscesses, intraosseous access, 67
Abuse, 338

  children, 207–8, 240, **240**
  definition, 173
  elderly patients, 356–7
Acceleration
  ambulances, 569
  effects of, 586, *586*
Accident and Emergency (A&E) consultants, 5
Acclimatization, 390–1, **391**
ACCOLC (ACCess OverLoad Control), 490, 660
Acetaminophen *see* Paracetamol
Achilles tendon injury, 318
Acid reflux in pregnancy, 421
Acidosis
  advanced life support, 50
  metabolic *see* Metabolic acidosis
Acids, poisoning, 186
Activated charcoal, 186
Active compression–decompression (ACD)
    CPR, 54, *54*
Active protein channels, 69
Active rewarming, 367
Active transport, 69
Acute abdomen, 139–48
  common causes, 143–6
  definition, 139
  history, 140–2
    constipation, 141
    diarrhoea, 141
    pain, 140–1
    time of onset, 141
    type of pain, 141
    vomiting, 141
  management, 147–8
  physical examination, 142–3
  reaching a diagnosis, 139, 146–7, **147**
Acute confusional states, 348
Acute radiation syndrome, 338
Acute respiratory distress syndrome (ARDS),
    546

Acute stress reaction, 291, 467
Acute tubular necrosis, hypothermia rewarming, 372
Adams-Stokes attack, 94
Adaptive response to radiation, 520
Adder bite, **187**, 193
Adelaide coma scale, 206
Adenosine
  atrial fibrillation, 113
  supraventricular tachycardia, 113
  tachycardia, 89, *90*, 91
Adenosine monophosphate (AMP), 188
Adhesions, bowel obstruction, 146
Adjustment disorders, 467
Adolescents, 197, **198**
  see also Children
Adrenaline
  action, 156–7
  advanced life support, 50
  anaphylaxis, 81
  asthma, 213
  autonomic response to shock, 77
  bradycardias, 108
  in children, 225, 226–7
  croup, 210
  neonates, 450
  pulseless electrical activity, 226–7
  unconscious patients, 135
Adrenocortical deficiency, 157
Adult learning, 672
Advanced Cardiac Life Support (ACLS) course, 11, 674
Advanced life support, 48–55
  advanced airway management and ventilation, 52
  alternative techniques in CPR, *54*, 54–5, *55*
  asystole, 51, *51*
  children, 11, *226*, 676
  defibrillation *see* Defibrillation
  definition, 48–9
  effect of time to starting, **49**
  electrocution injury, 409
  electromechanical disassociation (EMD), 51, *51*
  guidelines, 48, 49
  neonates, 450
  non VF-non-pulseless VT arrest, 51
  potentially reversible causes, **51**, 51–2
  training, 599, 672, 674
  VF-pulseless VT, 49–50, *50*
    see also specific condition; specific topic
Advanced Life Support Group, 494
Advanced Medical Priority Despatch System (AMPDS), 499, 600, 657, 658, 659, *659*
Advanced Trauma Life Support (ATLS), 11, 251, 598
  guidelines, abdominal injury, 300
  pregnant patients, 433
  training courses, 674–5
Adverse drug reactions, 356
Aeromedical evacuation, 572–80
  aircraft used in the UK, *578*, 578–9, *579*
  choice of aircraft, 577–8
  clinical care en route, 576
  data collection, 576
  equipment, 576
  fixed-wing operations, 573
  funding and planning, 575
  helicopter operations in the UK, 579
  hours of operation, 579
  indications, 573–4
  landing sites, 577
  medical crew configurations, 575–6
  mission planning, 576
  proof, 579–80
  rationale, 574–5
  regulation, 576–7
  rotary-wing operations, 573
  safety, 577
  safety at the scene, 577
  tasking, 575
Aerospatiale Dauphin, 578, *578*
Aerospatiale Squirrel, 577, 578, *578*
Affective problems, 175
Afferent fibres, 162–3
Age
  and diagnosing the acute abdomen, 146–7, **147**
  and sports injuries, 535–6
Aggressive patients *see* Violent/aggressive/ uncooperative patients
Agitation in children, 206
Agonists, 154, 163–4
  partial, 154, 164
Agranulocytosis, ionizing radiation, 338
Aid workers, 548–9
AIDS (acquired immunodeficiency syndrome), 144
Air composition, 398, 582
Air embolism
  blast injuries, 329, *329*
  central venous cannulation, 65
  peripheral venous cannulation, 63
Air Operator's Certificate (AOC), 576
Air pressure, 398–9
Air splints, gaseous expansion, 585
Airbags, 231
Aircraft *see* Aeromedical evacuation; Aviation medicine; *specific aircraft*
Airguns, 326
  see also Gunshot/missile wounds
Airwave digital system, 658
Airway
  during aeromedical transport, 587
  assessment, 27
    in children, 204
    detailed, 27
    fifteen-second, 27
    initial, 27
  basic adjuncts, **29**, 29–31, **30**, *30*, *31*, 222, 680
  basic life support, 18
  burns, 27
  with cervical spine control, 252
  differences in infants and children, 232
  equipment, 680–1
  head injury, 264
Laerdal pocket mask, **30**, 30–1, *31*
  major incidents, 491
  management, 26–41
    advanced, 31–8, 52
    basic, 27–31, *28*, **28**
  nasopharyngeal, 29–30, **30**, *30*
  near drowning/drowning, 386, 387
  obstruction *see* Airway obstruction
  oropharyngeal, 29, **29**
  paediatric life support, 198, 221–4, *223*, 232
  poisoning, 183
  in pregnancy, 420–1, **421**
  priority over cervical spine, 28–9
  respiratory emergencies, 118–19
  spasm, 591
  spinal injuries, 292–3, *293*
  surgical *see* Surgical airway
  tracheal intubation *see* Tracheal intubation
  trauma cases, 232, **252**, 252–3
  unconscious patients, 130–1, 132, **132**
  warming, 367, 370, *370*, *371*
    see also Upper airway
Airway obstruction, 26
  boxing and combat sports, 537
  causes, 26–7, 252
  in children, 204, 209–11
  intraoral swelling, 275
  laryngeal/tracheal trauma, 275
  lung injury, 339
  maxillofacial injuries, 272
  oxygen and brain injury, 261
  signs, 252
  tracheal intubation, 31
  trauma patients, 252
  unconscious patients, 132, **132**
    see also specific cause
Alanine aminotransferase (ALT), 395
Albumin, 79
Alcohol
  acute decompression illness, 401
  as an antidote, **187**
  dependence *see* Alcohol dependence
  effects/actions of ingestion, 174
  intoxication, 461
  poisoning, 137, 186, 189
  risk of hypothermia, 362
Alcohol dehydrogenase, 189
Alcohol dependence, 140, 142, 174–6
  delirium tremens, 176
  effects/actions of alcohol, 174
  emergencies related to, 176
  long-term consequences, 174–5
  prehospital management of alcohol-related disorders, 175–6
  prevalence, 174
  psychological problems, 175
  short-term consequences, 174
  social problems, 175
  withdrawal, 176
Alcohol gel, 414
Aldosterone, 77
Alfentanil, 166
Alkalinization of the urine, crush syndrome, 544

Alkalinizing agents, 50
Alkalis, poisoning, 186
Alkaloids, 191, **191**, 192
Allergic reactions
  drugs, 152
  methylprednisolone, 160
  non-steroidal anti-inflammatory drugs, 168
  treatment, 157
Alpha particles, 517
Alpha-1-antitrypsin deficiency, 124
Alternating current (AC), 406
Altitude, 582–6, *583*
  gaseous expansion, 584–6
  hypobaric (hypoxic) hypoxia, 584, **585**
  limitations for cardiorespiratory disease, 588,
    588
  pressure–volume relationship, *582*
Alveolar gas, 583, *583*, 584
Alveolar partial pressure of carbon dioxide
    ($P_A$co$_2$), 584, 588
Alveolar walls, collagen deposition, 124
Alveoli
  anatomy, 277
  gas exchange, 278, **278**
  neonates, 448
Alzheimer's disease, 348
Amanita phalloides, 192
Amatoxins, **192**
Ambu CardioPump™, 54, *54*
Ambulance service, 594–602
  as an NHS trust, 594–5, *595*
  in Australia, 12
  cardiac emergencies, 104–5
  contracting for, 599
  control and communications, 597–8
  emergency, 595
  in France, 10
  functions of, 595
  high-performance system, 600–1
  in Hong Kong, 13
  in Israel, 12–13
  major incident response, 595
  non-urgent patient transport, 595
  performance standards, 599–600
  receiving emergency calls, *656*, 656–8
  reserve, 629
  system design, 600
  thrombolytic therapy, 109
  training, 598–9
  in the UK, 4–5, 9
  in the USA, 11–12
  vehicles *see specific vehicle*
Ambulances, 569–70
  air, 597 (*see also* Aeromedical evacuation;
    Aviation medicine; Helicopters)
  despatching and priority-based despatch,
    600–1, 658
  emergency, 595, *596*
  high-performance system, 601
  locating, 598, 657, 658–9
  patient transport, 597
  science of locating, 600
  vehicle cleaning, 415
Ambulances volantes, 493, *493*

Amenorrhoea, ectopic pregnancy, 145, 426
American Civil War, 484
American College of Emergency Physicians, 109
American College of Surgeons Committee on
    Trauma (ACSCOT), 665, 666–7, 674
American football injuries, 536
American Psychiatric Association, 466
Amides, 170, **171**, 172
Aminophylline
  asthma, 123, 213
  respiratory failure, 125
Amiodarone
  supraventricular tachycardia, 113
  ventricular tachycardia, 114
Amitriptyline, 183
  overdose, 188–9
  post-traumatic disorders, 471
Amoxicillin, otitis media, 218
Amperes, 406
Amphetamines, 178, 179
AMPLE mnemonic, 653–4
Amputated parts, 320, *320*
Amygdalin, **191**
Amyl nitrate, 180, **187**
Anaesthesia
  general *see* General anaesthesia
  local *see* Local anaesthesia
  shocked patients, 152
  tracheal intubation, 35–6
Analgesia, **152**, 162–72
  acute abdomen, 148
  acute decompression illness, 403
  adverse reactions in elderly patients, **357**
  after head injury, 268
  agents/analgesics, 159, 163–72 (*see also
    specific analgesics*)
  cardiac emergencies, 107–8
  chest injuries, 288
  in children, 239
  extrication, 557
  flail chest, 282
  immobilization, 556
  neural transmission and modulation, 162–3
  paraquat poisoning, 190
  pharmacology of analgesics, 163
  in practice, 163
  prehospital practicalities, 163
  rib fractures, 285
  shocked patients, 152
  thermal injury, 341–2
  withholding, 162
Anaphylactoid reaction
  colloids, 71, **79**
  gelatins, 71
  local anaesthetics, 171
  presentation, 76
  vasogenic shock, 76
Anaphylaxis
  adrenaline, 157
  fluid maldistribution, 204
  insect bites, 193
  local anaesthetics, 171
  management, 80–1
  treatment, 157

unconscious patients, 135
Anatomical dead space, 278
Anatomical injury severity scores, 661, 665–6,
    666–7
  see also specific scoring system
Anger
  definition, 476
  as a trauma response, 469
    see also Violent/aggressive/uncooperative
      patients
Angina, 99, *99*, 105–6
  aims of management, 106
  chest pain, **105**
  definition, 105
  diagnosis, 106
  nitrates, 107
  pathophysiology, 105
  unstable, 105–6
Angiotensin II, 77
Animal bites and stings, 193–4
Ankle
  dislocation, 314
  fracture, 305, 314, *314*
  injuries, 319
  vein distribution, 58
Anorexia
  acute abdomen, 142
  appendicitis, 144
Antacids, 421
Antagonists, 154, 159
  see also specific drugs
Antecubital fossa, 58, *58*
Antepartum haemorrhage (APH), 428–9
Anthrax, **411**, 412
Antiarrhythmic drugs, 108, 112, **112**
Antibiotics
  adverse reactions in elderly patients, **357**
  barotrauma, 399
  hypothermia, 372
  meningitis, 217
  otitis media, 218
  pneumonia, 214
  respiratory failure, 125
  soft tissue injuries, 321
Anticholinergic syndrome, **184**
Anticonvulsants, 471
Antidepressants
  and bereavement, 473
  overdose, 183, 188–9
  tricyclic *see* Tricyclic antidepressants
Antidiuretic hormone (ADH), 77
Antidotes
  poisoning, 186, **187**
Anti-emetics, 159
  cardiac emergencies, 107–8
  motion sickness, 587
  opioid administration, 167
  paraquat poisoning, 190
  pulmonary oedema, 111
  radiation-induced vomiting, 526
    see also specific drugs
Antihistamines
  mountain rescue, 378
  and N-acetylcysteine, 187

Anti-inflammatory drugs, 167–9
Antilock braking systems (ABS), 247
Antimuscarinic alkaloids, **191**
Antipsychotic drugs, 458
Antipyretic drugs, 167–9
Anxiety
  disorders, 460, **460**
  elderly patients, 353
  post-traumatic stress disorder, 467
Aorta
  abdominal aneurysm *see* Abdominal aortic
    aneurysm
  anatomy, 298
  rupture, 284
Aortic aneurysm, abdominal *see* Abdominal
  aortic aneurysm
Aortic dissection, chest pain, **105**
Aortic stenosis, electrocardiography, 99, *99*
Aortoenteric fistula, 143
Apex beat assessment, 121
Apgar score, 442, **445**, 449, **449**
Apnoea
  in children, 203
  etomidate, 158
  grand mal convulsions, 132
  tracheal intubation, 31
Appendicitis, 143, 144
  pain, 141
  perforation, 144
  in pregnancy, 431
Arachidonic acid, 339
Arc burns, 407
Arm injuries, *309*, 309–11, *310*
Arm splints, 682
Armed conflict, 540–1, *542*
Armed forces, major incidents, 625, 626–8,
  627
Arrest (police), 618–19
Arrestable offences, 619
Arrhythmias, 111–12
  airway obstruction, 26
  antiarrhythmic drugs, 112, **112**
  blast injuries, 329
  central venous cannulation, 66
  in children, 221
  diagnosis, 111–12
  electrocution injury, 407, 409
  frequency of, within 4h of myocardial
    infarction, **106**
  in myocardial infarction, 108
  pathophysiology, 112
  pulmonary oedema, 110
  tracheal intubation complications, 32
  treatment, 111–12
  unconscious patients, 135
  see also specific arrhythmia
Arsenic, **187**
Arterial gas embolism, brain, 400
Arterial puncture, 65
Arthritis, **105**
As low as reasonably achievable (ALARA), 520
As low as reasonably practical (ALARP), 520
Ascending colon, 298
Aschermann® dressing, 282, *282*

Aspartate transaminase (AST), 395
Aspiration pneumonitis, 186
Aspirators *see* Suction units
Aspirin, 168
  cardiac emergencies, 108
  in children, 218
  mountain rescue, 378
  overdose, 186, 187–8
Assault
  home visits, 477, **478**
  in pregnancy, 436–7
  see also Violent/aggressive/uncooperative
    patients
Association football injuries, 536
Association of Emergency Medical Technicians,
  7
Association of Rally Doctors, 7
Asthma, 122–3
  acute severe, 123
  characteristics, 122
  in children, 211–14
    classification, 211–12
    life-threatening, 212, 213
    management, 212–13, **213**
    mild, 212
    moderate, 212, 213
    post-emergency treatment, 213–14
    severe, 212, 213
  classification, 211–12
  definition, 122
  diagnosis, 119
  life-threatening, 123, 212, 213
  management, 212–14, **213**
  mild, 212
  moderate, 123, 212, 213
  non-steroidal anti-inflammatory drugs, 168
  pathophysiology, 122–3
  pneumothorax, 127
  post-emergency treatment, 213–14
  in pregnancy, 431
  severe, 212, 213
  triggers, 122
  unconscious patients, 134
  volcanoes, 546
Asystole, 51, *51*
  in children, 221, 226–7
  drowning/near drowning, 384
  electrocution injury, 407
Atelectasis
  lung injury, 339
  in pregnancy, 421
Atenolol, 108
Atheroma, coronary artery, 105
Athletics injuries, 537
Atmosphere, 581–2
Atomic bombs, 520
Atoms, 515, *515*, 516
Atracurium, 36
Atrial fibrillation (AF), 91–2, *92*, 92–3, *93*
  common causes, **113**
  electrocution injury, 407
  in myocardial infarction, 108
  treatment, 113
Atrial flutter, 89, *89*, 92, 113

Atrial tachycardia, 88
Atrioventricular (AV) node
  block, 89–90, 94–5
    first-degree, 94, *94*, 108
    second-degree, 94, *95*, 108
    third-degree, 94, *95*, *96*, 108
  cardiac depolarization, 86
Atrioventricular nodal re-entrant tachycardia
  (AVNRT), 89
Atrioventricular re-entrant tachycardia
  (AVRT), 89
Atropine, 590
  action, 157
  as an antidote, 186, **187**, 188
  antidote for overdose, **187**
  basic life support, 51
  bradycardias, 108
  poisoning, **187**, 191, **191**
Audible warning devices, 680
Audit, research and, 655
Auscultation
  abdomen, 142, 146, 301
  chest, 119, 121, 256, **256**, 281
Australia, 12
Autochthonous bubbles, 402
Automated external defibrillators (AEDs), 53,
  227
Automatic vehicle location systems (AVLS),
  598, 657, 658–9
Autonomic hyperarousal, trauma response,
  469
Autonomic nervous system, response to shock,
  76–7
Autonomy, 636
AV block *see* Atrioventricular (AV) node,
  block
Aviation medicine, 581–92
  atmosphere, 581–2, *582*
  biodynamics of flight, 586–7
  clinical considerations during aeromedical
    transport, 587–92
  physiological effects of altitude, *582*, 582–6,
    583, *584*, **585**
  see also Aeromedical evacuation
Avoidant behaviour, trauma response, 469–70
AVPU scale, 131, **131**, 132, 257
  in children, 206, 236
  head injury, 264, **264**
  heatstroke, 393
  spinal injury, 293
  trauma in pregnancy, 435
Avulsion injuries
  digits/limbs, 320, *320*
  genitals, 304
  skin, 317
Azithromycin
  epiglottitis, 210
  otitis media, 218

B

Bacille Calmette-Guérin (BCG) vaccination,
  413
Back blows, choking, 22, 214
  in children, 204

Bad news, breaking, 473
Bag/valve/mask (BVM) device, 681
  advanced life support, 50
  injured children, 232, 234
  vs. Laerdal pocket mask, 30
Balance, elderly patients, 351–2
Barbiturates
  hypothermia, 372
  misuse, 181
  and *N*-acetylcysteine, 187
  overdose, 133, 186
Barosinusitis, 584
Barotitis, 584
Barotrauma, 399–400, 584
  ascent, 400
  descent, 399–400
Basal metabolic rate, 390
Basic life support (BLS), 17–24
  acute decompression illness, 403–4
  children *see* Paediatric life support
  choking, 22–3, *24*
  complications, 21
  continuation, 20
  contraindications, 18
  definition, 17
  effect of time to starting, **49**
  electrocution injury, 408
  indications, 17
  limitations, 17–18
  near drowning, 387
  physiology of, 20–1
  prolonged, 20
  recovery position, 21–2, *22*, *23*
  start time, 18
  technique, 18–20, **19**, *19–20*, **20**
  telephone instructions, 601, 660
  training, 672
  trauma in pregnancy, 435
    see also specific condition; specific topic
Basic Trauma Life Support (BTLS), 11
BASICS (British Association for Immediate
      Care), 494
  development of, *5*, 5–6
  immediate care definition, 3
  national accreditation, 6
  report form, 653, *654*
  structure of, 6
  training, 671, 673, 675
Basilic vein, 58, *58*, 61
Basket stretcher, 381
Battle fatigue, 466
Battle of Borodino, 8
Battle of Solferino, 8
Beck's triad, 52, 257, 283
Becquerel (Bq), 517
Bees, 193–4
Bell stretcher, 377, *379*
Bends, 400, 402
Beneficence, 636–7
Benzodiazepines
  antidote for overdose, **187**
  anxiety disorders, 460
  drug withdrawal, 461
  overdose, 136, 184–5, **187**, 189

post-traumatic disorders, 471
  tracheal intubation anaesthesia, 36
Bereavement *see* Grief
Beta particles, 517
Beta-2-agonists
  asthma, 212, 213, 214
  respiratory failure, 125
Beta-blockers
  adverse reactions in elderly patients, **357**
  antidote for overdose, **187**
  arrhythmias, 108
  cardiac emergencies, 108
  overdose, **187**, 188
  post-traumatic disorders, 471
  supraventricular tachycardia, 113
  tachycardia, 90
Beta-burns, 517
Bifascicular block, 97
Big toe dorsiflexion, 294
Bigeminal rhythm, 96
Bigeminy rhythm, 96
Biliary colic, 141, 144
Bilirubin, 395
Biological Effects of Ionizing Radiation (BEIR),
    519
Birdshot, 326
Birmingham Accident Hospital, 4, *4*
Bites and stings, 193–4
Black Talon®, 324
Bladder
  anatomy, 302
  injuries, 302–3
  pelvic fractures, 302
Blast injuries, 327–30, 335–6
  blast mechanisms, 327–8
  blast shock wave, 327–8, 329
  blast wind, 328, 329
  burn injury, 330
  chest, 280
  crush injury, 329
  effects of blast, **328**
  flash and conflagration, 328, 330
  fragmentation, 328
  initial assessment and early management,
    330
  management, 330
  patterns of injury, 328–30
  primary injury, 328–9, *329*
  psychological injury, 330
  secondary injury, 329
  tertiary injury, 329
  triage, 330
Blast shock wave, 327–8, 329
Blast wind, 328, 329
Bleeding
  non-steroidal anti-inflammatory drugs, 168
    see also Blood loss; Haemorrhage
Blood
  coagulation, 333
  fluid therapy, 70, 79–80
  grouping, 526
  infection transmission, 412, 413–14
  intravenous fluids, rewarming, 370–1
  loss *see* Blood loss; Haemorrhage

  rewarming, 371–2
  transfusion, shock, 79–80
  volume, 68–9
Blood glucose testing, 215
Blood loss
  in children, 203, 235
  femoral shaft fractures, 313
  from fractures, **79**
  head injury, 264
  pelvic and femoral injuries in children, 239
  reduction in immobilization, 556
    see also Haemorrhage
Blood pressure
  acclimatization, 391
  in children, **200**, 205
  monitoring, trauma, 256
  myocardial infarction, 106
  neonates, 449, **449**
  in pregnancy, 422, 429–30
  shock, 75, **75**
Blood products, 70, **79**, 79–80
  infection transmission, 412
Bloody show, 440
Blunt trauma
  abdominal, 299
  bladder, 302
  chest, 279–80
  genitals, 303
  kidneys, 303
  maxillofacial injuries, 272
  in pregnancy, 436–7
  spine, 291
  upper airway, 269
Body fluid compartments, 68–70
  extracellular fluid (ECF), 68–9
  intracellular fluid (ICF), 68–9
  movement of fluid between, 69, **69**
  Starling's forces, 69–70
Body fluids, infection transmission, 412,
    413–14
Body language, 476–7, **477**
Body space, 477
Body temperature
  core, 363, **365**, 390
  measurement, 393–4
  normal, 390
  oral, 365, **365**
  rectal, 365, **365**, 393–4
  regulation *see* Thermoregulation
Bohr concept, 515
Bolam test, 634–5, 636, 648–9
Bolam v. Friern Hospital Management
    Committee, 634
Bolin® seal, 282
Bolitho test, 649
Bolitho v. Hackney Health Authority, 634,
    649
Bolkow, 105, 577, *578*, 578–9
Bombs *see* Blast injuries
Bone marrow
  aspiration, 225
  embolism, intraosseous access, 67
  intraosseous access, 67
Bone trauma *see* Fractures; *specific bone*

Bowel(s)
blast injuries, 328, 329
obstruction, 141, 142, *142*, 146
in children, 216
sounds, 142
see also Large bowel; Small bowel
Box splint, 560–1, *561*
Boxer's fracture, 309
Boxing injuries, 537
Boyle's law, 399, 582–3, *583*, 584
Brachial artery, 58, *58*, 239
Brachial pulse, 205
Brachial vein cannulation, 225
Bradley report, 599
Bradycardias, 93–4
cardiac emergencies, 108–9
in children, 226–7
frequency of, within 4 h of myocardial
infarction, **106**
propofol, 158
sinoatrial nodal block, 94, *94*
sinus, 93
sinus arrest, 94, *94*
suxamethonium, 159
unconscious patients, 132
Bradypnoea, 132
Brain
acute decompression illness, 403
injury *see* Brain injury
swelling, secondary brain damage, 263
Brain injury
arterial gas embolism, 400
cerebral perfusion and oxygenation, 262
in children, 231, 236
depressed skull-vault fracture, 266
drowning/near drowning, 388
gunshot/missile wounds, 266
heat illness complications, 394–5
open and penetrating, 265–6, *266*
oxygen and, 261–2
pathophysiology of, 261–2
primary, 236, 261
raised intracranial pressure *see* Raised
intracranial pressure
secondary, 236, 261, **261**
preventing, 262–3
skull-base fractures, 265–6, **266**, *266*
and spinal cord injury, 291
stab wounds, 266
Brain-stem death in pregnancy, 437
Breaking bad news, 473
Breath sounds, 119, 127
Breathing
during aeromedical transport, 587–8
assessment, 204–5
basic life support, 18–19, *19*, **20**
in children, 204–5, 224, *224*
head injury, 264
hypothermia, 373
inspiration, 44
major incidents, 491
neonates, 448
noisy, 204
in pregnancy, **421**, 421–2

respiratory emergencies, 119
spinal injuries, 293
trauma patients, 253–6
unconscious patients, 130–1, 132, **132**
see also entries beginning Respiratory
Breathlessness *see* Dyspnoea
Breech delivery, 445
British Association for Immediate Care *see*
BASICS (British Association for
Immediate Care)
British Association of Ski Patrollers, 380
British 'dumdum,', 324
British Heart Foundation Working Group, 109
British National Formulary, 153, 155
British Red Cross, 625, 628–9
British Sub Aqua Club, 398
Broad arm sling, 560
Bronchi injury, 284
Bronchiectasis, 125, **125**
Bronchioles, 277
Bronchiolitis, 202, 210–11
Bronchitis, 124
Bronchodilators
airway spasm, 591
asthma, 123
Bronchopulmonary dysplasia, 202
Bronchospasm
lung injury, 339
opioids side-effects, 164
treatment, 119
Broselow tape, 155, 200, *202*, 231
Brucellosis, **411**, 412
Bruising pattern
chest, 256, **256**
fractures, 308
Bubbles, acute decompression illness, 401–2
Buckle fracture, 307
Buckshot, 326
Budesonide, 210, **210**
Buffeting, 586
Bullets, **323**, *323*, 323–5, *324*
fragmentation, 324–5
interaction with tissues, 324–5
patterns of injury, 325–6
temporary cavitation, 324
wound contamination, 325
yaw, 324, *324*
Bundle branch block, 97, *97*, *98*
Bundle of His
bundle branch block, 97, *98*
cardiac depolarization, 86
Bupivacaine, 172
Buprenorphine, 166
Burns *see* Thermal injury; *specific type*
Burns (flame), 335
assessment, 340–2, *341*
blast injuries, 330
in children, 198–9, *199*
cooling of, 334
guidelines for immediate care of, 336
heat loss and thermoregulation, 333–4
inflammatory response, 333, *333*
life-threatening, 332, *332*
maxillofacial injuries, 272

surface area, 340, *341*, *342*, 342–3
treatment, 332
wound, 333
Butane, 181
Butterfly fragment, fractures, 306, *307*
Butyl nitrate, 181
Butyrophenones, 458
BVM *see* Bag/valve/mask (BVM) device

C

Cadence braking, 247
Cadmium, **187**
Caesarean section, perimortem and
postmortem, 437–8
Café coronary, 26
Caffeine, 181
CAGE questionnaire, 176, **176**
Calcium disodium edetate, **187**
Calcium salts, 52
Caller line identification (CLI), 657
Cambridge cruciform triage card, 499, *499*, 654
Cambridge Immediate Care course, 675
Campylobacter, 203, **411**
Cannabis, 177–8
management, 178
psychological effects, 178
Cannula over needle, 59, *59*
Cannulas/catheters
central vein access, 64
fluid flow through, 67–8, **68**
peripheral vein access, 58–9, *59*
see also specific site
Capacity violation, 642
Capillary membrane, 70
Capillary refill time, 74–5, 495
in children, 205
Capillary walls, 69
Capnograph, 33
Car bomb, 327
Carbamazepine
and *N*-acetylcysteine, 187
overdose, 186
Carbohydrate metabolism disturbances, **349**
Carbon-14, 518
Carbon dioxide
detectors, tracheal intubation, 33
in fires, 338
respiratory pathophysiology, 278
retention, 42–3, 121
asthma, 123
Carbon monoxide
antidote for poisoning, **187**
in fires, 338–9
oxygen affinity, 41
poisoning, 182, **187**, 189–90, 335
Carboxyhaemoglobin (COHb), 127, 129, 189,
190
Cardiac activation sequence, *86*, 86–7, *87*
Cardiac arrest
adrenaline, 157
in children, 206, 220, 221
diagnosis, 21
drowning/near drowning, 384, 386–7, 388
electrocution injury, 405, 407

in hypothermia, 373
non-VF-non-pulseless VT, 51
occurrence, 48
prevention in children, 221
resuscitation *see* Advanced life support
trauma in pregnancy, 435
treatment, 157, 386–7
VF-pulseless VT, 48, 49–50, *50*
Cardiac causes of unconsciousness, 137
Cardiac compressions, 198
internal, 54
see also Chest compressions
Cardiac contusion, 234
Cardiac disease
in children, 202
in pregnancy, 431
Cardiac emergencies, 104–14
electrocardiography, 106–7
presentation, 104
treatment, 107–8
see also specific emergency
Cardiac enzymes, 106
Cardiac glycosides, **191**
Cardiac ischaemia, airway obstruction, 26
Cardiac monitoring, plant and fungi poisoning,
191
Cardiac output
acclimatization, 391
electrocution injury, 407
low, 41
in pregnancy, 422
Cardiac pacing, 54–5
in aeromedical transport, 589
asystole, 51
bradycardias, 108
electrocardiography, 102–3, *102–3*
external, 54–5, *55*
internal, 54
Cardiac pump theory, 21
Cardiac tamponade
chest injuries, 282–3, **283**
in children, 234
electromechanical dissociation, **51**, 52
signs, **283**
trauma, 257, **258**
Cardiogenic shock
classification, 76
management, 81
Cardiopulmonary bypass, rewarming, 371–2
Cardiopulmonary resuscitation (CPR) *see* Basic
life support (BLS)
CardioPump®, 21
Cardiorespiratory arrest, 17–18, 137
see also Cardiac arrest; Respiratory arrest
Cardiorespiratory disease, altitude limitations
for, 588, **588**
Cardiovascular monitoring, 107
pulmonary oedema, 111
tachycardia, 112
Cardiovascular system
adaptations to heat, 391
alcohol dependence, 175
considerations during aeromedical transport,
588, *588*, 588–9

effects of cold exposure, **362**
effects of near drowning, 385
electrocution injury, 407
heat illness complications, 395
local anaesthetic toxicity, 171
opioids side-effects, 165
in pregnancy, 422–3
unconscious patients assessment, 135
CARE (Central Accident Resuscitation
Emergency) team, 7
Carotid arteries, 273
Carotid pulse
in children, 205
palpation, 50
Carotid sinus massage, 89, *90*
atrial fibrillation, 113
supraventricular tachycardia, 113
Carpus fractures, 310
Casualty enquiry bureau, 624
Catecholamines
acute stress reaction, 291
response to shock, 77
Catheters *see* Cannulas/catheters
Cave rescue, 378–80
Cavitation, temporary from bullets, 324
C-CODES mnemonic, 124, **124**
CCTV, 478
CD34+ cells, 526
Ceftriaxone, 217
Cell membrane, 69
Cell salvage systems, 80
Cells, radiation effects, 518–19, *519*
Cellulitis
intraosseous access, 67
peripheral venous cannulation, 63
Cement burns, 336
Centers for Disease Control and Prevention,
396
Central Accident Resuscitation Emergency
(CARE) team, 7
Central nervous system (CNS)
acute intoxication, 174
alcohol dependence, 175
alcohol ingestion, 174
effects of cold exposure, **362**
electrocution injury, 407
heat illness complications, 394–5
local anaesthetic toxicity, 171
opioids side-effects, 165
resins, **192**
Central nervous system (CNS) syndrome, 519
Central rewarming, 367, *370*, 370–2, *371*
Central venous access/cannulation, 57, 63–6
anatomy, 63–4, *64*
in children, 224–5
complications, 65–6
equipment, 64
technique, 64–5
Centre for Research on the Epidemiology of
Disasters (CRED), 551
Cephalic vein, 58, *58*
Cephalosporins, 210
Cerebellum, acute decompression illness, 403
Cerebral blood flow (CBF), 262

Cerebral palsy, 202
Cerebral perfusion pressure (CPP), 262
Cerebrospinal fluid (CSF)
blood-stained, leaking from ear, 266, *266*
leak, 589
Cerebrovascular accident (CVA)
aeromedical transport considerations, 590
breathing patterns in unconscious patients,
132
definitions, 354
elderly patients, 354
epidemiology, 354
hospital admission, 354
toxic confusional states, **349**
unconscious patients, 135–6
Cervical collars, 558–9, *558–9*, 682
children, 233
remote industrial sites, 381
spinal injury, 294
Cervical dilatation, 440
Cervical immobilization, 557–9
cervical collars *see* Cervical collars
manual, 557–8
vacuum splints, 559, 566
Cervical spine injury, 260, 269–70
aeromedical transport considerations, 590
airway and, 252–3
airway priority over, 28–9
clinical assessment, 269–70
epidemiology, 260
general approach, 269
and head injury, 135
immobilization, 270
incidence, 290
tracheal intubation, 32, 34
transportation, 296
Chain of survival, 18, *18*
Chemical burns, 336–7
Chemical hazards, 249–50
Chemical incidents, 503–12
chemical burns, 336–7
chemical hazards, 249–50
chemicals involved in, 503, **504**
debriefing, 507–8
documentation, 507
evacuation, 506–7
exercises for major, 505
feedback, 507–8
fire service role, 611–13
management of casualties, 508–12
decontamination of casualties, 509–10
follow-up, 511–12
general considerations, 508
hospital care, 511
protection of emergency responders,
508–9
resuscitation, 510
specific treatment, 510
transfer to hospital care, 510–11
triage, 509
mnemonics, 506
operational management, 505–8
planning and preparation for, 504–5
preparedness, 504

Chemical incidents (*Continued*)
 prevention, 504
 reconnaissance and reporting, 505–6
 recovery, 504
 response, 504
 risk assessment, 507
 safety, 505
 shelter, 506–7
Chemicals
 airway obstruction, 27, 249–50
 poisoning, 186
Cherry red skin appearance, 190
Chest
 auscultation, 119, 121, 256, **256**, 281
 compressions *see* Chest compressions
 drains *see* Chest drains
 examination, 121, 256, **256**, **258**, 280–5,
  281
 hyperinflation *see* Hyperinflation of the chest
 immediately life-threatening conditions,
  281, 281–3
 injuries *see* Chest injuries
 pain *see* Chest pain
 palpation, 256, **256**
 paradoxical movement, 282
 percussion *see* Chest percussion
 silent *see* Silent chest
Chest compressions
 basic life support, 19–20, *20*
 in children, 207, 226
 choking, 214
 complications, 21
 effectiveness, 21
 external *vs.* internal cardiac compression, 54
 forward flow of blood, 21
 hypothermia, 373
 neonates, 450, *451*
 pulseless electrical activity, 226
 trauma in pregnancy, 435
 uncertainties, 21
Chest drains, 682, *682*
 complications, **287**
 equipment, 286
 insertion, 286–7, **287**, *287*
 massive haemothorax, 283
 open chest wound, 282
 pneumothorax, 284
 procedure, 286
 tension pneumothorax, 281
Chest injuries, 277–88
 and abdominal and pelvic injury, 300
 analgesia, 288
 anatomy, 277–8
 blast injuries, 280
 blunt trauma, 279–80
 chest drain insertion, 286–7, **287**, *287*
 in children, 234–5
 examination, 280–5
 immediately life-threatening, **256**
 mechanism of injury, 279–80
 needle thoracostomy, **285**, 285–6, *286*
 open wounds, **258**, 282, *282*
 penetrating trauma, 280, 300
 pericardiocentesis, **287**, 287–8

 practical procedures, 285–8
 respiratory assessment, 253–6
 respiratory pathophysiology, **278**, 278–9
 simple, 284–5
 sucking chest wound, 282
 thoracotomy, 288
Chest pain
 differential diagnosis, 104, **105**
 electrocardiogram during, 98–102
 myocardial infarction, 106
 pneumothorax, 127
Chest percussion, 119, 121
 chest injuries, 281
 pneumothorax, 127
 trauma, 256, **256**
Cheyne-Stokes breathing, 132
Chickenpox, **411**
Chief constable, 616
Chief fire officer, 604
Chief officers, 616
Childbirth, 439–46
 abnormal deliveries, 445
 birth before arrival, 440, 445–6
 concealed pregnancy, 440, 446
 Confidential Enquiry into Maternal and
  Child Health, 446
 emergency, 440
 first stage of labour, 440–1, *441*
 second stage of labour, *441*, 441–2, *442–4*
 third stage of labour, 442–5
Children
 abuse, 207–8, 240, **240**
 airway obstruction, 209–11
 asthma, 211–14
 and bereavement, 472
 burns, 198–9, *199*
 cardiac arrest, 157
 causes of death, **198**
 classification by age, 197, **198**
 comatose, 216
 consent, 643
 critically ill
  examination, 204–7
  history, 200–2, *202*
 definition, 197
 dehydration, **216**, 216–17, **217**
 development, 231
  neurological and emotional, 200
  physical, 197
 dextrose, 157
 drowning, 383
 drug dosage, 155
 electrocution injury, 405–6
 emergencies in, 209–19 (*see also specific
  condition*)
 epilepsy, 215
 fever, 218
 fractures, 199–200, 307
 history in critically ill, 200–2, *202*
 inhaled foreign body, 214
 injured *see* Injured children
 life support *see* Paediatric life support
 meningitis, 217
 metabolic emergencies, 215–16

 non-accidental injury (abuse), 207–8, 240,
  240
 normal, 197–200
  other differences, 199–200
  physiological differences, 200, **200**
  surface area, 198–9, *199*
 numerological and emotional development,
  200
 peak expiratory flow rate measurement, 211
 pneumonia, 214
 post-traumatic stress disorder, 467
 protection, 338
 pulse oximetry, 211–12
 safety and confidentiality, 646
 scalds, 334–5
 spinal immobilization, 295
 sudden death, 220
 thermoregulation, 390
 tracheal intubation, 35
 unwell, assessment, 207
 vomiting and diarrhoea, **216**, 216–17
  *see also specific age; entries beginning
   Paediatric*
Children Act 1989, 338
Chin lift, 18, *19*
 airway obstruction, 28, *28*
 in children, 204, 222
 trauma, 28
Chloramphenicol, 218
Chlordiazepoxide, 461
Chlorine gas, 503
Chlorpheniramine, 81
Chlorpromazine
 overdose, 133
 psychosis, 458
Chokes, the, 403
Choking, 22–3, *24*
 abdominal thrusts, 22–3, *24*
 back blows, 22
  see also Foreign bodies/material, inhaled
Cholangitis, 142
Cholecystitis, **105**, 143, 144
Cholera, **411**, 542
Cholinergic syndrome, **184**, 188
Chronic obstructive airways disease (COAD),
  42–3
Chronic obstructive pulmonary disease
  (COPD)
 respiratory failure, 124
 treatment, 125
Cicutoxin, **192**
Cigarette smoking *see* Smoking
Circulation
 advanced life support, 50
 assessment in children, 205
 basic life support, 18, 19–20, **20**
 in children, 203–4, 205, 224–5, 235
 equipment, 682
 injured children, 235
 major incidents, 491
 near drowning/drowning, 386
 neonatal, 448–9, *449*
 poisoning, 183
 and posture, 422–3

in pregnancy, **422**, 422–3
problems in children, 203–4
respiratory emergencies, 119–20
return of spontaneous, 21
spinal injuries, 293
trauma, 256–7
unconscious patients, 131, 132, **132**
Citrate toxicity, 80
Civil Aviation Authority (CAA), 576
Civil Contingencies Act 2004, 505, 625
Clapham train crash, 626
Clarithromycin
  epiglottitis, 210
  otitis media, 218
Clavicle
  dislocation, 311
  fracture, 311
Clinical audit, ambulance service, 601
Clinical waste disposal, 415
Clomethiazole, 461
Closed-circuit television (CCTV), 478
Clostridium tetani, 320
Clothing
  heat illness, 396
  mass gathering medicine, 532
  protective, 413, 414, **414**
  radiation incidents, 525
  removal, decontamination, 185
Co-amoxiclav, 214
Coastguard Service, 381
Cocaine, 178, 179
Codeine, 166
Cognitive changes, trauma response, 469
Cold
  body's response to, 363
  risk, 361, **362**
Coliforms, 214
Colitis, 141
Collagen deposition, alveolar walls, 124
Collateral ligaments, 319
College Fellowship in Pre-hospital Care, 5
Colles fracture, 310
Colloid osmotic pressure (COP), 69–70
Colloids, 68, 70, 71–2, **79**
  advantages, 73
  anaphylactic reactions, 71, **79**
  commonly used, **71**
  controversy, 72–3, 79
  dehydration, 217
  dextrans, 72
  gelatins, 71, **71**
  hydroxyethyl starch, **71**, 71–2
Colon *see* Large bowel
Coma *see* Unconscious patients
Combat exhaustion, 466
Combat sports injuries, 537
Combitube *see* Oesophageal-tracheal
    Combitube
Comfort following trauma, 470
Command
  chemical incidents, 611–12
  major incidents, **487**, 487–8, 610
Commanders, police, 616
Comminuted fractures, 306, *307*

Commissioners, police, 616
Common good and confidentiality, 646
Common law, 618
Communication
  elderly patients, 348
  major incidents, 488–90, **490**
  verbal and non-verbal, 476–7, **477**
Communications, 656–60
  ambulance service, 597–8
  armed forces, major incidents, 626–7
  confidentiality breach, 644
  disasters, 550–1
  equipment, 608, 683–4
  major incidents, 660
  receiving the emergency call, 656–7
Community reconstruction, major incidents,
    492
Compartment syndrome, 319–20
  gaseous expansion, 585
  tibia fracture, 314
Compassion fatigue, 473
*Competence and Curriculum Framework for the
    Emergency Care Practitioner*, 598
Complement activation, acute decompression
    illness, 402
Complex emergencies, 541
Complicated fractures, 306
Compound (open) fractures, 306, *307*, 309
Computer-aided despatch (CAD) systems,
    598, 657–8
Concealed pregnancy, 440, 446
Conduction, 390
Confidential Enquiry into Maternal and Child
    Health (CEMACH), 420, 439, 446
Confidentiality, 643–7
  after death, 648
  discussions and debriefings, 645
  information transmitted over the airwaves,
      644
  photography, 645–6
  police statements, 644
  press statements, 644–5
  record keeping at the scene, 644
  special circumstances requiring a doctor to
      breach obligations in respect of, 646–7
Confusional states, elderly patients, 348–9
Coniine, **191**
Conscious incompetent adults, consent, 640–1
Consciousness, assessing level of, 133–4
  in children, 206, 235
  see also Unconscious patients
Consent
  autonomy, 636
  beneficence, 636–7
  legal issues, 638–43
  obtaining, 638
  patient's best interests, 637
  psychiatric emergencies, 462–3
  refusal of, 642–3
  therapeutic privilege, 637–8
  treatment without, 638–41
    conscious incompetent adults, 640–1
    unconscious patients, 639–40
Constables, 616

Constipation
  acute abdomen, 141
  bowel obstruction, 146
  opioids side-effects, 165
Consulting rooms, 479, *479*
Contact burns, 336
Contamination
  chemical *see* Chemical incidents
  radiation, 516, 527, **527**
  from victim's mouth, BLS, 18
Contraceptive usage information, 424
Control, major incidents, 487, 611
Convection, 390, 394
Convulsions *see* Epilepsy; Seizures
Cooling, 393, 394
Coordination, major incidents, 487
Copper, **187**
Coprine, **192**
Cordons, 487, *487*, 609
  chemical incidents, 612
  fire service role, 612
  police service role, 622
Cornering safely, 247–8, *247–8*
Cornwall Drowning Study, 388
Coronary arteries
  air embolism, 329, *329*
  atheroma, 105
Coroners, 650
Corpses
  disposal, 651–2
  health risk of, 543–4
  identification, 623
  recovery of, 609
Corticosteroids
  adverse reactions in elderly patients, **357**
  hypothermia, 372
Cosmic radiation, 518
Costochondritis, **105**
Co-trimoxazole, **357**
Coughing
  croup, 210
  ventricular tachycardia, 114
Coumarin, **191**
Couplet ectopics, 96
Coupling rhythm, 96
Courses
  adult, 672–3
  developing, 672–3
  teaching, 676
    see also specific course
Crack cocaine, 179
CRAMS, 664, **664**
Craniotomy, aeromedical transport
    considerations, 589
CRASH trial, 268
Crepitus, 308
Cribriform plate penetration, nasopharyngeal
    airway, 30
Cricket injuries, 536
Cricoid pressure, 33, *34*
Cricothyroid membrane, 39, *39*
Cricothyroidotomy
  in children, 210, 223
  epiglottitis, 210

Cricothyrotomy, 38
  injured children, 232
  kit, 681
  needle, 39, **40**, 40–1, 223, 283
  needle *vs.* surgical, **40**, 40–1
  surgical, 39, **40**, 40–1
Criminal Investigation Department (CID), 617
Criminal Justice and Public Order Act 1994, 619
Criteria Based Despatch (CBD), 499, 575
Critical incident stress debriefing, 474
Criticality, radiation incidents, 522
Croup, 203, 209–10, **210**
Crowds *see* Mass gathering medicine
Crown Prosecution Service, 619
Cruciate ligaments, 319
Crush injuries
  blasts, 329
  earthquake, 544
  fractures, *307*
  treatment, 544
Crush syndrome, 329
  earthquake, 544
  treatment, 544
Crystalloids, 68, 70–1
  advantages, 73
  commonly used, **70**
  controversy, 72–3, 79
  dehydration, 217
  distribution of, 70
  hypertonic saline, 71
  injured children, 235
Cullen's sign, 142, 145
Cushing's response, 132, 236
Custody, police, 619
Cuts, 317
Cutting equipment, fire service, 608
Cyanide, 42
  antidote for poisoning, **187**
  in fires, 338, 339
  poisoning, **187**, 190
  remote industrial sites, 381
Cyanogenic glycosides, **191**
Cyanosis
  carbon monoxide poisoning, 190
  in children, 205
  injured children, 234
  pulse oximetry, 128
  tension pneumothorax, 281
Cyclizine, 167
Cyclones, 546–7, **547**
Cyclooxygenase, 168
Cyclopeptides, **192**
Cystic fibrosis, 202
Cytochrome oxidase, 190
Cytogenic dosimetry, radiation casualties, 526
Cytomegalovirus (CMV) transmission, 412
Cytosine, **191**

D
Dalton's law, 583, *583*
Damage, medical negligence, 649–50
Data collection, aeromedical evacuation, 576
Data Protection Act, 644

DC cardioversion
  atrial fibrillation, 113
  electrocution injury, 409
  hypothermia, 373
  ventricular tachycardia, 114
Deafness
  blast injuries, 329
  elderly patients, 348
Dealing with Disaster, 628
Death
  after rescue, hypothermia, 367
  confidentiality after, 648
  dealing with, 650–1
  diagnosis in hypothermia, 367
  duty of care termination, 648
  pronouncement and certification of, 650–1
Debriefing
  chemical incidents, 507–8
  and confidentiality, 645
  major incidents, 491–2
Decay chains, 516, **516**
Deceleration, ambulances, 569
Decompression, definition, 401
Decompression illness, acute, 400–4
  background, 400
  clinical features, **402**, 402–3
  incidence, 398
  infections, 404
  nitrogen narcosis, 404
  pathophysiology, 401–2
  predisposing factors, 400–1
  treatment, 403–4
Decongestants, 399
Decontamination, 185–6, 191–2
  chemical incidents, 508, 509–10
  radiation casualties, 526
Deep vein thrombosis, 431
Defibrillation, 49, 52–5
  in aeromedical transport, 589
  in ambulances, 570
  automated external defibrillators, 53
  in children, 227
  developments in, 53
  near drowning, 387
  paddle placement, 52, *52*
  safety, 52–3
  successful, 48
  technique, 53
Defibrillators, 683
Degloving injuries, 273, 317, *317*
Dehydration
  acute decompression illness, 401
  in asthma, 123
  in children, **216**, 216–17, **217**
  disasters, 542
  heat exhaustion, 392
  heat illness, **391**, 396
  hypovolaemic shock, 76
  toxic confusional states, **349**
Delirium, 169, 460, **461**
Delirium tremens (DTs), 176, 461
Delusions, 353, 457
Dementias, 348–9
Demonstrators, 673

Denial, trauma response, 468
Dental injuries, 274
Dentures, 274
Dependence, definition, 174
Depolarization, cardiac, 86
Depressed fractures, 266, 306
Depressed skull-vault fracture, 266
Depression, 459–60
  definition, 459
  elderly patients, 353–4
  post-traumatic stress disorder, 467
  signs and symptoms, **459**
  trauma response, 469
Deprivation, children, 208
Dermatomes, 141
Descending colon, 298
Desferrioxamine, **187**
Despatch, 494, 499, 575, 598, 600–1, 656–60, *659*
Detention in police custody, 619
Deterministic radiation effects, 518–19, *519*
Deuterium, 515
Dexamethasone, 210, **210**
Dexamphetamine, 179
Dextrans, 71, 72, **79**
Dextrose, **70**
  action, 157
  hypoglycaemia, 137, 215
Dextrose saline, **70**
Diabetes mellitus
  in children, 202, 215–16
  in pregnancy, 431
Diabetic emergencies, unconscious patients, 137
Diabetic ketoacidosis, 137
  abdominal pain, 146
  in children, 204, 216
  in pregnancy, 431
  unconscious patients, 132
Diagnostic and Statistical Manual, 466, **466**
Dialysis, crush syndrome, 544
Diamorphine, 165, 179
  acute abdomen, 148
  cardiac emergencies, 107
  head injury, 268
  pulmonary oedema, 111
  thermal injury, 342
Diaphoresis, 106
Diaphragm, 277
  anatomy, 298
  breathing, 44
  gunshot wounds, 299
  innervation, 44
  in pregnancy, 421
  rupture, 299, 300, 434
Diarrhoea
  acute abdomen, 141
  bloody, 141, 203
  in children, 203–4, 216–17
  disasters, 542
  infectious, **411**
  refugees, 547
Diazepam
  anxiety disorders, 460

eclamptic fits, 430
epilepsy, 215
fits after head injury, 238
rapid tranquillization, 464
seizures, 268
status epilepticus, 136
Diclofenac, 145, 148, 168
Diethylpropion, 179
Diffuse intravascular coagulation, 372
Diffusion, 69, 278–9
Digitalis, **191**
Digoxin
adverse reactions in elderly patients, **357**
antidote for poisoning, **187**
atrial fibrillation, 113
overdose, 186
tachycardia, 92
Digoxin specific Fab, **187**
Diltiazem, 92
Dimercaprol, **187**
Dioralyte®, 216
Diphtheria, **411**, 412
Diploma in Immediate Medical Care, 5, 6, 671, 674
Diploma of Pre-hospital Care, 5
Direct current (DC), 406
Disability
injured children, 236
respiratory emergencies, 120
spinal injury, 293
trauma, 257–8
Disasters, 484, 540–51
armed conflict, 540–1
communications, 550–1
complex emergencies, 541
the future, 551
impact of, 541–8
international medical aid, 548–9
man-made, 540, **541**
natural, 540, **541**
nature of casualties, 542–4
nature of events, 544–8
number of casualties, 541–2
preparation, practice and planning, 549–50
triage, 541–2
see also Major incidents *specific disaster*
Discussions and confidentiality, 645
Disease, disasters, 542
Dislocations, 308, 309
ankle, 314
clavicle, 311
elbow, 310
electrocution injury, 407
fingers, 309
hip, 312
shoulder, 311, *311*
Displaced fractures, *307*
Disseminated intravascular coagulation
electrical injury, 337
heat illness, 395
Dissociative disorders, 467
Diuretics, **357**
Diverticular disease, 146
Diverticulitis, 143, 146

Diving, 383
acute emergencies, 398–404
barotrauma, 399–400
decompression illness *see* Decompression illness, acute
physiology and physics, 398–9, *399*
Diving reflex, 364
DNA profiling, 621
Documentation, 653–5
chemical incidents, 507
disposal, 644
head injury, 267
mass gathering medicine, 532
respiratory emergencies, 122
at the scene, confidentiality breach, 644
Domesticated animal bites, 193
Donway traction splint, 563, *563*
Dorsal metacarpal veins, 58, *58*
Dorsalis pedis pulse, 205
Dothiepin, 183
Drink driving, 620
Drip stands, 682
Driving techniques, 246–9
cadence braking, 247
cornering safely, 247–8, *247–8*
overtaking, 248–9
safety, 246
stopping safely, 246–7
Droperidol, 458, 463
Drowning *see* Near drowning/drowning
Drug(s), 151–60
action, 154
aims of, 151
and bereavement, 473
choice of, 151–6
clinical condition of the patient, 152–3
contraindications, 154
dosage, 155
electromechanical dissociation, **51**, 52
experience and training of the practitioner, 152
illicit, intoxication, 461
legal classification, 155–6
misuse *see* Substance abuse
packs in use, 156
paramedic practice, 155–6
post-traumatic disorders, 471
pregnant patients, 152–3
routes of administration, **153**, 153–4
schedules, 155
shocked patients, 152
side effects, 154
speed of onset, **153**, 153–5
and the sportsperson, **538**, 538–9
suitability, 152
teratogenicity, 425
toxic confusional states, **349**
transportation, 156, 163
see also specific class; specific drug
DSM-IV, **466**
Ductus arteriosus, 448–9
Dunant, Jean Henri, 8–9, *9*
Duodenum, 298
Duty of care, 648–9

breach of, 648–9
termination, 648
Dysentery, **411**
Dyspnoea
during feeding, in children, 203, 204
pneumothorax, 127
potentially life-threatening causes of, **120**

E
Ear(s)
acute decompression illness, 403
barotrauma, 399, 400
blast injuries, 328, 329
gas expansion, 584
personal protection, 485
Earthquake, *544*, 544–5
Easton, Kenneth, 5, *5*
Ebola fever, **411**
Eclampsia, 429–30
ECPs
response vehicles, 597
training, 598
Ecstasy, 133, 180–1
Ectopic beats, ventricular, *96*, 96–7, *97*
Ectopic pregnancy, 142, 145, 426
management, 426
symptoms, 426
ED 2000, pelvic fractures, 312, *312*
Edinger-Westphal nucleus, 165
Education, 671–7
see also Training
EISEC, 657
Elapidae, 193
Elation, trauma response, 469
Elbow injuries, 310, *310*
Elderly patients, 347–57
access of emergency admissions to acute care, 357
accidents, 356
acute abdomen, 140
adverse drug reactions, 356, **357**
assessment, 347–8
communication, 348
delirium, 460
depression, 353–4
drowning, 383
examination, 348
falls, **352**, 352–3
fits and faints, 354–6
fractures, 356
history, 348
home environment, 348
immobility, 349–50
incontinence, 350–1, **351**
instability, 351–2
intellectual impairment, 348–9, **349**
nature of acute illness, 347–8
non-steroidal anti-inflammatory drugs, 168
physical abuse, 356–7
scalds, 335
stroke, 354
Elective treatment, 635
Electric current, 406
Electrical injuries *see* Electrocution injury

Electricity hazards, 249–50
Electrocardiogram (ECG), 85–103
  abnormalities of rate, 88
  atrioventricular block *see* Atrioventricular
    (AV) node, block
  basic principles, 85–6
  bipolar leads, 87, *87*
  bradycardias *see* Bradycardias
  broad QRS complexes, *90*, *93*, *95–8*, *96*, *97*
  cardiac emergencies, 106–7
  cardiac pacemakers, 102–3
  during chest pain, 98–102, *98–102*
  Diploma in Immediate Medical Care, 674
  electrical injury, 337
  electrode placement, *87*, 87–8
  heat illness, 394
  myocardial infarction, *100–1*, 100–2, 106–7
  near drowning, 385–6, 387
  sequence of cardiac activation, *86*, 86–7, *87*
  tachycardias *see* Tachycardia
  unipolar leads, 87–8
  VF-pulseless VT, 49
Electrocution injury, 337, 405–9
  domestic incidents, 405–6, 408
  immediate care, 407–9
  industrial/occupational incidents, 405, 408
  lightning strike, 406
  occurrence, 405–6
  pathophysiology of injury, 406–7
  in pregnancy, 437
  railway incidents, 408
  relevant electrical principles, 406
Electrolyte disorders
  heat exhaustion, 392
  toxic confusional states, **349**
Electromechanical disassociation (EMD), *51*,
    51–2
  in children, 226–7
  pneumothorax, 127
  potentially reversible causes, **51**, 51–2
Electronic monitoring devices, 683, *683*
Electrons, 515, *515*
Electrothermal burns, 406–7, 409
EM-DAT, 551
Emergency calls, 656–8
Emergency care courses, **245**
Emergency care practitioner *see* ECPs
Emergency medical despatch (EMD) systems,
    499
Emergency Medical Journal (EMJ), 6
Emergency Medical Services (EMS)
  components of a modern system, **11**
  USA, 11, **11**
Emergency medical technician (EMT), 607
Emergency planning, major incidents, 492
Emergency planning officer (EPO), 626
Emergency Reference Levels (ERLs), radiation,
    528, **528**
Emergency reserve channel (ERC), 660
Emergency services, 4
  see also specific service
Emergency treatment, 635–6
Emesis *see* Vomiting
Emotional debriefing, major incidents, 491–2

Emotional neglect, children, 208
Emphysema, 124
  chest compression complications, 21
  surgical airway complications, 39
Encephalitis, **411**
Endocrine disease
  air travel considerations, 592
  in children, 202
Endotracheal tubes, 680–1
  see also Tracheal intubation
Energy reserves, body's response to cold, 363
EnFlow®, 371
Entonox
  acute decompression illness, 403
  in children, 239
  complications, 169
  head injury, 268
  introduction, 4
  physical properties, 169
  remote industrial sites, 381
  thermal injury, 342
Entrapment, 556
  actual, 557
  fire service role, 605–7, 609
  pain relief, 557
  preparation and approach, 557
  relative, 557
  see also Extrication
Environmental control, 236–7
Ephedrine, 181
Epidural drug administration, **153**, 154
Epiglottitis, 203
  in children, 210, **210**
  vs. croup, **210**
Epilepsy
  aeromedical transport considerations, 589
  in children, 215
  in elderly patients, 354–6
  in pregnancy, 431
  respiratory depression in children, 203
  unconscious patients, 136
Epinephrine *see* Adrenaline
Epiphyseal plates, 199
Equipment, 246, 678–84
  aeromedical evacuation, 576
  cleaning, 415
  fire service, 607–9, **608**
  head injury, 267
  major incidents, 485–6
  mass gathering medicine, 532
  medical, 485, 486, **486**, 680–3
  personal protective, 413, **414**, 485–6
  safety, 250, 678–9
  sporting, 535
  susceptible to gaseous expansion, 585, **585**
Equity, 618
Erysipelas, **411**
Erythromycin
  otitis media, 218
  pneumonia, 214
Escherichia coli, 203, 217
Escorts, 246
Esmolol, 92, 113
Esters, 170, 172

Ethanol *see* Alcohol
Ethylene glycol, **187**, 189
Etomidate
  action, 158
  tracheal intubation anaesthesia, 36
Europe, 9–11
European Resuscitation Council (ERC)
  guidelines, 48, 49, *49*
  paediatric life support treatment algorithms,
    226
  paediatric resuscitation guidelines, 221
  Working Group on the Management of
    the Airway and Ventilation during
    Resuscitation, 222
European Society of Cardiology, 109
Eustachian tube, 584
Evacuation, chemical incidents, 506–7
Evaporation, 390, 394
Evisceration, abdominal injuries, 302
Examinations, 5
Exercise
  heat illness, 396
  rewarming, 368
Exhaustion
  drowning, 384
  heat, 392–3, **393**
  hypothermia, 364
Expiration, 277–8
Explosions *see* Blast injuries
Exposure
  injured children, 236–7
  spinal injury, 293
  trauma, 258
Exsanguination, gunshot wounds, 326
External carotid arteries, 273
External jugular vein
  cannulation, 57, 58, *59*, 60
    in children, 225
    near drowning/drowning, 386
  peripheral access, 50
Extracellular fluid (ECF), 68–9, **69**, 70
Extracorporeal blood warming, 367, 371–2
Extradural haemorrhage, 135
Extrapyramidal syndrome, **184**
Extravasation of fluid/drugs, 63
Extrication, 77, 294, 555
  basic principles, 556–7
  devices, 563–5, 682–3 (*see also specific device*)
  fire service role, 605, 606
  rapid, 565–6
  spinal injuries, 294
Eye contact, 477
Eye(s)
  air travel considerations, 591
  balance mechanisms, 351
  injuries, 274
  opening, unconscious patients, 134
  personal protection, 413, **414**, 485, 679

F

F v. West Berkshire Health Authority, 638, 639,
    640–1
Face
  examination in respiratory emergencies, 121

personal protection, 485
trauma *see* Facial trauma
Face masks, 413, 414, **414**
Facial artery, 273
Facial trauma, 272–6
    aeromedical transport considerations, 589
    airway obstruction, 29
    nasotracheal intubation, 35
    see also Maxillofacial injuries
Faculty of Immediate Care, 676–7
Faecal incontinence, 350–1, **351**
Fainting
    elderly patients, 354–6, *355*
    heat syncope, 392
Fallopian tubes torsion, 430
Falls, elderly patients, **352**, 352–3
Famine, 543
Fat embolism
    intraosseous access, 67
    reduction in immobilization, 556
Fatal accidents, confidentiality, 646
Fear, trauma response, 469
Feedback, chemical incidents, 507–8
Feeding
    breathlessness during, in children, 203
    bronchiolitis, 211
Femoral hernia, 143
Femoral injuries, 239
Femoral nerve blocks, 239
Femoral pulse, 205
Femoral vein
    anatomy, 64, *64*
    cannulation, 65, 225
Femur
    fracture
        neck, 312
        proximal, 356
        shaft, 312–13
    intraosseous access, 66, *66*
'Fend-off' position, 249, *249*
Fentanyl, 158, 165–6
Fetus
    assessment, 425
        during childbirth, 440
        in trauma in pregnancy, 434, 435–6
    heart rate, 425, 436
    labour, 442
    maternal burns, 437
    prehospital care, 423
    in road traffic accidents, 434
Fever
    acute abdomen, 142
    breathing, 204
    in children, 218
    diverticular disease, 146
    meningitis, 217
    thermal injury, 333–4
Fibrinolytic Therapy Trialists' Group, 109
Fibula fracture, 305–6, 314, *314*
Field sports injuries, 537
Filtration, 69
Fingerprints, 620–1
Finger(s)
    abduction/abduction, 294

dislocation, 309
    extension, 294
    fractures, *309*, 309–10
Fire, airway obstruction, 27
Fire hazards, 249
Fire Safety and the Safety of Places of Sport
        Act 1987, 530
Fire service, 603–13
    control room, 611
    equipment, 607–9, **608**
    medical training levels in, 607, **607**
    organization and structure, 603–5, *604*
    ranks, 604, *604*
    response, 609–10
    retained firefighters, 604
    role at incidents involving hazardous
            materials, 611–13
    role at major incidents, 609–11
    role at road traffic accident entrapments, 605–7
        extrication, 606
        full access, 606
        glass management, 606
        making the system work, 606–7
        scene assessment and safety, 605
        space creation, 606
        stabilization and initial access, 605–6
Fire Services Act 1947, 603, 604
Fire Services Act 1959, 603
First Aid for Lifeboat Crews, 381
First-aid kits, fire service, 607
First-pass effect, 153, 154
Fits *see* Seizures
Fixed-wing aircraft, 573
Flail chest
    aeromedical evacuation, 574
    chest injuries, 282, **283**
    in children, 234
    trauma, 256, **258**
Flame burns *see* Burns (flame)
Flashbacks, 469
Flashing lights, 246, 568, 680
Flight biodynamics, *586*, 586–7
Floods, 546
Fluid balance, body's response to cold, 363
Fluid insulators and warmers, 682
Fluid loss in children, 205
Fluid maldistribution in children, 204
Fluid overload, 157
Fluid retention, 168
Fluid therapy/replacement, 70–3
    abdominal injuries, 301
    acute abdomen, 147–8
    acute decompression illness, 403
    administration, 78
    blood and blood products, 70
    colloids *see* Colloids
    crystalloids *see* Crystalloids
    electrocution injury, 409
    equipment, 682
    fluid choice, **79**, 79–80
    future advances, 80
    heat exhaustion, 393
    heat illness, 394
    hypotensive resuscitation, 78–9

injured children, 235
    near drowning/drowning, 385, 386
    neonates, 450
    plant and fungi poisoning, 191
    poisoning, 183
    in pregnant patients, 437
    quantities, 80
    shock, 78, **79**, 79–80
    thermal injury, 340–2
    trauma in pregnancy, 435
Flumazenil
    as an antidote, **187**, 189
    benzodiazepines overdose, 136
Fluoxetine, 188
Flying ambulance, 8
Focal seizures, 268
Folate deficiency, **349**
Fontanelles, bulging, 217
Food poisoning, **411**
Foot
    fracture, 314
    plantar flexion, 294
Football injuries, 536
Football Licensing Authority, 530
Football Spectators Act 1989, 530
Forearm fractures, 310
Foreign bodies/material, inhaled
    airway obstruction, 26, 27
    in children, 214
    dental injuries, 274
    head injuries, 274
    maxillofacial injuries, 274
Formaldehyde, 189
Formic acid, 189, 191
Forward control point, 611
Frac® straps, 560
Fractures, 305–14
    blood loss from, 77
    buckle, 307
    butterfly fragment, 306, *307*
    children, 307
    in children, 199–200, 231
    classification, 306–7, *307*
    comminuted, 306, *307*
    complicated, 306
    compound (open), 306, *307*, 309
    crush, *307*
    deformity correction, 308
    depressed, 306
    diagnosis and assessment, 308, **308**
    displaced, *307*
    elderly patients, 356
    electrocution injury, 407
    falls, elderly patients, 352
    greenstick, 239, *307*, 310
    management, 308–9
    maxillofacial injuries, *273*, 273–4
    mechanism of injury, 305–6
    oblique, 306, *307*
    pathological, 306–7
    reduction *see* Reduction
    Salter-Harris classification, 199
    simple (closed), 306, *307*, 308–9
    ski patrolling, 380

Fractures (*Continued*)
spiral, 306, *307*
torus, 239, 307
transverse, *307*
    see also specific bones; specific types
Fragmentation, blasts, 328
France
aeromedical evacuation, 573, 575
prehospital care in, 9–10
French gauge (FG), 59
Frenzel manoeuvre, 584
Fresh frozen plasma (FFP), 80
Frontal bone fracture, 274
Frostbite, 380
Full blood count, radiation casualties, 526
Fuller's earth, **187**, 190
Fundal height, 435–6
Funding, aeromedical evacuation, 575
Fungi, poisonous, 190–2, **191–2**
Furanocoumarins, *192*
Furosemide
action, 157
pulmonary oedema, 111

G

Gallbladder
disease, 144
perforation, 144
Gallstones, 144
Gamma-glutamyl transferase ([3]-GT), 176
Gamma-rays, 517, 518
Gas exchange, 277, **278**, 278–9
Gas leaks, 335
Gaseous expansion, 584–6
Gastric inflation, 45
Gastric irritants, **191**
Gastric lavage, 185
Gastritis, 145
Gastroenteritis, 142, 143, **411**
abdominal pain, 141
in children, 216
at mass gatherings, 532
Gastrointestinal system
alcohol dependence, 174–5
heat illness complications, 395
non-steroidal anti-inflammatory drugs, 168
opioids side-effects, 165
Gelatins, 71, **71**
Gelofusine, 71, **71**, **79**
Gender and sports injuries, 535
General anaesthesia, drugs used for, 157–9
General practitioner-based immediate care, 5, 7
General practitioners (GPs)
cardiac emergencies, 104–5
drug packs in use, 156
mass gathering medicine, 532
thrombolytic therapy, 109
General sales list (GSL) medicines, 155
Genital injuries, 303–4
Genitourinary trauma, 302–4
management, **304**
and pelvic fractures, 299
    see also specific organ/site

Germany
aeromedical evacuation, 575
prehospital care in, 10
Gibson report, 530–1
Gissane, William, 4
Glandular fever, **411**
Glaser® safety slug, 324
Glasgow Coma Scale (GCS)
aeromedical transport considerations, 589
head injury, **264**, 264–5
paediatric scale, 206, 236, **236**
poisoning, 184
primary assessment, 131
secondary assessment, **133**, 133–4
trauma patients, 258, **259**, 662, **662**, 666
using, 265
Global positioning systems (GPS), 659
Gloves, protective, 413, 414, **414**, 679
Glucagon
as an antidote, **187**
beta-blockers overdose, 188
hypoglycaemia, 215
hypothermia, 372
Glucose
hypoglycaemia, 215
hypothermia, 372
mountain rescue, 378
neonates, 450–1
Glue, 181
Glutathione, 187
Glyceryl trinitrate
cardiac emergencies, 107
pulmonary oedema, 111
Glycoalkaloids, **191**
Glycosides, 191, **191**
Gold, **187**
Golden hour, 574
Gowns/overalls, protective, 413, 414, **414**
Grand mal convulsions
after head injury, 268
apnoea, 132
in children, 215
signs, 133
Gravel, 317
Gray (Gy), 517
Green beacons, 680
Green Guide, 530, 531
Greenstick fractures, 239, *307*, 310
Grey Turner's sign, 142, 145
Grief, 471–3
children and bereavement, 472
management of, 472–3
medication, 473
normal reactions, 472, **472**
pathological reactions, 472
poor prognostic indicators, 472, **473**
Griseofulvin, 187
Grunting in children, 204
Guardsman's fracture, 275
Guedel airway, 29, **29**, 222
Guidelines for Advanced Life Support, 48, 49, *49*
Guilt, trauma response, 469
Gunshot/missile wounds, 322–31

abdominal, 299–300
blast injury *see* Blast injuries
brain, 266
chest, 280
patterns of injury, 325–6
in pregnancy, 437
prevalence and epidemiology, 322–3
safety, immediate assessment and resuscitation, 326–7
shotguns and airguns, 326
wound ballistics, **323**, *323*, 323–5
high energy transfer, 325
interaction of bullets with the tissues, *324*, 324–5
low energy transfer, 325
Gut decontamination, 185–6, 191–2

H

Haemaccel, 71, **71**, **79**
Haemarthrosis, 319, *319*
Haematemesis, 141
abdominal aortic aneurysm, 143
in children, 203
Haematocrit, 79, 589
Haematological complications of heat illness, 395
Haematological investigations, radiation casualties, 526
Haematological problems, alcohol dependence, 175
Haematoma
airway obstruction, 26
central venous cannulation, 65
peripheral venous cannulation, 63
subcutaneous, 317
trismus, 276
Haematuria
acute abdomen, 141–2
bladder injury, 302
heat illness, 395
pelvic fractures, 302
renal calculus disease, 145
renal injury, 303
Haemoglobin (Hb), 583–4, *584*
in aeromedical transport, 589
dissociation curve, 128, *128*
oxygen affinity, 41
oxygenated *see* Oxygenated haemoglobin (HbO₂)
pulse oximetry, 127–8
Haemoglobin solutions, 80
Haemoglobinopathies, **184**
Haemolysis, hypothermia rewarming, 372
Haemolytic-uraemic syndrome, 203
Haemophilus influenzae, 214
meningitis, 217
resistance to antibiotics, 218
Haemophilus influenzae b (Hib), 210
Haemopoietic system in pregnancy, 423
Haemorrhage
abdominal vessels causing life-threatening, **299**
blood loss from fractures, **79**
in children, 203

crystalloid colloid controversy, 72
fluid administration, 78
gunshot wounds, 326
hypovolaemic shock, 75
injured children, 235–6
intra-abdominal *see* Intra-abdominal bleeding
intrathoracic, 77
major incidents, 491
maxillofacial injuries, 272, 274–5
pelvic, 77
pelvic fractures, 300
penetrating neck trauma, 269
postpartum, 445
in pregnancy, 423, 425, 436 (*see also*
    Antepartum haemorrhage (APH))
shock, 77
source of, 257
surgical airway complications, 38
trauma, 257
    see also specific site
Haemorrhagic shock
drugs in, 152
ectopic pregnancy, 145
Haemothorax
central venous cannulation, 65
chest injuries, 281
injured children, 234
massive, **258**, 283, **283**
Hagen-Poiseuille law, 67–8
Hallucinations
alcoholic, 175
depression, 353
fungi, 191
psychosis, 457
Hallucinogens, 180–1, 461
Haloperidol, 458, 463, 464
Hand signals, 490
Handguns
injuries *see* Gunshot/missile wounds
legislation, 322
Hand(s)
as a communication tool, 477, 490
examination in respiratory emergencies,
    121
extension, 294
fractures, 309–10
protection, 679
vein distribution, 57–8, *58*
washing, 414
Hard-tissue injury *see* Fractures
Hare traction splint, *561*, 561–2
Harmful use, definition, 173
Hartmann's solution, 70, **70**
    heat illness, 394
    shock, 79
    thermal injury, 340
Hazard assessment, fire service role, 609
Hazardous Area Response Teams (HARTs), 508
Hazardous materials *see* Chemical incidents;
    specific material
Hazardous use, definition, 173–4
Head
heat loss through, 362, 369
injury *see* Head injury

Head injury, 260–70
aeromedical transport considerations,
    589
airway, 253
analgesia, 268
breathing, 204
and cervical spine injury, 135
in children, 198, 236, 238, **238**
early seizures, 268
epidemiology, 260
examination priorities, 263–4
history, 263
horse riding, 536
hospital transfer, 266–7
ketamine, 158, 169
managing early deterioration, 267–8, **268**
neurological assessment
    primary survey, 264
    secondary survey, **264**, 264–5
primary survey, 264
respiratory depression in children, 203
secondary survey
    looking at the injuries, 265
    neurological assessment, **264**, 264–5
toxic confusional states, **349**
tracheal intubation, 31
unconscious patients, 135
using the Glasgow Coma Scale, 265
vomiting, in children, 203
    see also Brain injury
Head lamps, flashing, 680
Head tilt, 18, *19*
airway obstruction, 28, *28*
in children, 204, 222
Headache, subarachnoid haemorrhage,
    135–6
Health and Safety (First Aid) Regulations 1981
    Approved Code of Practice, 607
Health preservation procedures, 639, 640
Health Protection Agency (HPA), 503
Heart
auscultation *see* Heart auscultation
block *see* Heart block
failure *see* Heart failure
position in children, 198
in pregnancy, 421
rate *see* Heart rate
response to shock, 76
sounds *see* Heart sounds
    see also entries beginning Cardiac; *entries*
        beginning Cardio-Heart auscultation
myocardial infarction, 106
pulmonary oedema, 110
Heart block
AV block *see* Atrioventricular (AV) node,
    block
bundle branch block, 97, *97*, *98*
cardiac emergencies, 108–9
complete *see* Atrioventricular (AV) node,
    block
electrocution injury, 407
frequency of, within 4 h of myocardial
    infarction, **106**
SA block, 94, *94*

Heart failure
in children, 203
fluid maldistribution, 204
Heart rate
abnormalities, 88 (*see also specific*
    abnormality)
in children, **200**
fetus, 425
neonates, 449, **449**
in pregnancy, 422
Heart sounds
fourth, 106
respiratory emergencies, 121
third, 110
Heat exhaustion, 392–3, **393**
Heat illness, 389–96
acclimatization, 390–1, **391**
assessment, 393–4
complications, 394–5
cooling techniques, 394
education and awareness, 395
heat loss mechanisms, 390, **390**, **391**
heat production mechanisms, 390, **391**
identification of susceptible individuals,
    395–6
increased heat production, 392
major, 393, **394**
mass gatherings, 531
minor, 392–3, **393**
normal body temperature, 390
pathogenesis, 391
prevention, 395–6, **396**
recognition of risk factors, 396
reduced heat loss, 392
resuscitation, 394
risk factors for, **391**, 391–2
temperature regulation, 389–90, **390**
treatment, 394
Heat loss, 362
in children, 236–7
heat illness, **391**
mechanisms of, 390, **390**
neonates, 450
reduced, 392
thermal injury, 333–4
Heat production, 362
heat illness, **391**
increased, 392
mechanisms of, 390, **390**
Heat stress index, 396, **396**
Heat syncope, 392
Heatstroke, 393
differential diagnosis, **394**
inherited abnormalities, 396
signs and symptoms, **393**
vs. heat exhaustion, 392
Heavy hydrogen, 515
Heavy metals poisoning, 186, **187**
Heimlich manoeuvre, 22–3, *24*
in children, 214
contraindication in children, 198, 214
Helicopter Emergency Medical Service (HEMS),
    5, 6–7, 570, 575, 576–7, 579

Helicopters, 573, 597
  choice of, 577–8
  clinical rationale, 574–5
  mountain rescue, 377–8
  sea rescue, 381
  search and rescue, 381
  types of, *578*, 578–9, *579*
    see also Aeromedical evacuation
Helmets, 485, 679, *679*
Helplessness, trauma response, 469, 470
Hemlock, 191–2
Henoch-Schönlein purpura, 203
Henry's law, 399, 401
Heparin, atrial fibrillation, 113
Hepatitis A virus (HAV), **411**
Hepatitis B immunoglobulin (HBIG), 412
Hepatitis B virus (HBV), **411**
  classification, 410
  immunization, 412–13
  postexposure prophylaxis, 415–16
  risk to health-care workers, 411–12
  transmission, 411–12
Hepatitis C virus (HCV), **411**, 412
Hernias, bowel obstruction, 146
Heroin see Diamorphine
Herpes simplex, 412
Herpes zoster, **105**, **411**
Hetastarch, **71**, 71–2
Hidden Report, Clapham railway incident, 6
High arm sling, 560, *560*
High energy transfer wounds, 325
High-visibility clothing, 485–6, 678–9, *679*
Highway Safety Act, 11
Highway Traffic Safety Programme, 11
Hill walking, 537–8
Hillsborough Stadium tragedy, 484, 529
Hip
  dislocation, 312
  fracture, 356
  fractures around, 312
Histamine
  anaphylaxis, 76
  response to shock, 77
  stings, 194
History
  major incidents, 484
  triage, 493–4
  UK, 3–5, **6**
  worldwide, 8–9
History (patient)
  abdominal pain, 140–1
  acute abdomen see Acute abdomen, history
  childbirth, 440
  critically ill children, 200–2, *202*
  elderly patients, 348
  head injury, 263
  pregnancy, 424–5
  premature neonates, 202
  psychiatric patients, 456, **457**
  respiratory emergencies, 120
  soft-tissue injuries, 316
  unconscious patients, 131, 133
HLA typing, radiation casualties, 526
Hockey injuries, 536

Holmes-Adie pupils, 206
Home Office, 614, 615
Home Office Addicts Index, 177
Home visits, assault at, 477, **478**
Honey bees, 193–4
Hong Kong, 13
Hormesis, radiation, 520
Hormones, response to shock, 77
Horse riding injuries, 536
Hospital care, contaminated casualties, 511
Hospital Flying Squads, 6–7
Hospital information, radiation incidents, 527–8
Hot baths, rewarming, 369
H_2-receptor-blockers, 421
Hudson-type masks, 43, 422
Human immunodeficiency virus (HIV), **411**
  classification, 410
  postexposure prophylaxis, 415–16
  risk to health-care workers, 411–12
  transmission, 411–12
Human radiation levels, 518
Human reactions to trauma, 465–75
  anger, 469
  autonomic hyperarousal, 469
  avoidant behaviour, 469–70
  breaking bad news, 473
  children, 467
  chronicity of post-traumatic conditions, 468
  cognitive changes, 469
  depression, 469
  effect on staff, 473–4
  elation, 469
  fear, 469
  flashbacks, 469
  formal treatment methods, 471
  grief, 471–3, **472**, **473**
  guilt, 469
  helplessness, 469
  historical background, 465–6
  ICD-10, **466**, 466–7
  impaired sleep, 469
  interventions, 470–1
  irritability, 469
  normal reactions, **468**, 468–70
  numbness and denial, 468
  order out of chaos, 466
  pathological reactions and severe stress, **466**, 466–8
  prevalence of post-traumatic syndromes, 467
  prognostic factors, 468
  psychological first aid, 470, **470**
  psychological triage, 470–1
Humerus
  fracture, 310–11
  neck, fracture, 311
Hurricanes, 546–7, **547**
Hydration, 396
Hydrocarbons poisoning, 186
Hydrocephalus, 202
Hydrocortisone
  action, 157
  anaphylaxis, 81
  asthma, 123, 213

Hydrofluoric acid burns, 336, 337
Hydrogen radioactivity, *515*, 515–16
Hydrophiidae, 193
Hydrostatic pressure, 69, 110
Hydrostatic squeeze, 385
Hydroxyethyl starch (HES), **71**, 71–2, **79**
5-Hydroxytryptamine, **192**, 193, 194
Hyoscine, **191**
Hyoscyamine, **191**
Hyperarousal, trauma response, 469
Hyperbaric treatment, acute decompression illness, 402, 403
Hypercapnia
  opiates, 107
  opioids side-effects, 164
  respiratory pathophysiology, 278
Hypercarbia
  airway obstruction, 26
  injured children, 234
  secondary brain damage, 262, 267
  surgical airway complications, 38
Hyperglycaemia
  in children, 215–16
  diabetic patients, 137
  toxic confusional states, **349**
Hyperinflation of the chest, bronchiolitis, 211
Hyperkalaemia
  electromechanical dissociation, **51**, 51–2
  treatment, 157
Hypertension
  beta-blockers, 108
  ketamine, 158, 169
  in pregnancy, 429–30, **430**
  treatment, 157
  unconscious patients, 135
Hypertonic saline, 71
Hypertonic solutions, 69, 71, **79**
Hyperventilation
  anxiety disorders, 460
  management, 460
  pulmonary fibrosis, 125
Hypnotics, adverse reactions in elderly patients, **357**
Hypobaric (hypoxic) hypoxia, 584, **585**
Hypocalcaemia
  blood transfusion, 80
  electromechanical dissociation, **51**, 51–2
Hypocapnia, anxiety disorders, 460
Hypochondria, elderly patients, 353
Hypoglycaemia
  in children, 215
  diabetic patients, 137
  hypothermia, 372
  neonates, 450
  toxic confusional states, **349**
  treatment, 157
  unconscious patients, 131
Hypokalaemia
  asthma, 123
  hypertonic saline, 71
Hyponatraemia, toxic confusional states, **349**
Hypoperfusion, 74–5
Hypostop, 137

Hypotension
  abdominal aortic aneurysm, 143
  bradycardia and, 108
  fluid administration, 78
  heat illness, 394
  and nitrates, 111
  propofol, 158
  resuscitation, 78–9
  spinal injuries, 293
  supine hypotension syndrome, 422
  trauma, 257
  unconscious patients, 135
Hypothalamus, 361
Hypothermia, 361–73
  acute (immersion), 364
  basic life support, 20
  cold risk, 361
  death in, 366–7
  definition and classification, 362–4
  diagnosis, **365**, 365–6, *366*
  drowning/near drowning, 384
  effects of cold exposure, **362**
  electromechanical dissociation, **51**, 52
  late effects, 372
  mountain rescue, **377**, 378
  mountaineering and hillwalking, 537
  other treatment, 372
  practical management, 372–3
  regulation of body temperature, 361–2
  rescue from remote places, 376
  resuscitation, 373, **373**
  rewarming, 367–72
    active, 367
    central, *370*, 370–2, *371*
    combination treatment, 367–8
    correct diagnosis and, 365
    practical recommendations, 372–3
    spontaneous, 367, 368–9
    surface heating, 369–70
  ski patrolling, 380
  spinal injuries transportation, 296
  subacute (exhaustion), 364
  subchronic (urban), 364
  superacute (submersion), 364
  thermal injury, 334
  types of, 364–5
  unconscious patients, 133, 137
  watersports, 537
  wind-chill chart, **363**
Hypotonic solutions, 69
Hypoventilation, tracheal intubation, 31
Hypovolaemia
  aeromedical transport considerations, 591
  breathing, 204
  chest injuries, 277
  in children, 205, 206, 235
  earthquake, 544
  electromechanical dissociation, 51, **51**
  gunshot wounds, 326–7
  oxygen and brain injury, 261
  in pregnancy, 434
  respiratory emergencies, 120
  shivering, 369
  shock, 77

spinal injuries, 293
tachypnoea, 132
unconscious patients, 135
Hypovolaemic shock
  abdominal injuries, 301
  burns, 333
  classification, 75–6
  electrical injury, 337
  maxillofacial injuries, 272
Hypoxia
  airway obstruction, 26
  blood transfusion, 80
  carbon monoxide poisoning, 189
  causes, 41–2, **42**
  chest injuries, 277
  in children, 206, 220, 234
  definition, 41
  drowning/near drowning, 384, 385
  electromechanical dissociation, 51, **51**
  hypobaric (hypoxic), 584, **585**
  injured children, 234
  opiates, 107
  opioids side-effects, 164
  oxygen therapy, 41
  pneumothorax, 126–7
  poisoning, 183
  pulmonary fibrosis, 125
  pulse oximetry, 128
  respiratory emergencies, 120
  respiratory failure, 125
  respiratory pathophysiology, 278
  secondary brain damage, 262, 267
  signs and symptoms, **585**
  spinal injuries, 293
  surface heating, 369
  surgical airway complications, 38
  toxic confusional states, **349**
  tracheal intubation complications, 32
Hypoxic gap, 385

I
Ibotenic acid, **192**
Ibrox Park, 530
Ibuprofen, 169
ICD-10, **466**, 466–7
Identification cards, 679, *679*
Idioventricular rhythm, 97, 108
Illicit drug intoxication, 461
Immediate care
  current climate, 6–7
  definition, 3
  development of, 5
  doctors and standards of care, 634
  future, 7
  history
    UK, 3–5, **6**
    worldwide, 8–9
  legal issues, 634, 635–6
  in the UK, 3–7
  worldwide, 8–13
Immediate Care Course, 6
Immersion hypothermia, 364 *see also* Near drowning/drowning
Immobility, elderly patients, 349–50

Immobilization, 555
  basic principles, 556
  blood loss reduction, 556
  cervical spine injury, 270
  in children, 295
  fat emboli reduction, 556
  injured children, 233
  methods, 557–63 (*see also specific method*)
  pain relief, 556
  prevention of further injury, 556
  spinal injury, 294–5 *see also specific immobilization device*
Immunization
  aid workers, 550
  of prehospital health-care workers, 412–13
Immunocompromised patients, acute abdomen, 140
Immunoglobulin E (IgE)
  anaphylaxis, 76
  asthma, 122
Impaled objects removal, 301–2
Impetigo, **411**
Inborn errors of metabolism, 215
Incident control point (ICP), 250, 611
Incompetent adults, consent, 640–1, 642
Incontinence, elderly patients, 350–1, **351**
Induced abortion, 426
Induction agents, 36, 157–8 *see also specific drugs*
Industrial sites, remote, 381
Infants
  definition, 197, **198**
  surface area, 198
Infection(s), 410–16
  adoption of safe working practices, 413–15, **414**
  after miscarriage, 427
  air travel considerations, 592
  classification, 410, **411**
  divers, 404
  elderly patients, 347
  immunization of emergency health-care workers, 412–13
  intraosseous access, 67
  personal protective equipment, 413
  post exposure prophylaxis, 415–16
  respiratory depression in children, 203
  risk to BLS giver, 18
  risk to emergency health-care workers, 411–12
  surgical airway complications, 39
  toxic confusional states, **349**
Inferior vena cava
  anatomy, 298
  compression in pregnancy, 422–3
  obstruction, 422
  vascular access in children, 225
Inflammatory bowel disease, 141, 142
Inflammatory mediators, 333, *333*
Inflammatory response
  burns and scalds, 333, *333*
  smoke inhalation, 339
Inflatable splints, 560
Influenza immunization, 413
Informed consent *see* Consent

Inhalation drug administration, 153, **153**
Inhalation injury, 338–40, 339
  aeromedical transport considerations, 591
  blasts, 330
Injured children, 220, 221, 230–40
  abdominal injury, 238–9
  airway, 232, **232**
  analgesia, 239
  anatomical and physiological characteristics, 231
  breathing, **234**, 234–5
  circulation, 235–6
  disability and head injury, 236, **236**
  exposure and environmental control, 236–7
  extremity injury, 239
  future growth and development, 231
  head injury, 238
  immediate action on arrival, 230–2
  indications for hospital assessment, **238**
  mechanism of injury, 231
  non-accidental injury, 240, **240**
  pelvic and femoral injuries, 239
  primary survey and resuscitation, 232–7
  psychological implications, 231–2
  secondary survey and definitive care, **238**, 238–9
  spine control, 233, *233*
  transportation, 239–40
  triage, **237**, 237–8
Injury Minimization Programme for Schools (IMPS), 677
Injury Severity Score (ISS), 665–6, 666
In-line stabilization, spinal injuries, 292, *292, 293*
Insect bites/stings, 193–4
Inspiration, 44, 277
Instability, elderly patients, 351–2
Institute of Health Care Development (IHCD), 594, 598
Institute of Naval Medicine, 398
Insulin, hyperglycaemia, 216
Insurance companies, medical negligence, 647
Insurance reports, confidentiality, 647
Intellectual impairment, elderly patients, 348–9
Intercostal muscles, 277
  breathing, 44
  innervation, 44
Intermittent positive pressure ventilation (IPPV)
  pneumothorax, 127
  urban hypothermia, 364
Internal cardiac compression, 54
Internal carotid arteries, 121, 273
Internal jugular vein
  anatomy, 63, *63*
  cannulation, 65
    in children, 225
    pneumothorax, 127
Internally displaced people, **547**, 547–8
International Classification of Mental and Behavioural Disorders, **466**, 466–7
International Commission on Radiological Protection (ICRP), 519, **520**

International Consensus on Cardiopulmonary Resuscitation and Emergency Cardiovascular Care Science with Treatment Recommendations (COSTR), 220–1
International Liaison Committee on Resuscitation (ILCOR), 48, 220–1, 225–6
International medical aid, 548–9
International Programme on Chemical Safety, 503–4
International Red Cross, 628
Interstitial fibrosis, 124
Interstitial fluid, 68
Interstitial pulmonary oedema, 339
Intestinal worms, **411**
Intoxication
  alcohol, 461
  definition, 174
  spinal cord injury, 291
Intra-abdominal bleeding
  in children, 235
  hypovolaemic shock, 301
  treatment, 301
Intra-abdominal injury, stab wounds, 299
Intra-abdominal pressure increase, 299, 300
Intracellular fluid (ICF), 68–9, **69**
Intracranial haematoma
  pupils, 132
  secondary brain damage, 263
  time to removal, 574
Intracranial haemorrhage, toxic confusional states, **349**
Intracranial infection, secondary brain damage, 263
Intracranial pressure, 135
  ketamine, 158
  lowering, 236
  mannitol, 160
  normal mean, 262
  raised *see* Raised intracranial pressure
Intramuscular drug administration, 153, **153**, 167
Intranasal drug administration, 167
Intraoral swelling, 275
Intraosseous access, 57, 66–7
  anatomy, 66, *66*
  in children, 225, *225*, 235
  complications, 67, 225
  contraindications in injured patients, 235
  drug administration, 153, **153**
  equipment, 66–7, *67*, 682
  fluid flow through intraosseous needles, 68
  head injury, 267
  technique, 67
Intraperitoneal haemorrhage, 142, 144–5
Intraperitoneal organs, 298
Intrapleural space, 277
Intrathoracic haemorrhage, 77
Intrathoracic pressure, assisted ventilation, 44
Intrathoracic volume, 277
Intravascular fluid, 68
Intravenous access/cannulation, 57–73
  abdominal injuries, 301

  aeromedical evacuation, 576
  aeromedical transport considerations, 590
  chest injuries, 281
  in children, 235
  drug administration, 153, **153**, 167
  equipment, 682
  head injury, 267
  near drowning/drowning, 385, 386, 387
  neonates, 450
  in pregnancy, 425, 435
  rewarming, 370–1, 372
  shock, 78
  trauma, 257, 435
  unconscious patients, 131, 135
  see also specific route
Intussusception, 203
  bowel obstruction, 146
  in children, 204, 207, 216
  diarrhoea, 204
Ionization, 515, *515*
Ionizing radiation, 337–8, 514–15, 523, *523*
  see also Radiation; Radiation incidents
Ionizing Radiation Regulations (IRR) 1985, 520, 522
Ipratropium bromide
  asthma, 123, 213
  bronchiolitis, 211
Iron, antidote for poisoning, **187**
Irrigation of body cavities, rewarming, 367
Irritability, trauma response, 469
Ischaemia
  acute decompression illness, 403
  electrocution injury, 407
  limb, 318
  pain, 141
  tissue, drowning/near drowning, 384
  visceral pain, 140
Isolation following trauma, 470
Isotonic solutions, 69, 70, **79**
Israel, 12–13

J

J waves, 365, *366*
Jaundice, acute abdomen, 142
Jaw thrust, 18, *19*
  airway obstruction, 28, *28*
  in children, 204, 222
  spinal injuries, *293*
Jealousy, alcohol dependence, 175
Jellyfish, 193
Joint Aviation Authority (JAA), 576–7
Joint dislocations *see* Dislocations
Joint Royal Colleges and Ambulance Liaison Committee (JRCALC), 155
Jones, Sir Robert, 4, *4*
Journal of Accident and Emergency Medicine, 6
Journal of Pre-Hospital and Immediate Care, 5–6
Jugular veins *see* External jugular vein; Internal jugular vein
Jugular venous pulse (JVP)
  abnormalities, 121, **121**
  cardiac tamponade, 283
Justification, radiation protection, 520

K

Kelocyanor kit, 381
Kendrick extrication device (KED), 77, 294, 295, 312, 563–4
Ketamine, 169–70
  action, 158
  adverse effects, 169–70
  as an analgesic, 170
  asthma, 213
  in children, 239
  physiological effects, 169
  tracheal intubation anaesthesia, 36
  vs. midazolam, 158
Ketorolac, 168
Kidneys
  anatomy, 298
  blunt abdominal injuries, 299
  failure, toxic confusional states, **349**
  function, non-steroidal anti-inflammatory drugs, 168
  heat illness complications, 395
  injury, 299, 303, **303**
  see also entries beginning Renal
KILO code, 644
Kinins
  anaphylaxis, 76
  response to shock, 77
Knee
  acute swelling, 319, *319*
  extension, 294
  fractures, 313
  fractures around the, 313
  patella *see* Patella
  supracondylar fractures, 313
Knife injury *see* Stab wounds
Kussmaul respiration, 132
Kussmaul's sign, cardiac tamponade, 283

L

Labour
  Apgar score, 442
  baby, 442
  cord, 441–2
  crowning of the head, 441
  first stage, 440–1, *441*
  restitution, 441, *443*
  second stage, *441*, 441–2, *442*, *444*
  shoulders, 442
  third stage, 442–5
  see also Childbirth
Lactic acidosis
  alcohol ingestion, 174
  in hypothermia, 369
  shock, 77
Laerdal pocket mask, **30**, 30–1, *31*
  ventilation, 44, **45**
  vs. bag/valve/mask (BVM) device, 30
Land mines, 543
Landing site, aeromedical evacuation, 577
Landslide, 545–6
Laparotomy, intra-abdominal bleeding, 301
Large bowel
  gunshot wounds, 299
  obstruction, 141

stab wounds, 299
Larrey, Baron Dominique Jean, 8, *8*, 493
Laryngeal mask airway (LMA), *36*, 681
  advanced life support, 50
  advantages, 36
  in children, 222
  contraindications, 36
  disadvantages, 36–7
  indications, 36
  sizes, **36**
  using, 37
Laryngeal oedema, 591
Laryngoscope, 222, *223*, 681
Laryngotracheobronchitis, 203, 209–10, **210**
Larynx
  blunt trauma, 269
  direct trauma to, 275
  injuries, 269, 275, 283–4
  oedema, 338
Lassa fever, **411**
Lateral cutaneous nerve of the forearm, 58
Lava flows, 546
Law
  common, 618
  process of, 618–19
  road traffic, 619–20
  statute, 618
Law of Torts, The, 639
Le Fort fracture, 275
Lead, antidote for poisoning, **187**
Learning, 672
Lecturers, 672–3
Left ventricular failure
  atrial fibrillation, 113
  treatment, 157
Left ventricular hypertrophy, 99, *99*
Left-atrial pressure, 110
Legionellosis, **411**
Legislation/legal issues, 633–52
  autonomy, 636
  beneficence, 636–7
  Bolam test, 634–5, 636, 648–9
  confidentiality, 643–7
  consent
    conscious patients, 640–1
    obtaining, 638
    refusal of, 642–34
    treatment without, 638–43
    unconscious patients, 639–40
  dealing with death/disposing of corpses, 650–2
  elective treatment, 635
  emergency treatment/immediate care, 635–6
  immediate care doctor and standards of care, 634
  medical cover at mass gatherings, 530–1
  medical negligence, 647–50
  patient's best interests, 637
  therapeutic privilege, 637–8
  urgent treatment, 635
Leprosy, **411**
Leptospirosis, **411**
Leuconostoc mesenteroides, 72

Lidocaine, 172
  advanced life support, 50
  bradycardias, 108
  ventricular dysrhythmias, 189
  ventricular tachycardia, 114
Life support
  advanced *see* Advanced life support
  basic *see* Basic life support (BLS)
  paediatric *see* Paediatric life support
Lifeboats, 380–1
Life-saving procedures, 639, 640
Lifting equipment, fire service, 608
Ligaments
  definition, 315
  injuries, 315, 319, *319*
Lightning strike, 406, 408, 409
Lignocaine *see* Lidocaine
Limb immobilization, 559–63, 683
  box (Loxley) splint, 560–1, *561*
  Frac straps®, 560
  inflatable splints, 560
  manual methods, 559
  neighbour strapping, 560
  SAM® splint, 561
  simple methods, 559
  traction splint *see* Traction splints
  triangular bandage, 559–60, *560*
Limb ischaemia, 318
Limb trauma, 305–14
  in children, 239
  life-threatening, 305, *305*
  see also Fractures *specific injury*
Limit point technique, 247–8, *248*
Linear acceleration, 586, *586*
Listeria monocytogenes, 217
Listeriosis, **411**
Liver
  alcohol dependence, 175
  blunt abdominal injuries, 299
  failure, toxic confusional states, **349**
  gunshot wounds, 299
  heat illness complications, 395
  stab wounds, 299
  trauma, 21, 300
Lloyd airway warming equipment, 370, *370*, *371*
Local anaesthesia, 170–2
  agents (anaesthetics), **171**, 172
  characteristics of amide local anaesthetics, **171**
  in children, 239
  clinical considerations, 170
  complications, 171
  metabolism, 170
  pharmacology, 170
  prehospital considerations, 172
  and sportspeople, 538
Local authorities, major incidents, 625–6
Local infiltration of drugs, 153, **153**
Local irradiation, 526
Locard's law, 621
Lockerbie bombing, 626
Log books, 655
Log rolling, 292, 565

Long saphenous vein cannulation, 57, 58, *58*, 62
Long spinal boards, *564*, 564–5, *565*, 683
Long-duration accelerations, 586
Loop diuretics, 111
Lorazepam
  anxiety disorders, 460
  epilepsy, 215
  fits after head injury, 238
  rapid tranquillization, 463
  seizures, 268
  status epilepticus, 136
Low energy transfer wounds, 325
Lower limb fractures, 312–14
Loxley splint, 560–1, *561*
LSD (lysergic acid diethylamide), 180
Lund & Browder chart, 340, *341*
Lung(s)
  auscultation, pulmonary oedema, 110
  barotrauma, 400
  blast injuries, 328
  in hypothermia, 366, *366*
  injury in children, 234
  malignancy, chest pain, **105**
  mechanism of injury, 339
  neonates, 448–9
  in pregnancy, 421
  respiratory pathophysiology, 278–9
  respiratory portion, 277
  thermal injury, 338–40
    see also entries beginning Pulmonary
Lupinine, **191**
Lysergic acid diethylamide (LSD), 180

M

MAC A scheme, 627–8
Mackintosh blade, 222
McBurney's point, 144
McInnes stretcher, 377, *379*
Magen David Adom (MDA), 12–13
Magic mushrooms, 180
Magnesium
  asthma, 123
  pre-eclampsia, 430
  supraventricular tachycardia, 113
  tachycardia, 93
MAGPAS (Mid-Anglia General Practitioner
    Accident Service), 5
Major Incident Medical Management and
    Support (MIMMS) course, 250, 487,
    494, 676
Major incidents, 483–92
  ambulance service, 595
  armed forces, 626–8, *627*
  classification, 483–4, **484**
  command, *487*, 487–8
  communications, 660
  community reconstruction, 492
  compensated, 484
  compound, 483–4
  definition, 483, 622
  emergency planning, 492
  equipment, 485–6, **486**
  fire service role, 609–11
  history, 484

local authorities, 625–6
man-made, 483, **484**
natural, 483, **484**
operational and emotional debriefing, 491–2
phases, 623–4
planning, 484, 485, **485**
police service role, 622–4
preparation, 485–7
prevention, 484–5
recovery, 491–2
response, *487*, 487–91
role of other agencies, 625–30
safety, 488, **488**
simple, 483
structure, 488–91, *489*, **490**
training, 486–7, 675–6
triage, 491, 494
uncompensated, 484
voluntary services, 628–30, *630*
Major Trauma Outcome Study (MTOS), 5,
    655, 667
Malaria, **411**
  refugees, 547
  transmission, 412
Malignancy
  bowel obstruction, 146
  pathological fractures, 306
  radiation exposure, 519
Malnutrition, disasters, 542, 547
Manchester Ship Canal, 3, *4*
Mandible dislocation, 276
Mandibular fracture, 273, *273*
  airway obstruction, 29
  loss of tongue control, 275
Mania, 459–60
Man-made disasters, 540, **541**
Mannitol
  action, 160
  head injury, 236
Manual in-line stabilization (MILS), 292, *292*
Marburg disease, **411**
Marijuana *see* Cannabis
Marine animal bites, 193
Marrow embolism, intraosseous access, 67
Mask depression, 353
Mask squeeze, 400
Mass gathering medicine, 529–33
  clothing, 532
  documentation, 532
  equipment, 532
  legislation, 530–1
  medical skills, 531–2
Maternal death, **420**
Maxilla fracture, 273, *273*
  airway obstruction, 29
  posterior impaction of, 275
    see also Maxillofacial injuries
Maxillofacial injuries, 272–6
  airway management, 274–5
  classification of injury, *273*, 273–4
  dental injuries, 274
  eye injuries, 274
  haemorrhage management, 274
  hard-tissue injury, *273*, 273–4

mechanism of injury, 272–3
  soft-tissue injury, 273
  trismus and lower jaw dislocation, 276
*Maynard v. West Midlands Regional Health
    Authority*, 639
MDMA (Ecstasy), 133, 180–1
Mean arterial pressure (MAP), 262
Mean corpuscular volume (MCV), 176
Mean intracranial pressure (MICP), 262
Measles, **411**, 547
Mechanical ventilators, 45
Meckel's diverticulum, 203
Meconium aspiration, 451–2
Media, major incidents, 490, 624
Medial cutaneous nerve of the forearm, 58
Median nerve, 58
Median vein of the forearm, 58, *58*
Mediastinal bleeding, chest compression
    complications, 21
Medical Emergency Response Incident Teams
    (MERITs), 508
Medical Equestrian Foundation, 7
Medical equipment, 485, 486, **486**, 680–3
    see also specific item
Medical negligence, 647–50
  criteria for, 648–50
  damage, 649–50
  duty of care, 648–9
  reason for increase in, 647–8
Medical Priority Despatch, 575
Medical teams, disasters, 549
Medical transport, 568–9
MedicAlert® bracelets, 152
Medication *see* Drug(s)
Medicines Act 1968, 155
Memory, 672
Meningitis, 217, **411**
  in children, 203, 207, 216, 217, 218
  facemask ventilation, 44
  meningococcal, 218
  signs, 207
  vomiting, in children, 203
Meningococcal septicaemia, 205, 218
Meningococcus immunization, 413
Mental Health Act 1983, 456, 461–2
  section 2: admission for assessment, 461–2
  section 3: admission for treatment, 462
  section 4: admission in an emergency, 462
  section 5(2), 462
  section 135, 462
  section 136, 462
Mental illness *see* Psychiatric emergencies
Mental state examination, 456–7
Mental status, spinal cord injury, 292
Meptazinol, 166
Mercury, antidote for poisoning, **187**
Mesenteric infarction, 140, 143, 145
Mesentery, gunshot wounds, 299
Metabolic acidosis, 41
  blood transfusion, 80
  cyanide poisoning, 190
  drowning/near drowning, 384
  hypertonic saline, 71
  tachypnoea, 132

treatment, 157
Metabolic problems/emergencies
 alcohol dependence, 175
 in children, 215–16
Metacarpal fracture, 309, *309*
Methadone, 179
Methaemoglobin, 129, 190
Methaemoglobinaemia, 170, 172
Methicillin-resistant *Staphylococcus aureus*
 (MRSA), 410, **411**
Methionine, 187
Methyl alcohol, **187**, 189
Methylene blue, 172, **187**
Methylhydroxybenzoate, 170
Methylphenidate, 179
Methylprednisolone, 160
Metoclopramide
 antidote for poisoning, **187**
 vomiting, 107
Metoprolol, 108
Metropolitan police force, 614
Mettag labels, *498*, 498–9
Mid-Anglia General Practitioner Accident
 Service (MAGPAS), 675
Midazolam
 action, 158
 vs. ketamine, 158
Midwives, 439–40
Military antishock trousers (MAST), 563
Milk, caustic ingestions, 186
Miller Report, 4
Ministry of Defence, 627
Ministry of Defence Nuclear Accident
 Organization, 522
Miosis, 165
Mirtazapine, 471
Miscarriage, 426–7
 classification, *427*
 definition, 426
 differential diagnosis, 426
 features, 426
 incomplete, 424, 427
 induced, 426
 management, 426–7
 spontaneous, 426
 vaginal examination, 424
Misuse, definition, 173
Misuse of Drugs Act 1971, 155, **178**
Misuse of Drugs Regulations 1985, 155
Mobitz type 1 block, 94, *95*
Mobitz type 2 block, 94, *95*
Monoamine oxidase inhibitors, 471
Monomethylhydrazine, **192**
Morbid jealousy, alcohol dependence, 175
Moro reflex, 200
Morphine, 165
 action, 159
 acute abdomen, 148
 cardiac emergencies, 107
 head injury, 268
 lifeboats, 381
 mountain rescue, 378
 overdose, 159
 pulmonary oedema, 111

thermal injury, 342
 unwanted effects, 159
Morphine-6-glucuronide, 165
Motion sickness, 587
Motor response, 319
 head injury, 265
 spinal injury, 294
 unconscious patients, 134
Motor sports injuries, 537
Motorcycle helmet removal, 253, *254–5*
Mountain rescue, **377**, 377–8, **378**, *379*
Mountaineering, 537–8
Mouth-to-mouth resuscitation, infection
 transmission, 412
Movement, soft tissue injuries, 316–17
Mucous membranes in children, 207
Mud flows, 546
Multifocal ectopics, 96
Multi-infarct dementia, 348
Multiorgan damage in children, 231
Mumps, **411**
Munchausen's syndrome by proxy, 208
μ-receptor, 164
Murphy's sign, 143, 144
Muscarine, **192**
Muscimol, **192**
Muscle necrosis, electrocution injury, 407
Muscle relaxants, 36, 158–9
 see also specific drugs
Muscular injuries, 318, **362**
Musculoskeletal system, acute decompression
 illness, 402–3
Mycoplasma, 214
Myelinated nerve fibres, 162–3, 170
Myocardial contusion, chest compression
 complications, 21
Myocardial infarction, 105–6
 abdominal pain, 140, 146
 aeromedical transport, 588
 aims of management, 106
 airway obstruction, 26
 anti-arrhythmics, 108
 aspirin, 108
 bradycardia, 108–9
 chest pain, **105**
 definition, 105
 diagnosis, 106
 elderly patients, 347
 electrocardiography, *100–1*, 100–2, 106–7
 frequency of arrhythmias within four hours
 of, **106**
 heart block, 108–9
 pathophysiology, 105
 percutaneous coronary intervention, 109
 ventricular tachycardia in, 114
Myoglobinuria, 395

N

N-acetylcysteine, 187, **187**
Nalbuphine, 166
 action, 164
 cardiac emergencies, 108
 head injury, 268
 thermal injury, 342

Naloxone
 action, 159
 as an antidote, **187**
 hypercapnia, 107
 neonates, 451
 opiate overdose, 136, 167, 180, 186, 188
Napoleonic Wars, 465
Narcotic syndrome, **184**
Narcotics and sportspeople, 538, **538**
Nasal cannulae, 43
Nasal complex injuries, 273, 275, *275*
Nasal Epistats®, 275, *275*
Nasal sinuses, barotrauma, 399
Nasopharyngeal airway, 29–30, **30**, *30*
 in children, 222, 232
 contraindications, 222
 trauma cases, children, 232
Nasotracheal intubation (NTI)
 blind, 35
 drawbacks, 35
 vs. oral intubation, 35
National accreditation, 5, 6
National Arrangements for Incidents Involving
 Radioactivity (NAIR), 522–3
National Association of Air Ambulance
 Services, 575
National Blood Transfusion Service, 79
National Health Service Accreditation Agency,
 6
National Health Service Act, 4
National Health Service ambulance trusts,
 594–5, *595*
National Health Service Pathways, 657, 659
National Radiological Protection Board
 (NRPB), 519
National Training Centre for Scientific
 Support, 620
National Transportation Safety Board (NTSB),
 577
National Trauma Registry, 655
Natural disasters, 540, **541**
Nausea
 on aircrafts, 587
 bowel obstruction, 146
 diverticular disease, 146
 gallbladder disease, 144
 mesenteric infarction, 145
 opioids side-effects, 165, 167
 renal calculus disease, 145
Near drowning/drowning, 383–8
 aspects of rescue, 384–5, *385*
 conscious patient, 385–6
 exhaustion, 384
 hypothermia, 384
 immediate care, 385–6
 inability to swim, 384
 incidence, 383
 pathophysiology, 383–4
 results and prognosis, 387–8
 secondary drowning, 386
 transport to hospital, 387
 treatment of cardiac arrest, 386–7
 unconsciousness, 383, 386
 watersports, 537

Neck
  blunt trauma, 269
  examination, 121, 256, **256**
  injury *see* Cervical spine injury
  overextension in children, 222
  penetrating trauma, 269
  soft tissue injuries, 269
  stiffness, 217
  vein distribution, 58
NecLoc® collar, 558, 559, *559*
Needle cricothyroidotomy, 39, **40**, 40–1
  in children, 223
  laryngeal injuries, 283
Needle thoracocentesis, 285–6, *286*
  indications, **285**
  injured children, 234
  pneumothorax, 119, 127
  tension pneumothorax, 281
Needles, intraosseous access, 66–7, *67*
Needlestick injuries, 414–15
Neglect, elderly patients, 356–7
Negligence *see* Medical negligence
Neighbour strapping, 560
Neil Robertson stretcher, 380, *380*, 381
Neisseria meningitidis
  meningitis, 217
  transmission, 412
Neonates, 448–52
  Apgar score, 442, **445**, 449, **449**
  definition, 197, **198**
  meconium aspiration, 451–2
  normal physiological values, 449, **449**
  physiology, 448–9, *449*
  premature, 202
  resuscitation, 449–51, *451*
  surface area, 198
  transportation, 451–2
Nerve agent poisoning, 157
Nerve fibres, 162–3, 170
Neural transmission and modulation, 162–3
Neurogenic shock, 76
  air travel and, 590
  fluid maldistribution, 204
  management, 81
  spinal cord injuries, 293
  trauma, 257
Neuroleptic malignant syndrome, 180, 458, **459**
Neuroleptics, 458, 471
Neurological assessment
  head injury, **264**, 264–5
  unconscious patients, 131, **131**, 132, 134
Neurological considerations, air travel, 589–90
Neurological injuries, 171, 318–19
  acute decompression illness, 400
  aeromedical transport considerations, 589–90
Neurones, damaged, 261
Neutrons, 515, *515*, 516, *516*, 517
Nicotine, **191**
Nicotinic alkaloids, **191**
Night-stick injury, 310
Nineteenth century, 3–4, *4*, 8–9

Nitrates
  cardiac emergencies, 107
  pulmonary oedema, 111
Nitrites, **187**, 190
Nitrogen
  acute decompression illness, 401
  bubbles, 402
  narcosis, 404
  partial pressure, 401
Nitrous oxide
  cardiac emergencies, 107–8
  in oxygen *see* Entonox
  renal calculus disease, 145
Noise, aircraft, 587
Non-accidental injury (NAI) *see* Abuse
Non-rebreather reservoir mask, 43
Non-steroidal anti-inflammatory drugs (NSAIDs), 167
  adverse effects, 168–9, **357**
  commonly used, 168
  mountain rescue, 378
  thermal injury, 342
Non-verbal communication, 476–7, **477**
Noradrenaline, autonomic response to shock, 77
North Western Injury Research Unit (NWIRC), 667
Northern Ireland Fire Service, 604
Nostalgia, 465
Notartz, 569
Nuclear fission, 522
Nuclear Industry Road Transport Emergency Plan (NIREP), 522
Nuclear weapon accident, 521
Numbness, trauma response, 468

O
Oakley chart, 155, 200, *201*
Obesity, acute decompression illness, 401
Oblique fractures, 306, *307*
Observation, soft tissue injuries, 316
Obsessive compulsive disorder, 460
Obstetric haemorrhage, 436
  see also Antepartum haemorrhage (APH); Haemorrhage, in pregnancy
Occupational diseases, risks to health-care workers, 411–12
Occupational injuries in pregnancy, 437
Oedema
  airway obstruction, 27
  larynx, 338
  pharynx, 338
  pulmonary *see* Pulmonary oedema
Oenanthotoxin, **192**
Oesophageal-tracheal Combitube, *37*, 37–8, 681
  advanced life support, 50
  advantages, 38
  contraindications, 38
  disadvantages, 38
  indications, 37–8
Oesophagus
  body temperature measurement, 365
  detector devices, 33, *33*
  intubation, 31, 32

perforation, surgical airway complications, 39
  spasm, **105**
Off-line medical control, 12
Ohm's law, 406
Olecranon fracture, 310
Omentum, gunshot wounds, 299
Oncotic pressure, 69
Ondansetron, 167, 526
On-line medical control, 12, *12*
On-site operations and coordination centre (OSOCC), 548
Operational debriefing, major incidents, 491–2
Operations, police, 617
Ophthalmia neonatorum, 410, **411**
Opiate receptors, 163–4
Opiates
  acute abdomen, 148
  antidote for poisoning, **187**
  cardiac emergencies, 107
  in children, 239
  misuse, 179–80, **180**
  overdose, 132, 136, 159, **187**, 188, 206
  pulmonary oedema, 111
  tracheal intubation anaesthesia, 36
Opioids, 163–7
  administration, 164
  antiemetics, 167
  contraindications, 165
  dosage, 167
  overdose, 167
  physical properties, 164
  side-effects, 164–5
  see also specific drugs
Opium, 179
Optimization, radiation protection, 520
Oral drug administration, **153**, 153–4
Oral rehydration solution (ORS), 216–17, **217**
ORCON standards, 657
Organophosphates poisoning, **187**, 188
Organophosphorus poisoning, 157
Oropharyngeal airway, 29, **29**
  in children, 222
Orotracheal intubation
  technique, 32, 32–3
  vs. nasotracheal intubation, 35
Orthopaedic conditions, air travel considerations, 591
Orthopaedic infection in children, 218
Osmolality, 69
Osmosis, 69
Osmotic pressure, 69
Osteomyelitis, 67
Osteoporosis
  elderly patients, 356
  humeral neck fracture, 311
  pathological fractures, 306–7
Othello syndrome, 175
Otitis media, 218
Ovarian cystic tumour pain, 430
Ovarian cysts, 146, 424
Ovarian hyperstimulation syndrome, 424
Ovarian torsion, 146, 430
Overalls, 679
Overdose *see* Poisoning; *specific substance*

Overtaking, 248–9
Oxalates, **191**, **192**
Oxfordshire Community Stroke Project
    (OCSP), 354
Oxicams, 168
Oxygen, 681
  as an antidote, **187**
  carriage, 41
  consumption *see* Oxygen consumption
  cylinders, 42, **42**, 43
  dissociation curve, 583–4, *584*
  fire service, 607
  and the injured brain, 261–2
  masks, 681
  remote industrial sites, 381
  respiratory pathophysiology, 278
  saturation *see* Oxygen saturation
  storage, 42, **42**
  therapy *see* Oxygen therapy
  toxicity, acute, 404
Oxygen consumption
  heat production, 362
  in pregnancy, 423
  shivering, 369
Oxygen saturation, 583
  in asthma, 212
  pulse oximetry, 128
Oxygen therapy, 41–3, 681
  acute decompression illness, 402, 403
  during aeromedical transport, 587–8
  asthma, 123, 213
  bronchiolitis, 211
  carbon monoxide poisoning, 190
  cardiac emergencies, 107
  in children, 205, 206–7, 210, 224, *224*
  dangers, 42–3
  delivery systems, 43
  epiglottitis, 210
  flail chest, 282
  formula, 41
  head injury, 236
  hyperbaric, 402, 403
  hypothermia, 372
  injured children, 234
  Laerdal pocket mask, 31
  near drowning/drowning, 386
  neonates, 450
  in pregnancy, 421–2, 424
  pulmonary oedema, 111
  respiratory emergencies, 119
  respiratory failure, 125
  rib fractures, 285
  seizures, 268
  surgical airway, 39–41, **40**
  trauma patients, 253, 435
Oxygenated haemoglobin (HbO_2), 127
  dissociation curve, 128, *128*
  pulse oximetry, 128
Oxygen-powered resuscitators, 45

P

P_{450} cytochrome system, 187
P wave, 86, *87*, 89
Pacemakers *see* Cardiac pacing

Packed red cells, 79–80
Paediatric Advanced Life Support (PALS), 11,
    226, 599, 676
Paediatric life support, 220–7
  advanced, 11, *226*, 676
  airway, 222–4, *223*
  breathing, 224
  circulation, 224–5, *225*
  complications of resuscitation, 227
  non-ventricular fibrillation, 226–7
  prevention, 221
  pulseless ventricular tachycardia, 227
  survival, 221
  tachycardia, 226–7
  treatment algorithms, 225–6, *226*
  ventricular fibrillation, 227
Paediatric Trauma Score (PTS), 237, **237**,
    664–5, **665**
Pain
  abdominal *see* Abdominal pain
  breathing, 204
  neural transmission and modulation, 162–3
  parietal, 140–1
  referred, 141
  relief *see* Analgesia
  response to in unconscious patients, 133–4
  visceral, 140
Painful stimuli, unconscious patients, 133–4
Palpation
  abdomen, 143, 146, 301, 424, 429
  chest, 256, **256**
  soft tissue injuries, 316
Palpitation, sinus tachycardia, 88
Pancreas
  anatomy, 298
  haemorrhagic necrosis of, 144–5
Pancreatitis, 144–5
  abdominal pain, 140, 144
  hypothermia rewarming, 372
  referred chest pain, **105**
  vomiting, 141
Pancuronium
  action, 159
  tracheal intubation anaesthesia, 36
Panic attacks, 460
Paracetamol, 167, 168
  antidote for poisoning, **187**
  fever, 218
  overdose, 182, 186–7
Paradoxical breathing, 119, 256
Paraldehyde, 215
Paramedics
  drug administration, 155–6
  response vehicles, 597
Paranoia, 458
Paraquat
  antidote for poisoning, **187**
  poisoning, 190
Parasuicide, 458–9, **459**
Paratyphoid, **411**
Parietal pain, abdominal, 140–1
Parking at the scene, 249, *249*
Paroxetine, 471
Partial agonists, 154, 164

Partial pressure of carbon dioxide, 278, 583
Partial pressure of oxygen (Po_2), 278
Pasteurella multocida, 193
Patella
  dislocation, 313, *313*
  fracture, 313
Pathological fractures, 306–7
Pathological jealousy, alcohol dependence, 175
Patient report form, 653, *654*
Patient(s)
  assessment *see specific condition; specific
    situation*
  information, head injury, 267
  satisfaction, ambulance service, 601
  transfer vehicles, 569–70 (*see also specific
    vehicle*)
Patient's best interests, 637, 641
Peak expiratory flow rate (PEFR)
  asthma, 122, 211, 212
  measurement in children, 211
Peak inspiratory flow rate (PIFR), 43
Pelvic fractures, 312
  examination, 301
  and genitourinary injuries, 299
  haemorrhage, 257, 300 (*see also* Pelvic
    haemorrhage)
  and pelvic organ injury, 300
  in pregnancy, 434, 436
  stabilization, *312*
  treatment, 302
Pelvic haemorrhage, 77, 312
Pelvic inflammatory disease, 143, 146
Pelvic injuries
  and abdominal and chest injury, 300
  in children, 239
  examination, 301
Pelvic ligament pain, 430
Pelvis, 302
Penetrating trauma
  abdominal, 299–300, *301*
  bladder, 302
  chest, 280, 300
  genitals, 303
  kidneys, 303
  maxillofacial, 272
  neck, 269
  in pregnancy, 437
  spine, 291–2
  trachea, 284
  see also Stab wounds
Penicillin
  meningitis, 217
  meningococcal septicaemia, 218
  pneumonia, 214
Penicillin V, 218
Penis injury, 303, 304
Pentazocine, 166
Peptic ulcer disease, **105**, 145
Pepys, Samuel, 3
Percentage of inspired oxygen (F_iO_2), 588
Percussion, chest *see* Chest percussion
Percussion fist pacing, 51
Percutaneous coronary intervention (PCI),
    myocardial infarction, 109

Perfluorocarbons, 80
Pericardial bleeding, chest compression
    complications, 21
Pericardiocentesis, 287–8
    cardiac tamponade, 283
    complications, **287**
    equipment, 287
    indications, **287**
    procedure, 287–8
Pericarditis
    chest pain, **105**
    electrocardiography, 99
Perimortem caesarean section, 437–8
Perineum inspection, 424
Peripheral nervous system
    acute decompression illness, 403
    effects of cold exposure, **362**
    electrocution injury, 407
Peripheral perfusion assessment in shock, 74–5
Peripheral venous access/cannulation, 57–63
    advanced life support, 50
    anatomy, 57–8, *58*
    in children, 224–5
    complications, 62–3
    equipment, 58–9, *59*
    failed, 63
    shearing of the cannula, 63
    technique, 59–62, *60–2*
        percutaneous cannulation, 59–61, *60–1*
        Seldinger technique, 61, *61*
        venous cutdown, 61–2, *62*
Peritoneal cavity, 300
Peritoneum, 298
Peritonitis, 143
    abdominal pain, 141
    acute abdomen, 142
    appendicitis, 144
Personal protective equipment, 413, **414,**
        485–6, 678–9, *679*
    chemical incidents, 505, 508–9
    fire service, 608
    levels of protection, 509
Personal space, 477
Personality change, post-catastrophes, 467
Personality disorder, 461
Pest coaches, 3
Petechial rash, 205, 218
Pethidine, 148, 165
Petit mal seizures, 215
Pharmacodynamics, 154
Pharmacokinetics, 154
Pharmacological cardioversion, 114
Pharmacy-only (P) medicines, 155
Pharyngitis, 218, **411**
Pharynx
    oedema, 338
    soft-tissue obstruction in, 26
Phencyclidine, 169, 180
Phenelzine, 471
Phenobarbital, 215
Phenol burns, 336, 337
Phenyl acetic acids, 168
Phenytoin
    epilepsy, 215

and *N*-acetylcysteine, 187
    seizures, 268
Phobias, 460
Phosphorous burns, 336, 337
Photography
    and confidentiality, 645–6
    record keeping, 654
Photophobia, meningitis, 217
Phototoxins, 191, **192**
PHRASED mnemonic, 120, **121**
Physical abuse
    children, 207–8
    elderly patients, 356
Physical fitness, acute decompression illness,
        401
Physiological dead space, 278
Physiological injury severity scores, 661,
        662–5, 666–7
see also specific scoring system
Physostigmine, **187**
Piroxicam, 168
Placenta
    delivery of the, 442–5
    retained, 445
    in road traffic accidents, 434
Placenta praevia, 428, *428*, 429
Placental abruption, 428–9, *429*, 436, **436**
Plants and fungi, poisonous, 190–2, **191–2**
Plasma oncotic pressure, 110
Plasma volume, 68–9, 422
Plaster of Paris, 591
Platelets, 80
Pleura, 277
Pleurisy, **105**
Plutonium, 521, 527
Pneumatic antishock garment (PASG), 563
    chest injuries, 288
    gaseous expansion, 585
Pneumocephalus, 44
Pneumococcus, 210
Pneumomediastinum, 39
Pneumonia, **411**
    abdominal pain, 146
    chest pain, **105**
    in children, 214, 218
Pneumonic plague, **411**
Pneumothorax, 126–7, 278
    and altitude, 588
    assessment, 127
    assisted ventilation, 44
    asthma, 123, 127
    barotrauma, 400
    central venous cannulation, 65
    chest injuries, 281
    chest pain, **105**
    chest percussion, 256
    cocaine users, 179
    injured children, 234
    management, 127
    open chest wound, 282
    pathophysiology, 126–7
    primary, 127
    secondary, 127
    simple, 284

surgical airway complications, 39
    tension *see* Tension pneumothorax
Poikilothermic, 296
Poiseuille's law, 122
Poisoning, 182–94
    antidotes, 186, **187**
    bites and stings, 193–4
    breathing, 204
    decontamination, 185–6
        activated charcoal, 186
        caustic ingestions, 186
        emesis, 185
        gastric lavage, 185
    epidemiology, 182–3
    management priorities, 183–5
    plants and fungi, 190–2, **191–2**
    poison information services, 194, **194**
    poisons in victim's mouth, 18
    respiratory depression in children, 203
    specific poisons, 186–90 (*see also specific*
        poison)
    toxic syndromes, 183, **184**
    unconscious patients, 132, 136–7
    when to suspect, 183
    see also specific substance
Poisonous plants and fungi, 190–2, **191–2**
Police Act 1996, 615
Police and Criminal Evidence Act 1984, 618,
        619
Police authority, 615–16
Police Incident Commander, 505
Police service, 614–24
    civilianization, 617
    complaints and discipline, 617
    discipline code, 617
    image, 618
    major incidents, 622–4
    management, 615–16
    other police forces, 614, 618
    process of law, 618–19
    rank structure, *616*, 616–17, *617*
    road traffic law, 619–20
    scene of crime officers, 620–2
    specialized duties, 617
    statements, and confidentiality, 644
    statutory obligations, 618
Poliomyelitis, **411**, 412
Polydipsia, 204
Polyuria, 204
Portugal, 10–11
Portuguese man-of-war, 193
Positive end-expiratory pressure (PEEP)
    in children, 204
    mechanical ventilators, 45
Positrons, 517
Posterior tibial pulse, 205
Postmortem caesarean section, 437–8
Postpartum haemorrhage, 445
Post-traumatic stress disorder (PTSD), 466
    blasts, 330
    chemical incidents, 511–12
    in children, 467
    chronicity, 468
    formal treatment methods, 471

prevalence, 467
prognostic factors, 468
symptoms, 467
Posture, circulation and, 422–3
Potassium, 69, **69**
Potassium-40, 518
Potassium hydroxide, 186
Povey frame, 296
PR interval, 86, **87**
Practice
    anger and aggression prevention, 478–9
    closed-circuit television (CCTV), 478
    consulting room, 479, *479*
    waiting area, 479
Precordial thump, 49, 114
Precordium, palpation, 121
Prednisolone
    asthma, 123, 212, 213, **213**
    croup, 210, **210**
Pre-eclampsia, 429–30, **430**
Pre-excitation, 97–8
Pregnancy
    acute abdomen, 142
    airway changes, 420–1, **421**
    anatomical and physiological changes in,
        420–1, **421**, **422**, 434–5
    approach to victim, 424
    asthma in, 431
    breathing, **421**, 421–2
    cardiac disease in, 431
    categories of maternal death, **420**
    circulation, **422**, 422–3
    concealed, 440, 446
    deep vein thrombosis in, 431
    diabetes in, 431
    drugs in, 152–3
    ectopic *see* Ectopic pregnancy
    emergencies in, 419–32 (*see also specific
        condition*)
    epilepsy in, 431
    history taking, 424–5
    management of severe illness in, 423–5
    non-obstetric causes of abdominal pain,
        430–1
    perforated appendix, 144
    posture, 422–3
    pulmonary embolus in, 431
    resuscitation, 425
    specific emergency conditions, 425–30
    trauma in, 433–8
        anatomical and physiological change,
            434–5
        blunt trauma and assault, 436–7
        brain-stem death, 437
        burns, 437
        major obstetric haemorrhage, 436
        penetrating trauma, 437
        perimortem and postmortem caesarean
            section, 437–8
        primary survey, 435
        road traffic accidents, 434
        scope of the problem, 433–4, **434**
        secondary survey, 435–6
        sport, occupational and toxic injury, 437

uterine and fetal assessment, 435–6, **436**
    see also Childbirth
Pre-hospital Emergency Care Certificate, 5, 6
Pre-hospital Emergency Care (PHEC) courses,
    6, 251, 675
Pre-hospital Paediatric Life Support (PHPLS),
    599
Pre-hospital Trauma Life Support (PHTLS), 11
Pre-hospital Trauma Life Support (PHTLS)
    courses, 251, 598, 675
Premature neonates, 202
Pre-school children, **198**
Prescription-only medicines (POM), 155
Press statements and confidentiality, 644–5
Pressure, 398–9, *399*
Pressure sores
    spinal boards, 295, 565
    traction splint, 562
Preterm delivery, 445
Prevention of Terrorism Act, 646–7
Prilocaine, 170, 172
Primary survey *see* ABC/ABCDE, basic life
    support
Primitive reflexes, 200
Prioritized despatch, 494, 499, 660
Prochlorperazine, 159, 167
Procyclidine, **187**, 458
Prophylaxis, postexposure, 415–16
Propionic acids, 168
Propofol
    action, 157–8
    tracheal intubation anaesthesia, 36
Propranolol
    hypertension, 108
    tachycardia, 178
Proprioceptive balance mechanisms, 352
Prostacyclin, 168
Prostaglandins, 168
Protecting the Vulnerable, 639
Protective equipment, 413, **414**
Proteinuria
    heat illness, 395
    pre-eclampsia, 429
Protons, 515, *515*, 516, *516*, 517
Prozac, 188
Pruritus, acute decompression illness, 403
Pseudocoma, 137
Pseudodementia, 353
Pseudofit, 137
Psilocybin, 180
Psittacosis, **411**
Psoas abscess, 143
Psychiatric emergencies, 455–64
    aggressive and uncooperative patients, **463**,
        463–4, **464**
    air travel considerations, 592
    anxiety disorders, 460, **460**
    assessment, 456–7, **457**
    common law and informed consent, 462–3
    definition, 456, **456**
    depression and mania, 459–60
    Mental Health Act 1983, 456, 461–2
    mental state examination, 456–7
    organic causes, 457, **457**

parasuicide, 458–9, **459**
    personality disorder, 461
    physical causes of, 460–1, **461**
    physical examination, 457
    psychosis, 457–8
Psychiatric pseudocoma, 137
Psychological first aid, 470, **470**
Psychological implications
    of chemical incidents, 511–12
    of trauma in children, 231–2
Psychological injury, blasts, 330
Psychological triage, 470–1
Psychosis, 457–8
    antipsychotic drugs, 458
    assessment, 457–8
    dangerousness, 458
    delusions, 457
    hallucinations, 457
    illicit drugs, 461
    management, 458
    post-traumatic, 470
    psychotic behaviour, 457–8
Psychotherapy, post-traumatic, 471
Public protection, radiation incidents, 528
Puerperal fever, **411**
Pulmonary contusion, 285
Pulmonary embolism
    chest pain, **105**
    electrocardiography, 98, 98–9
    electromechanical dissociation, 52
    in pregnancy, 431
Pulmonary fibrosis, **124**, 124–5
Pulmonary oedema, 110–11
    airway obstruction, 26
    atrial fibrillation, 113
    crystalloid colloid controversy, 72
    diagnosis, 110–11
    interstitial, 339
    pathophysiology, 110
    treatment, 111, 157
    unconscious patients, 134
Pulmonary perfusion, 278
Pulse oximetry, 127–9
    in children, 211–12
    head injury, 267
    heat illness, 394
    limitations, 128–9
    misconceptions relating to, 129
    mountain rescue, 378
    near drowning, 386
    oxygen saturation, cyanosis and the
        oxyhaemoglobin dissociation curve,
        128, *128*
    practical applications, 128, **129**
    principles, 127
    pulse oximeter workings, 128
    trauma in pregnancy, 435
Pulse rate
    abnormalities, **121**
    in children, 205
    monitoring, trauma, 256
    myocardial infarction, 106
    respiratory emergencies, 120
    shock, 75

Pulseless electrical activity (PEA) *see*
    Electromechanical disassociation
    (EMD)
Pulse(s)
  abnormalities, **121**
  assessment in the unconscious patient, 131
  in children, 205
    see also specific pulse
Pulsus paradoxus, 283
Punch drunk, 537
Pupillary assessment
  in children, 206
  in trauma, 257–8
  in the unconscious patient, 131, 132, **133**, 134
Purkinje system, 86
Pyelonephritis
  acute abdomen, 142
  in pregnancy, 430
Pyloric stenosis, 204, 216
Pyrazoles, 168
Pyrexia *see* Fever
Pyrexia of unknown origin, **411**
Pyroclastic flows, 546

Q

Q fever, **411**
Q wave, 86
QRS complex, 86–7, *87*
  broad, 95–8
  irregular, broad tachycardia, *92*, 92–3, *93*
  irregular, narrow tachycardia, 91–2, *92*
  regular broad tachycardia, 91, *91*, *91*
  regular narrow tachycardia, 88–9, *89*, *90*
QS wave, 86
QT interval, *87*
Qualifications, 5
Quality, ambulance service, 601
Quinine, 186

R

R wave, 86
Rabies, **411**
Racquet sports injuries, 537
Radial acceleration, 586, *586*
Radial nerve damage, humeral fracture, 310–11
Radial pulse, 121
  in children, 205
Radiant heat, rewarming, 369
Radiation, 390
  annual limits of intake, 520–1, **521**
  categories, 527, **527**
  characteristics, 517, *517*
  and contamination, 516
  devices, 521
  dose, 517–18
  dosimeter, 517, *517*
  external contamination, 526
  hormesis, 520
  incidents *see* Radiation incidents
  internal contamination, 526–7
  local irradiation, 526
  and radioactivity, *515*, 515–16, **516**, *516*
  units, 517–18
  whole body irradiation, 525–6

Radiation incidents, 337–8, 514–28
  basic physics, 515–18
  biological effects, 518–20
  cell damage effects, 519, *519*
  cell death effects, 518–19, *519*
  classification of casualties, 525–7
  hormesis and adaptive response, 520
  human radiation levels, 518
  information to hospitals, 527–8
  ionization, 515, *515*
  Ionizing Radiation Regulations 1985, 522
  medical management of casualties, 525–7
  national arrangements, 522–3
  packages and source identification, *523*,
    523–4
  protection, 520–1, **521**
  public protection, 528, **528**
  radiation and contamination, 516
  radiation and radioactivity, *515*, 515–16,
    516, *516*
  radiation characteristics, 517, *517*
  radiation units, 517–18
  risk estimation, 519–20, **520**
  safety, 524–5
  transport plans, 522
  triage, 527–8
  types of accident, 521–2
Radiation sickness, 519
Radio systems, 658
Radioactive iodines, 525, 527
Radioactive material release, 521–2
Radioactivity, *515*, 515–16, 517
Radionuclides, 516, 518
Radiotherapy, 338
Radius fracture
  distal, 310
  head, 310
  neck, 310
Railway incidents, 408, **488**
Raised intracranial pressure, 165
  brain injury, 262, *262*
  breathing, 204
  oxygen and brain injury, 261
Rash
  acute decompression illness, 403
  petechial, 205, 218
Reading the wreckage, 250, 279
Rebound phenomenon, 174
Recall, 672
Record keeping *see* Documentation
Recovery
  chemical incidents, 503
  major incidents, 491–2
Recovery position, 21–2, *22*, **23**, *23*, 292, *292*
Rectal bleeding, diverticular disease, 146
Rectal drug administration, 153, **153**
Red Cross, 625, 628–9
Red degeneration of fibroids, 430
Reduction
  ankle fracture, 314
  closed fractures, 309
  open fractures, 309
Re-entry tachycardia, 90, 112
Reflux oesophagitis, **105**

Refugees, **547**, 547–8
Regulation, aeromedical evacuation, 576–7
Regurgitation
  during basic life support, 21
  tracheal intubation, 33
Remifentanil, 166
Remote industrial sites, 381
Remote places rescue *see* Rescue from remote
    places
Renal calculus disease, 145
Renal colic, 145, 148
Rendell-Baker-Suchet mask, 224
Renin, 77
Repetitive transcranial magnetic stimulation,
  471
Repolarization, cardiac, 86
Report into Trauma, 5
Rescue, near drowning, 384–5, *385*
Rescue from remote places, 376–81
  cave rescue, 378–80, *380*
  lifeboats, 380–1
  mountain rescue, **377**, 377–8, *378*, *379*
  remote industrial sites, 381
  search and rescue helicopters, 381
  ski patrolling, 380
Research and audit, 655
Resins, 191, **192**
Resistance (electric), 406
Respirator masks/filters, 508–9
Respiratory arrest
  drowning/near drowning, 384
  electrocution injury, 407
Respiratory assessment
  unconscious patients, 134–5
    see also Breathing
Respiratory depression
  in children, 203
  opioids side-effects, 164
Respiratory disease symptoms in children,
  202–3
Respiratory distress
  in children, 203
  injured children, 234, **234**
  signs, 234, **234**
Respiratory emergencies, 118–29
  documentation, 122
  immediately life-threatening (excluding
    trauma), **119**
  primary assessment, 118–20, **119**, **120**
  pulse oximetry *see* Pulse oximetry
  re-assessment, 121
  secondary assessment, 120–1, **121**
  transportation, 122
    see also specific emergency
Respiratory failure, 123–6
  acute, 123
  bronchiectasis, 125, **125**
  causes of treatment failure, **126**
  in children, 202
  chronic, 124, **124**
  chronic obstructive pulmonary disease, 124
  injured children, 234, **234**
  management, 125–6
  pathophysiology, 124–5

pulmonary fibrosis, **124**, 124–5
Respiratory rate
  in children, **200**, 204
  neonates, 449, **449**
  trauma patients, 253
Respiratory syncytial virus (RSV), 210
Respiratory system
  effects of cold exposure, **362**
  electrocution injury, 407
  heat illness complications, 395
  opioids side-effects, 164
  personal protection, 413
  in pregnancy, 421–2
Respiratory tract infections
  disasters, 542
  refugees, 547
Respiratory tract injury, 338–40, *339*
Response
  fire service, 609–10
  major incidents, 487–91
  times, 657
Responsiveness, unconscious patients, 130
Resting potentials, 86
Resuscitation
  acute abdomen, 147
  chemical incidents, 510
  heat illness, 394
  in hypothermia, 373, **373**
  neonates, 449–51, *451*
  poisoning, 184–5
  in pregnancy, 425
  respiratory emergencies, 119, 120
  shootings, 326–7
    see also Advanced life support; Basic life
      support (BLS)
Resuscitation Council, 7, 674
Resuscitation drugs, 156–7
  see also specific drugs
Resuscitators, 607, 681
Retained firefighters, 604
Retroperitoneal haemorrhage, 144–5
Retroperitoneal organs, 298, **299**
Retroperitoneal vasculature, 299
Revised Trauma Score (RTS), 663–4, **664**, 666
  see also Triage Revised Trauma Score
    (T-RTS)
Rewarming, 367–72
  active, 367
  central, *370*, 370–2, *371*
  combination treatment, 367–8
  correct diagnosis and, 365
  near drowning/drowning, 386
  practical recommendations, 372–3
  spontaneous, 367, 368–9
  surface heating, 369–70
Reye's syndrome, 218
Rhabdomyolysis, 183, 185
  crush injuries, 329
  earthquake, 544
  electrocution injury, 407
  heat illness, 395
Rib fractures
  chest compression complications, 21
  chest pain, **105**

in children, 234
identification, 256
in pregnancy, 434
simple, 284–5
RICE mnemonic, 317, 318, 536, 538
Rifampicin, 187
Rigors, 142
Ringer's lactate, **70**
  dehydration, 217
  electrocution injury, 409
  shock, 79
Risk assessment, chemical incidents, 507
Ritalin, 179
Road traffic accidents
  abdominal injuries, 299
  chest injuries, *279*, 279–80
  elderly patients, 356
  fire service role, 605–7
  glass management, 606
  involving children, 231
  law, 619
  maxillofacial injuries, 272–3
  ocular injuries, 274
  pelvic fractures, 302, 312
  pregnant patients, 433, 434, 436–7
  spinal injury, 290
Road Traffic Act 1976, 568
Road Traffic Act 1988, 620
Road traffic law, 619–20
Road Vehicles Lighting Regulations 1984, 680
R-on-T ectopics, 96, 108
Rooting reflex, 200
Rotary-wing aircraft, 573
  see also Helicopters
Routes of administration, drugs, **153**, 153–4
Rovsing's sign, 144
Royal Air Force, 381
Royal Flying Doctor Service, 12
Royal Humane Society, 4
Royal National Lifeboat Institution (RNLI),
    381
Royal Navy, 381
Rubella, **411**, 412, 413
Rugby injuries, 536
Rule of Nines, 340, *342*
Rupture, definition, 316, *316*
Russell extrication device (RED), 77, 294, 295,
    312, 563–4, *564*

S
S wave, 86
SA nodal block, 94, *94*
SAD CHALET mnemonic, 623–4
Safe Custody Regulations 1973, 155
Safety
  aeromedical evacuation, 577
  chemical incidents, 505
  electrocution injury, 407–8
  equipment, 678–9
  fire service at major incidents, 610–11
  major incidents, 488, **488**, 610–11
  personal protection from infection, 413–15
  radiation incidents, 514, 524–5
  scene *see* Scene safety/assessment

shootings, 326–7
  violent/aggressive/uncooperative patients,
    463–4
Safety at Sports Ground Act 1975, 530
Saffir/Simpson hurricane scale, **547**
Sager® traction splint, *562*, 562–3
St Andrew's Ambulance Association, 629
St John Ambulance Association, 4, 9, 625, 628
Salbutamol
  anaphylaxis, 81
  asthma, 123
  bronchiolitis, 211
  mountain rescue, 378
Salicylates, 168, 187–8
Saline
  dehydration, 217
  dextrose, **70**
  heat illness, 394
  hyperglycaemia, 216
  hypertonic, 71
  normal, **70**
  thermal injury, 340
Salivation, 169
Salmonella, 203, **411**, 543
Salpingitis, 143
Salter-Harris classification, 199
Salvation Army, 625, 630
SAM® splint, 561
Samaritans, 629–30
Saphenous vein cannulation, 225
Satellite technology, 551
Scabies, **411**
Scalds, 334–5
  guidelines for immediate care of, 335
  inflammatory response, *333*
  non-accidental, 338
  prevention, 335
Scalp haematoma, 265
Scalp injury, 265
Scaphoid fracture, 310
Scapular injuries, 312
Scarlet fever, **411**
SCBA (self-contained breathing apparatus),
    509
Scene of crime officers (SOCO), 620–2
Scene safety/assessment, 245–50
  aeromedical evacuation, 577
  approach, **245**, 245–6
  arrival, 249–50, *251*
  chemical incidents, 612
  chest injuries, 279, **279**
  driving techniques *see* Driving techniques
  emergency services liaison, 249
  equipment, 246, 249
  escorts, 246
  fire service role, 605, 612
  injured children, 230–1
  leaving for the scene, 246
  major incidents, 490–1
  parking, 249
  radiation incidents, 524
  training, 245
  trauma, 251
School age children, **198**

Sciatic nerve injury, 312
Scoop stretcher, 564
Scotland
    air ambulances, 573, **573**
    fire service in, 603–4
Scrotum injury, 303, 304
Sea King, 577, 579, *579*
Sea rescue, 380–1
Second World War, 466
Sedatives
    misuse, 181
    radiation-induced vomiting, 526
Seizures, 136, 184
    aeromedical transport considerations, 589
    after head injury, 238, 268
    in children, 202, 215
    diagnosis, 354–5
    eclamptic, 430
    elderly patients, 354–6, *355*
    management, 268
    secondary brain damage, 263
    types of, 355 (*see also specific type*)
Seldinger technique, 59, 61, *61*
Seldinger type cannula, 59, *59*, 61, *61*
Self-contained breathing apparatus (SCBA),
        509
Self-harm, 458–9
Self-inflating bag-valve device, 44–5
    in children, 224
Sellick's manoeuvre, 421
Semtex, 327
Septic abortion, 427
Septic shock, 76
    in children, 204
Septicaemia, 202
    fluid maldistribution, 204
    meningococcal, 205, 218
Serotonin, **192**, 193, 194
Serotonin re-uptake inhibitor antidepressants,
        471
Service d'Aide Medicale Urgente (SAMU),
        9–10, *10*, 494, 569
Service Mobile d'Urgence et de Réanimationé
        (SMUR), 10, *10*
Sexual abuse
    children, 208
    elderly patients, 356
Sharps, 414–15
Shell shock, 465
Shelter, chemical incidents, 506–7
Shigella, 203
Shigellosis, 532
Shivering, 365, 369, 378
Shock, 74–81
    abdominal aortic aneurysm, 143–4
    acute abdomen, 139
    burns, 333
    cardiogenic, 76, 81
    in children, 205
    classification, **75**, 75–6, 257
    crystalloid colloid controversy, 72
    definition, 74
    drugs in, 152
    fluid therapy

administration, 78
    fluid type, **79**, 79–80
    hypotensive resuscitation, 78–9
    quantity, 80
gunshot wounds, 326
haemorrhagic, 145, 152
hypotensive resuscitation, 78–9
hypovolaemic *see* Hypovolaemic shock
identification, 74–5, **75**
intravenous access, 78
management, 77–8, 80–1
mesenteric infarction, 145
neurogenic *see* Neurogenic shock
pathophysiology, 76–7
response to treatment, 76
secondary brain damage, 263
septic, 76
signs and symptoms, **258**
spinal, 76
unconscious patients, 135
vasogenic, 76
Short-duration accelerations, 586
Shotguns, 326
    see also Gunshot/missile wounds
Shoulder injuries, 311
Shunted blood, 278
Sicilian Gambit classification of antiarrhythmic
        drugs, 112
Sick cell syndrome, 77
Sick sinus syndrome, 94
Sickle cell anaemia, 589
Sidaway v. *Bethlem Royal Hospital Governors*,
        635
Sievert (Sv), 518
Silent chest, asthma, 123
Simmonds' test, 318, *318*
Simple (closed) fractures, 306, *307*, 308–9
Simple Triage and Rapid Treatment system
        (START), 496, *497*
Sinoatrial (SA) node, 93–4
    block, 94, *94*
    cardiac depolarization, 86
Sinus arrest, 94, *94*
Sinus bradycardia, 93, 108
Sinus tachycardia, 88, *89*, 407
Sirens, 246
Ski patrolling, 380
Skin
    acute decompression illness, 403
    electrocution injury, 406–7
    injuries, 317, *317*
    resistance, electric, 406
    rubbing, rewarming, 368
Skull fracture
    nasopharyngeal airways, 222
    nasotracheal intubation, 35
Skull-base fractures, 265–6, **266**
Skull-vault fracture, depressed, 266
Sleep impairment, trauma response, 469
Sling, 559–60, *560*
Slipped upper femoral epiphysis, 312
Small bowel
    anatomy, 298–9
    blunt abdominal injuries, 299

gunshot wounds, 299
    obstruction, 141
    stab wounds, 299
Smith's fracture, 310
Smoke inhalation injury, 338, 339
Smoking
    chronic obstructive pulmonary disease, 124
    emphysema, 124
Snake bites, **187**, 193
Sodium, 69, **69**
Sodium bicarbonate
    action, 157
    advanced life support, 50
    as an antidote, **187**, 188
    neonates, 451
Sodium channels, 170
Sodium chloride, **70**
Sodium hydroxide, 186
Sodium hypochlorite, 186
Sodium nitrate, **187**
Sodium thiosulphate, **187**
Soft-tissue injuries, 315–21
    see also specific injury; specific tissues
    amputated parts, 320, *320*
    antibiotic cover, 321
    compartment syndrome *see* Compartment
        syndrome
    definitions, 315–16
    examination, 316–17
    falls, elderly patients, 352
    history, 316
    management, 317
    maxillofacial, 273
    sports, 536
    tetanus prophylaxis, 320
    wounds *see* Wounds
Soldier's heart, 465
Solvent abuse, 181
Space blanket, 369
Space creation, fire service, 606
Special Constabulary, 618
Sphygmomanometer, 75
Spina bifida, 202
Spinal boards
    children, 233
    length of time spent on, 295
    long, *564*, 564–5, *565*, 683
    mountain rescue, 377–8
    spinal injury, 294–5
Spinal cord injury, 290
    aeromedical transport considerations, 590
    and brain injury, 291
    electrocution injury, 407
    hypotension, 257
    methylprednisolone, 160
    secondary, 290
    transportation, 296
    see also Spinal injury
Spinal injury, 290–6
    aeromedical transport considerations, 590,
        590
    blunt injury, 291
    in children, 233, *233*
    forces, 291, **291**

horse riding, 536
immediate management, 292–4
  positioning, 292, *292*
  primary survey and resuscitation, 292–3, *293*
  secondary survey, 293–4
immobilization, 233, *233*, 294–5
incidence, 290
in-line stabilization, 292, *292*, *293*
mountain rescue, 377–8
overlooked, 291–2
penetrating injury, 291–2
positioning, 292, *292*
primary survey and resuscitation, 292–3, *293*
recognition, **291**, 291–2
secondary survey, 293–4
transportation, 295–6
  see also Cervical spine injury
Spinal shock, 76, 293
Spine
  acute decompression illness, 403
  control in injured children, 233, *233*
  injury *see* Spinal injury
Spiral fractures, 306, *307*
Spleen
  blunt abdominal injuries, 299
  trauma, 300
Splinting, 683
  arm splints, 682
  closed fractures, 309
  fibular fracture, 314
  pain relief from, 268
  patellar fracture, 313
  pelvic and femoral injuries, 239, 312
  tibia fracture, 314
  see also specific type of splint
Spontaneous rewarming, 367, 368–9
Sporting events, 534–9
  cause of injury, 535–6
  drugs and the sportsperson, **538**, 538–9
  fatal accidents at, **534**
  injuries in pregnancy, 437
  injury profiles, 536–8
  management of injuries, 538
  nature of injuries, 536
  see also Mass gathering medicine
Sprains, 316
Spreading equipment, fire service, 608
ST segment, 87
Stab wounds
  abdominal, 299–300
  brain, 266
  chest, 280
  in pregnancy, 437
Staff
  training and education, violent/uncooperative patients, 480
  trauma care, emotions, 473–4
Standard wire gauge (SWG), 59
Standards of care, 634
Staphylococcus, 210
Staphylococcus aureus, 214, 335
Starling's forces, 69–70
Starling's law of the heart, 76

Station honorary medical adviser (SHMA), 381
Status asthmaticus, 165
Status epilepticus, 136, 356
Statute law, 618
Sternal fractures, 21
Steroids
  asthma, 123, 212, 213, **213**, 214
  croup, 210, **210**
  hypothermia, 372
  respiratory failure, 125
  response to shock, 77
  and sportspeople, 538
Stifneck® collar, *558*, 558–9, *559*
Stigmata, 121
Stimulants, 178–80
  see also specific stimulant
Stings, 193–4
Stochastic radiation effects, 518, 519, *519*
Stokes litter stretcher, 380, *380*
Stomach
  decompression, 238
  gas in, 585, 590
  injury, chest compression complications, 21
  in pregnancy, 421
  stab wounds, 299
  see also entries beginning Gastric
Stopping safely, 247
Storm surges, 546
Straight-blade laryngoscope, 222, *223*
Strains, 316
Streptococcal pharyngitis, **411**
Streptococcal tonsillitis, **411**
Streptococcus pneumoniae, 214, 217
Streptokinase, 108
Stress
  severe, post-traumatic, **466**, 466–7
  symptoms due to exposure to aggression, **477**
Stress reaction, acute, 467
Stretchers
  cave rescue, 380, *380*
  lifeboats, 381
  mountain rescue, 377–8, *379*
  remote industrial sites, 381
  scoop, 564
Stridor, 119, 203
Stroke *see* Cerebrovascular accident (CVA)
Stroke volume in pregnancy, 422
Strontium, radioactive, 527
Subarachnoid drug administration, **153**, 154
Subarachnoid haemorrhage, 135–6, 354
Subclavian artery damage, clavicular injury, 311
Subclavian vein
  anatomy, *63*, 64
  cannulation, 65
    in children, 225
    pneumothorax, 127
Subcutaneous drug administration, 153, **153**
Subcutaneous haematomas, 317
Subdural haematoma, 537
Subdural haemorrhage, 135
Subglottic stenosis, 39
Sublingual drug administration, 153, **153**
Submersion hypothermia, 364
Substance abuse, 133, 173–81

alcohol *see* Alcohol dependence
assessment, 177
commonly misused substances, 177–81
epidemiology, 177
management of non-alcohol substance misusers, 177
post-traumatic stress disorder, 467
prevalence, 177
psychiatric emergencies, 461
terminology, 173–4
  see also specific substance
Suction units, 253, 681, *681*
  neonates, 450
  spinal injuries, 292
Sudden infant death syndrome (SIDS), 220, 221
Sudden sniffing death, 181
Suicide, 353, 458–9, **459**
  alcohol dependence, 175
  drowning, 383
  post-traumatic, 470
  see also Poisoning
Sulph-haemoglobin, 129
Sulphuric acid, 186
Superior vena cava, 224–5
Supine hypotension syndrome, 422
Supplied air respirators (SARs), 509
Support vehicles, 597, 601
Supracondylar fracture
  in children, 239
  elbow, 310, *310*
  knee, 313
Supraventricular tachycardia (SVT), 88
  frequency of, within 4 h of myocardial infarction, **106**
  treatment, 112–13
Surface area of children, 198–9, *199*
Surface heating, 367, 369–70
Surfactant, 448
Surgical airway, 38–41
  anatomy, 39, *39*
  in children, *223*, 223–4, 232
  complications, 38–9
  contraindications, 38
  indications, 38
  injured children, 232
  needle vs surgical cricothyrotomy, **40**, 40–1
  oxygen delivery and ventilation systems, 39–41, **40**
  technique, 39
Surgical teams, disasters, 549
Suxamethonium
  action, 159
  tracheal intubation anaesthesia, 36
Suxamethonium chloride, 159
Sweating, 390, **390**
  myocardial infarction, 106
  renal calculus disease, 145
Swimming, 384
Sympathomimetic syndrome, **184**
Syncope *see* Fainting
Synometrine, 427
Syphilis transmission, 412
Systemic inflammatory response syndrome (SIRS), 333

T

T wave, 87
Tachycardia, 88–93, 111–12
  antiarrhythmic drugs, 112, **112**
  atrial, 88
  cannabis, 177–8
  in children, 226–7
  diagnosis, 111–12
  diverticular disease, 146
  irregular
    broad (QRS)-complex, 92, 92–3, *93*
    narrow (QRS)-complex, 91–2, *92*
  ketamine, 169
  pacemaker-mediated, 103
  pathophysiology, 112
  re-entry, 90, 112
  regular
    broad (QRS)-complex, 91, **91**, *91*
    narrow (QRS)-complex, 88–90, *89*, *90*
  respiratory emergencies, 120
  shock, 75
  sinus, 88, *89*
  supraventricular *see* Supraventricular
      tachycardia (SVT)
  tension pneumothorax, 281
  trauma, 257
  treatment, 111–12
  unconscious patients, 132, 137
  ventricular *see* Ventricular tachycardia
Tachypnoea, 119
  causes of, **121**
  tension pneumothorax, 281
  unconscious patients, 132
Taking Healthcare to the Patient, 657
Tamponade
  cardiac *see* Cardiac tamponade
  pelvic and femoral injuries, 239
Tasking, 575
Taylor, Lord Justice, 529–30
Taylor Report, 484
Teachers, 673
Teaching courses, 676
Teeth, injuries to, 274
Telecommunication, major incidents, 490
  see also Communications
Temazepam, 189
Tendonitis, 318
Tendons
  definition, 315–16
  injuries, 315–16, 318, *318*
Tenosynovitis, 318
Tension pneumothorax, 119
  aeromedical evacuation, 574, 576
  assessment, 127
  chest injuries, **281**, 281–2
  development, *126*
  electromechanical dissociation, **51**, 52
  injured children, 234
  management, 127
  pathophysiology, 126
  signs, 281, **281**
  trauma, 257, **258**
  treatment, 119
Tenuate, 179

Teratogenicity, 152–3, 425
Terrorism, 322, 327, 646–7
Testicular torsion, 142
Tetanus, **411**
  immunization, 412, 413
  prophylaxis, 320
Tetanus human immunoglobulin (TIG),
      320
Tetracycline, **357**
Tetrahydrocannabinoids (THCs), 177
Theophyllines, 186
Therapeutic privilege, 637–8
Therapeutic radiotherapy, 338
Therapeutics *see* Drug(s)
Thermal injury, 332–43
  aeromedical transport considerations, 591
  causes of, 334–40
  classification, 340
  electrocution *see* Electrocution injury
  fluid resuscitation, 340–2
  guidelines for immediate care of, 334
  pathophysiology, *333*, 333–4
  in pregnancy, 437
  specific considerations at major incidents,
      342–3
  wound assessment, 340–2, *341*
  see also specific injury
Thermoregulation, 361–2
  children, 390
  heat illness, 389–90, **390**
  thermal injury, 333–4
Thiamine deficiency, 189
Thiopental, 430
Thiopentone, 36
Thioridazine, 458
Thomas splint, 4
Thompson's test, 318, *318*
Thoracic duct injury, 65
Thoracic impedance, 53
Thoracic intervertebral disc disease, **105**
Thoracic pump theory, 21
Thoracotomy, 288
Thorium, 518
Thrills, 121
Thrombocytopaenia, 338
Thromboembolism, **51**, 52
Thrombolytic agents
  benefits, 109
  cardiac emergencies, 109
  heart block, 109
  indications and contraindications, **110**
  myocardial infarction, 106
  non-haemorrhagic stroke, 135
Thrombophlebitis, 63
Thromboxane A$_2$, 339
Thyroid disorders, **349**
Tibia
  fracture, 305–6, 313–14, *314*
  intraosseous access, 66, *66*
Tibial plateau fractures, 313
Tidal volume, 278
Tidal waves, 545
Toddlers, **198**
Toluene, 181

Tongue, loss of control in mandibular fracture,
      275
Tonsillitis, streptococcal, **411**
Torsade de pointes, 93, *93*
Torus fracture, 239, 307
Total body water (TBW), 68
  in pregnancy, 421
Towyn flood, 626
Toxic chemicals
  details of, 507, **507**
  testing, 511
  see also Chemical incidents
Toxic confusional states, 348, **349**, 460
Toxic shock syndrome, 427
  scalds, 335
  vaginal examination, 424
Toxic syndromes, 183, **184**
  in pregnancy, 437
Toxoplasmosis, **411**
Trac III traction splint, 561, 562
Trachea
  anatomy, 277
  blunt trauma, 269
  compression injury, 284
  deviation, 119, 121
  injuries, 275, 284
  intubation *see* Tracheal intubation
  palpation, 119, 121
  penetrating trauma, 284
  position, 256
  route of administration, 225
Tracheal intubation, 31–8
  advanced life support, 50, 52
  aeromedical evacuation, 576, 587
  anaesthesia, 35–6
  asthma, 213
  blunt trauma to the upper airway, 269
  burns patients, 338, *339*
  chest injuries, 288
  in children, 35, 204–5, 222–3, *223*, 232
  complications, 32
  contraindications, 32
  cricoid pressure, 33, *34*
  difficult, *34*, 34–5
  equipment, **32**
  indications, 31–2
  laryngeal injuries, 283
  laryngeal mask airway, 36, *36*, 36–7
  maxillofacial injuries, 275
  near drowning/drowning, 386, 387
  neonates, 450
  oesophageal-tracheal Combitube, *37*, 37–8
  oral *versus* blind nasotracheal intubation, 35
  in pregnancy, 421
  recognition of tube placement, 33, *33*
  spinal injuries, 293
  suxamethonium, 159
  technique, *32*, 32–3
  trauma cases
    children, 232
    in pregnancy, 435
  tube size, 222–3
  see also Nasotracheal intubation (NTI);
      Orotracheal intubation

Tracheostomy, 38
  in children, 210
  epiglottitis, 210
Traction
  closed fractures, 308–9
  spinal injuries transportation, 296
Traction splints, 561–3, 683
  Donway, 563, *563*
  Hare, *561*, 561–2
  Sager®, *562*, 562–3
Traffic department, police, 617
Training, 671–7
  adult courses, 672–3
  adult learning, 672
  adults as learners, 672
  ambulance service, 594, 598–9
  developing courses, 673
  Faculty of Immediate Care, 676–7
  future, 677
  lack of, 17–18
  major incidents, 486–7
  medical, in the fire service, 607, **607**
  scene approach, 245, **245**
  tracheal intubation, 31
  using drugs, 152 *see also specific courses*
Tramadol, 166–7
Tranquillization
  adverse reactions in elderly patients, **357**
  aggressive and uncooperative psychiatric
      patients, 463–4
  precautions, **464**
  rapid, 463–4, **464**
Transdermal drug administration, 153, **153**
Transient ischaemic attack (TIA), 354
Transportation, 568–71
  children, 239–40
  head injury, 266–7
  major incidents, 491
  medical transport, 568–9
  near drowning, 387
  neonates, 452
  patient transfer vehicles, 569–70
  pregnant patients, 424
  radiation incidents, 522
  respiratory emergencies, 122
  spinal injuries, 295–6
Transverse fractures, *307*
Trauma, 251–9
  aeromedical evacuation, 574
  airway obstruction, 27
  arrival at the scene, 251
  barotrauma *see* Barotrauma
  blunt *see* Blunt trauma
  in children *see* Injured children
  chin lift, 28
  disasters, 543
  human reactions to *see* Human reactions to
      trauma
  patient assessment and treatment,251–2
  penetrating *see* Penetrating trauma
  in pregnancy *see* Pregnancy, trauma in
  primary survey, 252–8 (*see also* Advanced
      life support; Basic life support (BLS);
      specific principles)

scoring *see* Trauma scoring
secondary survey, 258–9, **259**
unconscious patients, 135
    see also specific injury; specific site
Trauma Audit Research Network, 655
Trauma centres, 494
Trauma Injury Severity Score (TRISS),
    666–7
Trauma Score (TS), 501, 662–3, **663**, 666
    see also Paediatric Trauma Score; Revised
        Trauma Score (RTS); Triage Revised
        Trauma Score (T-RTS)
Trauma scoring, 499–501, *500*, 661–8
  anatomical injury severity scores, 665–6
  combined anatomical and physiological
      scores, 666–7
  good, 661–2
  need for, 661
  physiological injury severity scores, 662–5
  process of, 661
  UK Trauma Audit Research Network, 667
      see also specific scoring system
Trefoil sign, 523, *523*
Triage, 493–501
  aeromedical evacuation, 575
  blasts, 330
  categories, **495**
  chemical incidents, 509
  disasters, 541–2
  electrocution injury, 408
  expectant category, 496–7
  history, 493–4
  in history, 484
  injured children, **237**, 237–8
  labels, 486, 495, *498*, 498–9, *499*
  major incidents, 491, 494
  method, *495*, 495–6, **496**
  NHS Pathways, 657, 659
  primary, 491, 494
  prioritized despatch, 494, 499
  psychological, 470–1
  radiation incidents, 527–8
  secondary, 491
  sieve, 495, *495*
  sort, 488, 495–6, **496**
  thermal injury, 342–3
  trauma scoring, 499–501, *500*
Triage Decision Scheme, *500*, 501
Triage Revised Trauma Score (T-RTS), 237,
    495–6, **496**, 501, 664
Triage Trauma Score (TS), 501
Triangular bandage, 559–60, *560*
Tricyclic antidepressants
  adverse reactions in elderly patients, **357**
  antidote for poisoning, **187**
  overdose, 132, 136–7, 157, 186, 188
  post-traumatic disorders, 471
Trismus, 276
TRISS (Trauma Injury Severity Score), 666–7
Tritium, 515, 527
Tropical storms, 546–7, **547**
Troposphere, 582
Trypanosomiasis, 412
Tsunami, 545

Tuberculosis, **411**
  immunization, 412, 413
  transmission, 412
Twentieth century, 4–5, 9
Twin delivery, 445
Two-point discrimination test, 319
Tympanic membrane
  blast injuries, 329
  body temperature measurement, 365
  rupture, barotrauma, 399
Typhoid, **411**
Typhoons, 546–7, **547**

U
U wave, 87
UHF radio, 658
UK Office of Counter Terrorism, 503
UK Trauma Audit Research Network (UK
    TARN), 5, 655, 667
Ulna fracture
  distal, 310
  proximal, 310
Umbilical cord
  in labour, 441–2
  prolapsed, 423, 445
  replacement of prolapsed, 423
UN disaster assessment and coordination team
    (UNDAC), 549
UN High Commission for Refugees
    (UNHCR), 547
Unconscious patients, 130–8
  children, 216
  consent, 639–40
  drowning/near drowning, 383, 386
  heat illness, 395
  primary assessment, 130–3
    airway and breathing, 130–1, 132
    circulation, 131, 132
    diagnostic clues, **132**, 132–3
    external appearance, 133
    history, 131
    responsiveness, 130
    simple neurological assessment, 131, **131**,
        132, **133**
  secondary assessment, 133–5
    cardiovascular assessment, 135
    establishing conscious level, **133**, 133–4
    history, 133
    neurological assessment, 134
    respiratory assessment, 134–5
  specific syndromes, 135–7
  tracheal intubation, 31
Uncooperative patients *see* Violent/aggressive/
    uncooperative patients
Unifocal ectopics, 96
United Nations Scientific Committee on
    the Effects of Atomic Radiation
    (UNSCEAR), 519
United Nations (UN) *see entries beginning* UN
Unmyelinated nerve fibres, 162–3, 170
Upper airway blunt trauma, 269
Upper limb injuries, *309*, 309–11, *310*
Upper respiratory tract infection, 218
Uranium, 518, 521

Uranium decay chain, 516, **516**
Urban hypothermia, 364
Ureteric colic, 141, 142, 145
Ureters
    anatomy, 298
    injury, 303
Urethral injury, 302
Urgent treatment, 635
Urinary incontinence, elderly patients, 350–1, **351**
Urinary infection in children, 203, 216, 218
Urogenital system, opioids side-effects, 165
USA
    aeromedical evacuation, 573
    prehospital care in, 11–12, *11–12*
Uterine contractions, 436, 441
Uterine fibroids, 424
    red degeneration, 430
Uterus
    assessment in trauma in pregnancy, 435–6
    in pregnancy, 421
    in road traffic accidents, 434
    rupture, 436, **436**

V

Vacuum mattresses, 233, 566, *566*, 683
    mountain rescue, 377–8
    pelvic fractures, 312
    spinal injury transportation, 295–6
Vacuum splints, 559, 566
Vaginal bleeding
    ectopic pregnancy, 145, 426
    miscarriage, 426
    trauma in pregnancy, 436
Vaginal examination, 424
    antepartum haemorrhage, 428
    placental abruption, 429
    trauma in pregnancy, 435
Valsalva manoeuvre, 89, *90*, 113
Variable thoracic impedance, 53
Vascular access, 57–73
    in children, 224–5, 235
    gunshot wounds, 326
    neonates, 451
    tachycardia, 112 *see also specific route*
Vascular brain disease, 348
Vascular disruption, chest injuries, 284
Vascular injuries, 317–18
    abdominal stab wounds, 299
    electrocution injury, 407
    limb injuries/fractures, 308
Vascular responses to cooling, 363–4
Vasoconstriction, 278
    cold-induced, 363–4
    heatstroke, 393
    surface heating, 369
Vasoconstrictors, 170
Vasodilatation, alcohol ingestion, 174
Vasogenic shock, 76
Vaughan Williams classification of anti-arrhythmic drugs, 112, **112**
Vecuronium, 36
Vehicles
    cleaning, 415

    hazards, 249
    protection, 679–80 *see also specific vehicle*
Vein dilation devices, 682
Venous cutdown cannulation, 61–2, *62*
Ventilation, 43–5
    advanced life support, 52
    during aeromedical transport, 587–8
    assisted, 44
    asthma, 213
    basic life support, 20–1
    causes of inadequate, **44**
    in children, 206–7, 210, 224, *224*
    definition, 43
    epiglottitis, 210
    equipment, 681–2
    facemask, 44
    hypothermia, 373
    injured children, 232, 234
    Laerdal pocket mask, 44, **45**
    mechanical, 45
    near drowning/drowning, 386, 387
    neonates, 450
    oxygen-powered resuscitators, 45
    physiology, 44
    poisoning, 183
    respiratory pathophysiology, 278
    self-inflating bag-valve device, 44–5
    surgical airway, 39–41, **40**
    trauma in pregnancy, 435
Ventilation–perfusion (V/Q) mismatch
    asthma, 122–3
    pregnancy, 421
Ventilators, 681
Ventricular ectopics, 96, 96–7, 97
    electrocution injury, 407
    frequency of, within 4h of myocardial infarction, **106**
    in myocardial infarction, 108
Ventricular fibrillation, 48, 93
    after thrombolytic treatment, 109
    in children, 221
    defibrillation *see* Defibrillation
    electrocution injury, 407
    frequency of, within 4h of myocardial infarction, **106**
    hypothermia, 367, 373
    myocardial infarction, 108
    pulseless electrical activity, 227
    VF-pulseless VT, 48, 49–50, *50*
Ventricular flutter, 91, *92*
Ventricular heaves, 121
Ventricular standstill, 95, *96*
Ventricular tachycardia, 48, 91, **91**, *91*
    electrocution injury, 407
    frequency of, within 4h of myocardial infarction, **106**
    in myocardial infarction, 108, 114
    pulseless, in children, 227
    treatment, 114
    VF-pulseless VT, 48, 49–50, *50*
Venturi masks, 43
Verapamil
    supraventricular tachycardia, 113
    tachycardia, 91, 92

Verbal communication, 476–7
Verbal response
    head injury, 265
    unconscious patients, 134
Verminous infestations, **411**
Vestibular balance mechanisms, 351–2
VF-pulseless VT, 48, 49–50, *50*
VHF radio, 658
Vibration, aircraft, 586–7
Vibrio cholerae, 543
Vibrio metschnikovii, 532
Video recording, 654
Vietnam War, 466
Vigilance, trauma response, 469
Violence, definition, 476
Violent/aggressive/uncooperative patients, 476–80
    anger definition, 476
    following an incident, 479–80
    principles of assessment, 477–9
        in the home, 477, **478**
        in the practice, 478–9, *479*
        at the scene of an accident/incident, 477–8, **478**
    psychiatric patients, 463–4
    psychosis, 458
    rapid tranquillization, 463–4
    risk factors for, **463**
    staff training and education, 480
    verbal and non-verbal communication, 476–7, **477**
    violence definition, 476
Vipera berus, **187**, 193
Viperidae, 193
Viral haemorrhagic fever, **411**
Viral infections in children, 207
Visceral pain, abdominal, 140
Viscotoxins, 191, **191**
Viscus
    obstruction, 141
    perforation, 141
Vital signs
    in childbirth, 440
    tachycardia, 111–12
Vitamin B_{12} deficiency, **349**
Vocal cords, tracheal intubation, 32, *32*
Voice dysfunction, surgical airway complications, 39
Volatile solvents, 181
Volcanoes, 546, *546*
Voltage, 406
Volume replacement, crush syndrome, 544
Voluntary Rescue Association, 12
Voluntary services, 628–30
    see also specific service
Vomiting
    acute abdomen, 141
    after head injury, 238
    on aircrafts, 587
    during basic life support, 21
    bilious, 141
    bowel obstruction, 146
    cardiac emergencies, 107–8
    in children, 203–4, 216–17

diverticular disease, 146
gallbladder disease, 144
inducing in poisoning, 185, 191–2
meningitis, 217
mesenteric infarction, 145
myocardial infarction, 106
opiates, 107
opioids side-effects, 165, 167
pancreatitis, 144
projectile, 141, 203–4
radiation-induced, 526
renal calculus disease, 145

W
Wales Fire Service, 603
Wallace's Rule of Nines, 340, *342*
Wasps, 193–4
Waste disposal, 415
Wasting, 542
Watchful waiting, 471
Water immersion
    and diuresis, 363
    effects of, *368*
    hypothermia, 364
Water pressure, 399, *399*

Watersports injuries, 537
Waveforms, defibrillators, 53
Weather
    aviation medicine, 582
    mountaineering and hillwalking, 537
    and sports injuries, 535
Weaver fish, 193
Wenckebach block, 94, *95*
Wernicke's encephalopathy, 189
Wet bulb globe temperature (WBGT), 396
Wheezing, 119
    asthma, 122, 211
    unconscious patients, 134
    vs. stridor in children, 203
Whole blood, 70, 79–80
Whole body irradiation, 525–6
Whooping cough, **411**
Wind-chill, 362, **363**
Withdrawal states, 174, **184**, 461
Wolff-Parkinson-White syndrome, 89, *90*, 93,
        93, 97–8, 112
Women's Royal Voluntary Service (WRVS),
        625, 629
World War II, 466
Wound ballistics, **323**, *323*, 323–5

high energy transfer, 325
interaction of bullets with the tissues, *324*,
        324–5
low energy transfer, 325
Wounds, 317, *317*
    burn, 340–2, *341*
    contamination from bullets, 325
    healing in children, 200
Wrist
    fractures, 310
    tenosynovitis, 318

X
X-rays, 517, 521

Y
Yaw, 324, *324*
Yersinia pestis, 543

Z
Zagreb antivenom, **187**
Zinc, **187**
Zone of stasis, burns, 333
Zygomatic (malar) bone fracture, 273, 274
Zygomaticomaxillary complex fractures, 276